Textbook of Pediatric Gastroenterology and Nutrition

Textbook of Pediatric Gastroenterology and Nutrition

Edited by

Stefano Guandalini MD
Professor of Pediatrics
Chief, Section of Gastroenterology
University of Chicago Children's Hospital
Director, University of Chicago Celiac Disease Program
Chicago, IL
USA

CRC Press
Taylor & Francis Group
Boca Raton London New York

CRC Press is an imprint of the
Taylor & Francis Group, an **informa** business

CRC Press
Taylor & Francis Group
6000 Broken Sound Parkway NW, Suite 300
Boca Raton, FL 33487-2742

First published in 2004 by the Taylor & Francis Group.

ISBN-13: 978-1-841-84315-5 (hbk)
ISBN-13: 978-0-429-21226-0 (ebk)

DOI: 10.3109/9780203640456

A CIP record for this book is available from the British Library.

Library of Congress Cataloging-in-Publication Data available on application

Visit the Taylor & Francis Web site at
http://www.taylorandfrancis.com

Contents

Contributors

Fabio Albano
Department of Pediatrics
University of Naples 'Federico II'
Via S. Pansini 5
80131 Naples, Italy

Steven R Allen
University of Cincinnati College of Medicine
Cincinnati, OH 45229, USA

Jorge Amil Dias
Pediatric Gastroenterology Unit
Hospital S. João
4200 Porto, Portugal

Renata Auricchio
Department of Pediatrics
University of Naples 'Federico II'
Via S. Pansini 5
80131 Naples, Italy

Richard G Azizkhan
Cincinnati Children's Hospital Medical Center
Division of Pediatric Surgery
3333 Burnet Avenue
Cincinnati, OH 45229, USA

Mauro Batista de Morais
Division of Pediatric Gastroenterology
Escola Paulista de Medicina
Universidade Federal de São Paulo
São Paulo, Brazil

Adolfo Bautista Casasnovas
Section of Pediatric Surgery
Clinical University Hospital of Santiago de Compostela
Choupana s/n
15706 Santiago, Spain

Marc Benninga
Emma Kinderziekenhuis AMC
Department of Pediatrics
Postbus 22660
NL-1100 DD
Amsterdam, The Netherlands

Zulfiqar A Bhutta
Department of Paediatrics
The Aga Khan University
Stadium Road
Karachi 74800, Pakistan

Osvaldo Borrelli
Department of Pediatrics
Gastroenterology Service
University of Rome 'La Sapienza'
Viale Regina Elena 324
00161 Rome, Italy

Athos Bousvaros
Division of Gastroenterology and Nutrition
Children's Hospital
Boston, MA 02115, USA

David Brewster
Northern Territory Clinical School
Flinders University
Casuarina NT0811, Australia

Samy Cadranel
Queen Fabiola Children's Hospital
Department of Gastroenterology and Nutrition
Avenue J J Crocq 15
B-1020 Brussels, Belgium

Moti M Chowdhury
Department of Paediatric Surgery
Surgery Unit
Institute of Child Health
30 Guilford Street
London WC1N 1EH, UK

Virginie Colomb
Service de Gastroentérologie et Nutrition Pédiatriques
Hôpital Necker – Enfants Malades
149 Rue de Sèvres
75743 Paris, France

Salvatore Cucchiara
Department of Pediatrics
Gastroenterology Service
University of Rome 'La Sapienza'
Viale Regina Elena 324
00160 Rome, Italy

Luigi Dall'Oglio
Digestive Surgical and Endoscopic Unit
Ospedale Pediatrico Bambino Gesù-IRCCS
Viale S. Onofrio
00199 Rome, Italy

Paola De Angelis
Digestive Surgical and Endoscopic Unit
Ospedale Pediatrico Bambino Gesù-IRCCS
Viale S. Onofrio
00199 Rome, Italy

Mario De Curtis
Dipartimento Materno-Infantile
University of Palermo
90142 Palermo, Italy

Costantino De Giacomo
Unità Operativa di Pediatria
Ospedale Niguarda Cà Granda
Piazza Ospedale Maggiore 3
20162 Milano, Italy

Carlo Di Lorenzo
Division of Pediatric Gastroenterology
Children's Hospital of Pittsburgh
University of Pittsburgh Medical Center
3705 5th Avenue
Pittsburgh, PA 15213, USA

Ulysses Fagundes-Neto
Division of Pediatric Gastroenterology
Escola Paulista de Medicina
Universidade Federal de São Paulo
São Paulo, Brazil

Alessio Fasano
Mucosal Biology Research Center
University of Maryland School of Medicine
22 S. Greene Street
Baltimore, MD 21201, USA

Giovanni Federici di Abriola
Digestive Surgical and Endoscopic Unit
Ospedale Pediatrico Bambino Gesù-IRCCS
Viale S. Onofrio
00199 Rome, Italy

John Fell
Chelsea and Westminster Hospital
London, UK

Michael H N Golden
Department of Medicine and Therapeutics
University of Aberdeen
Scotland, UK

Olivier Goulet
Service de Gastroentérologie et Nutrition Pédiatriques
Hôpital Necker – Enfants Malades
149 Rue de Sèvres
75743 Paris, France

Stefano Guandalini
Section of Gastroenterology, Hepatology and Nutrition
University of Chicago
5839 S. Maryland Avenue
Chicago, IL 60637, USA

Alfredo Guarino
Department of Pediatrics
University of Naples 'Federico II'
Via S. Pansini 5
80131 Naples, Italy

Said Hachimi-Idrissi
Academische Ziekenhuis Kinderen
Vrije Universiteit Brussel
Laarbeeklaan 101
B-1090 Brussels, Belgium

Nigel Hall
Department of Paediatric Surgery
Institute of Child Health
30 Guilford Street
London WC1N 1EH, UK

Bruno Hauser
Academische Ziekenhuis Kinderen
Vrije Universiteit Brussel
Laarbeeklaan 101
B-1090 Brussels, Belgium

Leslie M Higuchi
Division of Gastroenterology and Nutrition
Children's Hospital
Boston, MA 02115, USA

Warren Hyer
Northwick Park and St Mark's Hospital
Middlesex, UK

Erika Isolauri
Department of Pediatrics
University of Turku
Kiinamyllynk. 4-8
FIN-20520 Turku, Finland

Carl-Christian A Jackson
University of Chicago Pritzker School of Medicine
5841 S. Maryland Avenue
Chicago, IL 60637, USA

Barbara S Kirschner
University of Chicago Pritzker School of Medicine
5841 S. Maryland Avenue
Chicago, IL 60637, USA

Jorma Kokkonen
Department of Pediatrics
University Hospital of Oulu
Oulu
FIN-90029, Finland

Kirsi Laiho
Department of Pediatrics
University of Turku
Kiinamyllynk. 4-8
FIN-20520 Turku, Finland

B UK Li
Department of Pediatrics
Northwestern University McGraw School of Medicine
Children's Memorial Hospital
Chicago, IL 60614, USA

Donald C Liu
Pediatric Surgery
University of Chicago Comer Children's Hospital
5841 S. Maryland Avenue
Chicago, IL 60637, USA

Erasmo Miele
Department of Pediatrics
University of Naples 'Federico II'
Via S. Pansini 5
80131 Naples, Italy

Peter J Milla
Gastroenterology Unit
Institute of Child Health
30 Guilford Street
London, WC1N 1EH, UK

Jacek Z Mrukowicz
Polish Institute for Evidence Based Medicine
Cracow, Poland

Simon Murch
Centre for Paediatric Gastroenterology
Royal Free Hospital and University College Medical School
Royal Free Campus
Rowland Hill Street
London, NW3 2PF, UK

Agostino Pierro
Department of Paediatric Surgery
Institute of Child Health
30 Guilford Street
London WC1N 1EH, UK

Michelle M Pietzak
Division of Gastroenterology and Nutrition
Children's Hospital of Los Angeles
4650 Sunset Boulevard
Los Angeles, CA 90027, USA

Lucia Quaglietta
Department of Pediatrics
University of Naples 'Federico II'
Via S. Pansini 5
80131 Naples, Italy

Jacques Rigo
Department of Pediatrics
Division of Neonatology
University of Liège
CHR Citadelle
4000 Liège, Belgium

Nigel C Rollins
Department of Paediatrics and Child Health
Nelson R Mandela School of Medicine
719 Umbilo Road
Congella 4013
Durban, South Africa

Frank M Ruemmele
Service de Gastroentérologie et Nutrition Pédiatriques
Hôpital Necker – Enfants Malades
149 Rue de Sèvres
75743 Paris, France

Silvia Salvatore
Academische Ziekenhuis Kinderen
Vrije Universiteit Brussel
Laarbeeklaan 101
B-1090 Brussels, Belgium

Miguel Saps
Division of Pediatric Gastroenterology
Children's Hospital of Pittsburgh
University of Pittsburgh Medical Center
3705 5th Avenue
Pittsburgh, PA 15213, USA

Michèle Scaillon
Queen Fabiola Children's Hospital
Department of Gastroenterology and Nutrition
Avenue J J Crocq 15
B-1020 Brussels, Belgium

Stig Somme
Louisiana State University School of Medicine
1542 Tulane Avenue
New Orleans, LA 70112, USA

Annamaria Staiano
Department of Pediatrics
University of Naples 'Federico II'
Via S. Pansini 5
80131 Naples, Italy

Bhanu Sunku
Department of Pediatrics
Northwestern University McGraw School of Medicine
Children's Memorial Hospital
Chicago, IL 60614, USA

Hania Szajewska
Department of Pediatric Gastroenterology and Nutrition
The Medical University of Warsaw
Dzialdowska 1
01-184 Warsaw, Poland

Jan Taminiau
Emma Kinderziekenhuis AMC
Department of Pediatrics
Postbus 22660
NL-1100 DD
Amsterdam, The Netherlands

Eunice Trindade
Pediatric Gastroenterology Unit
Hospital S. João
4200 Porto, Portugal

Yvan Vandenplas
Academische Ziekenhuis Kinderen
Vrije Universiteit Brussel
Laarbeeklaan 101
B-1090 Brussels, Belgium

Harland S Winter
Pediatric IBD Center
Department of Pediatrics
Massachusetts General Hospital for Children
55 Fruit Street
Boston, MA 02114, USA

Nelly Youssef
Service de Gastroentérologie et Nutrition Pédiatriques
Hôpital Necker – Enfants Malades
149 Rue de Sèvres Paris
75743 Paris, France

Qian Yuan
Pediatric IBD Center
Department of Pediatrics
Massachusetts General Hospital for Children
55 Fruit Street
Boston, MA 02114, USA

Preface

Our discipline is young. When I began focusing on pediatric gastroenterology, in the early 1970s, there were no textbooks available. My training was based on the teaching of outstanding mentors (such as Salvatore Auricchio and Armido Rubino, to whom I will always be indebted), on eager clinical work and on tireless research; and reading of adult gastrointestinal textbooks that were regarded as the necessary theoretical fundaments of knowledge. Then the Silvermann, Roy and Cozzetto book (*Pediatric Clinical Gastroenterology*. St Louis, MO: Mosby, 1971) came along, somewhat officially identifying our field as a free-standing subspecialty and heralding a new exciting era of educational tools directed at our discipline.

The knowledge then seems to have almost exploded, with technology rapidly introducing new investigative, diagnostic and therapeutic modalities; new acquisitions making old approaches quickly obsolete; and the sheer body of new information forcing us to become sub-subspecialists. Hepatologists (now rightly even *transplant* hepatologists), endoscopists, neurogastroenterologists and more 'ologists' have emerged and have gained or are gaining their cultural and operative independence.

In this scenario of ever-changing evolution, and in the Internet era, why another pediatric gastroenterology and nutrition book? I believe the answer lies in the progressive globalization that the Internet has certainly catalyzed and that we see occurring before our eyes. We are living more and more in a true global village, where educational resources need not only to be scientifically correct and updated, but also able to offer, in a comprehensive, cohesive package, information that is also reflective of the different realities that gastroenterological and nutritional problems take on in different parts of the world. Intentionally, this book does not cover any liver-related disorder. Hepatology has become a discipline in its own right, and authoritative, specific books addressing only pediatric hepatology have already appeared and are available. We felt that focusing on the two intertwined areas of gastroenterology and nutrition would serve better the needs of the pediatric gastroenterologist. However, the book has a rather ambitious goal: that of having a global 'flavor'. It is in fact born out of a new vision of worldwide co-operation among pediatric gastroenterologists, which is embodied by the recently created Federation of the International Societies of Pediatric Gastroenterology, Hepatology and Nutrition (FISPGHAN). I can only hope that its goal will be reached; certainly all the authors and I tried very hard. Happy Reading!

Stefano Guandalini, MD
Professor of Pediatrics
President of FISPGHAN

1 Microvillus inclusion disease and epithelial dysplasia

Olivier Goulet, Nelly Youssef and Frank M Ruemmele

Introduction

The definition, presentation and outcome of intractable diarrhea of infancy (IDI) have changed considerably over the past three decades, owing to major improvements in nutritional management, and a better understanding of the pathology of the small bowel mucosa.

Definition of protracted and intractable diarrhea of infancy

Originally, the syndrome of IDI was described by Avery et al in 1968, based on the following features: diarrhea occurring in a newborn younger than 3 months of age, lasting more than 2 weeks, with three or more negative stool cultures for bacterial pathogens.[1] Most cases were managed in hospital, using intravenous fluids while the diarrhea was persistent and intractable, with a high mortality rate from infection or malnutrition.[2] Recently, the term 'severe diarrhea requiring parenteral nutrition' was proposed.[3,4] Within this group of pathologies, two major subtypes can be differentiated. The first group is made up of patients with 'protracted diarrhea of infancy' (PDI), which subsides despite its initial severity. PDI can result from a specific immune deficiency, a sensitization to a common food protein (e.g. cow's milk or gluten), or it can be secondary to a severe infection of the digestive tract (post-enteritis syndrome). The second group is characterized by an 'intractable diarrhea of infancy', with onset within the first 2 years of life. In this second group, diarrhea persists sometimes for years, despite prolonged bowel resting and various therapeutic trials. In most cases, such as constitutive enterocyte disorders[5] or autoimmune enteropathy,[6] the situation becomes rapidly life threatening, and these patients depend on long-term parenteral nutrition (PN). Some of them are candidates for intestinal transplantation. Table 1.1 shows the diagnostic heterogeneity of 65 cases with severe diarrhea requiring PN for more than 1 month, as recently analyzed by a French multicenter study.[7] The so-called 'intractable ulcerating enterocolitis' of early onset is difficult to classify.[8] It is very important to distinguish between IDI and PDI, since children with PDI always recover, sometimes after only several weeks or months of parenteral and/or enteral nutrition. In contrast, patients with IDI never recover, and are dependent on life-long parenteral nutrition or – in the case of autoimmune enteropathy – life-long massive immunosuppressive medication.

Current classification

An attempt to classify intractable diarrhea according to villus atrophy was proposed, on the basis of immunohistological criteria emphasizing the role of activated T cells in the intestinal mucosa.[9] A multicenter survey from the European Society for Paediatric Gastroenterology, Hepatology and Nutrition (ESPGHAN) collected different cases of IDI and villus atrophy with precisely defined light microscopic characteristics, categorizing several types of IDI.[10] On histological analysis, two clearly different groups of IDI can be separated. The first one is characterized by a mononuclear cell infiltration of the lamina propria, and is considered to be associated with activated T cells. Within this group, two different clinical presentations can be distinguished. Patients presenting with additional extradigestive autoimmune symptoms (such as diabetes, arthritis, thyroiditis, dermatitis and nephrotic syndrome) tended to have a later onset

Table 1.1 Causes and outcomes of protracted and intractable diarrhea of infancy

Cause	Patients (*n*)	Deceased (*n*)
Protracted diarrhea	39	1
Multiple food intolerance	15	0
Infectious enteritis	14	0
Colitis (including two with CMV)	6	1
CDG syndrome	1	0
Ganglioneuroblastoma	1	0
Unknown	2	0
Intractable diarrhea	21	4
Abnormalities of the enterocyte		
intestinal epithelial dysplasia	6	1
microvillus atrophy	3	0
Autoimmune enteropathy	5	3
Phenotypic diarrhea	3	0
Undefined	4	0

CMV, cytomegalovirus; CDG, congenital disorders of glycosylation

of diarrhea, which was more abundant and more severe than in patients with isolated gastrointestinal symptoms and gut autoantibodies. The second histological pattern includes the early onset of severe intractable diarrhea with villus atrophy, without mononuclear cell infiltration of the lamina propria but specific histological abnormalities involving the epithelium. To date, several types of primary epithelial abnormality inducing IDI have been identified. The first described was microvillus atrophy or microvillus inclusion disease (MVID) and, more recently, tufting enteropathy or epithelial dysplasia.[11] Some patients are small for gestational age and present with phenotypic abnormalities corresponding to the previously described syndromatic diarrhea.[12]

Microvillus inclusion disease

In 1978, Davidson et al reported five infants with severe, persistent diarrhea beginning in the newborn period, in whom light microscopy revealed crypt hypoplastic villus atrophy.[13] Electron microscopic examination of small intestinal biopsies from three of the patients showed severe brush-border abnormalities and increased liposome-like bodies and, in one, intracytoplasmic cysts made up of brush border. Further children were reported with these characteristic cytoplasmic inclusions of the brush-border membrane.[5,14] From these first clinical and histological descriptions, MVID has been established as a distinct disease within the syndrome of IDI, based on the characteristic morphological features. MVID in its typical form is a congenital disorder of intestinal epithelial cells, presenting as intractable secretory diarrhea within the first days of life.[15]

Clinical expression

In general, infants develop severe secretory diarrhea within the first days after birth. Stool volumes reach 250–300 ml/kg body weight per day, with electrolyte concentrations similar to those seen in small-intestinal fluid. This disorder is life threatening, since massive diarrhea leads to rapid dehydration and electrolyte imbalance, with subsequent metabolic decompensation within a few hours.[13–15] Severe watery diarrhea persists despite bowel rest. The differential diagnosis may include congenital chloride diarrhea or sodium malabsorption diarrhea, which can be easily distinguished from MVID by blood and stool electrolyte assessment.[16,17] In contrast, clinical presentation of MVID may sometimes be atypical, in the form of a predominantly pseudo-occlusive syndrome, with full and distended small bowel and colon. Some newborns have been thought to present intestinal pseudo-obstruction syndrome, and unfortunately in some of them an ileostomy was created. The most common time of onset of diarrhea in MVID is within the first few days (early-onset or congenital form). However, in a few patients the onset of diarrhea is delayed (first month) and less severe (late-onset form).

Histological examination

Histological analysis of small bowel biopsies shows a variable degree of villus atrophy without any inflammatory infiltrate. Highly characteristic for this disorder is the accumulation of periodic acid Schiff (PAS)-positive secretory granules within the apical cytoplasm of enterocytes.[18–20] On the ultrastructural level, rare or absent microvilli on intestinal epithelial cells along with inclusions of microvilli in the cytoplasm of enterocytes are seen, which define this entity.[21]

Diagnosis may be easily performed from light microscopic examination of a duodenal or jejunal biopsy specimen. On hematoxylin–eosin staining, the mucosa appears flattened with hypoplastic villus atrophy. PAS staining reveals an abnormal brush-border pattern with positive-staining material within the apical cytoplasm of enterocytes (Figure 1.1). A valuable new tool for the light microscopic diagnosis of MVID was recently proposed.[22,23] CD-10 is a membrane-associated neutral peptidase, shown to have a linear brush-border staining pattern in normal small intestine. In contrast to this surface staining in different controls (normal intestine, celiac disease, autoimmune enteropathy, allergy), all MVID cases revealed prominent intracytoplasmic CD-10 immunoreactivity in surface enterocytes[22,23] (Figure 1.2). Similar results were obtained with PAS, polyclonal carcinoembryonic antigen and alkaline phosphatase, three stains known to show cytoplasmic staining of surface enterocytes in MVID.[23] On electron microscopy, surface epithelial cells show absent or grossly abnormal microvilli, as well as numerous vesicular bodies of various sizes, and the characteristic microvillus inclusions (Figure 1.3). Crypt cells are morphologically almost normal, but do not contain increased

(a) (b)

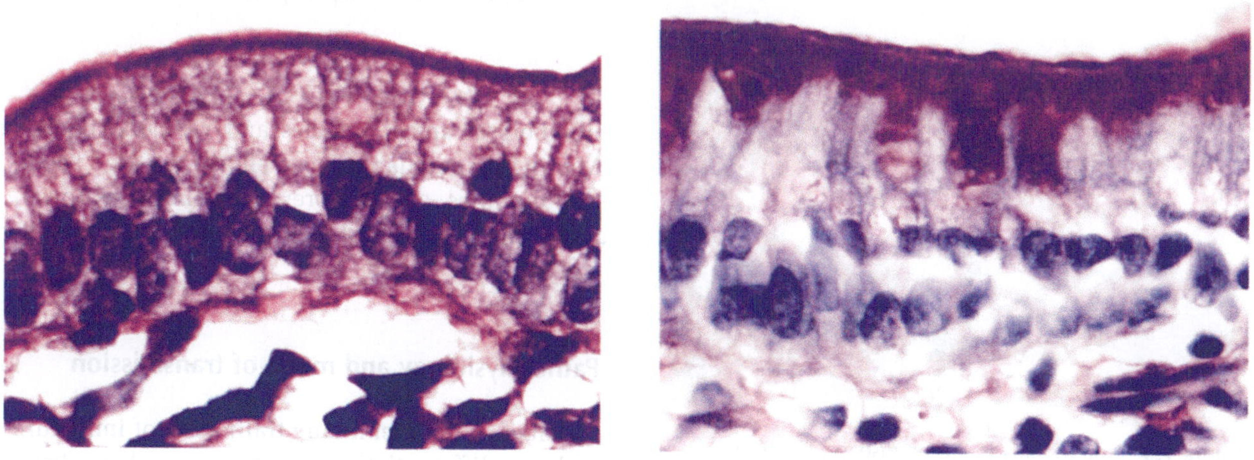

Figure 1.1 Microvillus inclusion disease: periodic acid-Schiff (PAS) staining. (a) Normal mucosa, normal PAS, brush-border staining; (b) abnormal accumulation of PAS, positive material in the apical cytoplasm of epithelial cells in microvillus inclusion disease.

(a) (b)

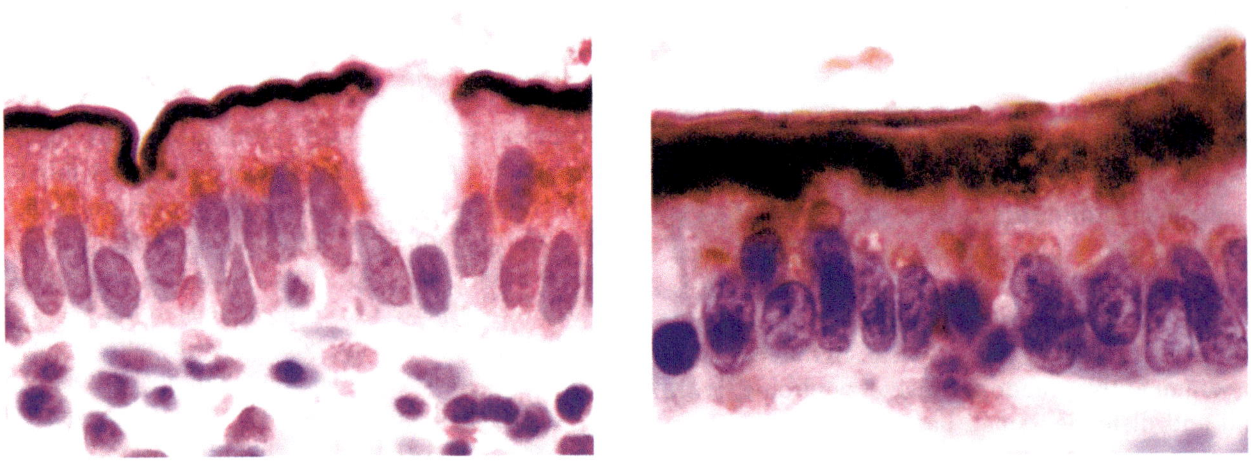

Figure 1.2 Microvillus inclusion disease: CD-10 immunostaining. (a) Normal mucosa, normal CD-10, brush-border immunostaining; (b) abnormal accumulation of positive material in the apical cytoplasm of epithelial cells in microvillus inclusion disease.

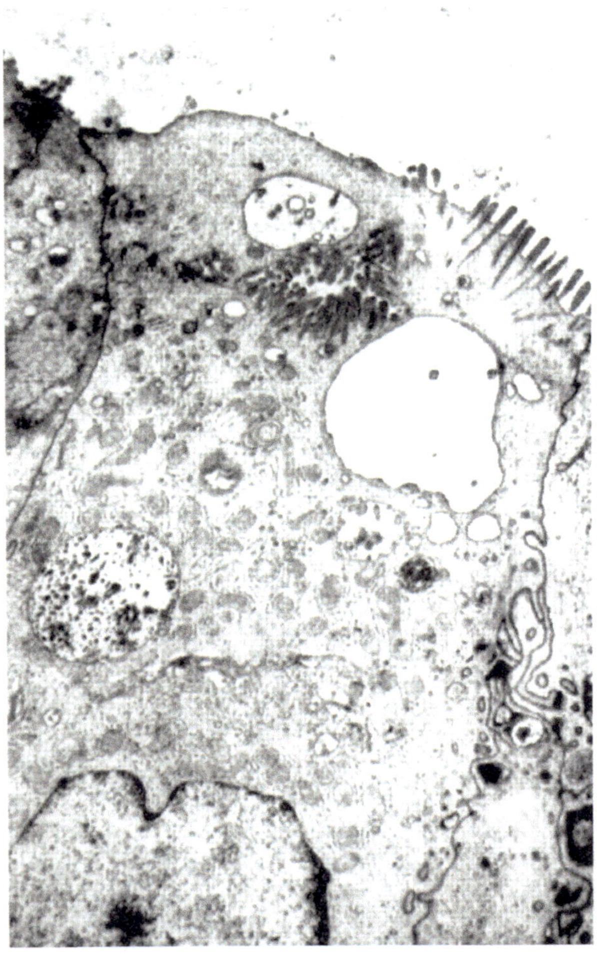

Figure 1.3 Microvillus inclusion disease. Electron microscopy of jejunal biopsy specimen. The brush border is almost absent. The cytoplasm contains a microvillus inclusion.

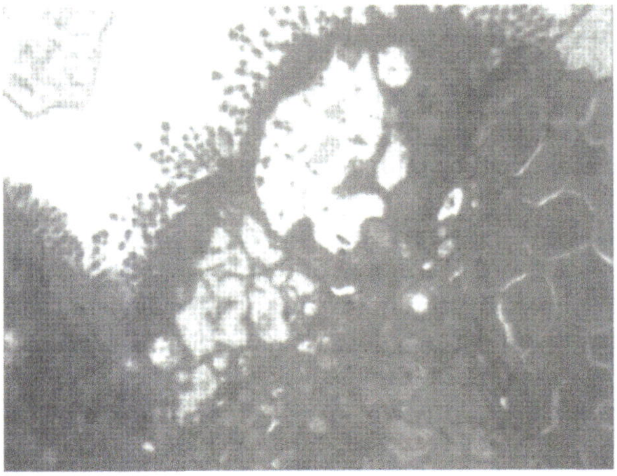

Figure 1.4 Microvillus inclusion disease. Electron microscopy of colonic biopsy specimen.

numbers of apical vesicles and vesicular bodies. Microvillus inclusions, as well as increased secretory granules, are also present in the large bowel, more easily accessible for biopsy, especially in early infancy (Figure 1.4).

Pathophysiology and mode of transmission

A defect in the membrane trafficking of immature and/or differentiating enterocytes has been discussed as an etiopathogenic mechanism in MVID.[20,21] This membrane defect results, as a direct functional consequence, in complete intestinal failure. It has been speculated that the disease is associated with a disorder of the enterocyte cytoskeleton, which produces an abnormal assembly of microvilli. Intestinal microvillus dystrophy was reported as being a hypothetic variant of MVID.[24] The underlying pathogenesis of MVID is still unclear, although a cytoskeletal myosin deficiency has been found.[25] When analyzing the turnover of sucrase-isomaltase, as a representative brush-border protein, there is clear evidence that the direct and indirect constitutive pathways are intact in MVID.[21] Therefore, a defect in endocytosis is rather unlikely. More recently, by investigating the glycobiological nature of the epithelial accumulation of PAS, Phillips et al[26] suggested that MVID involves a defect in exocytosis of the glycocalyx.[26] The absence of glycocalyx might impair normal cell functions.

Considering the number of cases with affected siblings, and the frequency of consanguinity among patients in families of affected infants, this disease appears to be transmitted as an autosomal recessive trait.[13,15,27] No candidate gene has been identified to date. MVID has been reported in a girl with autosomal dominant hypochondroplasia.[28] The gene defect of this disease was recently localized on the chromosome region 4p16.3, which might help in elucidating the genetic basis of MVID.

Long-term outcome

MVID is a congenital constitutive intestinal epithelial cell disorder leading, in its typical early-onset form, to permanent intestinal failure. The largest multicenter survey, of 23 MVID patients,[15] revealed an extremely reduced life expectancy with a 1-year survival rate of less than 25%. Most children died of septic complications, liver failure, or metabolic decompensation. Few cases of MVID, especially with the late-onset form, may survive with limited stool output and may require only partial PN.[29] Treatment with corticosteroids, colostrum or epidermal growth factor has not been successful, but octreotide has been used with partial success in one patient.[15] In contrast to the initial outcomes before the 1980s, PN now allows most infants and children to survive. However, complications related to inadequate PN do limit long-term survival. These include recurrent catheter-related sepsis, extensive thrombosis, fat overload syndrome and cholestasis. In addition, without evidence of an associated renal disease, some of these infants and children present chronic hydro-electrolytic imbalance and acidosis, with subsequent impaired length growth. Others, because of repeated dehydration episodes associated with unadapted phosphocalcic intakes, present with nephrocalcinosis. Finally, even with adequate long-term PN and normal growth, most children remain with high and uncomfortable stool output. This requires daily fluid replacement with the high risk of severe dehydration. Intestinal transplantation therefore became the only definitive treatment of this rare intestinal disease.[30–33]

Definitive treatment

Since the introduction of tacrolimus (originally FK506) as an immunosuppressive drug after organ transplantation in the early 1990s, the outcome of intestinal transplantation markedly improved. Several cases of successful transplantation for MVID have been reported.[30–35] Transplantation involved isolated intestine,[30–33] or intestine combined with the liver.[31,32] Following the report of these cases, there has been an ongoing discussion on whether or not the colon should be transplanted together with the small bowel.

We recently evaluated the possibility and outcome of intestinal transplantation in ten consecutive patients with early-onset congenital MVID at Necker-Enfants Malades Hospital (Paris) (Ruemmele et al, submitted for publication). Two patients died before they could be put on a waiting list for small-bowel transplantation; one patient is still waiting. We performed cadaveric intestinal transplantation in seven patients aged between 3 and 11 years by using tacrolimus, steroids and interleukin (IL-2) blockers. Three transplantations were performed with isolated intestine, and four with intestine associated with the liver. Right colon transplantation was performed in five cases (two with isolated intestine). One patient died during transplantation surgery from acute liver failure and hemodynamic shock, probably due to re-perfusion shock. The six others (86%) survived, with a median follow-up of 3 years (range 1–8 years). Graft rejections occurred in two patients (one with isolated intestinal transplantation, and one with intestine and liver), who responded favorably to methylprednisolone pulses. Complete weaning from PN was achieved in all patients: the five patients with an additional colon graft were off PN after a median of 36 days after surgery, as opposed to those without colonic transplant who obtained full intestinal autonomy several months after transplantation. Thus, intestinal transplantation alone or in combination with liver, offered MVID children for the first time a long-term perspective. In this series at Necker-Enfants Malades Hospital, additional colon grafting markedly improved outcome and quality of life after transplantation in MVID. These preliminary results of intestinal transplantation in this rare disease are very encouraging, and demonstrate that the prognosis of MVID has changed dramatically during the past decade.

Finally, in a child suspected of having MVID, a precise classification into one of three different subtypes (congenital–early-onset, late-onset or atypical) should be obtained as early as possible and confirmed by an experienced pathologist, according to clearly defined morphological criteria. Recently, Croft et al[34] reported a 5-year-old girl with a late-onset form of MVID who was weaned from total PN and is thriving on a normal unrestricted diet. This rare form of MVID probably has a better prognosis than the most frequent form of early-onset MVID, with a high mortality rate.[15] Given the high success rate of intestinal transplantation in MVID, we recommend transplantation, once the definitive diagnosis of early-onset MVID is made. In addition, the potential candidate for transplantation has to be in a eutrophic phase under total PN. This policy should allow avoidance of liver impairment. Conversely, patients with a late-onset or atypical form of MVID should not be automatically scheduled for small-bowel transplantation. The individual course of the disease will help in deciding whether or not a child with MVID is a candidate for intestinal transplantation.

Intestinal epithelial dysplasia (or tufting enteropathy)

In 1994, three cases of neonatal severe diarrhea with abnormal epithelial pictures were reported by Reifen et al under the name of 'tufting enteropathy'.[36] In our own series at Necker-Enfants Malades, we identified nine cases of severe neonatal diarrhea that were clearly different from MVID.[12] Further studies in these patients confirmed that intestinal epithelial dysplasia (IED) is a constitutive epithelial disorder involving both small intestine and colon.[37] In our experience, IED seems to be frequent in patients of Arabic origin, from the Middle-East or North Africa. Main characteristics of this disease are its clinical and histological heterogeneity and its association with malformations or other epithelial diseases.

Clinical expression

Typically, the patients present during the first weeks of life with severe diarrhea. Most have affected consanguineous parents and/or siblings, some of whom died during the first months of life with severe diarrhea of unknown origin. Most of the time, diarrhea persists despite bowel rest, but at a lower level when compared to MVID. Therefore, attempts at continuous enteral feeding with protein hydrolysates or amino acid-based formulas were performed in some patients. Unfortunately, most often the continuous enteral feeding exacerbated the diarrhea, and particularly the newborns with IED did not grow adequately. They rapidly developed failure to thrive, with severe protein energy malnutrition. Because of the early onset of diarrhea, MVID is often suspected in these children. However, morphological analysis of small- and large-bowel biopsies easily distinguishes these entities (see above). A major problem in the diagnosis of IED is its clinical and histological heterogeneity.

Histological features

Villus atrophy of variable severity is present. In the typical form, abnormalities are localized mainly in the epithelium and include a disorganization of surface enterocytes with focal crowding, resembling tufts (Figure 1.5). These characteristic 'tufts' of extruding epithelium first described by Reifen et al[36] are seen towards the villus tip, and may affect up to 70% of villi. The tufting process is not limited to the small intestine but also involves the colonic mucosa.[11] This picture can also be observed in crypt epithelium and, in addition,

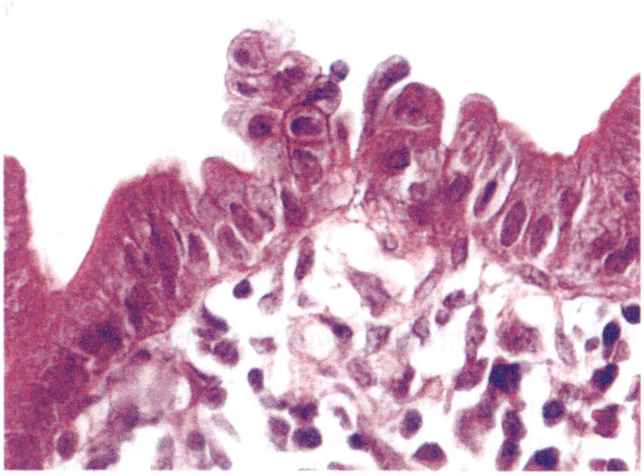

Figure 1.5 Epithelial dysplasia. Disorganization of surface epithelium showing tufts with apical rounding epithelial cells.

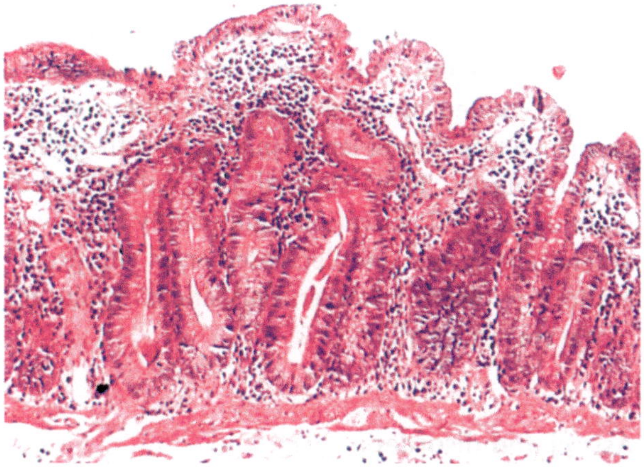

Figure 1.6 Epithelial dysplasia. Partial villus atrophy with crypt hyperplasia and/or pseudocystic crypt appearance, branching and disorganization of surface epithelium.

crypts often have an abnormal aspect with dilatations such as pseudocysts and abnormal regeneration with branching[11] (Figure 1.6). The study of basement membrane components demonstrated an abnormal laminin and heparan sulfate proteoglycan deposition at that level, compared to biopsy specimens from patients with celiac disease or autoimmune enteropathy.[11] Relative to the controls, there was faint and irregular laminin deposition at the epithelial–lamina propria interface, while heparan sulfate proteoglycan depositions were large and lamellar, suggestive of abnormal development of basement membrane at the origin of the epithelial abnormalities. On the other hand, we observed an increased immunohistochemical expression of desmoglein in IED, and ultrastructural changes of desmosomes, which were increased in length and number (Figure 1.7).[37]

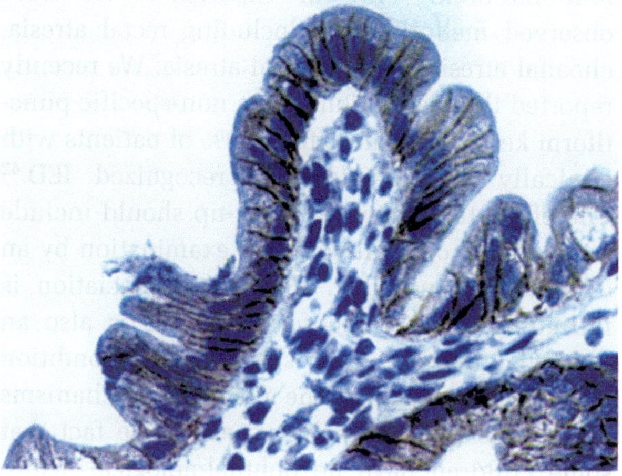

Figure 1.7 Desmoglein staining. Increased expression of desmoglein in the tight junctions.

Diagnosis

Diagnosis of IED is sometimes difficult for several reasons. The early onset of severe and permanent diarrhea and the lack of features diagnostic of microvillus inclusion disease are important diagnostic elements. However, the characteristic tufts of extruding epithelium may not be obvious, especially early on. At the onset of the clinical course, IED is most often suspected after elimination of MVID, and the final diagnosis is made rather late, by performing repeated intestinal biopsies which change from normal in early life (only non-specific villus atrophy with or without mononuclear cell infiltration of the lamina propria) to the characteristic tufts. In addition, it is difficult to show the rare, specific abnormalities of basement membrane components, integrins or desmosomes in part of the mucosa, in the absence of tufts.

Another difficulty is related to the infiltration of the lamina propria by T cells, a finding that would support the hypothesis of an immune-related enteropathy, especially when tufts are missing. One might speculate that defective cell adhesion increases intestinal permeability, with a subsequent inflammatory reaction. In a mouse model of dysfunctional E-cadherin, this primary disorder of epithelial integrity was responsible for secondary T-cell-mediated mucosal damage.[38] Murch et al[39] described this type of lesion in infants with epithelial dysplasia. They showed that inhibition of secondary T-cell activation significantly improved enteral absorption and decreased crypt cell proliferation, without, however, permanent resolution of the severe diarrhea.

Associated disorders

Several cases of IED have been reported as being associated with phenotypic abnormalities (e.g. Dubowitz syndrome or malformation syndromes).[40,41] An association between congenital IDI and choanal atresia was recently reported in four children.[40] In our experience, we have observed malformations including rectal atresia, choanal atresia or esophageal atresia. We recently reported the association with a non-specific punctiform keratitis in more than 50% of patients with clinically and histologically recognized IED.[42] Therefore, the diagnostic work-up should include a systematic ophthalmological examination by an experienced specialist. The latter association is intriguing, since punctiform keratitis is also an epithelial disease; thus, studying this condition might help to elucidate the molecular mechanisms of the intestinal epithelial disease. The fact that some children have no ophthalmological symptoms confirms the heterogeneity of the disease.

Interestingly, Lachaux et al have reported a case of a newborn presenting with pyloric atresia and intractable diarrhea.[43] Light microscopic examination showed extensive desquamation from fundus to rectum, with only a few epithelial cells remaining at the base of the crypts. Electron microscopy of the gut revealed normal desmosomes, but a cleavage located between the lamina propria and the basal pole of the enterocytes. This first-described disease is supposed to be related to congenital deficiency of $\alpha_6\beta_4$ integrin. This integrin is known to be defective in epidermolysis bullosa, in which gross epidermal shedding occurs, although the cutaneous expression of $\alpha_6\beta_4$ integrin appeared normal in this case of IDI. This is consistent with a mutation within an intestinal isoform of the $\alpha_6\beta_4$ integrin, or a deficiency of a related and immunohistochemically cross-reactive intestinal integrin.[44,45] Rather like epidermolysis bullosa, which shares several similarities with deficiency of $\alpha_6\beta_4$ integrin at the ultrastructural and possibly molecular level, there are likely to be several distinct mutations that can cause this phenotype.

Pathophysiology and mode of transmission

In infants with epithelial dysplasia with characteristic tufts, we have reported abnormal laminin and heparan sulfate proteoglycan deposition on the basement membrane, compared to biopsy specimens from patients with celiac disease or autoimmune enteropathy.[11] Basement membrane molecules are involved in epithelial–mesenchymal cell interactions, which are instrumental in intestinal development and differentiation.[46–49] Alterations suggestive of abnormal cell–cell and cell–matrix interactions were seen in patients with epithelial dysplasia without any evidence of abnormalities in epithelial cell polarization and proliferation.[37] Alterations included abnormal distribution of adhesion molecules $\alpha_2\beta_1$ integrin along the crypt–villus axis. The $\alpha_2\beta_1$ integrin is involved in the interaction of epithelial cells to various basement membrane components, such as laminin and collagen. To date, the pathophysiological mechanisms resulting in an increased immunohistochemical expression of desmoglein, and the ultrastructural changes of desmosomes remain unclear (Figure 1.7).[37] Tufts correspond to non-apoptotic epithelial cells at the villous tips that are no longer in contact with the basement membrane. It can be speculated that a defect of normal enterocyte apoptosis at the end of their lifespan, or an altered cell–cell contact, is responsible for this effect. The primary or secondary nature of the formation of tufts remains, however, to be determined.

To date, the genetic origin of this disorder is suspected from the clear association of parental consanguinity and/or affected siblings. These features suggest an autosomal recessive transmission. The gene involved in this congenital inherited autosomal recessive disease is not yet identified. This enteropathy appears more common than MVID, especially within the Middle-Eastern population.

Outcome

This neonatal diarrhea, which resists all treatments, requires permanent PN. However, it seems that some infants have a rather milder phenotype than others.[50] Thus, because of partial intestinal function and limited amount of stool output, some patients only need partial long-term PN, with three to four weekly infusions. Careful monitoring should be performed, in order to avoid progressive growth retardation. In most patients, the severity of intestinal malabsorption and diarrhea make them totally dependent on daily long-term PN with subsequent risk of complications. This is therefore another indication for intestinal transplantation.[51–53]

Other diseases of the intestinal epithelium

The classification of IDI is probably incomplete, since other forms with abnormal small-bowel mucosa have been described. These include mitochondrial DNA rearrangements; congenital enterocyte heparan sulfate deficiency, phosphomannose isomerase deficiency; and a carbohydrate-deficient glycoprotein syndrome with hepatic-intestinal presentation.[54–59] Rare diseases involving the immune system and small-bowel mucosa,[60] or severe intractable enterocolitis of infancy,[6] seem clearly different from the above-described diseases. The so-called 'phenotypic diarrhea' that is an IDI syndrome associated with phenotypic abnormalities and immune deficiency is one of these rare diseases recently reported. The patients present with diarrhea starting within the first 6 months of life (< 1 month in most cases), and have several features in common. They are small for gestational age and have an abnormal phenotype.[11] All have facial dysmorphism with prominent forehead, broad nose and hypertelorism. They have a distinct abnormality of hair, tricorrhexis nodosa, in which the hair is woolly, difficult to manage, easily pulled out and poorly pigmented, even in children of Middle-Eastern origin. Among the congenital forms of hair dysplasia, tricorrhexis nodosa is very common, and can be present in several pathological conditions.[61–64] In addition, the previously reported patients had defective antibody responses despite normal serum immunoglobulin levels, and defective antigen-specific skin tests despite positive proliferative responses *in vitro*.[12] Small-bowel biopsy specimens of the patients with diarrhea syndrome show moderate or severe villus atrophy with inconstant mononuclear cell infiltration of the lamina propria, and absence of epithelial abnormalities. Histologically, there are no specific abnormalities. The prognosis of this type of intractable diarrhea of infancy is poor, since most patients have died between the ages of 2 and 5 years – some of them with early onset of liver disease.[12] The cause of this diarrhea is unknown, and the relation between low birth weight, dysmorphism, severe diarrhea, trichorrhexis and immune deficiency is unclear. The coexistence of morphological, trichological and immunological abnormalities with early-onset intractable diarrhea disproportionate to the mucosal architectural abnormality (consistent with a primary enterocyte abnormality) suggests either mutation within several genes, inherited together by linkage disequilibrium, or, more probably, interference with a higher level of control, such as a patterning gene. The characteristic hair abnormalities may allow a more focused search for candidate mutations, as relatively few genes have been implicated in hair development.

REFERENCES

1. Avery GB, Villacivencio O, Lilly JR, Randolph JG. Intractable diarrhea in early infancy. *Pediatrics* 1968; **41**: 712–722.

2. Ricour C, Navarro J, Frederich A et al. La diarrhée grave rebelle du nourrisson (à propos de 84 observations). *Arch Fr Pediat* 1977; **34**: 44–59.

3. Guarino A, Spagnulo MI, Russo S et al. Etiology and risk factors of severe and protracted diarrhea. *J Pediatr Gastroenterol Nutr* 1995; **20**: 173–178.
4. Catassi C, Fabiani E, Spagnuolo MI et al. Severe and protracted diarrhea: results of the 3-year SIGEP multicenter survey. *J Pediatr Gastroenterol Nutr* 1999; **29**: 63–68.
5. Phillips AD, Jenkins P, Raafat F, Walker-Smith JA. Congenital microvillus atrophy: specific diagnostic features. *Arch Dis Child* 1985; **60**: 135–140.
6. Unsworth DJ, Walker-Smith JA. Auto-immunity in diarrheal disease. *J Pediatr Gastroenterol Nutr* 1985; **4**: 375–380.
7. Goulet O, Besnard M, Girardet JP, Lachaux A, Sarles J and the French Speaking Group of Hepatology, Gastroenterology and Nutrition. *Clin Nutr* 1998; **17**: 9 (A).
8. Sanderson IR, Risdon RA, Walker-Smith JA. Intractable ulcerating enterocolitis of infancy. *Arch Dis Child* 1991; **65**: 295–299.
9. Cuenod B, Brousse N, Goulet O et al. Classification of intractable diarrhea in infancy using clinical and immunohistological criteria. *Gastroenterology* 1990; **99**: 1037–1043.
10. Goulet O, Brousse N, Canioni D et al. Syndrome of intractable diarrhoea with persistent villus atrophy in early childhood: a clinicopathological survey of 47 cases. *J Pediatr Gastroenterol Nutr* 1998; **26**: 151–161.
11. Goulet O, Kedinger M, Brousse N et al. Intractable diarrhea of infancy: a new entity with epithelial and basement membrane abnormalities. *J Pediatr* 1995; **127**: 212–219.
12. Girault D, Goulet O, Ledeist F et al. Intractable diarrhea syndrome associated with phenotypic abnormalities and immune deficiency. *J Pediatr* 1994; **125**: 36–42.
13. Davidson GP, Cuiz E, Hamilton JR, Gall DG. Familial enteropathy: a syndrome of protracted diarrhea from birth, failure to thrive, and hypoplastic villus atrophy. *Gastroenterology* 1978; **75**: 783–790
14. Schmitz J, Ginies JL, Arnaud-Battandier F et al. Congenital microvillus atrophy, a rare cause of neonatal intractable diarrhea. *Pediatr Res* 1982; **16**: 1041a.
15. Phillips AD, Schmitz J. Familial microvillus atrophy: a clinicopathological survey of 23 cases. *J Pediatr Gastroenterol Nutr* 1992; **14**: 380–396.
16. Homberg C, Perheentupa J. Congenital chloride diarrhoea. *Ergeb Inn Med Kinderheilkd* 1982; **49**: 138–172.
17. Booth IW, Stange G, Murer H et al. Defective jejunal brush-border Na+/H+ exchange: a cause of congenital secretory diarrhoea. *Lancet* 1985; **1**: 1066-1069.
18. Phillips AD, Jenkins P, Raafat F, Walker-Smith JA. Congenital microvillus atrophy: specific diagnostic features. *Arch Dis Child* 1985; **60**: 135–140.
19. Bell SW, Kerner JA Jr, Sibley RK. Microvillus inclusion disease. The importance of electron microscopy for diagnosis. *Am J Surg Pathol* 1991; **15**: 1157–1164.
20. Phillips AD, Szfranski M, Man L-Y, Wall W. Periodic acid Schiff staining abnormality in microvillus atrophy: photometric and ultrastructural studies. *J Pediatr Gastroenterol Nutr* 2000; **30**: 34–42.
21. Phillips A, Fransen J, Hauri HP, Sterchi E. The constitutive exocytotic pathway in microvillus atrophy. *J Pediatr Gastroenterol Nutr* 1993; **17**: 239–246
22. Groisman GM, Amar M, Livne E. CD10: a valuable tool for the light microscopic diagnosis of microvillus inclusion disease (familial microvillus atrophy). *Am J Surg Pathol* 2002; **26**: 902–907.
23. Youssef N, Canioni D, Ruemmele F. CD-10 expression in microvillous inclusion disease. *J Pediatr Gastroenterol Nutr* 2003; **36**: 563(A).
24. Raafat F, Green NJ, Nathavitharana KA, Booth IW. Intestinal microvillus dystrophy: a variant of microvillus inclusion disease or a new entity? *Hum Pathol* 1994; **25**: 1243–1248.
25. Carruthers L, Dourmaskhin R, Phillips A. Disorders of the cytoskeleton of the enterocyte. *Clin Gastroenterol* 1986; **15** : 105–120.
26. Phillips A, Brown A, Murch S, Walker-Smith JA. Histochemical studies of microvillus atrophy: acetylated sialic acid residues accumulate in the epithelium. *J Pediatr Gastroenterol Nutr* 1999; **28**: 565 (abstract).
27. Nathavitharana KA, Green NJ, Raafat F, Booth IW. Siblings with microvillus inclusion disease. *Arch Dis Child* 1994; **71**: 71–73.
28. Heinz-Erian P, Schmidt H, Le Merrer M et al. Congenital microvillus atrophy in a girl with autosomal dominant hypochondroplasia. *J Pediatr Gastroenterol Nutr* 1999; **28**: 203–205.
29. Michail S, Collins JF, Xu H et al. Abnormal expression of brush-border membrane transporters in the duodenal mucosa of two patients with microvillus inclusion disease. *J Pediatr Gastroenterol Nutr* 1998; **27**: 536–542.
30. Oliva MM, Perman JA, Saavedra JM et al. Successful intestinal transplantation for microvillus inclusion disease. *Gastroenterology* 1994; **106**: 771–774.
31. Herzog D, Atkinson P, Grant D et al. Combined bowel–liver transplantation in an infant with microvillus inclusion disease. *J Pediatr Gastroenterol Nutr* 1996; **22**: 405–408.
32. Randak C, Langnas AN, Kaufman SS et al. Pretransplant management and small bowel–liver transplantation in an infant with microvillus inclusion disease. *J Pediatr Gastroenterol Nutr* 1998; **27**: 333–337.
33. Bunn SK, Beath SV, McKeirnan PJ et al. Treatment of microvillus inclusion disease by intestinal transplantation. *J Pediat Gastroenterol Nutr* 2000; **31**: 176–180.
34. Croft NM, Howatson AG, Ling SC et al. Microvillus inclusion disease: an evolving condition. *J Pediatr Gastroenterol Nutr* 2000; **31**: 185–189.
35. Goulet O, Michel JL, Jobert A et al. Small bowel transplantation alone or with the liver in children: changes by using FK506. *Transplant Proc* 1998; **30**: 1569–1570.
36. Reifen RM, Cutz E, Griffiths AM et al. Tufting enteropathy: a newly recognized clinicopathological entity associated with refractory diarrhea in infants. *J Pediatr Gastroenterol Nutr* 1994; **18**: 379–385.
37. Patey N, Scoazec JY, Cuenod-Jabri B et al. Distribution of cell adhesion molecules in infants with intestinal epithelial dysplasia (tufting enteropathy). *Gastroenterology* 1997; **113**: 833–843.
38. Hermiston ML, Gordon JI. Inflammatory bowel disease and adenomas in mice expressing a dominant negative N-cadherin. *Science* 1995; **270**: 1203–1207.
39. Murch S, Graham A, Vermault A et al. Functionally significant secondary inflammation occurs in a primary epithelial enteropathy. *J Pediatr Gastroenterol Nutr* 1997; **24**: 467.
40. Krantz M, Jansson U, Rectors S et al. Hereditary intractable diarrhea with choanal atresia. A new familial syndrome. *J Pediatr Gastroenterol Nutr* 1997; **24**: 470.
41. Abely M, Hankard GF, Hugot JP et al. Intractable infant diarrhea with epithelial dysplasia associated with polymalformative syndrome. *J Pediatr Gastroenterol Nutr* 1998; **27**: 348–352.
42. Djeddi D, Verkarre V, Talbotec C et al. Tufting enteropathy and associated disorders. *J Pediatr Gastroenterol Nutr* 2002; **34**: 446(A).
43. Lachaux A, Bouvier R, Loras I et al. a6b4 integrin deficiency. A new aetiology for protracted diarrhoea in infancy. *J Pediatr Gastroenterol Nutr* 1997; **24**: 470.

44. Beaulieu JF. Differential expression of the VLA family of integrins along the crypt–villus axis in the human small intestine. *J Cell Sci* 1992; **102**: 427–436.
45. Simon-Assmann P, Duclos B, Orian-Rousseau V et al. Differential expression of laminin isoforms and a6-b4 integrin subunits in the developing human and mouse intestine. *Dev Dynamics* 1994; **201**: 71–85.
46. Simon-Assmann P, Bouziges F, Vigny M, Kedinger M. Origin and deposition of basement membrane. Heparan sulfate proteoglycan in the developing intestine. *J Cell Biol* 1989; **109**: 1837–1848.
47. Simo P, Simon-Assmann P, Bouziges F et al. Changes in the expression of laminin during intestinal development. *Development* 1991; **112**: 477–487.
48. Simo P, Bouziges F, Lissitzky JC et al. Dual and asynchronous deposition of laminin chains at the epithelial mesenchymal interface in the gut. *Gastroenterology* 1992; **102**: 1835–1845.
49. Simon-Assmann P, Kedinger M. Heterotypic cellular cooperation in gut morphogenesis and differentiation. *Cell Biol* 1993; **4**: 221–230.
50. Cameron DJS, Barnes GL. Successful pregnancy outcome in tufting enteropathy. *J Pediatr Gastroenterol Nutr* 2003; **36**: 158.
51. Lacaille F, Cuenod B, Colomb V et al. Successful combined liver and small bowel transplantation in a child with epithelial dysplasia. *J Pediatr Gastroenterol Nutr* 1998; **2**: 230–233.
52. Goulet O. Intestinal transplantation. *Curr Opin Clin Nutr Metab Care* 1999; **2**: 315–321.
53. Paramesh AS, Fishbein T, Tschernia A et al. Isolated small bowel transplantation for tufting enteropathy. *J Pediatr Gastroenterol Nutr* 2003; **36**: 138–140.
54. Verloes A, Lombet J, Lambert Y et al. Tricho-hepato-enteric syndrome: further delineation of a distinct syndrome with neonatal hemochromatosis phenotype, intractable diarrhea, and hair anomalies. *Am J Med Gen* 1997; **68**: 391–395.
55. De Vries E, Visser DM, Van Dongen JJ et al. Oligoclonal gammopathy in 'phenotypic diarrhea'. *J Pediatr Gastroenterol Nutr* 2000; **30**: 349–350
56. Cormier-Daire V, Bonnefont JP, Rustin P et al. Mitochondrial DNA rearrangements with onset as chronic diarrhea with villus atrophy. *J Pediatr* 1994; **124**: 63–70.
57. Murch S, Winyard PJD, Koletzko S et al. Congenital enterocyte heparan sulphate deficiency with massive albumin loss, secretory diarrhoea and malnutrition. *Lancet* 1996; **347**: 1299–1301.
58. Jaeken J, Matthijs G, Saudubray JM et al. Phosphomannose isomerase deficiency: a carbohydrate-deficient glycoprotein syndrome with hepatic–intestinal presentation. *Am J Hum Genet* 1998; **62**: 1535–1539.
59. Oren A, Houwen RH. Phosphomannose isomerase deficiency as the cause of protein-losing enteropathy and congenital liver fibrosis. *J Pediatr Gastroenterol Nutr* 1999; **29**: 231–232.
60. Smith LJ, Szymanski W, Foulston C et al. Familial enteropathy with villus edema and immunoglobulin G2 subclass deficiency. *J Pediatr* 1994; **125**: 541–548.
61. Itin PH, Pittelkow MR. Trichothiodystrophy: review of sulfur-deficient brittle hair syndromes and association with the ectodermal dysplasia. *J Am Acad Dermatol* 1990; **22**: 705–717.
62. Happle R, Traupe H, Gröbe H, Bonsmann G. The Tay syndrome (congenital ichthyosis with trichothiodystrophy). *Eur J Pediatr* 1984; **141**: 147–152.
63. Stefanini M, Vermeulen W, Weeda G et al. A new nucleotide-excision-repair gene associated with the disorder trichothiodystrophy. *Am J Hum Genet* 1993; **53**: 817–821.
64. Mariani E, Facchini A, Honorati MC et al. Immune defects in families and patients with xeroderma pigmentosum and trichothiodystrophy. *Clin Exp Immunol* 1992; **88**: 376–382.

2 Congenital problems of the gastrointestinal tract

Nigel Hall and Agostino Pierro

Introduction

Congenital abnormalities of the gastrointestinal (GI) tract are relatively common. Owing to their nature, they frequently require surgical correction. On occasion this must be undertaken as a matter of emergency in order to avoid catastrophic intestinal ischemia and necrosis, resulting in loss of bowel or damage to a secondary organ system. It is not possible in the realms of one chapter to describe in detail all of the variants of congenital GI tract abnormalities that may be encountered and the precise nature of the treatment options available. Therefore, what follows is an overview of the most common conditions encountered and those which require intervention as a matter of urgency. For ease of understanding we commence with the upper GI tract and continue in a caudal direction.

Conditions affecting the upper gastrointestinal tract

Disorders of the mouth and oral cavity

Cleft lip and palate is one of the more common congenital anomalies with an incidence of about 1 in 600 live births.[1,2] The etiology is probably multifactorial: a genetic component is implicated as are a wide variety of exogenous factors and up to 50% of infants may have other associated anomalies.[3] The presentation may be during routine antenatal scans, although some cases do not become apparent until birth. Whilst the esthetic appearance may be the most obvious, respiratory and feeding difficulties associated with clefts carry greater medical significance and in some cases may require early intervention. The long-term management of these disorders is best in the setting of a specialist multidisciplinary team in order to achieve a satisfactory functional and cosmetic repair.

Esophageal atresia and tracheoesophageal fistula

This complex group of anomalies, with an incidence of 1 in 2440–4500 live births,[4,5] results from failure of correct division of the tracheal primordium from the esophagus during early embryonic development. The precise etiology is unknown with a number of embryological theories proposed to explain the different variants of this anomaly. There is a high incidence of co-existing abnormalities including the VACTERL syndrome, CHARGE association and isolated cardiovascular anomalies.[6]

Classification

A number of classification systems have been proposed over the years. The abbreviated list in Table 2.1 describes the most commonly encountered anatomical variants (Figure 2.1). The

Table 2.1 Classification of esophageal atresia (EA)/tracheoesophageal fistula (TEF) anomalies and frequency[6]

Type of lesion	Frequency (%)
EA and distal TEF	88.8
Isolated EA	7.3
H-type fistula	4.2
Distal and proximal TEF	2.8
Proximal TEF	1.1

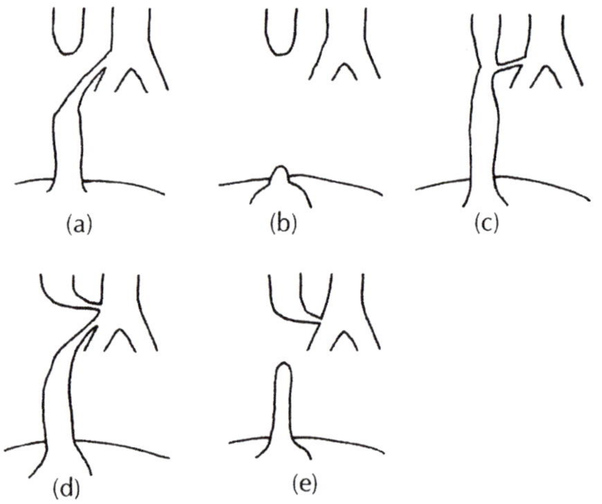

Figure 2.1 Common anatomical variants of esophageal atresia (EA)/tracheoesophageal fistula (TEF) anomalies. (a) EA with distal TEF; (b) isolated EA with no TEF; (c) H-type TEF; (d) proximal and distal TEF; (e) EA with proximal TEF.

Spitz classification[6] (Table 2.2), incorporating birth weight and presence of major congenital heart disease status, may be useful in predicting survival.

Clinical features

Esophageal atresia is commonly associated with maternal polyhydramnios. The diagnosis may be made in the antenatal period, particularly if there is no tacheoesophageal fistula. In the postnatal period, symptoms include excessive salivation, feeding difficulties, respiratory distress, and cyanotic episodes. Cases of esophageal atresia (with the exception of the rare esophageal atresia with double fistula) can be confirmed by failure of passage of a nasogastric tube into the stomach. Cases of tacheoesophageal fistula in the absence of esophageal atresia (i.e. H-type fistula) may present later, usually with recurrent episodes of respiratory distress or pneumonia.

Table 2.2 Spitz classification of esophageal atresia (EA)/tracheoesophageal fistula (TEF) anomalies and outcome[6]

Group	Clinical features	Survival (%)
I	BW ≥1500g with no major CHD	97
II	BW <1500g or major CHD	59
III	BW <1500g and major CHD	22

BW, birth weight; CHD, congenital heart disease

Treatment

The overall aim of surgical correction is early division of any fistula with the respiratory tract to protect the lungs and airway, and restoration and maintenance of esophageal continuity to allow normal feeding. Following diagnosis, a Replogle tube is placed in the upper esophageal pouch, allowing suction of secretions and minimizing of the risk of pulmonary aspiration. Surgical repair involves ligation and division of any fistula, and primary anastomosis of the two ends of the esophagus where possible. Infants in whom the gap between the two ends of the esophagus is too wide for primary anastomosis to be achieved pose a problem. These infants are initially fed by gastrostomy and the esophageal anastomosis is re-attempted after 6 weeks. If recurrent attempts at this remain unsuccessful, esophageal replacement alternatives including colonic interposition and gastric transposition are considered.

Outcome

The majority of patients do well following anastomosis, but a number of complications may occur and they require recurrent procedures. Complications include anastomotic leakage, anastomotic stricture, recurrent tacheoesophageal fistula, gastroesophageal reflux and disordered peristalsis.

The stomach

The most common abnormality of the stomach in the neonatal period is hypertrophic pyloric stenosis. Whether this is truly a congenital abnormality or an acquired disorder is questionable. It is further discussed in Chapter 35.

Other congenital conditions affecting the stomach, including congenital microgastria, gastric volvulus and congenital gastric outlet obstruction due to a pyloric web or atresia, are all extremely rare and are mentioned only for completeness.

Obstructive lesions of the duodenum, jejunum and ileum

The most common congenital conditions affecting the duodenum, jejunum and ileum all result in partial or complete gastrointestinal obstruction. The presenting features and investigations recommended to diagnose the underlying abnormality are similar for all conditions. The clinical features and investigations of these conditions are therefore presented first, followed by a description of each type of abnormality and the recommended treatment options.

Clinical features

Obstructive lesions of the small intestine from the pylorus down to the ileocecal valve may give rise to polyhydramnios in the antenatal period which is detectable by antenatal ultrasonography. As a general rule, the more proximal the lesion the more severe the degree of polyhydramnios; distal ileal lesions may be present in the absence of polyhydramnios.[7] The list of differential diagnoses giving rise to polyhydramnios is extensive, and it is rare for an obstructive lesion of the GI tract to be confirmed before birth.

Following birth, the most common and important clinical manifestation of obstructive lesions of the GI tract is bile-stained vomiting. Vomiting with truly bilious staining is abnormal in the neonatal period and always requires investigation. Lesions in the duodenum and jejunum usually result in bilious vomiting within hours. In addition, the abdomen may appear empty or even scaphoid and visible gastric peristalsis may be observed. Lesions lower in the ileum result in a distended abdomen if the obstruction is complete, and there may be failure to pass meconium. Obstructive lesions may also give rise to intestinal perforation in the neonatal period and occasionally antenatally. In all cases of neonatal intestinal obstruction, infants become progressively hypovolemic and are prone to circulatory and respiratory collapse. They require fluid resuscitation and may require ventilatory support. GI tract obstruction should therefore be considered in any infant who is dehydrated, especially if there is a history of vomiting.

Stenotic lesions of the small bowel in which the obstruction is incomplete may give rise to increased diagnostic difficulty. Affected infants often present with intermittent vomiting and episodes of partial obstruction. They eventually fail to thrive or develop complete obstruction, at which stage they are fully investigated and the diagnosis becomes apparent.

Intestinal malrotation is considered separately, as it may present with a spectrum of clinical scenarios depending on the degree of intestinal obstruction or midgut volvulus or both. The clinical pictures of all types of abnormal rotation are those of acute or chronic intestinal obstruction and/or acute or chronic abdominal pain suggestive of intestinal ischemia. True malrotation typically presents in the first year of life with symptoms of upper gastrointestinal tract obstruction including vomiting, which is usually bile-stained. A co-existing volvulus may be suspected by abdominal pain, peritonitis and hypovolemic shock associated with intestinal ischemia. However, these signs may be relatively non-specific in the young infant. Malrotation may also present later in life with similar symptoms.

Investigations

The aim of investigating cases of suspected obstruction of the small intestine is two-fold: first, to identify the nature and anatomical location of the lesion, to allow for planning of correct treatment; and second, to identify patients with malrotation in whom there is a risk of midgut volvulus and intestinal ischemia. These cases require urgent surgical intervention to reduce the risk of potentially catastrophic intestinal necrosis. The history and examination may give clues as to the location of the lesion as described above. An abdominal X-ray may simply confirm the presence of dilated intestinal loops but may also give further clues in some cases. A double-bubble appearance on abdominal X-ray with a lack of air in the distal intestine (Figure 2.2) is characteristic of duodenal obstruction. Multiple air-filled loops of proximal bowel often with air–fluid levels along with a paucity or complete absence of gas in the distal bowel is highly suggestive of obstruction of the ileum. Intestinal perforation if present will usually be apparent on abdominal X-ray, and in the rare cases of antenatal perforation there may be widespread or localized flecks of calcification representing calcified meconium within the peritoneum.

In cases in which the diagnosis is not clear on abdominal X-ray or in which midgut malrotation or volvulus is suspected, a limited upper gastrointestinal contrast study is indicated. The classical finding in cases of malrotation is that the duodenojejunal flexure lies to the right side of the spine instead of in its normal left-sided position (Figure 2.3). This finding should prompt urgent surgical treatment, because of the risk of co-existing midgut volvulus. The contrast study may also identify the presence of a stenotic segment or complete obstruction.

Cases of lower ileal stenosis or atresia are often more difficult to diagnose and a contrast enema is invaluable in distinguishing between ileal and colonic obstruction and could be therapeutic in cases of meconium ileus (see below).

Conditions affecting the duodenum

Duodenal atresia, duodenal stenosis and annular pancreas are the most common congenital conditions to affect the duodenum. All are capable of giving rise to duodenal obstruction. The incidence is reported to be between 1 in 5000 and 1 in 10 000 live births.[8]

Explanations of the etiology of duodenal atresias are not universally accepted. Unlike atresias of the ileum, they are not thought to be due to vascular accidents and the most widely accepted explanation is that of failure of recanalization of the intestinal lumen during early embryonic development.

Classification

There are four basic types of duodenal obstruction (Figure 2.4). In type 1 there is a stenosis of the duodenum resulting from a diaphragm or web partially or totally occluding the lumen. Owing to the incomplete nature of the obstruction, cases

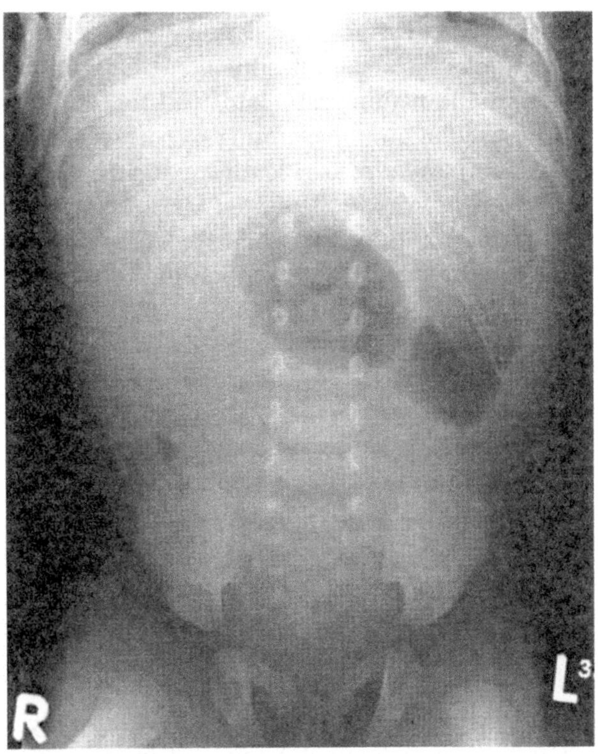

Figure 2.2 Abdominal X-ray of an infant with duodenal atresia showing the 'double bubble' appearance characteristic of duodenal obstruction.

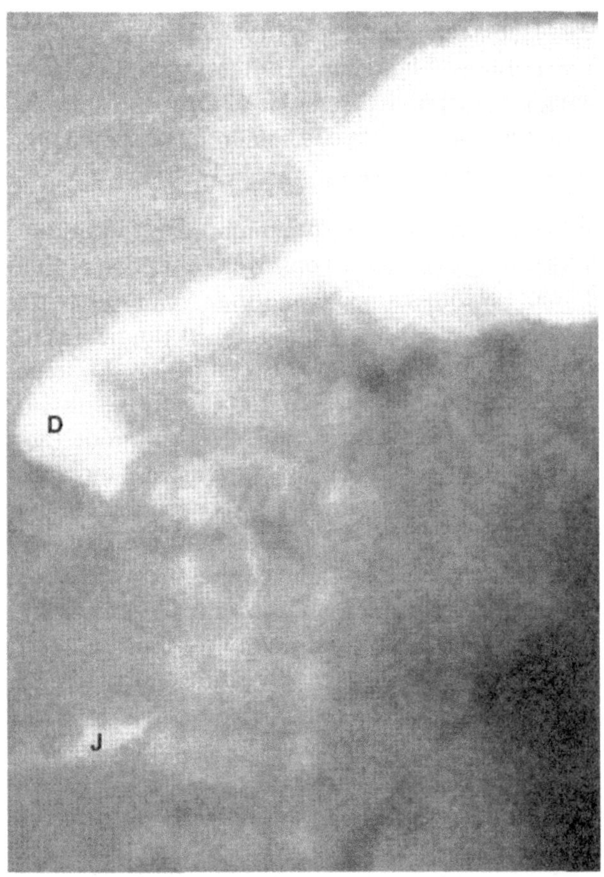

Figure 2.3 Upper gastrointestinal contrast study of a case of malrotation. The contrast is seen within the duodenum (D) and flowing into the upper jejunum (J), both of which lie completely to the right of the midline.

may present in childhood rather than in the neonatal period. In type 2 duodenal atresia, the proximal and distal segments end blindly but remain connected by a fibrous cord. There is complete separation of the bowel segments in type 3, and type 4 comprises extrinsic obstruction due to an annular pancreas although there may be an associated atretic segment. Multiple atresias are said to occur in approximately 15% of cases.[9]

Treatment

The principles of treatment are to restore intestinal continuity whilst avoiding interference with the ductal system draining the pancreas and biliary tree. This is best achieved using a duodenoduodenostomy in which the obstructed segment is bypassed by the proximal segment being joined directly to the distal segment. Following surgery the long-term gastrointestinal results are good.[10]

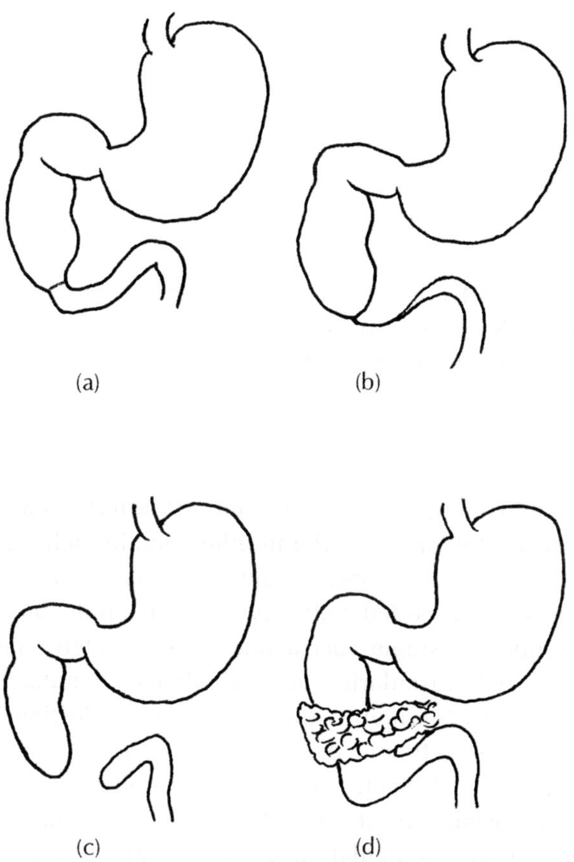

Figure 2.4 Variants of duodenal atresia. (a) Type 1 atresia due to an internal diaphragm; (b) type 2 atresia with blind-ending loops remaining connected by a fibrous cord; (c) type 3 atresia with blind ends completely separated; (d) type 4 – duodenal obstruction due to an annular pancreas.

Conditions affecting the ileum and jejunum

The main congenital problems directly affecting the small intestine from the duodenojejunal flexure down to the cecum are atresia and stenosis. Jejunoileal atresia occurs more commonly than its duodenal counterpart, with an incidence varying from 1 in 330 to 1 in 3000 livebirths.[11] Such lesions are one of the most common causes of neonatal intestinal obstruction. The major difference between atresias of the ileojejunum and those of the duodenum is in their etiology. It is postulated that atresia or stenosis of the jejunum and ileum is the result of a localized intravascular accident during intrauterine life. Subsequent ischemic necrosis and reabsorption of the affected segment or segments results in a contracted scarred bowel wall leading to stenosis at one end of the spectrum to a complete intestinal and mesenteric defect at the other. Fetal animal experiments have confirmed this hypothesis, at least in part,[12] and the absence of other congenital abnormalities found in association with jejunoileal stenoses and atresias supports the localized vascular accident theory.

Classification

Morphological classification of these lesions allows different surgeons and centers to compare outcomes and is also of therapeutic and prognostic value. The most commonly accepted system is that proposed by Louw[13] and modified by Grosfeld et al.[14] Whether the lesion is classified as ileal or jejunal is determined by the most proximal affected segment (Figure 2.5).

Stenosis is a localized narrowing of the lumen without any break in the continuity or mesenteric defect. The intestinal wall may be thickened and rigid at the stenotic site and there is a small, often minute, lumen. The overall intestinal length is not shortened. Type 1 atresia is the result of a membranous web occluding the lumen with no mesenteric defect and no intestinal shortening. The lumen is usually completely occluded and the proximal bowel is therefore dilated but remaining in continuity with the collapsed distal segment. Type 2

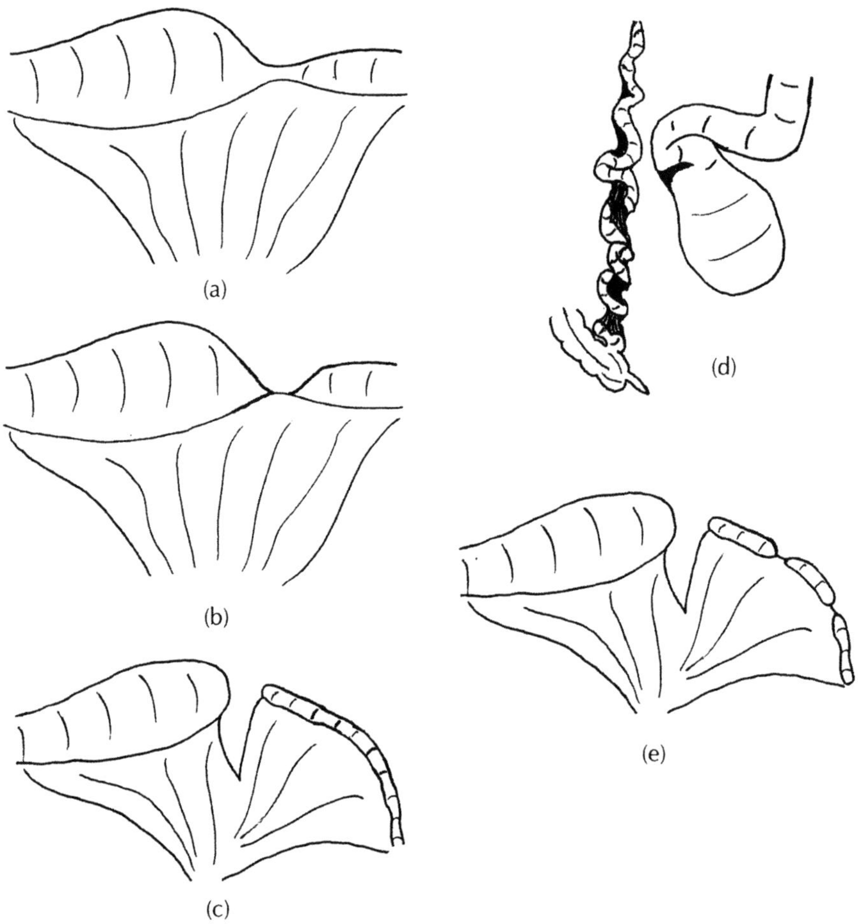

Figure 2.5 Variants of ileal atresia. (a) Type 1 due to an internal web (not shown) with no mesenteric defect; (b) type 2 atresia with blind ends joined by a fibrous cord; (c) type 3(a) – blind ends separated with a mesenteric defect; (d) type 3(b), in which the ileum is coiled like an 'apple peel' around a single vessel and completely separated from the proximal dilated duodenum; (e) type 4 or multiple atresias.

atresia arises from a complete obliteration of the intestinal segment into a fibrous cord, which joins two blind ends and runs in the free edge of the mesentery. There is no mesenteric defect and once again the total bowel length is usually normal. In both type 3(a) and type 3(b) atresia the intestine is likely to be shortened and this may have significant clinical consequences. Type 3(a) atresia consists of blind-ending proximal and distal bowel with no connection and an often large mesenteric defect. The blind ends are often physiologically abnormal with decreased or absent peristaltic activity, which may give rise to torsion, distension or perforation. Type 3(b) atresia, also known as apple peel atresia because of its gross morphology, may involve massive intestinal loss. It consists of intestinal atresia near the ligament of Treitz, obliteration of the superior mesenteric artery (SMA) beyond the origin of the middle colic branch and absence of the dorsal mesentery. The remaining intestine is coiled helically (like an apple peel) around a single perfusing vessel, often has impaired vascularity and is almost inevitably short. Furthermore, there may be additional segments of type 1 or 2 atresia within the apple peel segment. Such a configuration probably arises from occlusion of the SMA due to thrombus, embolus or strangulation as part of a midgut volvulus. In type 4 atresia there are multiple atretic segments and the intestine may resemble a string of sausages. Overall bowel length is usually shortened and the intestine grossly dilated. It has been proposed that the etiology of type 4 atresia may be due to failure of recanalization of solid epithelialization throughout the length of the intestine rather than from multiple single vascular events.

Whilst it is generally accepted that stenosis and atresia of types 1, 2 and 3(b) are the result of intrauterine vascular accidents, a genetic component has been suggested in types 3(b) and 4.

Treatment

The mainstay of surgical treatment for this type of lesion is resection of the atretic or stenotic segment and primary anastomosis, with closure of the mesenteric defect. The proximal intestinal segment is usually dilated and functionally abnormal with absent or ineffective peristalsis. This dilated proximal segment is excised along with a short segment distal to the stenosis or atresia. It is essential to establish patency of the distal bowel by irrigation or wash-out of the intestine and subsequently a primary anastomosis is performed. There is a balance to be struck between the length of the dilated proximal segment resected and the risk of leaving the infant with a short length of small bowel. It is almost inevitable that the caliber of the proximal bowel will be greater than that of the distal intestine, and a number of techniques including fishtailing and tapering exist to assist the anastomosis in such circumstances.

Outcome following intestinal atresia is dependent primarily on the length of remaining intestine and the presence of the ileocecal valve. Short bowel syndrome is defined as the presence of less than 75 cm of the small intestine or 30% of the predicted intestinal length in a premature infant.[15,16] Outcomes following short bowel syndrome vary and there is a high level of dependence on parenteral nutrition. However, intestinal adaptation can occur such that more than 80% of babies with short bowel syndrome do eventually become entirely enterally nourished.[17]

Intestinal malrotation

The incidence of intestinal malrotation is difficult to establish as not all affected patients develop symptoms, but autopsy studies estimate the incidence at approximately 1 in 500.

The traditional embryological basis for disorders of intestinal rotation is that of abnormal positioning of the intestinal loops in relation to one another as they return to the abdominal cavity from the yolk sac. During normal development the midgut rotates through 270° so that the duodenum lies posterior to the colon and the duodenojejunal flexure is to the left of the midline. A consistent finding in cases of malrotation is abnormal positioning of the duodenum. In 1995, an alternative hypothesis was proposed based on animal studies.[18] Kluth et al proposed that malrotation is the result of failure of localized growth of the duodenal loop rather than a disorder of rotation.

The term 'malrotation' covers a spectrum of anatomical abnormalities. In *non-rotation* the duodenojejunal flexure lies to the right of the spine along with most of the small intestine. The cecum and colon are typically on the left side of the abdominal cavity. Adhesions formed between loops of bowel or the intestine and abdominal wall are usually responsible for obstructive symptoms at presentation. In *malrotation* the distribution of intestinal contents within the abdominal cavity is such that the duodenum again lies to the right of the spine with the cecum anterior to it. Adhesions between these two structures (Ladd's bands) are often present and may result in partial or total occlusion of the second part of the duodenum. In addition the mesenteric attachment to the posterior aspect of the abdominal cavity is typically very short and there is a risk of volvulus with ensuing intestinal ischemia. Other forms of abnormal intestinal rotation (inverse rotation, malrotation with mesocolic hernia and malposition of the cecum) are all rare.

Treatment

There are two aspects to this disorder which require surgical intervention. The first and most important aspect is that of midgut volvulus. Any infant in whom malrotation is suspected based on clinical findings and radiological investigations should undergo laparotomy as a matter of urgency in order to minimize the risk of intestinal ischemia due to volvulus. At laparotomy blood-stained peritoneal fluid may indicate the presence of ischemic intestine. Any volvulus should be derotated (usually in the clockwise direction) and the intestine examined for viability. Non-viable bowel is resected and a primary anastomosis performed. If there is doubt about the viability of the remaining intestine a second-look laparotomy can be performed after 24 h.

In cases of malrotation not complicated by volvulus, the procedure of choice for most surgeons is the Ladd's procedure. This involves division of all adhesions or adhesive bands between the cecum, duodenum and parietal peritoneum, broadening of the mesenteric base around the superior mesenteric artery and repositioning of the intestine within the abdominal cavity so that the duodenum is on the right and the cecum lies in the left upper quadrant. It has become customary to perform an appendectomy, owing to the difficulties of diagnosis, should appendicitis develop later in life.

Meconium ileus

Meconium ileus is a common cause of neonatal intestinal obstruction and the most common cause of antenatal intestinal perforation.[19] It should be included in the differential diagnosis of infants presenting with GI tract obstruction. In approximately 80% of cases it is associated with cystic fibrosis.[20–22] The underlying defect in cystic fibrosis, an abnormality in a transmembrane chloride channel, results in the production of abnormally viscid and sticky meconium. This meconium sticks to the intestinal mucosa causing intestinal obstruction usually occurring late in gestation. Why some infants with cystic fibrosis do not develop meconium ileus is unclear. Meconium ileus can be classified as: 'uncomplicated', when it is limited to intraluminal obstruction caused by the abnormal meconium; or 'complicated', when it is associated with intestinal atresia, volvulus or meconium peritonitis.

Clinical features

In cases of uncomplicated meconium ileus, the infant usually presents shortly after birth with symptoms of lower gastrointestinal obstruction including abdominal distension and vomiting which may or may not be bile stained. The rectum may be empty and narrow and the infant does not pass meconium. If meconium ileus is complicated by volvulus, intestinal ischemia or perforation, the infant can be systemically unwell with acidosis, undergo hypovolemic shock and may require ventilatory support. Abdominal X-ray showing dilated intestinal loops and occasionally abundance of meconium in the right lower quadrant are supportive of the diagnosis, as is a gastrograffin contrast enema revealing a small collapsed colon (microcolon) and often inspissated pellets of meconium in the right lower quadrant.

Treatment

In some cases, the gastrograffin enema mentioned above may relieve the obstruction sufficiently to be curative. However, a number of uncomplicated cases and all complicated cases require surgery. The procedure performed depends on the findings during laparotomy. Atretic or grossly dilated segments of bowel may be resected, the inspissated meconium removed from the intestinal lumen and the distal bowel flushed through. Occasionally a stoma is formed to allow intestinal decompression. Outcome of surgical treatment is generally good and gastrointestinal complications are of lesser significance than the pulmonary disease caused by the underlying cystic fibrosis.

Meckel's diverticulum

Meckel's diverticulum is the most common omphalomesenteric remnant with a reported incidence of approximately 2%. Of these only a small proportion become clinically significant. The diverticulum originates from incomplete obliteration of the omphalomesenteric duct and exists as a free-lying diverticulum on the antimesenteric border of the ileum.

Clinical features

There are a variety of disease entities attributed to Meckel's diverticulum including gastrointestinal hemorrhage, intussusception, diverticulitis and perforation. The most common presenting symptom is that of gastrointestinal bleeding due to excessive acid and pepsin production from an ectopic gastric mucosa which may be present within the diverticulum. Bloody diarrhea in the absence of abdominal pain is the classical presenting picture. Other complications of Meckel's diverticulum are intussusception in which the diverticulum acts as a lead point, diverticulitis with symptoms similar to those of appendicitis and perforation.

Treatment

Management of all clinically significant cases of Meckel's diverticulum is resection of the diverticulum after adequate preoperative resuscitation. At operation the diverticulum and a wedge of ileum are resected. The ileal wedge is included, as ectopic tissue may not be entirely confined to the diverticulum. Following surgical excision the outcome is good.

Congenital hepatic, pancreatic and biliary abnormalities

Abnormalities of the hepaticopancreaticobiliary system are all extremely rare. They are included here as knowledge of their existence is important, as they form part of the differential diagnosis for infants with jaundice, malabsorption and hypoglycemia.

The most common lesions of the biliary tree are biliary atresia and congenital biliary dilatation. In biliary atresia the biliary tree is obliterated either completely or partially. Congenital biliary dilatation includes a variety of abnormalities of the biliary tree in which the dilated segment may be either intrahepatic or extrahepatic and either fusiform or cystic in nature. Dilatations of the extrahepatic biliary ducts are commonly known as choledochal cysts. The dilated bile duct is both anatomically and functionally abnormal, resulting in cholestasis. Infants with biliary atresia and severe cholestasis associated with biliary dilatation present in the neonatal period with prolonged jaundice due to accumulation of conjugated bilirubin. When the degree of obstruction to the biliary tree is not so severe, congenital biliary dilatation may present later in life with malabsorption, intermittent jaundice, abdominal pain or even pancreatitis. In addition, a choledochal cyst may present as an upper abdominal mass. Treatment of these lesions is centered around allowing drainage of the biliary tree into the intestine, and the surgery involved is often complex. The operation of choice for biliary atresia is the Kasai portoenterostomy.[23] The atretic remnants of the extrahepatic biliary ducts are removed and the porta hepatis is anastomosed to a defunctioned loop of jejunum. The timing of surgery is of paramount importance to avoid hepatocellular damage, but even with prompt diagnosis and early surgical intervention infants with biliary atresia often have residual hepatic impairment due to intrauterine cholestasis. In cases of choledochal cysts the dilated portion of the extrahepatic ducts are removed together with the gallbladder, and the common hepatic duct is anastomosed to the duodenum or a defunctioned loop of jejunum.

There are a number of congenital hepatic anomalies that give rise to structural and/or functional abnormalities of the liver parenchyma or the intrahepatic biliary tree. These include infantile and adult-type polycystic disease, congenital hepatic fibrosis, biliary hypoplasia and congenital tumors of the liver such as hamartomas and hemangiomas. Presentation is usually with one of hepatomegaly, portal hypertension or cholangitis. Treatment is that of resection of suitable lesions and prevention or treatment of hepatic disease.

Congenital lesions involving the pancreas are rare, the most common being annular pancreas (see the section on the duodenum p. 00). Other anatomical anomalies are seen including pancreatic ductal anomalies, pancreatic cysts and very rarely pancreatic agenesis. There are a group of infants who present in the neonatal period with hypoglycemia who are found to have inappropriately high levels of circulating insulin. The condition hyperinsulinemic hypoglycemia (previously commonly referred to as 'nesidioblastosis') is characterized by inappropriate endogenous insulin secretion in the presence of low blood glucose. It may result from an insulin-secreting tumor in the pancreas (a so-called 'insulinoma') but more commonly no tumor is identified and the disease is a result of a genetic defect in a membrane channel controlling insulin secretion. Infants require high glucose intake to maintain normoglycemia whilst they are investigated for the presence of an isolated secretory tumor. Treatment is by surgical excision of the tumor if present, otherwise a 90–95% subtotal pancreatectomy is performed.

Conditions affecting the lower gastrointestinal tract

Hirschsprung's disease

Hirschsprung's disease is the most common congenital malformation of the enteric nervous system with an incidence of approximately 1 in 5000 live births.[24–26] Whilst most cases are sporadic a positive familial occurrence exists in 3.6–7.8% of cases[27] and the presence of co-existing abnormalities including trisomy 21 suggests a genetic involvement (see also Chapter 17).

This condition is characterized by the absence of enteric neurons and hypertrophy of nerve trunks in the distal bowel always involving the rectum and for a variable distance proximally. There is an absence of peristaltic activity in this aganglionic segment resulting in symptoms of intractable constipation. The bowel proximal to the aganglionic segment contains ganglionated cells, and peristaltic activity is normal. However, in the so-called transitional zone, immediately proximal to the aganglionic segment, neuronal cells may exist but they are commonly of abnormal architecture and the intestinal peristalsis is abnormal. This zone is of fundamental importance when considering surgical treatment of this disorder.

Clinical features

In the neonatal period the disease should be considered in any infant who fails to pass meconium in the first 48 h of life. The usual presentation in the neonatal period is with constipation, abdominal distension and eventually vomiting during the first few days of life. More severe symptoms may be present in the neonatal period including those of gastrointestinal obstruction, enterocolitis (see below) and rarely perforation. Later in infancy symptoms of intractable constipation may signify the presence of Hirschsprung's disease.

Diagnosis

One of the most important factors in the management of Hirschsprung's disease is early diagnosis and appropriate treatment to avoid complications of the disease. Following clinical suspicion a number of investigations may be of use in making a diagnosis which must always be confirmed by histological examination of intestinal tissue. Plain abdominal X-ray will often show dilated proximal intestinal loops (Figure 2.6) prompting a lower GI contrast study to be performed to exclude intestinal atresia/stenosis or meconium ileus. This may show a prompt transition from narrow distal aganglionic bowel to dilated proximal bowel. A contrast enema is not necessary for diagnosis in many cases of Hirschsprung's disease. In addition, this investigation may be misleading in its indication of the length of intestinal aganglionosis.

The gold standard for diagnosis is the suction rectal biopsy. Characteristic histological findings are absence of ganglion cells and increase in acetylcholinesterase (AChE) staining in the parasympathetic nerve fibers. In cases where suction rectal biopsy fails to provide adequate information, a full-thickness rectal biopsy should be considered.

Treatment

Treatment in the first instance is aimed at decompression of the distal GI tract by regular rectal washouts. Subsequently a number of surgical options exist, all of which aim to remove the aganglionic segment and restore intestinal continuity by means of an anastomosis of ganglionated bowel to the rectal stump (so-called 'pull-through'). This may be performed either as a primary procedure or as a delayed procedure after initial colostomy formation

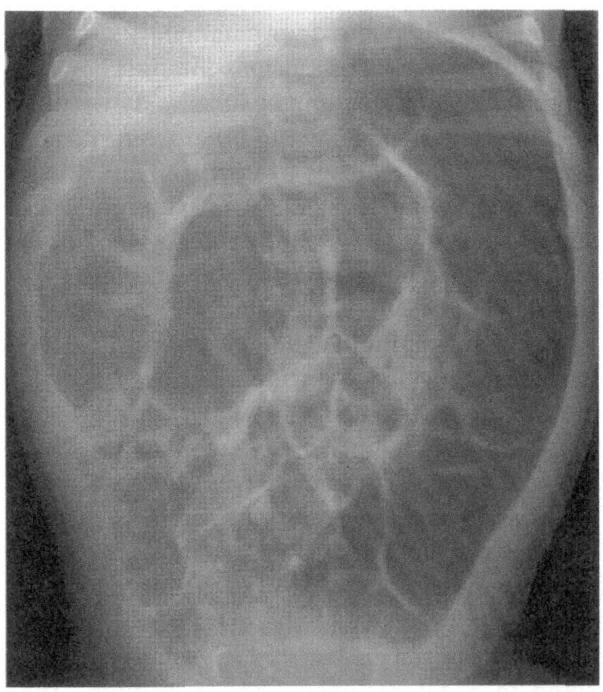

Figure 2.6 Plain abdominal X-ray of a child with rectosigmoid Hirschsprung's disease showing extensively dilated loops of bowel.

to allow distal intestinal decompression.[28] There are a number of surgical techniques, of which three are the most commonly used – the Swenson rectosigmoidectomy, the Duhammel retrorectal transanal pull-through and the endorectal pull-through of Soave. These techniques may also be carried out laparoscopically in suitable infants.

Of paramount importance in all surgical approaches is removal of the full length of aganglionic intestine. Failure to do so may result in recurrence of symptoms and complications of Hirschsprung's disease. To ensure normoganglionosis of the segment, pulled-through intraoperative biopsies are taken and rapidly examined histologically. Biopsies may be taken laparoscopically in infants undergoing a minimally invasive procedure. A number of authors have advocated laparoscopic colonic mapping prior to or during definitive surgery for exact characterization of the extent of the disease.[29,30] Recently there has been interest in infants who have retained a portion of the transition zone and have recurrent symptoms.[31,32] Attention has been drawn to the fact that the transition zone may not be linear around the circumference of the intestine, and it has been recommended that multiple circumferential biopsies be taken.[31,33]

Hirschsprung's enterocolitis

Despite appropriate treatment this serious complication of Hirschsprung's disease can develop at any stage and may be the presenting condition. Profuse, often bloody diarrhea with abdominal distension is the main presenting symptom. Vomiting and fever may be present and the child may become rapidly unwell and dehydrated. Treatment is initially with fluid resuscitation and intestinal decompression by means of a nasogastric tube. Rectal examination should be performed as it may produce an explosion of foul-smelling gas and stools which aids diagnosis and intestinal decompression. The bowel is rested, during which time parenteral nutrition may be considered. Our practice is to give enteral vancomycin, targeting *Clostridium* species which are often implicated.

Outcome

The results following surgery for Hirschsprung's disease are generally good. Long-term outcome may be difficult to assess fully, owing to the short follow-up periods reported in the literature. The incidence of incontinence is reported as ranging from zero to 82% and that of constipation from zero to 56%, these two complications probably having the greatest influence on quality of life.[34–36]

Whilst some patients may be relieved of their symptoms by surgery altogether, it should be remembered that, for some, lifelong symptoms persist particularly if the entire colon is involved by the disease.[34,36]

Anorectal anomalies

Congenital abnormalities of the anorectal region occur with an incidence of 1 in 4000 to 1 in 5000 live births.[37–39] A very small minority may be familial with the majority being isolated findings or part of a congenital syndrome such as the VACTERL syndrome. There are a number of different types of anorectal anomalies resulting from the complex embryological development of the anorectal region involving differentiation of the cloaca. The Wingspread classification[40] divides them into high, intermediate or low based on the relationship of the terminal bowel or any fistula arising from the bowel to the pelvic diaphragm. Precise definition of the abnormal anatomy is of paramount importance when planning corrective surgical treatment.

Clinical features

Abnormalities of the anorectal region are usually diagnosed on inspection during the newborn period, but surprisingly this is not always the case. In many cases the anus will be absent and meconium may be seen to originate from an abnormal site including a mucocutaneous fistula, the urethra in males or the vagina in females. Anomalies in which the anus is present but abnormally sited or stenosed may be more difficult to diagnose in the absence of adequate experience. The most complex abnormality in females is shown by the cloaca, represented by a single opening in the perineum with rectum, vagina and urethra joining a single channel.

Treatment

Treatment is aimed at preventing complications associated with the anomaly, including urinary tract infection and lower GI obstruction and subsequently restoring the anatomy to as near to normal a functional and cosmetic state as possible. In the majority of cases the initial surgery involves forming a colostomy in the descending or sigmoid colon to allow intestinal drainage and avoid dilatation of the lower bowel.[41] Following assessment, planning of surgery and growth of the infant reconstructive surgery is undertaken most commonly by the posterior sagittal approach.[42] Some anomalies also require a laparotomy to divide a high rectovesical fistula. Surgery of these cases and particularly of the cloaca is complex and should be performed by an experienced surgeon.

Outcome

In similarity to patients with Hirschsprung's disease, incontinence and constipation are the most significant long-term complications of surgically treated anorectal anomalies and often have a significant impact on quality of life. In one large series, soiling occurred in 57% of 387 cases. The incidence of fecal incontinence was 25% and constipation 43.1%.[42] Ongoing medical and, on occasion, surgical treatment is necessary to minimize disruption to a normal lifestyle.

Conditions which may occur at any point in the gastrointestinal tract

Gastrointestinal duplications

Duplication cysts of the GI tract are rare congenital abnormalities. They can occur at any point in the GI tract from mouth to anus, although they are most commonly found around the ileocecal region. Duplication cysts are defined according to strict criteria, as devised by Ladd and Gross; they are closely attached to some part of the GI tract, have a smooth muscle coat and have an epithelial lining that resembles some part of the alimentary canal.[43] Duplications may be spherical or tubular in macroscopic appearance, those that are tubular accounting for 10–20% and often having a communication with the bowel.

Clinical features

Between 25 and 30% present in the neonatal period and most have presented by the age of 10 years. Clinical features at presentation depend on anatomical site, size and secondary effects and include an oropharyngeal, abdominal or rectal mass, respiratory distress, GI bleeding, obstruction and intussusception. Duplication cysts may also be found as incidental findings at laparotomy and some lesions have been detected on antenatal ultrasound examination.[44,45]

Treatment

The recommended management of duplication cysts is complete surgical excision wherever possible, in order to prevent recurrence and complications secondary to ectopic gastric mucosa. When complete excision is not possible it is essential to remove the mucosal lining.

Conditions affecting the walls of the abdominal cavity

Whilst not truly conditions of the GI tract, there are a number of conditions that cause the abdominal contents to develop outside the abdominal cavity. These conditions are included as they have secondary effects which may significantly affect the GI tract and be a cause of GI dysfunction.

Congenital diaphragmatic hernia

The incidence of congenital diaphragmatic hernia varies from 1 in 3500 to 1 in 5000 live births.[46] Its etiology is unknown, although it is probably multifactorial. The essential anatomical defect is a breach in the continuity of the diaphragm which allows herniation of the abdominal viscera into the thoracic cavity. This has a secondary effect of impeding development of the lungs during intrauterine life. The resulting hypoplastic lungs are a cause of significant morbidity and mortality in this condition. Compression by misplaced abdominal contents does not explain the severity of lung disease seen and it is well recognized that lung development is markedly abnormal in infants with congenital diaphragmatic hernia.

Classification

A number of different defects can occur, owing to the complex development of the diaphragm. The majority of cases are of the Bochdalek type, in which the defect is posterolateral and most commonly on the left side. The defect can range in size from a small slit to involve almost the entire hemidiaphragm. Defects in the central tendon of the diaphragm result in Morgagni hernias, which are retrosternal in nature and most commonly on the right side. Finally, agenesis of the diaphragm may occur which is usually left sided and extremely rare.

Clinical features

In the current era, diaphragmatic hernia is often diagnosed during prenatal ultrasound scanning. The advantage of prenatal diagnosis is that delivery can be planned to take place in a unit with appropriate pediatric surgical and intensive care facilities. For those infants who avoid prenatal diagnosis, for whatever reason, the clinical features depend on the volume of abdominal contents within the thoracic cavity and the degree of lung hypoplasia. In the most severe cases, there will be severe respiratory distress and cyanosis from shortly after birth. At the other end of the spectrum are infants who have minimal if any respiratory symptoms or signs and in whom intestinal loops are noted to be in the abdomen on chest X-ray (Figure 2.7).

Treatment

Whilst the definitive treatment of diaphragmatic hernia is surgical closure, the timing of this is not of paramount importance and should be undertaken once the infant is stable from a cardiovascular and respiratory point of view. The respiratory management of these infants can be problematic owing to the severe lung hypoplasia and associated pulmonary hypertension. Most require conventional ventilatory support as a minimum and many require high-frequency oscillatory ventilation to ensure adequate oxygenation. Other measures to reduce pulmonary hypertension, including inhaled nitric oxide, adenosine or sildenafil, may be effective. Resistant cases may be candidates for extracorporeal membrane oxygenation, during which the infant is placed on a life-support system in the hope that the lungs and in particular the pulmonary vasculature will mature. Various criteria for extracorporeal membrane oxygenation exist[47] with the aim of

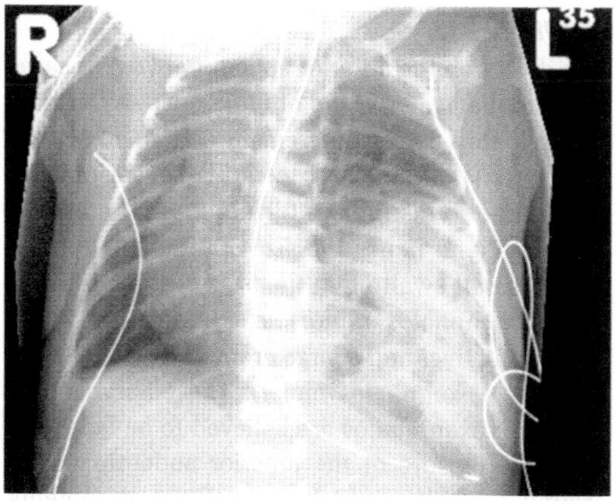

Figure 2.7 Chest radiograph of an infant with congenital diaphragmatic hernia. Loops of intestine are clearly seen within the left hemithorax and there is mediastinal shift to the right.

reserving it for those who have the most severe respiratory failure and those who are most likely to benefit. Unfortunately, there remain a number of infants with congenital diaphragmatic hernia whose lung disease presents too great a challenge and these do not survive.

Surgery

The principles of surgical repair are to return the abdominal contents to the abdominal cavity and repair the diaphragmatic defect. It may be possible to repair the defect by simply suturing the edges together. However, if the defect is large a patch repair may be undertaken using prosthetic material. The long-term outcome of congenital diaphragmatic hernia is dependent primarily on the degree of pulmonary hypoplasia. The main GI consequence appears to be gastroesophageal reflux, seen in up to 62% of cases.[48]

Anterior abdominal wall defects

Although separate clinical entities, the two conditions exomphalos and gastroschisis, which comprise anterior abdominal wall defects are grouped together, owing to similarity in their clinical appearance and the recommended course of management. In both conditions some portion of the viscera lies outside the abdominal cavity extruding through a defect in the anterior abdominal wall.

Exomphalos

The defect on the anterior abdominal wall in cases of exomphalos lies in the midline. Viscera herniate through this defect but remain contained within an avascular hernial sac comprising peritoneum and amniotic membrane (Figure 2.8). The size of the defect and hence the size of the sac may vary from a small swelling at the base of the umbilical cord (exomphalos minor) to a much larger sac containing liver and a large proportion of the small intestine (exomphalos major). The embryological origins of exomphalos are believed to be failure of complete closure of the anterior abdominal wall around a persistent body stalk. Visceral contents continue to develop within this body stalk and thus remain outside the abdominal cavity. Whilst the precise etiology of exomphalos is not clear, it is well recognized that exomphalos often co-exists with a number of other congenital abnormalities and this may suggest at least in part a genetic component. Associated abnormalities include Beckwith–Wiedemann syndrome, the trisomies 13, 18 and 21 and the upper and lower midline associations.

Gastroschisis

The anterior abdominal wall defect in cases of gastroschisis is of full thickness and typically to the right of the umbilical cord. Unlike exomphalos there is no sac covering the eviscerated intestine, which is usually dilated and inflamed (Figure 2.9). The liver is not herniated. The precise embryological basis of gastroschisis is unclear and a number of hypotheses have been proposed. The fact that gastroschisis is rarely associated with any other congenital abnormalities, with the exception of intestinal atresias and malrotation, suggests that it is most likely to have a separate embryological basis from the events resulting in exomphalos.

Treatment

It is now common for these two abnormalities to be detected in the antenatal period; delivery in a specialist center with pediatric surgical facilities is recommended. There is no consensus concerning the timing or mode of delivery of these babies and there is no convincing evidence to suggest that preterm or Cesarean section delivery confer any distinct advantage.[49–51] In gastroschisis, however, delivery is commonly induced at 37 weeks' gestation to avoid late-gestation fetal death. What is of paramount importance is protection of the intestine and prevention of fluid loss in cases of gastroschisis from the moment of delivery. In exomphalos the hernial sac confers a degree of protection to the intestine. In cases of gastroschisis the eviscerated intestine should be wrapped in clingfilm and adequate support provided to prevent fluid loss and ischemic damage to the bowel. Cases of exomphalos in which the hernial sac ruptures during delivery should subsequently be treated as for gastroschisis. Surgery and attempted closure should take place as

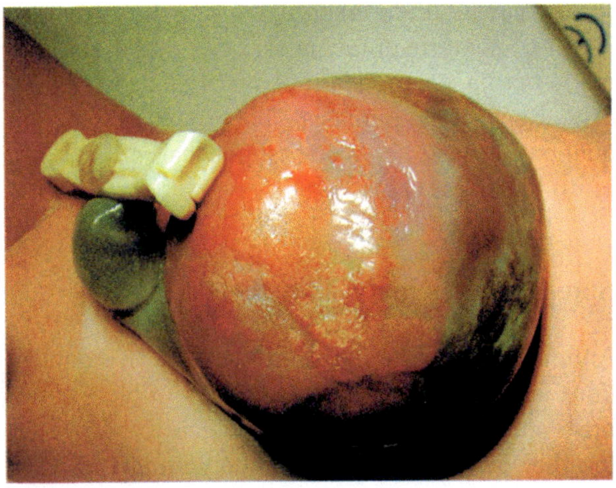

Figure 2.8 Clinical appearance of an infant with exomphalos. The abdominal contents are enclosed within an avascular hernial sac.

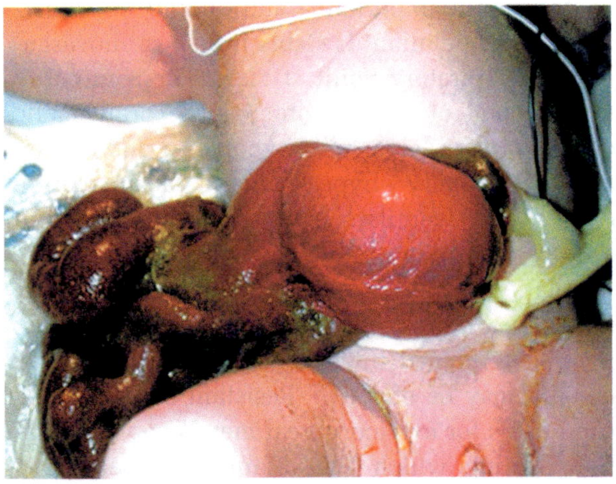

Figure 2.9 Clinical appearance of an infant with gastroschisis. There is no sac enclosing the herniated intestine, which is thickened and inflamed.

soon as possible following stabilization of the infant to prevent dehydration. Recent evidence suggests that a staged repair may result in favorable outcome when compared with primary closure.[52–54] Intestinal dysmotility is always present in neonates with gastroschisis requiring parenteral nutrition for a period of usually 2–3 weeks. Parenteral nutrition has significantly improved the survival of neonates with gastroschisis.

Surgical closure

The aim of surgery in both conditions is the return of abdominal contents to the abdominal cavity and closure of the overlying skin. In some cases this can be achieved in one surgical procedure (primary closure) but in many instances the abdominal cavity is not of sufficient volume to accommodate the eviscerated organs. In these cases a staged closure is performed in which a 'silo' is attached under the fascia around the base of the defect and completely encloses the eviscerated abdominal contents. This gives the intestine protection from dehydration and contains the bowel within a manageable sac, reducing the risk of intestinal damage. The silo is gradually reduced in size as the abdominal cavity allows and the skin is closed in a final operation. The prognosis for infants with both these conditions in the absence of co-existing abnormalities is good.

REFERENCES

1. Jensen BL, Kreiborg S, Dahl E et al, Cleft lip and palate in Denmark, 1976–1981: epidemiology, variability, and early somatic development. *Cleft Palate J* 1988; **25**: 258–269.
2. Womersley J, Stone DH. Epidemiology of facial clefts. *Arch Dis Child* 1987 **62**: 717–720.
3. Shprintzen RJ, Siegel-Sadewitz VL, Amato J et al. Anomalies associated with cleft lip, cleft palate, or both. *Am J Med Genet* 1985; **20**: 585–595.
4. Kyyronen P, Himminki K. Gastro-intestinal atresia in Finland in 1970–79, indicating time–place clustering. *J Epidemiol Community Health* 1988; **42**: 257–265.
5. Myers NA. Esophageal atresia: the epitome of modern surgery. *Ann R Coll Surg Engl* 1974; **54**: 277–287.
6. Spitz L, Kiely EM, Morecroft JA et al. Esophageal atresia: at-risk groups for the 1990s. *J Pediatr Surg* 1994; **29**: 723–725.
7. Pierro A, Cozzi F, Colarossi G et al. Does fetal gut obstruction cause hydramnios and growth retardation? *J Pediatr Surg* 1987; **22**: 454–457.
8. Sweed Y. Duodenal obstruction. In Puri P, ed. *Newborn Surgery*, 2nd edn. New York: Arnold, 2003: 423–433.
9. Menardi G. Duodenal atresia, stenosis and annular pancreas. In Freeman NV, Burge DM, Griffiths DM, Malone PSJ, eds. *Surgery of the Newborn*, 1st edn. Edinburgh: Churchill Livingstone, 1994: 107–115.
10. Stauffer UG, Irving I. Duodenal atresia and stenosis – long-term results. *Prog Pediatr Surg* 1977; **10**: 49–60.
11. Rode H, Millar AJW. Jejuno-ileal atresia and stenosis. In Puri P, ed. *Newborn Surgery*, 2nd edn. New York: Arnold, 2003: 445–456.
12. Louw JH, Barnard CN. Congenital intestinal atresia: observations on its origin. *Lancet* 1955; **2**:1065.
13. Louw JH. Congenital intestinal atresia and stenosis in the newborn. Observations on its pathogenesis and treatment. *Ann R Coll Surg Engl* 1959; **25**: 209.
14. Grosfeld JL, Ballantine TV, Shoemaker R. Operative mangement of intestinal atresia and stenosis based on pathologic findings *J Pediatr Surg* 1979; **14**: 368–375.
15. Rickham PP. Massive small intestinal resection in newborn infants. Hunterian Lecture delivered at the Royal College of Surgeons of England on 13th April 1967. *Ann R Coll Surg Engl* 1967; **41**: 480–492.
16. Touloukian RJ, Smith GJ. Normal intestinal length in preterm infants. *J Pediatr Surg* 1983; **18**: 720–723.
17. Hollwarth ME. Short bowel syndrome and surgical techniques for the baby with short intestines. In Puri P, ed. *Newborn Surgery*, 2nd edn. New York: Arnold, 2003; 569–576.

18. Kluth D, Kaestner M, Tibboel D et al. Rotation of the gut: fact or fantasy? *J Pediatr Surg* 1995; **30**: 448–453.
19. Farber SJ. The relation of pancreatic achylia to meconium ileus. *J Pediatr* 1944; **24**: 387–392.
20. Del Pin CA, Czyrko C, Ziegler MM et al. Management and survival of meconium ileus. A 30-year review. *Ann Surg* 1992; **215**: 179–185.
21. Fakhoury K, Durie PR, Levison H et al. Meconium ileus in the absence of cystic fibrosis. *Arch Dis Child* 1992; **67**: 1204–1206.
22. Murshed R, Spitz L, Kiely E et al. Meconium ileus: a ten-year review of thirty-six patients. *Eur J Pediatr Surg* 1997; **7**: 275–277.
23. Kasai M. Treatment of biliary atresia with special reference to hepatic porto-enterostomy and its modifications. *Prog Pediatr Surg* 1974; **6**: 5–52.
24. Passarge E. The genetics of Hirschsprung's disease. Evidence for heterogeneous etiologogy and a study of sixty-three families. *N Engl J Med* 1967; **276**: 138–143.
25. Orr JD, Scobie WG. Presentation and incidence of Hirschsprung's disease. *Br Med J (Clin Res Ed)* 1983: **287**: 1671.
26. Spouge D, Baird PA. Hirschsprung's disease in large birth cohort. *Teratology* 1985; **32**: 171–177.
27. Puri P. Hirschsprung's disease. In Oldham TO, Colombani PM, Foglia RP, eds. *Surgery of Infants and Children: Scientific Principles and Practice*. New York: Lippincott-Raven, 1997: 1277–1299.
28. Pierro A, Fasoli L, Kiely EM et al. Staged pull-through for rectosigmoid Hirschsprung's disease is not safer than primary pull-through. *J Pediatr Surg* 1997; **32**: 505–509.
29. Yamataka A, Yoshida R, Kobayashi H et al. Laparoscopy-assisted suction colonic biopsy and intraoperative rapid acetylcholinesterase staining during transanal pull-through for Hirschsprung's disease. *J Pediatr Surg* 2002; **37**: 1661–1663.
30. Carvalho JL, Campos M, Soares-Oliveira M et al. Laparoscopic colonic mapping of dysganglionosis. *Pediatr Surg Int* 2001; **17**: 493–495.
31. Ghose SI, Squire BR, Stringer MD et al. Hirschsprung's disease: problems with transition-zone pull-through. *J Pediatr Surg* 2000; **35**: 1805–1809.
32. Proctor ML, Traubici J, Langer JC et al. Correlation between radiographic transition zone and level of aganglionosis in Hirschsprung's disease: implications for surgical approach. *J Pediatr Surg* 2003; **38**: 775–778.
33. Farrugia M, Alexander N, Nicholls E et al. Does transitional zone pull-through in Hirschsprung's disease imply a poor prognosis? Presented at the *Pacific Association of Pediatric Surgeons 36th Annual Meeting*, Sydney, Australia 2003.
34. Ludman L, Spitz L, Tsuji H et al. Hirschsprung's disease: functional and psychological follow up comparing total colonic and rectosigmoid aganglionosis. *Arch Dis Child* 2002; **86**: 348–351.
35. Teitelbaum DH, Coran AG. Long-term results and quality of life after treatment of Hirschsprung's disease and allied disorders. In Holschneider AM, Puri P, eds. *Hirschsprung's Disease and Allied Disorders*, 2nd edn. Amsterdam: Harwood Academic, 2000: 457–465.
36. Tsuji H, Spitz L, Kiely EM et al. Management and long-term follow-up of infants with total colonic aganglionosis. *J Pediatr Surg* 1999; **34**: 158–161.
37. Brenner EC. Congenital defects of the anus and rectum. *Surg Gynecol Obstet* 1915; **20**: 579–588.
38. Santulli TV. Treatment of imperforate anus and associated fistulas. *Surg Gynecol Obstet* 1952; **95**: 601–614.
39. Trusler GA, Wilkinson RH. Imperforate anus: a review of 147 cases. *Can J Surg* 1962; **5**: 169–177.
40. Stephens FD, Smith ED. Classification, identification and assessment of surgical treatment of anorectal anomalies. *Pediatr Surg Int* 1986: **1**:200–205.
41. Patwardhan N, Kiely EM, Drake DP et al. Colostomy for anorectal anomalies: high incidence of complications. *J Pediatr Surg* 2001; **36**: 795–798.
42. Pena A. Anorectal anomalies. In Puri P, ed. *Newborn Surgery*, 2nd edn. New York: Arnold, 2003: 535–552.
43. Ladd WE, Gross RE. Surgical treatment of duplication of the alimentary tract; enterogenous cysts, enteric cysts, or ileum duplex. *Surg Gynecol Obstet* 1940; **70**: 295–307.
44. Duncan BW, Adzick NS, Eraklis A. Retroperitoneal alimentary tract duplications detected in utero. *J Pediatr Surg* 1992; **27**: 1231–1233.
45. Goyert GL, Blitz D, Gibson P et al. Prenatal diagnosis of duplication cyst of the pylorus. *Prenat Diagn* 1991; **11**: 483–486.
46. Robert E, Kallen B, Harris J. The epidemiology of diaphragmatic hernia. *Eur J Epidemiol* 1997; **13**: 665–673.
47. UK Collaborative ECMO Trial Group. UK collaborative randomised trial of neonatal extracorporeal membrane oxygenation. *Lancet* 1996; **348**: 75–82.
48. Kieffer J, Sapin E, Berg A et al. Gastroesophageal reflux after repair of congenital diaphragmatic hernia. *J Pediatr Surg* 1995; **30**: 1330–1333.
49. Quirk JG Jr, Fortney J, Collins HB et al. Outcomes of newborns with gastroschisis: the effects of mode of delivery, site of delivery, and interval from birth to surgery. *Am J Obstet Gynecol* 1996; **174**: 1134–1138.
50. Dunn JC, Fonkalsrud EW, Atkinson JB. The influence of gestational age and mode of delivery on infants with gastroschisis. *J Pediatr Surg* 1999; **34**: 1393–1395.
51. Sheth NP. Preterm and particularly, pre-labour cesarean section to avoid complications of gastroschisis. *Pediatr Surg Int* 2000; **16**: 229.
52. Jona JZ. The 'gentle touch' technique in the treatment of gastroschisis. *J Pediatr Surg* 2003; **38**: 1036–1038.
53. Kidd JN Jr, Jackson RJ, Smith SD et al. Evolution of staged versus primary closure of gastroschisis. *Ann Surg* 2003; **237**: 759–764.
54. Schlatter M, Norris K, Uitvlugt N et al. Improved outcomes in the treatment of gastroschisis using a preformed silo and delayed repair approach. *J Pediatr Surg* 2003; **38**: 459–464.

3 Infectious esophagitis

Salvatore Cucchiara and Osvaldo Borrelli

Epidemiology and predisposing conditions

In the recent years the spectrum of infectious esophagitis in childhood has expanded, owing to the emergence of new conditions, such as the acquired immunodeficiency syndrome (AIDS), the advancement in therapy and survival of patients transplanted and treated with immunosuppressive drugs, and the improvement in endoscopic and microbiological techniques. The most common infectious causes of esophagitis are fungal, viral, bacterial and, more rarely, protozoal. Primary esophageal infection is quite rare in otherwise normal subjects without permissive factors and most cases of infectious esophagitis are described in immunocompromised patients.

The immunocompetent subjects developing esophageal infections will have predisposing conditions that weaken defence mechanisms of the esophageal mucosa. Esophageal disorders that cause slowing of peristalsis and stasis of intraluminal content such as achalasia, systemic sclerosis, myopathies, neuropathies and esophageal strictures predispose to infections of the esophageal mucosa, usually candidiasis. Infections in the surrounding organs and structures may also involve the esophagus. Other conditions predisposing to esophageal infections are malnutrition and diabetes mellitus. The latter may derange esophageal peristalsis and emptying of intraluminal content, and may impair granulocyte function through hyperglycemia. Finally, antimicrobial drugs can alter the normal oropharyngeal flora leading to overgrowth of *Candida* organisms.

Conditions affecting both humoral and cellular immunological variables also lead to esophageal infections. This occurs in children with either genetic or acquired immunodeficiency as well as in the course of diseases promoting development of opportunistic infections. Transplant recipients are candidates for infectious esophagitis through different mechanisms: drug-induced immunosuppression, chemotherapy and neutropenia. Furthermore, whereas bacterial and fungal infections predominate in the early phases following transplantation, when granulocyte number and function are more compromised, the cytomegalovirus (CMV) infection occurs a few months after transplantation when T-cell function is more impaired.

In HIV-infected patients opportunistic infections develop and increase in frequency as immunodeficiency worsens. Esophageal and other opportunistic infections do not occur until immunodeficiency is severe, usually when the CD4 lymphocyte count is below 100–200/mm^3, according to references 1–3. More recently, however, the widespread availability of highly active antiretroviral therapy has been associated with an apparent decline in opportunistic infections in HIV-infected patients. The causes of esophageal disease in patients with HIV infection and AIDS are reported in Table 3.1. In contrast to the findings in other immunocompromised hosts, herpes simplex virus (HSV) esophagitis is uncommon, whereas by far the most common cause is *Candida*, accounting for about 50% of esophageal infections.[4,5] Esophageal candidiasis can also co-exist with other esophageal infections.[6]

Fungal infections

Candida species are the most common agents of infectious esophagitis. *Candida albicans* is the most common pathogen, but *C. tropicalis, C. parapsilosis and C. glabrata* have occasionally been reported. These organisms are usually

Table 3.1 Causes of esophageal disease in HIV infection and AIDS

Common	Uncommon	Rare
Candida	Herpes simplex virus	Neoplasm
Cytomegalovirus	Gastroesophageal reflux disease	Mycobacteria
Idiopathic		Protozoa

present in the normal oral flora, where their growth is controlled by commensal organisms. Conditions predisposing to esophageal candidiasis in immunocompetent subjects are inhaled or ingested corticosteroids, prolonged antibiotic administration, acid suppressive therapy, disorders of esophageal motility, malnutrition, diabetes mellitus and neck or head radiotherapy because of malignancy. All abnormalities in cellular immunity lead to esophageal candidiasis, whereas improved management of immunosuppressive therapies and antifungal prophylaxis have reduced the occurrence of esophageal candidiasis in solid-organ transplant recipients.[7]

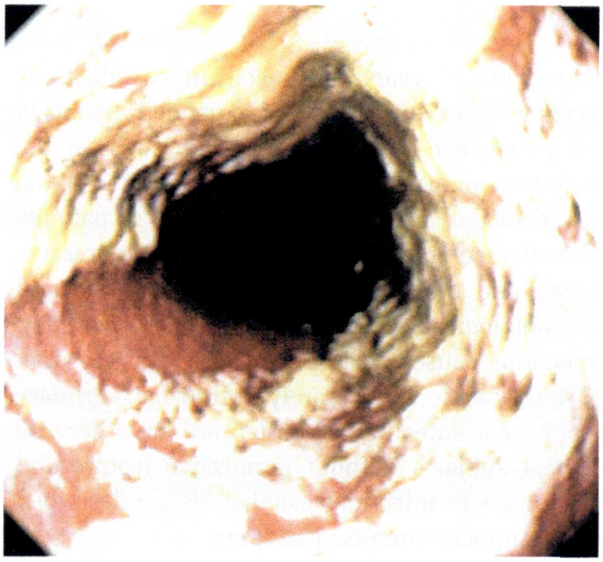

Figure 3.1 Esophageal candidiasis. White plaques coating the lower third of the esophageal mucosa.

Esophageal candidiasis has the classical appearance of white or yellow plaques coating the esophageal mucosa (Figure 3.1). These plaques can extend up to the proximal esophagus, are usually thick and, characteristically, cannot be washed or brushed off, unlike food or milk residues overlying esophageal mucosa. They include desquamated esophageal epithelial cells intermingled with inflammatory cells, bacteria and mycelia and spores typical for *Candida*.[8] The underlying squamous esophageal epithelium usually appears uninvolved, and ulcerations occur rarely.

Typical symptoms of esophageal candidiasis are painful swallowing (odynophagia) or dysphagia (difficulty in swallowing, described as food 'sticking') (Table 3.2).[3,9] Any patient with risk factors for esophageal infection and complaining of dysphagia should be suspected for esophageal candidiasis. The latter, however, can be detected by chance in asymptomatic subjects. When evaluating patients with esophageal complaints, an important part of the physical examination is a close inspection of the oropharynx. However, oral candidiasis is not predictive of esophageal involvement and the latter can occur in the absence of oral candidiasis even in the immunocompromised subject. Complications from esophageal candidiasis occur rarely. Hematemesis suggests underlying ulcerative esophagitis that occurs if the disease is severe and there is an associated coagulopathy.

Given that esophageal candidiasis is the most common of opportunistic infections of the esophagus in subjects with a predisposing condition (e.g. HIV infection, transplantation, immunosuppressive therapy), an empirical antifungal therapy has been proposed, with further diagnostic evaluation based on the clinical response (Figure 3.2). Interestingly, a prospective study comparing empirical fluconazole to endoscopy in HIV-infected adults has shown empirical fluconazole to be the best initial management strategy.[3] *Candida* esophagitis usually responds rapidly to fluconazole.[10]

Before the advent of upper endoscopy, a barium esophagram was used as the initial diagnostic tool. However, a number of studies have shown the rela-

Table 3.2 Symptoms and clinical signs in patients with esophageal infection

	Candida	Viruses	Bacteria	Parasites
Dysphagia	++++	+	+	+
Odynophagia	++	++++	+++	++
Heartburn	+	+	+	+
Chest pain	+	+++	++	+
Fever	-	+	+++	-
Hematemesis	+	++	+	+

(-), Not occurring; (+), rare; (++), occasional; (+++), common; (++++), always present

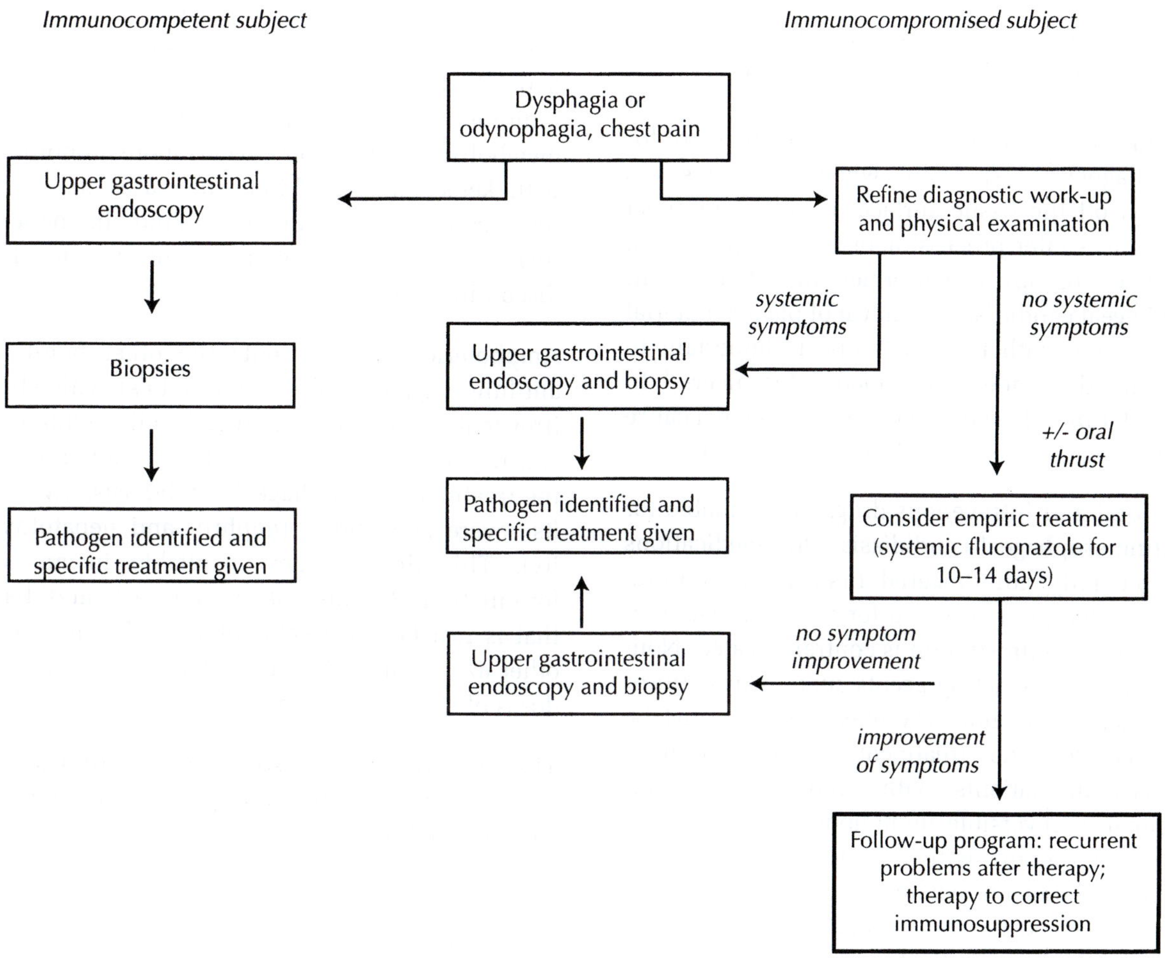

Figure 3.2 Algorithm for management of infectious esophagitis.

tive insensitivity and non-specificity of barium studies for evaluating esophageal mucosa infection. Commonly reported X-ray features in patients with esophageal candidiasis are plaque-like lesions in a linear configuration that, when severe, become confluent; a 'shaggy' aspect of the esophagus ensues.[11,12] However, a normal barium esophagram does not exclude esophageal candidiasis. It should be remarked that a well-circumscribed ulceration should not indicate *Candida* infection of the esophagus.

Non-invasive methods to diagnose esophageal infections without endoscopy are cytology brush and balloon devices. The latter consists of a tube with a ridged cytology balloon on the distal end: when inflated, it can be withdrawn from the esophagus and the brushings removed and submitted for cytological evaluation as well as viral culture. Whereas these methods are useful to identify *Candida*, they are less sensitive for viral disease and have no real advantage over empirical antifungal therapy.[13]

Endoscopy with biopsy is the gold standard for diagnosing esophageal candidiasis because mucosal biopsies can be performed. Despite the fact that gross endoscopic features can suggest a diagnosis of esophageal candidiasis, this is confirmed by the presence of hyphae in biopsies. Cytological specimens, which can be obtained at the time of endoscopy, are also a sensitive tool for the diagnosis, especially when organisms are washed off the tissue surface in mild superficial candidiasis after processing of bioptic specimens. When endoscopy is performed in patients with esophageal candidiasis, removal of plaque material by scraping with the endoscope is important to evaluate the underlying mucosa for ulcers.[6] In general, *Candida* should not be considered a cause of esophageal ulcers in HIV-infected patients.

Both oral and intravenous drugs are available for treating esophageal candidiasis. Oral medications are generally administered first, whereas intravenous therapy is reserved for refractory cases or when oral administration is contraindicated. Non-systemic locally acting agents such as nystatin or clotrimazole are not very effective and must be reserved for the treatment of oropharyngeal disease. In patients with mild disease, with minimal or reversible immunodeficiency, a short course of therapy with a systemically absorbed agent can be given, whereas in patients with HIV infection or with transplantation immunodeficiency, longer courses of azoles are best given. Patients with granulocytopenia, at risk for systemic *Candida* infection, require the use of systemically acting intravenous agents such as azoles or amphotericin B. All available oral agents (ketoconazole, fluconazole and itraconazole) are efficacious for the treatment of esophageal candidiasis (Table 3.3). Ketoconazole and itraconazole should be avoided in patients requiring anti-acid therapy, as an alkaline pH limits their bioavailability. Fluconazole appears to be more efficacious than itraconazole; a poor response to fluconazole suggests non-compliance, drug resistance or other causes for esophageal symptoms.[14] Randomized trials suggest that fluconazole is significantly more effective for the treatment of esophageal candidiasis in HIV-infected patients than ketoconazole and itraconazole.[14] Fluconazole is available in oral and intravenous preparations, is minimally metabolized, is highly water soluble and is slightly protein bound. The new oral suspension formulations of fluconazole and itraconazole may have superior efficacy over pills due to an additional local antifungal effect and improved absorption.[15] The adverse effects of ketoconazole, fluconazole and itraconazole are dose dependent and include nausea, hepatotoxicity, inhibition of steroid production and cyclosporin metabolism.[16] The latter effect is more pronounced with ketoconazole.[17] Minor increases in aminotransferases are commonly found in patients treated with oral azoles and do not require drug discontinuation.

Amphotericin B represents the other family of antifungal agents (polyene antibiotics), which bind irreversibly to sterol in fungal cell membranes, causing cell death. This drug has a limited use for the treatment of esophageal candidiasis, owing to its severe side-effects (nephro- and hepatotoxicity). This drug is now available in an oral formulation. Patients with esophageal candidiasis that is resistant to treatment with fluconazole or other azoles can be treated effectively with lower doses of intravenous amphotericin B.

The prophylaxis of esophageal candidiasis in malignancy and transplant patients has yielded controversial results.[18]

Viral infections

HSV and CMV are the most common viral agents involved in infectious esophagitis, although some cases have been ascribed to HIV infection of the esophagus. HSV (HSV I or, rarely, HSV II) esophagitis causes a self-limited disease in normal subjects, but it can be severe and prolonged in the compromised patients.

Table 3.3 Drugs for esophageal candidiasis

Drug/efficacy	Duration	Dosage	Remarks
Ketoconazole (<80%)	7–14 days	5–10 mg/kg/per day	Liver disorders can occur during therapy. The occurrence of liver disorders while on ketoconazole could be fatal unless properly recognized. Liver function tests should be performed before treatment, after 2 weeks and at periodic intervals during treatment in patients who are expected to be on prolonged therapy
Fluconazole (>80%)	7–14 days	3 mg/kg/per day for superficial infections; 6–12 mg/kg/per day for systemic infections	Nausea, vomiting, diarrhea and allergic reactions are most common adverse events. May cause clinical hepatitis, cholestasis and fulminant hepatic failure with underlying clinical conditions (e.g. AIDS, malignancy)
Itraconazole (approximately 80%)	7–14 days	3–5 mg/kg/per day	Caution in liver insufficiencies; nausea, vomiting, diarrhea and abdominal discomfort may occur; high doses may produce hypertension, hypokalemia or edema
Amphotericin B (>95%)	7 days	0.3–1.5 mg/kg/per day i.v. infused in 5% dextrose over 2–4 h	Infusion-related toxicity includes acute reactions occurring about 30–45 min after starting infusion; typically chills, fever and tachypnea may present; patients receiving any parenteral form of the drug must be monitored for renal and liver functions; normochromic normocytic anemia may develop, usually after 7–10 days of therapy
Amphotericin B, lipid formulations (>95%)	7 days	ABLC (amphotericin B lipid complex): 5 mg/kg/per day i.v. for 1–2 h; ABCD (amphotericin B colloidal dispersion): 3–6 mg/kg/per day i.v. for 1–2 h; L-AMB (liposomal amphotericin B): 1–7 mg/kg per day i.v. for 1–2 h	Novel lipid formulations of amphotericin B delivering higher concentrations of the drug with a theoretical increase in the therapeutic potential and decreased nephrotoxicity

HSV esophagitis occurs as a primary infection or as a reactivation of previously latent HSV, especially in the compromised patient. It is particularly common in patients receiving immunosuppression for solid organ or bone marrow transplantation,[19] whereas it is infrequently reported in HIV-infected patients.[4] HSV generally infects the squamous epithelium, where the earliest lesion is a vesicle. As vesicles enlarge and ulcerate, they tend to form larger lesions with a characteristic central ulceration and raised edges.

HSV esophagitis usually presents with a sudden onset of severe odynophagia, with inability to swallow liquids or solids. Herpes labialis and herpetic oropharyngeal ulcers can occur during the esophageal infection, whereas skin lesions are rarely present.[20]

A definite diagnosis of HSV esophagitis requires endoscopy and histology of the esophageal mucosa, even though contrast radiographic appearance of the esophagus may be suggestive by showing multiple vesicles and ulcers as stellate or volcano structures. Endoscopy usually reveals small, well-circumscribed ulcers (Figure 3.3), rarely vesicles, whereas deep ulcers, as seen with CMV, are rare.[21,22] Brushing or biopsies should be taken from the edge or periphery of ulcerations, given that HSV infects squamous epithelial cells.[23] Histology reveals intranuclear Cowdry type A inclusion bodies (eosinophilic material), ballooning degeneration cells, multinucleated giant cells, ground-glass-like nuclei and margination of chromatin.[24] Confirmation may require immunoperoxidase staining or positive viral culture.

Although HSV esophagitis has a spontaneous resolution in a normal host, antiviral therapy is commonly used both in immunocompetent and immunocompromised subjects. Several uncontrolled trials and clinical experience indicate the efficacy of acyclovir, a nucleoside analog, for the treatment of HSV esophagitis.[25] Parenteral acyclovir should be initiated until the patient can be converted to oral therapy (when dysphagia or odynophagia is resolved). Generally, patients are treated with acyclovir for 7–10 days. Because resistance to acyclovir has been reported, therapy with foscarnet should be considered in case of clinical failure with acyclovir.[25] Acyclovir is efficacious in prophylaxis for patients undergoing transplantation and those who are HSV-antibody-positive. Table 3.4 lists the available antiviral agents for treating viral esophagitis.

CMV is the most frequent infectious complication of organ transplantation, occurring in 60–70% of these patients. Esophagitis is one of the most common manifestations in this setting. CMV is by far the most frequent cause of esophageal ulcer in patients with advanced HIV infection and a CD4 count lower than 100 mm^3 (see reference 26). In contrast to HSV esophagitis, CMV esophagitis has rarely been detected in an immunocompetent host;[27] however, CMV and HSV are equally common organisms in transplant patients who do not receive antiviral prophylaxis.[28] Odynophagia is a constant feature and is typically severe; chest pain of esophageal origin, mainly occurring upon deglutition, is also described. Prior or co-existent

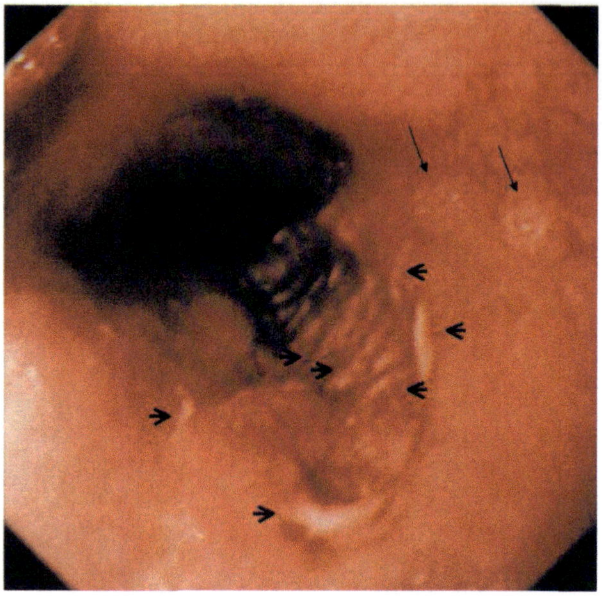

Figure 3.3 Herpes simplex virus esophagitis. Small, well-circumscribed ulcers (short arrows) and two small vesicles (long arrows) in the lower third of the esophageal mucosa.

CMV infection in other regions (e.g. retinitis, colitis) is not uncommonly found.[29]

As with HSV, a definite diagnosis of CMV esophagitis requires endoscopy and biopsy. Contrast X-ray examination of the esophagus reveals either focal or diffuse images of mucosal ulcerations. Ulcers may be vertical or linear with central umbilication, or may be diffuse and superficial;[30] they are usually deep and large in patients with advanced HIV infection. Endoscopy remains the definitive diagnostic tool for CMV esophagitis. The endoscopic appearance is variable and may include multiple shallow ulcers, solitary ulcers or diffuse superficial esophagitis (Figure 3.4). In contrast to *Candida* and HSV, brushing cytology has a poor sensitivity and multiple biopsies should be taken. Since the cytopathic effect of CMV occurs at the level of endothelial and mesenchymal cells in the granulation tissue, endoscopic biopsies must be taken from the base of the ulcer.[31] Histology typically shows large cells with intranuclear and intracytoplasmic inclusions having an eosinophilic appearance. Immunohistochemical stains can reveal more infected cells than routinely appreciated with hematoxylin and eosin staining. Mucosal biopsy is also more specific than viral culture as with other esophageal infections.[32]

The drugs available for treating CMV disease include ganciclovir, an acyclovir derivative, foscarnet and cidofovir. CMV esophagitis responds clinically and endoscopically to ganciclovir in approximately 75–80% of patients (Table 3.4).[29] Duration of treatment should be based on clinical and endoscopic variables, but there is wide agreement that a 2–4-week period is usually effective. Oral ganciclovir is not effective for treating active infection, owing to its low bioavailability (" 10%).[33] If an acute CMV infection occurs in transplant patients, ganciclovir should be given for about 1–2 months, until immunosuppressive drugs are reduced or discontinued. In patients receiving a protracted course of therapy, clinical and virological resistance to ganciclovir may occur.[34] In this condition foscarnet, a pyrophosphate analog inhibiting DNA polymerase and reverse transcriptase, is usually effective.[35] The relapse rate of CMV esophagitis in HIV-infected patients is approximately 50%,[29] but long-term ganciclovir maintenance therapy is not routinely recommended unless there is a co-existent retinitis.[33]

Ganciclovir and high-dose acyclovir have been used with moderate success for the prophylaxis of CMV infection in transplant patients. However, in this setting ganciclovir prophylaxis is limited to high-risk patients, i.e. CMV-seropositive patients, CMV-seronegative patients receiving CMV-seropositive organ or blood products, and patients treated with immunosuppressive drugs because of episodes of rejection.[36]

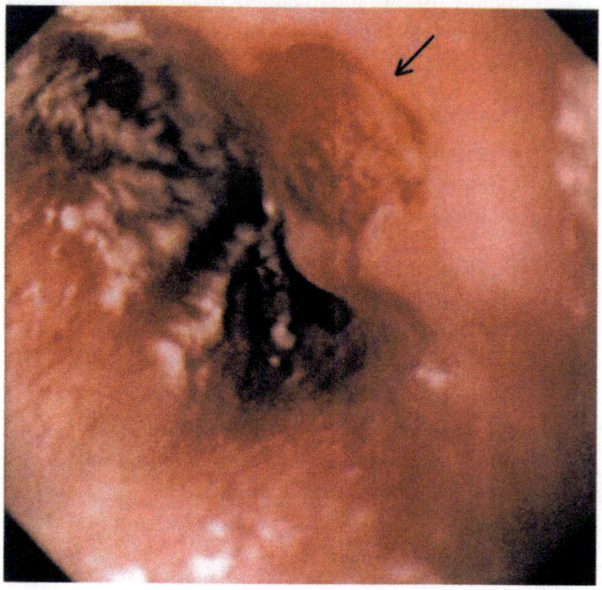

Figure 3.4 Cytomegalovirus esophagitis. A round, solitary deep ulcer is evident in the distal esophageal mucosa (arrow).

Other viral pathogens

Varicella zoster virus (VZV) is a relatively uncommon agent of infectious esophagitis in immunologically normal subjects, but it causes a severe esophagitis in immunocompromised patients, usually accompanied by other signs of systemic dissemination (e.g. pneumonitis, hepatitis, encephalitis).[37] The endoscopic appearance ranges from vesicles to necrotic ulcerations. Definite diagnosis requires biopsies both for routine histology (ballooning degeneration, multinucleated giant cells, intranuclear eosinophilic inclusion bodies) and for culture and immunohistochemical staining. The infection is treated with acyclovir or famciclovir; foscarnet is used for resistant viruses.

In a subject with clinical features consistent with infectious mononucleosis due to Epstein–Barr virus (EBV), the occurrence of nausea, dysphagia or hematemesis should raise the possibility of an infectious esophagitis. This however, develops only in a small minority of immunocompetent individuals, whereas in immunocompromised subjects, EBV-related infectious esophagitis has been reported.[38] Oral acyclovir may be a reasonable therapy, even if benefits of antiviral therapy in EBV-related esophagitis are unproven.

The human papillovirus, like HSV, usually infects squamous epithelial cells. The diagnosis requires histology[39] (multinucleated giant cells, koilocytosis, cellular atypia) and immunohistochemical staining. Endoscopy reveals non-specific lesions such as yellow plaques, small nodules or patches with small villous projections. The condition is generally asymptomatic, and specific treatment may be unnecessary

In specific HIV-related esophagitis, HIV is a well-known risk factor for many other infections. However, it is agreed that HIV itself can lead to esophageal ulcerations,[40] usually presenting as multiple, small and shallow lesions. This esophageal

Table 3.4 Drugs for viral esophagitis

Drug	Duration	Dosage	Remarks
Acyclovir	7–10 days	20 mg/kg per dose orally four times daily (80 mg/kg per day). Severe infections refractory to normal oral dosages or in which the patient is unable to swallow are treated with i.v. acyclovir, 15–30 mg/kg per day in 3 divided doses	A nucleoside analog available for both oral and intravenous administration. It is well tolerated; occasionally, rash, reversible renal failure or gastrointestinal symptoms occur. Dose adjustment should be made with renal impairment. Risk of renal insufficiency is reduced with adequate prehydration
Ganciclovir	14–28 days	5 mg/kg given intravenously twice per day	Drugs of first choice for the treatment of serious systemic CMV infections. The need for maintenance therapy of gastrointestinal CMV infection remains unclear. Dosage reduction is recommended in patients with renal impairment. Main side-effects are: neutropenia, thrombocytopenia, central nervous system symptoms, abnormal liver function tests, fever and rash. Simultaneous administration of G-CSF or GM-CSF can prevent ganciclovir-associated neutropenia
Foscarnet	14–28 days	HSV infection: 40 mg/kg of body weight given either every 8 or every 12 h. This dose is injected slowly into a vein by an infusion pump over at least 1 h. CMV infection: 60 mg/kg, as above	Second-line parenteral antiviral, reserved for treatment of HSV or CMV infections resistant to conventional therapy. Main side-effects are: nephrotoxicity, anemia, gastrointestinal toxicity, hyper- and hypocalcemia, hypomagnesemia, hyper- and hypophosphatemia, hypokalemia, seizures. It is mainly used in the treatment of acyclovir-resistant HSV infections and ganciclovir-resistant CMV infections
Famciclovir	7 days	In adults: 250 mg, three times daily orally	Consider with acyclovir resistance, but limited experience in infectious esophagitis. Use with caution in subjects with renal insufficiency. Main side-effects similar to those for acyclovir
Cidofovir	14 days	5 mg/kg i.v. once per week	A novel monophosphate nucleotide analog effective against CMV, HVS-1, HVS-2 and EBV. Parenteral antiviral recently approved to treat CMV retinitis. No reports on the treatment of CMV esophagitis. Generally reserved for patients with serious CMV disease for whom ganciclovir and/or foscarnet therapy has failed. Main side-effects are: nephrotoxicity, proteinuria, glycosuria, neutropenia and metabolic acidosis

CMV, cytomegalovirus; G, granulocyte; CSF, colony-stimulating factor; GM, granulocyte/macrophage; HSV, herpes simplex virus; EBV, Epstein–Barr virus involvement may occur in the setting of a mononucleosis-like illness that develops around the time of the primary HIV infoction. Biopsy specimens examined at electronic microscopy show enveloped virus-like particles with morphology compatible with that of retroviruses. In the later stages of HIV infection, when the CD4 lymphocyte count is below 100/mm^3, large esophageal ulcerations can be observed. These ulcers are commonly defined as idiopathic esophageal ulcers (IEU) and appear as uniformly well-circumscribed lesions, without histological features of a viral cytopathic effect. It has been observed that HIV-associated IEU are diagnosed when biopsy, cytology and cultures are negative. Electron micrographs from the margins of some superficial ulcers have revealed viral particles morphologically similar to retroviruses. The polymerase chain reaction (PCR) can identify the HIV genome in biopsy specimens, but it remains unclear whether HIV is pathogenic in esophageal ulcerations. Reports have revealed HIV histopathologically in esophageal biopsies from patients with *Candida*, HSV and CMV. It has been hypothesized that most esophageal disease in patients with advanced HIV infection is associated with specific pathogenic processes. However, HIV-induced ulcerations can occur and may require treatment with corticosteroids.[41] IEU present clinically in a fashion similar to CMV esophagitis; whereas bleeding is reported, strictures are rare. These ulcers usually respond well to oral corticosteroids or thalidomide. Despite the fact that these drugs may entail some risk for patients already immunosuppressed, this treatment is usually well tolerated.

Bacterial infections

The greatest risk factors for occurrence of bacterial infections of the esophagus are granulocytopenia (as seen in patients undergoing chemotherapy) and hypochlorhydria or acid suppression.[42] Despite often being unrecognized, bacterial esophagitis may have significant clinical relevance. Infection is usually polymicrobial and consists mainly of oral and upper respiratory flora (e.g. *Staphylococcus aureus, Staphylococcus epidermidis, Staphylococcus viridans*). It is possible that these organisms invade and colonize esophageal mucosa damaged by gastroesophageal reflux. Clinical presentation includes classical symptoms such as dysphagia, odynophagia and chest pain. Endoscopic pictures are non-specific and consist of ulcerations, discrete plaques, pseudomembranes and mucosal friability. Histology shows bacteria on Gram stain, but culture is not useful, since non-pathological bacteria can grow as well. The clinical course is usually mild and asymptomatic. At histology, features of bacterial invasion (either superficial or transmural) can be evident. Treatment consists of broad-spectrum antibiotics such as ampicillin–sulbactam or ticarcillin–clavulanic acid, which effectively treat both Gram-positive and -negative oropharyngeal flora. In patients systemically ill, combined therapy with a β-lactam/aminoglycoside or monotherapy with a carbapenem should be considered.

REFERENCES

1. Bacellar H, Munoz A, Hoover DR et al. Incidence of clinical AIDS conditions in a cohort of homosexual men with CD4+ cell counts < 100/mm3. Multicenter AIDS Cohort Study. *J Infect Dis* 1994; **170**: 1284–1287.
2. Bashir RM, Wilcox CM. Symptom-specific use of upper gastrointestinal endoscopy in human immunodeficiency virus-infected patients yields high dividends. *J Clin Gastroenterol* 1996; **23**: 292–298.
3. Wilcox CM, Alexander LN, Clark WS et al. Fluconazole compared with endoscopy for human immunodeficiency virus-infected patients with esophageal symptoms. *Gastroenterology* 1996; **110**: 1803–1809.
4. Bonacini M, Young T, Laine L. The cause of esophageal symptoms in human immunodeficiency virus infection. *Arch Intern Med* 1991; **151**: 1561–1572.

5. Connolly GM, Hawkins D, Harcourt-Webster JN et al. Oesophageal symptoms, their causes, treatment, and prognosis in patients with the acquired immunodeficiency syndrome. *Gut* 1989; **30**: 1033-1039.
6. Wilcox CM. A technique to examine the underlying mucosa in patients with AIDS and severe Candida esophagitis. *Gastrointest Endosc* 1995; **42**: 360–363.
7. Slavin MA, Osborne B, Adams R et al. Efficacy and safety of fluconazole prophylaxis for fungal infections after marrow transplantation – a prospective, randomized, double-blind study. *J Infect Dis* 1995; **171**: 1545–1552.
8. Wilcox CM, Schwartz DA. Endoscopic–pathologic correlates of Candida esophagitis in acquired immunodeficiency syndrome. *Dig Dis Sci* 1996; **41**: 1337–1345.
9. Lopez-Dupla M, Mora Sanz P, Pintado Garcia V et al. Clinical, endoscopic, immunologic, and therapeutic aspects of oropharyngeal and esophageal candidiasis in HIV-infected patients: a survey of 114 cases. *Am J Gastroenterol* 1992; **87**: 1771–1776.
10. Wilcox CM. Time course of clinical response to fluconazole for Candida oesophagitis in AIDS. *Alimentar Pharmacol Ther* 1994; **8**: 347–350.
11. Levine MS, Macones AJ Jr, Laufer I. Candida esophagitis: accuracy of radiographic diagnosis. *Radiology* 1985; **154**: 581–587.
12. Roberts L Jr, Gibbons R, Gibbons G et al. Adult esophageal candidiasis: a radiographic spectrum. *Radiographics* 1987; **7**: 289–307.
13. Brandt LJ, Coman E, Schwartz E et al. Use of a new cytology balloon for diagnosis of symptomatic esophageal disease in acquired immunodeficiency syndrome. *Gastrointest Endosc* 1993; **39**: 559–561.
14. Barbaro G, Barbarini G, Calderon W et al. Fluconazole versus itraconazole for Candida esophagitis in acquired immunodeficiency syndrome. *Gastroenterology* 1996; **111**: 1169–1177.
15. Laine L, Rabeneck L. Prospective study of fluconazole suspension for the treatment of oesophageal candidiasis in patients with AIDS. *Aliment Pharmacol Ther* 1995; **9**: 553–556.
16. Como JA, Dismukes WE. Oral azole drugs as systemic antifungal therapy. *N Engl J Med* 1994; **330**: 263–272.
17. Lewis JH, Zimmerman HJ, Benson GD et al. Hepatic injury associated with ketoconazole therapy. Analysis of 33 cases. *Gastroenterology* 1984; **86**: 503–513.
18. Wilcox CM, Darouiche RO, Laine L et al. A randomized, double-blind comparison of itraconazole oral solution and fluconazole tablets in the treatment of esophageal candidiasis. *J Infect Dis* 1997; **176**: 227–232.
19. Mosimann F, Cuenoud PF, Steinhauslin F et al. Herpes simplex esophagitis after renal transplantation. *Transplant Int* 1994; **7**: 79–82.
20. Baehr PH, McDonald GB. Esophageal infections: risk factors, presentation, diagnosis, and treatment. *Gastroenterology* 1994; **106**: 509–532.
21. McBane RD, Gross JB Jr. Herpes esophagitis: clinical syndrome, endoscopic appearance, and diagnosis in 23 patients. *Gastrointest Endosc* 1991; **37**: 600–603.
22. Agha FP, Lee HH, Nostrant TT. Herpetic esophagitis: a diagnostic challenge in immunocompromised patients. *Am J Gastroenterol* 1986; **81**: 246–253.
23. Ramanathan J, Rammouni M, Baran J Jr et al. Herpes simplex virus esophagitis in immunocompetent host: an overview. *Am J Gastroenterol* 2000; **95**: 2171–2176.
24. Feiden W, Borchard F, Burrig KF et al. Herpes oesophagitis. I. Light microscopical and immunohistochemical investigations. *Virchows Arch Pathol Anat Histopathol* 1984; **404**: 167–176.
25. Genereau T, Lortholary O, Bouchaud O et al. Herpes simplex esophagitis in patients with AIDS: report of 34 cases. The Cooperative Study Group on Herpetic Esophagitis in HIV Infection. *Clin Infect Dis* 1996; **22**: 926–931.
26. Wilcox CM, Schwartz DA, Clark WS. Esophageal ulceration in human immunodeficiency virus infection. Causes, response to therapy, and long-term outcome. *Ann Intern Med* 1995; **123**: 143–149.
27. Altman C, Bedossa P, Dussaix E et al. Cytomegalovirus infection of esophagus in immunocompetent adults. *Dig Dis Sci* 1995; **40**: 606.
28. Alexander JA, Brouillette DE, Chien MC et al. Infectious esophagitis following renal and liver transplantation. *Dig Dis Sci* 1988; **33**: 1121.
29. Wilcox CM, Straub RF, Schwartz DA. Cytomegalovirus esophagitis in AIDS: a prospective study of clinical response to ganciclovir therapy, relapse rate, and long-term outcome. *Am J Med* 1995; **98**: 169.
30. Balthazar EJ, Megibow AJ, Hulnick D et al. Cytomegalovirus esophagitis in AIDS: radiographic features in 16 patients. *Am J Roentgenol* 1987; **149**: 919.
31. Wilcox CM, Straub RF, Schwartz DA. A prospective evaluatuion of biopsy number for the diagnosis of viral esophagitis in patients with HIV infection and esophageal ulcer. *Gastrointest Endosc* 1996; **44**: 587.
32. Goodgame RW, Genta RM, Estrada R et al. Frequency of positive test for cytomegalovirus in AIDS patients: endoscopic lesions compared with normal mucosa. *Am J Gastroenterol* 1993; **88**: 338.
33. Crumpacker CS. Ganciclovir. *N Engl J Med* 1996; **335**: 721.
34. Erice A, Chou S, Biron KK et al. Progressive disease due to ganciclovir-resistant cytomegalovirus in immunocompromised patients. *N Engl J Med* 1989; **167**: 1184.
35. Blanshard C, Benhamou Y, Dohin E et al. Treatment of AIDS-associated gastrointestinal cytomegalovirus infection with foscarnet and gancyclovir: a randomized comparison. *J Infect Dis* 1995; **172**: 622.
36. Winston DJ, Wirin D, Shaked A et al. Randomised comparison of ganciclovir and high-dose acyclovir for long-term cytomegalovirus prophylaxis in liver-transplant recipients. *Lancet* 1995; **346**: 69.
37. Gill RA, Gebhard RL, Dozeman RL et al. Shingles esophagitis: endoscopic diagnosis in two patients. *Gastrointest Endosc* 1984; **30**: 26.
38. Kitchen VS, Helbert M, Francis ND et al. Epstein–Barr virus associated oesophageal ulcers in AIDS. *Gut* 1990; **31**: 1223.
39. Schechter M, Pannain VNL, de Oliveira AV. Papovavirus-associated esophageal ulceration in a patient with AIDS. *AIDS* 1991; **5**: 238.
40. Rabeneck L, Popovic M, Gartner S et al. Acute HIV infection presenting with painful swallowing and esophageal ulcers. *JAMA* 1990; **263**: 2318–2322.
41. Wilcox CM, Schwartz DA. A pilot study of oral corticosteroid therapy for idiopatic esophageal ulceration associated with human immunodeficiancy virus infection. *Am J Med* 1992; **93**: 131–134.
42. Ezzell JH, Bremer J, Adamec TA. Bacterial esophagitis: an often forgotten cause of odynophagia. *Am J Gastroenterol* 1990; **85**: 296.

4 Gastroesophageal reflux disease

Yvan Vandenplas, Silvia Salvatore and Bruno Hauser

Introduction

Gastroesophageal reflux (GER) is defined as the involuntary passage of gastric contents into the esophagus. GER is a physiological phenomenon, occurring in every individual. Most episodes of reflux are limited to the distal esophagus, and are brief and asymptomatic. The difference between physiological reflux and reflux disease is to a lesser extent defined by the frequency, duration and severity of the reflux episodes, than whether the reflux episodes result in the occurrence of symptoms, signs severe enough to impair the quality of life, or complications. GER disease (GERD) is reflux associated with mucosal damage or symptoms severe enough to impair quality of life.[1,2] When this occurs, and the forces overcome the defense, the esophagus may become damaged, with significant consequences for the affected individual.

Definitions

Regurgitation is defined as passage of refluxed gastric contents into the oral pharynx and the mouth and is accompanied by gastric content drooling out of the mouth. Spitting-up is synonymous with regurgitation. Vomiting is defined as expulsion of the refluxed gastric contents from the mouth.[3,4] Only a minority of reflux episodes is accompanied by regurgitation or vomiting. Rumination is characterized by the voluntary, habitual regurgitation of recently ingested food that is subsequently spitted up or re-swallowed.

Sometimes GER is a normal esophageal function, serving a protective role, e.g. during meals, or in the immediate postprandial period; if the stomach is overdistended, GER serves to decompress it. Regurgitation may be physiological in healthy, thriving, happy infants. Primary GER results from a primary disorder of function of the upper gastrointestinal tract. In secondary GER, reflux results from dysmotility occurring in systemic disorders such as neurological impairment or systemic sclerosis. It may also result from mechanical factors at play in chronic lung disease or upper airway obstruction, as in chronic tonsillitis. Other causes include systemic or local infections (urinary tract infection, gastroenteritis), food allergy, metabolic disorders, intracranial hypertension and medications such as chemotherapy. In some cases, secondary reflux results from stimulation of the vomiting center by afferent impulses from circulating bacterial toxins, or stimulation from sites such as the eye, olfactory epithelium, labyrinths, pharynx, gastrointestinal and urinary tracts, and testes.[3,4] These stimuli usually cause vomiting. The symptoms and signs of primary and secondary reflux are similar, but a distinction is conceptually helpful in determining a therapeutic approach. Secondary GER is not discussed further.

Epidemiology

Determination of the exact prevalence of GER and GERD at any age is virtually impossible because most reflux episodes are asymptomatic, show the absence of specific symptoms, undergo self-treatment and lack medical referral. In normal 3–4-month-old infants, three or four episodes of GER are detectable during 5 min of intermittent fluoroscopic evaluation,[5] and up to 31 ± 21 acid reflux episodes are recorded within a 24-h period with pH monitoring.[6]

The frequency of regurgitation varies according to age. Daily regurgitation is present in 50% of infants younger than 3 months and in more than 66% at 4 months, but only in 5% at 1 year of age.[7–9] Complete resolution of regurgitation is frequent and expected, by 10 months in 55%, by 18 months in 60–80% and by 2 years of age in 98%.[10] A prospective follow-up of 63 regurgitating infants reported in all subjects, before 12 months, a complete disappearance of symptoms, although accompanied by a significant increase in feeding refusal, duration of meals, parental feeding-related distress and impaired quality of life, even after the disappearance of symptoms.[11]

About 5–9% of infants have troublesome GERD.[6,12] According to parents, heartburn is present in 1.8% of 3–9-year-old healthy children and 3.5% of 10–17-year-old adolescents; regurgitation is said to occur in 2.3% and 1.4%, respectively, and 0.5% and 1.9% need anti-acid medication. In self-reports, adolescents complain about heartburn in 5.2% and regurgitation in up to 8.2%, while anti-acids are taken by 2.3% and histamine receptor antagonists (H_2RA) by 1.3%, suggesting that symptoms of GER are not rare during childhood and are underreported by the parents or overestimated by the adolescents.[13] In a Western population, GERD affected 4–30% of adults[14,15] and heartburn and regurgitation resolved within 3–10 years only in 12–33%, regardless of the presence of esophagitis at diagnosis.[1,16,17] In the absence of H_2RA or proton pump inhibitors (PPI), symptoms improved after 17–22 years in 60% but disappeared in only 12%.[18] Despite anti-secretory treatment, a 10-year follow-up of esophagitis showed that over 70% had persisting symptoms and 2% had strictures.[19]

Reflux esophagitis is reported in 2–5% of the general population.[12] Children with GER symptoms present esophagitis in 15 up to 62% of cases, Barrett's esophagus in 0.1–3% and refractory GERD requiring surgery in 6–13%.[20–24] In adults undergoing endoscopy, esophagitis is diagnosed in 15 up to 80% of cases.[1,17,25,26] The huge differences in incidence are determined by patient recruitment and availability of self-treatment.

Genetic and environmental factors

It has been demonstrated that physiological reflux, heartburn, acid regurgitation and severe GERD are more frequent in men than in women. Barrett's esophagus is in part genetically determined.[24] There is much information (in adults) demonstrating the aggravating effects of alcohol, smoking, drugs, dietary components, etc. on the incidence of GER. A detailed discussion on these environmental factors is beyond the scope of this chapter. Changes in lifestyle in men and women may result in the fact that the differences in incidence in GERD between both sexes may be disappearing. With pH monitoring, we could not demonstrate a male predominance in children. All forms of GERD affect Caucasians more often than African-Americans or Native Americans (adult data).[14] However, the same prevalence of troublesome infant regurgitation was found in Caucasian and Indonesian infants.[27] The importance of the genetic background was hypothesized by demonstrating that esophagitis and hiatus hernia were more common in a population with the same genetic background with dyspeptic symptoms in England than in Singapore.[28] Race, sex, body mass index and age were independently associated with hiatus hernia and esophagitis, race being the most important risk factor.[28] However, over-the-counter use of low-dose aspirin and non-steroidal anti-inflammatory drugs has a greater impact on severe GERD, such as esophageal stricture than age.[29]

Carre et al described the autosomal dominant inheritance of hiatal hernia by discovering familial hiatal hernia in a large five-generation family, but without demonstrating the link to GERD.[30] The genetic influence on GERD is supported by increased GER symptoms in relatives of GERD patients.[31] Moreover, the concordance for GER is higher in monozygotic than dizygotic twins.[32] A locus on chromosome 13q, between microsatellites D13S171 and D13S263, has been linked to severe GERD in five multiply affected families,[33] but not confirmed in another five families, possibly owing to the genetic heterogeneity of GERD and the different clinical presentations of patients.[34]

Pathophysiology

The pathophysiology of GER is complex and diverse, as it is influenced by factors that are genetic, environmental (e.g. diet and smoking), anatomic, hormonal and neurogenic (Figure 4.1 and Table 4.1). We have recently reviewed the

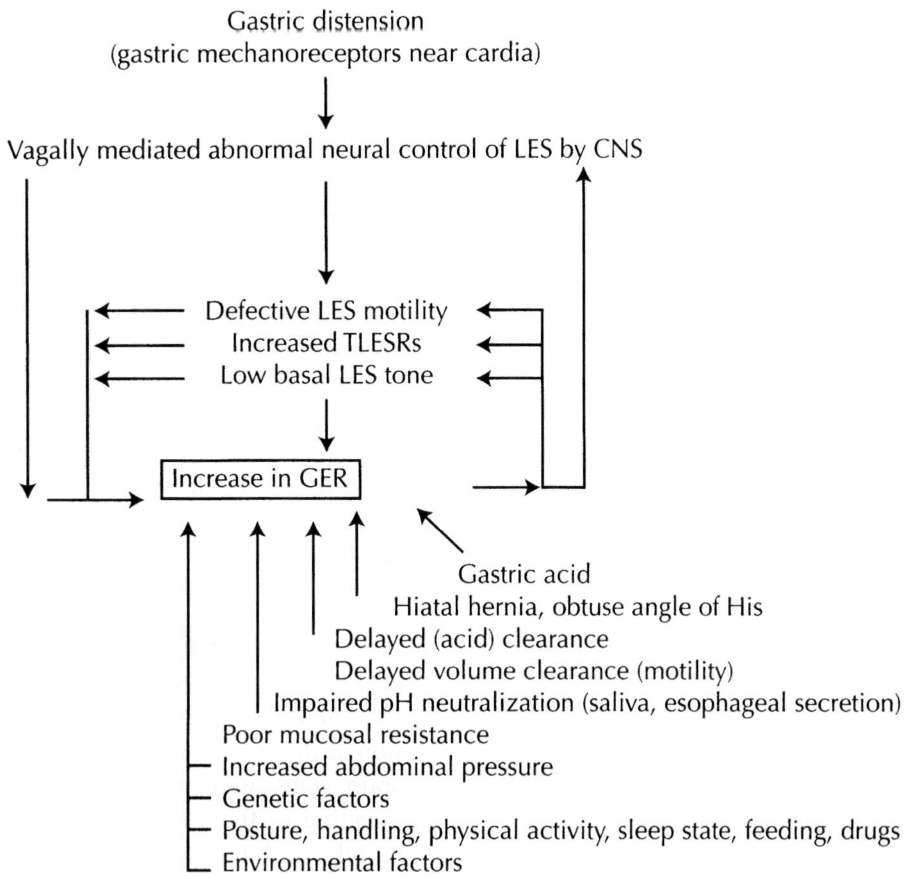

Figure 4.1 Illustration of multifactorial influences on gastroesophageal reflux (GER). LES, lower esophageal sphincter; CNS, central nervous system; TLESRs, transient lower esophageal sphincter relaxations.

pathophysiology of GER in infants and children.[35] The most relevant factors are gastric (gastric acid and non-acid content, gastric emptying, fundus tone, triggering of transient lower esophageal sphincter (LES) relaxations (TLESRs)), the anti-reflux barrier (LES basal pressure, TLESRs, hiatal hernia), the composition of the refluxate (air–liquid, acid, non-acid, bile), the esophageal tone and the esophageal clearance (volume and chemical clearance).[35,36] GER occurs during episodes of transient relaxation of the LES or inadequate adaptation of the sphincter tone to changes in abdominal pressure.

GERD was classically considered to be an acid peptic disease, although as a group, the majority of patients with reflux disease do not have a significant increase in gastric acid secretion. Three major tiers of defense serve to limit the degree of GER, and to minimize the risk of reflux-induced injury to the esophagus. The first line of defense is the 'anti-reflux barrier', consisting of the LES, and the diaphragmatic pinchcock and angle of His; this barrier serves to limit the frequency and volume of refluxed gastric contents. When this line of defense fails, the second, esophageal clearance, assumes greater importance, to limit the duration of contact between luminal contents and esophageal epithelium. Gravity and esophageal peristalsis serve to remove volume from the esophageal lumen, while salivary and esophageal secretions (the latter from esophageal submucosal glands), serve to neutralize acid. The third line of defense, 'tissue or esophageal mucosal resistance' comes into play when acid contact time is prolonged, such as when esophageal clearance is

Table 4.1 Parameters influencing the incidence of gastroesophageal reflux

Mastication, saliva secretion
Swallowing
Esophageal clearance
Esophageal innervation and receptors
Mucosal resistance
Lower esophageal sphincter pressure
Sphincter relaxation
Abdominal esophagus
Sphincter position
Angle of His
Gastric volume, gastric accommodation
Gastric emptying
Gastric acid output
Gastric acid feed buffering
Feeding regimen: type, frequency, volume
Pepsin/trypsin/bile salts
Helicobacter pylori
Intra-abdominal pressure
Genetic factors
Environmental factors
Posture
Physical activity
Sleep state
Respiratory disease
Medication (e.g. xanthines)

defective or not operative (motility disorders, sleep).[35]

Epidemiological data suggest that *Helicobacter pylori* plays a protective role in GERD, presumably by decreasing acid secretion. In adults, *Helicobacter pylori* and especially the cagA positive strains, which cause more severe gastric inflammation, are less prevalent in patients with esophagitis or Barrett's esophagus than in those with endoscopically negative reflux disease or in control patients.[37–41]

Recent detailed analysis of postprandial acidity in the gastroesophageal junction area suggests that local acid distribution rather than total gastric secretion might be more relevant to the pathogenesis of GERD.[42] Differences may exist in the degree of mixing of fundal contents leading to different distributions of acid in the stomach. Studies using pH monitoring and esophageal scintigraphy and gastric magnetic resonance imaging suggest that gastric mixing can be incomplete and different layers of viscosity within the stomach might therefore influence the distribution of the gastric contents. A collection of acid in the gastric part of the esophageal junction was shown in adults in a supine position, even in the postprandial period when the stomach content was neutralized by the meal.[43,44] This newly described mechanism is attractive as an explanation for postprandial distress in infants lying in the supine position.

TLESRs are the major mechanism of GER episodes, in premature infants and in adults.[35,45,46] TLESRs are a neural reflex, triggered mainly by the distension of the proximal stomach and organized in the brain stem, with efferent and afferent pathways traveling in the vagus nerve, activating an intramural inhibitory neuron which releases nitric oxide to relax the LES.[47,48] When investigated in the supine position, the incidence of TLESRs in healthy adults and those with GERD did not differ. In healthy adults, only 30% of the TLSERs were accompanied by acid reflux, but in patients with GERD the reflux occurred in 65% of the TLESRs. Thus adults, controls and GERD patients have the same incidence of TLESRs, but in patients with GERD these TLESRs are more than twice as frequently accompanied by acid GER.[36,49,50] The initial studies performed in the recumbent position found a higher frequency of TLSERs in patients with GERD than in normals.[51] These older studies in the recumbent position may be more relevant for infants.

Delayed gastric emptying may increase postprandial reflux possibly by increasing the rate of TLESRs and the likelihood of reflux during the TLESRs. A disturbed gastric accommodation to a meal and prolonged postprandial fundic relaxation where described in patients with GERD.[52] Both phenomena can influence postprandial fundic volume and pressure, which in turn may affect the rate of distension-induced triggerings of TLESRs and the volume of the refluxate. A recent study has shown that esophageal acid exposure in patients with GERD is directly correlated with the emptying time of the proximal stomach.[53] These new findings are especially of interest in infants with postprandial distress or regurgitation who are not responding to dietary treatment with thickened casein-predominant formula. This has a delayed gastric emptying time, and thus is related to an increased incidence of TLESRs.

Hiatal hernia increases the number of reflux episodes and delays esophageal clearance by promoting retrograde flow across the esophagogastric junction when the LES relaxes after a swallow. This mechanism underlies the so-called re-reflux phenomenon (acid reflux when the pH is still below 4).

The refluxate might be highly acid, moderately acid, or non-acid. Reflux may be a mixture of gas and liquid or pure liquid, and may or may not contain bile. More than half of the acid and non-acid reflux episodes are associated with reflux of gas.[36] Non-acid reflux also occurs predominantly during TLESRs. With liquid meals, patients with reflux disease had a similar total rate of reflux episodes but a higher proportion of acid reflux events than controls.[54] Non-acid reflux may be responsible for the remaining symptoms in patients under anti-secretory treatment.[55]

Acid reflux in patients with GERD is associated with an inhibition of tone in the esophageal body, whereas normals have an increased contractile activity. In order to have an effective volume clearance, motility of the esophageal body needs to be preserved. Acid is emptied from the esophagus with one or two sequences of primary peristalsis, then the residual acidity is neutralized by swallowed saliva.[35] Secondary peristalsis is the response to esophageal distension with air or water, and is more important during sleep, when peristalsis is reduced. Patients may have normal primary peristalsis but abnormal secondary peristalsis. Thus, non-acid reflux, as occurs in the postprandial period, may be inefficiently cleared and cause prolonged esophageal distension. The esophageal mucosal defense can be divided into pre-epithelial (protective factors in swallowed saliva and esophageal secretions containing bicarbonate, mucin, prostaglandin E_2, epidermal growth factor, transforming growth factor), epithelial (tight junctions, intercellular glycoprotein material) and post-epithelial factors.[35] There is a very important interindividual variation of reflux perception suggesting different esophagus-sensitive thresholds. The esophageal mucosa contains acid, and temperature- and volume-sensitive receptors. A widening of the intercellular spaces has been found in patients with esophagitis and in patients with endoscopy-negative disease. When esophagitis heals, esophageal sensitivity to acid decreases. The presence of fat in the duodenum increases the sensitivity to reflux. Hyposensitivity, as occurs in patients with Barrett's esophagus, is a secondary phenomenon.[56]

Clinical signs/symptoms

The most typical, although non-specific, symptoms of esophageal dysfunction are GER, regurgitation and vomiting. While reflux does occur physiologically at all ages, there is a continuum between physiological GER and GERD leading to significant symptoms and complications. GERD is a spectrum of diseases that can best be defined as the symptoms and/or signs of esophageal or adjacent organ injury secondary to the reflux of gastric contents into the esophagus or, beyond, into the oral cavity or airways.

Presentation may be with decreased food intake and aversive behavior around feeds. There is often clearly abnormal sucking and swallowing. Not surprisingly, the mother–child interaction is affected, making the situation less easily treated.[57] There may be poor weight gain. These infants have no apparent malformations, and may be diagnosed as 'non-organic failure to thrive' (NOFTT),[58] a 'disorder' that is sometimes attributed to social/sensory deprivation, socioeconomic or primary maternal–child problems. Primary GERD is but one root cause of 'feeding problems' in infancy, others being structural abnormalities of the mouth/pharynx/upper gastrointestinal tract, neurological conditions, primary behavior disorders, cardiorespiratory problems, or metabolic dysfunction. However, no matter what the cause, so-called 'feeding problems' are bio-behavioral conditions, i.e. disorders in which biological and behavioral causes interact.[59]

A wide spectrum of clinical presentations of GERD exists, with relevant differences within ages (Table 4.2). Regurgitation is the most common presentation of infantile GER, with occasional projectile vomiting.[7,60] In infants and young children, verbal expression of symptoms is often vague or impossible, and persistent crying, irritability, feeding and sleeping difficulties have been proposed as equivalents for heartburn in adults. Nevertheless, the descriptions for infants are non-specific and even functional. Therefore, poor weight gain, feeding refusal, back-arching, irritability and sleep disturbances have also been reported to be unrelated to GERD.[61,62] Esophageal pain and behaviors perceived by the caregiver (usually the mother) to represent pain (e.g. crying and retching) potentially affect the response of the infant to visceral stimuli and the ability to cope with these sensations, either painful or non-painful.[63] In addition, cow's milk allergy (CMA) may overlap with many symptoms of GER, and may coexist or complicate GERD in up to 40% of infants.[64–66]

Table 4.2 Spectrum of gastroesophageal reflux disease manifestations according to different ages

Symptoms and signs	Infants	Children	Adults
Vomiting	++	++	+
Regurgitation	+++	++	++
Heartburn/pyrosis	?	++	+++
Epigastric pain	?	+	++
Chest pain	?	+	++
Dysphagia	?	+	++
Excessive crying/irritability	+++	+	-
Anemia/melena/hematemesis	+	+	+
Food refusal/feeding disturbancies/anorexia	++	+	+
Failure to thrive/poor growth	++	+	-
Abnormal posturing/Sandifer's syndrome	++	+	-
Persisting hiccups	++	+	+
Dental erosions/halitosis/water brush	-	+	+
Hoarseness/globus pharyngeus	-	+	+
Persistent cough/aspiration pneumonia/wheezing	+	+	+
Laryngitis/ear problems	+	+	+
Laryngomalacia/stridor/croup	+	+	-
Laryngostenosis/resistant asthma/chronic sinusitis	-	+	+
Vocal nodule problems	-	-	+
ALTE/SIDS/apnea/desaturation	+	-	-
Bradycardia	+	?	?
Sleeping disturbancies	+	+	+
Impaired quality of life	?	?	+++
Esophagitis	+	+	++
Stenosis	-	(+)	+
Barrett's esophagus/esophageal adenocarcinoma	-	(+)	+

ALTE, apparent life-threatening events; SIDS, sudden infant death syndrome

+++ very common; ++ common; + possible; (+) rare; - absent; ? unknown

Compared to adults, children report more regurgitation and emesis and less heartburn, dysphagia and chest pain.[13,23,67] The younger the children are, the more difficult it is to describe and perceive these 'unpleasant sensations'. In 69 children with GERD, regurgitation and vomiting occurred in 72%, symptoms attributed to the esophagus (epigastric/abdominal pain, feeding difficulties, irritability and Sandifer–Sutcliffe syndrome) in 68%, failure to thrive in 28%, chronic respiratory symptoms in 13% and recurrent apnea in 12%, with more feeding difficulties in toddlers and more irritability in infants.[21] Clinical distinction is, however, not simple, as GERD may be occult or masquerade as respiratory or other manifestations co-existing at different ages.

GERD in adolescents is more adult-like. Heartburn is the predominant GER symptom, occurring weekly in 15–20%[15,68] and daily in 5–10% of subjects.[16] Atypical symptoms such as epigastric pain, nausea, flatulence, hiccups, chronic cough, asthma, chest pain, hoarseness and earache, account for 30–60% of presentations of GERD.[1,16] GERD is diagnosed in 50% of the adult patients with chest pain and in 80% presenting with chronic hoarseness and asthma.[69] The incidence of GERD in this group with atypical symptoms is determined by the selection (bias) of the patients.

Recent evidence has shown that GERD affects the quality of life significantly in adults, and probably also in children (and their parents), although quality of life is more difficult to evaluate in infants and young children. The developing nervous system of infants exposed to acid seems susceptible to pain hypersensitivity despite the absence of tissue damage.[70] The role of hypersensitivity to dietary allergens, both in exclusively breast-fed and formula-fed infants, is likely to be underestimated at present. The 'hygiene hypothesis' suggests that the Th2-predominant immune response at birth in the industrialized world is insufficiently skewed towards a well-balanced Th1/Th2 response.[71] Lack of controlled chronic or repetitive inflammation of the mucosa during the first months of life may account for the dramatic increase in atopic disease during infancy and childhood (which is a Th2 response) and the increase in autoimmune diseases such as diabetes and Crohn's disease in adolescents and adults (which are a Th1 response).[72] This hypothesis fits well with the observations that atopy is inversely related to family income and early attendance at a day-care center, and positively related to number of siblings and living on a farm. Repeated contacts with certain infectious organisms and endotoxins decrease the incidence of atopic disease. Infant distress and colic are now recognized as manifestations of food hypersensitivity during early childhood. Histology of the duodenal, gastric and esophageal mucosa reveals eosinophilic infiltration, characteristic of a Th2 type and thus allergic response, in many although not all infants.

Infants with GERD learn to associate eating with discomfort and thus subsequently tend to avoid eating, although behavioral feeding difficulties are common even in control toddlers.[11] In adults, impaired quality of life, notably regarding pain, mental health and social function, has been demonstrated in patients with GERD, regardless of the presence of esophagitis.[17] In an unselected population, 28% of the adults reported heartburn, almost half of them weekly, with a significant impact on the quality of life in 76%, especially if the symptoms were frequent and long-lasting. Despite that, only half of heartburn complainers sought medical help, although 60% were taking medications.[73] Thus, some adults 'learn to live with their symptoms', and acquire tolerance to long-lasting symptoms, while others accept living with an impaired quality of life.

The reason for the differences in presentation of GERD according to age remains unclear. The persistence of symptoms and progression to complications are unpredictable for a group of patients and for an individual patient. Alarm symptoms are similar in adults and children: weight loss, dysphagia, bleeding, anemia, chest pain and choking.[16,69] Additional alarm symptoms in children are failure to thrive, irritability/crying and feeding or sleeping difficulties.[74]

Gastroesophageal reflux disease and respiratory disease

Reflux may cause respiratory symptoms through different pathways, such as (micro-) aspiration or vagally mediated mechanisms. Many patients with chronic cough have gastrohypopharyngeal reflux.[35] A consequence of pulmonary aspiration of refluxed material may be the presence of an increased number of lipid-laden macrophages. Although simply observing the presence of lipid-laden alveolar macrophages is likely to be non-specific, it has been suggested that quantification would be a useful marker of silent aspiration.[75] Data are lacking and are therefore needed on the diagnostic accuracy, sensitivity and specificity of the detection and quantification of other substances in tracheal aspirates, such as lactose, pepsin and intrinsic factor.

In some patients it may not be GER that is causing respiratory disease, but the reverse. Respiratory difficulties cause greater respiratory breathing efforts and thus more pronounced negative intrathoracic pressure, and thus respiratory symptoms may provoke GER. However, the incidence of a direct temporal relation between reflux and cough episodes is relatively low.[76]

The relation between respiratory disease and GER may also be neurogenic, in this case designated as 'gastric asthma'.[77] The tracheobronchial tree and the esophagus have common embryonic foregut origins and share autonomic innervation through the vagus nerve.[78] In other words, it can be speculated that GER increases the irritability of the vagal nerve endings in the esophagus, and that as a result these nerve endings hyper-react together with the nerve endings in the airways because they have the same embryonic origin.

Complications

GERD is associated with severe complications such as esophagitis, Barrett's esophagus, strictures and esophageal adenocarcinoma. The severity of the complications is not clearly related to the duration or severity of symptoms, as severe histological changes are detectable at the first investigation. Differences in esophageal mucosal resistance and genetic factors may partially explain the diversity of lesions and symptoms.[16] Esophageal ulcers may be diagnosed in adults with dysphagia, odynophagia or esophageal bleeding, but are rarely seen in children.[20,74]

The incidence of congenital esophageal stenosis is approximately 1 in 25 000 to 1 in 50 000 live births, with associated esophageal atresia in one-third of cases.[79] More than 40 years ago, in the absence of reflux treatment, esophageal strictures were reported in about 5% of children with reflux symptoms.[80] Nowadays, except in Barrett's esophagus, esophageal stenosis and ulceration in children have become rare.[20] Esophageal stenosis may be related to the initial severity of the esophagitis and the persistence of symptoms, even during treatment.[16] Occasionally, esophageal stenosis is reported to have developed after an intervention for achalasia.[81]

Reflux esophagitis is reported in 2–5% of the general population.[82] Children with GER symptoms present esophagitis in 15–62%, Barrett's esophagus in 1.5–3% and refractory GERD requiring surgery in 6–13%.[20–24] In adults undergoing endoscopy, esophagitis is diagnosed in 15–80%.[1,17,25,26] The differences in incidence are determined by patient recruitment and availability of acid-blocking drugs over the counter (self-treatment). A 10-year follow-up of esophagitis showed that over 70% had persisting symptoms, and 2% had strictures.[19] Thus, esophagitis is not a necessary prerequisite for diagnosing GERD or starting therapy, either in children or in adults.

Abundant infiltration of the esophageal mucosa with eosinophils, as occurs in eosinophilic gastroenteritis and eosinophilic esophagitis, is increasing in prevalence and necessitates proper treatment (hypoallergenic feeding, corticoids, etc.). Patients with allergic esophagitis seem to have a younger age and common atopic features (allergic symptoms or positive allergy tests), but no specific symptoms. In children, eosinophilic esophagitis accounts for almost 1.0% of esophagitis in some selected series.[83] Atopic features are reported in more than 90% and peripheral eosinophilia in 50% of patients. At endoscopy, a pale, granular, furrowed and occasionally ringed esophageal mucosa may appear.[84] In reflux esophagitis, the distal and lower eosinophilic infiltrate is limited to less than 5 per high-power field (HPF) with 85% positive response to GER treatment, compared to primary eosinophilic esophagitis with >20 eosinophils per HPF.[83–85] In adults, allergic esophagitis and eosinophilic esophagitis are rarely found, suggesting an age-related regression or a possible underinvestigation. Patients with primary eosinophilic esophagitis may respond to dietary elimination, cromolyn sodium or steroids.[84] Recently, montelukast and fluticasone have also been reported to be of benefit.[86,87]

Barrett's esophagus is a premalignant condition with metaplastic columnar epithelium with goblet cells in the esophagus,[88] detectable in up to 5–10% of the endoscopies performed in adults,[16] but rarely seen in children. Children with severe reflux, as in those with neurological impairment, chronic lung disease (especially cystic fibrosis) and esophageal atresia, are at a higher risk of developing Barrett's esophagus.[24] In addition to severe reflux, a genetic component is also suggested.[20,24,88–91] In a series including 402 children with GERD without neurological or congenital anomalies, no case of Barrett's esophagus was detected.[20] In another series including 103 children with long-lasting GERD, and not previously treated with H_2-receptor antagonists or a proton pump inhibitor, Barrett's esophagus was detected in 13%. An esophageal stricture was present in five of the 13 patients with Barrett's esophagus (38%).[90] Reflux symptoms during childhood were not different in the adults without, than in the adults with, Barrett's esophagus.[88]

Peptic ulcer, esophageal and gastric neoplastic changes in children are extremely rare. In adults, over the past 30 years, a decreased prevalence of gastric cancer and peptic ulcer with an opposite increase of esophageal adenocarcinoma and GERD have been noted.[92] This has been attributed to independent factors amongst which are changes in dietary habits such as a higher fat intake, an increased incidence of obesity and a decreased incidence of *Helicobacter pylori* infection.[17,92] Nevertheless, the frequency, severity and duration of reflux symptoms are related to the risk of developing esophageal cancer. Among adults with longstanding and severe reflux the odds ratios are 43.5 for esophageal adenocarcinoma and 4.4 for adenocarcinoma at the cardia.[93] It is unknown whether mild esophagitis or GER symptoms persisting from childhood are related to an increased risk for severe complications in adults.

Diagnosis with differential

GERD is a primary motility disorder, mainly caused by reflux of gastric content during TLESRs inducing symptoms. None of the symptoms associated with GER and GERD are specific. Reflux disease can be a primary condition, or it can be the consequence of other abnormalities (such as neurological impairment, cystic fibrosis, pyloric hypertrophy) favoring GER. The long list of differential diagnoses is discussed under the other headings of this chapter, and depends on the age of the patient and the presenting symptom.

Because of lack of space, diagnostic procedures are not discussed in full detail. Detailed information regarding the techniques, indications and pitfalls of radiologic contrast studies, reflux scintiscanning, ultrasound, pH metry, endoscopy and manometry can be found in other textbooks or review papers. Interest will be focused on recent developments such as impedancometry. The development of a validated 'infant GERD questionnaire' is likely to be the development in diagnostic accuracy with the greatest impact.

Radiological contrast studies, scintiscanning and ultrasound are techniques evaluating postprandial reflux, and provide some information on gastric emptying. Normal ranges are not well established for any of the three procedures. Regarding gastric emptying, 13-C breath tests are more standardized (but the role of delayed gastric emptying in GER(D) is controversial). Scintiscanning may show pulmonary aspiration, although the sensitivity of the technique is extremely low. Contrast radiology is of importance to rule out anatomic abnormalities such as malrotation, duodenal web, stenosis and achalasia.

There are no age or weight limitations in performing endoscopy. Endoscopy shows anatomic malformations and esophagitis, not reflux. Endoscopy-negative reflux disease is common. Biopsies of duodenal, gastric and esophageal mucosa are mandatory to exclude eosinophilic infiltration.

Ambulatory 24-h esophageal pH monitoring measures the incidence and duration of acid reflux, and should be considered the 'silver standard'. It is the best method to measure the presence of acid in the esophagus, but not all reflux causing symptoms is acid. However, it is likely that the majority of GERD patients suffer acid reflux. Esophageal pH metry is useful in evaluating the effect of any therapeutic intervention on reducing esophageal acid exposure. Since medical treatment currently focuses on reducing gastric acid secretion, the technique offers the possibility of measuring intragastric and esophageal recording of pH simultaneously. Manometry does not demonstrate reflux, but is of interest in showing the pathophysiological mechanisms causing the reflux (by measuring the frequency and duration of TLESRs), and is indicated in specific situations such as achalasia. Ambulatory 24-h esophageal manometry, in combination with pH metry, is now technically feasible. Long-lasting investigations offer the opportunity of measuring events in upright and recumbent positions, awake and asleep. Results of pH monitoring depend on the hardware and the software used.[94] The correlation between results obtained with different types of electrodes, glass and antimony, is extremely poor.[95]

Impedancometry is a technique gaining more and more interest, although it has existed for many years. The technique measures electrical potential differences, and is therefore not pH-dependent. The technique offers the possibility of distinguishing between acid and non-acid reflux (in combination with pH metry), and between liquid and gas reflux. Interpretation of the recording is still quite laborious and necessitates sufficient experience. (This is of course true for any of the investigation techniques.) Impedancometry seems especially of interest in patients with endoscopic and pH metric-negative symptoms suggesting GERD.

Because reflux in infants is common, because there is no 'gold standard' investigation, and because investigations are invasive and expensive, interest has focused on the development of an 'infant GER-questionnaire'.[7] Recently, an improved questionnaire was developed.[96] The questionnaire offers the advantage of an objective, validated and repeatable quantification of symptoms suggesting GERD, and thus offers the possibility of measuring the impact of therapeutic intervention. However, although the correlation between the questionnaire and symptoms seems fair, the correlation between the questionnaire and results of investigations for reflux is poor.

Investigation methods for GER all test different aspects involved in the mechanisms and characteristics of reflux. Therefore, it is not unexpected that the correlation between different techniques is extremely poor; non-acid reflux can cause esophagitis, severe heartburn can exist without esophagitis, etc. Also, the correlation between questionnaires for GER symptoms and results of pH metry and endoscopy is quite poor.

Treatment options

Because symptoms suggesting GERD are frequent and non-specific, especially during infancy, and because there is no 'gold-standard' diagnostic technique, many infants are exposed to anti-reflux treatment. Therefore, attention in the paragraphs on therapeutic possibilities is focused on safety aspects. Therapeutic intervention should always be a balance between intended improvement of symptoms and risk for side-effects.

Complications of non-intervention

It is difficult to know the true natural history of GER in infants and children because most patients obtain treatment. Knowledge on the natural history in untreated patients from the initial studies, when effective treatment was unavailable, is extremely limited, because of the limited description and identification of the patients. The paucity of long-term reports, the presence of multiple pathogenic factors and the absence of pathognomonic symptoms for complications make it currently impossible to predict, on an individual basis, which child will continue to have GERD into and during adult life. However, we know that untreated GERD may be associated with severe complications such as esophagitis, failure to thrive in children, esophageal stricture and Barrett's esophagus.

Recent observations suggest a decreased quality of life in regurgitating infants and their parents, even if the regurgitation has disappeared. A 10-year follow-up of esophagitis showed that over 70% had persisting symptoms, and 2% had strictures.[19] Untreated or uncontrolled GERD is associated with severe complications such as esophagitis, Barrett's mucosa, stricture formation and esophageal adenocarcinoma. The frequency, severity and duration of reflux symptoms are related to the risk of esophageal cancer. It is not known whether mild esophagitis or GERD symptoms persisting from childhood into adulthood carry an increased risk for severe complications in adult life. Spontaneous improvement and healing of non-ulcerated esophagitis may exist. Nevertheless, complications and side-effects of medication have to be considered in relation to the natural evolution of untreated GERD.

Non-pharmacological and non-surgical therapies for gastroesophageal reflux

Non-pharmacological (and non-surgical) therapies for reflux do not have any proven efficacy on reflux, although some may decrease the incidence of regurgitation. Lifestyle changes (in adults) are rarely beneficial.[96] No significant difference was shown between the flat and head-elevated prone position. Despite gravity, the upright seated position leads to significantly more and larger reflux episodes than the simple prone and 30° elevated prone position, when the infant is awake or asleep.[97] This is likely to be due to increased abdominal or intragastric pressure. The supine (lying on the back) and lateral positions (lying on the left or right side) usually result in intermediate pH-metric GER values and do not appear to influence GER.[97,98] However, there is now ample evidence that the prone sleeping position is a risk factor in sudden infant death, independent of overheating, adult's smoking or way of feeding. The impact of pacifier ('dummy') use on reflux frequency was equivocal and dependent on infant position. The protein content of formula was not found to affect reflux. Another study suggested that the lower the osmolality, the less acid reflux. Larger food volume and higher osmolality increase the rate of transient LES relaxations and drifts in LES pressure; a reduction of the food volume results in a decrease in the number of regurgitations but no change in acid reflux.[99]

The data of ten randomized controlled trials of non-pharmacological and non-surgical GERD in healthy infants were recently reviewed.[100] Although no study demonstrated a significant reflux-reducing benefit of thickened formula compared to placebo, one study detected a significant benefit of formula thickened with carob bean gum compared with rice flour. Milk-thickening agents include bean gum preparations prepared from St John's bread, a galactomannan, carboxymethylcellulose, a combination of pectine and cellulose, cereals and starch from rice, potato, corn (maize), etc. There are as many different compositions of anti-regurgitation formulas as there are companies: some are casein-predominant, and others contain protein hydrolysates. Milk thickeners have been reported to reduce regurgitation in infants.[97] However, their effects on esophageal acid exposure are inconsistent. Increased coughing has also been demonstrated in infants receiving milk thickeners.[97] According to *in vitro* models testing the effect on one meal, bean gum may be associated with a malabsorption of minerals and micronutrients.[101] Studies of various thickening agents, including guar gum, carob bean gum and soybean polysaccharides, indicate the potential for decreased intestinal absorption of carbohydrates, fats, calcium, iron, zinc and copper.[102] Abdominal pain, colic and diarrhea may ensue from fermentation of bean gum derivatives in the colon. Carob bean gum induces frequent, loose, gelatinous stools. In some, but not all, animal studies, adding carob bean gum to the diet decreased growth.[102] However, growth and nutritional parameters in infants receiving a casein-predominant formula thickened with bean gum were normal.[103] Although rare, serious complications such as acute intestinal obstruction in newborns have been reported.[97] Milk thickeners are often wrongly considered as 'inexpensive'. Allergic reactions to carob bean gum have been reported in adults exposed to it at their workplaces and in infants after exposure to formula thickened with carob bean gum.[102] Nevertheless, in view of their safety and efficacy in decreasing regurgitation, milk thickeners remain a valuable first-line measure in relieving regurgitation in many infants. In contrast, their efficacy in GERD is questionable. Moreover, they are not devoid of side-effects.

Prokinetics

Prokinetic agents, e.g. metoclopramide, domperidone, erythromycin and cisapride, act on regurgitation through their effects on LES pressure, esophageal peristalsis or clearance and/or gastric emptying. Metoclopramide and domperidone also have anti-emetic properties, owing to their dopamine-receptor blocking action, while cisapride is a prokinetic mainly acting via indirect release of acetylcholine from the myenteric plexus.

Metoclopramide

Data supporting the efficacy of metoclopramide are contradictory, and positive results are limited to observations with intravenous administration.[104] Application in infants is limited because of severe adverse events that occur quite frequently (in more than 20% of patients) including central nervous system effects and interactions with the endocrine system.[104] The adverse effects regarding the central nervous system are mainly related to its dopamine-receptor blocking properties in the substantia nigra, and include extrapyramidal effects (dystonic reactions, irritability) and drowsiness, but also asthenia and sleepiness. Isolated cases of metoclopramide-induced methemoglobinemia and sulfhemoglobinemia have been reported.[104,105] Neuroendocrine side-effects such as galactorrhea do occur.[106] Also, metoclopramide has been reported to induce torsade de pointes.[107]

Domperidone

The studies supporting efficacy of domperidone in improving GER in infants are limited.[104] The ability of oral domperidone to increase the pressure of the LES or to promote healing of reflux esophagitis has not been demonstrated in placebo-controlled trials. Most studies have been performed in older children, or investigate the effects of domperidone co-administered with other anti-reflux agents.[104] Comparing domperidone to metoclopramide, elicited adverse effects on the central nervous system were more severe and more common with metoclopramide.[108] Because very little domperidone crosses the blood–brain barrier, reports of central nervous system adverse effects, such as dystonic reactions, are rare.[109] Domperidone is better tolerated than metoclopramide, since dystonic reactions (tremors) and anxiety are infrequent. Prolactin plasma levels may increase, owing to pituary gland stimulation.[110] Somnolence was acknowledged by 49% of patients after 4 weeks of metoclopramide treatment compared with 29% of patients after 4 weeks of domperidone.[108] A reduction in mental acuity was acknowledged by 33% of patients compared to 20% in the domperidone group. Akathisia, asthenia, anxiety and depression were also acknowledged less often, and at a lower severity after 4 weeks of domperidone, although these differences were not significant. Domperidone possesses cardiac electrophysiological effects similar to those of cisapride and class III antiarrhythmic drugs.[104] Intravenously administered domperidone clearly causes QT prolongation and ventricular fibrillation.[111,112]

Erythromycin

Erythromycin has a prokinetic activity if it is administered intravenously. Systemic administration of erythromycin in young infants increases the risk of the infants developing hypertrophic pyloric stenosis.[113] Similarly, a possible association exists with maternal macrolide therapy in late pregnancy.[113] Intravenous erythromycin is reported to cause QT prolongation and ventricular fibrillation.[97,114] The use of erythromycin at doses far below the concentrations necessary for an inhibitory effect on susceptible bacteria provides close to ideal conditions for the induction of bacterial mutation and selection.[115] Emergence of bacteria increasingly resistant to macrolide antibiotics has been reported.[116] New erythromycin-like molecules without the antibiotic properties are in development.

Cisapride

Critical evaluations of published reports on the efficacy of different prokinetics (cisapride, domperidone and metoclopramide) concluded that cisapride was the preferred agent.[117,118] According to these assessments, the vast majority of clinical trials on the efficacy of cisapride demonstrated that at least one of the end-points changed favorably as a result of the intervention.[117] Cisapride is more effective than metoclopramide.[118] A Cochrane review on cisapride in children analyzed data from seven trials, including 236 patients; they compared the effect of cisapride to that of placebo on symptom presence and improvement.[119] It was concluded that there was a statistical difference in the parameter symptoms 'present/absent' but that there was no statistically significant difference for 'symptom change' between placebo and cisapride. The Cochrane review also concluded that cisapride compared to placebo significantly reduced the number and duration of acid reflux episodes, since there was a significant decrease in reflux index, which is the percentage of time that esophageal pH is below 4.0.[119] In general, cisapride is well tolerated. The most common adverse events at therapeutic doses are transient diarrhea and colic (in about 2%). The effect of cisapride on relevant cardiac events such as QT prolongation and arrhythmia is related to dose and risk factors. More serious adverse events such as extrapyramidal reactions, seizures in epileptic patients, and cholestasis in very premature infants have been the objects of isolated reports.

The relation between cisapride, the P450 cytochrome and cardiac effects was considered in 1996.[120] The cytochrome P450 system and especially CYP3A4 metabolizes cisapride in the liver.[121] There is little doubt that cisapride has a QT-prolonging effect,[117] as do many other drugs or clinical situations.[122] Cisapride possesses class III antiarrhythmic properties and prolongs the action potential duration, delaying cardiac repolarization,[123] although many studies do not report an increase in duration of QTc, in neonates or in older children. Torsades de pointes have been reported with cisapride use, especially in those receiving high doses or macrolides.[124] Co-treatment of cisapride and macrolides such as clarithromycin and erythromycin clearly prolongs the QT duration.[125] Underlying cardiac disease, drug interactions and electrolyte imbalance are clearly interfering factors.[126] Cisapride causes prolongation of ventricular repolarization without causing increased heterogeneity of repolarization (QT dispersion), but all patients in the study remained asymptomatic without dysrhythmia.[127] The QT-prolonging effect of cisapride may be related to age.[128] The cytochrome P4503A4, which is involved in the metabolism of cisapride, is immature at birth and reaches adult activity by the age of 3 months. Cisapride accumulation occurs in newborns because of enzymatic immaturity. A significant QTc prolongation occurs, especially in infants younger than 3 months, but not in older infants.[129,130] This effect was related to higher plasma levels. A more frequent administration of lower doses (resulting in a recommended daily dose of 0.8 mg/kg per day) in premature infants results in lower peak levels.[131] Consumption of grapefruit juice also alters cisapride metabolism.[132] According to recent data, gene mutation may be the fundamental culprit.[133] Molecular screening may allow identification among family members of gene carriers potentially at risk if treated with I(Kr) blockers.[134]

Other molecules

From the pathophysiological point of view, prokinetics seems a logical therapeutic approach. However, efficacy data for the whole group of prokinetic drugs are disappointing. Cisapride was shown to have some efficacy in esophageal acid-exposure duration,[135] but it is now banned because of cardiac side-effects. Prucalopride, a 5-HT4 agonist, as been suggested has a possible option, but although the drug seems effective in adult constipation,[136] its use was prohibited for children because of the extrapyramidal side-effects. Ondansetron is a 5-HT3 receptor antagonist that accelerates gastric emptying, inhibits chemotherapy-induced emesis, but prolongs colonic transit time.[137] The most frequently reported adverse events of ondansetron were mild to moderate headache, constipation and diarrhea in patients receiving chemotherapy. Tegaserod is a partial 5-HT4 agonist that has been mostly studied in constipation-predominant irritable bowel syndrome in adults.[138] Tegaserod was shown to accelerate small intestinal transit time, and to increase proximal colonic emptying. Tegaserod also improves gastric emptying and decreases GER,[139] and may be a promising drug. However, to date there are no efficacy data published on the treatment of pediatric GER. Baclofen, 4-amino-3-(-chlorophenyl)-butanoic acid, is a γ-aminobutyric acid (GABA)-B receptor agonist, which is used in children with extreme spasticity. Given orally, it has been shown to decrease GER in healthy adults.[140] Administration in eight pediatric patients was reported to be safe.[141] Alosetron is a 5-HT3 antagonist that increases colonic compliance to distension, delays (ascending) colonic transit time and increases basal fluid absorption. Alosetron induces severe constipation and causes ischemic colitis.

(Alginate-) antacids

Experience with antacids is limited in infants. Their efficacy in buffering gastric acidity in infants is strongly influenced by the time of administration, and requires multiple administrations.

Alginate-antacids form a viscous fluid with surface-active properties, floating as a raft on the surface of the gastric contents, and hence forming an artificial protective barrier against reflux.[142] Their efficacy as monotherapy or in combination with prokinetics for reflux is not convincing. Important drug interactions with antacids include the prevention of the absorption of antibacterials such as tetracycline, azithromycin and quinolones.[143] Antacid ingestion decreased the bioavailability of famotidione, ranitidine and cimetidine by 20–25%, and the bioavailability of nizatidine by 12%.[144] Gaviscon® contains a considerable amount of sodium carbonate, so that its administration may increase the sodium content of the feeds to an undesirable degree (1g of Gaviscon contains 46mg of sodium and the suspension contains twice this amount). Algicon®, having a better taste than Gaviscon, has a lower sodium load, but a higher aluminium content.[142] Occasional formation of large bezoar-like masses of agglutinated intragastric material has been reported in association with Gaviscon. Side-effects include diarrhea with magnesium-rich preparations, and excessive absorption of aluminium in infants.[142] Dimethicone is used in some regions for regurgitation, although there are no reliable studies demonstrating its efficacy in the treatment of GER in infants. Although often classified as an antacid, it acts more as a feed thickener, as it contains more than 50% of bean gum and has hardly any acid-neutralizing properties.

H_2-receptor antagonists

Acid-suppressant therapy is recommended in severe esophagitis, but this does not rectify primary disordered motility, a major pathophysiological mechanism underlying GERD in children. Historically, cimetidine was the first H_2RA that became available. Ranitidine and nizatidine are the most popular and best studied (although quite poorly) H_2RAs in children.[145,146] Experience with other H_2RAs such as roxatidine or ebrotidine is very limited or non-existent in children. In general, H_2RAs are considered to be quite safe. Adverse events reported in clinical trials with ranitidine include headache, tiredness and mild gastrointestinal disturbances, but the incidence is not higher than that for placebo.[146] A high dose of cimetidine can cause reversible impotence and gynecomastia.[146] The endocrinological side-effects associated with long-term administration of cimetidine in adults essentially preclude its long-term use in children.[147] Fatigue, dizziness, headache, dyspepsia, nausea, abdominal pain, flatulence, constipation and diarrhea occur in 1–6% of patients.[148] H_2RAs have been reported to provoke central nervous system dysfunction, but these are poorly documented in children. Ranitidine enhances ischemic neuronal damage.[148] Ranitidine has occasionally been associated with acute interstitial nephritis in native and transplanted kidneys.[149] While ranitidine exhibits no clinically significant drug–drug interactions, cimetidine interacts with many drugs metabolized by cytochrome P450. Theophylline plasma levels were 25–32% higher if cimetidine was administered, compared to ranitidine. Neither ranitidine nor nizatidine increased theophylline levels.[144,150] H_2RAs, PPIs and prokinetic agents undergo metabolism by the cytochrome P450 system present in the liver and gastrointestinal tract.[143] Cimetidine is an inhibitor of CYP3A and it may cause significant interactions with drugs of narrow therapeutic range and low bioavailability that are metabolized by those enzymes.[143]

Whether ranitidine may exceptionally cause QT prolongation or not, is still debated.[151] If ranitidine is administered intravenously after autonomic blockade, the sinus cycle length is prolonged, and the systolic and diastolic blood pressures are decreased.[152] Thus, ranitidine has to be administered by a slow intravenous infusion in patients with sinus node dysfunction.[152] The altered cardiac sympathovagal balance after oral administration of the H_2RA ranitidine indicates a shift towards sympathetic predominance in the heart rate control.[153] Ranitidine modulates high-frequency power of heart rate, and this may be the underlying mechanism of cardiovascular side-effects.[154] Since H_2 receptors are present in the stomach and the heart, they have a trend towards decreasing the heart rate and cardiac contractility.

Nizatidine and ranitidine are susceptible to metabolism by colonic bacteria, but famotidine and cimetidine are not (see also the section on PPIs, below).[155] Ranitidine alters the gastrointestinal flora[156] and causes significantly more pneumonias in patients in intensive care units.[157] In the majority of patients on H_2RAs, there is a relatively important nocturnal breakthrough of acid secretion, sometimes limiting therapeutic efficacy, but on tho other hand minimizing side-effects related to long-term blockade of acid secretion as with PPIs. There is a rapid development of tachyphylaxis or tolerance to H_2RAs, limiting their long-term clinical use.[158]

The combination of ranitidine and pirenzipine, a muscarinic receptor antagonist, does not aid the healing of reflux esophagitis, but does improve symptom relief after 4 weeks.[159] However, side-effects were reported in nine of 75 patients in the ranitidine group and 19 of 76 patients in the ranitidine and pirenpizine group.[159]

Proton pump inhibitors

The suppression of gastric acid secretion achieved with H_2RAs has, however, proved to be suboptimal.[158] In this regard, the advent of the PPIs has been a major breakthrough. Drugs of this category have in fact been shown to be more effective than H_2RAs.[96] Esomeprazole seems to be the most effective PPI commercialized today.[160] Step-down treatment is recommended in adults.[161] Failure to control symptoms with high-dose PPI treatment raises the likelihood of non-acid-related causes for the symptoms.

The pharmacokinetics and tolerance of pantoprazole were similar in patients with moderate and severe hepatic impairment.[162] These were also evaluated for famotidine in 150 children.[163] Recent studies with lansoprazole showed its efficacy in reducing symptoms and healing esophagitis in children.[164] The availability of a syrup facilitates the use of this drug in children.[164] Zimmermann and colleagues reviewed the literature on the use and administration of omeprazole in children.[165] In uncontrolled trials and case reports, omeprazole was used at a dosage of 0.2–3.5 mg/kg per day for periods ranging from 14 days to 36 months, and found to be effective and well tolerated for the acute and chronic treatment of esophageal and peptic ulcer disease in children aged 2 months to 18 years.[165]

The following side-effects of PPI have been reported: headache (about 3%); neurological and psychiatric side-effects, especially fatigue, dizziness and confusion in patients with hepatic diseases and/or advanced age; cutaneous reactions, generally rash and urticaria; hemolytic anemia, leukopenia and agranulocytosis; gynecomastia; subacute myopathy; gastrointestinal side-effects such as flatulence, constipation, diarrhea (about 4%), dyspepsia and nausea (about 2%), vomiting and abdominal pain; hepatic disorders, especially moderate elevation of aminotransferases; and excessive urinary sodium loss.[97,142,166,167] The high cost of PPIs can also be considered an important albeit not medical 'side-effect'.

Omeprazole, esomeprazole, lansoprazole, rabeprazole and pantaprazole rarely exhibit clinically important interactions with other hepatically metabolized medications or pH-dependent drugs.[168] The absorption of drugs that are pH sensitive, as is the case with digoxin and ketoconazole, will be influenced by PPIs.[169]

The gastroparietal PPIs lansoprazole, omeprazole and pantoprazole are all primarily metabolized by a genetically polymorphic enzyme, CYP2C19, that is absent in approximately 3% of Caucasians and 20% of Asians.[143] These drugs may also interact with CYP3A, but to a lesser extent. Esomeprazole has the potential to interact with CYP2C19. The slightly altered metabolism of cisapride was also suggested to be the result of inhibition of a minor metabolic pathway for cisapride mediated by CYP2C19. Esomeprazole did not interact with the CYP3A4 substrates clarithromycin and quinidine.[169] Overall, the potential for drug–drug interactions with esomeprazole is low, and similar to that reported for omeprazole.[169] Salivary secretion is decreased with omeprazole. Prolonged use of PPIs can result in vitamin B_{12} deficiency as a consequence of impaired release of vitamin B_{12} from food in a non-acid environment. However, cystic fibrosis patients treated for at least 2 years with a PPIs and cystic fibrosis patients without PPI had higher vitamin B_{12} levels than healthy controls.[170]

The safety of long-term administration of acid-blocking medication needs to be considered in relation to potential consequences of prolonged acid suppression, including the risk of proliferation of gastric flora and the risk of developing enterochromaffin-like cell hyperplasia, which could, in turn, theoretically, lead to gastric malignancy. Hypergastrinemia occurs in nearly all patients treated with omeprazole, causing hyperplasia and pseudohypertrophy of the parietal cells, as recently shown in 93% of adult patients on long-term omeprazole. Patients on omeprazole therapy for 5–8 years remained without evidence of significant enterochromaffin cell hyperplasia, gastric atrophy, intestinal metaplasia, dysplasia or neoplastic changes.[171] Because of the excellent efficacy profile, these drugs tend to be overused.[172] Since PPIs could delay the diagnosis of gastric cancer, the long-term uncontrolled and unnecessary use of these drugs should be avoided. Bacterial proliferation in the gastric content may not only change colonic flora, but may also be a risk factor for the patient to develop nosocomial pneumonia.

Other drugs

Sucralfate causes bezoars, especially when given to patients in intensive care units, and diarrhea. Patients with renal failure treated with sucralfate are exposed to aluminium toxicity.[173–175] Other anti-emetic drugs such as batanopride also have a QTc-prolonging effect.[176] Octeotride is a long-acting somatostatin, that induces a phase 3-like migrating motor complex response, which is not inhibited by meals (differing from normal), and has an inhibitory effect on the gastric antrum (and is therefore indicated in dumping syndrome). Motilin agonists have been studied with inconsistent results in adults, and are not yet available for pediatric use.[177]

Therapeutic endoscopic procedures

During recent years, new endoscopic techniques intending to improve the function of the anti-reflux barrier have been developed. The first results of endoscopic gastroplasty (Endocinch® system), radiofrequency delivery at the cardia (Stretta® system) and injection therapy (Enteryx® procedure) in adults have been reported.[178–181] The first series in adolescents have been performed. Although experience is too limited to recommend broad use, the theoretical concept of these procedures is interesting. Further improvements to the techniques are still being introduced.

Surgery

While anti-reflux surgery in certain groups of children may be of considerable benefit, it also has a mortality and a failure rate.[184–187] Ninety per cent of patients remained free from significant reflux symptoms after a laparoscopic Nissen operation, although side-effects occurred in up to 22%.[186] After a median follow-up of 16 years, the Nissen–Rosetti procedure in 24 consecutive children without congenital or acquired anomalies of the esophagus except GERD showed a result that was considered excellent in only 75%, good in 21% and poor in 4%.[187] Failure rates of 5–20% have been found after objective postoperative follow-up.[187] A protective anti-reflux surgical procedure in neurologically impaired children needing a gastrostomy increased the morbidity and mortality rate of the gastrostomy procedure itself.[188]

Conclusion

GER and GERD are frequent conditions in infants, children and adolescents. Symptomatology differs with age, although the main pathophysiological mechanism, transient relaxations of the LES associated with reflux, is identical at all ages. Although infant regurgitation is likely to disappear with age, little is known about reflux. The majority of symptomatic reflux episodes are acid, but non-acid and gas reflux can also cause symptoms. Complications of reflux disease may be severe and even life threatening, such as esophageal stenosis and Barrett's esophagus. There is no gold standard for a diagnostic technique. A simple questionnaire may be among the best diagnostic aids in infants; non-acid reflux is best investigated with impedancometry. Primary GERD is mainly a motility disorder. Guidelines for treatment struggle with the fact that there is no prokinetic drug with a convincing efficacy profile. As a consequence, treatment of GERD focuses on anti-acid drugs, and particularly on PPIs. There is little or no information on how to organize follow-up.

REFERENCES

1. de Caestecker J. Oesophagus: heartburn. *BMJ* 2001; **323**: 736–739.
2. Dent J, Brun J, Fendrick AM. An evidence-based appraisal of the reflux disease management – The Genval Workshop Report. *Gut* 1999; **44**: S1–S16.
3. Rudolph CD, Mazur LJ, Liptak GS et al. Guidelines for evaluation and treatment of gastroesophageal reflux in infants and children. Recommendations of the North American Society for Pediatric Gastroenterology and Nutrition. *J Pediatr Gastroenterol Nutr* 2001; **32**(Suppl 2): S1–S31.
4. Vandenplas Y. *Oesophageal pH Monitoring for Gastro-oesophageal Reflux in Infants and Children*. Chichester, UK: John Wiley and Sons, 1992: 27–36.
5. Cleveland RH, Kushner DC, Schwartz AN. Gastroesophageal reflux in children: results of a standardized fluoroscopic approach. *Am J Roentgenol* 1983; **141**: 53–56.
6. Vandenplas Y, Goyvaerts H, Helven R. Gastroesophageal reflux, as measured by 24-hour pH-monitoring, in 509 healthy infants screened for risk of sudden infant death syndrome. *Pediatrics* 1991; **88**: 834–840.
7. Orenstein SR, Shalaby TM, Cohn J. Reflux symptoms in 100 normal infants: diagnostic validity of the Infant Gastroesophageal Reflux Questionnaire. *Clin Pediatr* 1996; **35**: 607–614.
8. Chouhou D, Rossignol C, Bernard F, Dupont C. Le reflux gastro-oesophagien dans les centres de bilan de santé de l'enfant de moins de 4 ans. *Arch Franc Ped* 1992; **49**: 843–845.
9. Nelson SP, Chen EH, Syniar GM. Prevalence of symptoms of gastroesophageal reflux in infancy. *Arch Pediatr Adolesc Med* 1997; **151**: 569–572.
10. Shepherd R, Wren J, Evans S. Gastroesophageal reflux in children. Clinical profile, course and outcome with active therapy in 126 cases. *Clin Pediatr* 1987; **26**: 55–60.
11. Nelson SP, Chen EH, Syniar GM. One year follow-up of symptoms of gastroesophageal reflux during infancy. *Pediatrics* 1998; **102**: e67.
12. Wienbeck M, Barnert J. Epidemiology of reflux disease and reflux esophagitis. *Scand J Gastroenterol* 1989; **24**: 7–13.
13. Nelson SP, Chen EH, Syniar GM, Christoffel KK. Prevalence of symptoms of gastroesophageal reflux during childhood. *Arch Pediatr Adolesc Med* 2000; **154**: 150–154.
14. Sonnenberg A, El-Serag HB. Clinical epidemiology and natural history of gastroesophageal reflux disease. *Yale J Biol Med* 1999; **72**: 81–92.
15. Isolauri J, Laippala P. Prevalence of symptoms suggestive of gastro-oesophageal reflux disease in an adult population. *Ann Med* 1995; **27**: 67–70.
16. The Jury of the Consensus Conference. French–Belgian Consensus Conference on adult gastro-oesophageal reflux disease 'Diagnosis and Treatment': report of a meeting held in Paris, France, on 21–22 January 1999. *Eur J Gastroenterol Hepatol* 2000; **12**: 129–137.
17. Nandurkar S, Talley NJ. Epidemiology and natural history of reflux disease. *Baillière's Clin Gastroenterol* 2000; **14**: 743–757.
18. Isolauri J, Luostarinen M, Isolauri E. Natural course of gastroesophageal reflux disease: 17–22 year follow-up of 60 patients. *Am J Gastroenterol* 1997; **92**: 37–41.
19. McDougall NJ, Johnston BT, Kee F. Natural history of reflux oesophagitis: a 10 year follow up of its effect on patient symptomatology and quality of life. *Gut* 1996; **38**: 481–486.
20. El-Serag HB, Bailey NR, Gilger M, Rabeneck L. Endoscopic manifestations of gastroesophageal reflux disease in patients between 18 months and 25 years without neurological deficits. *Am J Gastroenterol* 2002; **97**: 1635–1639.
21. Lee WS, Beattie RM, Meadows N, Walker-Smith JA. Gastro-oesophageal reflux: clinical profiles and outcome. *J Paediatr Child Health* 1999; **35**: 568–571.
22. Tolaymat N, Chapman DM. Gastroesophageal reflux disease in children older than two years of age. *West Virginia Med J* 1998; **94**: 22–25.
23. Treem W, Davis P, Hyams J. Gastroesophageal reflux in the older child: presentation, response to treatment, and long-term follow-up. *Clin Pediatr* 1991; **30**: 435–440.
24. Hassall E. Co-morbidities in childhood Barrett's esophagus. *J Pediatr Gastroenterol Nutr* 1997; **25**: 255–260.
25. Voutilainen M, Sipponen P, Macklin JP. Gastroesophageal reflux disease: prevalence, clinical, endoscopic and histopathological findings in 1,128 consecutive patients referred for endoscopy due to dyspeptic and reflux symptoms. *Digestion* 2000; **61**: 6–13.
26. Loof L, Gotell P, Elfberg B. The incidence of reflux oesophagitis. *Scand J Gastroenterol* 1993; **28**: 113–118.
27. Hegar B, Boediarso A, Firmansyah A, Vandenplas Y. Incidence of regurgitation and symptoms of gastroesophageal reflux in Indonesian infants. *Acta Gastroenterol Belg* 2003; Suppl:69 (abstr).
28. Kang JY, Ho KY. Different prevalences of reflux oesophagitis and hiatus hernia among dyspeptic patients in England and Singapore. *Eur J Gastroenterol Hepatol* 1999; **11**: 845–850.
29. Kim SL, Hunter JG, Wo JM et al. NSAIDs, aspirin, and esophageal strictures: are over-the-counter medications harmful to the esophagus? *J Clin Gastroenterol* 1999; **29**: 32–34.
30. Carre IJ, Johnston BT, Thomas PS, Morrisson PJ. Familial hiatal hernia in a large five generation family confirming true autosomal dominant inheritance. *Gut* 1999; **45**: 649–652.
31. Trudgill NJ, Kapur KC, Riley SA. Familial clustering of reflux symptoms. *Am J Gastroenterol* 1999; **94**: 1172–1178.
32. Cameron AJ, Lagergren J, Henriksson C. Gastroesophageal reflux disease in monozygotic and dizygotic twins. *Gastroenterology* 2002; **122**: 55–59.
33. Hu FZ, Preston RA, Post JC. Mapping of a gene for severe pediatric gastroesophageal reflux to chromosome 13q14. *JAMA* 2000; 284: 325–334.
34. Orenstein SR, Shalaby TM, Barmada MM, Whitcomb DC. Genetics of gastroesophageal reflux disease: a review. *J Pediatr Gastroenterol Nutr* 2002; **34**: 506–510.
35. Vandenplas Y, Hassall E. Mechanisms of gastroesophageal reflux and gastroesophageal reflux disease. *J Pediatr Gastroenterol* 2002; **35**: 119–136.
36. Sifrim D, Holloway R, Silny J et al. Acid, non-acid and gas reflux in patients with gastroesophageal reflux disease during 24 hr ambulatory pH-impedance recordings. *Gastroenterology* 2001; **120**: 1588–1598.
37. McNamara D, O'Morain C. Gastro-oesophageal reflux disease and *Helicobacter pylori*: an intricate relation. *Gut* 1999; **45**(Suppl 1) :S13–S17.
38. Graham DY, Yamaoka Y. Disease-specific *Helicobacter pylori* virulence factors: the unfulfilled promise. *Helicobacter* 2000; **5**(Suppl 1): S3–S9.

39. Wu JC, Sung JJ, Chan FK et al. *Helicobacter pylori* infection is associated with milder gastro-oesophageal reflux disease. *Aliment Pharmacol Ther* 2000; **14**: 427–432.
40. De Koster E. Adverse events of HP eradication: long term negative consequences of HP eradication. *Acta Gastroenterol Belg* 1998; **61**: 350–351.
41. Fallone CA, Barkin AN, Friedman G et al. Is *Helicobacter pylori* eradication associated with gastroesophageal reflux disease? *Am J Gastroenterol* 2000; **95**: 914–920.
42. Van Zanten SJ, Dixon MF, Lee A. The gastric transitional zones: neglected links between gastroduodenal pathology and helicobacter ecology. *Gastroenterology* 1999; **116**: 1217–1229.
43. Kuiken S, Van Den Elzen B, Tytgat G et al. Evidence for pooling of gastric secretions in the proximal stomach in humans using single photon computed tomography. *Gastroenterology* 2002; **123**: 2157-2158.
44. Fletcher J, Wirz A, Young J et al. Unbuffered highly acidic gastric juice exists at the gastroesophageal junction after a meal. *Gastroenterology* 2001; **121**: 775–783.
45. Dodds WJ, Dent J, Hogan WJ et al. Mechanisms of gastroesophageal reflux in patients with reflux esophagitis. *N Engl J Med* 1982; **307**: 1547–1552.
46. Omari TI, Benninga MA, Barnett CP et al. Characterization of esophageal body and lower esophageal sphincter motor function in the very premature neonate. *J Pediatr* 1999; **135**: 517–521.
47. Boulant J, Fioramonti J, Dapoigny M et al. Cholecystokinin and nitric oxide in transient lower esophageal sphincter relaxation to gastric distention in dogs. *Gastroenterology* 1994; **107**: 1059–1066.
48. Hirsch DP, Hollowy RH, Tytgat GNJ, Boeckxstaens GE. Involvement of nitric oxide in human transient lower esophageal sphincter relaxations and esophageal primary peristalsis. *Gastroenterology* 1998; **115**: 1374–1380.
49. Sifrim D, Tack J, Lerut T, Janssens J. Transient lower esophageal sphincter relaxations and esophageal body muscular contractile response in reflux esophagitis. *Dig Dis Sci* 2000; **45**: 1293–1300.
50. Mittal RK, McCallum RW. Characteristics and frequency of transient relaxations of the lower esophageal sphincter in patients with reflux esophagitis. *Gastroenterology* 1988; **95**: 593–599.
51. Holloway RH, Kocyan P, Dent J. Provocation of transient lower esophageal sphincter relaxations by meals in patients with symptomatic gastroesophageal reflux. *Dig Dis Sci* 1991; **36**: 1034–1039.
52. Penagini R, Hebbard G, Horowitz M et al. Motor function of the proximal stomach and visceral perception in gastro-oesophageal reflux disease. *Gut* 1998; **42**: 251–257.
53. Stacher G, Lenglinger J, Bergmann H. Gastric emptying: a contributory factor in gastro-oesophageal reflux activity? *Gut* 2000; **47**: 661–666.
54. Sifrim D, Holloway R. Transient lower esophageal sphincter relaxations: how many or how harmful? *Am J Gastroenterol* 2001; **96**: 2529–2532.
55. Vela MF, Camacho-Lobato L, Srinivasan R et al. Simultaneous intraesopahgeal impedance and pH measurement of acid and non-acid gastroesophageal reflux: effect of omeprazole. *Gastroenterology* 2001; **120**: 1599–1606.
56. Niemantsverdriet EC, Timmer R, Breumelhof R, Smout AJ. The role of excessive gastro-oesophageal reflux, disordered oesophageal motility and decreased mucosal sensitivity in the pathogenesis of Barrett's oesophagus. *Eur J Gastroenterol Hepatol* 1997; **9**: 515–519.
57. Mathisen B, Worall L, Masel J et al. Feeding problems in infants with gastro-oesophageal reflux disease: a controlled study. *J Pediatr Child Health* 1999; **35**: 163–169.
58. Black MM, Dubowitz H, Huctheson J. A randomized clinical trial of home intervention for children with failure to thrive. *Pediatrics* 1995; **95**: 807–814.
59. Burklow KA, Phelps AN, Schultz JR et al. Classifying complex pediatric feeding disorders. *J Pediatr Gastroenterol Nutr* 1998; **27**: 143–147.
60. Orenstein SR, Cohn JF, Shalaby T. Reliability and validity of an infant gastroesophageal questionnaire. *Clin Pediatrics* 1993; **32**: 472–484.
61. Heine RG, Jaquiery A, Lubitz L et al. Role of gastro-oesophageal reflux in infant irritability. *Arch Dis Child* 1995; **73**: 121–125.
62. Snel A, Barnett CP, Cresp TL. Behavior and gastroesophageal reflux in the premature neonate. *J Pediatr Gastroenterol Nutr* 2000; **30**: 18–21.
63. Hamilton AB, Zeltzer LK. Visceral pain in infants. *J Pediatr* 1994; **125**(Suppl): S95–S102.
64. Iacono G, Carroccio A, Cavataio F et al. Gastroesophageal reflux and cow's milk allergy in infants: a prospective study. *J All Clin Immunol* 1996; **97**: 822–827.
65. Salvatore S, Vandenplas Y. Gastroesophageal reflux and cow's milk allergy: is there a link? *Pediatrics* 2002; **110**: 972–984.
66. Hill DJ, Heine RG, Cameron DJ et al. Role of food protein intolerance in infants with persistent distress attributed to reflux esophagitis. *J Pediatr* 2000; **136**: 641–647.
67. Orenstein SR, Izadnia F, Khan S. Gastroesophageal reflux disease in children. *Gastroenterol Clin North Am* 1999; **28**: 947–969.
68. Locke GR, Talley NJ, Fett SL. Prevalence and clinical spectrum of gastroesophageal reflux: a population based study in Olmsted Country, Minnesota. *Gastroenterology* 1997; **112**: 1448–1456.
69. De Vault KR, Castell DO. Updated guidelines for the diagnosis and treatment of gastroesophageal reflux disease. *Am J Gastroenterol* 1999; **94**: 1434–1442.
70. Hyman PE. Gastroesophageal reflux: one reason why baby won't eat. *J Pediatr* 1994; **125**: S103–S109.
71. Holt PG. Parasites, atopy, and the hygiene hypothesis: resolution of a paradox? *Lancet* 2000; **356**: 1699–1701.
72. Van den Biggelaar AHJ, van Ree R, Rodrigues LC et al. Decreased atopy in children infected with *Schistosoma haematobium*: a role for parasite-induced interleukins-10. *Lancet* 2000; **356**: 1723–1727.
73. Louis E, DeLooze D, Deprez P. Heartburn in Belgium: prevalence, impact on daily life, and utilization of medical resources. *Eur J Gastroenterol Hepatol* 2002; **14**: 279–284.
74. Vandenplas Y. Reflux esophagitis in infants and children. A report from the Working Group of the European Society of Pediatric Gastroenterology and Nutrition on Gastro-oesophageal Reflux Disease. *J Pediatr Gastroenterol Nutr* 1994; **18**: 413–422.
75. Ahrens P, Noll C, Kitz R et al. Lipid-laden alveolar macrophages: a useful marker of silent aspiration in children. *Pediatr Pulmonol* 1999; **28**: 83–88.
76. Paterson WG, Murat BW. Combined ambulatory esophageal manometry and dual-probe pH metry in the evaluation of patients with chronic unexplained cough. *Dig Dis Sci* 1994; **39**: 1117–1125.
77. Bruno G, Graf U, Andreozzi P. Gastric asthma: an unrecognized disease with an unsuspected frequency. *J Asthma* 1999; **36**: 315–325.
78. Cunningham ET Jr, Ravich WJ, Jones B, Donner MW. Vagal reflexes referred from the upper aerodigestive tract: an infrequently recognized cause of common

cardiorespiratory responses. *Ann Intern Med* 1992; **116**: 575–582.

79. Murphy SG, Yazbeck S, Russo P. Isolated congenital esophageal stenosis. *J Pediatr Surg* 1995; **30**: 1238–1241.
80. Carre I. The natural history of the partial thoracic stomach ("hiatal hernia") in children. *Arch Dis Child* 1959; **34**: 344–353.
81. Karnak I, Senocak ME, Tanyel FC, Buyukpamukcu N. Achalasia in childhood: surgical treatment and outcome. *Eur J Pediatr Surg* 2001; **11**: 223–229.
82. Wienbeck M, Barnert J. Epidemiology of reflux disease and reflux esophagitis. *Scand J Gastroenterol* 1989; **156**: 7–13.
83. Liacouras CA, Wenner WJ, Brown K, Ruchelli E. Primary eosinophilic esophagitis in children: successful treatment with oral corticosteroids. *J Pediatr Gastroenterol Nutr* 1998; **26**: 380–385.
84. Orenstein SR, Shalaby TM, Di Lorenzo C. The spectrum of pediatric eosinophilic esophagitis beyond infancy: a clinical series of 30 children. *Am J Gastroenterol* 2000; **95**: 1422–1430.
85. Ruchelli E, Wenner W, Voytek T et al. Severity of esophageal eosinophilia predicts response to conventional gastroesophageal reflux therapy. *Pediatr Dev Pathol* 1999; **2**: 15–18.
86. Attwood SE, Lewis CJ, Bronder CS et al. Eosinophilic oesophagitis: a novel treatment using Montelukast. *Gut* 2003; **52**: 181–185.
87. Teitelbaum JE, Fox VL, Twarog FJ et al. Eosinophilic esophagitis in children: immunopathological analysis and response to fluticasone propionate. *Gastroenterology* 2002; **122**: 1216–1225.
88. Hassall E. Barrett's esophagus: new definitions and approaches in children. *J Pediatr Gastroenterol Nutr* 1993; **16**: 345–364.
89. Romero Y, Cameron AJ, Locke GR. Familial aggregation of gastroesophageal reflux in patients with Barrett's esophagus and esophageal carcinoma. *Gastroenterology* 1997; **113**: 1449–1456.
90. Krug E, Bergmeijer JH, Dees J. Gastroesophageal reflux and Barrett's esophagus in adults born with esophageal atresia. *Am J Gastroenterol* 1999; **94**: 2825–2828.
91. Dahms BB, Rothstein FC. Barrett's esophagus in children: a consequence of chronic gastroesophageal reflux. *Gastroenterology* 1984; **86**: 318–323.
92. Sonnenberg A, El-Serag HB. Clinical epidemiology and natural history of gastroesophageal reflux disease. *Yale J Biol Med* 1999; **72**: 81–92.
93. Lagergren J, Bergstrom R, Lindgren A, Nyrén O. Symptomatic gastroesophageal reflux as a risk factor for esophageal adenocarcinoma. *N Engl J Med* 1999; **340**: 825–831.
94. Vandenplas Y, de Pont S, Vandemaele C et al. Dependability of esophageal pH monitoring data on software. *J Pediatr Gastroenterol Nutr* 1996; **23**: 203–204.
95. Vandenplas Y, Helven R, Goyvaerts H. Comparative study of glass and antimony electrodes for continuous oesophageal pH monitoring. *Gut* 1991; **32**: 708–712.
96. Kaynard A, Flora K. Gastroesophageal reflux disease. Control of symptoms, prevention of complications. *Postgrad Med* 2001; **110**: 42–44.
97. Vandenplas Y, Belli D, Benhamou P et al. A critical appraisal of current management practicies for infant regurgitation – recommendations of a working party. *Eur J Pediatr* 1997; **156**: 343–357.
98. Ewer AK, James ME, Tobin JM. Prone and left lateral positioning reduce gastro-oesophageal reflux in preterm infants. *Arch Dis Child Fetal Neonatal Ed* 1999; **81**: F201–F205.
99. Khoshoo V, Ross G, Brown S, Edell D. Smaller volume, thickened formulas in the management of gastroesophageal reflux in thriving infants. *J Pediatr Gastroenterol Nutr* 2000; **31**: 554–556.
100. Carroll AE, Garrison MM, Christakis DA. A systematic review of nonpharmacological and nonsurgical therapies for gastroesophageal reflux in infants. *Arch Pediatr Adolesc Med* 2002; **156**: 109–113.
101. Bosscher D, van Caillie-Bertrand M, van Dyck K. Thickening of infant formula with digestible and indigestible carbohydrate availability of calcium, iron and zinc *in vitro*. *J Pediatr Gastroenterol Nutr* 2000; **30**: 373-378.
102. Aggett PJ, Agostoni C, Goulet O et al. Antireflux or antiregurgitation milk products for infants and young children: a commentary by the ESPGHAN Committee on Nutrition. *J Pediatr Gastroenterol Nutr* 2002; **34**: 496–498.
103. Levtchenko E, Hauser B, Vandenplas Y. Nutritional value of an 'anti-regurgitation' formula. *Acta Gastroenterol Belg* 1998; **61**: 285–287.
104. Vandenplas Y. Clinical use of cisapride and its risk–benefit in paediatric patients. *Eur J Gastroenterol Hepatol* 1998; **10**: 871–881.
105. Aravindhan N, Chisholm DG. Sulfhemoglobinemia presenting as pulse oximetry desaturations. *Anesthesiology* 2000; **93**: 883–884.
106. Cinquetti M, Bonetti P, Bertamini P. Current role of antidopaminergic drugs in pediatrics. *Pediatr Med Chir* 2000; **22**: 1–7.
107. Chou CC, Wu D. Torsade de pointes induced by metoclopramide in an elderly woman with preexisting complete left bundle branch block. *Chang Gubng Med J* 2001; **4**: 805–809.
108. Patterson D, Abell T, Rothstein R et al. A double-blind multicenter comparison of domperidone and metoclopramide in the treatment of diabetic patients with symptoms of gastroparesis. *Am J Gastroenterol* 1999; **94**: 1230–1234.
109. Barone JA. Domperidone: a peripherally acting dopamine 2-receptor antagonist. *Ann Pharmacother* 1999; **33**: 429–440.
110. Lu F, Wu H, Zhang K, Li D. Domperidone and hyperprolactinemia. *Human Yi Ke Da Xue Xue Bao* 1998; **23**: 100–102.
111. Drolet B, Rousseau G, Daleau P et al. Domperidone should not be considered a no-risk alternative to cisapride in the treatment of gastrointestinal motility disorders. *Circulation* 2000; **102**: 1883–1885.
112. Cameron HA, Reyntjes AJ, Lake-Bakaar G. Cardiac arrest after treatment with intravenous domperidone. *BMJ* 1985; **290**: 160.
113. Mahon BE, Rosenman MB, Kleiman MB. Maternal and infant use of erythromycin and other macrolide antibiotics as risk factors for infantile hypertrophic pylori stenosis. *J Pediatr* 2001; **139**: 380-384.
114. Mishra A, Friedman HS, Sinha AK. The effects of erythromycin on the electrocardiogram. *Chest* 1999; **115**: 983-986.
115. Guerin JM, Leibinger F. Why not use erythromycin in GI motility? *Chest* 2002; **121**: 301.
116. Gay K, Baughan W, Miller J. The emergence of *Streptococcus pneumoniae* resistant to macrolide antimicrobial agents: a 6-year population-based assessment. *J Infect Dis* 2000; **182**: 1417–1424.
117. Vandenplas Y, and the ESPGHAN Cisapride Panel. Current pediatric indications for cisapride. *J Pediatr Gastroenterol* 2000; **31**: 480–489.
118. Rode H, Millar AJW, Melis J, Cywes S. Esophageal assessment of gastroesophageal reflux in 18 patients and the effect of two prokinetic agents: cisapride and metoclopramide. *J Pediatr Surg* 1987; **22**: 931–934.

119. Augood C, MacLennan S, Gilbert R, Logan S. Cisapride treatment for gastro-oesophageal reflux in children. *Cochrane Database Syst Rev* 2000; **3**: CD002300.
120. Shulman RJ. Report from the NASPGN therapeutics subcommittee. Cisapride and the attack of the P-450s. *J Pediatr Gastroenterol Nutr* 1996; **23**: 395–397.
121. Desta Z, Zoukhova N, Mahal SK, Flockhart DA. Interaction of cisapride with the human cytochrome P450 system: metabolism and inhibition studies. *Drug Metab Dispos* 2000; **28**: 789–800.
122. Viskin S. Long QT syndromes and torsades de pointes. *Lancet* 1999; **354**: 1625–1633.
123. Tonini M, De Ponti F, Di Nucci A, Crema F. Review article: cardiac adverse effects of gastrointestinal prokinetics. *Aliment Pharmacol Ther* 1999; **13**: 1585–1591.
124. Hill SL, Evangelista JK, Pizzi AM et al. Proarrhythmia associated with cisapride in children. *Pediatrics* 1998; **101**: 1053–1056.
125. Ward RM, Lemons JA, Molteni RA. Cisapride: a survey of the frequency of use and adverse events in premature newborns. *Pediatrics* 1999; **103**: 469–472.
126. Levy J, Hayes C, Kern J et al. Does cisapride influence cardiac rhythm? Results of a US multicenter, double-blind, placebo controlled pediatric study. *J Pediatr Gastroenterol Nutr* 2001; **32**: 458–463.
127. Tutar HE, Kansu A, Kalayci AG et al. Effects of cisapride on ventricular repolarization in children. *Acta Paediatr* 2000; **89**: 820–823.
128. Semama DS, Bernardini S, Louf S et al. Effects of cisapride on QTc interval in term neonates. *Arch Dis Child Fetal Neonat Ed* 2001; **84**: F44-F46.
129. Benatar A, Feenstra A, De Craene T, Vandenplas Y. QTc interval in infants and serum concentrations. *J Pediatr Gastroenterol Nutr* 2001; **33**: 41–46.
130. Benatar A, Feenstra A, Decraene T, Vandenplas Y. Effects of cisapride on corrected QT interval, heart rate, and rhythm in infants undergoing polysomnography. *Pediatrics* 2000; **106**: E85.
131. Cools F, Benatar A, Bruneel E et al. A comparison of the pharmacokinetics of two dosing regimens of cisapride and their effects on corrected QT interval in premature infants. *Eur J Clin Pharmacol.* 2003; **59**: 17–22.
132. Kivisto KT, Lilja JJ, Backman JT, Neuvonen PJ. Repeated consumption of grapefruit juice considerably increases plasma concentrations of cisapride. *Clin Pharmacol Ther* 1999; **66**: 448–453.
133. Napolitano C, Schwartz PJ, Brown AM et al. Evidence for a cardiac ion channel mutation underlying drug-induced QT prolongation and life-threatening arrhythmias. *J Cardiovasc Electrophysiol* 2000; **11**: 691–696.
134. Walker AM, Szneke P, Weatherby LB et al. The risk of serious cardiac arrhythmias among cisapride users in the United Kingdom and Canada. *Am J Med* 1999; **107**: 356–362.
135. Augood C, Gilbert R, Logan S, MacLennan S. Cisapride treatment for gastro-oesophageal reflux in children. *Cochrane Database Syst Rev* 2002; **3**: CD002300.
136. Coremans G, Kerstens R, De Pauw M, Stevens M. Prucalopride is effective in patients with severe chronic constipation in whom laxatives fail to provide adequate relief. Results of a double-blind, placebo-controlled clinical trial. *Digestion* 2003; **67**: 82–89.
137. Culy CR, Bhana N, Plosker GL. Ondansetron: a review of its use as an antiemetic in children. *Paediatr Drugs* 2001; **3**: 441–79.
138. Wagstaff A, Frampton J, Croom K. Tegaserod: a review of its use in the management of irritable bowel syndrome with constipation in women. *Drugs* 2003; **63**: 1101–1120.
139. Kahrilas PJ, Quigley EM, Castell DO, Spechler SJ. The effects of tegaserod (HTF 919) on oesophageal acid exposure in gastro-oesophageal reflux disease. *Aliment Pharmacol Ther* 2000; **14**: 1503-1509.
140. Ciccaglione AF, Marzio L. Effect of acute and chronic administration of the GABA(B) agonist baclofen on 24 hour pH metry and symptoms in control subjects and in patients with gastro-oesophageal reflux disease. *Gut* 2003; **52**: 464–470.
141. Wiersma HE. Pharmacokinetics of a single oral dose of baclofen in pediatric patients with GERD. *Ther Drug Monitor* 2003; **25**: 93–98.
142. Vandenplas Y, Belli DC, Benatar A et al. The role of cisapride in the treatment of pediatric gastroesophageal reflux. The European Society of Pediatric Gastroenterology, Hepatology and Nutrition. *J Pediatr Gastroenterol Nutr* 1999; **28**: 518–528.
143. Flockhart DA, Desta Z, Mahal SK. Selection of drugs to treat gastro-oesophageal reflux disease: the role of drug interactions. *Clin Pharmacokinet* 2000; **39**: 295–309.
144. Bachmann KA, Sullivan TJ, Jauregui L et al. Drug interactions of H_2-receptor antagonists. *Scand J Gastroenterol* 1994; **206** (Suppl): 14–19.
145. Paul K, Redman CM, Chen M. Effectiveness and safety of nizatidine, 75 mg, for the relief of episodic heartburn. *Aliment Pharmacol Ther* 2001; **15**: 1571–1577.
146. Sabesin SM. Safety issues relating to long-term treatment with histamine H_2-receptor antagonists. *Aliment Pharmacol* 1993; **7**(Suppl 2): S35–S40.
147. Kelly DA. Do H_2 receptor antagonists have a therapeutic role in childhood? *J Pediatr Gastroenterol* 1994; **19**: 270–276.
148. Adachi N, Seyfried FJ, Arai T. Blockade of central histaminergic H_2-receptors aggravates ischemic neuronal damage in gerbil hippocampus. *Crit Care Med* 2001; **29**: 1189–1194.
149. Emovon OE, King JA, Holt CO, Browne BJ. Ranitidine induced acute interstitial nephritis in a cadaveric renal allograft. *Am J Kidney Dis* 2001; **38**: 169–172.
150. Boehning W. Effect of cimetidine and ranitidine on plasma theophylline in patients with chronic obstructive airways disease treated with theophylline and corticosteroids. *Eur J Clin Pharmacol* 1990; **38**: 43–45.
151. Alliet P, Devos E. Ranitidine-induced bradycardia in a neonate – secondary to a congenital long QT interval syndrome. *Eur J Pediatr* 1993; **152**: 933–934.
152. Hu WH, Wang KY, Hwang DS et al. Histamine 2 receptor blocker – ranitidine and sinus mode dysfunction. *Zhonghua Yi Xue Za Zhi* 1997; **60**: 1–5.
153. Nault MA, Milne B, Parlow JL. Effects of the selective H1 and H2 histamine receptor antagonists loretadine and ranitidine on autonomic control of the heart. *Anesthesiology* 2002; **96**: 336–341.
154. Ooie T, Saaikawa T, Hara M et al. H_2-blocker modulates heart rate variability. *Heart Vessels* 1999; **14**: 137–142.
155. Basit AW, Newaton JM, Lacey LF. Susceptibility of the H_2-receptor antagonists cimetidine, famotidine and nizatidine, to metabolism by the gastrointestinal microflora. *Int J Pharm* 2002; **237**: 23–33.
156. Cothran DS, Borowitz SM, Sutphen JL et al. Alteration of normal gastric flora in neonates receiving ranitidine. *J Perinatol* 1997; **17**: 383–388.
157. Messori A, Trippoli S, Vaiani M et al. Bleeding and pneumonia in intensive care patients given ranitidine and sucralfate for prevention of stress ulcer: meta-analysis of randomised controlled trials. *BMJ* 2000; **321**: 1103–1106.
158. Huang JQ, Hunt RH. Pharmacological and pharmacodynamic essentials of H(2)-receptor antagonists and proton

pump inhibitors for the practising physician. *Best Pract Res Clin Gastroenterol* 2001; **15**: 355–370.

159. Londong W, Phillips J, Johnson NJ, Wood JR. The effect of combined therapy with ranitidine and pirenzipine in the treatment of reflux esophagitis. *Aliment Pharmacol Ther* 1992; **6**: 609–618.
160. Vakil NB, Shaker R, Johnson DA et al. The new proton pump inhibitor esomeprazole is effective as a maintenance therapy in GERD patients with healed erosive esophagitis: a 6-month, randomized, double-blind, placebo-controlled study of efficacy and safety. *Aliment Pharmacol Ther* 2001; **15**: 927–935.
161. Jones R, Bytzer P. Acid suppression in the management of gastro-oesophageal reflux disease – an appraisal of treatment options in primary care. *Aliment Pharmacol Ther* 2001; **16**: 765–771.
162. Ferron GM, Preston RA, Noveck RJ et al. Pharmacokinetics of pantoprazole in patients with moderate and severe hepatic dysfunction. *Clin Ther* 2001; **23**: 1180–1192.
163. James LP, Kearns GL. Pharmacokinetics and pharmacodynamics of famotidine in paediatric patients. *Clin Pharmacokinetic* 1996; **31**: 103–110.
164. Scott LJ. Lansoprazole: in the management of gastroesophageal reflux disease in children. *Paediatr Drugs* 2003; **5**: 57–61.
165. Zimmermann AE, Walters JK, Katona BG et al. A review of omeprazole use in the treatment of acid-related disorders in children. *Clin Ther* 2001; **23**: 660-679.
166. Leufkans H, Claessens A, Heerdink E et al. A prospective follow-up study of 5669 users of lansoprazole in daily practice. *Aliment Pharmacol Ther* 1997; **11**: 887–897.
167. Castot A, Bidault I, Dahan R, Efthymiou ML. Evaluation of unexpected and toxic effects of omeprazole A90 – reported to the regional centers of pharmacovigilance during the first 22 postmarketing months. *Therapie* 1993; **48**: 469–474.
168. Berardi RR. A critical evaluation of proton pump inhibitors in the treatment of gastroesophageal reflux disease. *Am J Manag Care* 2000; **6**(9 Suppl): S491–505.
169. Andersson T, Hanssan-alin M, Hasselgren G, Rohss K. Drug interaction studies with esomeprazole, the (S)-isomer of omeprazole. *Clin Pharmacokinet* 2001; **40**: 523–537.
170. ter Heide H, Hendriks HJ, Heijmans H et al. Are children with cystic fibrosis who are treated with a proton-pump inhibitor at risk for vitamin B12 deficiency? *J Pediatr Gastroenterol Nutr* 2001; **33**: 342–345.
171. Singh P, Indaram A, Greenberg R et al. Long term omeprazole therapy for reflux esophagitis: follow-up in serum gastrin levels, EC cell hyperplasia and neoplasia. *World J Gastroenterol* 2000; **6**: 789–792.
172. Nuanton M, Peterson GM, Bleasel MD. Overuse of proton pump inhibitors. *J Clin Pharm Ther* 2000; **25**: 333–338.
173. Amaro R, Montelongo PC, Barkin JS. Sucralfate-induced diarrhea in an enterally fed patient. *Am J Gastroenterol* 1999; **94**: 2328–2329.
174. Guy C, Ollagnier M. Sucralfate and bezoars: data from the system of pharmacologic vigilance and review of the literature. *Therapie* 1999; **54**: 55–58.
175. Hemstreet BA. Use of sucralfate in renal failure. *Ann Pharmacother* 2001; **35**: 360–364.
176. Fleming GF, Vokes EE, McEvilly JM et al. Double-blind, randomized crossover study of metoclopramide and batanopride for prevention of cisplatin-induced emesis. *Cancer Chemother Pharmacol* 1991; **28**: 226–227.
177. Talley NJ, Verlinden M, Snape W et al. Failure of a motilin receptor agonist (ABT-229) to relieve the symptoms of functional dyspepsia in patients with and without delayed gastric emptying: a randomized double-blind placebo-controlled trial. *Aliment Pharmacol Ther* 2000; **14**: 1653–1661.
178. Mahmood Z, McMahon BP, Arfin Q et al. Endocinch therapy for gastro-oesophageal reflux disease: a one year prospective follow up. *Gut* 2003; **52**: 34–39.
179. Wolfsen HC, Richards WO. The Stretta procedure for the treatment of GERD: a registry of 558 patients. *J Laparoendosc Adv Surg Tech A* 2002; **12**: 395–402.
180. Johnson DA, Ganz R, Aisenberg J et al. Endoscopic, deep mural implantation of enteryx for the treatment of GERD: 6-month follow-up of a multicenter trial. *Am J Gastroenterol* 2003; **98**: 250–258.
181. Galmiche JP, Bruley des Varannes S. Endoluminal therapies for gastro-oesophageal reflux disease. *Lancet* 2003; **361**: 1119–1121.
182. Fonkalsrud EX, Bustorff-Silva J, Perez CA et al. Antireflux surgery in children under three months of age. *J Pediatr Surg* 1999; **34**: 527–531.
183. Pearl RH, Robie DK, Ein SH et al. Complications of gastroesophageal reflux surgery in neurologically impaired versus neurologically normal children. *J Pediatr Surg* 1990; **25**: 1169–1173.
184. Alexander F, Wyllie R, Jirousek K et al. Delayed gastric emptying affects outcome of Nissen fundoplication in neurologically impaired children. *Surgery* 1997; **122**: 690–697.
185. Spitz L, Roth K, Kiely EM et al. Operation for gastro-oesophageal reflux associated with severe mental retardation. *Arch Dis Child* 1993; **68**: 347–351.
186. Booth MI, Jones L, Stratford J, Dehn TC. Results of laparoscopic Nissen fundoplication 8 years after surgery. *Br J Surg* 2002; **89**: 476–481.
187. Bergmeijer JH, Harbers JS, Molenaar JC. Function of pediatric Nissen–Rosetti fundoplication followed up into adolescence and adulthood. *J Am Coll Surg* 1997; **184**: 259-261.
188. Burd RS, Price MR, Whalen TV. The role of protective antireflux procedures in neurologically impaired children: a decision analysis. *J Pediatr Surg* 2002; **37**: 500-506.

5 Achalasia

Carl-Christian A Jackson and Donald C Liu

Introduction

Diseases of the esophagus can generally be categorized into four types of abnormality: those of inadequate lower esophageal relaxation; those of uncoordinated contraction; those of hypercontraction; and those of hypocontraction.[1] Classic achalasia falls into this first category. Directly translated, achalasia means 'failure to relax', and describes a rare disease in which the lower esophageal sphincter (LES) remains constricted during swallowing and there is an absence of esophageal peristalsis. The first case of achalasia was reported in 1674 by Thomas Willis.[2] His patient was otherwise healthy, but suffered from frequent vomiting and regurgitation of food. Successful palliation was achieved through postprandial passage of a whalebone with a sponge attached to the tip, which accomplished both tamping of the food through the LES, as well as some degree of forceful dilatation. However, it was Sir Cooper Perry in 1913 who first used the term 'achalasia' to describe this disease.[3–5]

The exact etiology of achalasia is unknown, but certain factors remain consistent, namely inflammation of the myenteric plexuses with varying degrees of ganglion cell loss. When symptomatology suggests achalasia, the diagnosis is confirmed through radiographic and manometric studies. In treating children with achalasia, numerous modalities have been employed with varying degrees of success, including drug treatment, forceful dilatation and surgical esophagomyotomy. The purpose of this chapter is to provide an overview of this disease process, the tools with which to diagnose it and the available treatment options.

Epidemiology

Epidemiological studies of achalasia have been relatively few. A summary of the available investigations, which include both adults and children, shows an incidence of $0.4–1.2/10^5$ persons/year in Europe and North America.[6–11] The incidence in children is far lower. Approximately 4–5% of all cases of achalasia are diagnosed before the age of 15. More so than the adult form, childhood achalasia can occur with associated abnormalities, such as familial glucocorticoid deficiency, alacrima, autonomic system disorder, short stature, microcephaly and nerve deafness.[12–16] Contrary to the generally accepted view of a female predominance, achalasia actually appears to affect men and women equally.[17,18] Studies that exhibit higher rates in females, when adjusted for their higher population of women, show that the incidence of achalasia approaches that expected in the general population.[6,9]

Etiology

The etiology of achalasia remains uncertain. Proposed mechanisms for the disease include genetics, infectious agents, autoimmune destruction, and primary neural degeneration. Various case reports have identified instances of both horizontal and vertical 'transmission'.[19–24] The majority of these familial cases, however, occur in the setting of consanguinity. While this raises the possibility of a rare, recessive gene being expressed, a large-scale study of more than 1000 first-degree relatives of patients with achalasia showed no affected relatives – contrary to expected Mendelian genetics.[25]

Five per cent of patients with chronic Chagas' disease develop poor LES relaxation and mega-esophagus that mimics classic achalasia,[26] which suggests that an infectious etiology of achalasia is possible. The protozoan *Trypanosoma cruzi* which causes Chagas' disease acts through direct invasion of cells, toxin production or antigenic factors to cause degeneration of esophageal neurons. The mechanism of this process is also uncertain, and may be from direct injury to neurons of the esophagus, an inflammatory reaction or the generation of autoantibodies against these nerves.[27] Potential infectious candidates for idiopathic achalasia include measles and varicella viruses, but as yet no firm evidence exists to confirm this association.[25,28–31]

Pathology

While the etiology of achalasia remains unclear, the histopathological changes associated with it have been well described. Surgical specimens involving strips of esophageal muscle from esophagomyotomy or entire resected esophagi have formed the basis of study.[32–35] Gross examination of esophagectomy specimens from patients with severe/recurrent achalasia reveals the classic morphology of a dilated proximal esophagus, with distal tapering. The muscularis propria is frequently hypertrophied, and the mucosa exhibits exaggerated longitudinal folds.[32]

Upon microscopic examination, there is a range of associated changes in the esophagus. The most classic feature is an absence of myenteric ganglion cells, which is seen in specimens from patients with both early and late achalasia.[32,34–38] While there is no apparent association between the number of remaining ganglion cells and the degree of symptoms, there does seem to be a temporal relationship, i.e. patients with longstanding disease tend to exhibit fewer ganglion cells.[34,38] The most consistent histological feature, seen in all esophageal specimens, is inflammation.[32,35] The inflammation occurs in and around the myenteric nerves, predominantly involves lymphocytes and results in neural fibrosis. Goldblum et al made an interesting observation in their study of patients with early achalasia.[35] A woman with rapid onset of dysphagia and weight loss underwent esophagomyotomy only 2.5 months after the onset of symptoms. Histological examination was significant for mild myenteric inflammation, normal numbers of ganglion cells and an absence of fibrosis. These findings suggest that the earliest pathological feature of achalasia is myenteric inflammation.

Additional histological changes result from esophageal obstruction and the associated stasis. Esophageal obstruction leads to varying degrees of muscular hypertrophy of the muscularis propria, most notably in the inner circular layer.[32,36,39] Further findings include small leiomyomas of the inner circular layer, degenerative changes of the muscularis propria as well as focal fibrosis of the muscularis propria (again, predominantly in the inner circular layer).[32] Stasis of luminal contents results in both proximal and distal squamous hyperplasia, as well as changes similar to those seen in reflux esophagitis, namely papillomatosis and basal cell hyperplasia.[32] However, owing to the increased LES pressure limiting passage of gastric contents, these findings are unlikely to be due to true gastroesophageal reflux.

Extra-esophageal pathology accompanies achalasia, predominantly related to esophageal innervation. Both the vagus nerve and the vagal dorsal motor nucleus are affected. Electron microscopy of periesophageal vagal nerve biopsies reveals changes resembling Wallerian degeneration (i.e. secondary to nerve transaction), changes that are not seen on light microscopy.[33,38] Whether the affected nerves are motor, sensory or vagal-associated sympathetic nerves is unclear. Evaluation of the dorsal motor nucleus of the vagus, performed upon autopsy, also reveals degenerative changes, neuron loss and Lewy bodies.[40]

Pathophysiology

The resting state of the LES is one of contraction. Cholinergic neurons provide resting tone, whereas inhibitory neurons provide vagal-mediated relaxation[34,41,42] Vagal efferents contain both excitatory and inhibitory signals; however, the predominant effect of vagal stimulation is LES relaxation, as mediated by non-adrenergic, non-cholinergic (NANC) nerves.[43] In normal patients, stimuli from gastric, esophageal and pharyngeal sensory nerves are relayed to, and processed by, the dorsal motor nucleus of the vagus, which results in modulation of both excitatory and inhibitory impulses to the LES.[44]

Two strong candidates for mediation of LES relaxation are vasoactive intestinal polypeptide (VIP) and nitric oxide (NO). After it was realized that VIP was found in high concentrations in gut sphincters, subsequent investigations showed it to be a potent inhibitor of LES contraction *in vitro*.[45,46] Further association of VIP with sphincteric relaxation and achalasia is suggested by immunohistochemical studies that have shown decreased or absent VIP-containing neurons in LES specimens from patients with achalasia.[47–49] Human manometric studies have shown that the LES in patients with achalasia, as compared to normal controls, is hypersensitive to exogenous VIP, again supporting a role for VIP in LES relaxation.[44]

NO also figures prominently in gastrointestinal tract smooth muscle and sphincteric mechanisms.[50–57] The role of NO appears to be that of sphincter-muscle hyperpolarization, and therefore relaxation, and the loss of NO has been associated with conditions of persistent contraction, such as achalasia.[58–62] Preiksaitis et al elegantly demonstrated that blocking NO synthase prevents relaxation of LES muscles by NANC nerves, and that exogenous NO from sodium nitroprusside can overcome this inhibition.[57] Inhibitory regulation of gastrointestinal muscles by NANC transmitters was generally believed to be direct, until an intermediary, interstitial cell was proposed by Cajal (a cell that bears his name).[63] Recent work in both animal and human models confirms the relationship of interstitial cells of Cajal (ICC) to nitric oxide synthase (NOS)-positive neurons.[53,64] It is accepted that NO release results in sphincteric relaxation; however, the exact mechanism has not been fully elucidated. While evaluation of the LES in adults shows that ICC are altered, this may be a result of disruption of the interaction between NOS-positive neurons and ICC, because examination of the pediatric esophagus in achalasia (and therefore a shorter duration of disease) shows morphologically normal ICC, but disrupted contact with NOS-positive neurons.[53,54]

The precise cause of achalasia remains to be elucidated but the loss of NO- and/or VIP-associated neurons appears to be integral to the disease. By their destruction, these neurons permit unopposed contraction of the LES.

Signs and symptoms

Because the incidence of achalasia in children is so low, the majority of information regarding the diagnosis comes from adults. The earliest, and most common, symptom of achalasia is dysphagia. This dysphagia initially is for solids, but frequently progresses to dysphagia for liquids by the time treatment is sought.[65–67] The next most common symptom in adults is regurgitation, which is non-acidic and non-bilious, owing to the contracted LES, and most often occurs right after eating or during sleep. Patients often find ways to accommodate these dysfunctions, and will ameliorate symptoms by such methods as drinking large volumes of water with meals, holding their arms above the head or performing a Valsalva maneuver.[67–69] A summary of the most common presenting symptoms is provided in Table 5.1.

Table 5.1 Symptoms of achalasia (from reference 67)

Symptoms	Number of patients	Mean (%)	Mean range (%)
Dysphagia	1930	97	82–100
Regurgitation	1892	75	56–97
Weight loss	1675	58	30–91
Chest pain	1894	43	17–95
Heartburn	127	36	27–42
Cough	732	30	11–46

The presenting symptoms in children tend to correlate with patient age and can mimic those seen in adults, or they can be more vague, thus requiring a high degree of suspicion for diagnosis. Symptoms in older children (more than 7 years) tend to parallel those seen in adults, so dysphagia and regurgitation predominate, but with substernal chest pain and burning also appearing in about half the patients.[70] Children aged less than 6 years, particularly infants, more commonly present with respiratory symptoms, complaints, similar to those of gastroesophageal reflux disease (GERD), occasional emesis and failure to thrive.[12,71] Regurgitation and dysphagia are the most common symptoms, present in 83% and 71–80% of patients, respectively, followed by failure to thrive in 54–70%.[70,72] Especially in non-verbal children, a diagnosis of achalasia should be entertained when presented with a patient experiencing significant chronic respiratory symptoms, such as choking, recurrent pneumonia, severe asthma, chronic bronchitis or chronic cough, because these are seen in 25–100% of patients.[12,70] The physical examination tends to be unremarkable, but can reveal findings secondary to dysphagia (and a resultant decrease in oral intake) and food stasis, such as weight loss, malnutrition and halitosis.[67]

Laboratory and instrumental investigations

Radiographic studies

For patients in whom a diagnosis is uncertain, a plain chest radiograph may be the first available study. The classically described finding on upright chest X-ray is an absent gastric air-bubble. This finding, present in nearly all normal individuals, is absent in approximately half of patients with achalasia.[73,74] Additional findings include a widened mediastinum from esophageal dilatation, a posterior mediastinal air–fluid level from retained food/secretions and lung parenchymal abnormalities from chronic aspiration.[67,73,75]

Barium swallow, however, is the definitive radiographic study, and, in a review of the European experience with achalasia, it is the most commonly performed test.[76] On barium swallow, classic achalasia typically shows esophageal dilatation with distal narrowing at the gastroesophageal (GE) junction, the 'bird's beak' deformity (Figure 5.1). Also, retained food/secretions, absent peristalsis, tortuosity of the esophagus and, occasionally, an epiphrenic diverticulum can be seen.[67,73,75] Because a barium swallow is performed under fluoroscopy it is a dynamic study, and may also reveal back-and-forth sloshing of the barium boluses when the patient is in the supine position, owing to the esophageal dilatation and the ineffective peristalsis.[67,75,77] However, the diagnostic accuracy of barium swallow is approximately 85%, which can be due to a very early stage

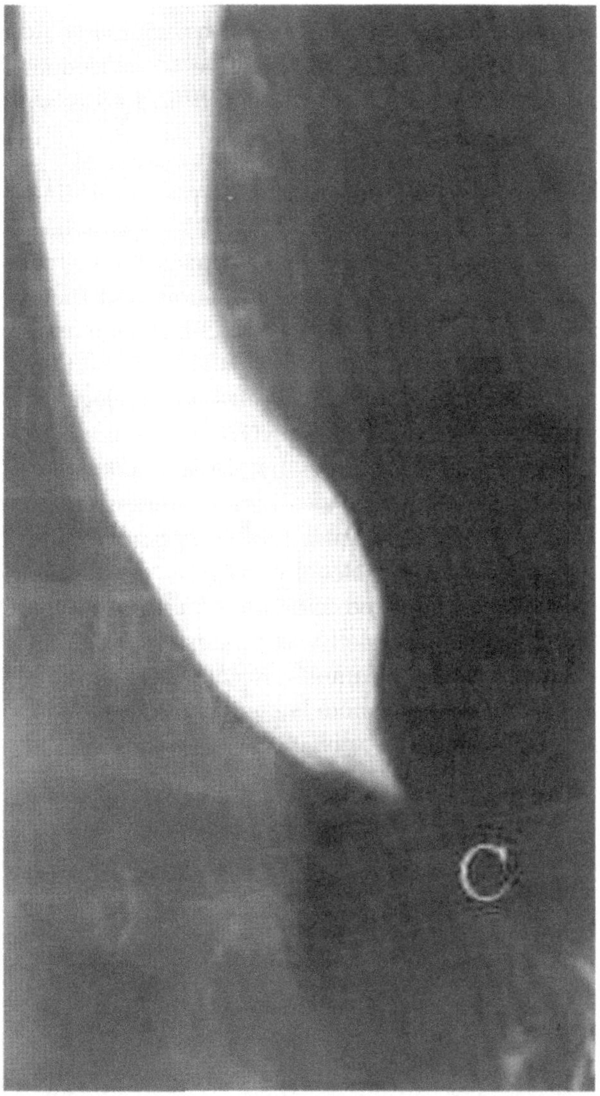

Figure 5.1 'Bird's beak' appearance characteristic of esophageal achalasia on esophogram (courtesy of Hans Björknäs, Gastrolabs, Finland).

of achalasia not showing the classic signs, due to a tumor of the GE junction mimicking achalasia or due to a peptic stricture.[67,73,76]

Computed tomography (CT) has no real role in the diagnosis of achalasia.[67] The findings are consistent with those already seen on plain X-ray or barium swallow, such as a dilated esophagus, esophageal air–fluid levels, and possibly displacement of mediastinal structures by a dilated esophagus. Furthermore, masses that may cause pseudoachalasia are infrequently identified on a CT scan.[78,79]

With the desire to limit radiation exposure, particularly in children, alternative means of diagnosis are sought. Radionuclide bolus transport has been evaluated as one such alternative, with achalasia diagnosed when esophageal emptying time is prolonged. When evaluating patients with manometrically diagnosed achalasia using radionuclide transport, Stacher et al found that sensitivity for this evaluation was 68%, with a specificity of 95%.[80] Their criteria were an esophageal emptying time of ≥ 20 s (the time for 95% of the bolus to enter the stomach), compared to a normal median time of 7.3 s (range 5.5–12.0 s). Because radionuclide bolus transport is a functional study with relatively low sensitivity (other esophageal motility disorders also show prolonged transit time), this study may be best suited for follow-up of patients after treatment, or in the few cases in which achalasia is suspected, despite normal LES pressure on manometry.[67,73,80]

Manometry

The gold standard for accurate diagnosis of achalasia remains esophageal manometry, using either a perfused-catheter or a solid-state system. The minimum information collected from manometry will include resting LES pressure, relaxed LES pressure and peristaltic function of the esophageal body. Depending on local protocol, upper esophageal sphincter (UES) pressure may also be assessed. Fluoroscopy may be used to assist in positioning of the sensors. Manometry is usually performed with a catheter containing multiple, evenly spaced sensors, which is passed by the oral or nasal route into the stomach. Resting gastric pressures are measured to provide a baseline. The catheter is slowly withdrawn until the sensor is measuring LES pressure. Under quiet respirations, resting LES pressure is measured at mid-respiration. Swallow-induced LES relaxation is measured with the patient taking several wet swallows using small volumes of liquid. The catheter is further withdrawn until the distal sensor is a few centimeters above the LES and the proximal sensors are spaced throughout the esophageal body. Esophageal peristalsis and wave progression are assessed during several more wet swallows.

Because achalasia affects the smooth muscles of the esophagus, the manometric findings involve the mid- and distal esophagus, sparing the proximal regions of predominantly striated muscle. The two manometric abnormalities found in all patients with achalasia are aperistalsis of the esophageal body and abnormal LES relaxation.[1,67–69] Simultaneous, low-amplitude contractions (< 40 mmHg) throughout the esophageal body are characteristic of the aperistalsis seen after wet swallows. Abnormal LES relaxation is characterized by either absent/incomplete relaxation (70–80% of patients) or normal relaxation of short, and therefore ineffective, duration – typically less than 6 s each (20–30% of patients).[69, 81] This latter finding commonly accompanies early stage achalasia.[68] Manometric findings associated with achalasia, but not required for diagnosis, include elevated resting LES pressure and resting esophageal body pressure exceeding baseline gastric pressure.[1] Table 5.2 summarizes normal and abnormal manometric findings.

Endoscopy

Despite radiographic and manometric evidence typical of achalasia, pseudoachalasia secondary to a tumor at the GE junction must be ruled out.[67,73] Findings consistent with achalasia may include a dilated, atonic esophageal body; mucosal thickening and/or erythema; and a puckered LES which fails to open with insufflation, but which is easily passed with the endoscope. If there is visual evidence of extrinsic compression or the endoscope fails to pass through the GE junction with gentle pressure, then a tumor must be excluded. Biopsies should be taken from suspicious areas seen above the GE junction or seen on retroflexion from within the stomach.

Table 5.2 Normal and abnormal manometric findings (from references 1, 67 and 68)

	Basal LES pressure	Swallow-induced LES relaxation	Peristaltic wave progression	Distal wave amplitude
Normal	10–45 mmHg	complete (less than 8 mmHg above gastric baseline, or 95% of LES baseline)	2–8 cm/s from UES to LES	30–180 mmHg
Achalasia	>45 mmHg (up to 40% of patients have normal values)	incomplete (more than 8 mmHg above gastric baseline, or 35% of LES baseline) Complete but of short duration (<6 s)	simultaneous	<40 mmHg

LES, lower esophageal sphincter; UES, upper esophageal sphincter

Treatment

Until such time as the primary cause of achalasia can be reversed, namely the loss of esophageal innervation by inhibitory neurons, treatment of achalasia must address the relief of symptoms. Since the primary disorders are aperistalsis and abnormal LES relaxation, the goal of non-invasive and invasive treatments is relief of the obstruction and its associated dysphagia. Medical treatment focuses on promoting LES relaxation, whereas endoscopic and surgical treatments address disruption of the LES muscle itself.

Medical options

Medical treatments have targeted improving LES relaxation through the use of anticholinergics, calcium channel blockers and nitrates. Anticholinergics were among the first drugs studied, but these generally showed no benefit.[82–84] Of the calcium channel blockers, nifedipine has shown the most promise.[85] A nifedipine dose of 10–30 mg prior to meals results in statistically significant decreases in mean LES pressure, as shown in a randomized, blinded trial by Traube et al.[86] Despite these statistically significant changes, nifedipine-lowered resting LES pressure remains sufficiently elevated for subjective symptoms to persist; furthermore, radionuclide transit studies fail to show significant improvement.[85,86] The side-effect profile of nifedipine includes peripheral edema, headache, flushing and hypotension, which are seen relatively frequently during chronic treatment.[82]

Nitrates have also been tried, given the role NO seems to play in the disease process. Administered sublingually prior to a meal, isosorbide dinitrate (a long-acting version of nitroglycerin) will reduce mean LES pressure for approximately 60 min.[87] A randomized, crossover trial evaluating sublingual isosorbide dinitrate and nifedipine showed both better subjective improvement and improved LES relaxation in the nitrate group versus the nifedipine group. However, side-effects (such as headache and hypotension) were greater, and radionuclide transport did not confirm improvement in four of eight patients reporting decreased symptoms.[88] Therefore, medical treatment does seem to offer some subjective benefit to a subset of patients, but at a cost of significant side-effects, and a general progression of the disease in up to 50% of patients.[82] The application of medical treatment seems relegated to those patients who are unwilling or medically unable to undergo more definitive treatment, or as a bridging measure until definitive treatment can be performed.[67,73,82,85,86]

Surgical options

The gold standard in treatment of achalasia is surgical esophagomyotomy – the modified Heller procedure. It is against this procedure that other surgical, and medical, treatments are compared. Surgical treatments include endoscopy with botulinum toxin injection, forceful dilatation, open Heller myotomy and laparoscopic Heller myotomy.

Endoscopic botulinum toxin injection

With endoscopy playing an important role in the work-up of achalasia, it seems attractive to initiate therapy concurrently. Botulinum toxin (BoTox) is a potent inhibitor of presynaptic acetylcholine release, and can be injected into the LES through an endoscope. After a pilot study had demonstrated efficacy, Pasricha et al undertook a randomized, blinded and controlled study of BoTox.[89] This study showed significant decreases in symptom scores, resting LES pressure and esophageal food retention. Approximately half of the injected patients, however, had no response or relapsed within 2 months of initial treatment and required either repeat injection or pneumatic dilatation. Subsequent studies in adults have shown that BoTox generally provides good initial results, but these improvements typically are not long-lasting.[90–92] Follow-up showed that 10–35% of patients had no initial response, 30–40% relapsed within 4 months, and 38–67% had 'lasting' effects to an average of 1.3–2.5 years.[90–92]

An initial experience with BoTox in an 11-year-old child showed encouraging initial results, with repeat injection required 1 year after initial therapy.[93] Two recent studies have evaluated the role of BoTox in a series of children.[94,95] In both, the mean duration of symptomatic relief was short-lived (3–7 months) and required repeat injections or eventual Heller myotomy. Among the limited patients who did not progress to surgical treatment, a few showed lasting benefit over several years, and some opted for frequent repeated injections rather than undergoing surgery. While BoTox is generally considered safe, complications such as gastroesophageal reflux, esophageal inflammation and ulceration with hemorrhage have been noted.[96] The consensus at this time relegates BoTox injection to patients who are unwilling or medically unsuitable for more invasive correction, or as a subsequent adjunct to patients who are symptomatic after myotomy or dilatation.[67, 90,91,94,95]

Esophageal dilatation

In contrast to the above-described treatments, esophageal dilatation addresses achalasia through forceful disruption of the LES muscle fibers. The largest experience with dilatation has been in adults, and current therapy involves the use of balloon dilators. The balloons are placed across the LES, rapidly inflated and then deflated after a period of 30 s to several minutes, depending on patient tolerance. As the procedure is performed under fluoroscopy, the dilatations are repeated until the waist of the LES is obliterated by the balloon. 'Excellent' to 'good' results, based on patient survey, are obtained in 65–93% of patients (this higher number was based on pooling results from multiple, graded dilatations).[82,97–99] With long-term follow-up, trends were seen in patients who either failed initial treatment or quickly relapsed, with the most significant in younger age (under 45 years).[73,100] While dilatation is relatively safe, early and late complications do occur. The most significant early complication is perforation (0–12%), which if recognized early can be treated conservatively with good effect.[73,82,101]

One of the major benefits of esophageal dilatations in adults is avoidance of general anesthesia, which is generally lost when treating children, making it a less attractive option. Despite showing some degree of success in a small series,[102] the typical experience is poor long-term response requiring frequent re-dilatation, and eventually surgery, particularly in younger children.[71,95,99,103] This requirement for multiple dilatations in children, as well as the need for monitored general anesthesia, also decrease the proposed benefit of lower hospital costs.[104] Given these results, balloon dilatation plays a minimal role in the treatment of children with achalasia. Balloon dilatation should be reserved for patients unwilling to undergo surgery, or as a treatment adjunct in patients with residual symptoms after surgery.

Esophagomyotomy

Surgical esophagomyotomy for achalasia was first performed in Germany by Ernest Heller, and involved a laparotomy with both an anterior and a posterior esophagomyotomy.[105] The procedure was modified by Zaaijer in 1923 to utilize only an anterior esophagomyotomy;[106] all surgery for achalasia now employs a variant of this procedure.[107] An example of the affected esophageal segment pre- and post-myotomy is shown in Figure 5.2. A consensus on the optimal surgical technique remains to be resolved. Traditional approaches have been through a standard midline laparotomy or a left thoracotomy, with equally good results.[108–111] A review of the literature by Ferguson showed that, regardless of operative approach, an open Heller procedure resulted in symptomatic improvement in 89% of patients, a mortality rate of 0.3%, a reoperative rate of 2.9% and a postoperative GERD incidence of 10%.[73]

The benefits of minimally invasive surgery, decreased pain, shorter hospital stay, and improved cosmesis have prompted surgeons to apply this approach to esophagomyotomy. As with open surgery, both thoracoscopic and laparoscopic approaches are in current use, and by nature of similar results to the open surgery, minimally invasive procedures are becoming the standard.[112–118] In addition to controversy over whether an abdominal or thoracic approach is better, there is no

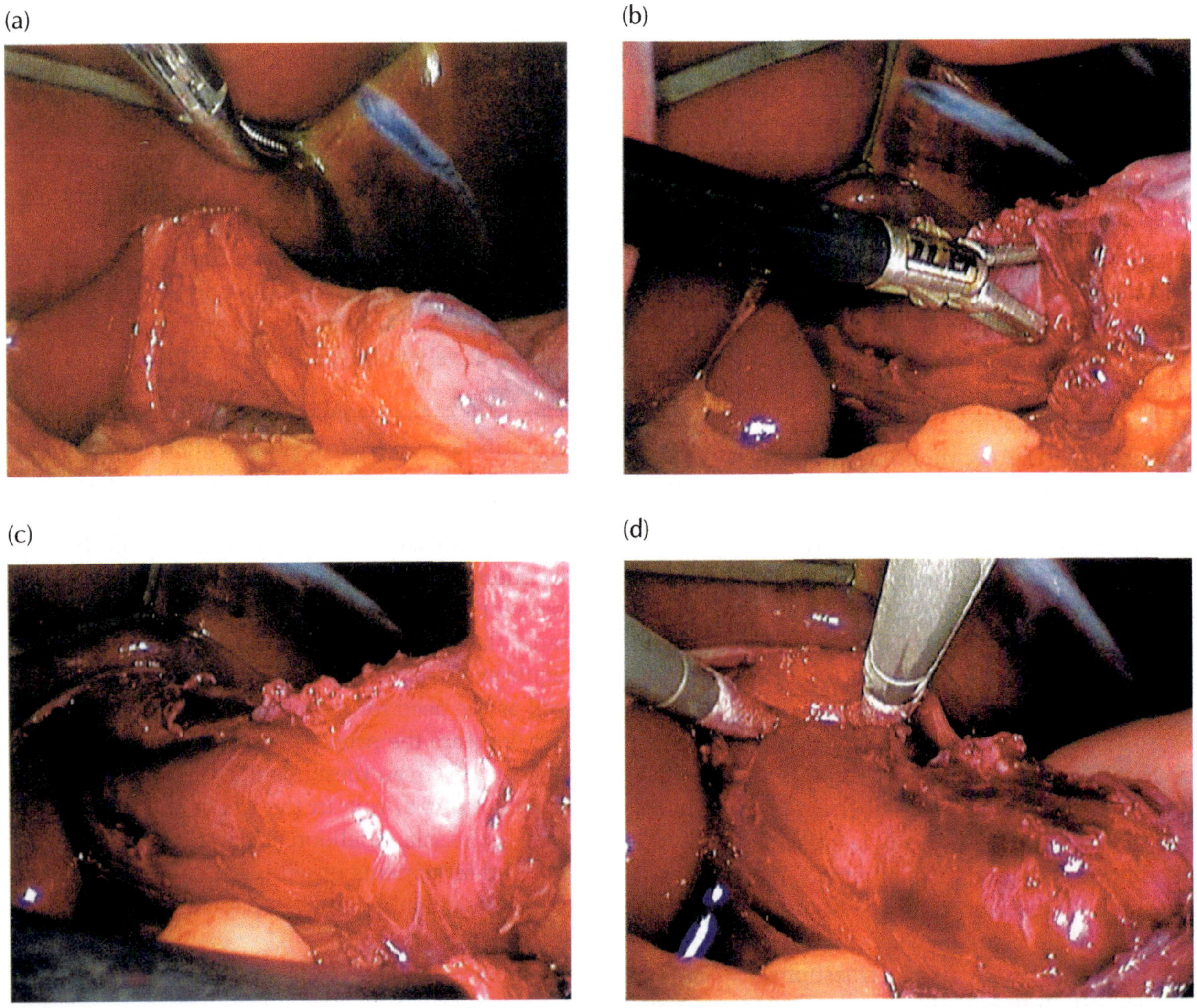

Figure 5.2 (a) Transition between dilated (normal) and narrowed (abnormal) segment of esophageal achalasia prior to myotomy. (b) Performing myotomy with an endoscopic spreader. (c) Myotomy completed to the gastroesophageal junction. (d) Completed myotomy including dissection onto the lesser curvature of the stomach (circularis muscle seen distally).

consensus on the benefit of performing a simultaneous fundoplication. For example, at our institution we do not routinely perform concomitant fundoplication. Proponents of a fundoplication cite increased risk of late GERD, whereas opponents state that limiting the gastric portion of the esophagomyotomy to less than 1 cm limits the incidence of GERD and that a fundoplication may actually result in pseudoachalasia from making an over-tight wrap.[73,119–124]

The complications of Heller myotomy include intraoperative perforation (treated by over-sewing the tear, and buttressing with gastric fundus), recurrence of symptoms (typically the result of incomplete myotomy or addition of a fundoplication that is too tight) and esophageal leak.[67,70,109,125] Concern exists about performing a Heller myotomy after previous non-surgical therapies, as this may incur a higher complication rate. While previous treatment by balloon dilatations or BoTox injection seems to result in scar formation,[126] it does not seem to affect subsequent esophagomyotomy.[127,128]

Conclusion

Achalasia presents a diagnostic challenge in children, given the varied presentations. High clinical suspicion is necessary, particularly when treating infants and young children. The mainstays of diagnosis are barium swallow and manometry, each with findings highly suggestive of achalasia. Once the diagnosis is made, the most efficacious treatment is surgical esophagomyotomy. As the operative experience in children progresses, laparoscopic Heller myotomy emerges as the surgical treatment of choice, with or without an added fundoplication. Balloon dilatation or BoTox injection should be reserved for addressing postoperative recurrence of dysphagia. Medical treatment with calcium channel blockers currently has only very limited application in children.

REFERENCES

1. Spechler SJ, Castell DO. Classification of oesophageal motility abnormalities. *Gut* 2001; **49**: 145–151.
2. Willis T. Pharmaceutice Rationalis sive Diatriba do Medicamentorum Operationibus in Humano Corpore. London: Hagae Comitis, 1674.
3. Hertz AF. The bismuth meal. *BMJ* 1913; **1**: 13.
4. Hertz AF. Achalasia of the cardia. *Q J Med* 1916; **8**: 300–308.
5. Mayberry JF, Probert CSJ, Sher KS et al. Some epidemiological and aetiological aspects of achalasia. *Dig Dis* 1991; **9**: 1–8.
6. Erlam RJ, Ellis FH, Nobrega FT. Achalasia of the esophagus in a small urban community. *Mayo Clin Proc* 1960; **44**: 478–483.
7. Galen EA, Switz M, Zfass AM. Achalasia: incidence and treatment in Virginia. *Va Med* 1982; **109**: 183–186.
8. Mayberry JF, Rhodes J. Achalasia in the city of Cardiff from 1926 to 1977. *Digestion* 1980; **20**: 248–252.
9. Mayberry JF, Atkinson M. Studies of incidence and prevalence of achalasia in the Nottingham area. *Q J Med* 1985; **56**: 451–456.
10. Mayberry JF, Atkinson M. Variations in the prevalence of achalasia over a decade in Great Britain and Ireland: an epidemiological study based on hospital admissions. *Q J Med* 1987; **62**: 67–74.
11. Mayberry JF, Mayall M. The epidemiology of achalsia in children. *Gut* 1988; **29**: 90–93.
12. Nihoul-Fekete C, Bawab F, Lortat-Jacob S et al. Achalasia of the esophagus in childhood. Surgical treatment in 35 cases, with special reference to familial cases and glucocorticoid deficiency association. *Hepatogastroenterol* 1991; **38**: 510–513.
13. Allgrove J, Clayden GS, Grant DB et al. Familial glucocorticoid deficiency with achalasia of the cardia and deficient tear production, *Lancet* 1978 **26**: 1284–1286.
14. Ehrich E, Aranoff G, Johnson WG. Familial achalasia associated with adrenocortical insufficiency, alacrima and neurologic abnormalities. *Am J Med Genet* 1987; **26**: 637–644.
15. Stuckey BG, Mastaglia FL, Reed WD et al. Glucocorticoid insuffiency, achalasia, alacrima with autonomic and motor neuropathy, *Ann Intern Med* 1987; **106**: 62–64.
16. El-Rayyes K, Hegab S, Besisso M. A syndrome of alacrima, achalasia and neurologic anomalies without adrenocortical insufficiency. *J Pediatr Ophthalmol Strabismus* 1991; **28**: 35–37.
17. Arber N, Grossman A, Lurie B et al. Epidemiology of achalasia in central Israel. Rarity of esophageal cancer. *Dig Dis Sci* 1993; **38**: 1920–1925.
18. Sonnenberg A, Massey BT, McCarty DJ et al. Epidemiology of hospitalization for achalasia in the United States. *Dig Dis Sci* 1993; **38**: 233–244.

19. Zimmerman FH, Rosenweig NS. Achalasia in a father and son. *Am J Gastroenterol* 1984; **79**: 506–508.
20. Bosher LP, Shaw A. Achalasia in siblings. Clinical and genetic aspects. *Am J Dis Child* 1981; **135**: 709–710.
21. Murphy MS, Gardner-Medwin D, Eastham EJ. Achalasia of the cardia associated with hereditary cerebellar ataxia. *Am J Gastroenterol* 1989; **84**: 1329–1330.
22. Chawla K, Chawla SK, Alexander LL. Familial achalasia of the esophagus in mother and son: a possible pathogenetic relationship. *J Am Geriatr Soc* 1979; **27**: 519–521.
23. Kilpatrick ZM, Milles S. Achalasia in mother and daughter. *Gastroenterology* 1972; **62**: 1042–1046.
24. Mackler D, Schneider R. Achalasia in father and son. *Dig Dis Sci* 1978; **23**: 1042–1045.
25. Mayberry JF, Atkinson M. A study of swallowing difficulties in first degree relatives of patients with achalasia. *Thorax* 1985; **40**: 391–393.
26. Pinotti HW, Felix VN, Zilberstein B et al. Surgical complications of Chagas' disease: megaesophagus, achalasia of the pylorus and cholelithiasis. *World J Surg* 1991; **15**: 198–204.
27. Kirchoff LV. *Trypanosoma* species (American trypanosomiasis, Chagas' disease): biology of trypanosomes. In Mandell GL, Bennett JE, Dolin R eds. In *Principles and Practice of Infectious Diseases*, 5th edn. Philadelphia: Churchill Livingstone, 2000: 2845-2851.
28. Robertson CS, Martin BA, Atkinson M. Varicella-zoster virus DNA in the oesophageal myenteric plexus in achalasia. *Gut* 1993; **34**: 299–302.
29. Jones DB, Mayberry JF, Rhodes J et al. Preliminary report of an association between measles virus and achalasia. *J Clin Pathol* 1983; **36**: 655–657.
30. Castex F, Guillemot F, Talbodec N et al. Association of an attack of varicella and achalasia. *Am J Gastroenterol* 1995; **90**: 1188–1189.
31. Niwatomto H, Okamoto E, Fujimoto J et al. Are human herpes viruses or measles virus associated with esophageal achalasia? *Dig Dis Sci* 1995; **40**: 859–864.
32. Goldblum JR, Whyte RI, Orringer MB et al. Achalasia: a morphologic study of 42 resected specimens. *Am J Surg Pathol* 1994; **18**: 327–337.
33. Cassella RR, Ellis FH, Brown AL. Fine-structure changes in achalasia of the esophagus. I: Vagus nerves. *Am J Pathol* 1965; **46**: 279–283.
34. Csendes A, Smok G, Braghetto I et al. Gastroesophageal sphincter pressure and histological changes in distal esophagus in patients with achalasia of the esophagus. *Dig Dis Sci* 1985; **30**: 941–945.
35. Goldblum JR, Rice TW, Richter JE. Histopathologic features in esophagomyotomy specimens from patients with achalasia. *Gastroenterology* 1996; **111**: 648–654.
36. Rake GW. A case of annular muscular hypertrophy of the esophagus. *Guy's Hosp Rep* 1926; **76**: 145–158.
37. Cross FS. Pathologic changes in megaesophagus (esophageal dystonia). *Surgery* 1952; **31**: 647–653.
38. Cassella RR, Brown AL, Sayre GP et al. Achalasia of the esophagus: pathologic and etiologic considerations. *Ann Surg* 1964; **160**: 474–487.
39 Cassella RR, Ellis FH, Brown AL. Fine-structure changes in achalasia of the esophagus. II: Esophageal smooth muscle. *Am J Pathol* 1965; **46**: 467–475.
40. Qualman SJ, Haupt HM, Yang P et al. Esophageal Lewy bodies associated with ganglion cell loss in achalasia. Similarity to Parkinson's disease. *Gastroenterology* 1984; **87**: 848–856.
41. Holloway RH, Dodds WJ, Helm JF et al. Integrity of cholinergic innervation to the lower esophageal sphincter in achalasia. *Gastroenterology* 1986; **90**: 924–929.
42. Goyal RK, Rattan S. Nature of the vagal inhibitory innervation to the lower esophageal sphincter. *J Clin Invest* 1975; **55**: 1119–1126.
43. Yuan C, Costa M, Brookes SJH. Neuronal pathways and transmission to the lower esophageal sphincter of the guinea pig. *Gastroenterology* 1998; **118**: 661–668.
44. Hornby PJ, Abrahams TP. Central control of lower esophageal sphincter relaxation. *Am J Med* 2000; **108**: 90S–98S.
45. Alumets J, Schaffalitzky De Muckadell O, Fahrenkrug J et al. A rich VIP nerve supply is characteristic of sphincters. *Nature* 1979; **280**: 155–156.
46. Goyal RK, Rattan S, Said SI. VIP as a possible neurotransmitter of non-cholinergic non-adrenergic inhibitory neurons. *Nature* 1980; **288**: 378–380.
47. Aggestrup S, Uddman R, Sundler F et al. Lack of vasoactive intestinal peptide nerves in esophageal achalasia. *Gastroenterology* 1983; **84**: 924–927.
48. Guelrud M, Rossiter A, Sourney PF et al. The effect of vasoactive intestinal polypeptide on the lower esophageal sphincter in achalasia. *Gastroenterology* 1992; **103**: 377–382.
49. Rattan S, Said SI, Goyal RK. Effect of vasoactive intestinal polypeptide on lower esophageal sphincter pressure. *Proc Soc Exp Bio Med* 1977; **155**: 40–43.
50. Aimi Y, Kimura H, Kinoshita T et al. Histochemical localization of nitric oxide synthase in rat enteric nervous system, *Neuroscience* 1993; **53**: 553–560.
51. Furness JB, Li ZS, Young HM et al. Nitric oxide synthase in the enteric nervous system of the guinea pig: a quantitative description. *Cell Tissue Res* 1994; **277**: 139–149.
52. Ward SM, Xue C, Sanders KM. Localization of nitric oxide synthase immunoreactivity in ileocolonic and pyloric sphincters. *Cell Tissue Res* 1994; **275**: 513–527.
53. Singaram C, Sengupta A, Sweet MA et al. Nitrinergic and peptidergic innervation of the human oesophagus. *Gut* 1994; **35**: 1690–1696.
54. Christensen J, Fang S, Rick GA. NADPH-diaphorase-positive nerve fibers in smooth muscle layers of opossum esophagus: gradients in density. *J Auton Nerv Sys* 1995; **52**: 99–105.
55. Lynn RB, Sankey SL, Chakder S et al. Colocalization of NADPH-diaphorase staining and VIP immunoreactivitiy in neurons in opossum internal anal sphincter. *Dig Dis Sci* 1995; **40**: 781–791.
56. Wang XY, Wong WC, Ling EA. Localization of nicotinamide adenine dinucleotide phosphate diaphorase (NADPH-d) activity in the gastrointestinal sphincters in the guinea pig. *J Auton Nerv Sys* 1996; **58**: 51–55.
57. Preiksaitis HG, Tremblay L, Diamant NE. Nitric oxide mediates inhibitory nerve effects in human esophagus and lower esophageal sphincter. *Dig Dis Sci* 1994; **39**: 770–775.
58. Conklin JL, Du C, Murray JA et al. Characterization and mediation of inhibitory junction potentials from opossum lower esophageal sphincter. *Gastroenterology* 1993; **104**: 1439–1444.
59. Bayguinov O, Sanders KM. Role of nitric oxide as an inhibitory neurotransmitter in the canine pyloric sphincter. *Am J Physiol* 1993; **264**: G975–G983.
60. Tottrup A, Ny L, Alm P et al. The role of the l-arginine/nitric oxide pathway for relaxation of the human lower oesophageal sphincter. *Acta Physiol Scand* 1993; **149**: 451–459.
61. Huang PL, Dawson TM, Bredt DS et al. Targetted disruption of the neuronal nitric oxide synthase gene. *Cell* 1993; **75**: 1273–1286.
62. Mearin F, Mourelle M, Guarner F et al. Patients with achalasia lack nitric oxide synthase in the gastro-

oesophageal junction. *Eur J Clin Invest* 1993; **23**: 724–728.
63. Ward SM, Morris G, Reese L et al. Interstitial cells of Cajal mediate enteric inhibitory neurotransmission in the lower esophageal and pyloric sphincters. *Gastroenterology* 1998; **115**: 314–329.
64. Watanabe Y, Ando H, Seo T et al. Attenuated nitrergic inhibitory neurotransmission to interstitial cells of Cajal in the lower esophageal sphincter with esophageal achalasia in children. *Pediatr Int* 2002; **44**: 145–148.
65. Howard PJ, Maher L, Pryde A et al. Five-year prospective study of the incidence, clinical features, and diagnosis of achalasia in Edinburgh. *Gut* 1992; **33**: 1011–1015.
66. Reynolds JC, Parkman HP. Achalasia. *Gastroenterol Clin North Am* 1989; **18**: 223–255.
67. Birgisson S, Richter JE. Achalasia: what's new in diagnosis and treatment? *Dig Dis* 1997; **15**(Suppl 1): 1–27.
68. Couturier D, Samama J. Clinical aspects and monometric criteria in achalasia. *Hepato-gastroenterol* 1991; **38**: 481–487.
69. Richter JE. Oesophageal motility disorders. *Lancet* 2001; **358**: 823–828.
70. Vane DW, Cosby K, West K et al. Late results following esophagomyotomy in children with achalasia. *J Pediatr Surg* 1988; **23**: 515–519.
71. Azizkhan RG, Tapper D, Eraklis A. Achalasia in childhood: a 20-year experience. *J Pediatr Surg* 1980; **15**: 452–456.
72. Myers NA, Jolley SG, Taylor R. Achalasia of the cardia in children: a worldwide survey. *J Pediatr Surg* 1994; **29**: 1375–1379.
73. Ferguson MK. Achalasia: current evaluation and therapy. *Ann Thorac Surg* 1991; **52**: 336–342.
74. Orlando RC, Call DL, Bream CA. Achalasia and absent gastric air bubble. *Ann Intern Med* 1978; **88**: 60–61.
75. Stewart ET. Radiographic evaluations of the esophagus and its motor disorders. *Med Clin North Am* 1981; **65**: 1173–1190.
76. Moreno Gonzalez E, Garcia Alvarez A, Landa Garcia I et al. Results of surgical treatment of esophageal achalasia. Multicenter retrospective study of 1856 cases. *Int Surg* 1988; **73**: 69–77.
77. Hewson EG, Ott DJ, Dalton CB et al. Manometry and radiology. Complementary studies in the assessment of esophageal motility disorders. *Gastroenterology* 1990; **98**: 626–632.
78. Tracey JP, Traube M. Difficulties in the diagnosis of pseudoachalasia. *Am J Gastroenterol* 1994; **89**: 2014–2018.
79. Vilgrain V, Mompoint D, Palazzio L. Staging of esophageal carcinoma: comparison of results with endoscopic sonography and CT. *Am J Roentgenol* 1990; **155**: 277–281.
80. Stacher G, Schima W, Bergmann H et al. Sensitivity of radionuclide bolus transport and videofluoroscopic studies compared with manometry in the detection of achalasia. *Am J Gastroenterol* 1994; **89**: 1484–1488.
81. Cohen S, Lipshutz W. Lower esophageal sphincter dysfunction in achalasia. *Gastroenterology* 1971; **61**: 814–820.
82. Tack J, Janssens J, Vantrappen G. Non-surgical treatment of achalasia. *Hepato-gastroenterol* 1991; **38**: 493–497.
83. Lobis JB, Fischer RS. Anticholinergic therapy for achalasia. A controlled study (abstract). *Gastroenterology* 1976; **70**: 976.
84. Christensen J. Effects of drugs on esophageal motility. *Arch Intern Med* 1976; **136**: 532–537.
85. Triadafilopoulos G, Aaronson M, Sackel S et al. Medical treatment of esophageal achalasia: double-blind crossover study with oral nifedipine, verapamil and placebo. *Dig Dis Sci* 1991; **36**: 260–267.
86. Traube M, Dubovik S, Lange RC et al. The role of nifedipine therapy in achalasia: results of a randomized, double-blind, placebo-controlled study. *Am J Gastroenterol* 1989; **84**: 1259–1262.
87. Gelfond M, Rozen P, Keren S et al. Effect of nitrates on LEOS pressure in achalasia: a potential therapeutic aid. *Gut* 1981; **22**: 312–318.
88. Gelfond M, Rozen P, Gilat T. Isosorbide dinitrate and nifedipine treatement of achalasia: a clinical, manometric and radionuclide evaluation. *Gastroenterology* 1982; **83**: 963–969.
89. Pasricha PJ, Ravich WJ, Hendrix TR et al. Intrasphincteric botulinum toxin for the treatment of achalasia. *N Engl J Med* 1995; **332**: 774–778.
90. Pasricha PJ, Rudra R, Ravich WJ et al. Botulinum toxin for achalasia: long-term outcome and predictors of response. *Gastroenterology* 1996; **110**: 1410–1415.
91. Neubrand M, Scheurlen C, Schepke M et al. Long-term results and prognostic factors in the treatment of achalasia with botulinum toxin. *Endoscopy* 2002; **34**: 519–523.
92. Bansal R, Nostrant TT, Scheiman JM et al. Intrasphincteric botulinum toxin versus pneumatic balloon dilation for treatment of primary achalasia. *J Clin Gastroenterol* 2003; **36**: 209–214.
93. Walton JM, Tougas G. Botulinum toxin use in pediatric esophageal achalasia: a case report. *J Pediatr Surg* 1997; **32**: 916–917.
94. Hurwitz M, Bahar RJ, Ament ME et al. Evaluation of the use of botulinum toxin in children with achalasia. *J Pediatr Gastroenterol Nutr* 2000; **30**: 509–514.
95. Hussain SZ, Thomas R, Tolia V. A review of achalasia in 33 children. *Dig Dis Sci* 2002; **47**: 2538–2543.
96. Eaker EY, Gordon JM, Vogel SB. Untoward effects of esophageal botulinum toxin injection in the treatment of achalasia. *Dig Dis Sci* 1997; **42**: 724–727.
97. Barnett JL, Eisenman R, Nostrant TT et al. Witzel pneumatic dilation for achalasia: safety and long-term efficacy. *Gastrointest Endosc* 1990; **36**: 482–485.
98. Kadakia SC, Wong RKH. Graded pneumatic dilation using Rigiflex achalasia dilators in patients with primary esophageal achalasia. *Am J Gastroenterol* 1993; **88**: 34–38.
99. Csendes A, Braghetto I, Henríquez A et al. Late results of a prospective randomized study comparing forceful dilatation and oesophagomyotomy in patients with achalasia. *Gut* 1989; **30**: 299–304.
100. Eckardt VF, Aignherr C, Bernhard G. Predictors of outcome in patients with achalasia treated by pneumatic dilation, *Gastroenterology* 1992; **103**: 1732–1738.
101. Nair, LA, Reynolds JC, Parkman HP et al. Complications during pneumatic dilation for achalasia or diffuse esophageal spasm: analysis of risk factors, early clinical characteristics, and outcome. *Dig Dis Sci* 1993; **38**: 1893–1903.
102. Babu R, Grier D, Cusick E et al. Pneumatic dilatation for childhood achalasia. *Pediatr Surg Int* 2001; **17**: 505–507.
103. Wilkinson AG, Raine PAM, Fyfe AHB. Pneumatic dilatation in childhood cardio-achalasia. *Pediatr Radiol* 1997; **27**: 60–62.
104. Parkman HP, Reynolds JC, Ouyang A et al. Pneumatic dilatation or esophagomyotomy treatment for idiopathic achalasia: clinical outcomes and cost analysis. *Dig Dis Sci* 1993; **38**: 75–85.

105. Heller E. Extramuköse Kardioplastik beim chronischen Kardiospasmus mit Dilatation des Oesophagus. *Mitt Grenzgeb Med Chir* 1914; **27**: 141–149.
106. Zaaijer JN. Cardiospasm in the aged. *Ann Surg* 1923; **77**: 615–617.
107. Crookes PF, DeMeester TR. Esophageal anatomy and physiology, and esophageal reflux. In Greenfield LJ, Mulholland MW, Oldham KT et al. eds. *Surgery: Scientific Principles and Practice*, 2nd Edn. Philadelphia: Lippincott-Raven, 1997: 653–694.
108. Ellis FH, Crozier RE, Watkins E. Operation for esophageal achalasia: results of esophagomyotomy without an antireflux operation. *J Thorac Cardiovasc Surg* 1984; **88**: 344–351.
109. Csendes A. Results of surgical treatment of achalasia of the esophagus. *Hepato-gastroenterol* 1991; **38**: 474–480.
110. Bonavina L, Nosadini A, Bardini R et al. Primary treatment of esophageal achalasia: long-term results of myotomy and Dor fundoplication. *Arch Surg* 1992; **127**: 222–227.
111. Mattioli S, DiSimone MP, Bassi F et al. Surgery for esophageal achalasia. Long-term results with three different techniques. *Hepato-gastroenterol* 1996; **43**: 492–500.
112. Wang PC, Sharp KW, Holzman MD et al. The outcome of laparoscopic Heller myotomy without antireflux procedure in patients with achalasia. *Am Surg* 1998; **64**: 515–521.
113. Pellegrini CA, Leichter R, Patti M et al. Thoracoscopic esophageal myotomy in the treatment of achalasia. *Ann Thorac Surg* 1993; **56**: 680–682.
114. Maher JW. Thoracoscopic esophagomyotomy for achalasia: maximum gain, minimal pain. *Surgery* 1997; **122**: 836–841.
115. Vogt D, Curet M, Pitcher D et al. Successful treatment of esophageal achalasia with laparoscopic Heller myotomy and Toupet fundoplication. *Am J Surg* 1997; **174**: 709–714.
116. Hunter JG, Trus TL, Branum GD et al. Laparoscopic Heller myotomy and fundoplication for achalasia. *Ann Surg* 1997; **225**: 655–665.
117. Ancona E, Anselmino M, Zaninotto G et al. Esophageal achalasia: laparoscopic versus conventional open Heller–Dor operation. *Am J Surg* 1995; **170**: 265–270.
118. Esposito C, Cucchiara S, Borrelli O et al. Laparoscopic esophagomyotomy for the treatment of achalasia in children. *Surg Endosc* 2000; **14**: 110–113.
119. Andreollo NA, Earlam RJ. Heller's myotomy for achalasia: is an added anti-reflux procedure necessary? *Br J Surg* 1987; **74**: 765–769.
120. Csendes A, Velasco N, Braghetto I et al. A prospective randomized study comparing forceful dilatation and esophagomyotomy in patients with achalasia of the esophagus. *Surgery* 1988; **104**: 469–475.
121. Anselmino M, Zaninotto G, Costantini M et al. One-year follow-up after Heller–Dor operation for esophageal achalasia. *Surg Endosc* 1997; **11**: 3–7.
122. Jamieson GG. Gastro-esophageal reflux following myotomy for achalasia. *Hepato-gastroenterol* 1991; **38**: 506–509.
123. Chen LW, Chughtai T, Sideris L. Long-term effects of myotomy and partial fundoplication for esophageal achalasia. *Dis Esophagus* 2002; **15**: 171–179.
124. Fernández AF, Martínez MA, Ruiz J et al. Six years of experience in laparoscopic surgery of esophageal achalasia. *Surg Endosc* 2003; **17**: 153–156.
125. Zaninotto G, Costantini M, Portale G et al. Etiology, diagnosis and treatment of failures after laparoscopic Heller myotomy for achalasia. *Ann Surg* 2002; **235**: 186–192.
126. Richardson WS, Willis GW, Smith JW. Evaluation of scar formation after botulinum toxin injection or forced balloon dilation to the lower esophageal sphincter. *Surg Endosc* 2003; **17**: 696–698.
127. Ferguson MK, Reeder LB, Olak J. Results of myotomy and partial fundoplication after pneumatic dilation for achalasia. *Ann Thorac Surg* 1996; **62**: 327–330.
128. Cosentini E, Berlakovich G, Zacherl J. Achalasia: results of myotomy and antireflux operation after failed dilatations. *Arch Surg* 1997; **132**: 143–147.

6 *Helicobacter pylori* gastritis and peptic ulcer disease

Costantino De Giacomo

Introduction

In adults, peptic disease (PD) is an important public health problem because of its clinical and economic implications. In children it is a well-known problem, but its prevalence and relative complications are less well defined.

PD includes some gastric and duodenal diseases characterized by the presence of the digestive symptoms of dyspepsia, the endoscopic appearance of mucosal lesions, and the histological features of chronic inflammation. However, these three characteristics might be expressed in different ways, producing a mix of clinical pictures, which range from the asymptomatic patient with normal endoscopic picture and mild gastritis, to the patient with a bleeding peptic ulcer.

Gastritis, duodenitis, gastric and duodenal ulcer are the definitive diagnoses of a patient who has gone through the appropriate endoscopic and histological investigation of the upper gastrointestinal tract. This means that most of the findings belonging to the pre-endoscopic era (in children, before 1980) are not reliable and not comparable with more recent data.

The strict link between the above-mentioned pictures is based on two major pieces of evidence. First, is the presence of mucosal inflammation and ulcer in the same patient. Even if gastroduodenitis and ulcer could be seen as a continuum in the natural history of PD, the evolution toward the crater (ulcer) is not mandatory, and the majority of patients with PD show only gastritis. Second, is the existence of a common etiological factor of both gastritis and ulcer in the majority of patients: the *Helicobacter pylori* (*H. pylori*) infection.

The history of the *H. pylori* infection begins in 1982, and it is one of the most exciting examples of how a fortuitous observation has produced one of the greatest impacts on our knowledge and treatment of an old disease. The oversight of cultures of antral biopsies taken from patients with PD during some days of vacation allowed two Australian investigators, Barry Marshall and Robert Warren, to observe and describe the growth of colonies of previously unknown bacteria.[1] As these Gram-negative, spiral bacteria had been isolated on *Campylobacter*-specific media, they were initially identified as *Campylobacter*-like organisms, but it soon became clear that *H. pylori* belonged to a new genus, taxonomically identified as *Helicobacter*, which, to date, consists of 19 zoonotic species with another ten potentially novel species. The official species differ in site of infection, which is the stomach in eight and the gut in 11, and in the host, but they show great homology in the analysis of 16S rRNA sequences (Table 6.1).[2]

During the past two decades, an impressive number of papers, consensus conferences, position documents and statements of the Gastroenterological Associations and Public Health Organizations (NIH) confirmed the existence of a strong association between *H. pylori* and PD. In particular, in 1994 a Consensus Conference of the NIH established the role of *H. pylori* in the pathogenesis and recurrence of peptic ulcer, emphasizing that the treatment of this condition should be considered the eradication of the *H. pylori* infection and not only the healing of the ulcer.[3] In the same year, the International Agency for Research on Cancer included *H. pylori* in the list of the carcinogenic factors of class I, as the main developing factor in gastric carcinoma [4]

Table 6.1 Natural hosts and usual site of isolation of *Helicobacter* species

***Helicobacter* species**	**Main host**	**Origin**
H. pylori	human	gastric
H. mustelae	ferret	gastric
H. nemestrinae	macaque monkey	gastric
H. felis	cat, dog	gastric
H. acinonychis	cheetah	gastric
H. bizzozeronii	dog	gastric
H. salomonis	dog	gastric
H. heilmannii	human, cat, dog, pig	gastric
H. cinaedi	human, hamster	intestinal
H. fennelliae	human, hamster	intestinal
H. muridarum	rat, mouse	intestinal
H. canis	dog	intestinal
H. pullorum	poultry	intestinal
H. pametensis	tern	intestinal
H. hepaticus	mouse	intestinal
H. bilis	mouse	intestinal
H. cholecystus	hamster	intestinal
H. trogontum	rat	intestinal
H. rodentium	mouse	intestinal

Epidemiology

Epidemiological data about peptic ulcer disease (PUD) are scanty and often related to series investigated by X-rays. Endoscopic data appeared after 1980 and showed a three-fold increase of cases of PUD over earlier findings.[5] A review of more than 1000 cases stated that the expected number of new PUD cases in a large children's hospital was evaluated as 3.5 per year.[6] Others found that the incidence of PUD was 4.4/10 000 children with a frequency of 3–6% in children who had undergone gastroscopy.[7]

However, there is now evidence that the incidence of PUD is decreasing in adults as well as in children. The progressive decrease of PUD is probably related to modifications in the epidemiology of *H. pylori* infection. The slow but continuous improvement of socioeconomic conditions, the diffuse use of antibiotics, and the decrease of the so-called ulcerogenic strains of *H. pylori* might reasonably explain this phenomenon.

H. pylori infection is one of the most diffuse infections in the world. There are areas at high risk of infection (in developing countries, such as those in the African or South American continents) and areas at low risk (such as Europe and North America).[8] In high-risk countries, the rate of infection is very high in the first 2 years of life, and older children and adults are almost totally infected. In a study on a cohort of 248 Gambian children aged 3–45 months, the prevalence of positive breath tests (a specific and non-invasive test to detect *H. pylori* infection, see below) rose from 19% at 3 months of age to 84% by the age of 30 months. Reversion to a negative breath test, in association with declining specific antibody levels, occurred in 20% of children, suggesting that in the first years of life children may acquire and clear the infection before ultimately being infected with a persistent strain.[9]

In developed countries, transverse serological studies have demonstrated that the rate of infection increases slowly and regularly by 10% with each decade of life.[8] In Italy, a recent epidemiological study showed that 11% of subjects from 6 to 18 years were infected,[10] while the prevalence rate in people of 50–60 years was 50–60%. Longitudinal studies demonstrated that this increase of infected subjects with aging was related to an effective decrease of infection in the youngest cohorts, rather than to an increase of new cases with aging.[11] This phenomenon is explained by the fact that each generation or cohort has a distinct and possibly unique environmental risk of exposure to the infection (cohort effect), linked to specific risk factors. These risk factors are well known and are socioeconomic, so that the cohort effect is considered to be the consequence of the improvement of socioeconomic conditions in the most recent decades. In Japan, a country that has had an impressive and fast economic development after the Second World War, epidemiological studies demonstrated a high prevalence rate of *H. pylori* infection in subjects born before the war, and a dramatic decrease in those born after the war and the industrial revolution.[12]

When the improvement of socioeconomic conditions was slow, but constant, as in the Netherlands, the decrease of the infection rate in childhood was continuous.[13]

The relationship between socioeconomic status and *H. pylori* infection has been emphasized by studies in subjects belonging to the same city or community, but with different socioeconomic conditions. Using family income as a measure of the socioeconomic class, the rate of acquisition of *H. pylori* in those children with family income less than $5000/year was twice that of those with incomes greater than $75 000/year in a study from Arkansas.[14] Absence of a fixed hot-water supply and domestic crowding in childhood were powerful independent risk factors for current infection with *H. pylori*. Among current living conditions, only the number of children living in the household was independently associated with *H. pylori* infection.[15] Different studies showed that the age of infection is in the first years of life.[16–18]

In a cohort of 224 children followed up retrospectively for 21 years by stored serum samples, the crude incidence rate per year was 1.4% for the whole cohort, ranging from 2.1% at 4–5 years and 1.5% at age 7–9 years to 0.3% at 21–23 years. The median age for seroconversion was 7.5 years. Nine of the 58 seropositive children cleared the infection during follow-up. The rate of seroreversion per year was 1.1%; it was highest among children at age 4–5 years (2.2% *vs* 0.2% at ages 18–19).[16] The finding that children infected before 5 years of age could eradicate the infection spontaneously, as well as be re-infected more easily than older children, has been confirmed by others.[14,17] A study of follow-up of 52 children successfully treated for *H. pylori* demonstrated that 11.5% of children who had eradicated the bacterium suffered reinfection, with the majority under 5 years of age. Only 4.3% of children older than 5 years were re-infected, even those living with *H. pylori*-positive parent in 81% of cases. The age of < 5 years was the major risk factor for re-infection.[17] In adults, the infection rate is approximately 0.3–0.5% per year and infection is rarely eradicated spontaneously, as demonstrated by longitudinal studies on stored samples.[19,20]

In addition to socioeconomic factors, genetic factors could play a role in the acquisition of the infection. A sibling study showed that the seroprevalence rate was similar in genetically identical twins living under different socioeconomic circumstances.[21] It should be acknowledged, however, that ethnic, genetic and socioeconomic factors are often intertwined and their various contributions are difficult to assess.

An important issue in the study of an infectious disease is its route of transmission. The absence of an animal reservoir, the demonstration of intrafamilial clustering,[22] as well as clustering of the infection among institutionalized children[23] suggests that person-to-person transmission is the most probable route. Approximately 90% of parents and 70% of siblings of *H. pylori*-positive children showed seropositivity for *H. pylori*.[22] In institutionalized children, including those living in a monastery, an inverse relationship between seroprevalence and age was demonstrated, with the increased rate of infection correlating with the age of entry more than the length of stay in the community.[23] Both vertical transmission (from mother to child as well as from father to child), and horizontal transmission from sibling to sibling, have been demonstrated.[24]

H. pylori has been isolated from saliva and dental plaque,[25] as well as from vomitus,[26] suggesting that the most diffuse routes of transmission between siblings or children in communities could be the oro-oral or gastro-oral. Epidemics of vomiting could easily diffuse the infection.

In developing countries, *H. pylori* has been identified in water[27] and in feces[28] by studies using the polymerase chain reaction (PCR). Clusters of infection independent of income, but strictly related to water source, have been demonstrated; the infection rate was 12-fold higher in children from high-income families using community wells rather than municipal water in a study in Peru.[27] The fecal-oral route of transmission typical of water-born diseases is quite possible, particularly in conditions where there is a lack of a municipal water supply.

Etiology

PUD is the progressive loss of the mucosal integrity up to the formation of a crater (ulcer). This is the final process of different etiological factors, which produce lesions by different mechanisms. These factors and mechanisms are not mutually exclusive and may co-operate to bring about their damage. The classical pathogenic theory was that an ulcer develops when the equilibrium is lost between defensive factors and aggressive factors. Defensive factors are the mucus layer, constituted by glycoproteins, bicarbonate and prostaglandins; and the gastric mucosa barrier, constituted by the epithelial layer, submucosal tissue and microcirculation. The best known aggressive factors are gastric acid, pepsins, gastrolesional substances, such as alcohol, drugs, non-steroidal anti-inflammatory drugs (NSAIDs) and, last to be identified, *H. pylori* infection). In primary ulcers (deep erosive lesions not secondary to other known causes) the most important factor was considered to be the acid output of the stomach. Both research and therapeutic interventional studies were directed towards evaluating and suppressing acid secretion (according to the theory 'no acid, no ulcer') until the discovery of *H. pylori*. The demonstration that duodenal ulcer is almost invariably associated with *H. pylori* infection, and recurrence depends on its persistence, established the importance of *H. pylori* as the main etiological factor in PUD.[3,29] Indeed, *H. pylori* infection has been demonstrated in 92% (33–100%) of children with duodenal ulcer in 14 studies, and in 25% (11–75%) of children with gastric ulcer in four studies.[30] Recurrence of ulcer after healing has been reported in 47% of children where *Helicobacter* was not eradicated, but it is rare, if not exceptional, in patients in whom eradication was achieved.[31] *H. pylori* is the main known etiological factor in chronic gastritis in adults as well as in children.[30]

H. pylori is a Gram-negative, unipolar flagellated bacterium with a spiral appearance (Figure 6.1). It was the first recognized bacterium of a new genus whose different species colonize the gastrointestinal tract of the human (*H. pylori* and *H. heilmannii*) and animals (all remaining species) (Table 6.1).[2]

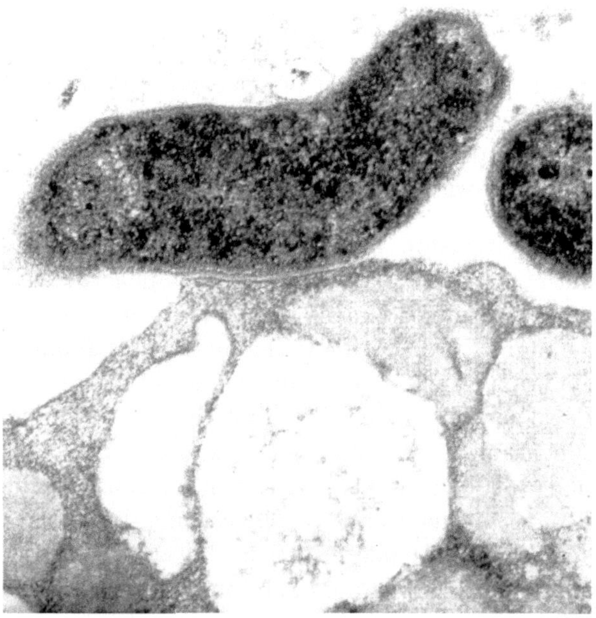

Figure 6.1 Electron micrograph of *Helicobacter pylori* attached to the cell membrane of gastric epithelial cells with evident cytoplasmic vacuolization.

H. pylori colonizes only the gastric mucosa, wherever it may be present: in the stomach or in heterotopic areas, as in Barrett's esophagus or in gastric metaplasia of the duodenum.[2] *H. heilmannii* is a rare (0.5% prevalence in humans) cause of dyspeptic symptoms and inflammation in adults, and its pathogenic role in children seems limited.[32]

The *H. pylori* genome (1.65 million bp) codes for about 1500 proteins and shows an extraordinary heterogeneity,[33] which could in part explain the wide spectrum of clinical pictures. Multiple strains may be present in the same patient, particularly in developing countries. Recombination and mutation between strains produces continuous changes of the genome during long-term gastric colonization in the same host.[34]

Pathogenesis

Role of acid and pepsinogen secretion

The bulk of our knowledge on acid secretion is derived from studies in adults. Gastric acid secretion begins in the newborn from the first day of life; it is not sensitive to gastrin, but rather to pentagastrin stimulation, which is the best way to evaluate it. Serum gastrin is usually elevated in the newborn period.[35,36]

Maximal acid output after pentagastrin stimulation increases from 0.031 mEq/kg per h at 1 month to 0.122 mEq/kg per h at 3 months, and up to 0.218 mEq/kg per h at 20 months, reflecting the increase of the mass of parietal cells.[37] In another study, maximal acid output values were demonstrated not to change from 3 months to 12 years of life.[38]

Basal acid output has been found to be normal in children with PUD in all[39–41] but one study.[42] Although children with PUD have been shown to have a higher average maximal acid output compared to age-matched controls, the occasional child with peptic ulcer may well have a completely normal maximal acid output. Similarly, control children may occasionally show increased maximal acid output.[39–42] This important overlap of values between children with or without ulcer is similar to that reported in adults. Interestingly, children with more severe PUD (requiring surgery, or presenting severe digestive bleeding) have been reported to have values of maximal acid output significantly higher than those with milder forms of disease or in remission.[40,42] Basal[41] or meal-stimulated serum gastrin[43] can be normal or slightly increased in children with ulcer.

Other disorders associated with severe gastric and duodenal ulcers secondary to increased gastric acid secretion are listed in Table 6.2. These situations are usually the consequence of an increased basal (Zollinger–Ellison syndrome, 'ZES') or stimulated (pseudo-ZES or antral G-cell hyperplasia/hyperfunction syndrome)[44] gastrin or histamine secretion.

Pepsins are proteolytic enzymes generated by the action of hydrochloric acid on their precursor pepsinogens. Pepsinogens are secreted by the principal cells of the gastric fundus (PGI) and by

Table 6.2 Causes of gastric acid hypersecretion
Zollinger–Ellison syndrome
Antral G-cell hyperplasia or hyperfunction
Mastocytosis
Chronic renal failure
Hypertrophic gastropathy
Small intestinal resection – short gut
Hyperparathyroidism

the mucous cells of the remaining stomach and part of the duodenum (PGII). Seven molecular forms (Pg1–Pg5 for PGI and Pg6–Pg7 for PGII) can be identified electrophoretically. Only traces of pepsins have been demonstrated in neonatal gastric juice, and their increase with age is slow.[37] In children with PUD, as well as in members of families with a high incidence of PUD, an increase of serum pepsinogen I has been demonstrated, and high serum pepsinogen I has been considered a marker of ulcerogenicity.[45]

Helicobacter pylori-related mechanisms

H. pylori may induce inflammation by two different pathways: direct toxicity mediated by secretion of specific toxins and other aggressive factors (Table 6.3); and immune-mediated toxicity secondary to stimulation of both innate and adaptive immune responses in the host.[46]

The gastric mucosa is a niche relatively resistant to bacterial infection. The main protective mechanism is the bactericidal activity of the gastric acid. However, *H. pylori* has developed some mechanisms to evade protection and to allow the colonization of the mucosa: urease production and motility. Urease activity is mediated by a unique pH-dependent urea channel, UreI, which works at low pH, and allows the influx of urea followed by hydrolysis into CO_2 and ammonia, which buffers acid conditions close to the bacterium.[47,48] By means of flagellar motility, *H. pylori* swims into the mucous layer, and attaches to epithelial cells by multiple bacterial-surface adhesins. The best characterized adhesin is Baba, a 78-kDa outer membrane protein, which binds to the fucosylated Lewis B blood-group antigen.[49]

Approximately half of the genomic variants of *H. pylori* are able to produce the thermolabile 95-kDa cytotoxin, called Vac-A, with a cytopathic effect induced by direct vacuolating action on epithelial cells (Figure 6.1).[50] The toxin inserts itself into the epithelial cell membrane, forming a channel through which bicarbonate and organic anions can reach the bacterium. Other mechanisms involved in the Vac-A-mediated epithelial damage are the release of cytochrome C from mitochondria, and apoptosis.[51] Even if the pathogenic role of Vac A is still under debate, it is relevant that Vac-A positive strains are isolated in 60% of patients with PUD, and in only 30% of patients with gastritis.[52]

Sixty-five to eighty per cent of strains of *H. pylori* have a chromosomal region called cag-PAI (37-kb genomic fragment containing 29 genes) which codifies a type IV secretory apparatus translocating the 120–128-kDa Cag-A protein inside the host cell.[53,54] At the cellular level, a direct proliferative response and cytokine production are induced. Cag-A-positive strains are usually isolated from 80–100% of patients with more severe peptic lesions and in 60–75% of patients with milder forms of disease.

Even if the majority of strains isolated from patients with PUD are positive for both Cag-A and Vac-A, it is not possible to distinguish ulcerogenic from non-ulcerogenic strains with certainty.

The second pathway involved in gastric injury is secondary to activation of an immune response. *H. pylori* produces gastric inflammation in virtually all infected persons.[55] This inflammatory response is triggered by bacterial attachment to epithelial cells, followed by recruitment of neutrophils, macrophages, T and B lymphocytes,

Table 6.3 Virulence factors demonstrated in *Helicobacter pylori* strains

Colonization factors	Toxicity factors
Urease (acidity inhibition)	vacuolizing cytotoxin (Vac-A)
Flagellins (motility)	*cag* pathogenicity island (*cag*-PAI)
Adhesins (adhesivity)	ammonium, lipopolysaccharide, phospholipase
Catalase, superoxide dismutase (phagocytosis resistance)	

and plasma cells. In the inflamed gastric epithelium, a high concentration of proinflammatory cytokines has been found. Increased production of interleukin (IL)-8, a potent neutrophil-activating cytokine, is induced by activation of NFKβ from Cag-A-positive, more than Cag-A-negative, strains.[56] IL-8 and other chemokines amplify the immune as well as the inflammatory response, producing severe epithelial damage. The multiplicity of possible pathogenic mechanisms is shown in Figure 6.2.

A systemic and mucosal immune response is elicited by *H. pylori* infection.[57] This does not lead to eradication, but it may contribute to further damage. Immunological studies have demonstrated that an IL-18-driven Th1 immune response, instead of the expected Th2, combined with Fas-mediated apoptosis of *H. pylori*-specific T-cell clones, may contribute to the persistence of the infection. Some patients produce autoantibodies against the H^+/K^+ ATPase of gastric parietal cells that play a role in the induction of gastric atrophy.[58]

In addition to the direct and inflammatory mechanisms of mucosal injury, *H. pylori* may play an ulcerogenic role by interfering with acid and pepsin secretion. In children, *H. pylori* infection seems to increase serum PGI[59] and in some, but not all, children with *H. pylori*, a meal-induced hypergastrinemia secondary to G-cell hyperplasia

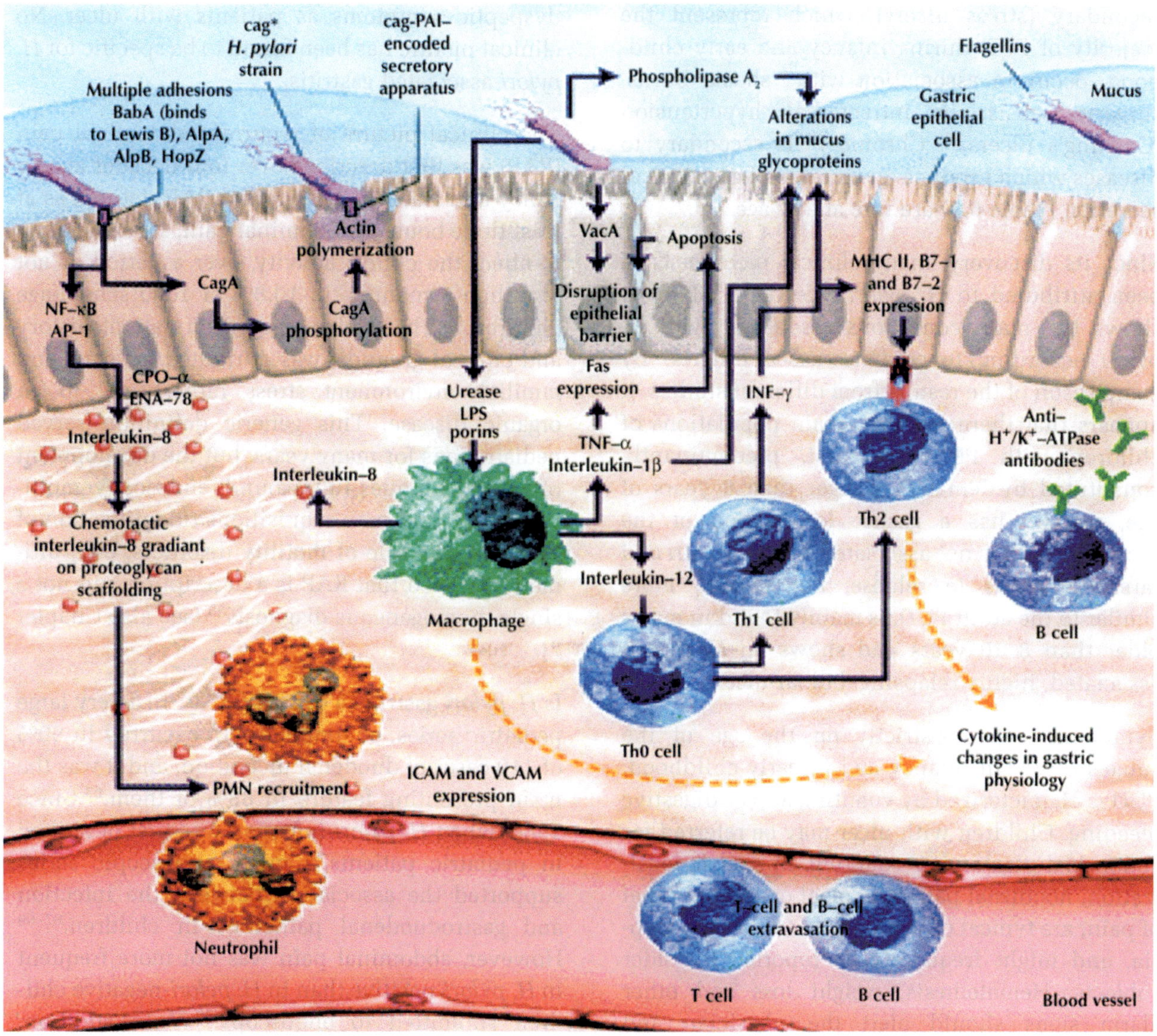

Figure 6.2 *Helicobacter pylori*-host interactions in the pathogenesis of mucosal lesions from reference 46, with permission.

has been reported. Eradication of *H. pylori* usually normalizes pepsinogen and gastrin secretion[59] as well as G- and D-cell hyperplasia.[60] *H. pylori* infection may interfere in the gastrin–HCl axis increasing gastric acid secretion, which in turn results in duodenal ulceration: in adults, an increased maximal acid output has been demonstrated to differentiate ulcer from non-ulcer *H. pylori*-positive patients.[61]

Table 6.4 Human digestive diseases associated with *Helicobacter pylori* infection

Acute gastritis
Chronic gastritis
Duodenal ulcer
Gastric ulcer
Gastric carcinoma
B-Lymphoma (MALToma)

Clinical aspects

Peptic ulcers are classified as either primary, when they occur in the absence of an underlying systemic disease, or secondary, when they are caused by medications or other diseases. Acute secondary (stress ulcers), which represent the majority of PUD during infancy and early childhood, occur in association with shock, burns, surgery, sepsis, or intracranial hypertension (Cushing's ulcers).[62] Chronic PUD secondary to diseases which produce an increase of gastric acid secretion (Table 6.2) are rare at any age.

Since its discovery, many clinical pictures have been attributed to *H. pylori* infection. Table 6.4 shows the main conditions associated with *H. pylori* according to evidence-based criteria. By comparison of the results from different studies, it appears that there are two main populations of children with PUD: the first, predominantly constituted by females younger than 8 years of age, usually has a gastric localization of the ulcer,[6,7] which is not associated with *H. pylori* and rarely proceeds to relapse; the second, more similar to the adult PUD, is mainly found in males older than 8–10 years and shows an *H. pylori*-associated, highly relapsing, bulbar ulcer.

Symptoms depend strictly on the age of the subjects.[6,62,63] In infancy and in early childhood, PUD is characterized by vomiting and/or digestive bleeding. Children with ulcer may be referred for abdominal pain and/or vomiting. Epigastric localization, nocturnal pain, and meal or antacid relief of pain, are typical of so-called 'ulcer-like' dyspepsia, and might frequently be reported by older subjects. Hematemesis, weight loss and other alarm signs should alert the physician and strongly suggest further evaluation.[62]

Children with *H. pylori*-associated gastritis without ulcer are asymptomatic in the majority of cases[10] or, rarely, they may suffer from the same dyspeptic symptoms as patients with ulcer. No clinical picture has been found to be specific for *H. pylori*-associated gastritis.

The clinical picture of recurrent abdominal pain (RAP) was first described over four decades ago by Apley and Naish.[64] They found RAP, defined as at least three bouts of abdominal pain, severe enough to affect the child's activity, over a period of not less than 3 months, in 10.8% of 1000 school-age children.[64] The etiology, based on patient history and clinical grounds, was attributed to social and familial environment stress rather than to an organic disease. This generic definition served pediatricians for many years, but the development of new techniques (ultrasound, endoscopy, motility probes) and new acquisitions (identification of *H. pylori*, the role of motility disorders, etc.) ultimately proved that RAP is a description and not a single, homogeneous diagnosis[65] (see also Chapter 7).

Is *H. pylori* gastritis a cause of RAP? In a very large pediatric series, abdominal pain occurred in 90% of 110 cases of duodenal ulceration, and it was the main presenting feature in 88% of them.[63] Since 1986, when *H. pylori* infection was first described in pediatric patients,[66] many endoscopic series supported the association between the infection and gastroduodenal pathology in children.[67–69] However, abdominal pain was not more frequent in *H. pylori*-positive than in *H. pylori*-negative children submitted to endoscopy.[70–72] In addition, eradication did not resolve symptoms in all cases, being very effective only in those rare cases with ulcer.[73]

Moreover, population-based studies failed to show any association between RAP and *H. pylori* infection in both school-aged and pre-school-aged populations.[10,74,75] Nevertheless, it is evident that discordant results may also be dependent on the heterogeneity of the clinical populations studied (endoscopic series vs. school populations), and the differences in the inclusion criteria (age, duration of the pain, etc.)[30]

A recent report from the Committee on Childhood Functional Gastrointestinal Disorders[76] states that 'it seemed more appropriate to apply the most specific diagnostic category to a symptomatic child', defining clinical criteria of functional dyspepsia as in adults. Gastroenterologists working on adults with upper gastrointestinal symptoms prefer to aggregate more symptoms in the complex picture of ulcer-like and dysmotility-like forms of dyspepsia. Recent studies have shown that a relationship between dyspeptic symptoms and some pathogenic factors (mainly *H. pylori* infection and motility disturbances) is apparent.[77] However, a large intervention study on adults failed to demonstrate that symptoms are dependent on *H. pylori* infection and, by extrapolation, on gastritis.[78] In the eradication trials, the summary odds ratio for improvement in dyspeptic symptoms in patients with non-ulcer dyspepsia in whom *H. pylori* was eradicated was 1.9 (1.3–2.6).

The presence of severe epigastric pain, associated with nocturnal pain, fasting pain and relief of pain after meal intake, characterizing the picture of ulcer-like dyspepsia in subjects aged over 10 years,[10] could be the clinical picture more suggestive of gastroduodenitis, suggesting the need for further evaluation.

Complications

The most frequent complication of PUD is digestive bleeding, with hematemesis and melena reported in more than half the cases.[6] Gastrointestinal bleeding may be present even in the absence of ulcer, if diffuse varioliform gastritis with erosions is present at endoscopy. Another complication of PUD is perforation (10%), which may result in peritonitis, if anterior, or in pancreatic penetration, if posterior. Pyloric stenosis as a consequence of a parapyloric ulcer is quite rare; a malignant ulcer is exceptional in children.

A vicious cycle between chronic diarrhea, malnutrition and *H. pylori* infection is evident, especially for children in developing countries.[79] Some other gastrointestinal disorders based on the presence of heterotopic gastric mucosa, such as Barrett's ulcer[80] and Meckel's diverticulum bleeding,[81] have been anecdotally associated with *H. pylori* infection, but further studies suggested that *H. pylori* did not play a causal role in their determination.

Extraintestinal manifestations have been controversially reported in patients with *H. pylori* infection; iron deficiency and sideropenic refractory anemia, short stature and growth failure, and sudden infant death are the most conflicting areas in childhood.[82]

Iron deficiency anemia may be a consequence of *H. pylori* infection in children. Case reports and series of children with sideropenic refractory anemia have been reported.[83] Iron deficiency without anemia has also been demonstrated in adults.[84] The efficacy of eradication in raising the hemoglobin level and in restoring ferritin values has been demonstrated in adults as well as in teenagers.[85] Potential mechanisms involved in producing iron deficiency are fecal occult blood loss, reduction in duodenal absorption and the iron-scavenging capability of the bacterium.

Some studies have reported the existence of an effect of the infection on the final height of the patient. *H. pylori*-positive children have been demonstrated to be shorter than those who are *H. pylori*-negative.[27] Growth velocity has been demonstrated to be decreased by 1.1 cm in affected females between 7 and 11 years of age.[86] However, this association has not been confirmed by other studies, which showed, instead, that reduced growth is related to genetic determinants, such as parental height, and to mixed genetic and environmental factors, such as birth weight. Low socioeconomic status was clearly relevant.[87]

Concerning the role of *Helicobacter* infection in causing infant deaths by sudden infant death syndrome (SIDS), one study detected *H. pylori* in lungs from 25 out of 32 SIDS cases.[88] However, a further study utilizing both histology and immunohistochemistry on 25 cases of infants with SIDS failed to confirm this hypothesis.[89]

Diagnosis

Diagnosis of ulcer is based on the endoscopic examination of the stomach and the duodenal bulb. Primary ulcers are often single and localized at the duodenal bulb (Figure 6.3) or in the distal part of the stomach (Figure 6.4) (antrum, lesser curvature); while secondary ulcers (NSAIDs, stress ulcer) can be located in all parts of the stomach and can be multiple. Endoscopy may show changes of the gastroduodenal mucosa typical of gastropathy. Dohil et al[90] have suggested an easy and quite useful endoscopic classification of gastropathies in erosive and non-erosive forms (Table 6.5). Even if some disorders may show both erosive and non-erosive lesions, each is classified by its most common clinical manifestation. The endoscopic picture of *H. pylori*-associated gastritis is characterized by the presence of micronodularity of the antral mucosa in more than 50% of cases (Figure 6.5).[90]

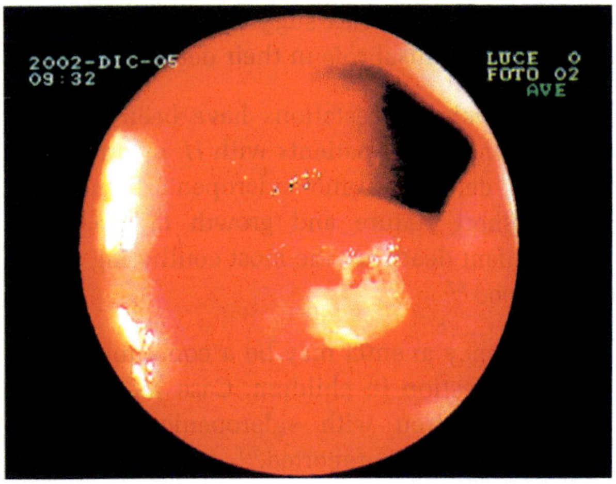

Figure 6.3 Endoscopic appearance of a *Helicobacter pylori*-associated peptic ulcer of the posterior wall of the duodenal bulb in an 11-year-old girl.

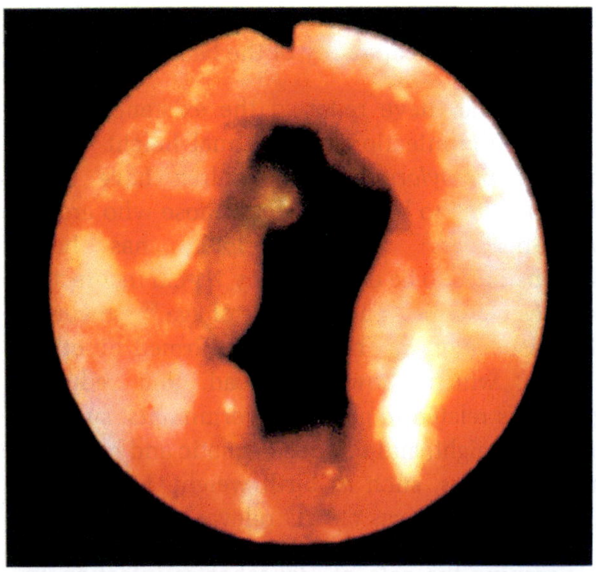

Figure 6.4 Endoscopic appearance of *Helicobacter pylori*-associated multiple peptic ulcers of the gastric body and hyperplastic regeneration of the surrounding mucosa in a 12-year-old girl.

Some endoscopic pictures might be suggestive of inflammation and/or be specific for a given etiology, but confirmation of the initial impression and definitive diagnosis is dependent on histological examination. For this reason, each endoscopic examination must be completed by biopsy sampling of both endoscopically abnormal and normal mucosa. At least two biopsies for *H. pylori* detection must be taken at the antral site. Further sampling from the fundus may be useful, especially after treatment, because of the tendency of the bacterial colonization to migrate proximally. Biopsies for other procedures (culture, urease test) should be considered after sampling for routine histology.

H. pylori-associated gastritis is the most frequent microscopic finding. It is predominantly an antral gastritis, but in some patients, and particularly in adults, inflammation may involve the entire stomach (pangastritis). In children, its severity is usually less, and features of activity (presence of polymorphonuclear leukocytes) are reported in 40% of cases.[69,90] The presence of lymphoid follicle hyperplasia (follicular gastritis) (Figure 6.6), suspected of being the histological counterpart of the nodular appearance of the gastric mucosa at endoscopy, has been reported in 20% of patients.[69,90] In adults, pangastritis may show gastric atrophy and/or focal intestinal metaplasia, particularly in association with gastric ulcers. In children, these findings are rarely reported (Figure 6.7).

Table 6.5 Classification of gastritis and gastropathy in children*[90]
Erosive and/or hemorrhagic gastritis or gastropathy
'Stress' gastropathy
Neonatal gastropathies
Traumatic gastropathy
Aspirin and other non-steroidal anti-inflammatory drugs
Other drugs
Portal hypertensive gastropathy
Uremic gastropathy
Chronic varioliform gastritis
Bile gastropathy
Henoch–Schönlein gastropathy
Corrosive gastropathy
Exercise-induced gastropathy or gastritis
Radiation gastropathy
Non-erosive gastritis or gastropathy
'Non-specific' gastritis
Helicobacter pylori gastritis
Crohn's gastritis
Allergic gastritis
Proton pump inhibitor gastropathy
Celiac gastritis
Gastritis of chronic granulomatous disease
Cytomegalovirus gastritis
Eosinophilic gastritis
Collagenous gastritis
Graft-versus-host disease
Ménétrier's disease
Pernicious anemia
Gastritis with autoimmune disease
Other granulomatous gastritides
Phlegmonous and emphysematous gastritis
Other infectious gastritides

*Although some disorders can present as either erosive or non-erosive, each is classified by its most common manifestation

In recent years, the importance of the histological diagnosis of gastritis, on the basis of routinely obtained antral and body biopsies, has increased enormously, particularly because of the discovery of *H. pylori*. The introduction of the Sydney system made it possible, for the first time, to grade histological parameters, to identify topographic distribution and, finally, to make a statement about

(a) (b)

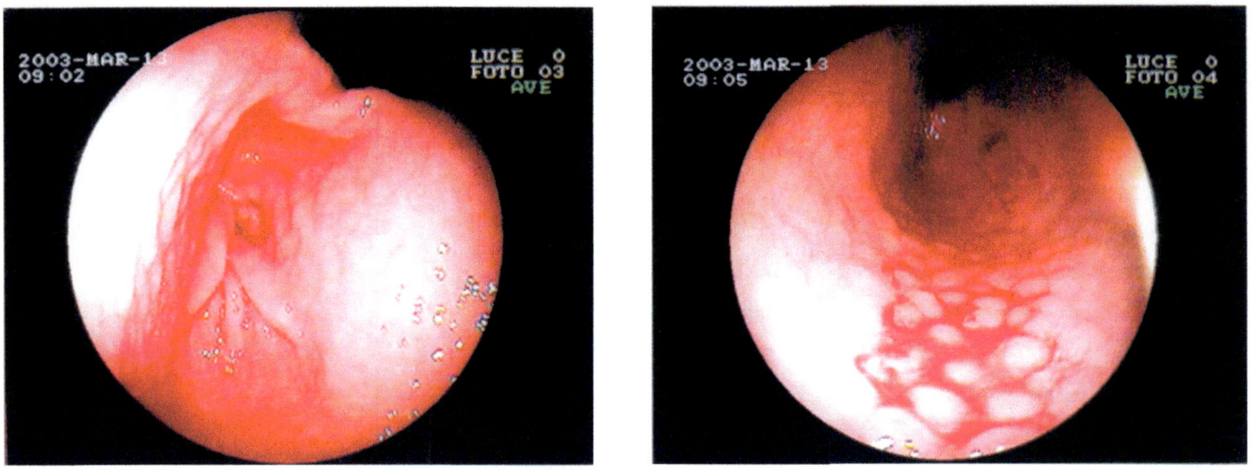

Figure 6.5 Endoscopic appearance of antral nodularity associated with *Helicobacter pylori* infection (a). After biopsy, mucosal bleeding enhances the evidence of the picture (b).

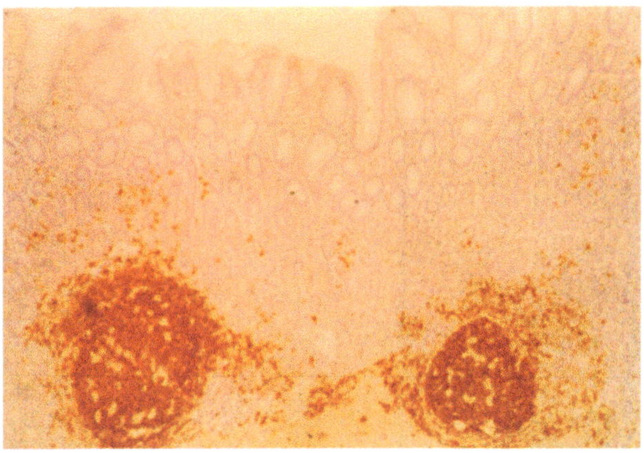

Figure 6.6 Immunohistochemical staining for B lymphocytes of a mucosa-associated lymphoid follicle in a child with *Helicobacter pylori*-associated antral nodularity.

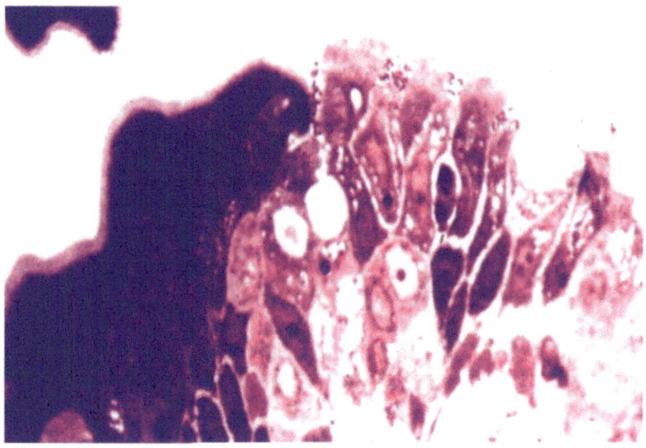

Figure 6.7 Giemsa-stained antral specimen showing, on the left side, typical intestinal metaplasia and, on the right side, *Helicobacter pylori*-associated chronic gastritis.

the etiopathogenesis of the gastritis in *H. pylori*- or non-*H. pylori*-associated gastritis.[91]

Multiple samplings from the antrum, the body and the fundus of the stomach allow further subdivision of the group of *H. pylori*-associated gastritis into forms of gastritis whose morphological distribution patterns usually identify them as sequelae of *H. pylori* infection. Moreover, the group of gastritis not associated with *H. pylori* can be differentiated into autoimmune, chemically induced reactive gastritis, ex-*H. pylori* gastritis, *H. heilmannii* gastritis, Crohn's gastritis and a number of special forms of gastritis (see Table 6.5).

Diagnosis of *H. pylori* infection is based on the demonstration of *H. pylori* by either direct (invasive) or indirect (non-invasive) methods. *H. pylori* can be demonstrated on the gastric mucosa specimen by staining with Warthin–Starry, Giemsa (Figure 6.7) or orange acridine stain, or it can grow in culture of gastric biopsies on specific media and in microaerophilic conditions.[2] Culture may be particularly useful for specific antibiotic sensitivity testing. An easy, diffuse and rapid test is the urease test, which is based on the color reaction induced by the presence of urease in the gastric specimen within 1 h.[92]

Indirect tests are based on the demonstration of an elevated titer of IgG or IgA antibodies against *H. pylori* in serum[22] or in saliva,[93] or the presence of a positive immunoassay for *H. pylori* in the stools.[94] For research purposes, *H. pylori* may be detected by PCR in some human samples, such as dental plaque or feces.[25,28] Results obtained using these diagnostic methods are variable, but among invasive tests, histology and culture are superior. If indirect tests are considered, the ^{13}C-urea breath test (UBT) and fecal antigen tests show the best accuracy. In a recent study comparing more tests on 53 children,[1] all the diagnostic tests except serology were excellent methods of diagnosing *H. pylori* infection. The diagnostic accuracy was 96.2% for the stool antigen test, 96.2% for the biopsy urease test, 98.1% for histology, 94.3% for PCR, 98.1% for culture, 100% for the ^{13}C-UBT and 84.9% for serology.[95]

The North American Society of Pediatric Gastroenterology, Hepatology and Nutrition (NASPGHAN) clinical practice guidelines (Table 6.6),[96] as well as the European (EPTFHP) (Table 6.6)[97] and Canadian[98] pediatric consensus conferences on *H. pylori* infection, recommend making a definitive diagnosis of *H. pylori* infection through endoscopy with multiple biopsies of the stomach. The role of non-invasive methods has to be reserved to the demonstration of eradication and for follow-up. For this purpose, the ^{13}C-UBT is the best validated method,[99] even though some problems may exist in patients younger than 6 years of age.

Treatment

One of the most debated problems is who should be treated for *H. pylori* infection. In adults, the most recent indications for *H. pylori* treatment are listed in the Table 6.7, derived from the Maastricht 2-2000 Consensus Report.[100]

Each of the three Pediatric Consensus Reports (North American, European and Canadian) outlined recommendations for the detection of *H. pylori* infection.[96–98] Regarding the *H. pylori*-positive subjects to be treated, the NASPGHAN supports the treatment only in case of PUD and MALToma.[96] The European Pediatric Task Force on *Helicobacter pylori* (EPTFHP) consensus statement suggests providing treatment for the infection if *H. pylori* is identified in a child at endoscopy (Table 6.6).[97]

Children with *H. pylori*-positive PUD must be submitted to eradicating treatment, because

Table 6.6 Guidelines for the management of *Helicobacter pylori* infection in children

Diagnosis	Evidence	Treatment	Evidence
North American Society of Pediatric Gastroenterology, Hepatology and Nutrition			
Endoscopy and histology	II	peptic ulcer disease	I
^{13}C-urea breath test	II	MALToma	III
		atrophic gastritis	
		I. metaplasia	III
		triple therapy for 1–2 weeks	
European Pediatric Task Force on *Helicobacter pylori*			
Endoscopy and histology		peptic ulcer disease	
^{13}C-urea breath test for follow-up		all *Helicobacter pylori*-positive children after endoscopy (information of the possibility of symptoms' persistence)	

Table 6.7 The Maastricht 2-2000 guidelines for the treatment of *Helicobacter pylori* infection in adults

Strongly recommended indications
Peptic ulcer disease
MALToma
Atrophic gastritis
Post-gastric cancer resection
First-degree relatives of gastric cancer patients
Patient's wishes (after physician consultation)
Advisable indications
Functional dyspepsia (subset of patients)
Gastroesophageal reflux disease (in patients requiring long-term proton pump inhibitor therapy)
Users of non-steroidal anti-inflammatory drugs

relapse after effective ulcer healing has been demonstrated in 47–80% of children with persistent *H. pylori* infection, and exceptionally in those in whom *H. pylori* has been eradicated.[31,37,97] Symptomatic relief of dyspeptic symptoms is usually achieved.[73]

H. pylori eradication in children with chronic active gastritis is associated with evident histological improvement,[69] but remission of symptoms does not necessarily follow.[73,97] However, if the infection is not treated, worsening of gastritis and of the clinical picture, particularly in males and in children infected with Cag-A-positive strains, has been documented in a close follow-up study.[101] In adults as well as in teenagers with iron-deficient anemia, *H. pylori* eradication was associated with a rise in hemoglobin levels and in ferritin values, suggesting that treatment should be considered.[82–85]

In adults with peptic esophagitis, the treatment of associated *H. pylori* infection is a question of debate.[102] Some authors have suggested that esophagitis and gastroesophageal reflux disease (GERD) may be exacerbated by eliminating the protecting buffering effect of *H. pylori* infection.[103] Nevertheless, a causal relationship between these phenomena remains unproven, and is mainly based on retrospective analyses or epidemiological hypothesis. The small number of prospective trials in adults has not consistently demonstrated an increased risk of GERD after *H. pylori* eradication.[104]

In a study planned to answer the question of whether eradication of *H. pylori* infection in children with RAP should result in clinical improvement, no correlation was seen between eradication and disappearance of RAP, after 3 or after 6 months of observation.[105]

To date, extrapolation of data from randomized controlled trials in adults has been the basic approach to treating children with *H. pylori* infection. A systematic review of the small published open trials in 870 children from 1987 to 2000 has recently been published.[106] A total of 79 children were treated with one drug (monotherapy); 345 were treated with dual therapy, including two antibiotics or one antibiotic plus bismuth compounds or H_2-receptor antagonists (H_2RA) or proton pump inhibitors (PPIs); and 446 with a bismuth- or PPI-based triple therapy plus two antibiotics. In pediatrics, the most frequently utilized antibiotics were amoxicillin, clarithromycin, and the nitroimidazoles, metronidazole or tinidazole. The reasons for the development of combined therapies were:

(1) Different strains with different antibiotic sensitivity may colonize the same patient. Sensitivity to amoxicillin, clarithromycin and nitroimidazoles is one of the key factors in the eradication rates. Unpublished data collected by the EPTFHP showed metronidazole, clarithromycin or double resistance before the first therapy in 24.5%, 20% and 7%, respectively, of 400 *H. pylori*-infected children aged under 15 years.

(2) Stability and efficacy of antibiotics are often impaired in the acid environment. This consideration prompted the combination of antibiotics with drugs able to increase the gastric pH (H_2RA or PPI).

In general, monotherapy with one antibiotic, or bismuth compounds, or H_2RA or PPI showed a very low eradication rate and it is not recommended. Combination of one antibiotic with PPI was not satisfactory (mean eradication rate of 39%), while combination of amoxicillin with nitroimidazole or one of the two antibiotics with bismuth salts was tried in 248 children, with a mean eradication rate of 73–76%.[106]

Triple therapy schedules did not work much better. A recent randomized clinical trial confirmed that 1 week of omeprazole–amoxicillin–clarithromycin resulted in successful eradication of *H. pylori* in 75% of 73 children <15 years old.[107] A higher efficacy was obtained with the combination of bismuth, metronidazole and clarithromycin, with an eradication rate of 95.5% in 22 children.[108] Data from two abstracts with a total of 58 children treated with omeprazole–amoxicillin–tinidazole schedules for 1 or 2 weeks showed 86% and 100% eradication rates, respectively.[106]

Concerning the duration of the different regimens, dual therapies with amoxicillin and nitroimidazole, or one of these two antibiotics and bismuth, reached better eradication rates (84% vs. 74%) when administered for 2 weeks rather than 1 week. In contrast, PPI-based triple therapies gave similar results when given for 1 or 2 weeks (75% vs. 77%).[106] Thus, it would appear that 1 week of PPI-based triple therapy with amoxicillin and clarithromycin or a nitroimidazole should be the first choice of treatment. If available, sensitivity data may help in making the final decision (Table 6.8).

Monitoring of the treatment should be based on non-invasive tests, and, among these, ^{13}C-UBT is

Table 6.8 Protocols of *Helicobacter pylori* treatment in children

First-line therapy
PPI (1 mg/kg per day up to 20 mg bid) plus Amoxicillin (50 mg/kg per day bid up to 1 g bid) plus Clarithromycin (15 mg/kg per day up to 500 mg bid) *or* Metro(ti)nidazole (20 mg/kg per day up to 500 mg bid) for 1 week
In case of failure to eradicate the bacterium: *Second-line therapy*
Amoxicillin + clarithromycin *or* metronidazole (based on antibiotic testing or, in the absence of testing, that not used in the first line) *plus*
PPI *or* bismuth salts (480 mg/1.73 m^2 of body surface up to 480 qid) for 2 weeks
Successive failures and retreatment need antibiotic testing and case-to-case evaluation

PPI, proton pump inhibitor; bid, twice a day; qid, four times a day the most recommended.[97] Recent data showed that fecal *H. pylori* antigen assays could be an effective alternative.[109] Re-infection after eradication is uncommon in children, and treatment of the affected family member at present is not supported.[17]

In the case of relapse, biopsy culture for antibiotic sensitivity testing should be proposed for a better chance of eradication. If culture is not available or if *H. pylori* does not grow, substitution of clarithromycin with a nitroimidazole (and vice versa) is the first step, because of the high probability of development of a resistance to either drug. A 2-week regimen should be offered to relapsing patients (Table 6.8).

Short- and long-term prognosis

In patients with *H. pylori*-associated PUD, successful eradication is followed by ulcer healing and usually evident clinical improvement. PUD does not relapse and reacquisition of the infection is rare after 5 years of age.[31,42,97] Children with abdominal complaints associated with chronic gastritis have a more unpredictable clinical outcome, even if *H. pylori* is eradicated.[73,97]

Among long-term complications of *H. pylori*-associated chronic gastritis, the most important is the multistep disease progression towards gastric atrophy, intestinal metaplasia, dysplasia and gastric cancer.[110] In general, this is a rare evolution, affecting no more than 1% of *H. pylori*-positive patients. This multifactorial process includes host, bacterial and dietary factors.

Family studies have shown that gastric cancer is significantly higher in first-degree relatives of gastric cancer patients.[111] Epidemiological case–control and cohort studies have demonstrated that *H. pylori* is strongly associated with non-cardia gastric carcinoma of both the intestinal and the diffuse type.[112,113] An extensive review on this topic showed the best estimate of the relative risk of non-cardia gastric cancer associated with *H. pylori* infection to be 5.9.[113] The odds ratio decreased significantly with aging, from 9.29 in patients with carcinoma at age 20–29 years, to 1 in those older than 70 years of age.[112] For some authors, the basis of the genetic predisposition lies either in genetic susceptibility to the infection[20] or in mechanisms of DNA repair and carcinogenesis.[114] Mutation in p53 is one of the most common genetic alterations found in human cancer, including gastric cancer.[115] Inhibition of apoptosis secondary to up-regulation of cyclo-oxygenase 2 by *H. pylori*-induced inflammation could play a role in inducing intestinal metaplasia. In a subgroup of gastric cancer, as well as in intestinal metaplasia, microsatellite instability, secondary to germline mutation of the DNA mismatch repair genes, has also been demonstrated. The mechanisms inducing intestinal metaplasia and carcinogenesis have recently been reviewed.[114]

Acid output has long been investigated as a key factor of ulcer development and gastric cancer. Indeed, patients with higher acid output are likely to have antral-predominant gastritis and eventually duodenal ulcer, but they do not show any predisposition towards gastric cancer.[116] Patients with lower acid output, on the other hand, are more likely to have a body-predominant gastritis, which predisposes to gastric ulcer and to the multistep progression of disease that, in rare cases, leads to gastric carcinoma. Polymorphisms of the IL-1β promoter have been linked to altered gastric acid secretion and pre-malignant histological features. Severity of the host response to *H. pylori* infection was related to individual ability to produce IL-1, which has been demonstrated to be a potent inhibitor of gastric acid secretion, as well as a proinflammatory cytokine.[117] The histological pathways of *H. pylori* infection and mechanisms involved in carcinogenesis are shown in Figure 6.8. Genetic as well as acquired (*H. pylori*-dependent) determinants co-operate, increasing the risk of gastric cancer up to 90-fold in patients with intestinal metaplasia.

Despite the strong causal link between *H. pylori* and gastric carcinoma, evidence that treatment for *H. pylori* infection may actually prevent gastric cancer is lacking. The long development time of gastric cancer is the main problem in performing such studies. It has been estimated that a trial with sufficient power to answer the question would have to recruit 100 000 infected subjects with a 20-year follow-up.[118] In addition, studies planned to investigate the regression of pre-malignant lesions after eradication gave conflicting results. The progression rate of intestinal metaplasia does not

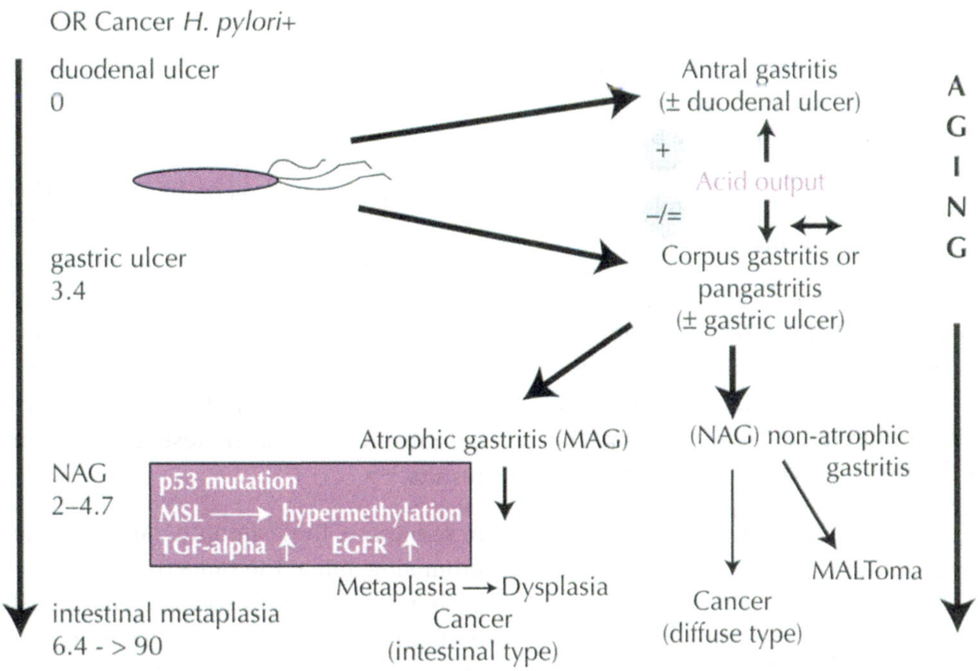

Figure 6.8 The natural history of *Helicobacter pylori* infection and associated diseases depends on aging, as well as genetic and bacterial factors (see text). Determinants of diseases are the acid output for the development of peptic ulcer, and the existence of carcinogenetic mechanisms which trigger the multistep gastric carcinogenesis pathway. On the left, are the odds ratios for gastric cancer associated with different clinical pictures. EGFR, epidermal growth factor receptor; MSL, microsatellite instability; TGF, transforming growth factor.

appear to be arrested by eradication; however, eradicating *H. pylori* leads to resolution of inflammation, elimination of DNA damage and reduction of proliferation, all changes possibly preventing gastric cancer.[114]

Another malignancy strongly associated with *H. pylori* infection is gastric B-cell lymphoma, known as MALToma. Even if the stomach is the most common site of the extranodal lymphomas, MALTomas are rare in adults (0.71 cases/100 000 per year in the USA) and definitely exceptional in children. The association of *H. pylori* infection and MALTomas is based on these considerations: *H. pylori* is found in more than 90% of cases;[119] *H. pylori* infection precedes the development of the malignancy; and eradicating the infection results in the regression of MALToma in approximately 70% of cases of low-grade disease (stage IE).[120] Thus, *H. pylori* infection in a patient with MALToma is a strong indication for eradication treatment.[100] Regression of MALToma after *H. pylori* eradication was described in a 14-year-old female.[121]

Prophylactic and therapeutic immunization

As we have seen, effective therapies against *Helicobacter* require the child to ingest multiple drugs several times a day for at least 1 week.[106] The common occurrence of adverse effects (nausea, diarrhea, abdominal pain and, more rarely, pseudomembranous colitis), the frequently observed low compliance and the high costs suggest the need to evaluate different approaches.

Despite the fact that patients infected with *H. pylori* have a systemic and local immune response,[57] this response does not resolve the infection. Studies on *H. pylori*-specific cellular immunity suggested that *H. pylori* induces a pro-inflammatory cascade and a Th1 response that contributes to the chronicity (Figure 6.2). Since 1993, several groups have developed animal models of *Helicobacter* infection.[122] Using the mouse model, oral immunization with *H. felis* lysates with cholera toxin (CT) as adjuvant resulted in 76–96% of protection. Others challenged the same models using *H. pylori* antigens such as Vac-A, Cag-A, catalase or urease B subunit. On the basis of the results of clinical therapeutic vaccination trials, it is likely that several antigens are needed for a subunit vaccine in humans.

Several groups administered the vaccine to infected animals for therapeutic and not for prophylactic use. Oral vaccination of *H. felis*-infected mice with either bacterial sonicate or *H. pylori* urease B subunit plus CT cured approximately half of the mice. Several groups have now developed murine models of *H. pylori* infection. Eradication in 70–92% was achieved by using recombinant Cag-A or Vac-A as oral antigens, respectively.

Studying the *H. mustelae* ferret model, which represents a natural host–pathogen disease, therapeutic immunization with *H. pylori* urease and CT achieved eradication in one-third of ferrets.

Recently, a clinical trial tested an oral therapeutic vaccine consisting of recombinant *H. pylori* urease apoenzyme coupled with *Escherichia coli* LT in humans; a significant reduction in gastric *H. pylori* density was achieved along with an increase of specific IgA-producing cells.[123]

A different approach was based on the development of attenuated recombinant enteric pathogens expressing *Helicobacter* antigens. Cloning of urease A and B subunits in an attenuated strain of *Salmonella typhimurium* achieved protection in mice. Recently, the safety and immunogenicity of live recombinant *Salmonella typhi* vaccine expressing urease A and B from *H. pylori* in human volunteers has been tested with encouraging results.[124]

In summary, these immunization studies are very promising, but at the same time indicate that many problems are still unsolved: what constitutes the best antigen, the safest adjuvant and the best route of administration? In spite of these uncertainties, it is evident that childhood vaccination could, in theory, prevent one of the most diffuse chronic infections in the world, avoiding consistent morbidity in adult life, and reducing the incidence of gastric cancer later in life.

REFERENCES

1. Marshall BJ, Warren JR. Unidentified curved bacilli in the stomach of patients with gastritis and peptic ulcerations. *Lancet* 1984; **1**: 1311–1315.
2. Windsor HM, O'Rourke J. Bacteriology and taxonomy of *Helicobacter pylori. Gastroenterol Clin North Am* 2000; **29**: 633–648.
3. NIH Consensus Development Panel on Helicobacter pylori in peptic ulcer disease. *JAMA* 1994; **272**: 65–69.
4. International Agency for Research on Cancer. *Monograph on the Evaluation of Carcinogenics Risks to Humans. Schistosomes, Liver Flukes and Helicobacter pylori.* Lyon, France: International Agency for Research on Cancer, 1994.
5. Drumm B, Rhoads JM, Sringer DA et al. Peptic ulcer disease in children: etiology, clinical findings and clinical course. *Pediatrics* 1988; **82**: 410–414.
6. Eastham EJ. Peptic ulcer. In Walker WA, Durie P, Hamilton JR et al, eds. *Pediatric Gastrointestinal Disease: Pathophysiology, Diagnosis, Management*, vol 1. Philadelphia: BC Decker, 1991: 438–451.
7. Nord KS, Rossi TM, Lebenthal E. Peptic ulcer in children: the predominance of gastric ulcers. *Am J Gastroenterol* 1981; **75**: 153–157.
8. Megraud F, Brassens-Rabbè MP, Denis F et al. Seroepidemiology of *Campylobacter pylori* infection in various populations. *J Clin Microbiol* 1989; **27**: 1870–1873.
9. Thomas JE, Dale A, Harding M et al. *Helicobacter pylori* colonization in early life. *Pediatr Res* 1999; **45**: 218–223.
10. De Giacomo C, Valdambrini V, Lizzoli F et al. A population-based survey on gastrointestinal tract symptoms and *Helicobacter pylori* infection in children and adolescents. *Helicobacter* 2002; **7**: 356–363.
11. Banatvala M, Mayo K, Megraud F et al. The cohort effect and *Helicobacter pylori. J Infect Dis* 1993; **168**: 219–221.

12. Fujisawa T, Kumagai T, Akamatsu T et al. Changes in sero-epidemiological pattern of *Helicobacter pylori* and hepatitis A virus over the last 20 years in Japan. *Am J Gastroenterol* 1999; **94**: 2094–2099.
13. Roosendaal R, Kuipers EJ, Buitenwerf J et al. *Helicobacter pylori* and the birth cohort effect: evidence of a continuous decrease of infection rates in childhood. *Am J Gastroenterol* 1997; **92**: 1480–1482.
14. Fiodorek SC, Malaty HM, Evans DL et al. Factors influencing the epidemiology of *Helicobacter pylori* infection in children. *Pediatrics* 1991; **88**: 578–582.
15. Mendall MA, Goggin PM, Molineaux N et al. Childhood living conditions and *Helicobacter pylori* seropositivity in adult life. *Lancet* 1992; **339**: 896–897.
16. Malaty HM, El-Kasabany A, Graham DY et al. Age at acquisition of *Helicobacter pylori* infection: a follow-up study from infancy to adulthood. *Lancet* 2002; **359**: 931–935.
17. Rowland M, Kumar D, Daly L et al. Low rates of *Helicobacter pylori* reinfection in children. *Gastroenterology* 1999; **117**: 336–341.
18. Klein PD, Gilman RH, Leon-Barua R et al. The epidemiology of *Helicobacter pylori* in Peruvian children between 6 and 30 months of age. *Am J Gastroenterol* 1994; **89**: 2196–2200.
19. Parsonnet J, Blaser MJ, Perez-Perez GI et al. Symptoms and risk factors of *Helicobacter pylori* infection in a cohort of epidemiologists. *Gastroenterology* 1992; **102**: 41–46.
20. Kuipers EJ, Pena AS, van Kamp G et al. Seroconversion for *Helicobacter pylori*. *Lancet* 1993; **342**: 328–331.
21. Malaty HM, Engstrand L, Pederson NL, Graham DY. *Helicobacter pylori* infection: genetic and environmental influences: a study of twins. *Ann Intern Med* 1994; **120**: 982–986.
22. De Giacomo C, Lisato L, Negrini R et al. Serum immune response to *Helicobacter pylori* in children: epidemiologic end clinical applications. *J Pediatr* 1991; **119**: 205–210.
23. Buckley M, Mitchell HM, Bolin TD et al. Impact of institutionalization on prevalence of *Helicobacter pylori* infection. *Gastroenterology* 2001; **120**: A735A735(abstract).
24. Drumm B, Rowland M. The epidemiology of *Helicobacter pylori*: where to from here? *J Pediatr Gastroenterol Nutr* 2003; **36**: 7–8.
25. Nguyen AMH, Engstrand L, Genta RM et al. Detection of *Helicobacter pylori* in dental plaque by reverse transciption-polymerase chain reaction. *J Clin Microbiol* 1993; **31**: 783–787.
26. Parsonnet J, Shmuely H, Haggerty T. Fecal and oral shedding of Helicobacter pylori from healthy infected adults. *JAMA* 1999; **282**: 2240–2245.
27. Klein P, Graham DY, Gaillour A et al. Water source as risk factor for *Helicobacter pylori* in Peruvian children. *Lancet* 1991; **337**: 1503–1506.
28. Thomas JE, Gibson GR, Darboe MK et al. Isolation of *Helicobacter pylori* from human feces. *Lancet* 1992; **340**: 1194–1195.
29. Marshall BJ, Goodwin CS, Warren JR et al. Prospective double-blind trial of duodenal ulcer relapse after eradication of *Campylobacter pylori*. *Lancet* 1988; **2**: 1437–1442.
30. Macarthur C, Saunders N, Feldman W. *Helicobacter pylori*, gastroduodenal disease, and recurrent abdominal pain in children. *JAMA* 1995; **273**: 729–734.
31. Oderda G, Forni M, Dell'Olio D, Ansaldi N. Cure of peptic ulcer associated with eradication of *Helicobacter pylori*. *Lancet* 1990; **335**: 1599.
32. Mention K, Michaud L, Guimber D et al. Characteristics and prevalence of *Helicobacter heilmannii* infection in children undergoing upper gastrointestinal endoscopy. *J Pediatr Gastroenterol Nutr* 1999; **29**: 533–539.
33. Tomb JF, White O, Kerlavage AR et al. The complete genome sequence of the gastric pathogen *Helicobacter pylori*. *Nature* 1997; **388**: 539-547. [Erratum, *Nature* 1997; **389**: 412]
34. Falush D, Kraft C, Taylor NS et al. Recombination and mutation during long-term gastric colonization by *Helicobacter pylori*: estimates of clock rates, recombination size, and minimal age. *Proc Natl Acad Sci USA* 2001; **98**: 15056–15061.
35. Euler AR, Byrne WJ, Cousins LM et al. Increased serum gastrin concentrations and gastric acid hyposecretion in the immediate newborn period. *Gastroenterology* 1977; **72**: 1271–1273.
36. Euler AR, Byrne WJ, Meis PJ et al. Basal and pentagastrin-stimulated acid secretion in newborn human infants. *Pediat Res* 1979; **13**: 36–37.
37. Agunod M, Yamaguchi N, Lopez R et al. Correlative study of hydrochloric acid, pepsin, and intrinsic factor secretion in newborns and infants. *Am J Dig Dis* 1969; **14**: 400–414.
38. Kopel FB, Barbero GJ. Gastric acid secretion in infancy and childhood. *Gastroenterology* 1967; **52**: 1101.
39. Christie DL, Ament ME. Gastric acid hypersecretion in children with duodenal ulcer. *Gastroenterology* 1976; **71**: 242–244.
40. Mohammed R, Hearns JB, Cream GP. Gastric acid secretion in children with duodenal ulceration. *Scand J Gastroenterol* 1982; **17**: 289–292.
41. Liebman WM. Gastric acid secretion and serum gastrin levels in children with recurrent abdominal pain, gastric and duodenal ulcers. *J Clin Gastroenterol* 1980; **2**: 243–246.
42. Tam PKH, Saing H. Gastric acid secretion and emptying rates in chidren with duodenal ulcer. *J Pediatr Surg* 1986; **21**: 129–131.
43. Christie DL, Ament ME. Gastrin response to a protein meal in children with duodenal ulcer. *Pediatr Res* 1976; **10**: 353.
44. De Giacomo C, Fiocca R, Villani L. Omeprazole treatment of severe peptic disease associated with antral G cell hyperfunction and hyperpepsinogenemia I in an infant. *J Pediatr* 1990; **117**: 898–993.
45. Habibullah CM, Alis MM, Ishaq M. Study of duodenal ulcer disease in 100 families using total serum pepsinogen as a genetic marker. *Gut* 1984; **25**: 1380–1383.
46. Suerbaum S, Michetti P. *Helicobacter pylori* infection. *N Engl J Med* 2002; **347**: 1175–1186.
47. Mobley HLT. *Helicobacter pylori* urease. In Achtman M, Suerbaum S, eds. *Helicobacter pylori: Molecular and Cellular Biology*. Wymondham, UK: Horizon Scientific Press, 2001: 155–170.
48. Weeks DL, Eskandari S, Scott DR, Sachs G. A H^+-gated urea channel: the link between *Helicobacter pylori* urease and gastric colonization. *Science* 2000; **287**: 482–485.
49. Ilver D, Arnqvist A, Ogren J et al. *Helicobacter pylori* adhesin binding fucosylated histo-blood group antigens revealed by retagging. *Science* 1998; **279**: 373–377.
50. Atherton JC, Cao P, Peek RM et al. Mosaicism in vacuolating citotoxin alleles of *Helicobacter pylori*. *J Biol Chem* 1995; **270**: 17771–17777.
51. Montecucco C, Papini E, de Bernard M et al. *Helicobacter pylori* VacA vacuolating cytotoxin and *H. pylori*-Nap neutrophil activating protein. In Achtman M, Suerbaum S, eds. *Helicobacter pylori: Molecular and*

Cellular Biology. Wymondham, UK: Horizon Scientific Press, 2001: 245–263.
52. Atherton JC, Peek RM Jr, Tham KT et al. Clinical and pathological importance of heterogeneity in vacA, the vacuolating cytotoxin gene of *Helicobacter pylori*. *Gastroenterology* 1997; **112**: 92–99.
53. Covacci A, Censini S, Bugnoli M et al. Molecular characterization of the 128 kDa immunodominant antigen of *Helicobacter pylori* associated with cytotoxicity and duodenal ulcer. *Proc Natl Acad Sci USA* 1993; **90**: 5791–5795.
54. Odenbreit S, Puls J, Sedlmaier B et al. Translocation of *Helicobacter pylori* CagA into gastric epithelial cells by type IV secretion. *Science* 2000; **287**: 1497–1500.
55. Crabtree JE. Mucosal immune responses to *Helicobacter pylori*. *Eur J Gastroenterol Hepatol* 1992; **4**(Suppl 2): S30–S32.
56. Naumann M, Wessler S, Bartsch C et al. Activation of activator protein 1 and stress response kinases in epithelial cells colonized by *Helicobacter pylori* encoding the cag pathogenicity island. *J Biol Chem* 1999; **274**: 31655–31662.
57. Perez-Perez GI, Dworkin BM, Chodos JE, Blaser MJ. *Campylobacter pylori* antibodies in humans. *Ann Intern Med* 1988; **109**: 11–17.
58. Negrini R, Savio A, Appelmelk BJ. Autoantibodies to gastric mucosa in *Helicobacter pylori* infection. *Helicobacter* 1997; **2**(Suppl 1): S13–S16.
59. Oderda G, Vaira D, Holton J et al. Amoxycillin plus tinidazole for *Campylobacter pylori* gastritis in children: assessment by serum IgG antibody, pepsinogen I, and gastrin levels. *Lancet* 1989; **1**: 690–692.
60. Queiroz DMM, Moura SB, Mendes EN et al. Effects of *Helicobacter pylori* eradication on G-cell and D-cell density in children. *Lancet* 1994; **343**: 1191–1193.
61. El-Omar EM, Penman IA, Ardill JES et al. *Helicobacter pylori* infection and abnormalities of acid secretion in patients with duodenal ulcer disease. *Gastroenterology* 1995; **109**: 681–691.
62. Nord KS. Peptic ulcer. In Lebenthal E, ed. *Textbook of Pediatric Gastroenterology and Nutrition*, 2nd edn. New York: Raven Press, 1989: 815–827.
63. Murphy MS, Eastham EJ, Jimenez M et al. Duodenal ulceration: review of 110 cases. *Arch Dis Child* 1987; **62**: 554–558.
64. Apley J, Naish N. Recurrent abdominal pains: a field survey of 1000 school children. *Arch Dis Child* 1958; **33**: 165–170.
65. Hyams JS, Hyman PE. Recurrent abdominal pain and the biopsychosocial model of medical practice. *J Pediatr* 1998; **133**: 473–478.
66. Czinn SJ, Dahms BB, Jacobs GH et al. *Campylobacter*-like organisms in association with symptomatic gastritis in children. *J Pediatr* 1986; **109**: 80–83.
67. Drumm B, Sherman P, Cutz E, Karmali M. Association of *Campylobacter pylori* on the gastric mucosa with antral gastritis in children. *N Engl J Med* 1987; **316**: 1557–1561.
68. Oderda G, Holton J, Altare F et al. Amoxycillin plus tinidazole for *Campylobacter pylori* gastritis in children: assessment by serum IgG antibody, pepsinogen I, and gastrin levels. *Lancet* 1989; **1**: 690–693.
69. De Giacomo C, Fiocca R, Villani L et al. *Helicobacter pylori* infection and chronic gastritis: clinical, serological, and histologic correlations in children treated with amoxicillin and colloidal bismuth subcitrate. *J Pediatr Gastroenterol Nutr* 1990; **11**: 310–306.
70. Glassman MS, Schwarz SM, Medow MS et al. *Campylobacter pylori*-related gastrointestinal disease in children. Incidence and clinical findings. *Dig Dis Sci* 1989; **34**: 1501–1504.
71. Blecker U, Hauser B, Lanciers S et al. Symptomatology of *Helicobacter pylori* infection in children. *Acta Paediatr* 1996; **85**: 1156–1158.
72. Mahony MJ, Wyatt JI, Littlewood JM. Management and response to treatment of *Helicobacter pylori* gastritis. *Arch Dis Child* 1992; **67**: 940–943.
73. Gormally SM, Prakash N, Durnin MT et al. Association of symptoms with *Helicobacter pylori* infection in children. *J Pediatr* 1995; **126**: 753–756.
74. O'Donohoe JM, Sullivan PB, Scott R et al. Recurrent abdominal pain and *Helicobacter pylori* in a community-based sample of London children. *Acta Paediatr* 1996; **85**: 961–964.
75. Bode G, Rothenbacher D, Brenner H, Adler G. *Helicobacter pylori* and abdominal symptoms: a population-based study among pre-school children in southern Germany. *Pediatrics* 1998; **101**: 634–637.
76. Rasquin-Weber A, Hyman PE, Cucchiara S et al. Childhood functional gastrointestinal disorders. *Gut* 1999; **45** (Suppl 2); II60–II68.
77. Tucci A, Corinaldesi R, Stanghellini V et al. *Helicobacter pylori* infection and gastric function in patients with chronic idiopathic dyspepsia. *Gastroenterology* 1992; **103**: 768–774.
78. Talley NJ. Dyspepsia management in the millennium: the death of test and treat? *Gastroenterology* 2002; **122**: 1521–1525.
79. Sullivan PB, Thomas JE, Wight DG et al. *Helicobacter pylori* in Gambian children with chronic diarrhoea and malnutrition. *Arch Dis Child* 1990; **65**: 189–191.
80. De Giacomo C, Fiocca R, Villani L et al. Barrett's ulcer and *Campylobacter*-like organisms infection in a child. *J Pediatr Gastroenterol Nutr* 1988; **7**: 766–768.
81. Hill P, Rode J. *Helicobacter pylori* in ectopic gastric mucosa in Meckel's diverticulum. *Pathology* 1998; **30**: 7–9.
82. Sherman P, Macarthur C. Current controversies associated with *Helicobacter pylori* infection in the pediatric population. *Frontiers Biosci* 2001; **6**: e187–192.
83. Barabino A, Dufour C, Marino CE. Unexplained refractory iron-deficiency anemia associated with *Helicobacter pylori* gastric infection in children: further clinical evidence. *J Pediatr Gastroenterol Nutr* 1999; **28**: 116–119.
84. Milman N, Rosenstock S, Andersen L et al. Serum ferritin, hemoglobin, and *Helicobacter pylori* infection: a seroepidemiologic survey comprising 2794 Danish adults. *Gastroenterology* 1998; **115**: 274–278.
85. Choe YH, Kwon YS, Jung MK et al. *Helicobacter pylori*-associated iron-deficiency anemia in adolescent female athletes. *J Pediatr* 2001; **139**: 100–104.
86. Patel P, Mendall MA, Khulusi S et al. *Helicobacter pylori* infection in childhood: risk factors and effect on growth. *BMJ* 1994; **309**: 1119–1123.
87. Oderda G, Palli D, Saieva C et al. Short stature and *Helicobacter pylori* infection in italian children: prospective multicentre hospital based case–control study. The Italian Study Group on Short Stature and *H. pylori*. *BMJ* 1998; **317**: 514–515.
88. Kerr JR, Al-Khattaf A, Barson AJ, Burnie JP. An association between sudden infant death syndrome (SIDS) and *Helicobacter pylori* infection. *Arch Dis Child* 2000; **83**: 429–434.
89. Elitsur Y. *Helicobacter pylori* and SIDS: the jury is in at last! *Am J Gastroenterol* 2002; **97**: 1576–1577.

90. Dohil R, Hassal E, Jevon G, Dimmick J. Gastritis and gastropathy of childhood. *J Pediatr Gastroenterol Nutr* 1999; **29**: 378–394.
91. Dixon MF, Genta RM, Yardley JH, Correa P. Classification and grading of gastritis. The updated Sydney system. *Am J Surg Pathol* 1996; **20**: 161–81.
92. Marshall BJ, Warren JR, Francis GJ et al. Rapid urease test in the management of *Campylobacter pylori*-associated gastritis. *Am J Gastroenterol* 1987; **82**: 200–210.
93. Luzza F, Oderda G, Maletta M et al. Salivary immunoglobulin G assay to diagnose *Helicobacter pylori* infection in children. *J Clin Microbiol* 1997; **35**: 3358–3360.
94. Oderda G, Rapa A, Ronchi B et al. Detection of *Helicobacter pylori* in stool specimens by non-invasive antigen enzyme immunoassay in children: multicentre Italian study. *BMJ* 2000; **320**: 347–348.
95. Ni Y-H, Lin J-T, Huang S-F et al. Accurate diagnosis of *Helicobacter pylori* infection by stool antigen test and 6 other currently available tests in children. *J Pediatr* 2000; **136**: 823–827.
96. Gold BD, Colletti RB, Abbott M et al. *Helicobacter pylori* infection in children: recommendations for diagnosis and treatment. [Medical Position Papers: The North American Society for Pediatric Gastroenterology and Nutrition]. *J Pediatr Gastroenterol Nutr* 2000; **31**: 490–497.
97. Drumm B, Koletzko S, Oderda S, on behalf of the European Pediatric Task force on *Helicobacter pylori*. *Helicobacter pylori* infection in children: a consensus statement. *J Pediatr Gastroenterol Nutr* 2000; **30**: 207–213.
98. Sherman P, Hassall E, Hunt RH et al. Canadian *Helicobacter* Study Group Consensus Conference on the Approach to *Helicobacter pylori* infection in Children and Adolescents. *Can J Gastroenterol* 1999; **13**: 553–559.
99. Bazzoli F, Cecchini L, Corvaglia L et al. Validation of the 13C-urea breath test for the diagnosis of *Helicobacter pylori* infection in children: a multicenter study. *Am J Gastroenterol* 2000; **95**: 646–650.
100. Malfertheiner P, Megraud F, O'Morain C et al. Current concepts in the management of *Helicobacter pylori* infection – the Maastricht 2-2000 Consensus Report. *Aliment Pharmacol Ther* 2002; **16**: 167–180.
101. Ganga-Zandzou PS, Michaud L, Vincent P et al. Natural outcome of *Helicobacter pylori* infection in asymptomatic children: a two-year follow-up study. *Pediatrics* 1999; **104**: 216–222.
102. Malfertheiner P, O' Connor HJ, Genta MR et al. Symposium: *Helicobacter pylori* and clinical risks – focus on gastro-esophageal reflux disease. *Aliment Pharmacol Ther* 2002; **16** (Suppl. 3): 1–10.
103. Labenz J, Blum AL, Bayerdorffer E et al. Curing *Helicobacter pylori* infection in patients with duodenal ulcer may provoke reflux esophagitis. *Gastroenterology* 1997; **112**: 1442–1447.
104. Moayyedi P, Bardhan C, Young L et al. *Helicobacter pylori* eradication does not exacerbate reflux symptoms in gastroesophageal reflux disease. *Gastroenterology* 2001; **121**: 1120–1126.
105. Wewer V, Andersen LP, Paerregaard A et al. Treatment of *Helicobacter pylori* in children with recurrent abdominal pain. *Helicobacter* 2001; **6**: 244–248.
106. Oderda G, Rapa A, Bona G. A systematic review of *Helicobacter pylori* eradication treatment schedules in children. *Aliment Pharmacol Ther* 2000; **14** (Suppl 3): 59–66.
107. Gottrand F, Kalach N, Spyckerelle C et al. Omoprazolo combined with amoxicillin and clarithromycin in the eradication of *Helicobacter pylori* in children with gastritis: a prospective randomized double-blind trial. *J Pediatr* 2001; **139**: 664–668.
108. Walsh D, Goggin N, Rowland M et al. One week treatment for *Helicobacter pylori* infection. *Arch Dis Child* 1997; **76**: 352–355.
109. Roggero P, Bonfiglio A, Luzzani S et al. *Helicobacter pylori* stool antigen test: a method to confirm eradication in children. *J Pediatr* 2002; **140**: 775–777.
110. Correa P. Human gastric carcinogenesis: a multistep and multifactorial process. First American Cancer Society Award Lecture on Cancer Epidemiology and Prevention. *Cancer Res* 1992; **52**: 6735–6740.
111. Woolf CM. A further study on the familial aspects of carcinoma of the stomach. *Am J Hum Genet* 1956; **8**: 102–109.
112. Huang J-Q, Sridhar S, Chen Y et al. Meta-analysis of the relationship between *Helicobacter pylori* seropositivity and gastric cancer. *Gastroenterology* 1998; **114**: 1169–1179.
113. Helicobacter and Cancer Collaborative Group. Gastric cancer and *Helicobacter pylori*: a combined analysis of 12 case control studies nested within prospective cohorts. *Gut* 2001; **49**: 347–353.
114. Leung WK, Sung JJY. Intestinal metaplasia and gastric carcinogenesis. *Aliment Pharm Ther* 2002; **16**: 1209–1216.
115. Shiao YH, Rugge M, Correa P et al. p53 alteration in gastric precancerous lesions. *Am J Pathol* 1994; **144**: 511–517.
116. Hansson LE, Nyren O, Hsing AW et al. The risk of stomach cancer in patients with gastric or duodenal ulcer disease. *N Engl J Med* 1996; **335**: 242–249.
117. El-Omar EM, Carrington M, Chow WH et al. Interleukin-1 polymorphisms associated with increased risk of gastric cancer. *Nature* 2000; **404**: 398–402.
118. Forman D. Should we go further and screen and treat? *Eur J Gastroenterol Hepatol* 1999; **11**(Suppl 2): S69–S71.
119. Parsonnet J, Hansen S, Rodriguez L et al. *Helicobacter pylori* infection and gastric lymphoma. *N Engl J Med* 1994; **330**: 1267–1271.
120. Bayerdorffer E, Neubauer A, Rudolph B et al. Regression of primary gastric lymphoma of mucosa-associated lymphoid tissue type after cure of *Helicobacter pylori* infection. *Lancet* 1995; **345**: 1591–1594.
121. Blecker U, McKeithan TW, Hart J, Kirschner BS. Resolution of *Helicobacter pylori*-associated gastric lymphoproliferative disease in a child. *Gastroenterology* 1995; **109**: 973–977.
122. Blanchard TG, Czinn SJ. Immunology of *Helicobacter pylori* and prospects for vaccine, *Gastroenterol Clin North Am* 2000; **29**: 671–685.
123. Michetti P, Kreiss C, Kotloff KL et al. Oral immunization with urease and *Escherichia coli* heat-labile enterotoxin is safe and immunogenic in *Helicobacter pylori*-infected adults, *Gastroenterology* 1999; **116**: 804–812.
124. Bumann D, Metzger WG, Mansouri E et al. Safety and immunogenicity of live recombinant *Salmonella enterica* serovar Typhi Ty21a expressing a urease A and B from *Helicobacter pylori* in human volunteers *Vaccine* 2001; **20**: 845–852.

7 Other gastritides

Salvatore Cucchiara and Osvaldo Borrelli

Introduction

Epithelial damage, mucosal inflammation and epithelial cell regeneration represent the histological response of the stomach to injury. The term 'gastritis' implies the microscopic evidence of inflammation, in which all processes of mucosal response to injury are present, whereas the term 'gastropathy' is used for conditions in which epithelial injury is associated with cellular regeneration and the inflammation is not the prominent feature.[1] The definite diagnosis of gastritis is thus exclusively based on histological assessment of biopsy specimens, whereas gastropathies are occasionally diagnosed on endoscopic appearance. For this reason, great confusion has been generated by the inappropriate use of the term gastritis.

Gastritis and gastropathy were previously classified either as primary (idiopathic) or secondary on the basis of the underlying etiology.[2] It is now clear that most cases of unexplained gastritis are caused by previously unrecognized *Helicobacter pylori* (*H. pylori*) infection. Recently, an endoscopic classification of gastritis and gastropathy, has been proposed, that differentiates between erosive and/or hemorrhagic gastritis or gastropathy and non-erosive gastritis or gastropathy.[3] The confounding aspect lies in the fact that some disorders can be either erosive or non-erosive. The most common causes of gastritis are summarized in Table 7.1.

Infectious gastritides

Bacterial gastritides

Helicobacter heilmannii

Although *H. pylori* is by far the most common agent in bacterial gastritides (discussed in detail in Chapter 6), a spirochete-like organism, *Helicobacter heilmannii* (formerly *Gastrospirillum hominis*), has been found to infect the human stomach. H. *heilmannii* is closely related to *Helicobacter* types found in dogs and cats, such as *Helicobacter felis*. In a pediatric population, Oliva et al found a prevalence of infection of 0.3%, whereas in domestic cats and dogs the frequency of infection was up to 100%.[4,5] *H. heilmannii* infection is thought to be a zoonosis, and a fecal–oral route of transmission is suggested. Recently, van Loon et al found an identical *H. heilmannii* strain in a 5-year-old boy and his cats.[6]

Histology shows a typical chronic inflammation, milder than *H. pylori* gastritis, and the presence of a spiral organism with four to six coils per cell and up to 12 flagella at each pole. The bacterium is usually recognized focally and in small groups in the foveola, maintaining a large distance from the surface epithelium. Endoscopic features such as erosions, peptic ulcerations and antral nodularity have rarely been reported. Eradication treatment, as with *H. pylori* infection, should be considered in both humans and animals.

Tuberculosis gastritis

Tuberculosis infection of the stomach is very rare and usually occurs in patients with immune deficiency or after transplantation.[7] In adults, gastric tuberculosis typically involves the antrum and extends to the lesser curvature, although in patients with AIDS it may also involve the esophagogastric junction. Endoscopic features include hypertrophic nodular lesions and multiple ulcers, whereas outlet obstruction, caused by prepyloric narrowing or mass effect, has rarely been described. Histology can show both caseous and non-caseous granulomas. Culture of biopsy specimens is essential to establish the diagnosis,

Table 7.1 Common causes of gastritis and gastropathy

Infectious gastritis	
Bacteria	*Helicobacter pylori*
	Helicobacter heilmannii
	Mycobacterium tuberculosis,
	Mycobacterium avium-intracellulare
Viruses	cytomegalovirus
	herpes simplex virus
	varicella zoster virus
Fungi – Protozoa	*Candida albicans*
	Histoplasma, Mucormycosis
	Anisakis simplex
	Giardia lamblia
	Cryptosporidium
Drugs and other agents	
Aspirin and other non-steroidal anti-inflammatory drugs	
Corticosteroids	
Potassium chloride, calcium	
Chemotherapeutic agents, antibiotics, prostaglandin E_1	
Ethanol, cocaine, methamphetamines	
Gastrostomy tubes	
Endoscopic procedures	
Foreign-body ingestion	
Stress	
Ménétrier's disease	
Bile reflux gastropathy	
Portal hypertensive gastropathy	
Zollinger–Ellison and pseudo-Zollinger–Ellison syndrome	
Lymphocytic gastritis	
Chronic varioliform gastritis	
Celiac gastritis	
Helicobacter pylori lymphocytic gastritis	
Crohn's disease	
Chronic granulomatous disease	
Eosinophilic gastritis	
Collagenous gastritis	
Proton pump inhibitor gastritis	
Pernicious anemia	
Gastritis associated with other autoimmune diseases	
Graft-versus-host disease	

because the organism may not be seen microscopically.

Organisms of the *Mycobacterium avium*–intracellular complex are common pathogens in immunosuppressed patients, and mainly occur in the small and large intestines. However, the stomach may occasionally be involved, with refractory gastric ulcerations.[8]

Viral gastritides

Viral infections of the stomach typically affect immunocompromised or severely debilitated children. Their frequency substantially increases in such children, whereas they are quite rare in healthy subjects. Rare cases of gastric involvement by herpes simplex virus (HSV) or disseminated varicella zoster virus (VZV) infections have been reported.[9,10] Bleeding from hemorrhagic gastropathy has been described in children with influenza A infection.[11] Cytomegalovirus (CMV) is the main recognizable viral agent, occurring in both healthy and immunodeficient children, and has been involved as an etiologic agent in Ménétrier's disease.

Fungal and protozoan gastritides

Fungal infections, such as *Candida albicans*, histoplasmosis and mucormycosis, rarely affect the stomach, although bleeding, gastric ulcers and perforation during disseminated infections have been described in preterm or sick neonates, as well as in malnourished or immunodeficient children.

In adults, acute gastric anisakiasis frequently occurs in countries where the consumption of raw or undercooked fish is high. It is caused by ingesting the organism's larvae. Because humans represent an aberrant host, it is a dead-end infection characterized by an intense acute eosinophilic inflammation. Acute gastrointestinal symptoms, such as upper abdominal pain, nausea and vomiting occur within a few hours, and acute anaphylactic reactions have been described in patients previously exposed to the organism.[12] Endoscopic findings include multiple erosions, edema and single or multiple worms, while histology shows an acute eosinophilic inflammation. The removal of worms with endoscopic forceps induces rapidly symptomatic relief.

Gastric colonization of *Giardia lamblia* has been reported in 0.3% of adults undergoing upper gastrointestinal endoscopy.[13] Because giardiasis is associated with intestinal metaplasia of the stomach, some authors suggest that this organism is not a gastric pathogen.

Gastric outlet obstruction due to enteric cryptosporidiosis has been reported in immunocompromised patients.[14]

Gastropathies due to drugs, toxins and other agents

Acetylsalicylic acid and other non-steroidal anti-inflammatory drugs

It is well known that acetylsalicylic acid and other non-steroidal anti-inflammatory drugs (NSAIDs) can cause gastric injury including gastritis, gastric ulcers and gastrointestinal hemorrhage. Gastroduodenal damage can be seen at endoscopy in 20–40% of adults taking NSAIDs, and the overall risk for peptic complications (hemorrhage and perforation) in these patients is about three times greater than in controls.[15] There are no data on the frequency of upper gastrointestinal injury in children related to NSAID use. Because of the risk of Reye syndrome and the availability of different types of antipyretic drugs, the use of acetylsalicylic acid and NSAIDs in children has significantly diminished.

The routine use of these drugs in different clinical conditions is associated with severe complications such as mucosal erosions and ulceration, and gastrointestinal bleeding. Endoscopic features include hemorrhagic gastric erosions (most often in the corpus) and gastric ulcers (mainly in the antrum). Histology shows foveolar hyperplasia, edema, vascular dilatation and congestion, increased smooth muscle fibers in the lamina propria and, characteristically, a relative paucity of inflammation. The term 'chemical gastritis' is usually employed for this condition.

Several mechanisms are thought to play a role in the pathogenesis of NSAID-induced injury, including inhibition of prostaglandin (PG) synthesis, increased platelet-activating factor, platelet dysfunction, increased oxygen free radicals, increased neutrophil adherence, decreased mucosal blood flow and topical irritant effects.[16] Endogenous PGs are well-known mucosal defense factors, protecting the gastric mucosa against injury caused by a variety of toxic stimuli. PGs are synthesized through cyclo-oxygenase (COX), which is the target of NSAIDs. Two isoforms of COX molecules (COX-1 and COX-2) have been recognized. COX-1 is a constitutively expressed enzyme in many tissues, including the gastrointestinal tract, and is usually active, while COX-2 is an inducible enzyme predominantly expressed at the site of inflammation. It has been shown that the side-effects of NSAIDs are related to COX-1 affinity, while their therapeutic effects are dependent on activity against COX-2.[17]

Corticosteroids

The association between peptic ulcer disease and corticosteroids has never been accepted unequivocally. Ng et al described two cases of gastric perforation in preterm babies treated with dexamethasone for bronchopulmonary dysplasia.[18] A meta-analysis of 71 controlled studies performed by Messer et al demonstrated an increased risk for gastrointestinal ulceration and hemorrhage among adult patients who had received corticosteroids, and the risk was correlated with the dosage employed.[19] Although to date there are no similar studies in childhood it is commonly agreed that, when steroids are administered to children for long periods, prophylactic therapy for gastric mucosal damage should be started concomitantly (see p.109).

Other agents

Gastropathies can be caused by a variety of drugs including potassium chloride, calcium, valproic acid, chemotherapeutic agents and antibiotics, such as penicillin, chloramphenicol, sulphonamides, tetracyclines and cephalosporins. In neonates the administration of PGE_1 can induce gastric outlet obstruction due to antral hyperplasia.[20]

In experimental animals, exposure to a high concentration of ethanol rapidly produces grossly evident focal hemorrhagic erosions. Chronic ingestion of alcohol may also result in human gastric pathology. Endoscopic findings include subepithelial hemorrhages ('blood under plastic wrap'), usually in the fundus and corpus, and small white-based erosions.[21] Histology reveals areas of subepithelial hemorrhage, associated with superficial and deep epithelial damage, and marked edema of the surrounding mucosa. Inflammatory cell infiltrate is usually minimal. Experimental studies in animals have shown that alteration of the mucosal microcirculation might be an early event in the evolution of ethanol-induced gastric injury, as suggested by the occurrence of focal damage of mucosal capillaries and increased permeability within 1 or 2 min after intragastric instillation of a high concentration of ethanol.[22]

Gastric ulcerations have been reported in association with cocaine and methamphetamine abuse. In children requiring enteral nutrition, ulcers and small multiple erosions, usually localized in the proximal stomach, have been described after placement of gastrostomy feeding tubes. Subepithelial hemorrhages and focal erosions are commonly detected after ingestion of a foreign body or endoscopic procedures.

Stress gastropathy

Although the overall prevalence is unknown, most critically ill infants and children are prone to develop stress-related gastropathy. In infants, stress gastropathy is usually related to traumatic delivery, respiratory or cardiac failure, sepsis, hypoglycemia or dehydration, while in older children it is related to severe life-threatening illness (e.g. respiratory or cardiac failure), intracranial lesion, trauma, burns, coagulopathy, or vasculitis.[23] Endoscopic features include isolated gastroduodenal erosions, usually in the fundus and proximal body, and, in severe cases, mucosal ulcerations occurring at multiple sites within the stomach and duodenum (Figure 7.1). The majority of patients develop erosions and ulcers within minutes to hours after the initial insult, and the most common presenting symptoms are hematemesis and melena rather than abdominal

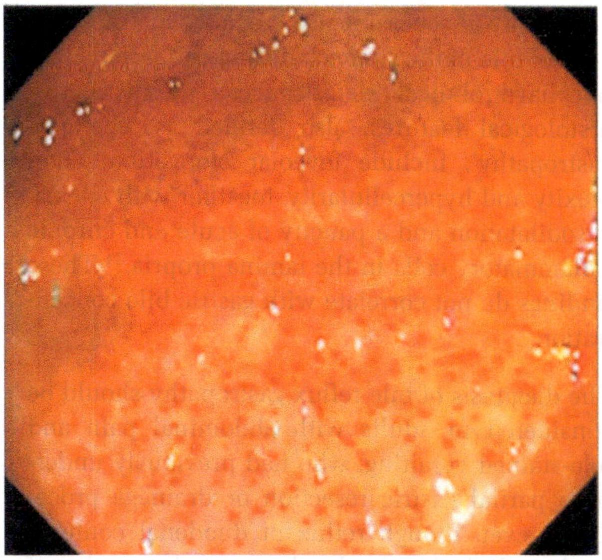

Figure 7.1 Congested gastric mucosa in an infant with stress hemorrhagic vomiting. The mucosa shows non-confluent cherry red spots on a finely granular background.

pain. Recently, Chaibou et al showed that more than 10% of children admitted to an intensive care unit experienced upper gastrointestinal bleeding, but the bleeding was clinically significant in only 1.6% of them.[24]

Alterations of the mucosal microcirculation and mucosal ischemia have been implicated in the pathogenesis of stress-induced gastropathy, even though other mechanisms have been suggested, such as increased acid output, decreased production of mucus and impairment of local prostaglandin synthesis.

Ménétrier's disease

Ménétrier's disease, a rare disorder of unknown etiology, is characterized by enlarged gastric folds due to mucosal thickening in the gastric body. To date, fewer than 100 pediatric cases have been described. Significant differences between adult and pediatric disease in terms of onset, presentation, course and prognosis have been observed.[25,26] In children, the disease often begins abruptly and is usually self-limited, with resolution of clinical features within weeks or months. In contrast, in adults, Ménétrier's disease is a persistent and more severe condition often associated with gastrointestinal bleeding, in most cases requiring surgical resection.

Although this disease has also been reported in the neonatal period, the mean age of onset is 5 years (ranging from 2 days to 17 years). Common features include vomiting, abdominal pain, anorexia, hypoproteinemia and, in some cases, eosinophilia and raised IgE levels. Several studies have confirmed that hypoproteinemia is due to a non-selective increased loss of proteins through the gastric mucosa, occurring in a paracellular fashion via widened tight junctions.[27] In childhood, hematemesis and melena occur rarely, whereas in adults the incidence of gastrointestinal bleeding ranges from 20 to 40%.

The etiology of Ménétrier's disease is unknown, although its acute presentation and self-limited clinical course in childhood suggest an infectious cause. Nearly 30% of affected children show evidence of CMV infection, either through the presence of characteristic inclusion bodies and CMV antigen in the gastric tissue or by serology.[25] It has also been proposed that an increase in both serum IgE levels and the number of peripheral blood eosinophils might be an idiosyncratic antibody-mediated response to the penetration of the gastric mucosa by allergens after the cytopathic effect of CMV on the gastric mucosa.

H. pylori infection has also been reported in children with enlarged gastric folds and protein-losing enteropathy, and its eradication has resulted in disease resolution.[28] However, the classic clinical and histological features of Ménétrier's disease were absent in all reported cases.

Insights into the disease pathogenesis have been gained through the investigation of the mediators of gastric mucosal growth and function, such as transforming growth factor-α (TGFα). The latter stimulates gastric epithelial cell proliferation and mucin secretion, and inhibits parietal cell acid production, in transgenic mice reproducing many altered mucosal features of Ménétrier's disease. As in adult patients, elevated levels of TGFα have been found in gastric mucosal biopsies taken from children with Ménétrier's disease, suggesting a role for this polypeptide in the development and progression of the disease.[29]

Upper gastrointestinal X-ray series identifies the characteristic gastric rugae hypertrophy, predominantly in the fundus and in the corpus of the stomach. Thickened gastric mucosal folds have also been demonstrated by additional diagnostic imaging modalities, such as ultrasound and computed axial tomography. Endoscopy and histology should be performed in all patients to confirm the diagnosis, to search for the pathogen and to exclude different diagnoses, such as eosinophilic gastritis, primary gastric lymphoma, gastric carcinoma, Crohn's disease of the stomach and other conditions in which hypertrophic gastric rugae occur. Endoscopy shows swollen gastric folds predominantly in the greater curvature of the stomach or within the entire body region of the stomach, large quantities of gelatinous mucus and, less commonly, multiple areas of focal erosions in the fundus. Histology usually shows considerable elongation and complexity of the superficial epithelium, so-called foveolar hyperplasia (gastric pit), with reduction of chief and parietal cell glands and often with cystic dilatation, which may extend into the submucosa. An inflammatory infiltrate of eosinophils, neutrophils, lymphocytes and, occasionally, plasma cells is found in the edematous lamina propria.

Bile reflux gastropathy

This is also known as alkaline gastritis and describes an ongoing, chronic condition in which bile-containing intestinal contents reflux into the stomach. In animal studies it has been shown that bile salts and other intestinal contents, such as lysolecitin, break down the gastric mucosal barrier, leading to back-diffusion of H^+ ions and histological injury. Bile acid salts are also potent releasers of histamine and other mediators from mast cells and induce non-specific cytotoxicity.[30]

Duodenogastric bile reflux is thought to be a physiological event during the second phase of the interdigestive motor complex and during the postprandial phase, but it is rapidly flushed out during the third phase of the interdigestive period. It may be considered abnormal when it is frequent, when it is abundant or when it is associated with delayed gastric emptying.

Typical endoscopic findings are 'beefy' redness or erythema and, occasionally, erosions, but the presence of bile in the stomach during endoscopy does not have clinical significance. The distinctive histological features, also defined as 'chemical gastropathy', include foveolar elongation, complexity and hypercellularity, together with edema, vasodilatation and a paucity of acute and chronic inflammatory cells in the lamina propria.[31] These findings do not correlate with gastric bile concentration.

The diagnosis of bile reflux gastropathy should be considered in adults with abdominal pain and bile-stained vomiting, who had previously undergone partial gastric resection or drainage procedures, even though reflux of duodenal contents has been linked to the development of a number of pathological gastric conditions, such as non-specific gastritis, gastric ulcer, gastric carcinoma and non-ulcer dyspepsia. In adults, an association between bile reflux and intestinal metaplasia in the gastric and cardiac mucosa has been reported, suggesting that the latter represents a defense response against a sustained adverse environment, in the same way that gastric metaplasia develops in the duodenum when subjected to a high acid load.[32]

Portal hypertensive gastropathy

Involvement of the gastric mucosa is common in children with intrahepatic or extrahepatic causes of portal hypertension.[33] Endoscopic findings vary from mild involvement, including a snake-skin mosaic pattern of the mucosa, a fine pink speckling and superficial erythema (scarlatina-type rash), to a severe gastropathy, defined by cherry red spots with a diffuse confluence of reddened areas and a hemorrhagic appearance. These patterns seem to be specific for portal hypertensive gastropathy and have not been found in any of 500 endoscopic examinations performed in children without hepatic disease. The fundus and corpus are usually involved, although antral involvement is occasionally observed. Histologically, portal hypertensive gastropathy is characterized by ectasia of mucosal capillaries and venules and by submucosal venous dilatation, with no acute or chronic inflammation.

Hemodynamic disturbances are thought to be involved in the pathogenesis of portal hypertensive gastropathy, because gastric perfusion alterations parallel the severity of mucosal involvement and previous endoscopic sclerotherapy of esophageal varices both in adults and children may exacerbate mucosal congestion and the severity of gastropathy.[34]

Zollinger–Ellison and pseudo-Zollinger–Ellison syndromes

It is intuitive that excessive acid production can result in multiple erosions and frank ulcers in the stomach, duodenum and jejunum. Although rare, this condition may arise from a gastrinoma (Zollinger–Ellison syndrome (ZES)) or from antral gastrin cell hyperfunction with or without hyperplasia (pseudo-Zollinger–Ellison syndrome (PZES)).

ZES is the most frequent ulcerogenic syndrome associated with increased gastrin levels and, in adults, represents the most common of the malignant islet cell tumors.[35] ZES is characteristically associated with increased levels of serum gastrin (hypergastrinemia), which, in turn, causes an overproduction of gastric acid and results in complicated ulcer disease. As would be expected, the most common presenting signs are abdominal pain, nausea, vomiting, hematemesis and melena. Diarrhea occurs less commonly in childhood than in adulthood. ZES can be sporadic or associated with multiple endocrine neoplasia type I (MEN I). ZES-associated MEN-I patients often become symptomatic in childhood and at an earlier age than those with the sporadic form. Thus, if patients show severe peptic ulceration, kidney stones, watery diarrhea and malabsorption with a positive family history of endocrinopathy, MEN-I and nephrolithiasis, ZES should be strongly suspected. The diagnosis of ZES is made if the patient shows an elevated fasting serum gastrin level, gastric acid hypersecretion and either a positive secretin test or a histologically proven gastrinoma.[36] Typically, patients have fasting serum gastin levels of > 100 pg/ml, even though adult patients usually show a level greater than 500 pg/ml, a level greater than 1000 pg/ml is nearly diagnostic of the disease. The basal acid output (BAO) is generally more than 10 mEq/h. The secretin provocative test (2 units/kg, intravenously) has a high diagnostic value; in adults, a rise in the serum gastrin level of 200 pg/ml above the fasting concentration is considered a positive diagnosis. Endoscopic findings are characterized by multiple peptic ulcers, most of which are localized in the duodenum, but the stomach and jejunum are involved less commonly. Recent developments of both radiological and nuclear medicine studies have increased the capability for identifying neoplastic lesions in the majority of patients with ZES. Recommended imaging procedures are computed tomography (CT), magnetic resonance imaging (MRI) and somatostatin receptor scintigraphy (octreoscan); more recently, endoscopic ultrasound has been proposed as the most sensitive imaging modality.[37]

'PZES' is usually used for two distinct entities: antral G-cell hyperplasia, described as an increased number of G cells, and antral G-cell hyperfunction, in which hypergastrinemia occurs in the absence of detectable G-cell hyperplasia.[38] The clinical manifestation of PZES varies from vague features, such as non-specific abdominal pain, vertigo, anemia and occult bleeding, to severe gastrointestinal bleeding. The differentiation between ZES and PZES is based on the response to provocative tests. PZES is characterized by exaggerated serum gastrin release in response to a feeding test, and unchanged or even depressed serum gastrin values after injection of secretin.

Lymphocytic gastritis

Lymphocytic gastritis is characterized by an increase of intraepithelial lymphocytes in surface and foveolar epithelium, together with a variable amount of inflammation in the lamina propria of the gastric mucosa, which ranges from a predominantly lymphocytic pattern to a mixed chronic active pattern. The generally accepted criterion for the diagnosis of lymphocytic gastritis is the finding of 25 or more lymphocytes per 100 epithelial cells.[39]

Lymphocytic gastritis is thought to be a histologic response of the gastric mucosa to several antigens. The main interest comes from its association with

Table 7.2 Conditions associated with lymphocytic gastritis

Varioliform gastritis
Celiac disease
Helicobacter pylori infection
Ménétrier's disease
Drug administration (ticlopidine)

seemingly diverse groups of disorders (Table 7.2), among them celiac disease, where this type of gastritis is very prevalent (see below).

Chronic varioliform gastritis

Chronic varioliform gastritis is a rare disorder of unknown origin, commonly affecting middle-aged and elderly men. To date, few cases have been reported in the pediatric literature. In children, clinical signs arise insidiously, are often subacute or chronic and include epigastric pain, nausea and vomiting, anorexia, weight loss, anemia, protein-losing enteropathy and, in some cases, peripheral eosinophilia and increased serum IgE levels.[40]

The endoscopic features of chronic varioliform gastritis are enlarged and thickened rugal folds bearing erosions and widespread small nodules frequently surmounted by an umbilicated central crater or small rounded erosions (aphthoid nodules). According to the topography of the lesions, three forms can be distinguished: diffuse, when the whole stomach is involved; corporeal, when the lesions are limited to the fundus and proximal body of the stomach; and antral, when they are present only in the antrum. Histology shows a focal or diffuse infiltrate of intraepithelial lymphocytes in the surface and foveolar epithelium. Throughout the lamina propria an inflammatory infiltrate consisting of IgE plasma cells, lymphocytes, neutrophils and eosinophils is observed.

The etiology of chronic varioliform gastritis is still unsettled. An immunological mechanism related to food antigens is suggested by raised serum IgE levels and increased numbers of IgE staining plasma cells. However, owing to a decreased incidence of the disorder and to the fact that the histological pattern is highly reminiscent of celiac gastritis (see below), it has been suggested that chronic varioliform gastritis is only a crude endoscopic expression of a disease that has the characteristic features of lymphocytic intraepithelial infiltration. The macroscopic appearance might appear only at some periods in the evolution of the disease.

Celiac gastritis

An association between lymphocytic gastritis and celiac disease has been reported in both adults and children. Lymphocytic gastritis is found in up to 45% of adults with celiac disease, with a range of prevalence from less than 10% to 45%. Wolberg et al identified ten of 22 adult patients with lymphocytic gastritis characterized by marked infiltration of the surface and superficial pit epithelium by lymphocytes, primarily T cells, with sparing of the deep glandular epithelium both in the antrum and in the body. The lamina propria showed an infiltrate of plasma cells, lymphocytes and rare neutrophils.[41] Recently, it has been shown that the pattern of involvement of the gastric mucosa is predictive of duodenal villous atrophy. Patients with corpus-predominant lymphocytic gastritis are unlikely to have duodenal pathology, whereas those with an antrum-predominant or a diffuse pattern have a 50% chance of coexistent villous atrophy.[42] In a study of 60 children with chronic gastritis, De Giacomo et al found lymphocytic gastritis in nine of 25 children with celiac disease, but in none of 35 children without gluten-sensitive enteropathy. Children with celiac gastritis showed an average of 40 lymphocytes per 100 epithelial cells, compared with an average of three to five in control subjects or patients with *H. pylori*-associated gastritis. Interestingly, at endoscopy, all children showed resolution of the lymphocytic infiltrate after strict adherence to a gluten-free diet.[43]

Recently, some authors have suggested that celiac lymphocytic gastritis may represent an abnormal immunological response to gliadin. It is now recognized that there is a spectrum of gluten-induced intestinal changes, ranging from the classic 'celiac' lesions of total and/or subtotal villous atrophy to more subtle manifestations, such as an abnormal density and subtype distribution of intraepithelial lymphocytes in the small intestinal mucosa. It is conceivable that lymphocytic gastritis, such as lymphocytic colitis, is another manifestation of a mucosal immune response to a luminal antigen, which is maximally expressed in the small intestine.[44] Thus, it is believed that the presence of lymphocytic gastritis in dyspeptic children may be used as an indication to perform a small-bowel biopsy to rule out covert celiac disease.

Helicobacter pylori lymphocytic gastritis

Some authors have suggested that lymphocytic gastritis may represent an idiosyncratic immune response to some local antigen, such as *H. pylori*, although the relationship is still not clear. It has been shown that many cases of lymphocytic gastritis are associated with *H. pylori* infection, and that the eradication brings about significant reduction in the gastric intraepithelial lymphocytic infiltration and dyspeptic symptoms. On the other hand, in adults and pediatric series, *H. pylori* has been detected in a minority of patients with lymphocytic gastritis, whereas the infection was more frequent in control biopsy specimens.

Crohn's disease

Although Crohn's disease (CD) most commonly affects the terminal ileum and/or the colon, involvement of the upper gastrointestinal tract is frequently found in both adults and children. Symptoms such as epigastric pain, early satiety, nausea, vomiting, weight loss and, less frequently, hematemesis and melena are commonly reported in these patients and have previously been related to reflex inhibition of foregut motility secondary to inflammation and partial obstruction of the distal small bowel. It has been shown that macroscopic and/or histological abnormalities are found in up to 70% of adults and 90% of children with CD.[45] Endoscopic findings include patchy or streaky mucosal reddening, edema, single or multiple nodularities, a cobblestone appearance, rigidity of the antrum wall, narrowing of the lumen, aphthoid erosions and linear or serpiginous ulcers (Figure 7.2). Histological diagnosis of gastric CD is best achieved by the detection of epithelioid granulomas and giant cells in biopsy specimens, although focal, non-specific gastritis containing a mixed inflammatory cell infiltrate is observed in a high percentage of patients. Endoscopic and/or histological gastric involvement in CD may be present in the absence of upper gastrointestinal symptoms and may precede diagnostic findings in the small and large bowel. The prevalence of granulomas in bioptic specimens of adult patients is highly variable, ranging from 7 to 83%, whereas in children it is up to 40%.[46] Table 7.3 lists the most common causes of granulomatous gastritis in children. In

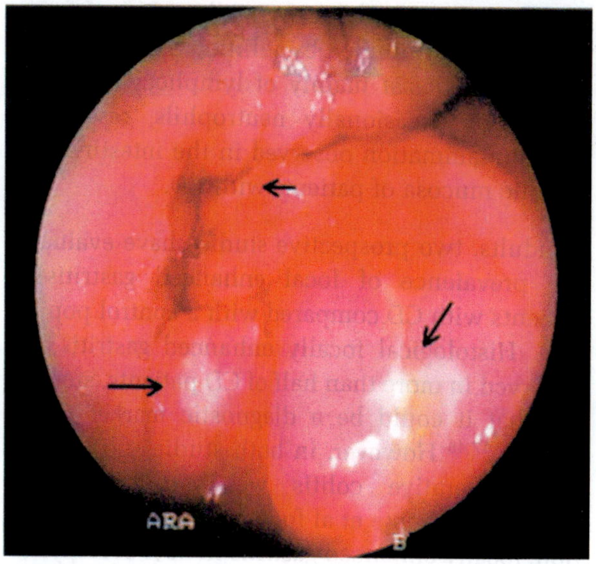

Figure 7.2 Small pre-pyloric ulcers (arrows) in a 14-year-old girl with Crohn's disease.

Table 7.3 Causes of granulomatous gastritis in children

Systemic disease
Crohn's disease
Chronic granulomatous disease
Sarcoidosis
Other vasculitides
Infectious causes
Tuberculosis
Helicobacter pylori
Histoplasmosis
Syphilis
Parasites
Isolated
Idiopathic
Foreign substances

recent years a characteristic pattern of inflammation, the so-called focal enhanced gastritis, has caused great interest, because of the observation that it is quite common and is certainly seen with greater frequency than granulomas in both adults and children. It is found more commonly in the antrum than in the body and is characterized by at least one foveola/gland or small groups of foveolae/glands surrounded by infiltrated inflammatory cells that consist mainly of lymphocytes, monocytes and occasionally neutrophils, resembling focal inflammation observed in the intestinal and colonic mucosa of patients with CD.

In adults, two prospective studies have evaluated the prevalence of focal enhanced gastritis in patients with CD compared with a control population. Histological focally enhanced gastritis was observed in more than half of CD patients, suggesting that it could be a diagnostic marker of the disease.[47,48] However, in both studies no patients with ulcerative colitis were included. Subsequently, Parente et al found, in an adult population, focally enhanced gastritis in 43% of *H. pylori*-negative CD patients, 12% of ulcerative colitis (UC) patients and 19% of controls with no inflammatory bowel disease (IBD). The authors reported a specificity and positive predictive value of focally enhanced gastritis for CD of 84% and 71%, respectively.[49] These results have been confirmed in two pediatric studies. Sharif et al showed that focally enhanced gastritis was present in 65.1% of children with CD, 20.8% of children with UC and 2.6% of children without IBD.[50] More recently, Kundhal et al found focally enhanced gastritis in 52% of children with CD and 8% of patients with UC.[51] This suggested that, although this histological finding was highly suggestive of CD, it could not be seen as a specific diagnostic marker.

Chronic granulomatous disease

Chronic granulomatous disease is a rare group of inherited disorders characterized by impaired phagocyte oxidative metabolism caused by missing components or subunits of the NADPH oxidative complex, resulting in defective intracellular killing of catalase-positive micro-organisms. The most common form of chronic granulomatous disease is inherited as an X-linked recessive trait, although autosomal-type mutations have been described. The disease usually appears during the first two years of life with symptoms and signs of recurrent pyogenic infections, although milder forms of the disease have been described, with onset occurring in adulthood. Characteristic granulomas may develop in any organ system, including the skin, lungs, genitourinary, bone and reticoloendothelial systems. Gastrointestinal involvement has commonly been described. Narrowing of the gastric antrum, with signs of gastric outlet obstruction, such as vomiting, weight loss and epigastric pain, is a rare but distinctive feature of chronic granulomatous disease.[52] Endoscopic features are usually not specific, whereas histology shows mild edema of the lamina propria, chronic inflammatory cells and granulomas characterized by phagocytes, giant cells and lipid-containing histiocytes. Upper gastrointestinal series reveal gastric rugae hypertrophy and narrowing of the antral lumen. Recent developments of nuclear medicine studies have increased the capability of evaluating thickness and inflammatory involvement of the gastric wall.

Eosinophilic gastritis

Eosinophilic gastritis is a component of eosinophilic gastroenteropathy, a rare disease characterized by prominent eosinophilic infiltration of the gastrointestinal tract. The cause is unknown and the mechanisms responsible for gastrointestinal infiltration by eosinophils remain poorly understood. Recently, it has been shown that the production of eotaxin, a protein with 73 amino acid residues and a member of the chekines family, at the site of inflammation promotes recruitment and aggregation of eosinophils in the tissue by up-regulating integrins and enhancing eosinophilic adhesion to endothelial cells. Finally, it may contribute to tissue damage by stimulating the release of highly cytotoxic granular proteins.[53] It has been suggested that food allergy might be a triggering factor in childhood. Associations between eosinophilic gastritis and parasitic infection of the stomach have been described.

Any part of the gastrointestinal tract, from the esophagus to the rectum, can be affected, even though the stomach seems to be the most frequent site.[54] Eosinophilic infiltration may involve the mucosa, the muscularis propria and the serosa. On the basis of the predominant affected layer, the enteropathy has been classified into three different forms: mucosal, which produces clinical features of inflammatory diseases; submucosal, usually producing obstruction; and serosal, producing eosinophilic ascites. The clinical picture depends on the site and depth of the inflammatory involvement. Gastric involvement is commonly associated with abdominal pain, bloating, growth failure, weight loss, nausea and non-bilious vomiting secondary to gastric outlet obstruction. Gastric perforation has also been reported. Patients with associated small bowel involvement may develop protein-losing enteropathy, malabsorption and iron-deficiency anemia. In some patients, an elevated circulating eosinophilic count and raised serum IgE level can be found, although their clinical significance remains unclear.

Endoscopy and biopsy are the main ways to establish the diagnosis. Endoscopic findings, when present, are non-specific and include erythema, antral nodular lesions, ulcers and, rarely, a narrowed lumen. In mucosal involvement, histology is diagnostic in more than 80% of patients, revealing a striking eosinophilic infiltrate of the lamina propria and penetration of eosinophils into the epithelium. Although eosinophils may be a prominent inflammatory component in other types of gastritis, such as *H. pylori* gastritis and chemical gastropathy, the diagnosis can be made in almost all cases through multiple biopsies. Rarely, laparoscopy and full-thickness biopsies are needed to confirm the suspicions.

Collagenous gastritis

Collagenous gastritis is an extremely rare disorder of unknown etiology, To date, fewer than ten cases have been reported in the literature. The condition is characterized by deposition of a subepithelial collagen band greater than 10 μm in thickness. The disorder was originally described by Colletti and Trainer in a 15-year-old girl with refractory *H. pylori*-negative chronic gastritis.[55] It has been reported either as an isolated entity or with synchronous collagenous colitis, collagenous duodenitis, lymphocytic colitis or celiac disease. Clinical features, such as epigastric pain, vomiting, anorexia, postprandial fullness and weight loss are reported. Endoscopic findings include diffuse nodularity, patchy or diffuse erythema, erosions and frank ulcers with hemorrhage. The diagnosis relies on mucosal histology, usually of the fundus and corpus, sharing discontinuous subepithelial collagen deposition with entrapped capillaries and fibroblasts, in association with mild glandular atrophy and mixed inflammatory infiltrate in the lamina propria, including lymphocytes, neutrophils, degranulating eosinophils and mast cells.[56] Depending on the extension of the inflammatory infiltrate, the corresponding surface epithelium may show an increased number of intraepithelial lymphocytes and degenerative changes.

Three major pathogenic theories have been proposed for the increased subepithelial collagen deposition: inflammatory origin, abnormality of the pericryptal collagen sheath and autoimmune injury. It has been suggested that an initial stimulus caused by an infective agent, drug or food allergen may damage the mucosal surface and, in susceptible individuals, determine subepithelial collagen deposition irrespective of the course of gastritis in the rest of the mucosa. However, this theory remains to be demonstrated.

Proton pump inhibitor gastritis

Omeprazole, a proton pump inhibitor (PPI) is now widely used for severe erosive esophagitis in both adults and children. Long-term omeprazole treatment is associated with increased levels of serum gastrin (hypergastrinemia) and gastric mucosal change, including parietal cell hypertrophy, an increased number of antral G cells and an increased number of argyrophil cells.

Pashankar and Israel found gastric nodules or polyps in seven of 31 children receiving omeprazole for more than 6 months.[57] At histology, nodules, ranging from 2 to 4 mm, showed only mucosal edema and disappeared spontaneously during treatment, whereas gastric polyps, of hyperplastic or fundic gland types, persisted during ongoing therapy. Two different pathogenetic mechanisms for polyp formation have been suggested: it has been proposed that glandular obstructions and dilatation may be caused by increased viscosity of gland secretion, because of decreased gastric acid and fluid output; it has also been speculated that hypertrophy of parietal cells, induced by omeprazole therapy, may increase outflow resistance and induce dilatation of the gland.

This gastropathy seems to be benign, but a careful endoscopic follow-up is suggested in children receiving long-term omeprazole therapy.

Pernicious anemia

Pernicious anemia is an autoimmune disorder caused by production of autoantibodies against the parietal cell antigen, H^+/K^+-ATPase, and against the parietal cell secretory product, intrinsic factor, resulting in the loss of parietal cells in the fundus and body of the stomach. The loss of these cells is associated with achlorhydria, vitamin B_{12} deficiency and megaloblastic anemia.[58]

Macroscopically, it is characterized by loss of mucosal folds and thinning of the gastric mucosa. Histology shows a marked infiltration into the submucosa by mononuclear cells, including autoantibody-containing plasma cells, T and B cells, which can extend into the lamina propria between the glands. Cellular infiltration of the mucosa is accompanied by degenerative change in parietal cells. In the fully established lesion, as mentioned, there is a marked reduction in number of gastric glands and the parietal cells are replaced by mucus-containing cells. Recently, studies in murine models of autoimmune gastritis have suggested that macrophages and $CD4^+$ T cells might play a role in the pathogenesis of the disease and that the interaction between the Fas antigen on the target cells and its ligand on the effector cells might be responsible for target cell destruction.[59]

In children the 'adult form' of pernicious anemia has been reported in association with other autoimmune diseases, such as thyroiditis and diabetes mellitus, and with precancerous and malignant lesions. In childhood, pernicious anemia has been attributed to dietary lack of cobalamin, to absence of cobalamin in the ileum or to so-called juvenile pernicious anemia. The last is characterized by absent or very low levels of intrinsic factor in the gastric juice, in the absence of achlorhydria and the absence of intrinsic factor or H^+/K^+-ATPase autoantibodies.[58] It has been suggested that this defect could be due to abnormal synthesis and biological elaboration in the gastric lumen of intrinsic factor.

Gastritis associated with other autoimmune disease

Gastritis with or without atrophy has been described in association with several autoimmune diseases, such as connective tissue disorders, autoimmune thyroiditis and vitiligo. Histological gastritis has been reported in 25 of 27 diabetic children undergoing gastroscopy for upper gastrointestinal symptoms; only half of them had evidence of macroscopic involvement of the gastric mucosa, including erosion and ulcers.[60] A teenage girl with scleroderma and atrophic gastritis has been reported.[3]

Graft-versus-host disease

Acute graft-versus-host disease (GVHD) begins 3 or 4 weeks after transplantation with mucositis, dermatitis, enteritis and hepatic dysfunction. Upper non-specific gastrointestinal symptoms, such as nausea, vomiting, bloating and food intolerance, occur in a large proportion of patients, even in the absence of lower gastrointestinal symptoms.[61] These symptoms seem to be more frequent than those arising from lower involvement and are thought to represent an early manifestation of GVHD. Endoscopic findings vary considerably, ranging from normal-appearing mucosa to exensive mucosal sloughing. Histological findings are diagnostic, including gastric epithelial cell apoptosis and a marked lymphocytic infiltrate in the lamina propria. Upper gastrointestinal GVHD appears to be highly responsive to immunosuppressive therapy.

Clinical assessment

Symptoms of gastritis and gastropathy are usually not specific. The most common presenting clinical features are upper gastrointestinal bleeding and abdominal pain, which can also characterize other clinical conditions (Table 7.4). In very young children, abdominal pain is usually poorly localized and in some cases may manifest as feeding refusal or irritability, whereas in older children and adolescents, the site of pain is more often defined and a mealtime relationship may be present. Rarely, acute abdominal pain, resulting from ulcer perforation, may dominate the clinical presentation. Gastric blood losses can be revealed by chronic signs such as iron deficiency anemia or, alternatively, by acute hemorrhage, with hematemesis and/or melena. Severe bleeding and perforation may occur, resulting in a high mortality rate.

Diagnosis

Both single- and double-contrast barium studies show poor sensitivity in documenting gastritis and gastropathy, although in some conditions they may be helpful. Double-contrast studies of the upper gastrointestinal tract can reveal an irregular mucosal profile, nodularity, ulceration, lumen narrowing or mass effect in almost 50% of children with Crohn's disease.[62] A double-contrast upper gastrointestinal tract series in varioliform gastritis revealed multiple, well-defined, circular filling defects, 3–10 mm in diameter, with central punctate flecks of barium reflecting central superficial ulceration, usually located on antral and/or gastric body hypertrophied rugae.[40] In patients with Ménétrier's disease, upper gastrointestinal series identified the characteristic gastric ruga hypertrophy, localized predominantly in the fundus and proximal corpus. However, in the evaluation of children with suspected organic abdominal pain, a radiology study of the upper gastrointestinal tract is performed to exclude anatomic abnormalities such as malrotation, duodenal bands or antral web.

Upper gastrointestinal endoscopy represents the first-line procedure for investigating gastric mucosal pathology. Endoscopic features have been previously discussed in each section. Although upper gastrointestinal endoscopy is the most reliable method for identifying the bleeding source, defining the lesions and localizing the anatomic site of mucosal damage, the ability to make a definitive diagnosis based on endoscopic appearance alone is limited, because of a poor correlation between endoscopic abnormalities and histological findings. The diagnosis and definition of gastritis and gastropathy are primarily established by histology. A sampling strategy dealing with number and size of specimens taken during endoscopy is recommended. Biopsy specimens should be taken from both endoscopically visible lesions and normal-appearing sites, adjacent to the lesions. Ideally, at least two specimens from each site should be taken. Visualization and knowledge of endoscopic and histological findings of other sites of the gastrointestinal tract (esophagus, duodenum and colon) can be helpful for a correct assessment of the gastric mucosa.

Treatment

Stress-associated gastric ulcer

Controlled data on management and outcome of acute upper gastrointestinal bleeding in children are lacking. Generally, therapy should start by replacing the depleted blood volume with human albumin, saline or Ringer's lactate. If patients have massive bleeding, blood transfusion should be started within a few hours. The use of a nasogastric tube to decompress the stomach, remove

Table 7.4 Differential diagnosis of gastritis and gastropathy

Upper abdominal pain
Esophagitis
Non-ulcer dyspepsia
Cholelithiasis
Cholecystitis
Pyelonephritis
Urolithiasis
Ureteropelvic junction stricture
Spinal cord lesion
Colitis involving transverse colon
Pancreatitis
Gastrointestinal bleeding
Non-gastrointestinal sources
nasopharynx
chest
maternal blood
Munchausen's syndrome by proxy
Gastrointestinal sources
esophagitis
Mallory–Weiss tear
erosions/ulcerations
hematobilia
duodenitis
structural lesions
ectopic pancreas
duplication
polyp
duplication cyst
pancreatitis
Vascular causes
hemangioma (Klippel–Trenaunay–Weber syndrome, blue rubber bleb nevus syndrome)
arteriovenous malformation
connective tissue disorders
bleeding diathesis

gastric secretions and stop the bleeding with saline lavage is routinely recommended, although the efficacy of the gastric lavage has not been confirmed. PPIs have been shown to be effective in the treatment of active bleeding from gastric and duodenal ulcers in adults, and they are widely used in children as well, although scarce data are available. While in adults therapeutic endoscopy is effective in reducing further bleeding and lowering mortality, its efficacy in children has not been formally addressed. However, it is conceivable that endoscopic treatment by an experienced endoscopist might be effective in the treatment of highly selected children with active gastrointestinal bleeding. Surgery should be performed when medical treatment has not stopped the bleeding. (See also Chapter 36).

The use of prophylactic treatment remains controversial. Although in adults the results of a recently published meta-analysis indicated a decreased frequency of stress-associated gastrointestinal bleeding with prophylaxis using the H_2-receptor antagonist, the prophylactic use of cimetidine in a pediatric intensive care unit has not been shown to be effective in preventing gastrointestinal bleeding episodes.[63,64] However, prophylactic treatment with PPIs or sucralfate can be suggested in patients with severe life-threatening illness.

Other gastritis or gastropathy

Two major issues confront clinicians using NSAIDs: prevention of induced ulcers, especially in high-risk groups, and their treatment. In adults, patients at high risk for gastrointestinal hemorrhage and perforation from aspirin and NSAIDs should be considered for prophylactic treatment.[65,66] Risk factors include a history of gastrointestinal complications, age > 60 years, high dosage, concurrent use of corticosteroids and concurrent use of an anticoagulant. Several randomized controlled trials have shown that concomitant use of the PGE_1 analog misoprostol is effective in preventing NSAID-related gastropathy. In a retrospective study, the use of misoprostol during NSAID therapy resolved symptoms in 82% of arthritic children with gastrointestinal complaints, while 18% had recurrence of symptoms after initial improvement.[67] However, no controlled trials are available in childhood and the concerns raised about its use do not support widespread prophylactic treatment at this time. PPIs are certainly a good alternative for prevention of NSAID-related complications. It has been shown in three large randomized controlled trials in adults that omeprazole significantly reduced the total number of NSAID-related ulcers when compared with placebo and ranitidine, and was also more effective than misoprostol in preventing duodenal ulcers and equally so in reducing gastric ulcers.[66]

NSAID-related ulcers may be treated effectively with any approved therapy for peptic ulcer disease. In patients who develop severe dyspeptic symptoms during NSAID use it is preferable to discontinue the therapy. A PPI is the drug of choice for a large ulcer or if NSAIDs must be continued. Despite the fact that several epidemiological studies have shown little interaction between *H. pylori* and NSAIDs in the development of ulcer disease, it has been shown that eradication of *H. pylori* before NSAID therapy can reduce the incidence of peptic disease, suggesting that the organism should be eradicated in any infected patients before they start NSAIDs.[66]

A new class of agents, the so-called selective COX-2 inhibitors, are thought to be associated with greater short-term and long-term gastrointestinal safety compared to regular NSAIDs (non-selective COX inhibitors).[17] These newly introduced drugs, by sparing the COX-1 enzyme and its physiological function, reduce PG-dependent inflammation while leaving protective gastric mucosal PG synthesis intact. Although in adulthood initial studies have shown that they are associated with fewer ulcer complications compared to non-selective NSAIDs and they have already been approved for arthritis treatment, prospective clinical data are still needed to establish the short- and long-term safety profiles in childhood.

In patients with Ménétrier's disease, treatment is generally supportive, with the majority of patients (about 90%) responding to a high-protein diet, diuretic drugs, intravenous albumin transfusion, and salt and fluid restriction.[25–27] Some patients can require an 8-week course of antisecretory agents (H_2-receptor antagonist or PPIs). In rare cases, parenteral nutrition, due to enteral feeding intolerance, or gastric resection for controlling protracted hemorrhage, is necessary.

In ZES, although the occurrence of peptic acid disease can be significantly reduced with an adequate control of gastric acid secretion, through appropriate doses of PPIs, surgical resection of a neoplastic lesion is recommended for any patient. In patients with PZES, antrectomy was usually suggested before the advent of antisecretory drugs. Currently, however, the treatment of choice has become the long-term maintenance of acid suppression by PPIs.[35]

Crohn's disease gastritis usually responds to systemic anti-inflammatory therapies, even though PPIs are effective for symptomatic relief. Gastric-outlet obstruction in chronic granulomatous disease has been successfully managed with prolonged antimicrobial therapy, corticosteroids and immunosuppressive drugs, such as cyclosporin.[68] In eosinophilic gastritis, although an elemental amino acid-based diet occasionally appears helpful, corticosteroids remain the mainstay of therapy in patients. The use of sodium cromoglycate is very controversial, whereas montelukast, a selective leukotriene receptor antagonist, has been successfully used in a 13-year-old girl with acute gastrointestinal disease.[69] In celiac disease the lymphocytic infiltrate usually resolves after strict adherence to a gluten-free diet.[43] The standard treatment for pernicious anemia is regular monthly intramuscular injection of vitamin B_{12} to correct the vitamin deficiency.[58]

REFERENCES

1. Yardley JH, Hendrix TR. Gastritis, gastropathy, duodenitis and associated ulcerative lesions. In Yamada T, eds. *Textbook of Gastroenterology*, 3rd edn. Philadelphia: Lippincot Williams & Wilkins, 1999: 1463–1499.
2. Drumm B, Rhoad JM, Stringer DA et al. Peptic ulcer disease in children: etiology, clinical findings, and clinical course. *Pediatrics* 1988; **82**: 410–414.
3. Dohil R, Hassall E, Jevon G et al. Gastritis and gastropathy of childhood. *J Pediatr Gastroenterol Nutr* 1999; **29**: 378–394.
4. Oliva MM, Lazenby AJ, Perman JA. Gastritis associated with *Gastrosporillum hominis* in children: comparison with *Helicobacter pylori* and review of the literature. *Mod Pathol* 1993; **6**: 513–515.
5. Norris CR, Marks SL, Eaton KA et al. Healthy cats are commonly colonized with '*Helicobacter heilmannii*' that is associated with minimal gastritis. *J Clin Microbiol* 1999; **37**: 189–194.
6. van Loon S, Bart A, den Hertog EJ et al. *Helicobacter heilmannii* gastritis caused by cat to child transmission. *J Pediatr Gastroenterol Nutr* 2003; **36**: 407–409.
7. Subei I, Attar B, Schmitt G et al. Primary gastric tuberculosis: a case report and literature review. *Am J Gastroenterol* 1987; **82**: 769–72.
8. Bodmer T, Miltner E, Bermudez LE. *Mycobacterium avium* resists exposure to the acidic conditions the stomach. *FEMS Microbiol Lett* 2000; **182**: 45–49.
9. Howiler W, Goldberg HI. Gastroesophageal involvement in herpes simplex. *Gastroenterology* 1976; **70**: 775–778.
10. McGluggage WG, Fox JD, Baillie KEM et al. Varicella zoster gastritis in a bone marrow transplant recipient. *J Clin Pathol* 1994; **47**: 1054–1056.
11. Armstrong KL, Fraser DK, Faoagali JL. Gastrointestinal bleeding with influenza virus. *Med J Aust* 1991; **154**: 180–182.
12. Alonso A, Daschner A, Moreno-Ancillo A. Anaphylaxis with *Anisakis simplex* in the gastric mucosa. *N Engl J Med* 1997; **337**: 350–354.
13. Doglioni C, De Boni M, Cielo R et al. Gastric giardiasis. *J Clin Pathol* 1992; **45**: 964–967.
14. Garone MA, Winston BJ, Lewis JH. Cryptosporidiosis of the stomach. *Am J Gastroenterol* 1986; **81**: 465–470.
15. Gabriel SE, Jaakkimainen L, Bombardier C. Risk for serious gastrointestinal complications related to use of nonsteroidal anti-inflammatory drugs. A meta-analysis. *Ann Intern Med* 1991; **115**: 787–796.
16. Wallace JL. Nonsteroidal anti-inflammatory drugs and gastroenteropathy: the second hundred years. *Gastroenterology* 1997; **112**: 1000–1016.
17. Vane JR. Towards a better aspirin. *Nature* 1994; **367**: 215–216.
18. Ng PC, Brownlee KG, Dear PRF. Gastroduodenal perforation in preterm babies treated with dexamethasone for bronchopulmonary dysplasia. *Arch Dis Child* 1991; **66**: 1164–1166.
19. Messer J, Reitman D, Sacks HS et al. Association of adrenocorticosteroid therapy and peptic-ulcer disease. *N Engl J Med* 1983; **309**: 21–24.
20. Peled N, Dagan O, Babyn P et al. Gastric-outlet obstruction induced by prostaglandin therapy in neonates. *N Eng J Med* 1992; **327**: 505–510.
21. Laine L, Weinstein WM. Histology of alcoholic hemorrhagic 'gastritis': a prospective evaluation. *Gastroenterology* 1988; **94**: 1254–1262.
22. Trier JS, Szabo S, Allan CH. Ethanol-induced damage to mucosal capillaries of rat stomach. Ultrastructural features and effects of prostaglandin F_{2b} and cysteamine. *Gastroenterology* 1987; **92**: 13–22.
23. Grjboski JD. Peptic ulcer disease in children. *Med Clin North Am* 1991; **75**: 899–902.
24. Chaibou M, Tucci M, Dugas MA et al. Clinically significant upper gastrointestinal bleeding acquired in a pediatric intensive care unit: a prospective study. *Pediatrics* 1998; **102**: 933–938.
25. Occena RO, Taylor SF, Robinson CC et al. Association of cytomegalovirus with Ménétrier's disease in childhood: report of two new cases with a review of literature. *J Pediatr Gastroenterol Nutr* 1993; **17**: 217–224.
26. Eisenstat DDR, Griffiths AM, Cutz E et al. Acute cytomegalovirus infection in a child with Ménétrier's disease. *Gastroenterology* 1995; **109**: 592–595.
27. Kelly DG, Miller LJ, Malagelada J-R et al. Giant hypertrophic gastropathy (Ménétrier's disease): pharmacologic effects on protein leakage and mucosal ultrastructure. *Gastroenterology* 1982; **83**: 581–589.
28. Bayerdörffer E, Ritter MM, Hatz R et al. Healing of protein losing hypertrophic gastropathy by eradication of *Helicobacter pylori* – Is *Helicobacter pylori* a pathogenic factor in Ménétrier's disease. *Gut* 1994; **35**: 701–704.
29. Sferra TJ, Pawel BR, Qualman SJ et al. Ménétrier's disease of childhood: role of cytomegalovirus and

trasforming growth factor alpha. *J Pediatr* 1996; **128**: 213–219.

30. Bechi P, Amorosi A, Mazzanti R et al. Reflux-related gastric mucosal injury is associated with increased mucosal histamine content in human. *Gastroenterology* 1993; **104**: 1057–1063.
31. Dixon MF, O'Connor HJ, Axon ATR et al. Reflux gastritis: distinct histopathological entity? *J Clin Pathol* 1990; **39**: 524–530.
32. Dixon MF, Mapstone NP, Neville PM et al. Bile reflux gastritis and intestinal metaplasia at the cardia. *Gut* 2002; **51**: 351–355.
33. Hyams JS, Treem WR. Portal hypertensive gastropathy in children. *J Pediatr Gastroenterol Nutr* 1993; **17**: 13–18.
34. Yachha SK, Ghoshal UC, Gupta R et al. Portal hypertensive gastropathy in children with extrahepatic portal venous obstruction: role of variceal obliteration by endoscopic sclerotherapy and *Helicobacter pylori* infection. *J Pediatr Gastroenterol Nutr* 1996; **23**: 20–23.
35. Pisegna JR. The effect of Zollinger-Ellison syndrome and neuropeptide-secreting tumors on the stomach. *Curr Gastroenterol Rep* 1999; **1**: 511–517.
36. Hirschowitz BI. Zollinger–Ellison syndrome: pathogenesis, diagnosis and management. *Am J Gastroenterol* 1997; **92** (S): 44S–48S.
37. Modlin IM, Tang LH. Approaches to the diagnosis of gut neuroendocrine tumors: the last word (today). *Gastroenterology* 1997; **112**: 583–590.
38. Annibale B, Bonamico M, Rindi G et al. Antral gastric cell hyperfunction in children: a functional and immunocytochemical report. *Gastroenterology* 1991; **101**: 1547–1551.
39. Haot J, Hamichi L, Wallez L et al. Lymphocytic gastritis: a newly described entity: a retrospective/endoscopic and histological study. *Gut* 1988; **29**: 1258–1264.
40. Couper R, Laski B, Drumm B et al. Chronic varioliform gastritis in childhood. *J Pediatr* 1989; **115**: 441–444.
41. Wolberg R, Owen D, DelBuono L et al. Lymphocytic gastritis in patients with celiac sprue or spruelike intestinal disease. *Gastroenterology* 1990; **98**: 310–315.
42. Hayat M, Arora DS, Wyatt JI et al. The pattern of involvement of the gastric mucosa in lymphocytic gastritis is predictive of the presence of duodenal pathology. *J Clin Pathol* 1999; **52**: 815–819.
43. De Giacomo C, Gianatti A, Negrini R et al. Lymphocytic gastritis: a positive relationship with celiac disease. *J Pediatr* 1994; **124**: 57–62.
44. Verkarre V, Asnafi V, Lecomte T et al. Refractory coeliac sprue is a diffuse gastrointestinal disease. *Gut* 2002; **52**: 205–211.
45. Schmidt-Sommerfeld, Kirschner B, Stephens J. Endoscopic and histologic findings in the upper gastrointestinal tract of children with Crohn's disease. *J Pediatr Gastroenterol Nutr* 1990; **11**: 448–454.
46. Tobin JM, Sinha B, Ramani P et al. Upper gastrointestinal mucosal disease in pediatric Crohn disease and ulcerative colitis: a blinded, controlled study. *J Pediatr Gastroenterol Nutr* 2001; **32**: 443–448.
47. Oberhuber G, Puspok A, Oesterreicher C et al. Focally enhanced gastritis: a frequent type of gastritis in patients with Crohn's disease. *Gastroenterology* 1997; **112**: 698–706.
48. Meining A, Bayerdorffer E, Bastlein E et al. Focally inflammatory infiltrations in the gastric biopsy specimens are suggestive of Crohn's disease. *Scand J Gastroenterol* 1997; **32**: 813–818.
49. Parente F, Cucino C, Bollani S et al. Focal gastric inflammatory infiltrates in inflammatory bowel disease: prevalence, immunohistochemical characteristics, and diagnostic role. *Am J Gastroenterol* 2000; **95**: 705–711.
50. Sharif F, McDermott M, Path MRC et al. Focally enhanced gastritis in children with Crohn's disease and ulcerative colitis. *Am J Gastroenterol* 2002; **97**: 1415–1420.
51. Kundhal PS, Stormon MO, Zachos M et al. Gastral antral biopsy in the differentiation of pediatric colitides. *Am J Gastroenterol* 2003; **98**: 557–561.
52. Dikerman JD, Colletti RB, Tampas JP et al. Gastric outlet obstruction in chronic granulomatous disease of childhood. *Am J Dis Child* 1986; **140**: 567–570.
53. Daneshjoo R, Talley NJ. Eosinophilic gastroenteritis. *Curr Gastroenterol Rep* 2002; **4**: 366–372.
54. Kelly KJ. Eosinophilic gastroenteritis. *J Pediatr Gastroenterol Nutr* 2000; **30**: S28–S35.
55. Colletti RB, Trainer TD. Collagenous gastritis. *Gastroenterology* 1989; **97**: 1552–1555.
56. Pulimood AB, Ramakrishna BS, Mathan MM. Collagenous gastritis and collagenous colitis: a report with sequential histological and ultrastructural findings. *Gut* 1999; **44**: 881–885.
57. Pashankar DS, Israel DM. Gastric polyps and nodules in children receiving long-term omeprazole therapy. *J Pediatr Gastroenterol Nutr* 2002; **35**: 658–662.
58. Toh BH, van Driel IR, Gleeson PA. Pernicious anemia. *N Engl J Med* 1997; **337**: 1441–1448.
59. Nishio A, Katakai T, Oshima C et al. A possible involvement of Fas–Fas ligand signaling in the pathogenesis of murine autoimmune gastritis. *Gastroenterology* 1996; **111**: 959–967.
60. Burghen GA, Murrell LR, Whitington GL et al. Acid peptic disease in children with type I diabetes mellitus: a complicating relationship. 1992; **146**: 718–722.
61. Weisdorf DJ, Snover DC, Haake R. Acute upper gastrointestinal graft-versus-host disease: clinical significance and response to immunosoppressive therapy. *Blood* 1990; **76**: 624–629.
62. Ruuska T, Vaajalahati P, Arajarvi P et al. Prospective evaluation of upper gastrointestinal mucosal lesions in children with ulcerative colitis and Crohn's disease. *J Pediatr Gastroenterol Nutr* 1994; **19**: 181–186.
63. Cook DJ, Reeve BK, Guyatt GH et al. Stress ulcer prophylaxis in critically ill patients: resolving discordant meta-analyses. *JAMA* 1996; **275**: 308–314.
64. Lacroix J, Nadeau D, Laberge S et al. Frequency of upper gastrointestinal bleeding in a pediatric intensive care unit. *Crit Care Med* 1992; **20**: 35–42.
65. Goldstein JL, Brown RD. NSAID-induced ulcers. *Curr Treat Options Gastroenterol* 2000; **3**: 149–157.
66. Lanza FL. A guideline for the treatment and prevention of NSAID-induced ulcers. *Am J Gastroenterol* 1998; **93**: 2037–2046.
67. Gazarian M, Berkovitch M, Koren G et al. Experience with misoprostol therapy for NSAID gastropathy in children. *Ann Rheum Dis* 1995; **45**: 277–280.
68. Rash JR, Tang HB, Mayer L et al. Treatment of intractable gastrointestinal manifestations of chronic granulomatous disease with cyclosporine. *J Pediatr* 1995; **126**: 143–145.
69. Neustrom MR, Friesen C. Treatment of eosinophilic gastroenteritis with montelukast. *J Allergy Clin Immunol* 1999; **104**: 506.

8 HIV and the intestine

Nigel C Rollins

Introduction

It was estimated that at the end of 2002 there were 42 million people worldwide with HIV-1 infection, over 29 million of whom were living in sub-Saharan Africa. Despite some encouraging signs that the rate of new infections is stabilizing, there are still about 3 million children under 15 years of age living with HIV. As a case in point, approximately 68 000 children with HIV infection were born in South Africa in 2002, and AIDS-related complications now account for 60–80% of pediatric admissions there and 70% of hospital deaths. Gastrointestinal disease, mainly diarrhea, accounts for about a third of these admissions.

Pathophysiology: transmission and progression of HIV disease

The gut, more than any other organ in the body, plays a critical role in the vertical transmission and progression of HIV infection. This reflects not only its nutritional function but also its central activity in immune programming and regulation. More than half the body's total lymphoid tissue is found in the bowel; as HIV infects lymphocytes with CD4 or other co-receptors, this makes the bowel an ideal target for primary infection and a site for viral replication and seeding.

Intestinal lymphoid tissue is organized into distinct structures including the tonsils, Peyer's patches (mainly in the ileum) and mesenteric lymph nodes, and is also diffusely spread throughout the mucosal epithelium and lamina propria. Activation of both the organized and diffuse elements of the gut immune system depends on presentation of antigens to T and B lymphocytes lying beneath the epithelium. M cells are specialized epithelium found in the follicle-associated epithelium (FAE) that overlies Peyer's patches in the small intestine and lymphoid follicles in the rectum, and are also found in rich supply in the tonsils. These are capable of transporting macromolecules and micro-organisms, including viruses such as polio, to macrophages or possibly dendritic cells in the lamina propria. These latter cells are the professional antigen-presenting cells that facilitate presentation of antigens to activated and possibly non-activated T cells. However, intestinal epithelium itself can also generate antigen-specific responses and may be able to function as antigen-presenting cells. Complementing these responses are intraepithelial lymphocytes, interspersed throughout the mucosa, that produce cytokines which support humoral and cell-mediated responses. Finally, the lamina propria throughout the gut contains the bulk of the immune effector cells including T and B lymphocytes, plasma cells, macrophages, mast cells and some eosinophils and neutrophils.

Primary infection with ingested HIV depends on the virus gaining access to the lamina propria, where, in early infection, it replicates primarily in lymphocytes.[1,2] The exact mechanism for entry to the lamina propria is not fully understood, but may be through a variety of routes, and is likely to be a complex process modified by viral characteristics, gut mucosal receptors and the factors that promote or impede the interaction.

Direct passage through disruptions in mucosa or between immature mucosal junctions is possible. However, longitudinal gut permeability studies in children born to HIV-infected mothers do not support this mechanism.[3] Rather, increased permeability, without clinical symptoms, may be present soon after children become infected.

Recent work shows that gut mucosa does not express the familiar CD4 binding sites that the HIV-1 gp120 protein commonly uses for attaching to and thereby infecting mononuclear cells.[4] Rather, early infection is dependent on HIV strains binding to alternative sites, namely the primary receptor galactosyl ceramide (GalCer) and the CCR5 co-receptor, which are expressed on upper gastrointestinal epithelium.[5] This is supported by the observation that HIV-1 isolates from acutely infected persons are predominantly R5 viruses, i.e. macrophage-tropic HIV that require CCR5 for cell entry (in contrast to R4 viruses, which are lymphocyte-tropic requiring the CXCR4 chemokine co-receptor).[6] Once attached, the virus is probably translocated across the epithelial cell and presented to T lymphocytes that express the same CCR5 co-receptor. The lamina propria now becomes a potent site for viral replication. M cells, in mouse and rabbit *ex vivo* systems, can transport HIV-1 to mononuclear cells, but human M cells have not been shown to take up and transport HIV in the same way.[7]

The gut has a number of defense mechanisms against primary infection apart from maternal factors. The rapid passage of ingested amniotic fluid or maternal blood limits contact time with M cells expressed on the surface of the tonsils. Gastric acid would normally inhibit HIV in the stomach, but this is reduced in neonates and young infants. Mucin produced by goblet cells and the rapid turnover of the intestinal mucosa provide additional mechanical barriers to HIV attachment.

However, mother-to-child transmission of HIV through breast feeding depends on a number of risk factors other than the susceptibility of the gut to HIV. Increased viral load in breast milk is correlated with high plasma viral load and decreased CD4 count in the mother, and is associated with higher transmission.[8–10] These conditions are found in the early stages of new infection or in advanced disease. It is not clear, however, whether it is cell-associated or cell-free virus that is more important for transmission. Other breast-milk factors such as HIV-1-specific IgG and secretory leukocyte protease inhibitor (SLPI) have HIV-1 inhibitory activity *in vitro*.[11] SLPI acts on the target cell rather than the virus and inhibits internalization of HIV-1 rather than initial binding.[12]

Infant feeding practices may significantly influence the way in which these non-intestinal factors interact: exclusive breast feeding results in a greater volume of milk being ingested and hence increases the HIV load presented to the infant gut. However, it also increases the protective breast-milk factors reaching the infant and that promote the development and maintain the integrity of the mucosa and which may have direct anti-HIV effects.[13] Exclusive breast feeding is associated with fewer breast health problems, e.g. clinical and subclinical mastitis that are associated with increased breast-milk viral load.[14] Infant feeding practices also contribute to the establishment of different enteric microflora that might significantly affect the priming or responses of intestinal lymphoid cells or dendritic cell.[15–17] This could, theoretically, modify adherence or facilitate infection of HIV, although this interesting concept has not been explored to date. Innate responses such as lactoferrin and lysozymes that are secreted by exocrine glands onto mucosal surfaces are bactericidal, but their protective capacity in HIV is unknown. There is also renewed interest around secretory IgA and IgM that can inhibit transcytosis of HIV-1 across enterocytes in *in vitro* models.[18,19] Passive immunization of macaque monkeys with monoclonal antibodies against the HIV-1 gp120 protein, given either orally or applied locally, protected against mucosal challenges with HIV-1.[20] This raises the possibility of a vaccine strategy, similar to that used against hepatitis B, of combining active and passive immunization to induce effective mucosal protection against HIV-1.

Once HIV infection is established the gut serves as a major reservoir for viral amplification. CD4 lymphocytes in the lamina propria are infected and progressively depleted;[21] this precedes the eventual decrease in CD4 counts in the peripheral circulation and other sites.[22,23] IgA-secreting plasma cells, especially the IgA2 subclass, are lost early in disease, resulting in reduced secretory IgA, thereby predisposing the gut to infection with enteric pathogens.[24–27] Responses to oral vaccines may also be impaired, raising concern about the effectiveness of putative rotavirus vaccines in areas of high HIV seroprevalence.[28] Local cytokine responses have been extensively reported, although it is still not entirely clear whether they influence the development of AIDS or HIV enteropathy or are simply the consequence of the latter.[29,30] These responses may be the consequence of opportunistic infections or the direct effect of HIV on the mucosa.

Diarrhea

Persistent and recurrent diarrheas are amongst the most frequent manifestations of HIV/AIDS in both children and adults, especially in developing countries, where diarrhea is associated with growth failure, weight loss and death. In Zaire, 85% of adults admitted with persistent diarrhea had HIV infection.[31] Among children presenting to a primary health care facility in South Africa, a history of persistent diarrhea in the preceding 3 months strongly predicted HIV infection (odds ratio 4.8; CI 2.5–9.3 and positive predictive value of 63%). In South Africa, the profile of children admitted with diarrheal diseases has changed, with increasing prevalence of persistent diarrhea and loss of seasonal peaks of acute diarrhea. HIV-infected children admitted to hospital with diarrhea have more severe symptoms than children uninfected by HIV;[32] they frequently have severe co-infections such as pneumonia, pseudomonal skin sepsis and tuberculosis (TB). These result in longer periods of admission and case fatality rates in the order of 27%. In Zaire, children with HIV and persistent diarrhea had an 11-fold increased risk of death compared with uninfected controls. Hence, in developing countries, HIV-related diarrheal diseases represent a major burden on both caregivers and health resources. The availability of antiretroviral drugs in North America and Europe has dramatically altered the natural history of HIV infection and has reduced the incidence of gastrointestinal disease due to opportunistic infections.[33,34] This has shifted much of the scientific interest and research funding to other complications such as lipodystrophy.

Although there is considerable knowledge of the pathophysiology and management of diarrhea in adults with AIDS, less is known about this problem in children. Opportunistic infections and fat malabsorption are common causes of prolonged and recurrent diarrhea in infected adults.[35,36] Among children with HIV, carbohydrate intolerance is common and may follow acute infections with rotavirus or other common enteropathogens.[37–39] In resource-poor settings, the optimal management of HIV-related diarrhea remains largely unexamined. Even after 25 years of the epidemic, fewer than 40% of countries with a high HIV seroprevalence have published national recommendations for the management of HIV-associated diarrhea.[40]

Mucosal structure and function in HIV-related diarrhea

A number of intestinal mucosal structural and functional abnormalities have been described in HIV-infected children with diarrhea. Their pathogenesis is multifactorial and includes the direct effect of pathogens, other inflammatory processes, malnutrition and the direct effect of HIV itself. Variable degrees of villous atrophy, crypt hyperplasia and increased inflammatory cells in the lamina propria are found in the small intestine of children with diarrhea (Figure 8.1), although these can be present without symptoms, and are often diffusely spread throughout the upper duodenum and jejunum.[41,42] Even when the mucosa appears normal on conventional histology, short and irregular microvilli may be evident on electron microscopy and tubuloreticular inclusions may be seen in endothelial cells.[43] In the large bowel, loss

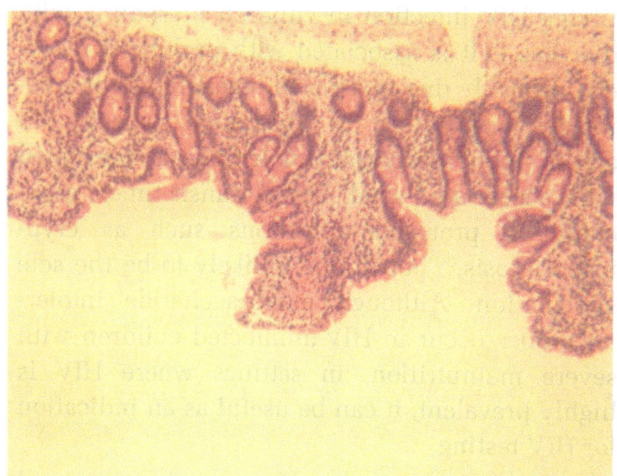

Figure 8.1 Villous blunting with crypt hyperplasia and increased inflammatory cells in the lamina propria are evident in this small-intestinal biopsy of an HIV-infected child.

of mucin-producing cells is accompanied by an increase in inflammatory cells, especially mast cells; crypt abscesses and apoptosis are also detected. Although up to 75% of adult HIV-related diarrhea has been attributed to enteric pathogens, causal agents have not been demonstrated with the same frequency in children.[44] This may be explained by the difficulty of obtaining appropriate specimens from small children or identifying pathogens such as microsporidia; in addition, alternative pathways of diarrhea may be involved, as seen in other causes of severe malnutrition.

Carbohydrate malabsorption is commonly found in HIV-infected children with persistent diarrhea.[37] This may be the consequence of preceding enteric infection but in most cases the precipitant is unknown. Intestinal biopsies in these children do not always demonstrate villous atrophy.[45,46] An abnormal breath H_2 analysis in the presence of relatively normal mucosal architecture suggests a non-specific brush-border disorder rather than a specific enzyme deficiency.[37,46] Gut permeability, measured by the dual sugar absorption test, is increased, especially in patients with more advanced disease;[41] however, this may also be increased in asymptomatic patients and early in disease.[3,47] Furthermore, lactose malabsorption is not always associated with clinical symptoms such as diarrhea or growth failure.[48] Monosaccharide intolerance has been described in African children with HIV and severe diarrhea, and has an 87% positive predictive value for identifying HIV infection in children presenting with diarrhea.[49] It is associated with prolonged recovery, probably due to delayed regeneration of enterocytes and return of absorptive capacity. In adults, monosaccharide intolerance is associated with accelerated small bowel transit times, especially in protozoal infections such as cryptosporidiosis,[50] but this is unlikely to be the sole explanation. Although monosaccharide intolerance does occur in HIV-uninfected children with severe malnutrition, in settings where HIV is highly prevalent, it can be useful as an indication for HIV testing.

Other macronutrients and micronutrients may not be adequately absorbed or there may be increased losses in stools. Bile salt and fat malabsorption are associated with low-grade enteropathies in adult patients with AIDS,[51] but are not consistent findings in HIV-infected children.[39,52] Protein maldigestion and malabsorption are seen in children with severe carbohydrate malabsorption and indicate a profound disruption of normal gastrointestinal function and absorptive capacity. Enteric cytomegalovirus or bacterial infections, and occasionally intestinal Kaposi's sarcoma, may present in adults as a protein-losing enteropathy.[53,54] In children, protein-losing enteropathy, suggested by increased fecal α_1-antitrypsin, has also been reported, but specific enteric pathogens were not identified.[39] Iron malabsorption has been reported in children with symptomatic HIV with decreased D-xylose absorption, suggesting a general loss of absorptive capacity rather than a specific iron transport defect.[55] Vitamin A is absorbed even in the presence of severe diarrhea;[56] health-care personnel should aim, therefore, to provide vitamin A supplements, according to the WHO/UNICEF Integrated Management of Childhood Illnesses protocol, to all children presenting with persistent diarrhea at primary health-care facilities.[57]

Host responses and susceptibility

The relationship between the risk and type of enteric infection and HIV-viral activity, or host immune competence as measured by CD4 counts, has been established in HIV-infected adults in developed countries, and to a limited extent in developing countries. The rapid and pronounced loss of CD4 T-helper cells in gut mucosa that precedes losses in the peripheral blood might explain the loss of local defenses to opportunistic infections. In Uganda, HIV-infected adults with lower CD4 counts were at greater risk of non-typhi salmonellae septicema and other opportunistic infections[58] (Figure 8.2).

Children with reduced CD4 counts have more severe diarrhea, i.e. higher fluid losses and more prolonged disease; this is often due to cryptosporidiosis.[45,59] Local gut immunity may also play an important role in both local susceptibility and disease progression. Total IgA in stool is decreased in symptomatic children with severe diarrhea; elevated serum IgA, which may be due to selective increase of the IgA1 subclass, is related to decreased CD4 counts.[26,60] These changes occur early in pediatric HIV infection and reflect the disturbance of the gut mucosal immune system.

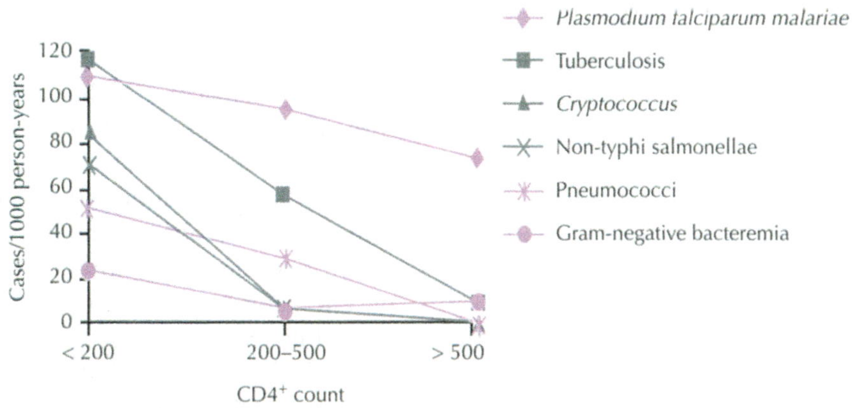

Figure 8.2 CD4 counts in HIV-infected adults presenting with specific infections in Uganda.

HIV enteropathy

HIV enteropathy is typified by weight loss, diarrhea and characteristic endoscopic and pathological appearances without any identifiable enteric pathogens.[61] These include reduced villous height, increased crypt length, focal enterocyte vacuolization, and hyporegeneration and dysmaturation of intestinal cells.[62,63] Several hypotheses have been proposed to explain these findings, including a mucosal immune reaction to HIV-infected cells[64] or to signals from regulatory T cells, the effect of bacterial overgrowth or bile salt malabsorption,[65,66] unidentified enteric pathogens, or direct small-intestinal damage by HIV itself. The latter hypothesis is supported by the finding of HIV-infected mononuclear cells in the gut, epithelial hypoproliferation, altered intestinal cell differentiation[67] and reduced apoptotic lymphoid cells following the onset of antiretroviral therapy.[68] Intestinal cell lines directly infected with HIV clade B strains have reduced brush-border enzyme activity and altered calcium responses, suggesting that direct infection of enterocytes with HIV may modify absorptive and secretory function.[69] Some of these effects may be due to activation of the HIV-1 transactivating factor protein gene (*Tat*) which is an early immediate regulatory gene that is essential for virus integration and protein expression.[70] Circulating cytokines and lymphokines such as interleukin-1β and tumor necrosis factor-α may have a role in diarrhea due to bacteria, protozoa, cytomegalovirus or where there is no identifiable infection.[30,53] These may produce diarrhea through their secretory effects in the colon rather than by altering mucosal barriers. There are isolated reports of collagenous colitis in adults with chronic watery diarrhea, but none in children.[71]

Enteric infections in HIV-infected children

Surprisingly little is known about the patterns of enteric infection in HIV-infected children, timing of their acquisition, their individual effects on children's health and nutrition, and their relationship to HIV activity and host immune status. There is reasonable consistency between the few studies that have been conducted in Africa describing the pathogens isolated in children presenting with HIV and diarrhea.[44,72] Enteric pathogens that commonly cause acute diarrhea in children uninfected by HIV also frequently result in diarrhea in HIV-infected children.[73] Adenovirus 40/41 and astrovirus have been identified in children with persistent diarrhea, but their relative contribution to the burden of diarrheal disease in HIV infection is not known.[74–76] Only a few pathogens seem to be opportunistic in HIV-infected children with diarrhea. The most prevalent of these are *Candida*, *Cryptosporidium parvum* and cytomegalovirus (CMV); these usually cause oropharyngeal lesions and invasive lesions elsewhere in the gut or persistent diarrhea. Additional pathogens, which occasionally cause diarrhea or other symptoms in children with symptomatic HIV disease, may include herpes simplex virus and *Mycobacterium avium* intracellulare. *Mycobacterium tuberculosis* may be isolated from stools in both adults and children with no evidence of pulmonary TB. Perhaps surprisingly, there is little to suggest any association between shigellosis and HIV. One study from North America described an increase in prevalence in HIV-infected homosexuals; however, numerous reports from the African continent do not support this finding. It may be that the virulence of *Shigella* readily overcomes even the intact mucosal defense system and so the immunocompromised individual is not at any greater risk. Another possibility is that because *Shigella* must be taken up by enteric immune cells in order to be invasive, an immune system that is not competent may, paradoxically, be protective. *Isospora belli*, a significant enteric pathogen in HIV-infected adults[77–79] has not been commonly reported amongst HIV-infected children in Africa.[72,80] Little is known about the role of the *Microsporidia* spp and the newly recognized protozoan enteric pathogen *Cyclospora cayetanensis* in AIDS-associated diarrhea in children.[81–83] Laboratory identification of several of these infections may be very difficult, requiring special stains or techniques that are expensive or unavailable in most developing countries. In children, the proportion of diarrhea cases due to infective agents may, therefore, be underestimated.

Cryptosporidium parvum

C. parvum is a common cause of diarrhea in both HIV-infected and uninfected children, but in the immunocompromised child it results in prolonged disease and high fluid losses.[84–86] It may be responsible for up to 25% of persistent diarrhea in HIV-infected children in sub-Saharan Africa.[59,72] Infection is usually through person-to-person contact, food contamination (e.g. unwashed raw vegetables or fruit) and contaminated water. Two distinct genotypes cause clinical disease in HIV-infected children: human and bovine (calf) types.[87] The clinical and epidemiological differences between these genotypic variations is unclear, but the human genotype may be associated with a less severe clinical course in HIV-infected adults. Identifying *C. parvum* is difficult on direct microscopy; without experienced laboratory staff and appropriate stains, the diagnosis is easily missed.[88] In most developing countries, enzyme-linked immunosorbent assay (ELISA) or immunofluorescence methods to enhance identification rates are not routinely available. Shedding of the parasite is sporadic, and several stools should be examined to confirm or reject the diagnosis. Endoscopy and duodenal biopsy and aspirate examination further enhance the diagnostic yield.[45]

The most common site of infection is the duodenum, where it causes marked, though sometimes patchy, villous atrophy and reactive epithelial changes. Co-infection with CMV may exacerbate these responses. Other sites of infection include the stomach and colon (where cryptitis and apoptosis may occur) and the bile tract (which may be associated with pancreatitis).[89] Gut permeability may be markedly increased and fat malabsorption may be significant.[90,91] Protracted, or even intractable, secretory diarrhea with high fluid losses follows. It is often associated with weight loss, and up to 2–4% loss of body weight has been reported.[36] In HIV-infected children infection and a higher case fatality rate are more common in those with a lower CD4 count.[59]

In developing countries management is largely supportive to prevent severe dehydration and to recover lost weight through extended nutritional support. Several antimicrobial agents including spiromycin, parmomycin, azithromycin and nitazoxanide, and other approaches such as oral bovine immunoglobulin have been used with limited benefit.[92–94] The most effective treatment by far remains highly active antiretroviral treatment, which restores gut mucosal CD4 cells with eradication of opportunistic infections including *C. parvum*.[95]

Candida

Oral thrush is one of the most characteristic signs in young children with HIV/AIDS, appearing as white–yellow plaques that cannot be easily scraped off the buccal mucosa. It is not, however, reliable or specific as an indicator of HIV infection; recurrent episodes are better markers of HIV-infection in both children and adults. Thrush is often reported as a risk factor for breast-feeding transmission of HIV, presumably by inducing mucosal breaks facilitating viral entry, but the direction of causality is unclear from the available data.[96,97] Gut colonization follows oral infection with *Candida* species. Candidiasis of the mouth and esophagus is associated with poor appetite and weight loss. Esophageal inflammation is reported in up to 40% of children with AIDS and can be severe;[45,98] occasionally a necrotizing esophagitis which may bleed or even perforate can occur. The main differential diagnosis is herpes, CMV and *Mycobacterium avium* intracellulare. *Candida* may also produce inflammation and erosions in the gastric mucosa and the large and small intestines. The parasite can occasionally cause local abscesses, which may disseminate resulting in generalized candidiasis. Endoscopy and biopsy are generally required to diagnose invasive *Candida*, but in developing countries a high index of suspicion may be all that is available. Fluconazole is generally effective, although resistance does occur and higher doses are sometimes needed.

Cytomegalovirus

Gastrointestinal CMV infection in children most commonly presents with fever and persistent diarrhea.[99,100] CMV-associated disease including retinitis, pneumonia, encephalitis and gastrointestinal involvement is estimated to affect up to 40% of adult AIDS patients, but is probably less frequent in children.[101] Symptomatic infection is more common and severe in HIV-infected children less than 12 months of age and with low age-corrected CD4 counts.[99] In children the colon is the most common site of gastrointestinal infection, followed by the small intestine and then the esophagus. Mucosal ulceration may sometimes result in massive hemorrhage and perforation of the large bowel, and strictures may follow CMV infection of the esophagus.[102] Diagnosis can be difficult. The virus may remain latent for long periods of time and neither serological tests nor positive urine cultures necessarily imply active disease. Children with chronic diarrhea, fever and no other identifiable pathogen should be investigated for CMV infection with lower gastrointestinal endoscopy and biopsy. CMV DNA quantification (CMV viral load) by polymerase chain reaction (PCR) can be used to decide when to offer prophylactic or active treatment. Prophylaxis and treatment with ganciclovir can prevent complications and significantly reduce morbidity, although the infection is not eradicated and relapses are still frequent.[103] Multiple pinpoint perforations or near perforations of the bowel may occur in the small bowel, ascending colon or both.[104] The prognosis is poor with or without ganciclovir.

Rotavirus

Studies in sub-Saharan Africa show that rotavirus is a common cause of diarrhea in HIV-infected children.[105] It is not, however, found more commonly, shed for longer or associated with greater clinical severity than in children uninfected by HIV in similar settings; nor do children with more advanced HIV disease demonstrate any additional susceptibility.[106] Rotavirus was not associated with changes in viral load or CD4 counts in a small study in Malawi.[107] The pending availability of two new live oral rotavirus vaccines highlights the importance of understanding the relationship, and potential interaction, between these two viral infections. Clinical trials are necessary to ensure that any vaccine is safe and immunogenic in this population.

Microsporidia spp

Intestinal microsporidiosis is increasingly being reported in patients with HIV.[83,108] These intracellular protozoa are able to infect most animal species and, in humans, five genera (*Enterocytozoon*, *Encephalitozoon*, *Septata*, *Pleistophora* and *Nosema*) are associated with pulmonary, ocular, muscular, renal, intestinal and hepatic clinical disease. In Thailand, *Enterocytozoon bieneusi* was diagnosed in 25% and 15% of HIV-infected and uninfected children presenting with diarrhea, respectively.[81] In Uganda, however, it was found in 17% of children of unknown HIV status attending hospital out-patient clinics for conditions other than diarrhea.[82] In contrast, microsporidiosis in HIV-infected adults produces chronic watery diarrhea and wasting, suggesting that responses in children may be quite different.[82,109] Villous atrophy and reduced brush-border enzyme activity may cause lactose intolerance.[110]

Diagnosis is made on stool microscopy using a modified trichrome stain, but this requires considerable technical skill to identify organisms correctly. Identification of parasites in stool or biopsy can be optimized by using PCR methods or electron microscopy on upper gastrointestinal biopsy.[111] Albendazole is an effective treatment for *Encephalitozoon* spp infections.[77]

Management of diarrhea and nutritional support

HIV infection in children is often thought to be a rapidly and uniformly lethal disease. In Rwanda, however, 40% of children with perinatal infection survive for 5 years without antiretroviral treatment, and there are many children in sub-Saharan Africa with vertically acquired HIV infection attending schools and growing into adolescence.[112] Optimizing the quality of life for these children is a necessary challenge, especially when the option of effective antiretroviral therapy is absent. The approaches outlined below are intended for developing countries.

Diarrhea

In most clinical settings in southern Africa it is not possible to investigate children presenting with recurrent or persistent diarrhea extensively. Using a syndromic approach for managing diarrhea in both HIV-infected and uninfected children is therefore appropriate. The WHO/UNICEF Integrated Management of Childhood Illnesses (IMCI) recommends that children with a history of persistent diarrhea and/or reported weight loss in the previous 3 months should be assessed for possible HIV infection.[113] Where there are no specific guidelines for HIV-infected children, the WHO guidelines for the management of severe malnutrition, including persistent diarrhea, are helpful.

An approach for resource-poor countries would be:

(1) Assess for and correct dehydration, hypoglycemia, hypothermia and electrolyte disturbances, especially K^+ deficiency;

(2) Treat concurrent bacterial infections, e.g. pneumonia, *Pneumocystis carinii* pneumonia (PCP) and urinary tract infection, and exclude TB. This often means giving antibiotics empirically, e.g. cefuroxime, gentamycin and cotrimoxazole;

(3) Start low lactose (< 3.2 g/kg) containing feeds such as F-75 (WHO) and porridge;

(4) Provide vitamin A, zinc and multivitamins, including folate. See below for comment on zinc supplements;

(5) If diarrhea persists then test stools for lactose intolerance using Clinitest® tablets;

(6) If Clinitest is positive then exclude all lactose from diet – use milks containing maltodextran as the main carbohydrate;

(7) If Clinitest is negative then send repeat stools for routine microbiological assessment, including for *Shigella*, non-typhi *Salmonella*, *Cryptosporidium*, microsporidia and TB. Treat accordingly. Cryptosporidia may be shed intermittently; three stools should be sent to exclude diagnosis. Experienced staff are required to identify cryptosporidia and microsporidia on routine stool analysis. Prolonged fluid and nutritional support is often required for patients with cryptosporidiosis;

(8) If no pathogen is identified then treat for bacterial overgrowth, e.g. cholestyramine for 5 days and neomycin for 3 days;

(9) If diarrhea persists check for monosaccharide intolerance; test for glucose in stool using Clinitest or Glucostix®. If positive, check for excessive intake of oral rehydration solution (ORS). Use maltodextran (glucose polymer) containing feeds and deliver milk by continuous slow infusion through a nasogastric tube. Use plain boiled water for oral rehydration rather than ORS. Only revert back to bolus feeds once the stool becomes formed again and glucose is not present. This takes longer in children who are more wasted or who have severe diarrhea;

(10) Where resources are available, perform upper gastrointestinal endoscopy to increase the microbiological diagnostic yield. If visible or microscopic blood is present in stools then perform sigmoidoscopy for biopsy and culture;

(11) Where there is persistent pyrexia consider CMV colitis and exclude TB;

(12) If no cause for persisting diarrhea is evident then consider antimotility drugs such as loperamide (HIV enteropathy is a diagnosis of exclusion);

(13) Older children should be asked about abdominal pain and on these occasions underlying opportunistic infections such as TB, *Cryptosporidium* or CMV should be excluded; opiates such as codeine phosphate may be helpful;

(14) Attention must be given in the weeks following discharge to restoring, as much as possible, any weight loss that has occurred. It is often very difficult to achieve this during hospitalization, and in busy hospitals significant weight gain cannot be used as a criterion for discharge (see Nutrition, below).

Parenteral nutrition is not generally feasible in most developing countries because of the risk of systemic infection and metabolic complications.

Terminal care

When children are admitted with evidence of clinically advanced HIV infection such as diarrhea and severe wasting, clinicians and carers must consider what is reasonable and right for the child. The first admission with diarrhea often results in HIV testing. Many mothers discover for the first time that both she, and her child, are HIV-infected. In this situation it is appropriate to use all resources available to ensure that the child recovers and is able to go home. However, the treatment paradigm and objectives for care often change when the child has suffered several admissions, and the family has had some time to adapt to the diagnosis. In the absence of antiviral drugs, relieving discomfort becomes the overriding priority, and being less aggressive when complications such as concurrent severe bacterial infections intervene may be more caring for the child.

In resourced settings

While the same principles apply, the use of invasive diagnostic methods, i.e. upper and lower intestinal endoscopy, should be used early to determine whether a treatable enteric pathogen is present. Parenteral feeding may be a safe option if severe malabsorption is present. Antiretroviral drugs should be initiated if the child has not been previously treated.

Micronutrients and HIV-related diarrhea

Multiple micronutrient deficiencies have been reported in both HIV-infected adults and children with, or without, diarrhea. Biochemical indicators of vitamin and trace element status may be misleading and reflect redistribution or acute-phase responses rather true body depletion. A few studies have shown that micronutrient supplementation in HIV-infected or exposed children is associated with improved morbidity or immune function.[114–116] In children uninfected with HIV, zinc supplementation reduces the incidence, duration and severity of acute and chronic diarrhea and promotes recovery of the mucosal lining.[117,118] This effect has not so far been demonstrated in HIV-infected children.

Vitamin A does not seem significantly to influence the course of acute or persistent diarrhea in uninfected children, but does decrease the severity and likelihood of recurrence.[119] HIV-infected children with persistent diarrhea should receive vitamin A (0–6 months, 50000IU; 6–12 months, 100000 IU; >12 months, 200000IU daily for 2 days), zinc sulfate or gluconate 2 mg/kg for 2 weeks and multivitamin preparations including folate for 2–4 weeks.

Nutrition

Much of the impact of diarrheal illnesses and repeated opportunistic infections on the health of HIV-infected children is mediated by its effect on nutrition. Loss of lean body tissue is consistently seen in adults and children with advanced disease and is a strong predictor of death.[120] Resting energy expenditure (REE) in adults increases by about 10% once they are infected with HIV, but this does not been seem to be the case in children.[53,121] However, even if REE increases modestly, total energy expenditure may not increase, because of inactivity. Rather, weight loss is most likely to be due to decreased energy intake, especially during the recovery period from opportunistic infections. Nutritional interventions, however, have generally only reversed weight loss through gain of fat rather than lean body tissue. There is work to suggest that different opportunistic infections may have differential effects on nutrition with some being capable of impairing anabolism and effective utilization of energy from food.

WHO currently recommends that infected children should increase their overall energy intake by about 10% in order to maintain normal health, growth and activity. In chronic illness such as TB infection or chronic lung disease, energy intake should increase by 25–30%. During acute illnesses, particularly when recovering from acute weight loss, these requirements may increase to 50–100% extra energy. Protein should represent about 10–15% of energy. These goals should ideally be achieved through dietary approaches rather than by specialized supplements which may not be available or affordable in most developing countries.[122]

Surgical aspects of HIV infection

The prevalence of HIV disease among pediatric surgical patients in southern Africa has increased dramatically and is frequently considered as part of the differential diagnosis. Abdominal pain is not uncommon in adults with HIV, but there are no data on children. An underlying pathological cause can be identified in most cases[123] and include TB abdomen, cryptosporidia and CMV. There are four common surgical manifestations of gastrointestinal HIV disease: destructive lesions, opportunistic infections, primary peritonitis and tumors.

Destructive lesions

Rectovaginal fistulae are an extremely common presentation of HIV disease in female infants.[124,125] In the past this was treated with a defunctioning colostomy followed by closure of the fistula. Recurrence was frequent. Antiretroviral therapy may improve surgical results, but in the absence of such treatment it is generally better to leave the fistula alone.[126] In males, there is the less common presentation of a rectourethral fistula which always requires surgical repair.

Occasionally stricture formation may follow sclerosis of the lower esophagus after repeated ulcerative disease such as CMV or invasive candidiasis.

Opportunistic infections

Intestinal perforations due to CMV are described above.[104] HIV occasionally presents as cancrum oris, where early treatment with penicillin and metronidazole may help, but excision and reconstruction may be required for large areas of full-thickness skin and tissue loss.

Primary peritonitis

This is sometimes seen in the older child who presents with a clinical picture suggestive of appendicitis. At surgery an odorless pus is found in the abdomen; pneumococcus is often isolated.

Tumors

Kaposi's sarcoma in the gut may present with rectal bleeding, and other less common smooth-muscle tumors may rarely present as an intussusception and intestinal obstruction.[127,128]

Condyloma accuminata that may vary in size from isolated lesions to large pancake lesions can cover the perineum and genitalia. The more extensive lesions cause severe discomfort and problems with local hygiene. Isolated lesions may respond to podophyllin, but diathermy results in annular scarring and anal stenosis. Treatment with interferon may be helpful.

Sialadenitis is a frequent complaint. Parotid size may increase and decrease intermittently, and pain may be due to superimposed bacterial infection, TB, bleeding into cysts or malignant change. Acute pain should be treated with antibiotics and analgesia; if the parotid continues to enlarge and is painful, then fine-needle or open biopsy should be performed to exclude TB or malignant change. Corticosteroids may be helpful.

REFERENCES

1. McDougal JS, Mawle A, Cort SP et al. Cellular tropism of the human retrovirus HTLV-III/LAV. I. Role of T cell activation and expression of the T4 antigen. *J Immunol* 1985; **135**: 3151–3162.
2. Lapenta C, Boirivant M, Marini M et al. Human intestinal lamina propria lymphocytes are naturally permissive to HIV-1 infection. *Eur J Immunol* 1999; **29**: 1202–1208.
3. Rollins NC, Filteau SM, Coutsoudis A, Tomkins AM. Feeding mode, intestinal permeability, and neopterin excretion: a longitudinal study in infants of HIV-infected South African women. *J Acquir Immune Defic Syndr* 2001; **28**: 132–139.
4. Meng G, Wei X, Wu X et al. Primary intestinal epithelial cells selectively transfer R5 HIV-1 to CCR5+ cells. Nat Med 2002; **8**: 150-156.
5. Poles MA, Elliott J, Taing P et al. A preponderance of CCR5(+) CXCR4(+) mononuclear cells enhances gastrointestinal mucosal susceptibility to human immunodeficiency virus type 1 infection. *J Virol* 2001; **75**: 8390–8399.
6. Wolinsky SM, Wike CM, Korber BT et al. Selective transmission of human immunodeficiency virus type-1 variants from mothers to infants. *Science* 1992; **255**: 1134–1137.
7. Amerongen HM, Weltzin R, Farnet CM et al. Transepithelial transport of HIV-1 by intestinal M cells: a mechanism for transmission of AIDS. *J Acquir Immune Defic Syndr* 1991; **4**: 760–765.
8. Dunn DT, Newell ML, Ades AE, Peckham CS. Risk of human immunodeficiency virus type 1 transmission through breastfeeding. *Lancet* 1992; **340**: 585–588.
9. Lewis P, Nduati R, Kreiss JK et al. Cell-free human immunodeficiency virus type 1 in breast milk. *J Infect Dis* 1998; **177**: 34–39.
10. Leroy V, Karon JM, Alioum A et al. Postnatal transmission of HIV-1 after a maternal short-course zidovudine peripartum regimen in West Africa. *AIDS* 2003; **17**: 1493–1501.
11. Hocini H, Bomsel M. Infectious human immunodeficiency virus can rapidly penetrate a tight human epithelial barrier by transcytosis in a process impaired by mucosal immunoglobulins. *J Infect Dis* 1999; **179**(Suppl 3): S448–S453.
12. McNeely TB, Dealy M, Dripps DJ et al. Secretory leukocyte protease inhibitor: a human saliva protein exhibiting anti-human immunodeficiency virus 1 activity *in vitro*. *J Clin Invest* 1995; **96**: 456–464.
13. Janoff EN, Scamurra RW, Sanneman TC et al. Human immunodeficiency virus type 1 and mucosal humoral defense. *J Infect Dis* 1999; **179**(Suppl 3): S475–S479.
14. Willumsen JF, Filteau SM, Coutsoudis A et al. Breastmilk RNA viral load in HIV-infected South African women: effects of subclinical mastitis and infant feeding. *AIDS* 2003; **17**: 407–414.
15. Fearon DT, Locksley RM. The instructive role of innate immunity in the acquired immune response. *Science* 1996; **272**: 50–53.
16. Medzhitov R, Janeway CA Jr. Innate immunity: impact on the adaptive immune response. *Curr Opin Immunol* 1997; **9**: 4–9.
17. Kalliomaki M, Salminen S, Arvilommi H et al. Probiotics in primary prevention of atopic disease: a randomised placebo-controlled trial. *Lancet* 2001; **357**: 1076–1079.
18. Devito C, Broliden K, Kaul R et al. Mucosal and plasma IgA from HIV-1-exposed uninfected individuals inhibit HIV-1 transcytosis across human epithelial cells. *J Immunol* 2000; **165**: 5170–5176.
19. Alfsen A, Iniguez P, Bouguyon E, Bomsel M. Secretory IgA specific for a conserved epitope on gp41 envelope glycoprotein inhibits epithelial transcytosis of HIV-1. *J Immunol* 2001; **166**: 6257–6265.
20. Veazey RS, Shattock RJ, Pope M et al. Prevention of virus transmission to macaque monkeys by a vaginally applied monoclonal antibody to HIV-1 gp120. *Nat Med* 2003; **9**: 343–346.
21. Lim SG, Condez A, Lee CA et al. Loss of mucosal CD4 lymphocytes is an early feature of HIV infection. *Clin Exp Immunol* 1993; **92**: 448–454.
22. Schneider T, Jahn HU, Schmidt W et al. Loss of CD4 T lymphocytes in patients infected with human immunodeficiency virus type 1 is more pronounced in the duodenal mucosa than in the peripheral blood. Berlin Diarrhea/Wasting Syndrome Study Group. *Gut* 1995; **37**: 524–529.
23. Clayton F, Snow G, Reka S, Kotler DP. Selective depletion of rectal lamina propria rather than lymphoid aggregate CD4 lymphocytes in HIV infection. *Clin Exp Immunol* 1997; **107**: 288–292.
24. Kotler DP, Scholes JV, Tierney AR. Intestinal plasma cell alterations in acquired immunodeficiency syndrome. *Dig Dis Sci* 1987; **32**: 129–138.
25. Schneider T, Zippel T, Schmidt W et al. Secretory immunity in HIV infection. *Pathobiology* 1998; **66**: 131–138.
26. Kakai R, Bwayo JJ, Wamola IA et al. Effect of human immunodeficiency virus on local immunity in children with diarrhoea. *East Afr Med J* 1995; **72**: 699–702.
27. Bard E, Laibe S, Clair S et al. Nonspecific secretory immunity in HIV-infected patients with oral candidiasis. *J Acquir Immune Defic Syndr* 2002; **31**: 276–284.
28. Chadwick EG, Chang G, Decker MD et al. Serologic response to standard inactivated influenza vaccine in human immunodeficiency virus-infected children. *Pediatr Infect Dis J* 1994; **13**: 206–211.
29. Olsson J, Poles M, Spetz AL et al. Human immunodeficiency virus type 1 infection is associated with significant mucosal inflammation characterized by increased expression of CCR5, CXCR4, and beta-chemokines. *J Infect Dis* 2000; **182**: 1625–1635.
30. Bode H, Schmitz H, Fromm M et al. IL-1beta and TNF-alpha, but not IFN-alpha, IFN-gamma, IL-6 or IL-8, are secretory mediators in human distal colon. *Cytokine* 1998; **10**: 457–465.
31. Colebunders R, Francis H, Mann JM et al. Persistent diarrhea, strongly associated with HIV infection in Kinshasa, Zaire. *Am J Gastroenterol* 1987; **82**: 859–864.
32. Chintu C, DuPont HL, Kaile T et al. Human immunodeficiency virus-associated diarrhea and wasting in Zambia: selected risk factors and clinical associations. *Am J Trop Med Hyg* 1998; **59**: 38–41.
33. Monkemuller KE, Call SA, Lazenby AJ, Wilcox CM. Declining prevalence of opportunistic gastrointestinal disease in the era of combination antiretroviral therapy. *Am J Gastroenterol* 2000; **95**: 457–462.
34. Nannini EC, Okhuysen PC. HIV1 and the gut in the era of highly active antiretroviral therapy. *Curr Gastroenterol Rep* 2002; **4**: 392–398.

35. Kotler DP, Francisco A, Clayton F et al. Small intestinal injury and parasitic diseases in AIDS. *Ann Intern Med* 1990; **113**: 444–449.
36. Carbonnel F, Beaugerie L, Abou RA et al. Macronutrient intake and malabsorption in HIV infection: a comparison with other malabsorptive states. *Gut* 1997; **41**: 805–810.
37. Yolken RH, Hart W, Oung I et al. Gastrointestinal dysfunction and disaccharide intolerance in children infected with human immunodeficiency virus. *J Pediatr* 1991; **118**: 359–363.
38. Miller TL, Orav EJ, Martin SR et al. Malnutrition and carbohydrate malabsorption in children with vertically transmitted human immunodeficiency virus 1 infection. *Gastroenterology* 1991; **100**: 1296–1302.
39. The Italian Paediatric Intestinal/HIV Study Group. Intestinal malabsorption of HIV-infected children: relationship to diarrhoea, failure to thrive, enteric microorganisms and immune impairment. *AIDS* 1993; **7**: 1435–1440.
40. Lepage P, Spira R, Kalibala S et al. Care of human immunodeficiency virus-infected children in developing countries. International Working Group on Mother-to-Child Transmission of HIV. *Pediatr Infect Dis J* 1998; **17**: 581–586.
41. Keating J, Bjarnason I, Somasundaram S et al. Intestinal absorptive capacity, intestinal permeability and jejunal histology in HIV and their relation to diarrhoea. *Gut* 1995; **37**: 623–629.
42. Kotler DP, Reka S, Chow K, Orenstein JM. Effects of enteric parasitoses and HIV infection upon small intestinal structure and function in patients with AIDS. *J Clin Gastroenterol* 1993; **16**: 10–15.
43. Fontana M, Boldorini R, Zuin G et al. Ultrastructural changes in the duodenal mucosa of HIV-infected children. *J Pediatr Gastroenterol Nutr* 1993; **17**: 255–259.
44. Thea DM, St Louis ME, Atido U et al. A prospective study of diarrhea and HIV-1 infection among 429 Zairian infants. *N Engl J Med* 1993; **329**: 1696–1702.
45. Miller TL, McQuinn LB, Orav EJ. Endoscopy of the upper gastrointestinal tract as a diagnostic tool for children with human immunodeficiency virus infection. *J Pediatr* 1997; **130**: 766–773.
46. Oktedalen O, Skar V, Dahl E, Serck-Hanssen A. Changes in small intestinal structure and function in HIV-infected patients with chronic diarrhoea. *Scand J Infect Dis* 1998; **30**: 459–463.
47. Pernet P, Vittecoq D, Kodjo A et al. Intestinal absorption and permeability in human immunodeficiency virus-infected patients. *Scand J Gastroenterol* 1999; **34**: 29–34.
48. Taylor C, Hodgson K, Sharpstone D et al. The prevalence and severity of intestinal disaccharidase deficiency in human immunodeficiency virus-infected subjects. *Scand J Gastroenterol* 2000; **35**: 599–606.
49. Rollins NC, Wittenberg DF, Coovadia HM. Trends in HIV prevalence outcome and monosaccharide intolerance in a paediatric diarrhoea unit in South Africa. *Commonwealth Congress on Diarrhoea and Malnutrition*, Karachi, Pakistan, 1997.
50. Sharpstone D, Neild P, Crane R et al. Small intestinal transit, absorption, and permeability in patients with AIDS with and without diarrhoea. *Gut* 1999; **45**: 70–76.
51. Kotler D, Haroutiounian G, Greenberg R. Increased bile salt deconjugation in AIDS. *Gastroenterology* 1985; **88**: 1455.
52. Sentongo TA, Rutstein RM, Stettler N et al. Association between steatorrhea, growth, and immunologic status in children with perinatally acquired HIV infection. *Arch Pediatr Adolesc Med* 2001; **155**: 149–153.
53. Sharpstone DR, Ross HM, Gazzard BG. The metabolic response to opportunistic infections in AIDS. *AIDS* 1996; **10**: 1529–1533.
54. Laine L, Garcia F, McGilligan K et al. Protein-losing enteropathy and hypoalbuminemia in AIDS. *AIDS* 1993; **7**: 837–840.
55. Guarino A, Tarallo L, Guandalini S et al. Impaired intestinal function in symptomatic HIV infection. *J Pediatr Gastroenterol Nutr* 1991; **12**: 453–458.
56. Rollins NC, Filteau SM, Elson I, Tomkins AM. Vitamin A supplementation of South African children with severe diarrhea: optimum timing for improving biochemical and clinical recovery and subsequent vitamin A status. *Pediatr Infect Dis J* 2000; **19**: 284–289.
57. Gove S. Integrated management of childhood illness by outpatient health workers: technical basis and overview. The WHO Working Group on Guidelines for Integrated Management of the Sick Child. Bull. *World Health Organ* 1997; **75**(Suppl 1): 7–24.
58. Brink AK, Mahe C, Watera C et al. Diarrhea, CD4 counts and enteric infections in a community-based cohort of HIV-infected adults in Uganda. *J Infect* 2002; **45**: 99–106.
59. Rollins NC, Pent M, Kindra G et al. CD4 count, HIV viral load and enteric pathogens in HIV-infected children with persistent diarrhea in Durban, South Africa. *Pediatric Academic Societies & American Academy of Pediatrics Joint Meeting*, Boston, 2000: Poster abstr 1620.
60. Quesnel A, Moja P, Blanche S et al. Early impairment of gut mucosal immunity in HIV-1-infected children. *Clin Exp Immunol* 1994; **97**: 380–385.
61. Kotler DP, Gaetz HP, Lange M et al. Enteropathy associated with the acquired immunodeficiency syndrome. *Ann Intern Med* 1984; **101**: 421–428.
62. Kelly P, Davies SE, Mandanda B et al. Enteropathy in Zambians with HIV related diarrhoea: regression modelling of potential determinants of mucosal damage. *Gut* 1997; **41**: 811–816.
63. Zeitz M, Ullrich R, Schneider T et al. HIV/SIV enteropathy. *Ann NY Acad Sci* 1998; **859**: 139–148.
64. Batman PA, Miller AR, Forster SM et al. Jejunal enteropathy associated with human immunodeficiency virus infection: quantitative histology. *J Clin Pathol* 1989; **42**: 275–281.
65. Wilcox CM, Waites KB, Smith PD. No relationship between gastric pH, small bowel bacterial colonisation, and diarrhoea in HIV-1 infected patients. *Gut* 1999; **44**: 101–105.
66. Bjarnason I, Sharpstone DR, Francis N et al. Intestinal inflammation, ileal structure and function in HIV. *AIDS* 1996; **10**: 1385–1391.
67. Delezay O, Yahi N, Tamalet C et al. Direct effect of type 1 human immunodeficiency virus (HIV-1) on intestinal epithelial cell differentiation: relationship to HIV-1 enteropathy. *Virology* 1997; **238**: 231–242.
68. Kotler DP. Characterization of intestinal disease associated with human immunodeficiency virus infection and response to antiretroviral therapy. *J Infect Dis* 1999; **179**(Suppl 3): S454–S456.
69. Asmuth DM, Hammer SM, Wanke CA. Physiological effects of HIV infection on human intestinal epithelial cells: an *in vitro* model for HIV enteropathy. *AIDS* 1994; 8: 205–211.
70. Canani RB, Cirillo P, Mallardo G et al. Effects of HIV-1 Tat protein on ion secretion and on cell proliferation in human intestinal epithelial cells. *Gastroenterology* 2003; **124**: 368–376.
71. Otegbayo JA, Oluwasola AO, Akang EE. Collagenous colitis in an adult patient with chronic diarrhoea: case report. *East Afr Med J* 2001; **78**: 272–274.

72. Chintu C, Luo C, Baboo S et al. Intestinal parasites in HIV-seropositive Zambian children with diarrhoea. *J Trop Pediatr* 1995; **41**: 149–152.
73. Powell KR. Guidelines for the care of children and adolescents with HIV infection. Approach to gastrointestinal manifestations in infants and children with HIV infection. *J Pediatr* 1991; **119**: S34–S40.
74. Yan Z, Nguyen S, Poles M et al. Adenovirus colitis in human immunodeficiency virus infection: an underdiagnosed entity. *Am J Surg Pathol* 1998; **22**: 1101–1016.
75. Pollok RC. Viruses causing diarrhoea in AIDS. *Novartis Found Symp* 2001; **238**: 276–283.
76. Orenstein JM, Dieterich DT. The histopathology of 103 consecutive colonoscopy biopsies from 82 symptomatic patients with acquired immunodeficiency syndrome: original and look-back diagnoses. *Arch Pathol Lab Med* 2001; **125**: 1042–1046.
77. Kelly P, Baboo KS, Wolff M et al. The prevalence and aetiology of persistent diarrhoea in adults in urban Zambia. *Acta Trop* 1996; **61**: 183–190.
78. Bini EJ, Weinshel EH, Gamagaris Z. Comparison of duodenal with jejunal biopsy and aspirate in chronic human immunodeficiency virus-related diarrhea. *Am J Gastroenterol* 1998; **93**: 1837–1840.
79. Sewankambo N, Mugerwa RD, Goodgame R et al. Enteropathic AIDS in Uganda. An endoscopic, histological and microbiological study. *AIDS* 1987; **1**: 9–13.
80. Pavia AT, Long EG, Ryder RW et al. Diarrhea among African children born to human immunodeficiency virus 1-infected mothers: clinical, microbiologic and epidemiologic features. *Pediatr Infect Dis J* 1992; **11**: 996–1003.
81. Wanachiwanawin D, Chokephaibulkit K, Lertlaituan P et al. Intestinal microsporidiosis in HIV-infected children with diarrhea. *Southeast Asian J Trop Med Public Health* 2002; **33**: 241–245.
82. Tumwine JK, Kekitiinwa A, Nabukeera N et al. *Enterocytozoon bieneusi* among children with diarrhea attending Mulago Hospital in Uganda. *Am J Trop Med Hyg* 2002; **67**: 299–303.
83. Drobniewski F, Kelly P, Carew A et al. Human microsporidiosis in African AIDS patients with chronic diarrhea. *J Infect Dis* 1995; **171**: 515–516.
84. Enriquez EJ, Avila CR, Santos JI et al. *Cryptosporidium* infections in Mexican children: clinical, nutritional, enteropathogenic and diagnostic evaluations. *Am J Trop Med Hyg* 1997; **56**: 254–257.
85. Newman RD, Sears CL, Moore SR et al. Longitudinal study of *Cryptosporidium* infection in children in northeastern Brazil. *J Infect Dis* 1999; **180**: 167–175.
86. Cegielski JP, Ortega YR, McKee S et al. *Cryptosporidium*, enterocytozoon, and cyclospora infections in pediatric and adult patients with diarrhea in Tanzania. *Clin Infect Dis* 1999; **28**: 314–321.
87. Leav BA, Mackay MR, Anyanwu A et al. Analysis of sequence diversity at the highly polymorphic Cpgp40/15 locus among *Cryptosporidium* isolates from human immunodeficiency virus-infected children in South Africa. *Infect Immun* 2002; **70**: 3881–3890.
88. Mayer HB, Wanke CA. Diagnostic strategies in HIV-infected patients with diarrhea. *AIDS* 1994; **8**: 1639–1648.
89. McGowan I, Hawkins AS, Weller IV. The natural history of cryptosporidial diarrhea in HIV-infected patients. *AIDS* 1993; **7**: 349–354.
90. Lima AA, Silva TM, Gifoni AM et al. Mucosal injury and disruption of intestinal barrier function in HIV-infected individuals with and without diarrhea and cryptosporidiosis in northeast Brazil. *Am J Gastroenterol* 1997; **92**: 1861–1866.
91. Guarino A, Castaldo A, Russo S et al. Enteric cryptosporidiosis in pediatric HIV infection. *J Pediatr Gastroenterol Nutr* 1997; **25**: 182–187.
92. Hicks P, Zwiener RJ, Squires J, Savell V. Azithromycin therapy for *Cryptosporidium parvum* infection in four children infected with human immunodeficiency virus. *J Pediatr* 1996; **129**: 297–300.
93. Amadi B, Mwiya M, Musuku J et al. Effect of nitazoxanide on morbidity and mortality in Zambian children with cryptosporidiosis: a randomised controlled trial. *Lancet* 2002; **360**: 1375–1380.
94. Greenberg PD, Cello JP. Treatment of severe diarrhea caused by *Cryptosporidium parvum* with oral bovine immunoglobulin concentrate in patients with AIDS. *J Acquir Immune Defic Syndr Hum Retrovirol* 1996; **13**: 348–354.
95. Schmidt W, Wahnschaffe U, Schafer M et al. Rapid increase of mucosal CD4 T cells followed by clearance of intestinal cryptosporidiosis in an AIDS patient receiving highly active antiretroviral therapy. *Gastroenterology* 2001; **120**: 984–987.
96. Embree JE, Njenga S, Datta P et al. Risk factors for postnatal mother-child transmission of HIV-1. *AIDS* 2000; **14**: 2535–2541.
97. Ekpini ER, Wiktor SZ, Satten GA et al. Late postnatal mother-to-child transmission of HIV-1 in Abidjan, Cote d'Ivoire. *Lancet* 1997; **349**: 1054–1059.
98. Haller JO, Cohen HL. Gastrointestinal manifestations of AIDS in children. *Am J Roentgenol* 1994; **162**: 387–393.
99. Chandwani S, Kaul A, Bebenroth D et al. Cytomegalovirus infection in human immunodeficiency virus type 1-infected children. *Pediatr Infect Dis J* 1996; **15**: 310–314.
100. Ukarapol N, Chartapisak W, Lertprasertsuk N et al. Cytomegalovirus-associated manifestations involving the digestive tract in children with human immunodeficiency virus infection. *J Pediatr Gastroenterol Nutr* 2002; **35**: 669–673.
101. Kitchen BJ, Engler HD, Gill VJ et al. Cytomegalovirus infection in children with human immunodeficiency virus infection. *Pediatr Infect Dis J* 1997; **16**: 358–363.
102. Kahn E, Greco MA, Daum S. Pathology of the gastrointestinal tract in pediatric AIDS. *Surg Pathol* 1994; **5**: 239–252.
103. Wilcox CM, Straub RF, Schwartz DA. Cytomegalovirus esophagitis in AIDS: a prospective evaluation of clinical response to ganciclovir therapy, relapse rate, and long-term outcome. *Am J Med* 1995; **98**: 169–176.
104. Shaik AS, Hadley GP. Surgically significant CMV enterocolitis in children. 25th Biennial Congress of the South African Paediatric Association, and the South African Association of Paediatric Surgeons, 20–24 Oct, 2002 (abstr).
105. Oshitani H, Kasolo FC, Mpabalwani M et al. Association of rotavirus and human immunodeficiency virus infection in children hospitalized with acute diarrhea, Lusaka, Zambia. *J Infect Dis* 1994; **169**: 897–900.
106. Cunliffe NA, Gondwe JS, Kirkwood CD et al. Effect of concomitant HIV infection on presentation and outcome of rotavirus gastroenteritis in Malawian children. *Lancet* 2001; **358**: 550–555.
107. Jere C, Cunliffe NA, Hoffman IF et al. Plasma HIV burden in Malawian children co-infected with rotavirus. *AIDS* 2001; **15**: 1439–1442.
108. Brasil P, Sodre FC, Cuzzi-Maya T et al. Intestinal microsporidiosis in HIV-positive patients with chronic unexplained diarrhea in Rio de Janeiro, Brazil: diagnosis, clinical presentation and follow-up. *Rev Inst Med Trop Sao Paulo* 1996; **38**: 97–102.

109. Hautvast JL, Tolboom JJ, Derks TJ et al. Asymptomatic intestinal microsporidiosis in a human immunodeficiency virus-seronegative, immunocompetent Zambian child. *Pediatr Infect Dis J* 1997; **16**: 415–416.
110. Schmidt W, Schneider T, Heise W et al. Mucosal abnormalities in microsporidiosis. *AIDS* 1997; **11**: 1589–1594.
111. van den Bergh Weerman MA, van Gool T, Eeftinck Schattenkerk JK, Dingemans KP. Electron microscopy as an essential technique for the identification of parasites in aids patients. *Eur J Morphol* 1993; **31**: 107–110.
112. Spira R, Lepage P, Msellati P et al. Natural history of human immunodeficiency virus type 1 infection in children: a five year prospective study in Rwanda. *Pediatrics* 1999; **104**: 56.
113. Horwood C, Liebeschuetz S, Blaauw D et al. Diagnosis of paediatric HIV infection in a primary health care setting using a clinical algorithm. *Bull World Health Organ* 2003; **81**: 858–866.
114. Coutsoudis A, Bobat RA, Coovadia HM et al. The effects of vitamin A supplementation on the morbidity of children born to HIV-infected women. *Am J Public Health* 1995; **85**: 1076–1081.
115. Villamor E, Mbise R, Spiegelman D et al. Vitamin A supplements ameliorate the adverse effect of HIV-1, malaria, and diarrheal infections on child growth. *Pediatrics* 2002; **109**: E6.
116. Fawzi WW, Mbise R, Spiegelman D et al. Vitamin A supplements and diarrheal and respiratory tract infections among children in Dar es Salaam, Tanzania. *J Pediatr* 2000; **137**: 660–667.
117. Bahl R, Bhandari N, Saksena M et al. Efficacy of zinc-fortified oral rehydration solution in 6- to 35-month-old children with acute diarrhea. *J Pediatr* 2002; **141**: 677–682.
118. Bhandari N, Bahl R, Taneja S et al. Substantial reduction in severe diarrheal morbidity by daily zinc supplementation in young north Indian children. *Pediatrics* 2002; **109**: E86.
119. Faruque AS, Mahalanabis D, Haque SS et al. Double-blind, randomized, controlled trial of zinc or vitamin A supplementation in young children with acute diarrhoea. *Acta Paediatr* 1999; **88**: 154–160.
120. Berhane R, Bagenda D, Marum L et al. Growth failure as a prognostic indicator of mortality in pediatric HIV infection. *Pediatrics* 1997; **100**: E7.
121. Arpadi SM, Cuff PA, Kotler DP et al. Growth velocity, fat-free mass and energy intake are inversely related to viral load in HIV-infected children. *J Nutr* 2000; **130**: 2498–2502.
122. WHO Technical Advisory Group on Nutrition and HIV/AIDS. *Nutrient Requirements for People Living with HIV/AIDS.* Summary report of a Technical Consultation. Geneva, Switzerland: World Health Organisation, 2003.
123. O'Keefe EA, Wood R, Van Zyl A, Cariem AK. Human immunodeficiency virus-related abdominal pain in South Africa. Aetiology, diagnosis and survival. *Scand J Gastroenterol* 1998; **33**: 212–217.
124. Borgstein ES, Broadhead RL. Acquired rectovaginal fistula. *Arch Dis Child* 1994; **71**: 165–166.
125. Oliver MJ. Spontaneously occurring rectovaginal fistulae in children and adults with HIV infection. *East & Central Afr J Surg* 1995; **1**: 23–25.
126. Wiersma R. HIV-positive African children with rectal fistulae. *J Pediatr Surg* 2003; **38**: 62–64.
127. Wang NC, Chang FY, Chou YY et al. Intussusception as the initial manifestation of AIDS associated with primary Kaposi's sarcoma: a case report. *J Formos Med Assoc* 2002; **101**: 585–587.
128. Chadwick EG, Connor EJ, Hanson IC et al. Tumors of smooth-muscle origin in HIV-infected children. *JAMA* 1990; **263**: 3182–3184.

9 Viral diarrhea

Alfredo Guarino and Fabio Albano

Epidemiology and etiology

While infectious gastroenteritides are the second most common diseases in childhood worldwide, viruses are the most frequent agents of infectious diarrhea. Viral infections of the gastrointestinal tract cause 2 billion cases of diarrhea in children per year, resulting in 18 million hospitalizations and as many as 3 million deaths.[1]

Acute diarrhea is thus an enormous problem both in developing and in industrialized countries, but with two distinct consequences. In the former, enteric infections are extremely frequent, as the incidence of diarrhea is estimated at 3.8 episodes/child per year in infants and 2.1 episodes/child per year in children 1–4 years of age.[2] A cumulative incidence of 2.5–3 million deaths each year has been estimated, corresponding to 25% of all deaths in childhood up to 5 years of age. In the developing world, one out of 40 children will die because of diarrhea.[3]

In industrialized countries, on the other hand, the incidence of diarrhea is approximately 1–2 episodes/child per year in subjects younger than 3 years. The case/fatality ratio is far from the figures in poor countries, but not negligible. In the USA, 150–300 infants or younger children die each year because of acute diarrhea, and substantial resources are needed for hospitalizations and medical visits. Diarrhea was associated with an annual average of 35 hospitalizations per 10 000 children younger than 5 years, corresponding to 4% of all hospitalizations.[4] It was estimated that 1 in 57 children would be hospitalized by 5 years of age for diarrhea-associated illness. The rate of outpatient visits was 943/10 000 children, corresponding to 2% of all visits. Rotavirus is the leading agent of infectious diarrhea, being responsible for approximately 40% of all cases of diarrhea in the USA.[4] Similar figures have been recorded in Europe,[5] with rotavirus consistently playing a leading role in younger subjects.[6] The estimated average costs for an episode of diarrhea requiring hospital admission may be as high as US$ 2300. Costs for acute diarrhea are not negligible even in less severe cases, particularly when the so-called societal costs are considered. It has been estimated that the cost of an episode of diarrhea requiring an office visit in the USA averages approximately $300,[7] half of which is related to the loss of working days by the parents of sick children.

During the past three decades, there has been a dramatic increase in the number of newly recognized etiological agents of gastroenteritis. Before 1970, a pathogen could be identified in fewer than 10% of patients hospitalized with diarrhea; the remaining 90% of cases represented a 'diagnostic void' consisting of various idiopathic, poorly defined conditions. Since 1970, more than 20 different micro-organisms – bacteria, parasites and viruses – have been recognized as etiological agents, and most cases of gastroenteritis are now presumed to have an infectious etiology. Nevertheless, a pathogen is currently identified in only a small proportion of cases. Although numerous viruses have been identified in fecal samples of patients with diarrhea, causal relationships have been determined for relatively few (Table 9.1). Most children are infected with viruses belonging to four distinct families: rotaviruses, caliciviruses, astroviruses and enteric adenoviruses. Other viruses, such as the toroviruses, picornaviruses (the Aichi virus), and enterovirus 22, play a minor epidemiological role. Finally, selected viruses induce diarrhea only in children at risk. These include cytomegalovirus, Epstein–Barr virus and picobirnaviruses. Recent evidence suggests that

Table 9.1 Etiological role of viruses in childhood diarrhea

Conclusively established	Probable	Possible in selected children
Rotavirus	Torovirus	HIV
Adenovirus	Aichi virus	Cytomegalovirus
Astrovirus	Enterovirus 22	Epstein–Barr virus
Calicivirus		Picobirnavirus

HIV-1 virus may directly induce diarrhea through the production and release of TAT, its transactivating transfer factor.[8]

Enteric infections are usually associated with diarrhea and, less frequently, with vomiting. Diarrhea usually lasts a few days and resolves spontaneously without any major problem. However, in selected cases it may be severe, leading to dehydration, requiring hospital admission and possibly even resulting in fatal outcome.

The impact of viral diarrhea is related to the specific strain, but occasionally also to the epidemiological setting, the host baseline features and the efficacy of early medical intervention (Table 9.2). Viral diarrhea may have a major impact in closed communities such as day-care centers and hospitals. It may be severe in malnourished or immunocompromized children, but also in children not belonging to groups at risk. Finally, diarrhea may become severe if rehydration is not initiated in the initial phases of the disease.

Pathophysiology of viral diarrhea

In the classic and simple view, the pathogenesis of diarrhea may be divided into osmotic and secretory (Figure 9.1). Viral diarrhea was originally believed to be caused by cell invasion and epithelial destruction by enteropathogenic agents, therefore being the result of endoluminal fluid accumulation osmotically driven by non-absorbed nutrients. It is now known that several mechanisms are responsible for diarrhea, depending on the specific agents and the host features. In addition, selected viruses possess multiple virulence pathways that act synergistically to induce diarrhea.

The mechanisms of diarrhea induced by group A rotaviruses have been extensively investigated and provide a paradigm of the pathophysiology of viral diarrhea. Rotavirus has tissue- and cell-specific tropisms, infecting the mature enterocyte of the small intestine. The first step is virus binding to specific receptors located on the cell surface, the GM1 ganglioside. However, different rotavirus strains bind in either a sialic acid-dependent or an -independent fashion.[9] Most rotaviruses, including all human strains, infect polarized enterocytes through both the apical and the basolateral side, in a sialic acid-independent manner, suggesting the presence of different receptors.[10] The early stages of rotavirus binding involve the viral protein (VP)4 spike attachment and cleavage. This outer capsid protein contains ligand sequences for $\alpha2\beta1$ and $\alpha4\beta1$ integrins, and for complement receptor 4, located on the enterocyte surface. After binding, the rotavirus enters into the cell by a multistep process that requires both VP7 and VP4 proteins. The route of internalization remains controversial. Two mechanisms have been proposed: direct penetration through the cell membrane, which could be mediated by the VP5 cleavage product of VP4, or a receptor-primed calcium-dependent endocytosis.

Infection of the villous enterocyte leads to cell lysis, compromising nutrient absorption and driving water into the intestinal lumen through an osmotic mechanism (Figure 9.1). However, the destruction of villus-tip cells induces a compensatory proliferation of crypt cells. These immature enterocytes physiologically maintain a secretive tone, thus contributing to diarrhea with ion secretion, as the result of the imbalance between absorptive villous and secretory crypt cells. Thus, the cytopathic action by rotavirus results in both osmotic and secretory diarrhea.

Table 9.2 Epidemiological features and associated impact of viral diarrhea in specific settings

Setting	Features	Impact	Viruses
Developing countries	high frequency	high mortality	rotavirus
Industrialized countries	high frequency	high costs	all
Day-care centers	high frequency	high costs for the society	rotavirus + others
Seasonal pattern	major outbreaks	↑ winter/early spring	rotavirus
Food-related transmission	food poisoning	massive attack rates	calicivirus, rotavirus, Aichi virus
Age	maximal incidence in children <5 years	increased severity in younger infants	rotavirus
Children at risk	severity increased in immunocompromised malnourished, other chronic diseases	poor outcome	rotavirus, CMV, EBV, adenovirus, astrovirus, picornavirus
Protection	neonates, breast-fed infants, previous infections	protected from severe clinical course more than infection	rotavirus
Persistent diarrhea	occasional (prolonged shedding described)	more frequent in malnourished/ immunocompromised children	rotavirus, CMV
Intractable diarrhea	rare (but described) in industrialized countries	high case/fatality ratio in children at risk but also with no risk	rotavirus
Nosocomial	second most frequent cause of nosocomial infections	increase in hospital stay and associated costs	rotavirus (group B), calicivirus, astrovirus

CMV, cytomegalovirus; EBV, Epstein–Barr virus

Histological changes induced by rotavirus infection occur within 24 h of infection in animal models.[11,12] The proximal small intestinal wall appears thinner with villous atrophy, blunting and conversion to a cuboidal epithelium, without extensive pathological changes. This observation led to the hypothesis of a neurovascular mechanism with a role of a local villous ischemia induced by a vasoactive agent from rotavirus-infected neuronal cells.[13] The enteric nervous system may also play a direct role in inducing fluid secretion, similar to that induced by cholera toxin and other intestinal secretagogs.[14]

The molecular mechanisms of fluid secretion have also been investigated. Rotavirus induces an increase in intracellular calcium levels,[15] which is responsible for the disassembly of microvillar F-

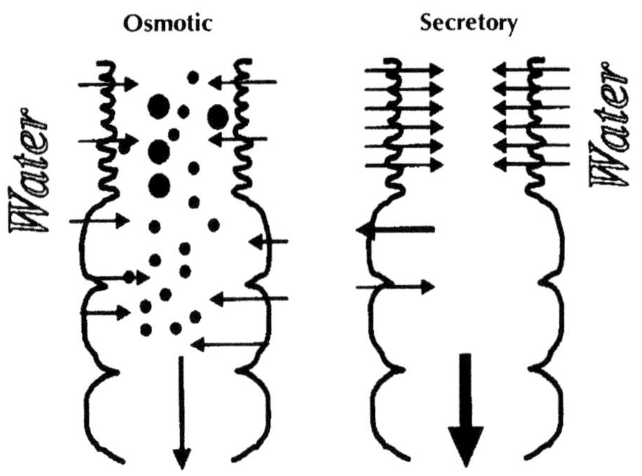

Figure 9.1 Diagram of osmotic and secretory mechanisms of viral diarrhea. The arrows indicate the water's movements and their volumes. In osmotic diarrhea, water is driven into the intestinal lumen by the osmotic force of non-absorbed nutrients. In secretory diarrhea, ions are actively pumped within the lumen and are passively followed by water. From Guandalini S. Acute diarrhea. In Walzer WA et al. *Pediatric Gastrointestinal Disease*, 3rd edn. Hamilton, Ontario: BC Decker Inc. 2000, with permission.

actin, the perturbation of cellular protein trafficking, the damage of tight-junctions, with disruption of cell–cell interaction and cytolysis.[16,17] This is reflected by the loss of epithelial integrity, as shown by the progressive decrease in tissue resistance measured in Caco-2 cell monolayers mounted in Ussing chambers[18] (Figure 9.2).

In children with rotavirus infection, the onset of diarrhea is abrupt and occurs in the absence of histological changes, even if oral feeding is withdrawn, suggesting that a secretory pathway is responsible for diarrhea, at least in the initial phases of infection. A major advancement in the understanding of rotavirus pathophysiology came from the identification of the non-structural protein NSP4 as a viral enterotoxin, defined by its ability to cause fluid secretion, but not epithelial changes.[19]

NSP4 is a multifunctional virulence factor, as it possesses the following features (Figure 9.3):

(1) It is released from infected cells;[20]

(2) It enters the cells through a specific receptor;[21–24]

(3) It causes calcium-dependent chloride secretion, with an age-dependent pattern;[19]

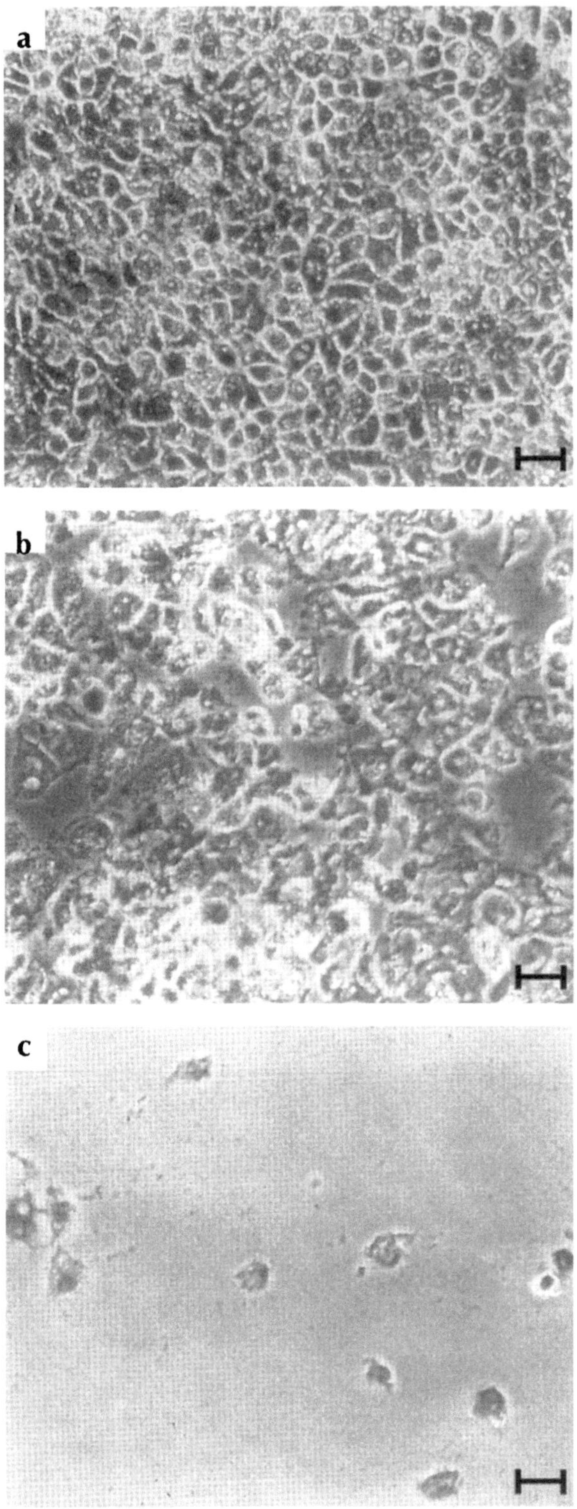

Figure 9.2(a) Cytopathic effects induced by rotavirus (5 PFU/cell) in a model based on the morphology of Caco-2 cell monolayers. a, Uninfected Caco-2 cell monolayers; b, Caco-2 cells at 48 h post-infection: cellular vacuolization, opening of intracellular junction and spotting cell detachments are observed; c, Caco-2 cells at 96 h post-infection: extensive cellular detachment is observed with only a few picnotic cells yet present. From reference 18.

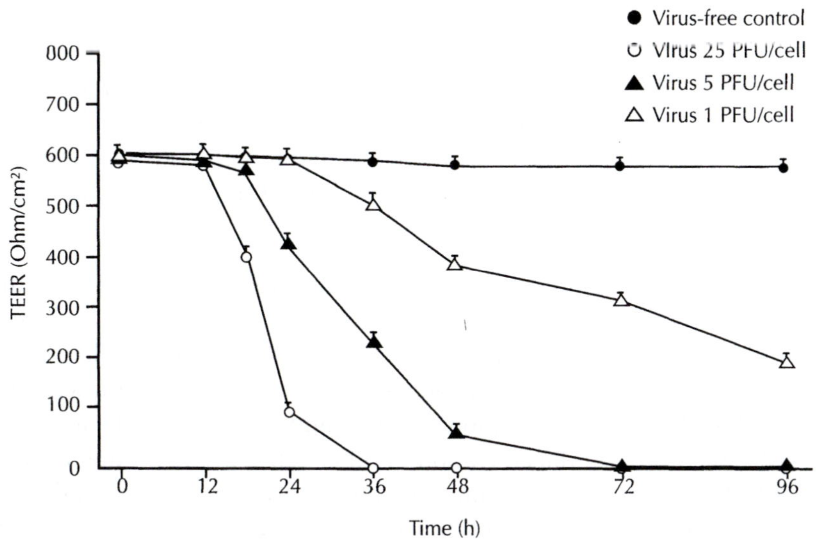

Figure 9.2(b) Cytopathic effects of rotavirus infection in a Caco-2 cell model, as measured by transepithelial electrical resistance (TEER). The decrease of TEER reflects progressive cell damage, which is shown in Figure 9.3. Increasing loads of virus induce an earlier and steeper fall of TEER, with a clear relationship with virus multiplicity. The TEER value decreases below a detectable level within approximately 36 h postinfection with 25 PFU/cell, 60–72 h post-infection with 5 PFU/cell, and 96 h post-infection with 1 PFU/cell. From reference 18.

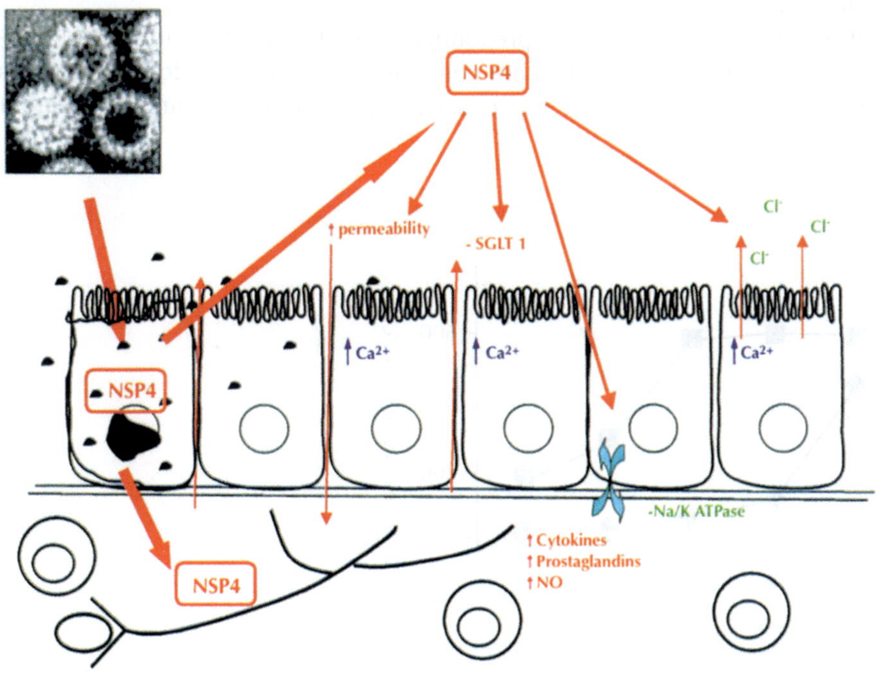

Figure 9.3 Combined effects by NSP4 in the pathophysiology of rotavirus diarrhea. Rotavirus infects epithelial cells of the small intestine, replicates, and induces cell lysis. NSP4 is released by infected cells and functions as a Ca^{2+}-dependent enterotoxin triggering Cl^- secretion. It decreases fluid and electrolyte transport by inhibiting Na–glucose symport SGLT1 and, possibly Na–K ATPase. It also impairs disaccharidase expression. Furthermore, rotavirus and/or NSP4 may diffuse underneath the intestinal epithelium activating secretory reflexes in the enteric nervous system. Late during the infection, an inflammatory response in the lamina propria may be detected, and the production of inflammatory substances and cytokines may further contribute to the increase of intestinal permeability and diarrhea.

(4) It alters plasma membrane permeability and is cytotoxic;[25–27]

(5) It is sensitive to specific antibody, which prevents or reduces diarrhea;[28,29]

NSP4 is the only rotavirus gene product capable of eliciting intracellular calcium mobilization.[30] NSP4 was demonstrated to stimulate a calcium-dependent chloride secretion, in mouse small intestinal mucosa sheets mounted in Ussing chambers, suggesting that this enterotoxin triggers diarrhea in the early phase of infection in animal models.[14,31] NSP4 further contributes to diarrheal pathogenesis by directly altering enterocyte actin distribution and paracellular permeability.[32] Finally, NSP4 plays a role in the inhibition of the Na^+-dependent glucose transporter SGLT-1.[33] Glucose absorption is impaired in rotavirus diarrhea as well as disaccharidase activities, whereas the Na/amino acid co-transporters are not involved.

Rotavirus diarrhea may also have an inflammatory component. The induction of cytokines is important in developing an inflammatory and immune response, especially in intestinal infection caused by bacteria. In rotavirus infection, limited inflammation is detected by histological studies, suggesting that cytokines are effective in inducing a host immune response to rotavirus diarrhea. However, it has been shown that the rotavirus-infected enterocyte activates NF-κB and the production of chemokines interleukin (IL)-8, Rantes and GRO-a, and of cytokines interferon (IFN)α and granulocyte/macrophage–colony-stimulating factor (GM-CSF).[34,35]

In conclusion, the primary target of rotavirus is the enterocyte, which is induced to secrete fluids and is subsequently destroyed. On the other hand, the enterocyte acts as a sensor to the mucosa with the production of viral and endogenous factors and the activation of other cell types including nerves. Thus, rotavirus-induced diarrhea is a multistep and multifactorial event, in which fluid secretion and cell damage are observed in sequence, as shown in an intestinal cell line-based experimental model (Figure 9.4). A summary of the multiple mechanisms involved in the rotavirus–intestine interaction is given in Table 9.3.

Clinical signs and symptoms

The predominant symptoms of vomiting and diarrhea are common to enteric infections, regardless of the causative role of more than 20 different

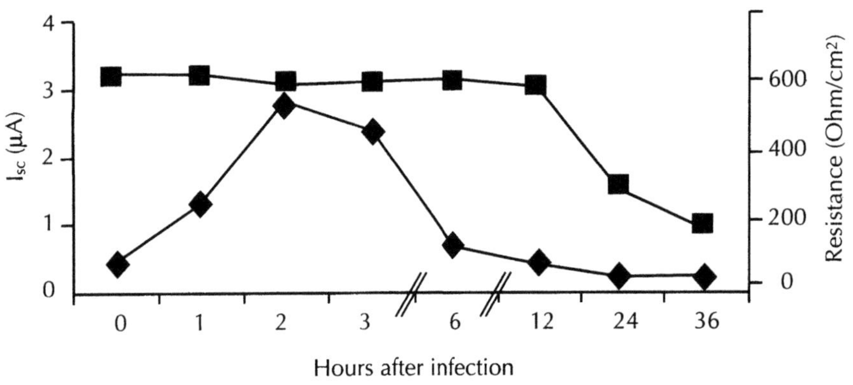

Figure 9.4 Biphasic effect of rotavirus in Caco-2 cells. Rotavirus induces a biphasic response, in an *in vitro* model of infection in Caco-2 enterocytes mounted in Ussing chambers. An early secretion is evident in the first few hours of infection, with a peak at 2 h post-infection, as shown by the increase in short circuit current (I_{sc}, -◆-). Subsequently, rotavirus exerts a cytotoxic effect with a loss of tissue integrity, as demonstrated by the fall of transepithelial resistance (Ohm/cm^2, -■-) which is evident at 24 h post-infection. The results suggest that rotavirus diarrhea is initially the result of an early secretory mechanism and of a subsequent osmotic pathway, due to cell damage and loss of functional absorptive surface, leading to nutrient malabsorption. From G. De Marco et al, unpublished data.

Table 9.3 Pathogenesis of rotavirus diarrhea

Key process	Pathway	Consequences
Villous cell destruction	cytoskeleton disruption, cell lysis	nutrient malabsorption, osmotic diarrhea
Crypt cell proliferation	compensatory secretory cell proliferation	secretory diarrhea
NSP4 enterotoxin	increase in intracellular calcium, chloride secretion	secretory diarrhea
NSP4-induced glucose malabsorption	inhibition of SGLT-1	osmotic diarrhea
Neuromediated vascular ischemia	neurotransmitter microcirculation impairment	secretory diarrhea
Inflammation	NF-κB, IL-8, Rantes	osmotic/secretory diarrhea

microbial agents, including bacteria, parasites and viruses.

Usually, viral diarrhea lasts for 3–5 days. In selected cases, viral diarrhea may be persistent and even become life-threatening. In a series of children with intractable diarrhea syndrome, rotavirus was detected in five out of 38 children who had no evident risk factors.[36]

The history may provide valuable clinical information. Diarrheal onset may be abrupt or progressive. The child's age, admission to a day-care center, the time of year, exposure to diarrheal contacts, previous antibiotic courses, and ingestion of contaminated food such as eggs or water should be evaluated to define the origin of diarrhea. Risk factors for severe diarrhea include malnutrition, immune derangement and AIDS, and history of repeated episodes of diarrhea. Recent weaning from breast milk or introduction of feedings other than milk may be associated with a more severe course of the disease (Table 9.2).

Dehydration is the key symptom to define the severity of the disease and the need for fluid replacement. The degree of dehydration should be evaluated at first observation and followed up to evaluate the ongoing losses and the efficacy of fluid intake to replace them. The gold standard for determining dehydration is acute weight loss. Because a patient's pre-illness weight is rarely known, an estimate of fluid deficiency is made on clinical grounds.

Vomiting may be associated with diarrhea and induce additional fluid losses. In addition, vomiting may prevent oral rehydration, thus requiring parenteral fluid replacement.

Body temperature may be elevated, as a consequence of dehydration or reflecting an inflammatory response. Abdominal pain is not frequent and suggests colonic involvement, but may also indicate a surgical problem.

Stool characteristics should be carefully considered: large volumes of watery stools indicate small bowel involvement and are frequently associated with dehydration, whereas frequent outputs of a small amount of mucus or bloody stools are associated with colitis. In severe cases the entire intestine is involved.

Colonic involvement is more often associated with bacterial rather than viral etiology. Some features may help in distinguishing viral from bacterial diarrhea (Table 9.4).[37] Viral diarrhea is more frequently associated with vomiting and dehydration. It affects younger children compared to

Table 9.4 Main clinical features associated with the most frequent enteric pathogens (modified from reference 37)

	Salmonella species	*Campylobacter* species	Rotavirus	NLV	*Giardia lamblia*
Fever	++++*	++++*	++++*	+	+
Blood in stool	++	++++*	+	++	+++
Abdominal cramps	++++*	++	-*	+	+
Vomiting	+	+	++++ *	++++*	+
>6 stools per day	+	++++*	++	+	+
Duration of symptoms (days)	7	7	<4	<4	>7

NLV, Norwalk-like virus
*$p<0.05$

Table 9.5 Individual symptoms and signs of acute gastroenteritis according to etiological agents in subjects younger than 2 years; mixed infections excluded (modified from reference 38)

	Rotavirus (n=189)	Adenovirus (n=35)	Astrovirus (n=34)	NLV (n=115)	SLV (n=44)
Duration of diarrhea (days)	4	5	1	2	3
Maximum number of diarrhea episodes in 24h	6	5	4	4	4
Duration of vomiting (days)	2	1	1	1	1
Maximum number of vomiting episodes in 24h	3	1	1	4	1
Temperature (°C)	38.8	38.4	37.9	37.9	37.8
Severity score	10	7	5	8	6

Data are medians of findings
NLV, Norwalk-like virus; SLV, Sapporo-like virus

bacterial diarrhea. Selected features are more frequently associated with specific enteric viruses (Table 9.5).[38] However, signs and symptoms in the individual child do not reliably allow identification of specific etiological agents of gastroenteritis.

Diagnosis

Although acute diarrhea is generally the manifestation of an enteric infection, it may be associated with other illnesses, such as food poisoning or intolerance, extraintestinal infections or surgical disease.[39] Acute diarrhea may be a side-effect of various drugs including antibiotics. History and clinical evaluation may aid in the differential diagnosis. However, close follow-up is required.

Generally, microbiological investigations are not necessary in children with acute gastroenteritis. Several studies have reported a low yield and cost/efficacy ratio per identified agent even in hospitalized children. Microbiological examination should be considered: in cases of persistent diarrhea; when a specific antimicrobial treatment is considered, such as for children belonging to a group at risk; when an intestinal infection must be excluded in order to support a different etiology; and to investigate an outbreak.

The search for enteric viruses is made by several techniques, including culture in sensitive cells, electron microscopy, immune-based assays and molecular probes (Table 9.6). Virus culture is the gold standard, but it is cumbersome and the results are available only with delay, limiting its clinical applications. Immune-based methods are widely used, but a progressive increase in the use of polymerase chain reaction (PCR) techniques is leading to a shift of diagnostic techniques. The choice of a specific technique is based on the clinical need, the availability of technical skills and the efficacy ratio. In most clinical institutions, immune-based assays are available to detect rotavirus and less frequently enteric adenovirus. The search for other viruses is generally available in reference centers or research institutions.

However, trying to identify the etiology may not be clinically useful, as treatment of diarrhea is relatively independent of the responsible agent. Rather, it is the evaluation of the child's clinical condition that provides information for case management.

Features of specific etiologies and virology

Rotaviruses

Reovirus-like particles were first identified in 1973 by electron microscopy in duodenal biopsies from children with acute diarrhea.[40] This led to a cascade of clinical and laboratory studies that have established the rotavirus as the single most common agent causing diarrhea in childhood.

Table 9.6 Etiological diagnosis of viral infections of the gastrointestinal tract

Viruses	Antigen detection	EM	PCR	Preferred test method
Rotavirus	EIA, latex agglutination	++++	RT-PCR	EIA
Calicivirus	EIA	+	RT-PCR	RT-PCR
Astrovirus	EIA	+	RT-PCR	EIA RT-PCR
Adenovirus	EIA	+++	RT-PCR	EIA
Cytomegalovirus			PCR	histology, immunohistochemistry
Picornavirus	EIA		RT-PCR	EIA
Epstein–Barr virus			PCR	histology, immunohistochemistry

EM, electron microscopy; PCR, polymerase chain reaction; EIA, enzyme immunoassay; RT, reverse transcriptase; +, detectable with low sensitivity by a skilled microscopist; +++, visible; ++++, easily visible

The global illness and deaths caused by rotavirus in children were recently estimated by reviewing studies between 1985 and 2000. Rotavirus caused 111 million episodes of gastroenteritis requiring home treatment, 25 million clinic visits, 2 million hospitalizations and 350–600 000 deaths in children less than 5 years of age, worldwide. All children were expected to be infected with rotavirus within 5 years of age, one in five children were expected to need a clinic visit and one in 65 to be hospitalized. Finally, one out of 293 children would die because of rotavirus infection, 84% in the poorest countries.[41]

Also, in countries with high economic standards, rotaviruses are a major problem. In industrialized countries, the estimates were: a total of 7 122 000 episodes of rotavirus gastroenteritis requiring only home care in children less than 5 years of age, a total of approximately 1 781 000 clinic visits and a total of 223 000 rotavirus-associated hospitalizations.[41] There are an estimated 3.5 million cases annually among children less than 5 years of age in the USA, leading to 500 000 office visits, 50 000 hospitalizations, and approximately 20 deaths.[42] These numbers translate into costs, resulting in US$ 1 billion/ year.[43]

Infection is widespread throughout the world. Rotavirus infection may occur repeatedly in humans from birth to old age. The first infection is predominant among children aged 6–24 months, although cases may occur in older children. Neonatal infections appear to be nosocomial in origin, because they are rarely seen in babies born at home or at village health centers. Approximately 90% of children in both developed and developing countries experience rotavirus infection by 3 years of age. The cumulative incidence of rotavirus illness by the age of 5 years approaches 0.8 episodes/child per year.

Several factors are responsible for the high spreading of rotavirus. Rotavirus shedding averages 6 days per episode, but may be persistent. Asymptomatic carriers contribute to infection spreading. Infected children develop a protective immunity and, although repeated infections generally occur in growing children, their clinical severity decreases.[44] Despite differences among studies in geographical areas, years and age groups, an increase in rotavirus cases is consistently reported in the winter months, with a peak in February to April. In tropical areas, rotaviruses are identified throughout the year.

Transmission occurs through the fecal–oral route. However, droplet transmission has been suggested to explain the rapidity with which the rotavirus can spread through a community.[45]

Virology

Rotavirus is a double-stranded RNA virus belonging to the Reoviridae family. The virion, 70–75 nm, is composed of a three-layered protein capsid that encloses 11 distinct segments of genomic RNA, each coding for a different capsid or non-structural protein. The internal core contains viral proteins (VP) 1, 2 and 3; the inner capsid contains VP4; the two outer capsid proteins encoded by genes 4 and 7, namely VP4 and VP7, represent the only established neutralization antigens of the virus. The protective role of antibodies directed at these proteins has been confirmed both in experimental animal models and in humans. A possible role has been suggested for antibodies directed at the inner capsid protein VP6, which is not associated with *in vitro* neutralization. The non-structural proteins NSP1, NSP2 and NSP4 are virulence factors in mice.

Rotavirus groups A–F have been described, but only groups A, B and C have been identified in humans. Most human infections are caused by group A rotaviruses that are classified into serotypes by a dual classification system based on neutralizing antigens on two outer capsid proteins, VP7 (G serotype) and VP4 (P serotype). To date, 10 G types and almost as many P types have been identified in infected humans. There is great genetic diversity within each G and P type, as shown by gel electrophoretic analysis of gene patterns (electropherotypes). Epidemiological and molecular studies in many countries show complex changes from year to year in the serotypes and electropherotypes that cause diarrhea in children from the same geographical areas.[46,47] The majority of severe diseases have been caused by serotypes G1 to G4, P1A and P1B, worldwide.[48] Epidemiological studies in Bangladesh,[49] Brazil,[50] India,[51] Kenya[48] and the USA[52] show that other G and P types (G5 to G10, P2A and P8) can be common and may be of emerging importance in communities.[53] Specific strains may express stronger virulence factors, which could be related to the severity of symptoms. More severe diseases may also be related to the reintroduction of strains in areas where they have been previously absent.[54]

Astroviruses

Human astroviruses (HAstVs) were first identified in 1975 in an outbreak of diarrhea in infants, and were named astrovirus because of the distinctive five- or six-pointed stars seen at electron microscopy.[55]

Recent studies have established that astrovirus is the third most frequent cause of diarrhea in children and the second in selected settings. The reported infection rates depend on detection methods. These include electron microscopy (EM), enzyme immunoassay (EIA) or reverse transcriptase-polymerase chain reaction (RT-PCR).[56] Incidence rates also depend on the population under study. The reported incidence of HAstV diarrhea ranges from 2% of children seeking medical care in Baltimore, to 17% of children with persistent diarrhea in Bangladesh.[57] Younger infants are at greater risk of developing diarrhea than older children. In a child-care center, attack rates among infants and toddlers ranged between 11 and 89%.[58]

HAstV may be an important agent of diarrhea in immunocompromised hosts such as those infected with HIV[59] and bone marrow transplanted patients.[60,61] Current evidence supports food-borne, water-borne and person-to-person transmission. The incidence peaks in winter months in temperate climates.

Virology

HAsVs are non-enveloped, single-stranded RNA viruses with a distinctive star appearance and a smooth particle edge. The genomic organization is unique among positive stranded RNA and warrants classification of astroviruses as a separate family, the Astroviridae.[62] Eight antigenic types have been identified. The complete genomic sequence of types 1 and 2 and the sequence of the capsid gene of types 3, 4, 5, 6, 7 and 8 have been obtained.[63]

HAstV-1 is the dominant genotype followed by HAstV-2. It is not known whether infection with one serotype confers protection against subsequent infection with other serotypes.

Caliciviruses

In 1972, the 'Norwalk agent' was discovered in fecal specimens during a gastroenteritis outbreak in an elementary school in Norwalk, Ohio.[64,65] This was the first discovered viral agent of gastroenteritis in humans using EM. Subsequently, a large number of other small round structured viruses (SRSVs) were detected. These agents appeared morphologically indistinguishable from the Norwalk virus by EM, but they were antigenically distinct by immune EM. SRSVs were discovered during investigations of gastroenteritis outbreaks and were named for the investigation site (e.g. Bristol, Hawaii, Snow Mountains, etc.). In addition, a morphologically distinct SRSV, defined as 'classic human calicivirus', was first described in the UK,[66] and the prototype strain – the Sapporo agent – was subsequently identified in Japan.[67]

This rather confusing classification system of these viruses has been recently revised and is now based on genetic sequences of the viruses and of their genomic organization. All viruses belong to the family Caliciviridae, and fall into two provisionally named genera: 'Norwalk-like viruses' (NLV) and 'Sapporo-like viruses' (SLV).

Molecular epidemiological studies showed that caliciviruses are the main cause of non-bacterial gastroenteritis outbreaks causing over 90% of outbreaks of acute, non-bacterial gastroenteritis in the USA.[68] They are spread by the fecal–oral route, but outbreaks are often caused by contaminated food or water.[69] Contaminated surfaces carry calicivirus in detectable amounts, thereby providing another important substrate for explosive outbreaks.[70] Droplets or person-to-person transmission explain outbreaks in which other spreading routes cannot be identified.[71] Infections rates increase in cold seasons,[72] almost disappearing in the warm summer months. NLVs have been found in 5–20% of stool specimens from sporadic cases of diarrhea using RT-PCR.[73] SLVs cause predominantly diarrheal diseases, while NLVs cause 'winter vomiting disease' in young children.[74]

Virology

Caliciviruses are single-stranded, positive sense RNA viruses closely related to picornaviruses.

Based on morphology, typical and atypical caliciviruses have been described. SLVs have the typical calicivirus morphology, with a six-pointed star appearance similar to those of many animal caliciviruses. In contrast, the surface structure of NLVs is rather smooth, leading to the designation 'small round structured viruses'.

The family Caliciviridae encompasses four distinct virus genera. Two, the NLVs and SLVs, contain the human calicivirus (previously referred to as small round structured viruses) and the classic human caliciviruses, respectively. Phylogenetic analyses of sequences in the RNA polymerase and the capsid regions of the genome revealed that currently identified NLVs and SLVs can be divided into genogroups and genetic clusters. The NLV genus includes two genogroups (I and II) and at least 15 genetic clusters.[75] The SLV genus has fewer members, with a total of 4–5 genetic clusters.

Enteric adenoviruses

There are six different groups of adenovirus, but only group F, including serotypes 40 and 41, are referred to as enteric adenoviruses. Both cause endemic diarrhea and outbreaks in hospitals, orphanages and day-care centers.

The enteric adenoviruses are non-enveloped particles, containing double-stranded DNA.[76]

These viruses infect children more than adults; more than 50% of children are seropositive by years 3–4 of life.[77] Enteric adenoviruses are detected in 1.5–4% of children with diarrhea and are isolated throughout the year with no specific seasonal distribution.[78,79] Transmission is fecal–oral. The incubation lasts from 3 to 10 days. Adenovirus diarrhea lasts for 6–9 days and may be associated with vomiting and fever. Stools are watery, without blood or fecal leukocytes. EM initially was used to detect enteric adenoviruses, but commercial enzyme-linked immunosorbent assays are now widely available.

Toroviruses

Toroviruses include the Breda virus of cattle and Berne virus of horses,[80–82] and were first documented in 1984 by EM in humans with gastroenteritis.[83] These enveloped RNA viruses contain a tightly coiled tubular nucleocapsid that generally assumes a 'donut' torus shape in the virion.[80] Toroviruses were classified on the basis of the Berne virus genome sequence as members of the family Coronaviridae, which together with the family Arteriviridae are now classified in the order Nidovirales.[84–86]

Study of torovirus infections in calves indicates that Breda viruses infect differentiating crypt cells, expecially in the large intestine.[81,82]

The incidence of torovirus infection remains relatively constant throughout the year. Early studies indicated that toroviruses infect school-age children, and are responsible for nosocomial infections, more frequently in immunocompromised patients.[87]

The clinical manifestations of torovirus infection are similar to those of rotavirus or astrovirus, except that children with torovirus infection had less vomiting and bloodier diarrhea.[83,87] Symptom duration is similar to that of rotavirus infection, but toroviruses more frequently induce persistent diarrhea.[87] Further epidemiological studies are needed to determine its frequency in the community.

Picornaviruses (the Aichi virus)

In 1989, a cytopathic small round virus was isolated from a patient with oyster-associated gastroenteritis.[88] Genetic analyses of this virus, named Aichi virus, led to its classification into the Picornavirus family. It is distinct from any other genus such as the enterrhino-, cardio-, aptho-, hepato- and parechovirus group.[89] The Aichi virus is presently an unassigned species in the Picornavirus family.[90] Recently, it has been proposed to assign the Aichi virus to a new genus named Kobuvirus.[91]

The Aichi viruses cause acute gastroenteritis outbreaks. The main clinical symptoms are diarrhea (59%), abdominal pain (83%), nausea (92%), vomiting (71%) and fever (58%).[92]

Coronaviruses

Coronaviruses are large enveloped single-stranded RNA viruses related to toroviruses. These viruses are a well-documented cause of gastroenteritis in animals and of the common cold in humans. Coronaviruses have been identified in the stools of children with diarrhea, but their role as a cause of diarrhea is unknown. They have been detected more commonly in the diarrheal stools of older children and young adults. The prolonged virus excretion makes it difficult to assess their etiological role. Recently, coronavirus mutants have been implicated in the severe acute respiratory syndrome (SARS).[93]

Picobirnaviruses

These viruses have icosahedral symmetry with triangulation number (T) equal to 3.[94] They have been detected in diarrheic as well as non-diarrheic animals, and occasionally in children and in humans with HIV infection. Their etiological role in immunocompetent children is unknown.

Treatment

For the cornerstone of treatment of acute diarrhea, i.e. the restoration of fluid and electrolyte homeostasis[95,96] see Chapter 39.

For children hospitalized with severe rotavirus diarrhea, passive immune treatment should be considered. Several studies have shown that oral administration of human serum immunoglobulin is associated with an effective antiviral effect. Human immunoglobulin, including pooled gammaglobulin, bovine colostrums, or human milk, may decrease the frequency and duration of diarrhea.[97] Human immunoglobulin was initially used to treat children with life-threatening rotavirus diarrhea.[98] In a double-blind, placebo-controlled study oral administration of human serum immunoglobulin, in a single bolus of 300 mg/kg body weight, resulted in faster recovery and early discharge of immunocompetent children admitted to hospital with severe rotavirus diarrhea, without adverse effects[99] (Figure 9.5). The same treatment was given to children with AIDS and severe rotavirus infection, and led to rapid remission of diarrhea and permanent clearance of the virus.[100] We currently give human immunoglobulin to children hospitalized with severe rotavirus infection and to patients at risk of a poor outcome.[101]

Human immunoglobulin, although expensive, is widely available. Its efficacy might be related to high titers of specific neutralizing antibodies to rotavirus. Specific titers are consistently detected in preparations commercially available for intravenous use, because of the high frequency of rotavirus infection and the consequent widespread immune response. The efficacy of immunoglobulin is probably related to dose- and time-related direct neutralization of rotavirus, which prevents enterocyte infection and cell death.[18] Preliminary experimental evidence indicates that immunoglobulin prevents both the cytotoxic and the enterotoxic effect induced by rotavirus in human enterocytes.[102] Thus, immunoglobulin should be administered orally early in the course of the disease for maximum efficacy.

This information may be of practical relevance, while awaiting the development of safer vaccines that will hopefully be effective, for normal or compromised immune function.

Vaccine development

Rotavirus

A review of the global prevalence of rotavirus disease was published in 1985, showing that rotavirus accounted for 6% of diarrhea episodes and 20% of deaths caused by diarrhea in children less than 5 years of age in developing countries.[103] The incidence of rotavirus disease was similar in both industrialized and developing countries, suggesting that adequate control may not be achieved by improvements in water supply,

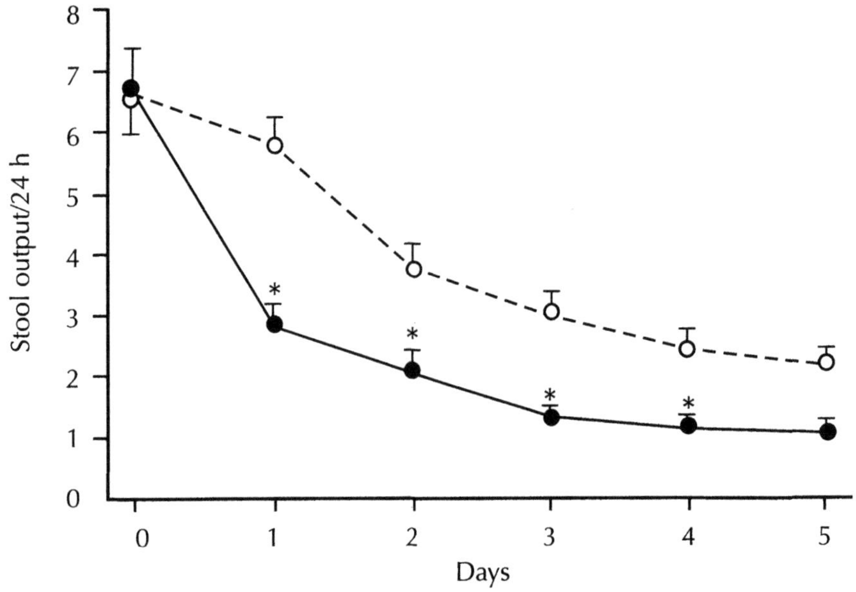

Figure 9.5 Stool frequency (stools/24 h) in children hospitalized because of Rotavirus treated with human serum immunoglobulin administered per oral route in a single dose of 300 mg/kg body weight (•) and control children (o). Values are means ± SEM. *p <0.05 (from reference 118).

hygiene and sanitation. Based on the results of a recent paper, rotavirus is still a major threat to child health worldwide.[40]

After more than 15 years of basic research and clinical trials, a live-attenuated rhesus rotavirus-tetravalent vaccine (RRV-TV), was licensed by the Food and Drug Administration. However, the life-span of the RRV-TV was short. After initial marketing and after nearly 1.5 million doses already administered in 9 months, the Centers for Disease Control withdrew the vaccine recommendation because of the possible association of the vaccine with intestinal intussusception, and the RRV-TV was removed from the market.[104] This event represented a major drawback and introduced new complications in producing a safe and effective vaccine for children, particularly in the developing world, where the vaccine is mostly needed to reduce high mortality rates.

Recent epidemiological surveillance of circulating rotavirus strains, performed to follow the impact of the RRV-TV vaccine, raised questions about whether the RRV-TV would be effective in all settings. Rotavirus strains are characterized into glycoprotein (G) serotypes based on the antigenic properties of their VP7 surface protein. The reassortant RRV-TV vaccine contained G serotypes 1 to 4. In developed countries, more than 80% of rotavirus strains circulating in humans belongs to G serotypes 1 to 4. In the developing world, unusual rotaviruses (G5, G8, G9, or G10) are detected with increasing prevalence. The detection of unusual G9 strains in several developed countries indicates the appearance of more G serotypes in the developed world as well. Thus, vaccine formulations may need to be modified to encompass the diversity of rotavirus strains in particular geographic regions.

Development of alternative vaccination strategies, e.g. virus-like particles (VLPs), vector-expressed proteins, and DNA immunization, continues to be pursued. Among these, preclinical data are strongest for VLPs, because these non-replicating particles are immunogenic and are able to induce protective immunity in several animal models. A number of other candidate rotavirus vaccines have been developed. A summary of vaccines currently in human trials is given in Table 9.7.[105] The development of new vaccines is complicated by a lack of understanding of which proteins are essential to prevent diarrhea in children. Thus, even

Table 9.7 Live, attenuated, oral rotavirus vaccines currently in human trials (modified from reference 105)

Product	Company	Concept
LLR	Lanzhou Institute of Biological Products (China)	monovalent lamb strain (P[12]G10)
Rotateq	Merck (USA)	WC-3 based multivalent human-bovine reassortant
Rotarix (89-12)	GlaxoSmithKline (Belgium)	monovalent human strain (P[8]G1)
UK-reassortant vaccine	Wyeth Ayerst/NIH (USA)	UK-based multivalent human–bovine reassortant
RV3	University of Melbourne (Australia)	neonatal strain (P[6]G3)
116E	Bharat Biotech (India)	neonatal strain (P[11]G9)
I321	Bharat Biotech (India)	neonatal strain (P[11]G10)

though a rotavirus vaccine was licensed, correlates of protective immunity remain relatively unclear.

'Norwalk-like viruses'

Some human study volunteers never become infected after challenge with NLV, perhaps reflecting the recent finding that NLVs recognize human histoblood group antigens as receptors, defining host susceptibility. Immunity to NLV infections is believed to be short lived, as volunteers were re-infected with the same strain within months of previous challenge.

Self-assembled recombinant capsid proteins of Norwalk virus (rNV) into VLPs have been tested as oral immunogens.[106] Preclinical studies in mice and phase I studies in healthy adult volunteers have shown that these VLPs are immunogenic in the absence of adjuvant, and high doses (250 mg) delivered orally were safe and elicited antibody responses in all volunteers. The positive results obtained with oral delivery of rNV VLPs have stimulated new vaccine developments, including the expression of rNV in tobacco and potato tubers.[107] RNV VLPs expressed in potato tubers were also immunogenic when given to volunteers orally.[108] The protective efficacy of these candidate vaccines in human volunteers is currently under study.

Conclusions/summary

Viral diarrhea still represents a major threat to childhood health, worldwide. It has an immense, but distinct, impact in poor and rich countries, being responsible for a substantial number of deaths in the former and of heavy money loss in the latter. Rotavirus is the leading agent and its pathophysiology involves multiple mechanisms, several of which are triggered by NSP4 enterotoxin. Diarrhea is the hallmark of viral diarrhea and is usually self-limiting. However, it may run a severe course and have a fatal outcome in children with malnutrition or immune impairment and in those who have no access to rehydration. Diagnosis is usually based on clinical grounds, and investigations are not necessary. Treatment is based on carbohydrate and electrolyte solution administered through the oral or parenteral route. Selected probiotics may be effective in reducing the duration of symptoms, whereas, in severe cases in which rotavirus is involved, oral administration of human serum immunoglobulin may be effective. Efforts towards vaccine development have been hampered by withdrawal of anti-rotavirus vaccine, because of its association with intussusception, but novel vaccines are currently under investigation.

REFERENCES

1. Taterka JA, Cuff CF, Rubin DH. Viral gastrointestinal infections. *Gastroenterol Clin North Am* 1992; **21**: 303–330.
2. Kosek M, Bern C, Guerrant RL. The magnitude of the global burden of diarrhoeal disease, as estimated from studies published between 1992 and 2000. *Bull World Health Organ* 2003; **81**:197–204.
3. Glass RI, Bresee J, Jiang B et al. Gastroenteritis viruses: an overview. *Novartis Found Symp* 2001; **238**: 5–25.
4. Zimmermann CM, Bresee JS, Parashar UD et al. Cost of diarrhea-associated hospitalizations and outpatient visits in an insured population of young children in the United States. *Pediatr Infect Dis J* 2001; **20**: 14–19.
5. Fruhwirth M, Karmaus W, Moll-Schuler I et al. A prospective evaluation of community acquired gastroenteritis in paediatric practices: impact and disease burden of rotavirus infection. *Arch Dis Child* 2001; **84**: 393–397.
6. de Wit MAS, Koopmans MPG, van der Blij JF et al. Hospital admission for rotavirus in the Netherlands. *Clin Infect Dis* 2000; **31**: 698–704.
7. Avendano P, Matson DO, Long J et al. Costs associated with office visits for diarrhea in infants and toddlers. *Pediatr Infect Dis J* 1993; **12**: 897–902.
8. Berni Canani R, Cirillo P, Mallardo G et al. Effects of HIV-1 Tat protein on ion secretion and on cell proliferation in human intestinal epithelial cells. *Gastroenterology* 2003; **124**: 368–376.
9. Ciarlet M, Estes MK. Human and most animal rotavirus strains do not require the presence of sialic acid on the cell surface for efficient infectivity. *J Gen Virol* 1999; **80**: 943–948.
10. Ciarlet M, Crawford SE, Estes MK. Asymmetric infection of epithelial cell lines of sialic-acid-dependent rotaviruses. *Gastroenterology* 2000; **118**: A101.
11. Reynolds D, Hall G, Debney T et al. Pathology of natural rotavirus infection in clinically normal calves. *Res Vet Sci* 1985; **38**: 264–269.
12. Collins J, Benfield D, Duimstra J. Comparative virulence of two porcine group A rotavirus isolates in gnotobiotic pigs. *Am J Vet Res* 1989; **50**: 827–835.
13. Osborne MP, Haddon SJ, Worton KJ et al. Rotavirus-induced changes in microcirculation of intestinal villi of neonatal mice in relation to the induction and persistence of diarrhea. *J Pediatr Gastroenterol Nutr* 1991; **12**: 111–120.
14. Lundgren O, Timar Peregrin A, Persson K et al. Role of the enteric nervous system in the fluid and electrolyte secretion of rotavirus diarrhea. *Science* 2000; **287**: 491–495.
15. Ruiz MC, Cohen J, Michelangeli F. Role of Ca^{2+} in the replication and pathogenesis of rotavirus and other viral infections. *Cell Calcium* 2000; **28**: 137–149.
16. Obert G, Peiffer I, Servin AL. Rotavirus-induced structural and functional alterations in tight junctions of polarized intestinal Caco-2 cell monolayers. *J Virol* 2000; **74**: 4645–4651.
17. Brunet JP, Cotte-Laffitte J, Linxe C et al. Rotavirus infection induces an increase in intracellular calcium concentration in human intestinal epithelial cells: role in microvillar actin alteration. *J Virol* 2000; **74**: 2323–2332.
18. Guarino A, Casola A, Bruzzese E et al. Human serum immunoglobulin counteracts rotaviral infection in Caco-2 cells. *Pediatr Res* 1996; **40**: 881–887.
19. Ball JM, Tiam P, Zeng CQ-Y et al. Age-dependent diarrhoea is induced by a viral nonstructural glycoprotein. *Science* 1996; **272**: 101–104.
20. Zhang M, Zeng CQ-Y, Morris AP et al. A functional NSP4 enterotoxin peptide secreted from rotavirus infected cells. *J Virol* 2000; **74**: 11663–11670.
21. Au KS, Chan WK, Burns JW et al. Receptor activity of rotavirus nonstructural glycoprotein NS28. *J Virol* 1989; **63**: 4553–4562.
22. Meyer JC, Bergmann CC, Bellamy AR. Interaction of rotavirus cores with nonstructural glycoprotein NS28. *Virology* 1989; **171**: 98–107.
23. Taylor JA, O'Brien JA, Lord VJ et al. The RER-localized rotavirus intracellular receptor: a truncated purified soluble form is multivalent and binds virus particles. *Virology* 1993; **194**: 807–814.
24. Bergmann CC, Maass D, Poruchynsky MS et al. Topology of the non-structural rotavirus receptor glycoprotein NS28 in the rough endoplasmic reticulum. *EMBO J* 1989; **8**: 1695–1703.
25. Tian P, Hu Y, Schilling WP et al. The nonstructural glycoprotein of rotavirus affects intracellular calcium levels. *J Virol* 1994; **68**: 251–257.
26. Tian P, Estes MK, Hu Y et al. The rotavirus nonstructural glycoprotein NSP4 mobilizes Ca2+ from the endoplasmic reticulum. *J Virol* 1995; **69**: 5763–5772.
27. Newton K, Meyer JC, Bellamy AR et al. Rotavirus nonstructural glycoprotein NSP4 alters plasma membrane permeability in mammalian cells. *J Virol* 1997; **71**: 9458–9465.
28. Richardson SC, Grimwood K, Bishop RF. Analysis of homotypic and heterotypic serum immune responses to rotavirus proteins following primary rotavirus infection by using the radioimmunoprecipitation technique. *J Clin Microbiol* 1993; **31**: 377–385.
29. Johansen K, Hinkula J, Espinoza F et al. Humoral and cell-mediated immune responses to the NSP4 enterotoxin of rotavirus. *J Med Virol* 1999; **59**: 369–377.
30. Estes MK, Morris AP. A viral enterotoxin. A new mechanism of virus-induced pathogenesis. *Adv Exp Med Biol* 1999; **473**: 73–82.
31. Salim AF, Phillips AD, Walker-Smith JA et al. Sequential changes in small structure and function during rotavirus infection in neonatal rats. *Gut* 1996; **36**: 231–238.
32. Ciarlet M, Estes MK. Rotaviruses and calicivirus infections of the gastrointestinal tract. *Curr Opin Gastroenterol* 2001; **17**: 10–16.
33. Halaihel N, Lievin V, Alvarado F et al. Rotavirus infection impairs intestinal brush-border membrane Na^+-solute cotransport activities in young rabbits. *Am J Physiol Gastrointest Liver Physiol* 2000; **279**: G587–G596.
34. Casola A, Estes MK, Crawford SE et al. Rotavirus infection of cultured intestinal epithelial cells induces secretion of CXC and CC chemokines. *Gastroenterology* 1998; **114**: 947–955.
35. Rollo EE, Kumar KP, Reich NC et al. The epithelial cell response to rotavirus infection. *J Immunol* 1999; **163**: 4442–4452.
36. Guarino A, Spagnuolo MI, Russo S et al. Etiology and risk factors of severe and protracted diarrhea. *J Pediatr Gastroenterol Nutr* 1995; **20**: 173–178.
37. de Wit MAS, Koopmans MPG, Kortbeek LM et al. Etiology of gastroenteritis in sentinel general practices in the Netherlands. *Clin Infect Dis* 2001; **33**: 280–288.

38. Pang XL, Honma S, Nakata S et al. Human caliciviruses in acute gastroenteritis of young children in the community. *J Infect Dis* 2000; **181**: S288–S294.
39. Capano G, Guandalini S, Guarino A et al. Enteric infections, cow's milk protein intolerance and parenteral infections in 118 consecutive cases of acute diarrhea in children. *Eur J Pediatr* 1984; **142**: 281–285.
40. Bishop RF, Davidson GP, Holmes IH et al. Virus particles in epithelial cells of duodenal mucosa from children with viral gastroenteritis. *Lancet* 1973; **2**: 1281–1283.
41. Parashar UD, Hummelmann E, Brese JS et al. Global illness and deaths caused by Rotavirus disease in children. *Emerg Infect Dis* 2003; **9**: 565–572.
42. Glass RI, Kilgore PE, Holman RC et al. The epidemiology of rotavirus diarrhea in the United States: surveillance and estimates of disease burden. *J Infect Dis* 1996; **174**: S5–11.
43. Ho MS, Glass RI, Pinsky PF et al. Rotavirus as a cause of diarrheal morbidity and mortality in the United States. *J Infect Dis* 1988; **158**: 1112–1116.
44. Velasquez FR, Matson DO, Calva JJ et al. Rotavirus infection in infants as protection against subsequent infections. *N Engl J Med* 1996; **335**: 1022–1028.
45. Prince DS, Astry C, Vonderfecht S et al. Aerosol transmission of experimental rotavirus infection. *Pediatr Infect Dis* 1986; **5**: 218–222.
46. Bishop RF. Natural history of rotavirus infection. In AZ Kapikian, ed. *Viral Infections of the Gastrointestinal Tract*, 2nd edn. New York: Marcel Dekker, 1994; 131–167.
47. Gentsch JR, Woods PA, Ramachandran M et al. Review of G and P typing results from a global collection of rotavirus strains: implications for vaccine development. *J Infect Dis* 1996; **174**: S30–S36.
48. Nakata S, Gatheru Z, Ukae S et al. Epidemiological study of the G serotype distribution of group A rotaviruses in Kenya from 1991 to 1994. *J Med Virol* 1999; **58**: 296–303.
49. Unicomb LE, Podder JR, Gentsch PA et al. Evidence of high-frequency genomic reassortment of group A rotavirus strains in Bangladesh: emergence of type G9 in 1995. *J Clin Microbiol* 1999; **37**: 1885–1891.
50. Santos N, Lima RCC, Pereira CFA et al. Detection of rotavirus types G8 and G10 among Brazilian children with diarrhea. *J Clin Microbiol* 1998; **36**: 2727–2729.
51. Aijas S, Gowda K, Jagannath HV et al. Epidemiology of symptomatic human rotaviruses in Bangladore and Mysore, India from 1988 to 1994 as determined by electropherotype, subgroup and serotype analysis. *Arch Virol* 1996; **141**: 715–726.
52. Ramachandran M, Gentsch JR, Parashar UD et al. Detection and characterization of novel rotavirus strains in the United States. *J Clin Microbiol* 1998; **36**: 3223–3229.
53. Gouvea V, Santos N. Rotavirus serotype G5: an emerging cause of epidemic childhood diarrhea. *Vaccine* 1999; **17**: 1291–1292.
54. Cascio A, Vizzi E, Alaimo C et al. Rotavirus gastroenteritis in Italian children: can severity of symptoms be related to the infecting virus? *Clin Infect Dis* 2001; **32**: 1126–1132.
55. Madeley CR, Cosgrove BP. Virus in infantile gastroenteritis. *Lancet* 1975; **2**: 451–452.
56. Glass RI, Noel J, Mitchell D et al. The changing epidemiology of astrovirus-associated gastroenteritis: a review. *Arch Virol Suppl* 1996; **12**: 287–300.
57. Unicomb LE, Banu NN, Azim T et al. Astrovirus infection in association with acute, persistent and nosocomial diarrhea in Bangladesh. *Pediatr Infect Dis J* 1998; **17**: 611–614.
58. Mitchell DK, Monroe SS, Jiang X et al. Virologic features of an astrovirus diarrhea outbreak in a day care center revealed by reverse transcriptase-polymerase chain reaction. *J Infect Dis* 1995; **172**: 1437–1444.
59. Grohmann GS, Glass RI, Pereira HG et al. Enteric viruses and diarrhea in HIV-infected patients. Enteric Opportunistic Infections Working Group. *N Engl J Med* 1993; **329**: 14–20.
60. Cox GJ, Matsui SM, Lo RS et al. Etiology and outcome of diarrhea after marrow transplantation: a prospective study. *Gastroenterology* 1994; **107**: 1398–1407.
61. Cubitt WD, Mitchell DK, Carter MJ et al. Applications of electronmicroscopy, enzyme immunoassay, a RT-PCR to monitor an outbreak of astrovirus type 1 in a paediatric bone marrow transplant unit. *J Med Virol* 1999; **57**: 313–321.
62. Wyatt RG, Dolin R, Blacklow NR et al. Comparison of three agents of acute infectious nonbacterial gastroenteritis by cross-challenge in volunteers. *J Infect Dis* 1974; **129**: 709–714.
63. Monroe SS, Jiang B, Stine SE et al. Subgenomic RNA sequence of human astrovirus supports classification of Astroviridae as a new family of RNA viruses. *J Virol* 1993; **67**: 3611–3614.
64. Adler JL, Zickl R. Winter vomiting disease. *J Infect Dis* 1969; **119**: 668–673.
65. Kapikian AZ, Wyatt RG, Dolin R et al. Visualization by immune electron microscopy of a 27 nm particle associated with acute infectious nonbacterial gastroenteritis. *J Virol* 1972; **10**: 1075–1081.
66. Madeley CR, Cosgrove BP. 28 nm particles in faeces in infantile gastroenteritis. *Lancet* 1975; **2**: 451–452.
67. Chiba S, Sakuma Y, Kogasaka R et al. An outbreak of gastroenteritis associated with calicivirus in an infant home. *J Med Virol* 1979; **4**: 249–254.
68. Fankhauser RI, Noel JS, Monroe SS et al. Molecular epidemiology of 'Norwalk-like viruses' in outbreaks of gastroenteritis in the United States. *J Infect Dis* 1998; **178**: 1571–1578.
69. Lopman BA, Reacher MH, van Duijnhoven Y et al. Viral gastroenteritis outbreaks in Europe, 1995–2000. *Emerg Infect Dis* 2003; **9**: 90–96.
70. Brown DWG. The pattern and burden of disease due to human calicivirus infections in the UK (abstract S1-2). In *Proceedings of the International Workshop on Human Caliciviruses*, Atlanta GA, 29–31 March 1999. Atlanta: Centers for Disease Control and Prevention,1999.
71. Sawyer LA, Murphy JJ, Kaplan JE et al. 25 to 30 nm virus particle associated with a hospital outbreak of acute gastroenteritis with evidence for airborne transmission. *Am J Epidemiol* 1988; **127**: 1261–1271.
72. Mounts AW, Ando T, Koopmans M et al. Cold weather seasonality of gastroenteritis associated with Norwalk-like viruses. *J Infect Dis* 2000; **181**: S284–S287.
73. Jiang Xi, Pickering LK. Update on caliciviruses and human acute gastroenteritis. *Pediatr Infect Dis J* 2002; **21**: 1069–1070.
74. Zahorsky J. Hyperemesis hiemis or the winter vomiting disease. *Arch Pediatr* 1929; **46**: 391.
75. Green J, Vinje J, Gallimore CI et al. Capsid protein diversity among Norwalk-like viruses. *Virus Genes* 2000; **20**: 227–236.
76. Favier AL, Schoehn G, Jaquinod M et al. Structural studies of human enteric adenovirus type 41. *Virology* 2002; **293**: 75–85.
77. Kotloff KL, Losonsky GA, Morris JG et al. Enteric adenovirus infection and childhood diarrhea: an epidemiologic study in three clinical settings. *Pediatrics* 1989; **84**: 219–225.

78. Soares CC, Volotao EM, Albuquerque MC et al. Prevalence of enteric adenoviruses among children with diarrhea in four Brazilian cities. *J Clin Virol* 2002; **23**: 171–177.
79. Waters V, Ford-Jones EL, Petric M et al. Etiology of community-acquired pediatric viral diarrhea: a prospective longitudinal study in hospitals, emergency departments, pediatric practices and child care centers during the winter rotavirus outbreak, 1997 to 1998. The Pediatric Rotavirus Epidemiology Study for Immunization Study Group. *Pediatr Infect Dis J* 2000; **19**: 843–848.
80. Weiss M, Horzinek MC. The proposed family, Toroviridae: agents of enteric infections. *Arch Virol* 1987; **92**: 1–15.
81. Woode GN, Reed DE, Runnels PL et al. Studies with an unclassified virus isolated from diarrheic calves. *Vet Microbiol* 1982; **7**: 221–240.
82. Woode GN, Saif LJ, Quesanda M et al. Comparative studies on three isolates of Breda virus of calves. *Am J Vet Res* 1985; **46**: 1003–1010.
83. Beards GM, Green J, Hall C et al. An enveloped virus in stools of children and adults with gastroenteritis resembles the Breda virus of calves. *Lancet* 1984; **1**: 1050–1052.
84. Snijder E, Horzinek MC. Toroviruses: replication, evolution and comparison with other members of the coronavirus-like family. *J Gen Virol* 1993; **74**: 2305–2316.
85. Cavanagh D, Horzinek M. Genus Torovirus assigned to the Coronaviridae. *Arch Virol* 1993; **128**: 395–396.
86. Cavanaugh D. Nidovirales: a new order comprising Coronaviridae and Arteriviridae. *Arch Virol* 1997; **142**: 629–633.
87. Jamieson FB, Wang EEL, Bain C et al. Human Torovirus: a new nosocomial gastrointestinal pathogen. *J Infect Dis* 1998; **178**: 1263–1269.
88. Yamashita T, Kobayashi S, Sakae K et al. Isolation of cytophathic small round viruses with BS-C-1 cells from patient with gastroenteritis. *J Infect Dis* 1991; **164**: 954–957.
89. Yamashita T, Sakae K, Tsuzuki H et al. Complete nucleotide sequence and genetic organization of Aichi virus, a distinct member of Picornaviridae associated with acute gastroenteritis in humans. *J Virol* 1998; **72**: 8408–8412.
90. King AMQ, Brown F, Christian P et al. Picornaviridae. In van Regenmortel MHV, Fauquet CM, Bishop DHL, et al., eds. *Virus Taxonomy: Seventh Report of the International Committee on Taxonomy of Viruses*. San Diego: Academy Press, 2000: 657–678.
91. King AMQ, Brown F, Christian P et al. Picornavirus taxonomy: a modified species definition and proposal for three new genera. *XIth International Congress of Virology*, Sidney, Australia, 1999.
92. Yamashita T, Ito M, Tsuzuki H et al. Identification of Aichi virus infection by measurement of immunoglobulin responses in a enzyme linked immunosorbent assay. *J Clin Microbiol* 2001; **39**: 4178–4180.
93. Stohr K. A multicentre collaboration to investigate the cause of severe acute respiratory syndrome. *Lancet* 2003; **361**: 1730–1733.
94. Chandra R. Picobirnavirus, a novel group of undescribed viruses of mammals and birds: a minireview. *Acta Virol* 1997; **41**: 59–62.
95. Guarino A, Albano F, Guandalini S et al. Oral rehydration solution: toward a real solution. *J Pediatr Gastroenterol Nutr* 2001; **33**: S2–S12.
96. Guarino A, Albano F. Guidelines for the approach to outpatient children with acute diarrhoea. *Acta Paediatr* 2001; **90**: 1087–1095.
97. Guarino A, Berni Canani R, Russo S. Developments in the treatment of rotaviral gastroenteritis: oral therapy with immunoglobulins and prospects for a vaccine. *Clin Immunother* 1995; **3**: 476–484.
98. Guarino A, Guandalini S, Albano F et al. Enteral immunoglobulin for treatment of protracted Rotaviral diarrhea. *Pediatr Infect Dis J* 1991; **10**: 612–614.
99. Guarino A, Berni Canani R, Russo S et al. Oral immunoglobulins for treatment of acute rotaviral gastroenteritis. *Pediatrics* 1994; **93**: 12–16.
100. Guarino A, Russo S, Castaldo A et al. Passive immunotherapy for Rotavirus-induced diarrhoea in children with HIV infection. *AIDS* 1996; **10**: 1176–1178.
101. Guarino A, Albano F, Berni Canani R et al. HIV, fatal rotavirus infection, and treatment options. *Lancet* 2002; **359**: 74.
102. De Marco G, Bruzzese E, Di Nardo G et al. Rotavirus induces a galanin-dependent chloride secretion which is inhibited by human immunoglobulin in a Caco-2 experimental model. *J Pediatr Gastroenterol Nutr* 2003; **36**: 521(abstr).
103. De Zoysa I, Feachem RG. Interventions for the control of diarrhoeal disease among young children: rotavirus and cholera immunization. *Bull World Health Organ* 1985; **62**: 569–583.
104. Rennels MB. The rotavirus vaccine story: a clinical investigator's view. *Pediatrics* 2000; **106**: 123–125.
105. Cunliffe NA, Bresee JS, Hart CA. Rotavirus vaccines: development, current issues and future prospects. *J Infect* 2002; **45**: 1–9.
106. Ball JM, Graham DY, Opekun AR et al. Recombinant Norwalk-like particles given orally to volunteers: phase I study. *Gastroenterology* 1999; **1117**: 40–48.
107. Mason H, Ball JM, Shi J et al. Expression of Norwalk virus capsid protein in transgenic tobacco and potato and its oral immunogenicity in mice. *Proc Nat Acad Sci USA* 1996; **93**: 5335–5340.
108. Tacket C, Mason H, Losonsky G et al. Human immune responses to a novel Norwalk virus vaccine delivered in transgenic potatoes. *J Infect Dis* 2000; **182**: 302–305.

10 Bacterial infections

Alessio Fasano

Enteric infections exact a heavy toll on human populations, particularly among children. Despite the explosion of knowledge on the pathogenesis of enteric diseases experienced during the past decade, the number of diarrheal episodes and childhood deaths reported worldwide remains of apocalyptic dimensions. In the next 15 s, a child somewhere in the world will die from diarrhea. Worldwide, it is estimated that 6–60 billion cases of gastrointestinal illness occur annually, the vast majority being severe enough and affecting so many unprivileged populations to pose a serious global health burden. In overpopulated developing countries, poor sanitation and hygiene, unsafe water supplies and limited education contribute to the propagation of diarrheal diseases. In industrialized nations, diarrhea had been thought of as more of an inconvenience rather than a serious cause of illness, but recent attention to food contamination by pathogens such as *Salmonella* and *Escherichia coli*, in combination with a growing population of immunosuppressed patients, has led to increased recognition of their impact. The situation is further complicated by the recent escalation of international terrorism that is raising the risk of epidemics of enteric pathogens beyond the boundaries of natural endemic areas.

The appreciation of these multifaceted aspects of the problem is pivotal for full comprehension of the threat that diarrheal diseases pose to public health and for appropriate allocation of resources and efforts to tackle them. However, there are a series of obstacles that have historically hampered this process, including non-standardized definitions of disease and symptoms; failure to identify a causative agent in many, if not most, cases of disease; failure to report episodes to health authorities; and the existence of incompatible reporting systems. Most of all, the lack of long-term commitment of rich countries to finance sanitation campaigns to treat and prevent diarrheal diseases in endemic areas has been a key limiting factor in tackling the burden of gastrointestinal diseases. Nevertheless, bacterial genome sequencing and better understanding of the pathogenic mechanisms involved in the onset of diarrhea, particularly concerning the elaboration of toxin (Figure 10.1), are finally leading to preventive interventions, such as enteric vaccines, that may have a significant impact on the magnitude of this human plague.

The majority of acute infectious diarrheal illnesses in both children and adults in developing countries are due to bacteria (Table 10.1). The risk factors for transmission of these pathogens are higher in these countries, owing to increased exposure to the organisms (by contact with feces, water, food and fomites) and increased susceptibility of the host due to malnutrition.

Cholera

Of all enteric pathogens, *Vibrio cholerae* is responsible for the most rapidly fatal diarrheal disease in humans.[1] Although cholera is rare in developed countries, it remains a major cause of diarrheal morbidity and mortality in many parts of the developing world.[2] However, with the occurrence of both natural (e.g. earthquakes) and human-generated calamities (such as ethnic wars), the spreading of cholera infection in refugee camps, where sanitary conditions resemble those in cholera endemic areas, represents a significant threat worldwide. Vibrios (from the Greek for 'comma') are single, short, curved Gram-negative rods, with a single, long, polar flagellum that allows for the organism's characteristic motility.

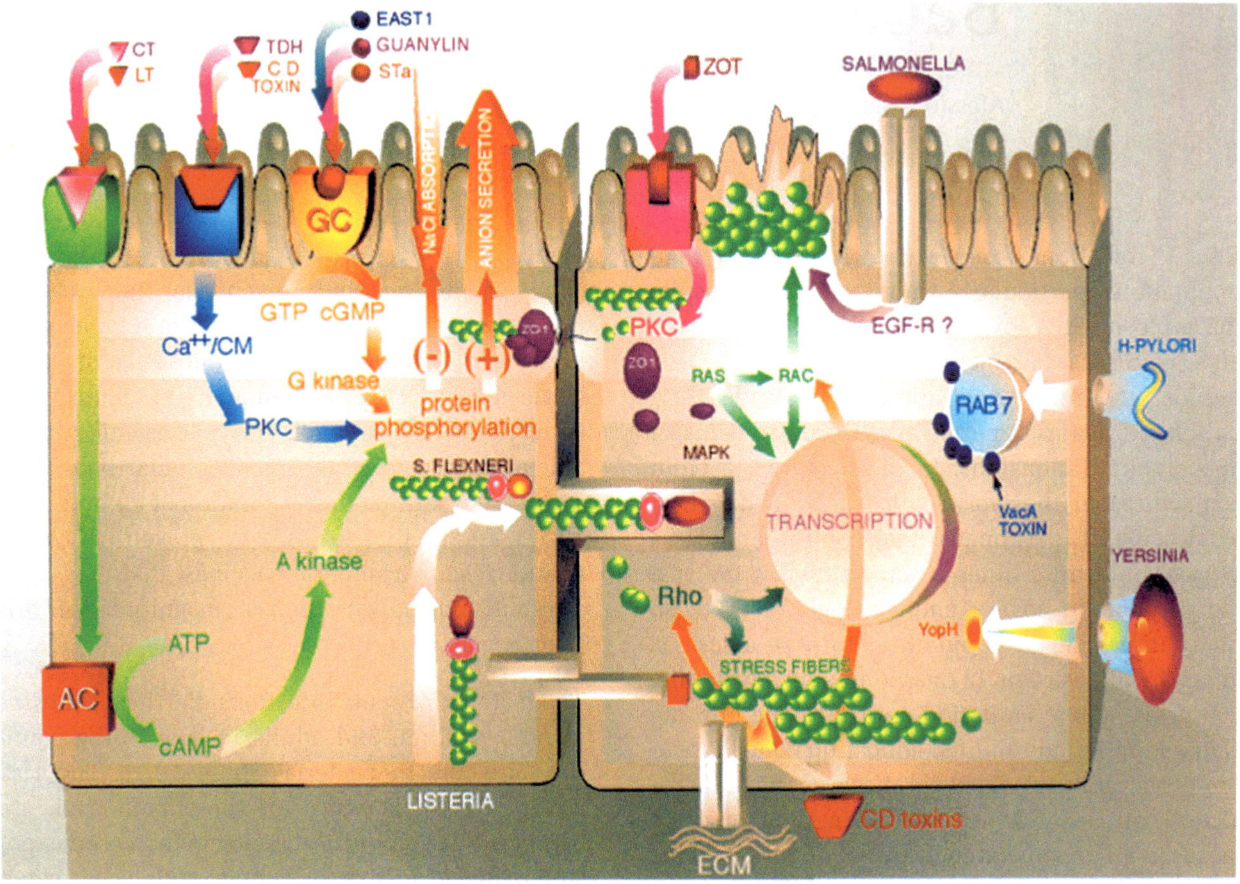

Figure 10.1 Enterocyte intracellular signaling leading to intestinal secretion. Four main pathways seem to be involved in the intestinal secretion of water and electrolytes: cAMP, cGMP, Ca and the cytoskeleton. These pathways are activated by several enteric pathogens, either directly or through the elaboration of enterotoxic products. CT, cholera toxin; LT, heat-labile enterotoxin; TDH, thermostable direct hemolysin; C.D., *Clostridium difficile*; EAST1, enteroaggregative *Escherichia coli* heat stable toxin 1; STa, heat stable toxin a; AC, adenylate cyclase; GC, guanylate cyclase; CM, calmodulin; PKC, protein kinase C; ZOT, Zonula Occludens Toxin; EGF-r, epidermal growth factor receptor; ECM, extracellular matrix.

Table 10.1 Percentage of identified bacterial pathogens in symptomatic patients from industrialized and developing countries

Agent	Industrialized countries (%)	Developing countries (%)
Vibrio cholerae	<1	0–3
Non-O1 *Vibrio* species	—	?
Salmonella	3–7	4–6
Shigella	1–3	5–9
Campylobacter	6–8	7–9
Yersinia	1–2	?
Escherichia coli	2–5	14–17
Clostridium difficile	?	?
Aeromonas, Plesiomonas, and *Edwardsiella*	0–2	4–5

Vibrio cholerae O1 is transmitted by the fecal–oral route and is spread through contaminated food and water, with a period of incubation of a few hours to 5 days. The vast majority of subjects infected remain asymptomatic or experience mild disease with watery stools, rare nausea or vomiting, and no significant dehydration. Stools are classically described as 'rice water' due to the presence of mucus in clear stools. In cholera gravis, profuse watery diarrhea and vomiting lead to massive fluid and electrolyte loss that can occur at a rate of 1 litre/h, and can reach a total volume loss of 100% of body weight. Vibrios can be easily identified from the stool by Gram stain.

Cholera has been a recognized human plague for over two millennia. The study of this disease has spanned from ancient Greece, and the Roman Empire, to the famous John Snow's tracing of an outbreak to a water pump in Broad Street, London, in 1854. Thirty years later Robert Koch proposed that the agent responsible for cholera produced 'a special poison' acting on the intestinal epithelium and that the symptoms of cholera could be 'regarded essentially as a poisoning'. Considerable time elapsed before the existence of this hypothesized toxin was demonstrated in 1959. Ten years later, cholera toxin (CT) was purified to homogeneity. It was only recently, however, that we learned that vibrios produce a variety of other extracellular products that enable these microorganisms to activate different intracellular signaling in the host mammalian cells, all leading to diarrhea. One of the most intriguing new toxins discovered in *V. cholerae* is zonula occludens toxin (Zot),[3] an enterotoxin that increases the intestinal permeability by interacting with a mammalian cell receptor, with subsequent activation of intracellular signaling leading to the disassembly of the intercellular tight junctions (Figure 10.2).

The introduction of oral rehydration solutions (ORS) decreased the mortality from this illness from over 50% to less than 1%. The use of antibiotics has limited indications, but has been demonstrated to reduce the volume and duration of diarrhea by half and reduce the duration of excretion to one day. Tetracycline (500 mg/dose, given four times per day) is the most widely used antibiotic, but large outbreaks of tetracycline-resistant organisms have been reported. Furazolidone (1.25 mg/kg four times per day), trimethoprim (TMP, 5 mg/kg twice per day), sulfamethoxazole (SMX, 25 mg/kg twice per day), and erythromycin (10 mg/kg three times per day) have been suggested for children.

Both killed whole-cell and live attenuated cholera vaccines have been proposed as a preventive intervention for cholera.[3] A large double-blind field trial of the killed vaccine showed 85% efficacy for a period of 4–6 months, dropping to 50% over 3 years of follow-up.[4] A locally produced killed vaccine in Vietnam provided a 66% protection against El Tor cholera during an outbreak occurring 8–10 months after vaccination.[5] A genetically engineered attenuated cholera vaccine (CVD 103-HgR), obtained by deleting the active subunit of cholera toxin (see below) from a *V. cholerae* O1 classic biotype, was well tolerated when administered to volunteers. This vaccine elicited a high level of protection (82–100%) against homologous challenge with a strain of the same biotype.[6] Protection across biotypes was also observed, albeit to a lesser extent,[7] lasting for at least 6 months after a single oral dose.[8] Live attenuated *V. cholerae* O139 vaccines have been developed, with promising preliminary results.[9,10]

Non-01 *Vibrio* species

V. parahaemolyticus, V. fluvialis, V. mimicus, V. hollisae, V. furnissii and *V. vulnificus* cause sporadic cases of gastroenteritis, and are present in coastal and estuarine areas throughout the world.[11] Virtually all cases of non-O1 *Vibrio* infections in the USA are associated with eating raw shellfish,[12] and the gastroenteritis can range from a mild illness to profuse, watery diarrhea comparable to that seen in epidemic cholera. Diarrhea, abdominal cramps and fever are the most common symptoms, with nausea, vomiting and bloody stools occurring less frequently.[11] As with *V. cholerae* O1, the mainstay of therapy for diarrheal disease is oral rehydration. In cases of septicemia (which typically occur in immunocompromised patients), supportive care and correction of shock are essential interventions associated with the antibiotic treatment (tetracycline). In countries such as the USA non-O1 infections can be prevented by not eating raw or undercooked seafood, particularly during the warm months.

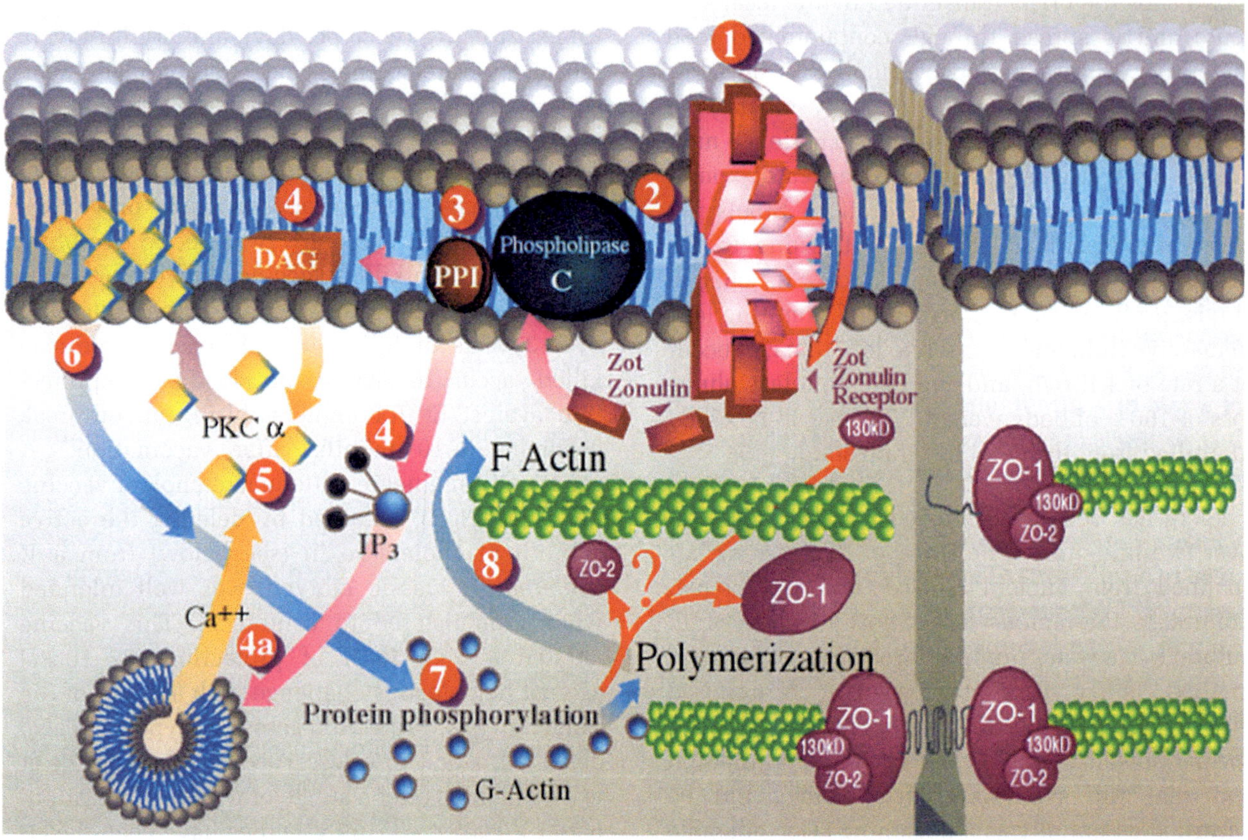

Figure 10.2 Proposed zonula occludens toxin (Zot) intracellular signaling leading to the opening of intestinal tight junctions. Zot interacts with a specific surface receptor (1) whose distribution within the intestine varies. The protein is then internalized and activates phospholipase C (2) that hydrolyzes phosphatidyl inositol (PPI) (3) to release inositol 1,4,5-tris phosphate (IP_3) and diacylglycerol (DAG) (4). Protein kinase Cα (PKCα) is then activated (5), either directly (via DAG) (4) or through the release of intracellular Ca^{++} (via IP_3) (4a). PKCα catalyzes the phosphorylation of target protein(s), with subsequent polymerization of soluble G actin in F actin (7). This polymerization causes the rearrangement of the filaments of actin and the subsequent displacement of proteins (including ZO1) from the junctional complex (8). As a result, intestinal tight junctions become looser.

Salmonella

Salmonella typhi and *S. paratyphi* are Gram-negative, motile bacilli that colonize only humans. Therefore, disease is acquired through close personal contact or through the ingestion of water or food contaminated with human excrement. Typhoid fever continues to represent a global health problem, with more than 12.5 million annual cases, and subequatorial countries reporting mortality rates of up to 32% despite antibiotic treatment.[13] In the USA, substantial progress has been made in their eradication, with better sanitation, food-handling and water treatment. These bacteria cause systemic illnesses characterized by fever, gastrointestinal symptoms and occasionally psychosis, confusion or rose spots on the trunk.[14] The incubation period varies between 5 and 21 days (depending on the inoculum ingested), and chills, headache, cough, weakness and muscle pain are frequent prodromes. Most symptoms resolve by the 4th week without antimicrobial treatment. However, some patients relapse with high fever, abdominal pain from inflammation of Peyer's patches, and intestinal microperforation followed by secondary bacteremia with normal enteric flora. The definitive diagnosis of enteric fever requires the isolation of *S. typhi* or *S. paratyphi* from blood, stool, urine, rose spots, bone marrow, or gastric or enteric secretions. Chloramphenicol is the treatment of choice and has been shown to reduce the duration of fever and mortality.

In contrast to *S. typhi*, the cases of infection with non-typhoidal salmonellae infections have been increasing in the developed world. Patients as higher risk for infection include those with immunodeficiencies, age younger than 3 months, alterations in intestinal defenses (achlorhydria, antacids, rapid gastric emptying post-gastrectomy), impaired reticuloendothelial function, (sickle cell and hemolytic anemias) and ingestion of antibiotics to which the organism was resistant. Reservoirs include a wide range of domestic and wild animals, including poultry, swine, cattle, rodents and reptiles. *S. enteriditis* is the leading reported cause of food-borne disease outbreaks in the USA, with eggs and contaminated raw fruits and vegetables identified as vehicles.[15] Transmission from person to person and from pets has also been reported. The incubation period is 6–48 h, after which fever, headache, vomiting, abdominal pain and watery diarrhea (which may contain blood, mucus, and leukocytes) occur for about 1 week. Severe extraintestinal infections can range from life-threatening sepsis to focal infections in the meninges, bones and lungs. The micro-organism is easily isolated from fresh stools or blood culture. Antimicrobials are not indicated to treat asymptomatic carriage or uncomplicated infections in the normal host, as they may prolong excretion or induce relapse. Although efficacy is unproven, it is common clinical practice to administer oral or parenteral antibiotics to high-risk patients or to those who have an extraintestinal focus of infection. Increasing resistance to commonly used antibiotics is seen, so the choice of regimens should be guided by susceptibility data. Suggested therapies include TMP–SMX (Bactrim®, Septra®, Sulfatrim®), ampicillin (10–20% of isolates in the USA are resistant), cefotaxime, ceftriaxone or chloramphenicol.

Hygienic practices for preventing food-borne transmission is the most efficient prevention for non-typhoidal *Salmonella* infections, since the vast majority of outbreaks and sporadic cases result from culinary practices that allow the organisms to survive and multiply in food. Parents should be instructed to avoid serving food containing raw or undercooked eggs and meat (especially poultry). Food should be thawed in the refrigerator, microwave, or under cold water but not at room temperature, because surface bacteria begin to multiply when the outer layers warm. Eggs should be cooked until both the yolk and the white are firm, and meats must reach an internal temperature of at least 74°C (165°F). Frequent hand washing is important. High-risk pets (especially chicks, ducklings and reptiles) are not advisable for young children.

An extremely problematic situation is the management of an infected child who is attending day care. Excretion can go on for weeks and create a hardship to working parents if the child must be excluded from day care. While the decision to admit such a child must be made in concert with day care and public health officials, it is generally recommended that the infected children be excluded from day care if they are symptomatic or if adequate hygiene cannot be ensured. There is no vaccine to prevent non-typhoidal salmonellosis.

Enteric fever

The definitive diagnosis of enteric fever requires the isolation of *S. typhi* or *S. paratyphi* from the patient. Cultures of blood, stool, urine, rose spots, bone marrow and gastric and enteric secretions may all be useful in establishing the diagnosis. Chloramphenicol has been the treatment of choice since its introduction, given its low costs and its high efficiency after oral administration. Treatment with chloramphenicol reduced typhoid fever mortality from approximately 20 to 1% and reduced the duration of the fever from 14–28 days to 3–5 days.[16]

The most effective attenuated vaccine for typhoid fever currently available, Ty21a, has proved to be free of adverse reactions in large-scale efficacy field trials involving almost 600 000 pediatric subjects.[17] When administered as a liquid suspension, Ty21a protected both young (82% vaccine efficacy) and older children (69% vaccine efficacy).[17] Currently, there are three new-generation attenuated vaccines, genetically engineered by deleting different pathogenic factors, that are undergoing extensive phase II trials.

Shigella

Kiyoshi Shiga first isolated *Shigella dysenteriae* type 1 during a severe dysentery epidemic in Japan in 1896, when more than 90000 cases were described with a mortality rate approaching 30%.[18] Shigellae are Gram-negative, non-lactose fermenting, non-motile bacilli, with *S. sonnei* the main type found in industrialized countries, and *S. flexneri* and *S. dysenteriae* predominating in underdeveloped countries. Humans are the only natural hosts and transmission occurs by fecal–oral contact. The low infectious inoculum (as few as ten organisms)[19] renders shigellae highly contagious. *Shigella* causes 250 million cases of diarrhea and 650 000 deaths worldwide.[20] In the USA, *S. dysenteriae* infection is seen almost exclusively among travelers. After an incubation of 1–4 days, shigellosis begins with fever, headache, malaise, anorexia and occasional vomiting and watery diarrhea with progression to dysentery within hours to days. Unusual extraintestinal manifestations may occur, including hemolytic uremic syndrome (HUS) in children and thrombotic thrombocytopenic purpura in adults. Most episodes of shigellosis in otherwise healthy individuals resolve within 7 days. Shigellae are extremely fastidious and are best isolated from fresh stool rapidly inoculated onto selective culture plates incubated immediately at 37°C. Appropriate antibiotics (ampicillin or TMP–SMX) given for 5 days significantly decrease the duration of fever, diarrhea, intestinal protein loss and pathogen excretion. However, *Shigella* strains that are resistant to one or both drugs have been identified. Several promising *Shigella* mutants with deletions in virulence genes have entered clinical trials as oral vaccine candidates.

Campylobacter

These organisms are small, microaerophilic, spiral-shaped Gram-negative organisms that enjoy a widespread reservoir in the intestines of both wild and domestic animals.[21] It is the most frequently identified bacterial cause of diarrhea in the USA. Common vehicles are poultry, unpasteurized milk and contaminated water.[22–24] After an incubation of 3–6 days, enteritis begins abruptly with cramps and watery diarrhea, which may progress to blood-containing stools. The abdominal pain may mimic appendicitis. Diarrhea usually lasts 4–5 days, with the duration of fecal excretion 1 month. The micro-organism can be identified only from stool. Indications for antibiotics remain controversial, with some studies showing a shortened course of diarrhea, and others no clear benefit. It is advisable to reserve antibiotics for patients in high-risk groups with severe symptoms. Erythromycin remains the drug of choice. *Campylobacter* vaccine development has proceeded cautiously, because of concerns about post-exposure arthritis or Guillain–Barré syndrome. However, a monovalent, formalin-inactivated, *C. jejuni* whole-cell vaccine with a mucosal adjuvant has entered human trials.

Yersinia

Yersinia enterocolitica and *Y. pseudotuberculosis* are two important human enteropathogens distributed widely in the environment, with swine serving as the major reservoir. The incubation period is 3–7 days, with food-borne transmission the suspected route for most infections. *Yersinia*'s preference for cool temperatures makes this pathogen more common in Northern Europe, Scandinavia, Canada, the USA and Japan, where it is responsible for up to 8% of sporadic diarrhea episodes. *Yersinia* enterocolitis occurs most often in children younger than 5 years[25] and is characterized by fever, vomiting, exudative pharangitis, cervical adenitis, abdominal pain and watery diarrhea, which may contain blood.[26,27] Diarrhea typically lasts for 14–22 days but fecal excretion may persist for 7 weeks or longer. Abdominal complications include appendicitis, pseudoappendicitis, diffuse ulceration of the intestine and colon, intestinal perforation, peritonitis, ileocecal intussusception, toxic megacolon, cholangitis and mesenteric vein thrombosis. Bacteremic spread may result in abscess formation and granulomatous lesions in the liver, spleen, lungs, kidneys and bone, as well as mycotic aneurysms, meningitis and septic arthritis. Infection can also be associated with immunopathological sequela including reactive arthritis, uveitis, Reiter's syndrome and erythema nodosum.[28] It may be isolated from stool or pharyngeal exudate on commonly used selective media, and appears as gram-negative colonies after 48 h of growth at 25–28°C. Most uncomplicated cases resolve without treatment, which is reserved for patients with severe symptoms, extraintestinal infections and immunocompromised hosts. Production of β-lactamases generally renders all but third-generation cephalosporins, aztreonam and imipenem ineffective. Treatment is generally 2–6 weeks, with an initial intravenous antibiotic (third-generation cephalosporin often in combination with aminoglycosides), followed by an oral agent to which the clinical isolate is sensitive.

Escherichia coli

An extremely heterogeneous group of micro-organisms, *Escherichia coli* encompasses almost all features of possible interactions between intestinal microflora and the host, ranging from a role of mere harmless presence to that of a highly pathogenic organism. In fact, the *E. coli* species is made up of many strains that profoundly differ from each other in terms of biological characteristics and virulence properties.[29]

Escherichia coli is a Gram-negative, lactose-fermenting motile bacillus of the family Enterobacteriaceae. Currently, 171 somatic (O) and 56 flagellar (H) antigens are recognized. Six distinct categories of *E. coli* are currently considered enteric pathogens (based on either outbreak data or volunteer studies) (Table 10.2). The diagnosis of diarrheagenic *E. coli* relies on isolation from stool and subsequent differentiation from commensal *E. coli* either by using genetic probes or by phenotypic assays. With the exception of *E. coli* O157:H7, assays for detection are not routinely available in clinical laboratories.

Table 10.2 Pathogenic *Escherichia coli*

Enteropathogenic *E. coli* (EPEC)
Enterotoxigenic *E. coli* (ETEC)
Enteroinvasive *E. coli* (EIEC)
Enterohemorrhagic *E. coli* (EHEC)
Diffusely adherent *E. coli* (DAEC)
Enteroaggregative *E. coli* (EAggEC)

Enteropathogenic *E. coli*

This was the first group of *E. coli* serotype shown to be pathogens for humans and has been responsible for devastating outbreaks of nosocomial neonatal diarrhea and infant diarrhea in virtually every corner of the globe. Strains of enteropathogenic *E. coli* (EPEC) are distinguished from other *E. coli* strains by their ability to induce a characteristic attaching and effacing lesion in the small-intestinal enterocytes and by their inability to produce Shiga toxins. Between the 1940s and the 1960s, EPEC was associated with infant diarrhea in summertime and nursery outbreaks of diarrhea in the USA and other industrialized countries. Since then, it has become extremely uncommon in industrialized countries, although it is occasionally reported in child-care settings.[30] However, EPEC persists as an important cause of infantile diarrhea in many developing countries.[31] In nursery outbreaks, transmission was thought to occur via the hands of caregivers and via fomites. In less developed countries, contaminated formula and weaning foods have been incriminated. Volunteer studies and epidemiological observations suggest that the infective dose for EPEC is high (approximately 10^9 colony-forming units (CFU)).[32] EPEC causes a self-limited watery diarrhea with a short incubation period (6–48 h). There may be associated fever, abdominal cramps and vomiting, and EPEC is a leading cause of persistent diarrhea (lasting 14 days or longer) in children in developing countries.[33] Although few data exist to guide antibiotic therapy of EPEC diarrhea, administration of appropriate antibiotics seems to diminish morbidity and mortality. A 3-day course of oral, non-absorbable antibiotics such as colistin or gentamicin (if available) has been shown to be effective.[34] Some clinicians also advocate the use of oral neomycin; however, this drug causes diarrhea in about 20% of people. In a placebo-controlled trial among Ethiopian infants with severe EPEC diarrhea, TMP–SMX and mecillinam resulted in significant clinical and bacteriological cure rates by the third day, as compared with placebo.[35] Strategies for the prevention of EPEC infection include efforts to improve social and economic conditions in developing countries, efforts to encourage breast feeding and prevention of nosocomial infections.

Enterotoxigenic *E. coli*

Strains of enterotoxigenic *E. coli* (ETEC) are an important cause of diarrheal disease in humans and animals worldwide. The clinical importance of these micro-organsims was first outlined in the 1970s by epidemiological studies in India that identified them as a major cause of endemic diarrhea.[36] Their pathogenicity is related to the elaboration of one or more enterotoxins that are either heat stable (ST) or heat labile (LT) (see Pathogenesis section) without invading or damaging intestinal epithelial cells. Together with rotavirus, ETEC is the leading cause of dehydrating diarrheal disease among weaning infants in the developing world. These children experience 2–3 episodes of ETEC diarrhea in each of the first 2 years of life. This represents over 25% of all diarrheal illness[37] and results in an estimated 700000 deaths each year.[38] In industrialized countries, ETEC does not contribute to endemic disease, but is notorious for being the leading agent of travelers' diarrhea, accounting for about half of all episodes.[39] Transmission occurs by ingestion of contaminated food and water, with peaks during the warm, wet season. Like EPEC, ETEC requires a relatively high inoculum[40] and a short incubation period (14–30 h). The cardinal symptom is watery diarrhea, sometimes with associated fever, abdominal cramps and vomiting. In its most severe form, ETEC can cause cholera-like purging, even in adults. The illness is typically self-limited, lasting for less than 5 days and with few cases persisting beyond 3 weeks. Infection with ETEC has also been associated with short- and long-term adverse nutritional consequences in infants and children.

Most diarrheal illnesses due to ETEC are self-limited and do not require specific antimicrobial therapy. Empirical therapy is reserved for those whose diarrhea is moderate to severe despite rehydration and supportive measures. Antibiotic regimens that have been efficacious in clinical trials, shortening the duration of illness by 1–2 days, include doxycycline, TMP–SMX, ciprofloxacin, quinolones, and furazolidone.[41] In the past, the drug of choice for children has been TMP–SMX; however, except in Central Mexico,[42] a large proportion of ETEC is now resistant. An alternative regimen for children is furazolidone.

Prevention of ETEC infection is based on avoiding contaminated vehicles. Although antibiotics are effective as prophylactic agents, their use is not recommended. Some experts advocate the use of bismuth subsalicylate to diminish the risk of travelers' diarrhea.[43] The development of vaccines against ETEC has received a great deal of attention because of its disease burden. Oral vaccines for ETEC are being developed by five different strategies, including killed whole cells, toxoids, purified fimbriae, living attenuated strains and live carrier strains elaborating ETEC antigens. A killed whole-cell *Vibrio cholerae* vaccine given with cholera toxin B (CTB) provided 67% protection against LT-producing ETEC diarrhea for 3 months.[44] A formalin-inactivated whole-cell oral vaccine consisting of ETEC strains bearing colonization factor antigens (CFAs) in combination with CTB has entered field trial.[45]

Enteroinvasive *E. coli*

This group consists of invasive *E. coli* strains that are genetically, biochemically and clinically nearly identical to *Shigella*. This section will serve only to highlight relevant characteristics that distinguish this pathogen. Strains of enteroinvasive *E. coli* (EIEC) are endemic in developing countries, where they exhibit similar epidemiology to *Shigella* and cause an estimated 1–5% of diarrheal episodes among patients visiting treatment centers.[46] The occurrence of EIEC in industrialized countries is limited to rare food-borne outbreaks.[47] From volunteer studies, it appears that the infectious inoculum contains more organisms than that required to cause shigellosis.[48] Like *Shigella*, EIEC can produce dysentery, but watery diarrhea is more common.[49] The rare episodes for which treatment is desired are treated with antibiotics recommended for shigellosis. The same general preventive measures used for *Shigella* infections apply to EIEC-associated diarrhea.

Enterohemorrhagic *E. coli*

These *E. coli* strains produce either one or both phage-encoded potent cytotoxins termed Shiga-like toxin I (SLT I) (which is neutralized by antisera to Shiga toxin produced by *S. dysenteriae* type 1) or Shiga-like toxin II (SLT II) (which is not neutralized) and can cause diarrhea or HUS. *E. coli* O157:H7 is the prototypic (but not the exclusive) enterohemorrhagic *E. coli* (EHEC) serotype, since it is the predominant SLT-producing *E. coli*, the one most commonly associated with HUS in North

America and the type most readily identified in stool specimens.[50] In 1982, a multistate outbreak of hemorrhagic colitis that was linked to the consumption of hamburgers at the same fast-food restaurant led to the identification of EHEC.[51] The causative organism was *E. coli* O157:H7, a serotype not previously recognized as a human pathogen. Soon after, Canadian investigators uncovered an association between O157:H7 and other SLT-producing strains of *E. coli* and HUS.[52] EHEC is now recognized as a global health problem; in 1996, an outbreak in Japan linked to eating radish sprouts affected over 6000 persons.[53] One the most severe EHEC outbreaks in the USA took place in New York State in 1999, with more than 1000 ascertained cases, two HUS-related casualties, and eight children in dialysis because of renal failure. Most of the infected individuals attended a fair whose underground water supply was contaminated by cow manure from a nearby cattle barn. The predominant mode of transmission is ingestion of contaminated, undercooked ground beef. However, the spectrum of vehicles is widening to include raw fruits (including apple juice) and vegetables,[54,55] raw milk,[56] processed meats,[57] and drinking[58] or swimming[59] in contaminated water. The uncooked food vehicles are usually contaminated with manure from infected animals during growth or processing. Person-to-person transmission is the mode of spread in day-care outbreaks, where secondary transmission rates of 22% have been reported.[60]

EHEC also causes sporadic diarrhea. Isolation from stools of unselected patients is low (< 1%), but isolation from stools of patients with bloody diarrhea may be as high as 20–30%.[61] A USA national laboratory-based study demonstrated that infection was more frequent in northern states and that it peaked from June to September.[61] The highest age-specific isolation rates are in patients 5–9 and 50–59 years of age. A population-based incidence rate based on stool samples submitted to a large health maintenance organization laboratory in the state of Washington was eight per 100000 person-years.[62] Illness with EHEC follows 3–9 days after ingestion of as few as 100 organisms.[63] Crampy abdominal pain and non-bloody diarrhea are the first symptoms, sometimes associated with vomiting. By the 2nd or 3rd day of illness, diarrhea becomes bloody in about 90% of cases, and abdominal pain worsens.[64] Bloody diarrhea lasts for 1–22 days (median 4 days). Unlike other infectious causes of bloody diarrhea, fever is usually absent or remains low-grade. Younger children appear to excrete the organisms for longer (median 3 weeks) than older children and adults.[65]

In outbreaks, approximately 25% of patients are hospitalized, 5–10% develop HUS and 1% die.[66,67] Intestinal complications include rectal prolapse, appendicitis, intussusception, and pseudomembranous colitis.[68,69] Extraintestinal complications are rare.

The most frightening complication of EHEC infection is HUS. It is usually diagnosed 2–14 days after the onset of diarrhea.[52] Risk factors include young and old age, bloody diarrhea, fever, an elevated leukocyte count and treatment with antimotility agents.[68,70] Two-thirds of patients who develop HUS are no longer excreting the organism at presentation.[71] The most widely accepted indication for seeking a clinical diagnosis of *E. coli* O157:H7 infection is a patient with bloody diarrhea, in whom an accurate diagnosis may avoid unnecessary medical procedures because a surgical abdomen (such as appendicitis or intussusception) is suspected. A multicenter study found that, when the presence of fecal blood was used as the sole criterion for culturing O157 strains, only 3% of stools would be cultured to detect 63% of infections.[70,71] Diagnosis may also be helpful in patients with HUS or with any type of diarrhea in a patient in contact with HUS. *E. coli* O157:H7 is not detected by routine stool culture. A relatively inexpensive method exploits the inability of *E. coli* O157 rapidly to ferment sorbitol after 24 h of incubation on sorbitol-MacConkey agar, in contrast to about 90% of commensal *E. coli*. The 'sorbitol-negative' colonies can then be screened for the presence of the O157 antigen, using commercially available antisera. These strains should be considered pathogenic pending the determination of the H type in a reference laboratory. Although data are not available from prospective randomized double-blind trials, there is considerable evidence to suggest that patients who receive antibiotics to which the offending *E. coli* O157:H7 is sensitive have either the same or a poorer outcome when compared with untreated patients.[68,72,73] Therefore, antibiotic therapy is not recommended for EHEC infection. As mentioned above, antimotility agents have been identified as a risk factor for the development of HUS and should be avoided.

Prevention of *E. coli* O157:H7 is a complex process. From a public health standpoint, control measures at the level of farms, slaughterhouses and processing plants can decrease the risk of colonization of cattle and contamination of beef. Since these procedures are unlikely to achieve complete success, regulations governing proper processing and cooking of contaminated foods are also required. Advice to consumers should include recommending complete avoidance of raw foods of animal origin. Hamburger should be cooked until no pink remains and until the juices are clear.

Because of the severity of disease, there has been a recent focus on vaccine development for EHEC infection. Efforts have concentrated on three approaches: parenteral toxoids and live oral carrier strains elaborating the B subunit of Shiga toxin;[74] vaccines expressing the adhesin intimin, designed to prevent intestinal colonization;[75] and a parenteral O157 polysaccharide protein conjugate.[76]

Diffusely adhering *E. coli*

Until recently, diffusely adhering *E. coli* (DAEC) was considered a non-pathogenic *E. coli*, since early studies failed to find an association between this micro-organism and diarrheal disease.[77–79] However, more recent studies have demonstrated such an association, particularly in children older than 2 years of age. A community-based case–control study in southern Mexico revealed that DAEC was significantly associated with diarrhea in children less than 6 years of age.[80] Prospective cohort studies in Chile[81] and Bangladesh[81] also demonstrated a diarrheagenic role for DAEC that peaked in the 48–60-month age group.[81] This micro-organism was more frequently isolated from cases of prolonged diarrhea,[82] and it showed a seasonal pattern similar to that of ETEC, occurring more frequently in the warm season.[81] The gastrointestinal symptoms that characterize DAEC infection are practically indistinguishable from those caused by ETEC, with self-limiting watery diarrhea rarely associated with vomiting and abdominal pain. The diagnosis is mainly based on the DNA probe technique and on the pattern of adherence of the micro-organism to HE-2 cells. Given the technical challenge of both assays, their use is limited to epidemiological surveys rather than the diagnosis of single individuals.

Enteroaggregative *E. coli*

Enteroaggregative *E. coli* (EAggEC) are diarrheagenic *E. coli* defined by a characteristic aggregating pattern of adherence to HEp-2 cells and the intestinal mucosa. They have been particularly associated with cases of persistent diarrhea in the developing world. It has been hypothesized that the aggregating pattern of adherence may be a result of non-specific, possibly hydrophobic interaction, and therefore, not all organisms meeting the definition of EAggEC may be pathogenic in humans. Moreover, since epidemiological studies have not uniformly implicated EAggEC as pathogenic, some investigators have questioned the virulence of all EAggEC isolates. Volunteer studies performed to address both of these questions[82] confirmed that at least some EAggEC strains are genuine human pathogens but that virulence is not uniform among isolates. More recently, EAggEC pathogenicity has also been proven in several outbreaks.

From the earliest epidemiological reports, EAggEC was most prominently associated with persistent cases of pediatric diarrhea (i.e. lasting ≥ 14 days),[84] a condition that represents a disproportionate share of diarrheal mortality. On the Indian subcontinent, several independent studies have demonstrated the importance of EAggEC in pediatric diarrhea.[85] These studies include hospitalized patients with persistent diarrhea,[78] outpatients visiting health clinics,[85] and cases of sporadic diarrhea detected by household surveillance.[77] In Fortaleza, Brazil, Fang et al have demonstrated a consistent association between EAggEC and persistent diarrhea;[86] in this area, EAggEC accounts for more cases of persistent diarrhea than all other causes combined.[86] EaggEC have been implicated as a cause of sporadic diarrhea in other developing countries (including Mexico, Chile, Bangladesh, Congo and Iran) as well as in industrialized countries such as Germany and England.[87] Besides being responsible for sporadic cases of diarrhea, EAggEC has also been associated with outbreaks in India,[88] Serbia,[89] Japan[90] and the UK.[69]

The clinical features of EAggEC diarrhea are becoming increasingly well defined in outbreaks, in sporadic cases and in the volunteer model. Typically, illness is manifested by a watery, mucoid, secretory diarrheal illness with low-grade fever and little or no vomiting.[77,91] However, in epidemiological studies, grossly bloody stools have been reported in up to one-third of patients with EAggEC diarrhea.[92] This phenomenon may well be strain-dependent. In volunteers infected with EAggEC strain 042, diarrhea was mucoid, of low volume, and notably, without occult blood or fecal leukocytes; all patients remained afebrile. In such volunteers, the incubation period of the illness ranged from 8 to 18 h.[82]

Perhaps even more significant than the association of EAggEC with diarrhea are the recent data from Brazil that link EAggEC with growth retardation in infants.[92] In this study, the isolation of EAggEC from the stools of infants was associated with a low z-score for height and/or weight, irrespective of the presence of diarrheal symptoms. Given the high prevalence of asymptomatic EAggEC excretion in many areas,[84,93] such an observation may imply that the contribution of EAggEC to the human disease burden is significantly greater than is currently appreciated. Colonization of EAggEC is detected by the isolation of *E. coli* from the stools of patients and the demonstration of the aggregative pattern in the HEp-2 assay. Implication of EAggEC as the cause of the patient's disease must be cautious, given the high rate of asymptomatic colonization in many populations.[84,93] If no other organism is implicated in the patient's illness and EAggEC is isolated repeatedly, then EAggEC should be considered a potential cause of the patient's illness. A DNA-fragment probe has proven highly specific in the detection of EAggEC strains. A polymerase chain reaction (PCR) assay using primers derived from the aggregative probe sequence shows similar sensitivity and specificity.[94]

The optimal management of EAggEC infection has not been studied. Acute diarrhea is apparently self-limiting; however, more persistent cases may benefit from antibiotic and/or nutritional therapy. Given the high rate of antibiotic resistance among EAggEC,[95] susceptibility testing is recommended when available.

Clostridium difficile

Even though *Clostridium difficile* is now recognized as the single most common cause of bacterial diarrhea in hospitalized patients, its role as a pathogen had not been established as recently as the late 1970s. *C. difficile* has the ability to become established in the gastrointestinal tract once the natural microflora have been modified by antibiotic therapy. The organism causes intestinal disease ranging from mild diarrhea to fatal pseudomembranous colitis (PMC). While *C. difficile* is associated with almost all cases of PMC, only 25% of antibiotic-associated diarrheas are due to this pathogen. *C. difficile* is a Gram-positive anaerobe that forms spores, making this micro-organism very difficult to remove from the hospital environment. Unlike some toxigenic clostridia, the production of spores is not associated with toxin production. *C. difficile* spreads from patient to patient[96] and tends to persist in the environment because of the formation of spores. The micro-organism is not only present in the infected patient and soiled linens but can be isolated from bookshelves, curtains and floors of rooms of infected patients where it can persist for as long as 5 months.[96–98] The organism is spread primarily by health-care workers; up to 60% of personnel attending patients infected with *C. difficile* in one study had the organism on their hands.[96] The isolation of *C. difficile* toxins from the feces of asymptomatic normal-term neonates and (in higher proportion) those admitted into neonatal intensive care units,[99] further support the concept of the nosocomial spreading of the infection.

Several outbreaks of *C. difficile* infection have been reported in the USA and throughout the world, and the incidence continues to rise. Whether this increase represents a true increment or represents an increased awareness of the disease is not clear at this stage. Infections with *C. difficile* range in severity from asymptomatic forms to clinical syndromes, such as severe diarrhea, PMC, and toxic megacolon, and can even lead to death.[100] The onset of symptomatic forms usually begins several days after antibiotic therapy is started up to 2 months following cessation of treatment. Diarrhea and abdominal cramps are usually the first symptoms, followed by the development of fever and chills in severe cases. Mild forms of colitis, with bloody stools and mucus, particularly if they are preceded by antibiotic treatment, should be considered suspicious for *C. difficile* infection. Clinical microbiologists face an array of methods and commercial tests when considering what procedure to use for the detection of *C. difficile* and its toxins. Culturing of the organism, latex agglutination, tissue culture assay and enzyme-linked immunosorbent assay (ELISA) are all used as aids for the diagnosis of *C. difficile* infection.

In many instances, *C. difficile* disease is self-limiting, and the patient may respond simply to the withdrawal of the offending antibiotic. In more severe forms, particularly if complicated by PMC, antibiotic treatment with either oral vancomycin[101] (5–10 mg/kg, maximum 500 mg, given every 6 h for 7 days) or metronidazole[102] (5–10 mg/kg, maximum 500 mg, given every 8 h for 7 days) is recommended. Despite pharmacological treatment, the rate of relapse is significant (up to 40–50% of cases). In these complicated cases, the use of probiotics, particularly *Lactobacillus* GG[103] and *Saccharomyces boulardii*,[104] has been associated with a significant eradication of *C. difficile* and a substantial decrease in the recurrence of the infection.

Evaluation of diarrheal diseases

The patient's history, signs and symptoms should direct the diagnostic evaluation of the patient with acute infectious diarrhea. With a history of travel to developing nations, *E. coli*, *Salmonella*, *Shigella*, *Campylobacter*, cholera, *Entamoeba histolytica*, and *Giardia lamblia* should be high on the differential. Vomiting after the ingestion of fast foods, canned products, or raw seafood and meats should prompt the clinician to look for toxin-producing enteropathogens associated with food poisoning, such as *Staphylococcus aureus* and *Bacillus cereus*, as well as hepatitis A, parasites (tapeworms, flukes, trichinae), *Salmonella* and *E. coli*. The hospitalized patient may experience diarrhea not only from *C. difficile*, but also from procedures and medications (such as antibiotics, antacids, and medications with a high osmolality). The immunocompromised host presents a special challenge in the work-up of acute diarrhea, in the face of polypharmacy and malabsorpsion due to enteropathy and pancreatic insufficiency (see Chapter 8). With potential multiple pathogens, gastrointestinal endoscopy with biopsy and aspiration of fluid and fecal contents may give the highest yield of diagnosis in the immunocompromised patient.

Direct examination of the stool for the presence of mucus, blood, or leukocytes may be helpful in classifying infectious agents. For example, profusely watery stools without mucus, blood or leukocytes are characteristic of cholera, *Salmonella*, ETEC, *C. parvum*, *Giardia* and most viral agents. The presence of mucus, blood and leukocytes in the stool are more consistent with inflammatory infections such as *Campylobacter*, EIEC, *Shigella*, *C. difficile*, *Yersinia*, *Entamoeba* and cytomegalovirus.

General guidelines for treatment of diarrheal diseases

As outlined in the various sections of this chapter (see also Chapter 37), the treatment of the majority of infectious diarrheal episodes is supportive, with ORS representing the cardinal intervention to minimize life-threatening dehydration, particularly in young children.[105] Breast feeding should be continued, as it may confer protection. Intravenous rehydration should be reserved for high-risk patients who are unable to tolerate enterals due to recurrent vomiting or diminished mental status. The use of antimotility agents, such as bismuth subsalicylate (Pepto-Bismol®), loperamide (Imodium®), and atropine sulfate with diphenoxylate hydrochloride (Lomotil®) should be discouraged, owing to the possible risk of salicylate intoxication, ileus, toxic megacolon, bowel perforation, and HUS in subjects infected with EHEC. Probiotics, such as *Lactobacillus* GG, have been recently shown to be effective both in the prevention, and in the treatment of viral (rotavirus) and antibiotic-associated (*C. difficile*) diarrheas, as well documented by two recent meta-analyses.[106,107]

REFERENCES

1. Barua D, Greenough WB III. *Cholera*, 1st edn. New York: Plenum Publishing, 1992.
2. Wachsmuth IK, Blake PA, Olsvik O. *Vibrio cholerae and Cholera: Molecular and Perspectives*, 1st edn. Washington, DC: American Society for Microbiology, 1994.
3. Nataro JP, Levine MM. Enteric bacterial vaccines, *Salmonella*, *Shigella*, cholera, *Escherichia coli*. In Ogra P et al, eds. *Mucosal Immunology*, 2nd edn. San Diego: Academic Press, 1999: 851–866.
4. Clemens JD, Sack DA, Harris JR et al. Field trial of oral cholera vaccines in Bangladesh. *Lancet*. 1986: **2**: 124–127.
5. Trach DD, Clemens JD, Ke NT et al. Field trial of a locally produced, killed, oral cholera vaccine in Vietnam. *Lancet* 1997; **349**: 231–235.
6. Levine MM, Kaper JB, Herrington D et al. Safety, immunogenicity, and efficacy of recombinant live oral cholera vaccines, CVD103 and CVD103-HgR. *Lancet* 1988; **2**: 467–470.
7. Suharyono PM, Simanjuntak C, Witham N et al. Safety and immunogenicity of single-dose live oral cholera vaccine CVD103-HgR in 5–9-year-old Indonesian children. *Lancet* 1992; **340**: 689–694.
8. Tacket CO, Losonsky G, Nataro JP et al. Onset and duration of protective immunity in challenged volunteers after vaccination with live oral cholera vaccine CVD103-HgR. *J Infect Dis* 1992; **166**: 837–841.
9. Tacket CO, Losonsky G, Nataro JP et al. Initial clinical studies of CVD112 *Vibrio cholerae* O139 live oral vaccine: safety and efficacy against experimental challenge. *J Infect Dis* 1995; **172**: 883–886.
10. Coster TS, Killeen KP, Waldor MK et al. Safety, immunogenicity, and efficacy of live attenuated *Vibrio cholerae* O139 vaccine prototype. *Lancet* 1995; **345**: 949–952.
11. West PA, Brayton PR, Twilley RR, et al. Numerical tazonom of nitrogen-fixing 'decarboxylase-negative' *Vibrio* species isolated from aquatic environments. *Int J Syst Bacteriol* 1985; **35**: 198–205.
12. Morris JG Jr, Wilson R, Davis BR et al. Non-O group 1 *Vibrio cholerae* gastroenteritis in the United States: clinical, epidemiologic and laboratory characteristics of sporadic cases. *Ann Intern Med* 1981; **94**: 656–658.
13. Edelman R, Levine MM. Summary of an international workshop on typhoid fever. *Rev Infect Dis* 1986; **8**: 329–349.
14. Hoffman TA, Ruiz CJ, Counts GW. Water-borne typhoid fever in Dade County, FL: clinical and therapeutic evaluations of 105 bacteremic patients. *Am J Med* 1975; **59**: 481–487.
15. Centers for Disease Control and Prevention: Surveillance for foodborne-disease outbreaks, United States, 1988–1992. *Morbid Mortal Weekly Rep* 1996; **45**: 1S–66S.
16. Woodward TE, Smadel JE, Ley HL et al. Preliminary report on the beneficial effect of chloromycetin in the treatment of typhoid fever. *Ann Intern Med* 1948; **29**: 131–134.
17. Levine MM, Ferreccio C, Cryz S, Ortiz E. Comparison of enteric-coated capsules and liquid formulation of Ty21 a typhoid vaccine in randomized controlled field trial. *Lancet* 1990; **336**: 891–894.
18. Shiga K. Ueber den Dysenteriebacillus (*Bacillus dysenteriae*). *Zentralbl Bakteriol Parasit Kde Abt I Orig* 1898; **24**: 817–824.
19. DuPont HL, Levine MM, Hornick RB, Formal SB. Inoculum size in shigellosis and implications for expected mode of transmission. *J Infect Dis* 1989; **159**: 1126–1128.
20. Institute of Medicine. The prospects for immunizing against *Shigella* spp. In *New Vaccine Development. Establishing Priorities: Diseases of Importance in Developing Countries*, vol 2. Washington DC: National Academy Press, 1986: 329–337.
21. Blaser MJ, Reller LB. *Campylobacter* enteritis. *N Engl J Med* 1981; **305**:1444–1452.
22. Deming MS, Tauxe RV, Blake PA et al. *Campylobacter* enteritis at a university: transmission from eating chicken and from cats. *Am J Epidemiol* 1987; **126**: 526–534.
23. Wood RC, Macdonald KL, Osterholm MT. *Campylobacter* enteritis outbreaks associated with drinking raw milk during youth activities: a 10-year review of outbreaks in the United States. *JAMA* 1992; **268**: 3228–3230.
24. Mentzing LO. Waterborne outbreaks of *Campylobacter* enteritis in central Sweden. *Lancet* 1981; **2**: 352–354.
25. Metchock B, Londway DR, Carter GP et al. *Yersinia enterocolitica*: a frequent seasonal stool isolate from children at an urban hospital in the southeast United States. *J Clin Microbiol* 1991; **29**: 2868–2869.
26. Marks MI, Pai CH, Lafleur L et al. *Yersinia enterocolitica* gastoenteritis: a prospective study of clinical, bacteriologic and epidemiologic features. *J Pediatr* 1980; **96**: 26–31.
27. Tacket CO, Davis BR, Carter GP et al. *Yersinia enterocolitica* pharyngitis. *Ann Intern Med* 1983; **99**: 40–42.
28. Cover TL. *Yersinia enterocolitica* and *Yersinia pseudotuberculosis*. In Blaser MJ et al, eds. *Infections of the Gastrointestinal Tract*. New York: Raven Press, 1995: 811–823.
29. Levine MM. *Escherichia coli* that cause diarrhea: enterotoxigenic, enteropathogenic, enteroinvasive and enteroadherent. *J Infect Dis* 1987; **155**: 377–389.
30. Paulozzi LJ, Johnson KE, Kamahele LM et al. Diarrhea associated with adherent enteropathogenic *Escherichia coli* in infant and toddler center, Seattle, Washington. *Pediatrics* 1986; **77**: 296–300.
31. Donnenberg MS, Kaper JB. Enteropathogenic *Escherichia coli*. *Infect Immun* 1992; **60**: 3953–3961.
32. Levine MM, Bergquist EJ, Nalin DR et al. *Escherichia coli* strains that cause diarrhoea but do not produce heat-labile or heat-stable enterotoxins and are non-invasive. *Lancet* 1978; **1**: 1119–1122.
33. Clausen CR, Christie DL. Chronic diarrhea in infants caused by adherent enteropathogenic, *Escherichia coli*. *J Pediatr* 1982; **100**: 358–361.
34. Nelson JD. Duration of neomycin for enteropathogenic *Escherichia coli* diarrheal disease: a comparative study of 113 cases. *Pediatrics* 1971; **48**: 248–258.
35. Thoren AL. Antibiotic sensitivity of enteropathogenic *Escherichia coli* to mecillinam, trimethoprim–sulfamethoxazole and other antibiotics. *Acta Pathol Microbiol Scand* 1980; **88**: 265–268.
36. Gorbach SL, Banwell JG, Chatterjee BD et al. Acute undifferentiated human diarrhea in the tropics, vol 1. Alterations in intestinal microflora. *J Clin Invest* 1971; **50**: 881–889.
37. Black RE, Merson MH, Huq I et al. Incidence and severity of rotavirus and *Escherichia coli* diarrhoea in

rural Bangladesh: implications for vaccine development. *Lancet* 1981; **1**: 141–143.
38. Institute of Medicine. *New Vaccine Development: Establishing Priorities*, vol 2, *Diseases of Importance in Developing Countries*. Washington, DC: National Academy Press, 1986.
39. Sack RB. Travelers' diarrhea: microbiologic bases for prevention and treatment. *Rev Infect Dis* 1990; **12**: 59S–63S.
40. Black RE, Levine MM, Clements ML et al. Treatment of experimentally induced enterotoxigenic *Escherichia coli* diarrhea with trimethoprim, trimethoprim–sulfamethoxazole or placebo. *Rev Infect Dis* 1982; **4**: 540–545.
41. DuPont HL, Ericsson CD. Prevention and treatment of traveler's diarrhea. *N Engl J Med* 1993; **328**: 1821–1827.
42. Bandres JC, Mathewson JJ, Ericsson CD, Dupont HL. Trimethoprim/sulfamethoxazole remains active against enterotoxigenic *Escherichia coli* and *Shigella* species in Guadalajara, Mexico. *Am J Med Sci* 1992; **303**: 289–291.
43. Wolfe MD. Protection of travelers. *Clin Infect Dis* 1997; **25**: 177–184.
44. Peltola H, Siitonen A, Kyronseppa H et al. Prevention of travellers' diarrhoea by oral B-subunit/whole-cell cholera vaccine. *Lancet* 1991; **338**: 1285–1289.
45. Svennerholm AM, Ahren C, Jertborn M. Vaccines against enterotoxogenic *Escherichia coli* infections: I. Oral inactivated vaccines against enterotoxigenic *Escherichia coli*. In Levine MM et al, eds. *New Generation Vaccines,* 2nd edn. New York: Marcel Dekker, 1997: 865–873.
46. Echeverria P, Sethabutr O, Pitarangsi C. Microbiology and diagnosis of infections with *Shigella* and enteroinvasive *Escherichia coli*. *Rev Infect Dis* 1991; **13**: 220S–225S.
47. Macdonald KL, Eidson M, Strohmeyer C et al. A multistate outbreak of gastrointestinal illness caused by enterotoxigenic *Escherichia coli* in imported semisoft cheese. *J Infect Dis* 1985; **151**: 716–720.
48. DuPont HL, Formal SB, Hornick RB et al. Pathogenesis of *Escherichia coli* diarrhea. *N Engl J Med* 1971; **285**: 1–9.
49. Snyder JD, Wells JG, Yashuck et al. Outbreak of invasive *Escherichia coli* gastroenteritis on a cruise ship. *Am J Trop Med Hyg* 1984; **33**: 281–284.
50. Tarr PI. *Escherichia coli* O157:H7 clinical, diagnostic and epidemiological aspects of human infection. *Clin Infect Dis* 1995; **20**: 9–10.
51. Riley LW, Remis RS, Helgerson SD et al. Hemorrhagic colitis associated with a rare *Escherichia coli* serotype. *N Engl J Med* 1983; **308**: 681–685.
52. Karmali MA, Petric M, Lim C et al. The association between idiopathic hemolytic uremic syndrome and infection by verotoxin-producing *Escherichia coli*. *J Infect Dis* 1985; **151**: 775–782.
53. Centers for Disease Control and Prevention. Isolation of *E. coli* 157:H7 from sporadic cases of hemorrhagic colitis, United States. *Morbid Mortal Weekly Rep* 1997; **46**: 700–704.
54. Besser RE, Lett SM, Weber JT et al. An outbreak of diarrhea and hemolytic uremic syndrome from *Escherichia coli* O157:H7 in fresh-pressed apple cider. *JAMA* 1993; **269**: 2217–2220.
55. Watanabe H, Guerrant RL. Summary: Nagasaki enterohemorrhagic *Escherichia coli* meeting and workshop. *J Infect Dis* 1997; **176**: 247–249.
56. Keene WE, Hedberg K, Herriott DE et al, A prolonged outbreak of *Escherichia coli* O157:H7 infections caused by commercially distributed raw milk. *J Infect Dis* 1997; **176**: 815–818.
57. Tilden J Jr, Young W, McNamara AM et al. A new route of transmission for *Escherichia coli*: infection from dry fermented salami. *Am J Public Health* 1996; **86**: 1142–1145.
58. Swerdlow DL, Woodruff BA, Brady RC et al. A waterborne outbreak in Missouri of *Escherichia coli* O157:H7 associated with bloody diarrhea and death. *Ann Intern Med* 1992; **117**: 812–819.
59. Keene W, McAnulty JM, Hoesly FC et al. A swimming-associated outbreak of hemorrhagic colitis caused by *Escherichia coli* O157:H7 and *Shigella sonnei*. *N Engl J Med* 1994; **331**: 579–584.
60. Belongia EA, Osterholm MT, Soler JT et al. Transmission of *Escherichia coli* O157:H7 infection in Minnesota child day-care facilities. *JAMA* 1993; **269**: 883–888.
61. Slutsker L, Ries AA, Greene KD et al. *Escherichia coli* O157:H7 diarrhea in the United States: clinical and epidemiologic features. *Ann Intern Med* 1997; **126**: 505–513.
62. Macdonald KL, O'Leary MJ, Cohen ML et al. *Escherichia coli* O157:H7, an emerging gastrointestinal pathogen: results of a one-year, prospective, population-based study. *JAMA* 1988; **59**: 3567–3570.
63. Griffin PM et al. Large outbreak of *Escherichia coli* O157:H7 infections in the western United States: the big picture. In Karmali MA, Goglio AG, eds. *Recent Advances in Verocytotoxin-producing Escherichia coli Infection*. Amsterdam: Elsevier Science BV, 1994: 7–12.
64. Griffen PM, Ostroff SM, Tauxe RV et al. Illnesses associated with *Escherichia coli* O157:H7 infections: a broad clinical spectrum. *Ann Intern Med* 1988; **109**: 705–712.
65. Pai Ch, Ahmed N, Lior H et al. Epidemiology of sporadic diarrhea due to verocytotoxin-producing *Escherichia coli*: a two-year prospective study. *J Infect Dis* 1988; **157**: 1054–1057.
66. Boyce TG, Swerdlow DL, Griffin PM. *Escherichia coli* O157:H7 and the hemolytic-uremic syndrome. *N Engl J Med* 1995; **333**: 364–368.
67. Uc A, Mitros FA, Kao SC, Sanders KD. Pseudomembranous colitis with *Escherichia coli* O157:H7. *J Pediatr Gastroenterol Nutr* 1997; **24**: 590–593.
68. Pavia AT, Nichols CR, Green DP et al. Hemolytic-uremic syndrome during an outbreak of *Escherichia coli* O157:H7 infections in institutions for mentally retarded persons: clinical and epidemiologic observations. *J Pediatr* 1990; **116**: 544–551.
69. Smith HR, Cheasty T, Rowe B. Enteroaggregative *Escherichia coli* and outbreaks of gastroenteritis in UK. *Lancet* 1997; **350**: 814–815.
70. Cimolai N, Carter JE, Morrison BJ, Anderson JD. Risk factors for the progression of *Escherichia coli* O157:H7 enteritis to hemolytic-uremic sydrome. *J Pediatr* 1990; **116**: 589–592.
71. Tarr PI, Neill MA, Clausen CR et al. *Escherichia coli* O157:H7 and the hemolytic uremic syndrome: importance of early cultures in establishing the etiology. *J Infect Dis* 1990; **162**: 553–556.
72. Proulx F, Turgeon JP, Delage G et al. Randomized, controlled trial of antibiotic therapy for *Escherichia coli* O157:H7 enteritis. *J Pediatr* 1992; **121**: 299–303.
73. Carter AO, Borczyk AA, Carlson JA et al. A severe outbreak of *Escherichia coli* O157:H7-associated hemorrhagic colitis in a nursing home. *N Engl J Med* 1987; **317**: 1496–1500.
74. Bosworth BT, Samuel JE, Moon HW et al. Vaccination with genetically modified Shiga-like toxin IIe prevents edema disease in swine. *Infect Immun* 1996; **64**: 55–60.

75. Butterton JR, Ryan ET, Acheson DW, Calderwood SB. Coexpression of the B subunit of Shiga toxin 1 and EaeA from enterohemorrhagic *Escherichia coli* in *Vibrio cholerae* vaccine strains. *Infect Immun* 1997; **65**: 2127–2135.
76. Konadu E, Robbins JB, Shiloach J et al. Preparation, characterization and immunological properties in mice of *Escherichia coli* O157 O-specific polysaccharide-protein conjugate vaccines. *Infect Immun* 1994; **62**: 5048–5054.
77. Bhan MK, Raj P, Levine MM et al. Enteroaggregative *Escherichia coli* associated with persistent diarrhea in a cohort of rural children in India. *J Infect Dis* 1989; **159**: 1061–1064.
78. Bhan MK, Khoshoo V, Sommerfelt H et al. Enteroaggregative *Escherichia coli* and Salmonella associated with nondysenteric persistent diarrhea. *Pediatr Infect Dis J* 1989; **8**: 499–502.
79. Cravioto A, Tello A, Navarro A et al. Association of *Escherichia coli* Hep-2 adherence patterns with type and duration of diarrhoea, *Lancet* 1991; **337**: 262–264.
80. Giron JA, Jones T, Millan-Velasco F et al. Diffuse-adhering *Escherichia coli* (DAEC) as a putative cause of diarrhea in Mayan children in Mexico. *J Infect Dis* 1991; **163**: 507–513.
81. Levine MM, Ferreccio C, Prado V et al. Epidemiologic studies of *Escherichia coli* diarrheal infections in a low socioeconomic level peri-urban community in Santiago, Chile. *Am J Epidemiol* 1993; **138**: 849–69.
82. Baqui AH, Sack RB, Black RE et al. Enteropathogens associated with acute and persistent diarrhea in Bangladeshi children < 5 years of age. *J Infect Dis* 1992; **166**: 792–796.
83. Nataro JP, Deng Y, Cookson S et al. Heterogeneity of enteroaggregative *Escherichia coli* virulence demonstrated in volunteers. *J Infect Dis* 1995; **171**: 465–468.
84. Henry FJ, Udoy AS, Wanke CA, Aziz KMA. Epidemiology of persistent diarrhea and etiologic agents in Mirzapur, Bangladesh. *Acta Paediatr Suppl* 1996; **381**: 27–31.
85. Bhatnagar S, Bhan MK, Sommerfelt H et al. Enteroaggregative *Escherichia coli* may be a new pathogen causing acute and persistent diarrhea. *Scand J Infect Dis* 1993; **25**: 579–583.
86. Fang GD, Lima AA, Martins CV et al. Etiology and epidemiology of persistent diarrhea in northeastern Brazil: a hospital-based, prospective, case–control study. *J Pediatr Gastroenterol Nutr* 1995; **21**: 137–144.
87. Nataro JP. Enteroaggregative *Escherichia coli*. *Alpe Adria Microbiol J* 1998; **7**: 265–273.
88. Pai M, Kang G, Ramakrishna BS et al. An epidemic of diarrhoea in south India caused by enteroaggregative *Escherichia coli*. *Indian J Med Res* 1997; **106**: 7–12.
89. Cobeljic M, Miljkovic-Selimovic B, Paunovic-Todosijevic D et al. Enteroaggregative *Escherichia coli* associated with an outbreak of diarrhoea in a neonatal nursery ward. *Epidemiol Infect* 1996; **117**: 11–16.
90. Itoh Y, Nagano I, Kunishima M, Ezaki T. Laboratory investigation of enteroaggregative *Escherichia coli* O untypeable:H10 associated with a massive outbreak of gastrointestinal illness. *J Clin Microbiol* 1997; **35**: 2546–2550.
91. Paul M, Tsukamoto T, Ghosh AR et al. The significance of enteroaggregative *Escherichia coli* in the etiology of hospitalized diarrhoea in Calcutta, India and the demonstration of a new honey-combed pattern of aggregative adherence. *FEMS Microbiol Lett* 1994; **117**: 319–326.
92. Steiner TS, Lima AAM, Nataro JP, Guerrant RL. Enteroaggregative *Escherichia coli* produce intestinal inflammation and growth impairment and cause interleukin-8 release from intestinal epithelial cells. *J Infect Dis* 1998; **177**: 88–96.
93. Bouzari S, Jafari A, Farhoudi-Moghaddam AA et al. Adherence of non-enteropathogenic *Escherichia coli* to HeLa cells. *J Med Microbiol* 1994; **40**: 95–97.
94. Schmidt H, Knop C, Franke S et al. Development of PCR for screening of enteroaggregative *Escherichia coli*. *J Clin Microbiol* 1995; **33**: 701–705.
95. Yamamoto T, Echeverria P, Yokota T. Drug resistance and adherence to human intestines of enteroaggregative *Escherichia coli*. *J Infect Dis* 1992; **165**: 744–749.
96. McFarland LV, Mulligan ME, Kwok RYY, Stamm WE. Nosocomial acquisition of *Clostridium difficile* infection. *N Engl J Med* 1989; **320**: 204–210.
97. Kaatz GW, Gitlin SD, Schaberg DR et al. Acquisition of *Clostridium difficile* from the hospital environment. *Am J Epidemiol* 1988; **127**: 1289–1294.
98. McFarland LV, Surawicz CM, Stamm WE. Risk factors for *Clostridium difficile* carriage and *C. difficile*-associated diarrhea in a cohort of hospitalized patients. *J Infect Dis* 1990; **162**: 678–684.
99. Donta ST, Myers MG. *Clostridium difficile* toxin in asymptomatic neonates, *J Pediatr* 1982; **100**: 431–434.
100. Borriello SP. Pathogenesis of *Clostridium difficile* infection. *J Antimicrob Chemother* 1998; **41**: 13–19.
101. Batts DH, Martin D, Holmes R et al. Treatment of antibiotic-associated *Clostridium difficile* diarrhea with oral vancomycin. *J Pediatr* 1980; **97**: 151–153.
102. Bolton RP, Culshaw MA. Maecal metronidazole concentrations during oral and intravenous therapy for antibiotic colitis due to *Clostridium difficile*. *Gut* 1986; **27**: 1169–1172.
103. Gorbach SL, Chang T-W, Foldin B. Successful treatment of relapsing *Clostridium difficile* colitis with *Lactobacillus* GG. *Lancet* 1987; **2**: 1519.
104. Surawicz CM, Elmer GW, Speelman P et al. Prevention of antibiotic-associated diarrhea by *Saccharomyces boulardii*: a prospective study. *Gastroenterology* 1989; **96**: 981–988.
105. Guandalini S. The treatment of acute diarrhea in the third millennium: a pediatrician's perspective. *Acta Gastroenterol Belgn* 2002; **65**: 33–6.
106. Huang JS, Bousvaros A, Lee JW et al. Efficacy of probiotic use in acute diarrhea in children: a meta-analysis. *Dig Dis Sci* 2002; **47**: 2625–2634.
107. D'Souza AL, Rajkumar C, Cooke J, Bulpitt CJ. Probiotics in prevention of antibiotic associated diarrhoea: meta-analysis. *BMJ* 2002; **324**:1361–1366.

11 Intestinal parasites

David Brewster

Introduction

The parasites of humans are classified into five major divisions: Protozoa (amebae, flagellates, ciliates, sporozoans, coccidia, microsporidia); Platyhelminths (cestodes, trematodes), Acanthocephela (thorny headed worms); Nematodes (roundworms) and Arthropods (insects, spiders, mites, ticks). Geohelminths are a sub-group of soil-transmitted intestinal nematodes with similar epidemiological characteristics. They include *Strongyloides*, hookworm, *Ascaris* and *Trichuris*.[1] In this chapter, we focus on the common protozoa, nematodes and trematodes which affect the intestine (Table 11.1). Out of the large numbers of children infected by these parasites in the developing world, most are asymptomatic and do not present to the health services for treatment.

The World Health Organization (WHO) estimates that some 3.5 billion people worldwide are infected by intestinal parasitic and protozoan infections, including 350 million with morbidity from ascariasis, 220 million from trichuris and 150 million from hookworm.[2] A nationwide survey of intestinal parasites in China during 1988–92 on 1.5 million people reported a prevalence of 62.6%, of whom 43.3% had multiple parasites. The five common parasites were *Ascaris lumbricoides* (47.0%), *Enterobius vermicularis* (26.4%), *Trichuris trichiura* (18.8%), *Giardia lamblia* (2.5%) and *Entamoeba histolytica* (0.9%).[3] In sub-Saharan African schoolchildren, on the other hand, estimates of the prevalence of helminth infections were: hookworms 32.1%, *Ascaris* 30.2%, *Trichuris* 29.5% and *Schistosoma mansoni* 14.0%.[4] These prevalence rates have been fairly stable over the past 50 years with only a modest decrease in ascariasis. However, higher rates have been reported, such as surveys reporting that only 14% of Tanzanian and 37% of Ghanaian children were free from worm infections.[5] Intestinal parasites also occur in industrialized countries, with a third of 5792 fecal specimens positive for parasites in the USA in 2000, peaking between July and October.[6]

The peak age for intestinal parasites tends to be school-age children but overt sickness from them is the exception. A large Tanzanian morbidity survey of schoolchildren found that no sign or symptom was significantly associated with any helminth infection, only blood in stool and hepatomegaly with *Schistosoma mansoni*.[7] The major determinant of morbidity from parasitic diseases is the intensity of infection, but this is rarely reported in children. A Zairean study found that the highest mean intensities (measured as eggs per gram of feces (epg)) of *Ascaris* and *Trichuris* were among 2–4-year-olds, whereas school-age children excreted the most hookworm ova.[8] Using disability-adjusted life years lost (DALY), WHO estimated that intestinal helminthiasis caused 39 million DALYs, with 57% attributed to hookworm, 27% to ascariasis and 16% to trichurasis.[2]

The most common symptoms of intestinal parasites are diarrhea and/or failure to thrive from anorexia and malabsorption. The protozoa *Giardia lamblia* and *Cryptosporidium parvum* are common causes of diarrhea in children, but other protozoa such as *Cyclospora cayetanensis*, *Entamoeba histolytica*, and *Microsporidia* species may also cause diarrhea, and these include *Isospora belli* in immunodeficient (e.g. HIV-seropositive) patients. Only five helminthic parasites are associated with diarrheal disease: *Strongyloides stercoralis*, *Trichuris trichiura*, *Schistosoma mansoni*, *Trichinella spiralis* and *Capillaria philippinensis*.[9] Strictly intraluminal worms (e.g. *Ascaris lumbricoides*) only rarely affect intestinal function

Table 11.1 Classification of intestinal parasites

Infection	Other name	Symptoms	Transmission	Alternative treatments	Treatment of choice
PROTOZOA					
Intestinal amebae					
Entamoeba histolytica	amebiasis	dysentery	fecal–oral		metronidazole
Entamoeba dispar		asymptomatic	fecal–oral		nil
Flagellates					
Giardia lamblia (duodenale or intestinalis)	giardiasis	chronic diarrhea, malabsorption	fecal–oral	metronidazole	tinidazole
Ciliates					
Balantidium coli		asymtomatic	fecal–oral		nil
Coccidia					
Cryptosporidium parvum	cryptosporidiosis	persistent diarrhea	fecal–oral		nitazoxanide*
Cyclospora cayetanensis	cyclosporiasis	diarrhea	fecal–oral		co-trimoxazole
Isospora belli	isosporiasis	diarrhea with AIDS	fecal–oral		co-trimoxazole
NEMATODES					
Ascaris lumbricoides	roundworm	intestinal obstruction	fecal–oral	levamisole, pyrantel	albendazole†
Enterobius vermicularis	pinworm, threadworm	nocturnal anal pruritis	fecal–oral	levamisole, pyrantel	albendazole†
Ancylostoma duodenale	hookworm	iron deficiency anemia	percutaneous	levamisole, pyrantel	albendazole†
Necator americanus	hookworm	iron deficiency anemia	percutaneous	levamisole, pyrantel	albendazole†
Strongyloides stercoralis	strongyloidiasis	diarrhea	percutaneous	albendazole	ivermectin
Trichuris trichiura	whipworm, trichuriasis	dysentry, rectal prolapse (rare)	fecal–oral	levamisole, pyrantel	albendazole†
CESTODES					
Hymenolepis nana	dwarf tapeworm	asymptomatic	fecal–oral	praziquantel	nitazoxanide*
TREMATODES					
Schistosoma mansoni	bilharzia	melena, portal hypertension	percutaneous	oxamniquine	praziquantel
Fasciolopsis buski	giant intestinal fluke		percutaneous		praziquantel

*Nitazoxanide is the drug of choice (if available) where treatment is indicated; †or mebendazole adversely when the intensity of infection is high. Infections such as giardiasis, cryptosporidiosis and severe trichuriasis may contribute to growth failure via malabsorption, so their resolution or treatment should lead to catch-up growth. Malnutrition appears to predispose children to an acute diarrheal syndrome in strongyloidiasis, which may then exacerbate the nutritional status through anorexia and enteropathy.[10] Owing to the prolonged carriage of many parasites, only *Strongyloides* and *Cryptosporidium* have a consistently significant association with diarrheal disease when compared to non-diarrheal controls (Table 11.2).

Giardiasis

Introduction

Giardia lamblia (also called *intestinalis* or *duodenale*) is a flagellate protozoan with two stages: motile trophozoites (Figure 11.1) and cysts.

Life cycle

Infection may result from ingesting cysts, which release trophozoites in the upper small intestine, attaching to the mucosa by a ventral disc. *Giardia* trophozoites undergo significant biological changes to survive outside the host by differentiating into infective cysts, which is promoted by exposure to conjugated bile salts and

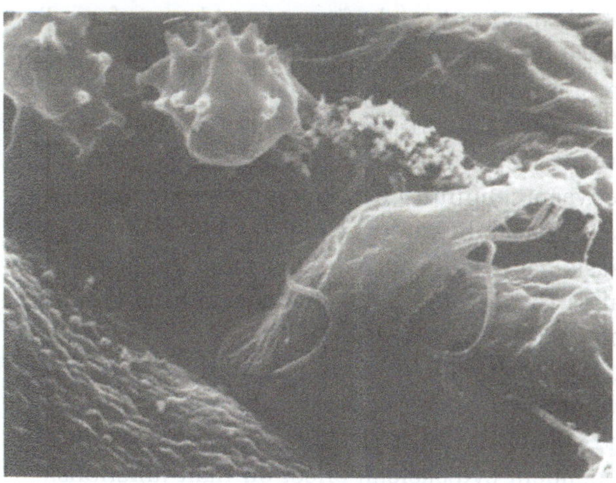

Figure 11.1 *Giardia lamblia* trophozoite. Courtesy of UK Tropical International Health.

Table 11.2 Parasites in diarrhea in children: case–control studies

	Guinea-Bissau[16]		Bangladesh[207]		Five Countries†[208]		Tropical Australia[10]		South Africa[209]		Total	
	Cases	Controls	Cases	Controls	Cases	Controls	Cases	Controls	Cases	Controls	Cases	Controls
n	1219	511	814	814	3640	3279	290	85	373	371	6336	5060
Giardia	233	128	7	23	109	98	9	5	24	22	6.0%	5.5%
*Cryptosporidium**	69	11	11	3			20	1	9	2	4.0%	1.0%
*Strongyloides**	54	15					21	2			5.0%	2.9%
Entamoeba	50	31	5	1	11	3	0	0	1	0	1.1%	0.7%
Ascaris	7	1					0	0	40	53	2.5%	5.6%
Hookworm	31	28					1	0			2.1%	4.7%
Trichuris	5	2					22	4	13	23	2.1%	3.0%
Hymenolepis	2	0					2	4	1	3	0.3%	0.7%

*Significantly associated with diarrhea, odds ratio 4.4 (95% CI 2.6–7.6) for *Cryptosporidium* and 1.8 (95% CI 1.0–3.3) for *Strongyloides*
†China, India, Mexico, Myanmar, Pakistan

low levels of cholesterol.[11,12] A specific proteolytic event caused by a constitutively expressed membrane-associated dipeptidyl peptidase IV is necessary for encystation.[13] The incubation period is 1–2 weeks.

Epidemiology

Giardia lamblia is one of the most common parasitic infections in humans with a prevalence of 2–5% in industrialized countries, and high transmission rates in day-care center outbreaks among 12–36-month-old children who are not toilet trained.[14,15] In developing countries, prevalences of 20–30% occur with up to 60% of children infected at some time during childhood. Since cysts are excreted for prolonged periods, community studies often find higher rates of infection in children without diarrhea than in diarrheal cases.[16] *Giardia* accounts for about 5% of travelers' diarrhea and is more common in children with immunodeficiency, although not HIV infection. The main routes of transmission are water, food and fecal–oral. Infection may occur after the ingestion of only 10–100 cysts and unfiltered water has been a common source of outbreaks in developed countries.

A Brazilian 4-year cohort study of 157 children from an urban slum documented substantial morbidity from giardiasis, with a similar frequency between diarrheal and non-diarrheal cases (9.7% vs. 7.4%), an association with persistent diarrhea (20.6% of episodes) and recurrent or relapsing infections (46%) and poorer nutritional status for those with symptomatic infections.[17] A study of a rural Egyptian cohort of 152 infants documented 4.5 episodes per child-year with a mean duration of excretion of 7.2 weeks, and reduced risk in breast-fed infants, particularly for symptomatic illness.[18] A Kenyan cohort study of 84 rural children aged 10–28 months reported a 44.7% prevalence, an estimated incidence of 2.8 episodes per year and a duration of 75.3 days per child for giardiasis.[19]

Pathophysiology

Despite intensive investigations, the exact mechanisms by which *Giardia* causes diarrhea and malabsorption are still unclear. There is evidence of a secretory mechanism, malabsorption, decreased brush-border surface area and interference with intraluminal digestion. Another possible mechanism for diarrhea is small-bowel bacterial overgrowth, but mucosal invasion is uncommon. Duodenal morphology may be normal, but partial or even total villus atrophy may occur, as well as a mucosal inflammatory response with increased intraepithelial lymphocytes. *Giardia* parasites are able to adhere to the gut mucosa and may cause a direct effect on intestinal function by disrupting the brush border and its enzymatic system.

The effect of giardiasis on intestinal structure and function is quite variable, but animal and *in vitro* studies have documented villus atrophy, malabsorption, increased paracellular permeability and reduced brush-border enzymes.[20,21] *Giardia* trophozoites are known to produce glycosidase enzymes which may affect the barrier function of mucins secreted by mucosal epithelial cells.[22] An Italian study of 61 children with symptomatic giardiasis documented lactose malabsorption on breath testing, resulting in intolerance to cows' milk but not to yogurt.[23] However, a breath hydrogen study in asymptomatic Mexican children with giardiasis did not find significant carbohydrate malabsorption.[24] Another study found only modest effects of *Giardia* treatment on biopsy changes, absorptive studies and bile salt conjugation, suggesting that the parasite's effect was synergistic with other organisms in contributing to tropical enteropathy.[25]

A Danish study of 29 children with chronic diarrhea from giardiasis documented enteropathy in 20, vitamin B_{12} malabsorption in nine, folate malabsorption in only five, no evidence of small-bowel bacterial overgrowth (SBBO) or iron malabsorption and more severe manifestations in those who acquired giardiasis overseas.[26] A study of 210 urban Nepali children found no association between helminth infection and growth or intestinal permeability, but the eight children with giardiasis had significantly higher mean permeability ratios (L : M ratio 0.43) than for either helminth infected (0.27) or uninfected (0.25).[27] A Canadian study in a mouse model showed that *Giardia* trophozoites increase small-intestinal permeability, mediated by a myosin light chain kinase-dependent cytoskeletal effect on tight junctions.[28] This disrupted enterocyte barrier function was T-cell independent and did not affect the stomach or colon. It is still unclear whether it is these effects or other mechanisms that cause the T-cell-dependent shortening of the brush-border microvilli with reduced disaccharidases and impaired absorptive function.

The immune response to *Giardia* involves both humoral and cellular mechanisms.[29] Humans produce IgG, IgM, IgA and IgE responses including cytotoxic antibodies and an important intestinal IgA response to acute infection. Nevertheless, there is still no direct evidence that antibodies control infection. A Gambian study of six children with giardiasis, persistent diarrhea and malnutrition who failed to clear infection after treatment had raised only *Giardia*-specific IgM antibodies, so poor serum and secretory IgA response may be a marker for ineffective parasite clearance.[30] Children with agammaglobulinemia, but not HIV-infected children, are susceptible to giardiasis and it is difficult to eradicate. Breast feeding provides protection from symptomatic disease, but not from infection.[31]

An association between giardiasis and allergy has been suggested based on the hypothesis that increased antigen penetration through damaged intestinal mucosa enhances sensitization to food antigens. One study documented allergy symptoms in 70% of children with giardiasis who had mean IgE levels of 1194 IU/ml compared to 43% and 822 IU/ml, respectively, for controls.[32] The giardiasis group also had higher levels of specific serum IgE antibodies to food allergens compared both to controls and to other parasitic infections, whereas IgE responses to house dust mite were similar.

Clinical features

The clinical manifestations of *Giardia* infection vary from asymptomatic passage of cysts to chronic diarrhea with malabsorption and weight loss. The usual clinical syndrome is characterized by watery diarrhea, foul-smelling stools, bloating and abdominal cramps. Only about half of patients develop symptoms following ingestion of cysts, with 15% passing cysts asymptomatically and the remainder showing no trace of infection. Although older children may be asymptomatic, infection early in life usually causes acute symptoms with watery diarrhea, anorexia, abdominal distension and foul stools which persist untreated and may result in malabsorption. The course of giardiasis is frequently prolonged and, although many eventually resolve without treatment, some go on to syndromes of chronic diarrhea or frequent relapses. The severity of disease may be determined by strain-dependent virulence factors in the parasite, as well as age, nutritional status and immunocompetence of the host.[33] Young children are more likely to be severely affected, with failure to thrive, hypokalemia and malabsorption (fat, vitamins A and B_{12}, protein and lactose). Children in the developing world with chronic diarrhea and malnutrition often have giardiasis, but it is not always clear how much *Giardia* is contributing to the illness, since they are often co-infected with other enteric pathogens. The results of a small Venezuelan trial suggested that the therapeutic control of giardiasis could be important in programs to combat anemia in children living in settings with high prevalence.[34]

Diagnosis

The diagnosis of giardiasis relies upon stool microscopy finding trophozoites or cysts. The sensitivity of a single stool is only 50–70% but increases to 90% if three stools are examined. Commercial assays for *Giardia* antigen are more sensitive and use polyclonal or monoclonal antibody directed against cyst or trophozoite antigens, usually as an enzyme-linked immunosorbent assay (ELISA) or immunofluorescent assay. These antigen detection assays are most useful for population screening such as children at day-care centers. Duodenal aspirates or biopsies are invasive, so are not justified exclusively to diagnose giardiasis, but when done for other reasons are reliable, particularly in the immunocompromised subject.

Prevention

Giardia is waterborne and cysts are highly resistant to chlorine and ozone, so filtration provides the best protection against transmission through tap water.[35] Hygiene measures to prevent fecal–oral transmission need to focus on young children. The drug treatment of choice for symptomatic disease (not just cyst excretors) is tinidazole (see p.183).

Ascariasis

Introduction

Ascaris lumbricoides is a large, 15–35 cm long white roundworm that is specific to humans. *Ascaris* is one of 63 species of nematode infecting humans, and the adult roundworm has a biologically inert surface, so the main antigenic stimuli to the host are excretory and secretory antigens from the orifices. *A. suum* is the related pig species which may migrate through human tissues in the larval stage,[36] but cannot complete its life cycle in man.

Life cycle

The female *Ascaris* worm produces about 200 000 eggs/day, which embryonate in soil in about 3 weeks to become infectious, but are sensitive to excessive heat, drying and sunlight. Ingested eggs moult to form larvae (0.2 mm long) which penetrate blood vessels or lymphatics and travel to the lung via the portal vein or thoracic duct to pulmonary capillaries and alveoli, where they moult, grow in size, migrate up the airways and down the esophagus, and mature and reproduce in the small intestine. Adult *Ascaris* are large white roundworms (females 2–4 cm long) which, unlike hookworm and *Trichuris,* do not attach to the mucosa but live free in the small-intestinal lumen. The duration of the life cycle from ingestion of *Ascaris* ova to new egg excretion in feces by the mature worm takes about 2 months. Adult worms are expelled from the intestine after about 18 months.

Epidemiology

Ascariasis is one of the most prevalent infections in the world affecting approximately 1400 million people (23% of the world population) with 59 million (mostly children) at risk of morbidity, including 95% of the population of Africa and 45% of inhabitants of Central and South America.[37] Highest prevalences are found in countries where sanitation is deficient, and children have higher mean worm loads than adults. There is some evidence of a predisposition to high infestation of *Ascaris* worms due to a genetic or immunological predisposition. Morbidity is related to worm load, which is indirectly assessed by egg concentration per gram (epg) of feces (e.g. light infection, < 5000 epg, heavy infection, $> 50\,000$ epg). Community prevalence levels greater than 70% are associated with high worm burdens, likelihood of morbidity and rapid reinfection, so warrant antihelminthic control programs (see below).[38] Geophagy (eating soil) is a risk factor for ascariasis in African schoolchildren.[39,40]

Immunology of helminths

An important principle of helminth immunology is that very few responses elicited by infection are likely to be functionally *protective* and some have severe *pathological* consequences for the host. Immune responses can also be divided into innate (immediate response on exposure with little memory and broad molecular specificity not involving lymphoid cells) and adaptive (lymphocyte-mediated and antigen-specific with memory).[41] Although immune responses in the intestinal mucosa are similar to systemic responses, an important difference is the predominance of IgA antibodies.

Immune responses against helminth invasion rarely eliminate them directly. Effective immunity against reinfection is also difficult to demonstrate for helminth infections, since worms persist in the face of specific immune responses, although age-related declines in infection rates do occur in endemic areas. However, detailed epidemiological and animal model studies have demonstrated that acquired protective immunity is important for control of hookworm, *Trichuris* and schistosomiasis.[41] *Ascaris* produces the lipid-binding protein ABA-1 which can stimulate IgE antibodies, high levels of which correlate with protection against *Ascaris.*[42]

The traditional view of the host immune response was that with time it reduced their fecundity and survival via mechanisms such as induction of intestinal mast cells and eosinophils. More recent evidence suggests that other indirect host responses may result in parasite starvation or depletion of energy sources for defending itself against the host's immune responses, leading to reduced fecundity or survival.[43] However, there is also a cost to the host from mounting an immune response to the parasite, particularly on nutritional status in children. For example, zinc deficiency may prolong nematode survival in the host by its known effect on mucosal immune function.[44] In addition, many helminths release immunomodulatory molecules which inactivate components of the host's immune response, but this may also predispose the host to other infections such as tuberculosis (TB) or AIDS. There is also evidence that ascariasis impairs immune responses to vaccines in that albendazole treatment increased the seroconversion rate and antibody titers after cholera immunization, mediated by suppression of interleukin (IL)-2 responses.[45,46] Moreover, treatment of helminths in HIV-infected individuals was associated with significant reductions in viral load.[47]

Immune-mediated inflammation occurs in most parasitic infections, particularly involving IgE antibodies, eosinophils, cytokines and T cells, but there are important differences between helminths and protozoa. First, although protozoa may be phagocytosed by macrophages, cell-mediated immunity against helminths involves attachment to its surface with antibody or complement-mediated mechanisms and release of mediators which damage its surface. Second, whereas protozoa tend to elicit T-helper lymphocytes with activation of macrophages, cytokines (IL-12) and specific IgG antibodies (Th1 responses), helminths elicit Th2 responses with IL-4 stimulating IgE antibodies and inflammatory cells (e.g. eosinophils and mast cells). Thus, compared to controls, cytokine responses in *Ascaris*-infected subjects involved mononuclear cell IL-4 and IL-5 stimulation with no difference in IL-10 and interferon-γ responses, consistent with a highly polarized Th2 cytokine response.[48]

Helminth infections are characterized by increased mast cells and eosinophils. The key function of IL-5, which is produced by activated CD4 T cells, is control of eosinophils, although early differentiation of eosinophils is controlled by granulocyte-macrophage–colony-stimulating factor (GM-CSF) and IL-3. It is now recognized that eosinophils, together with antibody and complement, have a role in the killing of infective larval stages of most helminths, but not of adult worms. Recent studies in mice suggest that the effect of IL-5 and eosinophils differs for each parasite species, but they do have a role in host protection which is not yet clearly defined.[49,50]

IgE antibodies are an important component of host-protective immune responses against helminthic parasites, including both parasite-specific IgE and non-specific polyclonal IgE mediated by IL-4. Excessive polyclonal stimulation of IgE synthesis by helminths, which is prevented by anthelminthic treatment, suppresses allergic reactivity by saturating mast cell receptors and inhibiting specific IgE antibodies (e.g. to inhaled antigens such as house dust mite) and skin test reactivity.[51] Compared to urban children, rural Kenyan children's total IgE and *Ascaris*-specific IgE antibodies were much higher, and evidence of atopy (skin testing, bronchial hyper-reactivity) were much lower.[52] A Venezuelan study examined two groups of children with comparable living conditions and *Ascaris* prevalence but with very different prevalences of allergic disease.[53] Those in the atopic group had an intrinsic propensity for specific over polyclonal IgE responses to the parasite and had significantly lower intensities of infection than the non-atopic group, suggesting that the atopic state conferred a selective evolutionary advantage.

Immune responses are useful as a means of diagnosing infection by ELISA tests. The major drawback of antibody-based tests is that a positive test does not prove current infection in an endemic area, although use of particular classes of antibody (e.g. IgG4, IgM) may improve the specificity. Newer diagnostic tests by antigen-capture ELISA for coproantigens in feces are becoming available, which are highly sensitive and specific.

Clinical features

Ascaris infection is not associated with mucosal damage, increased intestinal permeability or lactose malabsorption,[54,55] since 85% of infected individuals have light infections which remain asymptomatic. Heavy infection (ingestion of > 2000 eggs) may induce a pneumonitis from migrating pulmonary larvae, with cough, wheeze, eosinophilia and transient patchy infiltrates which may be difficult to differentiate from pneumonia, asthma or bronchitis. This syndrome of tropical pulmonary eosinophilia (Loeffler's) is rarely recognized clinically in children with *Ascaris* or hookworm, but is more often symptomatic with filariasis or toxocara infections.[56]

The most common clinical feature of ascariasis is intestinal obstruction from a bolus of worms, which occurs in 0.2% of infections in children, accounting for 72% of all complications of *Ascaris*.[57] The mean age of cases is under 5 years and the case fatality rate about 5.7%. Surgical management can invariably be avoided with experience with this syndrome, and daily nasogastric administration of anthelminthics with supportive therapy until the bolus is passed. Worms are often vomited or passed in stool on presentation of febrile children with severe malaria or bacterial infections, which invariably prompts comments from health workers about them 'abandoning a sinking ship'. Fever, acute phase reactants and certain irritants (e.g. carbon tetrachloride, a former hookworm therapy) are associated with worm expulsion or aberrant migration. Less frequent complications of migrating *Ascaris* worms are biliary colic, pancreatitis, appendiceal abscess and appearance through a surgical abdominal wound.

Diagnosis

The diagnosis of ascariasis is based upon identification of the characteristic eggs on microscopy of stool or identification of the adult worm passed spontaneously or after treatment. Eggs are plentiful in feces since each female produces a mean of 200 000 daily, although the correlation between eggs per gram of feces and intensity of infection is imperfect.

Prevention

If human feces are used as fertilizer for growing vegetables, they need to be stored at 30°C for 40 days to ensure destruction of ova. A number of reports have examined environmental risk factors for ascariasis. A Brazilian study, for example, gave the following relative risks with 95% CI for ascariasis intensity: over crowding 2.2 (1.0–4.5), poor household water availability 2.4 (1.1–5.0), poor hygiene 2.4 (1.0–5.6), less than 4 years' schooling 5.9 (2.6–14.3) and no recent anthelminthic treatment 2.0 (1.0–4.0).[58] A Kenyan study found that household overcrowding and the absence of latrines increased the risk of hookworm infection, whereas a lack of soap and other household children under 5 years increased the risk of *Ascaris* infection.[59] Since the lack of latrines and soap usage were identified as risk factors for infection, helminth control interventions should focus on these. Mass chemotherapy campaigns for geohelminths is discussed below.

Hookworm

Introduction

The two major species of hookworms are *Ancylostoma duodenale* and *Necator americanus* (Figure 11.2). They will be considered together here, because they have similar life cycles and disease. However, *Ancylostoma* tends to be more virulent than *Necator*, and adult females are larger (10–13 vs. 9–11 mm), survive for a shorter time in the host (1 vs. 4 years), produce more eggs (10 000–30 000 vs. 5–10 000/day), cause greater blood loss (0.2 vs. 0.02 ml/day) and their larvae can rest dormant and infect via oral ingestion (unlike *Necator*).

Life cycle

The gravid female hookworm produces about 5000–30 000 eggs/day (60 μm long) in feces, which require a moist shady environment to hatch into

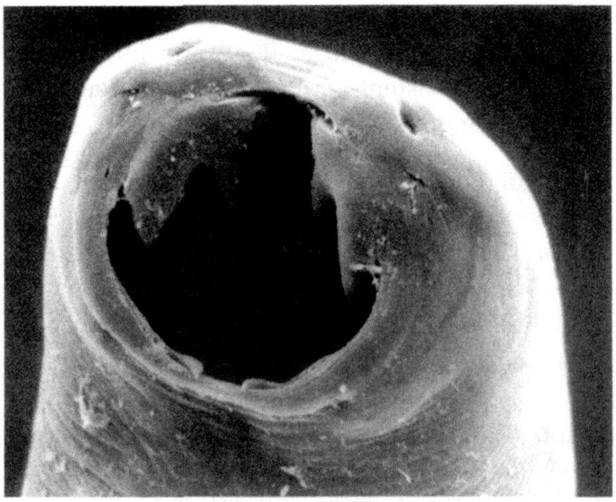

Figure 11.2 *Necator americanus* hookworm. Courtesy of UK Tropical International Health.

rhabditiform larvae (300 μm long) which grow to become infective larvae (600 μm) and enter the host's venules or lymphatics, usually when walked upon with bare feet. The larvae then migrate into the lungs and ascend up the respiratory tract and descend to the small intestine, where they attach and mature in the jejunum. The time from infection to egg production is almost 2 months.

Epidemiology

Hookworm is probably the second most prevalent intestinal parasite after ascariasis, with 1200 million people infected worldwide (two-thirds by *Necator*), including 90–130 million with morbidity. *Necator* predominates in Central and South America (New World), and *Ancylostoma* in India, China, North Africa and tropical Australia, but mixed infections occur in many regions of Asia, Africa, Central America and the South Pacific. *Ancylostoma* extends into more temperate regions than *Necator* (e.g. North Africa, China and Europe) because its ova are more resistant to cold. In an urban Nigerian study of 862 schoolchildren with hookworm, 72.0% had *Necator* alone, 4.5% *Ancylostoma* alone and 23.4% both species of hookworm, but with *Necator* in higher numbers.[60]

Unlike *Ascaris* and *Trichuris*, hookworm transmission is closely associated with rural farming rather than urban slums. There are several other species of dog and cat helminths (e.g. *Toxocara* species) which can cause eosinophilic enteritis, cutaneous larva migrans or viscera larva migrans in humans. For example, studies in tropical Australia have described eosinophilic enteritis with abdominal pain caused by *Ancylostoma caninum*, a dog hookworm.[61]

Pathophysiology

Hookworms attach to the mucosa with teeth (*Ancylostoma*) or cutting plates (*Necator*) and release anticoagulant polypeptides and neutrophil inhibitory factor which down-regulate the inflammatory response of the host. They also release hydrolytic enzymes which damage mucosal capillaries and exacerbate the blood loss. Hookworm larvae release *Ancylostoma*-secreted proteins (ASPs) during the early stages of infection, which are highly antigenic. The indirect evidence of reduced hookworm burdens in adults suggests an effect of host immunity, but humoral antibodies and cell-mediated immune responses correlate poorly with resistance to infection. The possibility of a hookworm vaccine to ASPs is under investigation.[62]

Clinical features

Hookworm larvae entering skin can result in a papulovesicular rash at the site of entry (ground itch) or cutaneous larvae migrans for animal hookworms. Although eosinophilia accompanies the larval migration phase, pneumonitis is mild and rarely recognized in children. The main morbidity from hookworm is iron deficiency anemia, particularly with heavy infections. It was not uncommon in Caribbean and Pacific islands to have school children presenting in congestive heart failure with loud hemic murmurs and hemoglobin levels of <20 g/l from hookworm. Blood transfusions are indicated only for heart failure, so can be avoided in most cases of hookworm infection in endemic areas due to its chronic anemia (unlike more acute malarial anemia). Heavy infections may result in hypoalbuminemia as well as anemia, but malabsorption or severe enteropathy do not appear to be common features of hookworm infection, unlike strongyloidiasis. Infantile hookworm infection occurs in China with severe manifestations, presumably due to *Ancylostoma* transmission transplacentally or via breast milk.[63]

Diagnosis

The diagnosis of hookworm infection is based upon identifying hookworm eggs on microscopy of feces. The intensity may be gauged from a quantitative egg count, which is mostly used for epidemiological studies. Differentiation between eggs of *Ancylostoma* and *Necator* requires culture to the infective larval stage or newer polymerase chain reaction (PCR) techniques, but adult worm identification is easier (except after benzimidazole treatment, which may affect morphology). Eosinophilic enteritis due to animal hookworm may require endoscopy for definitive diagnosis, since stool microscopy will be negative. Charcot–Leydan crystals in stool reflect breakdown of eosinophils, which is a non-specific feature of early infection.

Prevention

Measures to prevent hookworm include ceasing the use of human feces as fertilizer, use of toilets, wearing shoes and generally improving living standards. Mass treatment programs with albendazole have a transient effect, but need to be combined with improved sanitation and health education to prevent high reinfection rates.[64] Iron supplementation has no effect on either reinfection rates or helminth intensities in children.[65] In high prevalence areas of hookworm infection and schistosomiasis, regular mass deworming campaigns with albendazole and praziquantel are effective in reducing anemia rates.[66,67]

Trichuriasis

Introduction

Trichuris trichiuria, meaning 'hairy tail', is actually a misnomer, since it is the proximal end that is hairlike. The popular name is whipworm, with the whip as the long thin pharynx (stichostome) and the whip handle as the posterior end with reproductive organs and intestine (Figure 11.3).

Life cycle

A mature female worm produces up to 20 000 eggs/day, which are 50 µm long and not infectious until the larval stage develops in the soil over 2–4 weeks. Warm damp soil is ideal for embryonation, and environmental exposure is associated with poor hygiene practices. Once ingested, larvae penetrate the epithelium of the mucosal crypt in the cecum, where they moult and the hair-like stichosome remains attached while the broader distal end extends into the lumen. The adult worm is 4 cm long and survives for 1–2 years in the host.

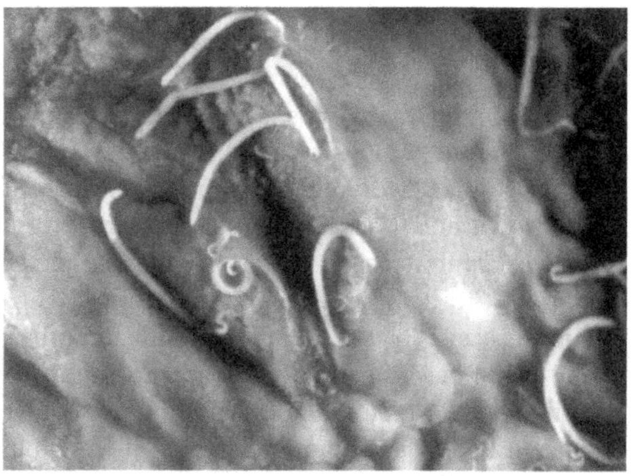

Figure 11.3 *Trichuris trichiura* worms attached to the colon. Courtesy of UK Tropical International Health.

Epidemiology

Trichuriasis is a very common infestation with an estimated 1049 million cases worldwide, including 114 million preschool and 233 million school-age children.[68] Most of these infections are asymptomatic, but children suffer greater morbidity than adults. There appears to be a genetic or immunological predisposition to heavy infection, which may be HLA group-mediated.[69] There also appears to be some epidemiological 'synergism' between ascariasis and trichuriasis in that high-intensity infections occur together more often than by chance.[70]

Pathophysiology

With severe infection, the cecal mucosa becomes inflamed and edematous, but there are only minor changes in histology (increased IgM lamina propria plasma cells and calprotectin-secreting cells, crypt epithelial cell proliferation, distended goblet cells).[71] The cytokine response in colonic mucosa involves both interferon-γ (Th1) and IL-4 (Th2), but results in neither worm expulsion nor obvious protection from reinfection. There may be a protein-losing enteropathy proportional to the worm burden.[72] There is an acute-phase response with intense trichuriasis, including increases in plasma tumor necrosis factor (TNF)-α, C-reactive protein (CRP), globulins, viscosity and fibronectin with decreased insulin-like growth factor (IGF)-I[73–75]. There is also development of an IgE-mediated immediate hypersensitivity reaction in the colon,[76] usually, but not always, with systemic eosinophilia.

Clinical features

Most infections in children are light (< 20 adult worms) and asymptomatic, with symptoms developing in < 10% of infected children. Occult blood in feces is uncommon even with heavy infestations, although even light infections incite a local inflammatory response involving eosinophils and neutrophils in the colon.[77,78] With heavy infestations, frequent watery or mucous stools occur, sometimes with frank blood. Rectal prolapse can occur with heavy infestations.[79,80] A very small minority of heavily infected children (> 200 worms in the rectum, colon and often terminal ileum) develop the *Trichuris* dysentery syndrome,[81,82] characterized by chronic dysentery, stunting, anemia and finger clubbing.

Diagnosis

The diagnosis is based on finding eggs on stool microscopy, with more than 10 000 epg generally associated with heavy infection, although there is considerable individual variation in eggs to worm load. *Trichuris* dysentery in children must be differentiated from amebic and bacilliary causes. Most cases of rectal prolapse in malnourished children are not due to trichuriasis.

Prevention

The use of proper latrines, good hygiene with handwashing and washing of vegetables will interrupt the life cycle. Overcrowded urban slums with limited water supply and heavily fecally contaminated soil for growing vegetables place children at particular risk. Mass chemotherapy is highly effective, but reinfection occurs rapidly in this setting.

Cryptosporidiosis

Introduction

The protozoa *Cryptosporidium parvum*, *Isospora belli*, *Cyclospora cayetanensis* and *Sarcocystis hominis* all belong to the group of intestinal coccidial infections, which cause diarrhea. They have come into prominence in recent years due to causing severe and protracted diarrhea in AIDS or cell-mediated immune deficiency and infecting piped water supplies due to the chlorine resistance of oocysts. The opportunistic protozoal infections which affect HIV-infected patients include *Cryptosporidium*, *Microsporidia*, *Cyclospora* and *Isospora belli*. *Cryptosporidium* also causes persistent diarrhea and proximal small-intestinal enteropathy in children with normal immune function.[10,83]

Life cycle

Cryptosporidiosis is transmitted by a 3–6 μm acid-fast thick-walled oocyst shed in stool which encysts in the lumen of the small bowel after ingestion and produces four sporozoites. These penetrate the microvillus border and develop into trophozoites, which cause disease and can reproduce asexually, releasing eight merozoites, which invade nearby cells and redevelop into trophozoites to continue the infection. The life cycle is completed by asexual reproduction of trophozoites to schizonts, which develop progressively into male microgametes or female macrogametes, combining to form zygotes and then oocysts, which pass into the stool. After ingestion of oocysts, encystation takes place in the upper small intestine and sporozoites invade the absorptive epithelial cells causing inflammation, partial villus atrophy, malabsorption and diarrhea. About 20% of oocysts are thin-walled and can autoinfect the host, which explains how a small number of ingested oocysts can cause severe disease, especially in immunocompromised patients. Fecal oocysts can survive for at least 2 days, and the incubation period from cyst ingestion to diarrhea in humans is 2–14 days. The major difference from *Plasmodium* species (malaria) is that *Cryptosporidium* completes its life cycle in a single host without the mosquito vector.

Epidemiology

Cryptosporidium causes diarrheal disease in children of developing countries, in travelers and in immunocompromised patients; there have been waterborne outbreaks in developed countries. Transmission is from person to person and from animals to people by ingestion of fecally contaminated food or water. *C. parvum* infects numerous mammals, including man and cattle, and although there is a human-specific form, animal forms may also cause disease in humans. Oocysts are highly infectious, with ingestion of a median of 132 cysts found to be infectious in adult volunteers. Infected

AIDS patients excrete millions of oocysts daily. Person-to-person transmission is common, occurring in 19% of infected children and is especially common in day-care center settings. Oocysts are relatively resistant to conventional chlorination and filtering, but 1-μm filters, heating (72°C for a minute) and freezing are effective.

Cryptosporium has been reported to occur in 6.1% of diarrheal cases vs. 1.5% of controls in developing world subjects compared to 2.2% vs. 0.2%, respectively, in the developed world. For AIDS patients, these rates increase to 24% vs. 5%, respectively, in the developing world and 14% vs. 0% in the developed world. A Peruvian periurban study found a peak cryptosporidiosis incidence of 0.42 episodes/year in 1-year-olds (mean childhood incidence of 0.20), with the rainy season and lack of toilets as risk factors.[84] In Zambian periurban children, cryptosporidial infection appeared to be predominantly waterborne with a prevalence among diarrheal cases of 18%, and no association with home animals, nutritional status or parental education.[85]

In community studies of children in Guinea-Bissau, *Cryptosporidium* was found in 5.8–7.4% of diarrheal episodes and 2.0% without diarrhea, with peak prevalences in the early rainy season (17.6% in May), in young children (e.g. 12.6% in infants < 6 months) and with persistent diarrhea (15%).[86–88] Additional risk factors were pigs and dogs in the household, prolonged storage of cooked food and male sex, but not impaired immunity.[89] According to the authors, the epidemiology of infection was consistent with a small infective dose, airborne transmission and slow development of protective immunity. In Kuwait, *C. parvum* oocysts were found in 10% (51 cases) of childhood diarrhea, but more older children were affected (73% > 2 years).[90] A Gambian study of 1200 children documented *Cryptosporidium* in 8.8% of diarrheal cases vs. 2.8% of controls ($p < 0.001$), with peak incidence during the rainy season and among infants (6–11 months).[91] A Mexican study of 403 children with diarrhea had a 6.4% prevalence of *Cryptosporidium*, which was associated with young age, malnutrition and lack of breast feeding.[92] A Brazilian case–control study showed that children who acquired symptomatic cryptosporidiosis before 1 year of age had a higher burden of subsequent diarrheal disease.[93]

A major waterborne cryptosporidiosis outbreak in Milwaukee, USA in 1993 increased IgG antibody responses from 15% to 82% over a 5-week period in the area served by the water treatment plant, demonstrating that *C. parvum* infection had been much more widespread than was previously appreciated from stool testing.[94] During this outbreak, *Cryptosporidium*, as the sole pathogen, was identified in stools from only 23% of affected children suggesting that stool tests for *Cryptosporidium* were insensitive early in the course of illness.[95] Although secondary transmission undoubtedly took place in child-care facilities, the presence of children with asymptomatic *Cryptosporidium* infections did not result in an increased risk of diarrhea.[96]

Pathophysiology

It is paradoxical that *Cryptosporidium* can produce such profound inflammatory mucosal damage without invasion. It has no known cytotoxins or enterotoxins, but some of the damage may be cytokine-mediated (TNF-α, IL-8), contributing to the malabsorption. *C. parvum* sporozoites produce a mucin-like surface glycoprotein which may help in parasite attachment to enterocytes.[22] Animal studies have revealed that cryptosporidiosis impairs glucose-stimulated sodium absorption at the villus without affecting cyclic AMP-mediated chloride secretion by the crypt epithelium.[97,98] The inflammatory response in the lamina propria does not appear to enhance active transport processes such as chloride secretion, but diarrhea is related to loss of villus epithelium and glucose-facilitated sodium transport.

Severe disease occurs in agammaglobulinemia, so humoral immunity provides important protection, but cell-mediated immunity is also important in clearing infection. An antibody response to *Cryptosporidium* develops in the ileal mucosa which is responsible for termination of the infection.[99] Interferon-γ, produced by the Th1 subset of CD4 intraepithelial lymphocytes, is also important in combating cryptosporidiosis, as are TNF-α and IL-1β but without any synergistic effect.[100,101] The mechanisms of action of interferon-γ *in vitro* are prevention of penetration of host enterocytes by the parasite and retardation of development of intracellular parasites, which were independent of nitric oxide-mediated killing of parasites, although interferon-γ may also up-regulate nitric oxide synthesis in enterocytes.[100]

Parasite expulsion and immune-mediated enteropathic changes appear to be mediated by T-cell function, dependent upon TNF, inducible nitric oxide synthase (iNOS) and IL-4 cytokines (Th2 responses).[102,103] Thus, Th2 cytokines (e.g. IL-4) are involved in protection but may also produce a pathological response in the intestinal mucosa, which had been attributed to Th1 cytokines, and does not occur in TNF-α- and interferon-γ-deficient subjects. Both severe intestinal inflammation with enteropathy and protective immune responses to intestinal parasites are dependent upon IL-4, but immune protection can be acquired without enteropathy.[102] A neonatal mouse model of cryptosporidiosis documented increased inducible nitric oxide (NO) production with infection, which was worsened by NO inhibition and antioxidant administration, suggesting a protective role for NO.[104,105] The severity of nutrient malabsorption, villus atrophy and abnormal intestinal permeability with *Cryptosporidium* infection in AIDS is proportional to the number of infecting organisms.[106]

Clinical features

Cryptosporidial infection causes watery diarrhea with low-grade fever, vomiting and often cramps, severe dehydration and hypokalemia. Among Aboriginal children in Darwin, it was found in the stool of 7.4% of admissions with diarrheal disease with a mean age of 12.2 (9.6–15.5) months and mean admission serum potassium level of 2.7 (2.4–3.0) mmol/l. It was associated with the most severe and prolonged mucosal damage and inflammation on permeability and NO testing, but showed less lactose intolerance than rotavirus.[10] A retrospective hospital study of 109 cases in London, 92% had watery and offensive stools with blood and mucus only occasionally, 50% had persistent diarrhea (> 14 days, and 33% > 21 days), 51% had vomiting, 21% had significant abdominal pain and 23% were underweight.[83] Biopsies in nine cases with prolonged diarrhea and failure to thrive showed a mild to moderate enteropathy with *Cryptosporidium* adhering to the villus epithelium, reduced villus height, reduced disaccharidases and increased intraepithelial lymphocytes. Key risk factors for cryptosporidiosis in this European setting were travel to a developing country and itinerant parents living in caravan sites. There have been two community growth studies in Peru and Guinea-Bissau, both suggesting an adverse long-term effect of cryptosporidiosis on growth.[107,108]

Cryptosporidium causes more prolonged and severe diarrhea, which may be fulminant, in immunocompromised patients. In an Italian study of HIV-infected children with cryptosporidiosis, the median duration of diarrhea was 32 days compared to only 4 days for other causes.[109] It was also associated with loss of 5–30% of body weight. A Peruvian hospital case–control study found an association between *C. parvum* infection and malnutrition, and high nosocomial spread in the hospital context.[110] In a follow-up study, they documented that a first symptomatic infection resulted in a mean (with 95% CI) of 342 g (167–517) weight deficit whereas asymptomatic infection (which was twice as common) led to a 162g (27–297) deficit during the first month of infected cases compared to uninfected non-diarrheal cases.[111]

Diagnosis

Cryptosporidiosis is diagnosed by finding oocysts in stool using an acid-fast stain. This is sensitive with more than 10 000 cysts/g in diarrheal cases, but 50 times less sensitive without diarrhea. Immunofluorescent and ELISA techniques are more sensitive, and PCR may be even more sensitive for detecting low numbers of oocysts in stool specimens.[92] Serological testing for cryptosporidial antibodies is useful for epidemiological surveys, but not for clinical diagnosis in endemic areas. A Peruvian study has questioned whether cryptosporidiosis is caused by a single species by identifying both human (in 81% of children) and zoonotic genotypes of *Cryptosporidium* (bovine, dog, *C. meleagridis* and *felis*) in HIV-negative children, with only duration of oocyst shedding longer in the human genotype.[112]

Prevention

The high infectivity and ubiquitous oocysts in the environment make prevention by water, hygiene and sanitation programs very difficult, indeed impossible, in the developing world, where up to 95% of children in some areas have positive serology by the age of 2 years. Precautions for travelers include washing hands, boiling water, avoiding animals, proper cooking of food, peeling fruit and avoiding uncooked food in contact with unboiled water (e.g. salads).

Strongyloidiasis

Introduction

Although not a major cause of morbidity worldwide, the nematode *Strongyloides stercoralis* is unique in its ability to persist indefinitely within the host through autoinfection, and cause disseminated disease with the prolonged use of corticosteroids or other causes of immunosuppression.

Life cycle

Adult females are about 2.5 mm in length and are attached to the lamina propria of the duodenum or proximal jejunum (Figure 11.4). Their eggs, which hatch into rhabditiform larvae (250 μm long) and pass via feces into the external environment, where they moult into the infective filariform larvae (550 μm long) which infect by penetrating the skin, like hookworms (see above) or become tissue-penetrating infective larvae by penetrating the colonic wall or perianal skin, becoming re-established as mature female worms in the small intestine (autoinfection). Larvae are sensitive to drying, excessive heat (> 40°C) and cold (< 8°C), but may survive for about 2 weeks in soil. Rhabditiform larvae in feces may also moult in moist warm soil to form free-living adult males and females, who mate. The females produce eggs which develop into infective larvae to continue their life cycle in man. The time from skin penetration to mature worms producing eggs is approximately 28 days.

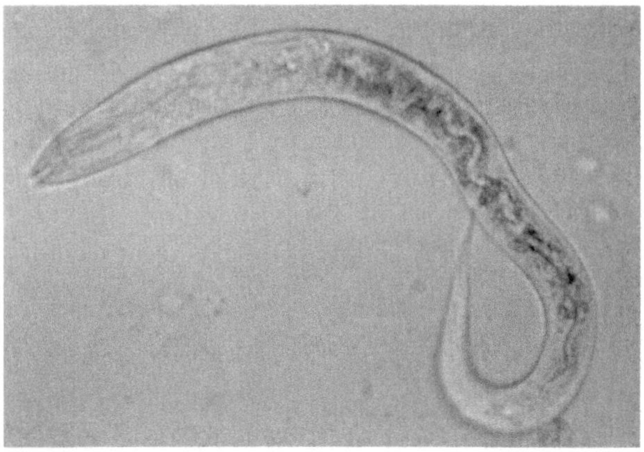

Figure 11.4 *Strongyloides stercoralis* lava. Courtesy of UK Tropical International Health.

Epidemiology

S. stercoralis is present in virtually all tropical and subtropical regions, but estimates of worldwide prevalence vary widely (3–100 million) with the best estimate probably around 30 million people in 70 countries.[113] It is known to be prevalent among children in Cambodia, Laos, India (Bihar), Guinea-Bissau, Kenya, Sierra Leone, Brazil and the Caribbean. A large study in a Peruvian Amazon community found a 19.5% prevalence of stool larvae, including 25% in preschool children who also had high rates of other parasites.[114] Strongyloidiasis accounted for 7.8% of 269 acute diarrheal admissions in Australian Aboriginal children in Darwin, with a mean age of 23.3 (18.1–30.1) months, which was significantly older than the mean age of 12.7 (11.8–13.7) months for other diarrheal admissions.[10]

Prevalence rates vary with climate, geographical region, environmental conditions, soil characteristics and socioeconomic status, but also with modifiable risk factors such as quality of housing, hygiene standards and high population density. In endemic areas, most affected individuals have a low intensity of infection, but a few are heavily infected. Household aggregation of infection has been documented in Bangladesh, with risk factors being older age (7–10 years), lack of a home latrine and low socioeconomic status.[115,116] *S. fuelleborni* is a more virulent infection affecting young children in Papua New Guinea, which may be transmitted via breast milk.[117]

Pathophysiology

Malabsorption was recognized as a feature of strongyloidiasis in a 1965 Jamaican study using iron, folate and xylose absorption tests along with jejunal biopsies.[118] SBBO and abnormal intestinal permeability to ^{51}Cr-ethylenediaminetetra-acetic acid (EDTA) has also been documented in Brazilian adults with strongyloidiasis and symptoms of abdominal pain, diarrhea and weight loss.[119,120] The suggested mechanisms for abnormal permeability were enhanced mucus secretion, increased enterocyte turnover with impaired paracellular barrier function, and protein-losing enteropathy. The latter was documented by means of increased fecal α_1-antitrypsin excretion in 17% (5/29) of Gambian children with persistent diarrhea and malnutrition, including two of six with *Strongyloides* and two of 17 *Giardia* cases.[121]

Small-bowel biopsy studies have reported normal histology in some mild infections, but most show thickening of the bowel wall with edema or fibrosis in what has been described as catarrhal, edematous or ulcerative enteritis.[122] In severe cases of autoinfection, larvae hatching from deposited eggs burrow through the lumen causing superficial damage to the mucosa with excess mucus production, larvae in the lymphatics lead to a granulomatous lymphangitis, and parasites in the submucosa cause edematous and atrophic changes with fibrosis. As with other intestinal nematodes, *Strongyloides* infection elicits Th2-dependent antibodies. Immunoglobulin responses to *S. stercoralis* indicate that IgA affects larval output, IgE regulates autoinfection and IgG4 blocks IgE responses.[123] These immune responses appear to offer little protective immunity, and the relative contributions of genetic versus environmental factors to heavy infections is still unclear. Preexisting malnutrition (wasting) is a risk factor for hospitalization with the acute diarrheal syndrome compared to other causes of diarrhea, increasing the risk 6.5-fold even after adjusting for confounding factors.[10]

Clinical features

As with hookworm, larval migration may affect the lungs (eosinophilic pneumonitis) or skin ('ground itch' on the foot or 'larva currens' on the buttocks) but these are not usually recognized in children. Larvae from species infecting other mammals may penetrate the skin of humans, causing only local irritation, but cannot complete their life cycle. The most common manifestation of *S. stercoralis* infection in children is an acute diarrheal illness with foul stools with a typical musty odor which can be recognized by experienced staff in high-prevalence areas. Severe dehydration is uncommon, but hypokalemia and malabsorption commonly occur. Eosinophilia (5–15% of total white blood cell (WBC) count) is a common but not universal finding. A syndrome of partial intestinal obstruction with strongyloidiasis has been described in Aboriginal children in the Northern Territory of Australia.[124,125]

S. fuelleborni in infants is associated with abdominal swelling, ascites, pleural effusions and a high mortality.[126] In contrast to hookworm, with which it is commonly associated in infants in Papua New Guinea, the intensity of infection peaks by about 12 months of age.[117,127] A similar *S. fuelleborni* species affects monkeys and humans in central Africa, causing less virulent disease with fever, lymphadenitis, abdominal pain and eosinophilia.[41]

Disseminated strongyloidiasis (hyperinfection) occurs with impaired cell-mediated immunity, as in children treated with prolonged courses of steroids (although not from short courses of steroids for asthma) or malignancy (e.g. lymphoma, leukemia) or on immunosuppressive drugs (except cyclosporin, which is antiparasitic). Eradication of *Strongyloides* is essential before immunosuppressive therapy is commenced. Disseminated infection is always a serious complication with high mortality, usually affecting the bowel, lungs and central nervous system (CNS) and often accompanied by sepsis. Although strongyloidiasis is not a common opportunistic infection in AIDS, there is an increased frequency of larvae with HTLV-I infection, possibly due to suppression of the host IgE response.[128]

Diagnosis

The diagnosis is established by identification of larvae on stool microscopy, which is very reliable with acute diarrhea, but less reliable with chronic or asymptomatic infection, because rhabditiform larva excretion is irregular and the parasite load is often low. In this situation, a single stool examination may detect larvae in only 30% of cases of latent infections, although this can be increased to

50% with three stool specimens or various concentration techniques. There are a number of culture methods which are particularly useful if no larvae are found on stool microscopy in the face of clinical suspicion. The agar plate technique has a 96% sensitivity, which identifies larval tracks (*Strongyloides* larvae lash like a whip, whereas hookworm larvae move like a snake).[41,129] In an immunocompromised child with suspected overwhelming infection, rapid diagnosis can be made from a duodenal aspirate, although larvae are abundant with hyperinfection so diagnosis is less difficult than with latent infection. *S. fuelleborni* infection can be diagnosed from abundant eggs shed in the feces.

Owing to the unreliability of stool microscopy and the importance of detecting even low levels of infection, various serological tests are available. An ELISA test for IgG is available, but there is still controversy about its reliability, because of its low specificity and positive predictive value.[130,131] The main problems with antibody tests are differentiating current from past infection, cross-reactivity with other helminth infections and false negatives on presentation of acute diarrheal disease in children (when stool is more reliable). Improved diagnostic tests are being developed using more specific antigens and specialized techniques, which have better potential to detect a risk of hyperinfection with immunosuppressive therapy.[129]

Prevention

Disposal of human excreta, wearing of shoes, treatment of cases and improved hygiene reduce the risk of transmission of strongyloidiasis in communities. Regular mass chemotherapy programs against all geohelminths (e.g. albendazole) may have a modest impact on strongyloidiasis, but less than for the other helminths.

Amebiasis

Introduction

Recent molecular and immunological techniques have demonstrated two distinct species of *Entamoeba* that are morphologically identical. *E. histolytica* is pathogenic, causing symptomatic disease in 10% of infections whereas *E. dispar* causes only asymptomatic colonization. In addition to the *E. histolytica* strain, other risk factors for invasive disease are interaction with bacterial flora, host genetic susceptibility, malnutrition, male sex, young age and immunodeficiency. *Entamoeba coli* and *E. hartmanni* are also non-pathogenic morphologically distinct members of the genus.

Life cycle

The *E. histolytica* life cycle consists of an infective cyst (10–15 μm in diameter) and an invasive trophozoite (10–60 μm in diameter). Cysts are resistant to chlorination, gastric acidity and desiccation and can survive in a moist environment for several weeks. For transmission of *E. histolytica*, cysts are ingested from fecally contaminated food and water and encystation occurs in the intestine, transforming the cyst into eight trophozoites. Mucosal invasion by trophozoites leads to colonic ulcers with migration of parasites to the liver via the portal vein.

Epidemiology

It is estimated that 500 million people are infected with *E. histolytica* in the world with 50 million per year developing invasive disease and 50 000–100 000 deaths. The case/fatality rate is 1 per 500–1000 diagnosed cases, but in a hospital setting, the case/fatality ratio in children is higher, with 9% mortality and 27% morbidity. Liver abscess and extra-abdominal amebiasis has a much higher mortality rate of 10–40% or up to 90% for cerebral amebiasis.

The epidemiology of amebiasis has been complicated by the difficulty of identifying two genetically identical but morphologically distinct species, *E. histolytica* and *E. dispar*. It is estimated that 10% of the population is colonized by *Entamoeba* but 90% of these are with non-pathogenic *E. dispar*. Although *E. dispar* distribution is worldwide, *E. histolytica* infection occurs predominantly in Central and South America, Africa and the Indian subcontinent. Prevalence studies based on stool parasites measure predominantly *E. dispar*, whereas serological surveys reflect the incidence of *E. histolytica*, since *E. dispar* does not cause seroconversion.

A Bangladeshi study of urban children found the prevalence of *E. histolytica* to be 4.2% compared to 6.5% for *E. dispar* with the highest prevalence of *E. histolytica* infection in children with diarrhea aged 6–14 years.[132] A Mexican national survey reported an 8.4% seropositivity to *E. histolytica*, peaking at 11% in the 5–9-year-old age group, with 4.2% of diarrheal cases due to *E. histolytica* infection, and 6.5% with *E. dispar*.[132] Children 6–14 years of age with diarrhea had the highest incidence of *E. histolytica* infection (8%), whereas rural asymptomatic children had a 1% prevalence of *E. histolytica* and 7% prevalence of *E. dispar*. *Shigella* (*dysenteriae* and *flexnerii*) were also more frequent in children with diarrhea who also had *Entamoeba* infection. A West African study in school children found a ratio of *E. histolytica* : *E.dispar* of 1 : 46 (compared to 1 : 3–9 in Asian studies), suggesting that the vast majority of *Entamoeba* infections in this region are not pathogenic.[133] A Brazilian study documented a 10.6% colonization rate for *E. histolytica* (excluding *E. dispar*), affecting predominantly those of poor socioeconomic status, hygiene and nutritional status, but most infections were asymptomatic and self-limited (clearing within 30–45 days) and reinfection rates were low.[134]

Pathophysiology

Amebic disease occurs when trophozoites invade colonic tissue, which is initiated by prior adherence to mucins lining the surface of the large bowel followed by enzymatic destruction of the basement membrane and underlying tissue. The resulting inflammatory response contributes further to tissue destruction. The stages of amebic infection include: adherence to bacteria (especially *Escherichia coli*) and intestinal epithelial cells via galactose-binding lectin, which protects the parasite by blocking complement; activation of virulence factors in parasites such as cysteine proteinases; stimulation of intestinal epithelial cells to produce cytokines and inflammatory mediators by activation of NF-κB; the resulting release of chemokines leading to neutrophil influx; mediators greatly contributing to the destruction of host tissues by lytic necrosis and apoptosis, enabling amebic invasion.[135]

Cell-mediated immunity limits the extent of invasive amebiasis and protects the host from recurrence, including trophozoite killing by activated macrophages and cytotoxic lymphocytes. Cytokines such as TNF-α and interferon-γ contribute to immunocompetent cell activation. Innate resistance to infection in children is linked to the absence of serum anti-trophozoite IgG, which is inherited, whereas acquired resistance is linked to intestinal IgA and serum antibodies to a parasite lectin.[136,137]

The initial colonic lesion in amebiasis is a small intraglandular ulcer of only 1 mm, which extends only to the muscularis mucosa. Margins may be hyperemic with slight edema of the surrounding mucosa. The next stage involves deeper buttonhole ulcers which are up to 1 cm in diameter and extend into the sub-mucosa. In young children this can progress to a fulminant necrotizing colitis associated with transmural necrosis. Amebomas are uncommon in children but involve the formation of granulation tissue with a fibrous outer wall, which may result in stricture or obstruction to the lumen. Dissemination to the liver occurs in a high proportion of patients with fulminant disease.

Clinical features

The carrier state is the most common form of amebic infestation with all *E. dispar* infections and up to 90% of *E. histolytica* infections remaining asymptomatic with only cysts in the feces. Amebic dysentery is the most common form of symptomatic disease, with gradual onset of symptoms over 3 or 4 weeks after infection with increasingly severe diarrhea with abdominal pain such that an acute abdomen is often suspected. Stools contain blood and mucus, fever occurs in about half, and a small proportion develop abdominal distension with dehydration. Occasionally, young children present in a more fulminant manner with intussusception, perforation, peritonitis or necrotizing colitis. Rarely, children with amebic dysentery may present with an abdominal mass that has an 'apple-core' appearance on radiographs, similar to colonic carcinoma. Amebic liver abscess and extra-abdominal amebiasis are much less common in children than in adults.

Diagnosis

The diagnosis of amebiasis should be considered in any child with blood or mucus in the stools, particularly if associated with abdominal pain or distension. Stool microscopy will yield cysts in < 30% of infected individuals, owing to the intermittent nature of cyst shedding, although multiple examinations increase the diagnostic yield to 60–70% with amebic colitis but to under half of amebic hepatic abscesses.

Serology can be helpful with invasive amebiasis since asymptomatic infections with *E. dispar* do not usually elicit a serological response. The gold standard remains culture or iso-enzyme analysis, but stool antigen detection tests are now commercially available which are more reliable than microscopy. A PCR-based amplification technique is now available for stool samples; infecting isolates are genetically diverse, with differences between those associated with intestinal and hepatic disease.[138] The major problem with serological tests is that they remain positive for years after an episode of amebiasis, so they may not be useful in endemic areas.

Wet preparations of material aspirated or scraped from the base of ulcers on colonoscopy can be examined for motile trophozoites and tested for *E. histolytica* antigen. The appearance of amebic colitis resembles inflammatory bowel disease with a granular, friable and diffusely ulcerated mucosa. It is preferable for biopsy specimens to be taken from the edge of ulcers, but the sensitivity of this method of diagnosis appears variable.

Prevention

Prevention requires interruption of the fecal–oral spread of the infectious cyst stage of the parasite by improved hygiene, sanitation and water treatment. This is of course very difficult in the developing world. Current efforts towards a vaccine are focusing on the adherence lectin, which may prevent colonization. This would lead to elimination of the parasites if effective, since humans are the only significant reservoir of *E. histolytica* infection.

Other parasites

Hymenolepiasis

Hymenolepis nana is the dwarf tapeworm and the only human tapeworm that does not require an intermediate host. Nevertheless, rodent strains for *H. nana* are infectious for humans including pet rodents such as rats, mice and hamsters. It occurs worldwide, with high childhood prevalences (> 10%) reported from Argentina, Peru, Brazil, Egypt, Pakistan and Zimbabwe.[41] Transmission is mostly fecal–oral, either from person to person or in food and water, with high rates in children from orphanages.[139]

Adult worms are only 15–45 mm in length with the spherical/ovoid eggs measuring 30–45 μm in diameter, which do not survive beyond 11 days and are sensitive to heat and drying. In children who ingest eggs, the larval stage develops in the intestinal villi in 4–5 days, then break into the lumen and develop into adult worms, which produce ova in the feces within a month or less. The larval stage of *H. nana* is a cyst-like structure about 250 μm in diameter and is called a cysticercoid. As for other intestinal parasites, transmission is enhanced by poor hygiene and overcrowding, but control programs have found mass treatment more effective than improved hygiene.[41]

Most infected children are asymptomatic. High worm burdens of over 3000 may be associated with abdominal pain, loose stools and growth retardation. Disseminated larval infection has been described but is rare. Diagnosis is based on the characteristic eggs in stool. A single dose of praziquantel 20 mg/kg is effective. Niclosamide 60–80 mg/kg per day for 5 days or paromomycin 45 mg/kg per day for 7 days are alternatives, but compliance is more difficult to ensure. Retreatment 10 days later may be necessary to ensure eradication of cysticercoids in tissues.

Enterobiasis

Enterobius vermicularis is the common pinworm or threadworm of the large bowel. Unlike most other helminthic infection, enterobiasis may be more common in temperate, developed countries than in poor, tropical, developing countries. For example, rates in Australian schoolchildren have been reported as 43% compared to 12% in India. However, it is worldwide in distribution and is almost exclusively transmitted person to person. The organism is a small white roundworm with the adult female worm 9–12 mm long with the male worm only 2.5 mm long and rarely observed. The worm's lifespan is 5–13 weeks for females and only 7 weeks for males, but reinfection is common. The oval eggs laid by the gravid female on the anus are 50 x 25 µm and the diagnosis is based on observation of these typical eggs from sticky tape applied to the perianal skin and then examined under a microscope. Adult pinworms or their eggs are rarely found in the feces, so this tape test for demonstrating pinworm eggs on the perianal skin is the most reliable technique.

Humans are the only host for *E. vermicularis*, and worms inhabit the lumen of the cecum and appendix. The gravid adult female migrates to the perianal skin where she deposits her eggs resulting in intense anal pruritus, itching of the perianal skin leads to the contamination of the fingernails with the infective eggs. Each mature female worm can produce up to 11 000 eggs. Most infections are asymptomatic, but perianal pruritus is the most common symptom of enterobiasis. Eosinophilia is uncommon, since the organism does not generally invade tissues. The incubation period is 3–4 weeks.

There is no definitive evidence that pinworms cause appendicitis, since most pinworms encountered in the appendix are an incidental finding, occurring in as many normal as inflamed appendices after surgery. However, it is impossible to exclude the possibility that chronic inflammatory changes due to local pinworm infection may contribute to some cases of appendicitis. Large numbers of larval pinworms have been shown to cause eosinophilic enterocolitis in an adult.[140] The most common site of infection (86.5%) is the lumen of the appendix, where the worms invoke no histological reaction. Other sites of infection include the abdominal and pelvic peritoneum and female genital tract.[141] Little girls sometimes present with ectopic pinworm infection of the vagina, which can cause hysterical reactions.

The treatment of choice is albendazole or mebendazole, but ivermectin, pyrantel and levamisole are also effective. Since reinfection is very common, it is wise to readminister the drugs 2 weeks later and treat all household members, particularly children. Prevention of enterobiasis rests largely on treating infected children, keeping nails short and possibly improving personal hygiene, although infection is not an indicator of poor hygiene.

Schistosomiasis

There are seven human species of this trematode, including *S. haematobium* which affects the renal tract and *S. mansoni* the gastrointestinal tract. It has been estimated that 220 million people in 74 countries are infected by schistosomiasis, and 20 million have severe disease. Eggs of *S. mansoni* are passed in the feces, and hatch in warm water; the ciliated larvae swim and penetrate fresh-water snails (*Biomphalaria*). After a sporocyst stage, by 4–5 weeks of infection, the larval phase results in thousands of cercariae (300 x 60 µm) which penetrate human skin in water and enter peripheral lymphatics or veins and are carried to the lungs and mature in portal vessels. Adult worms migrate to the liver and mesenteric veins, where they may survive for 2–5 years or longer, producing eggs 25–28 days after cercarial infection.

Eggs cause granuloma formation resulting in localized colitis and hepatitis. The acute phase of *S. mansoni* infection may cause allergic symptoms (Katayama syndrome) which are rarely recognized in children. Most chronic infections are light and asymptomatic, but with heavy infections up to half of the eggs become trapped in the mucosa and submucosa of the colon, resulting in granulomatous reactions with significant blood loss. The host's inflammatory reaction to eggs carried to the liver in the portal veins leads to portal hypertension. Severe disease with hepatosplenomegaly affects about 10% of *S. mansoni* cases in endemic areas, taking 5–15 years to develop.

Diagnosis is based on finding eggs in the feces, but stool concentration methods and numerous immunological techniques (ELISA, immunoblotting) are more sensitive for milder infections. Treatment is with praziquantel 40 mg/kg as a single dose. Prevention involves avoidance of water sources containing cercariae and promotion of latrine use. Control programs for schistosomiasis involve mass chemotherapy, destruction of snails, environmental sanitation, prevention of water contact, health education and the future development of vaccines.

Fasciolopsiasis

The giant intestinal fluke *Fasciolopsis buski* is a class of flatworm called trematodes, which includes schistosomes. It is estimated that more than 40 million people have food-borne trematode infections. Those affecting the liver and lungs will not be considered here. The adult worm of *F. buski* measures up to 7.5 cm in length and attaches to the mucosa of the proximal small intestine. It has a lifespan of about 6 months and begins producing eggs about 3 months after infection. These are excreted in the stool and measure 130 μm in length. Up to 25 000 eggs may be excreted daily.

After several weeks in fresh water, the larvae hatch from the eggs and penetrate snails, where they undergo further development. Cercariae emerge from the snail after 1–2 months and encyst on a wide variety of aquatic vegetation. When humans ingest these raw, they develop infection, which lodges in the duodenum. The severity of symptoms correlates with the number of parasites, but heavy infections may cause nausea, vomiting, abdominal pain, edema, eosinophilia and poor nutrition. The diagnosis of fasciolopsiasis is based upon stool microscopy identifying the eggs. These are indistinguishable from those of the liver fluke, *Fasciola hepatica*. However, the intestinal fluke has a short lifespan and infection does not persist beyond 9 months from the time of departure from and endemic area.

The treatment of choice is praziquantel 25 mg/kg three times daily for 1 day. The prognosis is generally excellent, except for heavy infection in children with intestinal obstruction of edematous malnutrition. The infection can be prevented by cooking aquatic vegetation or immersing plants or nuts in boiling water. The use of human feces as fertilizer in aquaculture is a major cause of human infection.

Trichostrongylus

Species of *Trichostrongylus* (wireworms) mostly affect ruminants, but they affect humans in close proximity to cattle, particularly in Africa, Australia, India, Iran and South America. The small adult worms (5–10 mm long) attach to the wall of the duodenum and jejunum after ingestion, and excrete eggs similar to those of the hookworm. Light infections are asymptomatic, but abdominal pain, diarrhea and eosinophilia may occur with heavy infections. Treatment is as for hookworm, and prevention involves thorough washing or cooking of vegetables.

Parastrongylus costaricensis

This nematode was discovered in Costa Rica in 1971 and appears to be mainly confined to Latin America and the Caribbean. The natural host is the cotton rat but adult worms (20 mm long) have been found in the cecum of children with appendicitis-like illnesses with eosinophilia. Infection occurs by ingesting infected slugs. Diagnosis before surgery is based upon eosinophilia, radiology or serology, but larvae are not excreted in stool and no chemotherapy is effective.

Cyclospora cayetanensis

Cyclospora has emerged recently as an important protozoal pathogen causing diarrheal disease.[142] It appears to be endemic in most parts of the Americas, Africa and Asia, with infections occurring in travelers, as well as waterborne and food-borne outbreaks.[143–145] Children in tropical areas appear to have a high prevalence, and the disease peaks in the hot rainy season.[146,147] A Venezuelan study documented prevalences in adult AIDS patients and children with diarrhea of 9.8% vs. 5.3%, which was more common than *S. stercoralis* (4.2% vs. 1.5%, respectively) but less common than *C. parvum* (35.2% vs. 9.8%, respectively) and had a peak prevalence in children between 2 and 5 years of age.[148] Other childhood diarrheal prevalences have been similar in Nepal and Guatemala, but higher in Peru and Haiti (up to 18–20%). The incidence in Peruvian periurban children was 0.21–0.28 episodes/child-years.[84] A Haitian study found a prevalence of 11% in AIDS diarrhea, with symptoms identical to isosporiasis and cryptosporidiosis.[149]

Since other pathogens are often found, it is difficult to characterize the illness exactly, but prolonged watery diarrhea with weight loss is typical, often associated with fever. Mucosal biopsies show inflammatory changes with partial villus atrophy with crypt hyperplasia.[150] Stool oocytes are sparse in infected immunocompetent children with diarrhea (< 10/field) but may be higher in AIDS patients. The modified Ziehl–Neelson stain of the acid-fast trichrome technique is used for diagnosis.[151] Oocysts have been found in the environment in sewage, vegetable washings and animal feces.[152,153] A Peruvian study in childhood found that only 20% of cases with oocysts were symptomatic and co-trimoxazole treatment for 3 days decreased excretion from 12.1 to 4.8 days.[154] An adult Nepali trial of travelers confirmed this, but suggested that 7 days of co-trimoxazole was more effective (clearance rate of 94% for 7 days vs. 29% for 3 days).[155]

Drug treatment

The drugs recommended by WHO for soil-transmitted helminthiasis are albendazole, mebendazole, levamisole, pyrantel and ivermectin; and for schistosomiasis they are praziquantel and oxamniquine for *S. mansoni* (Table 11.3).[2]

Benzimidazoles

The benzimidazoles, albendazole and mebendazole, have broad-spectrum activity against roundworm, whipworm, hookworm, pinworm and wireworm species. The action of albendazole on the parasite is to bind to tubulin, inhibit microtubule assembly, decrease glucose absorption and inhibit

Table 11.3 Drugs for the treatment of soil-transmitted helminthisasis and schistosomiasis (from reference 2)

Drug and formulation	Therapeutic activity	Pediatric dosage
Albendazole (tablets 200 and 400 mg, suspension 100 mg/5 ml)	ascariasis +++ trichuriasis ++ hookworm infection +++ strongyloidiasis ++	400 mg stat dose (200 mg if < 10 kg) (daily for 3 days)
Ivermectin (tablets 6 mg)	ascariasis +++ trichuriasis + strongyloidiasis ++	200 μg/kg stat dose
Levamisole (tablet 40 mg, syrup 40 mg/5 ml)	ascariasis +++ trichuriasis + hookworm infection ++	2.5 mg/kg stat dose (repeat after 7 days)
Mebendazole (tablets 100 mg and 500 mg suspension 100 mg/5 ml)	ascariasis +++ trichuriasis ++ hookworm infection ++	500 mg stat dose 100 mg twice a day for 3 days (or 500 mg stat dose)
Pyrantel (tablets 250 mg, suspension 50 mg/5 ml)	ascariasis +++ hookworm infection ++	10 mg/kg stat dose (repeat daily for 4 days)
Praziquantel (tablet 600 mg)	schistosomiasis +++ (all species)	40–60 mg/kg stat dose or in divided doses
Oxamniquine (capsules 250 mg, syrup 250 mg/ml)	schistosomiasis +++ (*S. mansoni* only)	20 mg/kg stat dose (or 20–60 mg/kg divided doses)

fumarate reductase. It is poorly soluble in water, but well absorbed with a fatty meal. It is rapidly metabolized in the liver to the active form, albendazole sulfoxide, which has a serum half-life of 8–9 h, and is excreted by the kidneys. It is usually very well tolerated as a single dose or daily for 3 days, with gastrointestinal symptoms (e.g. pain, diarrhea, nausea or vomiting) in only 1.3% of courses.[156] Worm migration is uncommon with albendazole treatment, but prolonged therapy may cause alopecia, reversible marrow suppression or hepatocellular damage. Albendazole should be avoided in pregnancy and in children under 6 months of age.

Albendazole 400 mg (200 mg if < 10 kg) as a single dose or mebendazole 200 mg (100 mg if < 10 kg) daily for 3 days are the treatments of choice for ascariasis, but pyrantel pamoate, piperazine tartrate and levamisole are equally effective and may be cheaper in the context of the developing world. The benzimidazoles and pyrantel have potential teratogenicity so should be used with caution in infancy. The first-line treatment for hookworm is albendazole 400 mg as a single dose (200 mg if < 10 kg) or mebendazole 100 mg twice daily for 3 days (or single dose of 500 mg if over 2 years of age). Alternatives are pyrantel pamoate or levamisole, but ivermectin is ineffective and bephenium is no longer recommended.

For clinically significant *Trichuris* infections, the treatment of choice is albendazole 400 mg (or mebendazole 200 mg) daily for 3 days. Half of these doses are used for children < 10 kg, but clinical judgment must be used to assess risk–benefit in this age group. Single doses are used for mass campaigns or 3–6 months of prophylaxis, but ivermectin, pyrantel, levamisole and piperazine are mostly ineffective against *Trichuris*. Treatment of heavy infections associated with malnutrition should result in catch-up growth. A community-based Mexican trial of 622 children with asymptomatic trichuriasis followed their growth for 12 months after treatment with albendazole 400 mg daily for 1 or 3 days, or pyrantel 11 mg/kg as a single dose.[157] Although children with heavy pretreatment worm loads had improved catch-up growth on 3 days of albendazole compared to pyrantel, those with low infection had worse growth parameters, so the authors suggest that 3-day albendazole may have 'toxic effects' on growth. This resulted in discouragement of its routine use in children under 2 years, but such an effect has not been confirmed in Tanzania, so there has been a recent call for reinstitution of antihelminthic treatment in children under 24 months.[158]

A recent adult study of albendazole (800 mg twice daily for 14 days) in HIV-related persistent diarrhea showed 46% clearance rates of protozoa at 3 weeks and 39% clinical resolution and mucosal recovery at 6 weeks.[159] A review of albendazole studies in adults and children calculated overall cure rates after standard treatment (single 400 mg dose, except for *S. stercoralis*, *H. nana* and *Taenia* requiring 3 days) of 98% for pinworm, 95% for *Ascaris*, 85% for *Taenia* species, 78% for hookworm, 68% for *H. nana*, 62% for *Strongyloides* and 48% for *Trichuris*.[156] Egg reduction rates after albendazole treatment were also high for *Ascaris* (99%), hookworm (88%) and *Trichuris* (75%). The cure rates for hookworm in children differed by species with rates of 91% for *A. duodenale* but only 67% for *N. americanus*.[156] Heavy *Trichuris* infections require at least 3 days of albendazole for high cure rates in children, but a Filipino study found that a combination of single-dose albendazole plus ivermectin gave high cure rates for single-dose therapy.[160] Albendazole 400 mg daily for 5 days is an alternative treatment for giardiasis.[161] Albendazole 400 mg daily for 3 days and repeated a week later is also highly effective in acute strongyloidiasis in children, but parasitological cure rates are only 45–75% so all larvae may not be eradicated.

A Turkish study randomized 162 school children with halitosis to mebendazole vs. placebo and documented a significant improvement in their chronic bad breath in the treatment group for those with intestinal parasites (pinworm, roundworm, giardiasis, *Taenia* or whipworm).[162]

Pyrantel

Pyrantel is a depolarizing neuromuscular blocking agent which paralyses worms until they are expelled in feces. Pyrantel pamoate is active against *Ascaris* and *Enterobius*, only partially effective against hookworm and ineffective against *Trichuris* and *Strongyloides*. It is given as a single dose of 20 mg/kg up to 750 mg orally (repeat after 7 days if heavy infection) or 10 mg/kg daily for 3 days for hookworm.

Levamisole

Levamisole is an immune stimulant which is effective against *Ascaris* and hookworm, and may be more effective for intestinal obstruction from roundworms, since it acts by paralyzing the myoneural junction of the worm. The dosage is 3 mg/kg as a single dose.

Ivermectin

Ivermectin has broad-spectrum activity against helminths and filariasis, but is the drug of choice against strongyloidiasis. Ivermectin is well absorbed orally, accumulating in adipose tissue, metabolized in the liver, highly protein bound with a serum half-life of 12 h and excreted in stool. It is generally well tolerated, with occasional abdominal distension, chest tightness or wheezing. In a Tanzanian study of children, ivermectin was found to be more effective than albendazole for curing *Strongyloides*, equally effective for *Ascaris*, less effective for *Trichuris* and ineffective against hookworm infections.[163] Another African study of ivermectin in intestinal nematode infections found little effect on either prevalence or intensity of *N. americanus* hookworm or *Trichuris*, and only a modest effect on *Ascaris*.[164]

Ivermectin 200 µg/kg as a single dose has a reported cure rate of 83% for *Strongyloides*. In complicated or disseminated infection, ivermectin should be repeated on days 2, 15 and 16 to decrease relapse. In immunosuppressed patients, treatment is not always successful, and may need to be repeated at monthly intervals, or a longer course given. An adult open-label study of 60 patients with strongyloidiasis compared single-dose ivermectin with albendazole for 3 days and found higher cure rates with the former (83% vs. 38%).[165] Another adult study comparing ivermectin with thiabendazole documented high cure rates for both drugs but the adverse effects were much greater for thiabendazole (e.g. disorientation, fatigue, nausea and anorexia).[166] A comparative trial in 301 children from Zanzibar with *S. stercoralis* larvae in stool had cure rates of 82.9% with single-dose ivermectin compared to only 45.0% with 3 days of albendazole.[163] Disseminated disease has a high mortality, so may require ivermectin over 3–4 weeks.

Metronidazole

Metronidazole is used for giardiasis and amebiasis. It is activated by reduction of its 5-nitro group, is concentrated in anaerobic organisms and interacts with DNA to cause microbial death. It is not well tolerated, with anorexia and gastrointestinal upset occurring after several days' treatment.[167] The dose of metronidazole has been controversial, but a computer simulation study using the conventional 30 mg/kg per day regime calculated that steady state was reached at 24 mg/kg per day in rehabilitated children and at 12 mg/kg per day in severely malnourished children using the twice daily dosage.[168] Patients with immunodeficiency may require treatment for 6–8 weeks for giardiasis. The American Academy of Pediatrics and Centers for Disease Control recommend that asymptomatic *Giardia* infections not be treated.[169,170] Asymptomatic cyst excretors, even at day-care centers, do not warrant treatment.[170,171]

Amebic colitis or dysentery should be treated with metronidazole plus a luminal agent such as diloxanide furoate, paromomycin or iodoquinol. Although improvement usually occurs within 3–4 days of treatment, metronidazole should be continued for a minimum of 10 days to eliminate intestinal colonization with risk of relapse. Treatment of asymptomatic cyst passers is inappropriate for *E. dispar*, but is warranted for *E. histolytica* in developed countries but probably not practical in most of the developing world where the disease in endemic. The dosage for treatment of acute amebic colitis is metronidazole 35–50 mg/kg per day in three divided doses for 10 days. The intraluminal agents are used for eradicating cyst passage. The dosages are: iodoquinol 30–40 mg/kg per day in three divided oral doses for 20 days, or diloxanide furoate 20 mg/kg per day in three divided doses, or paromomycin 25–35 mg/kg per day in three divided doses for 7 days.

Tinidazole

Tinidazole is another 5-nitroimidazole with a similar mechanism of action to that of metronidazole but a convenient single dosage. A Cochrane review of 34 trials on drugs for treating giardiasis concluded that tinidazole 50 mg/kg in a single dose had a higher clinical cure rate than a short course of treatment with metronidazole, albendazole or secnidazole.[172]

Nitazoxanide

Nitazoxanide is a new broad-spectrum antimicrobial agent with activity against nematodes, trematodes, anaerobic bacteria and protozoal parasites such as *Cryptosporidium*. It is metabolized in blood to tizoxanide, which inhibits the key enzyme pyruvate ferredoxin oxidoreductase of target organisms, and is excreted in urine and feces. Adverse effects tend to affect the gastrointestinal tract, but appear to be mild and transient.[173] A 3-day course of 100–200 mg 12-hourly in children (adults 500 mg) is effective against giardiasis, amebiasis, *Blastocystis hominis, Balantidium coli, Isospora belli, Ascaris, Trichuris,* hookworm and *Hymenolepis nana*.[168] In view of this wide spectrum of action, single-dose therapy in combination with other drugs is under investigation for community treatment programs.

Two Egyptian randomized placebo-controlled trials of diarrheal subjects have shown that nitazoxanide was associated with resolution of the diarrhea within 7 days in about 80% of cases of giardiasis, amebiasis or cryptosporidiosis compared to about 40% in the placebo group.[174,175] A Mexican study of 275 children with helminth or protozoan infections documented a higher (but non-significant) parasite eradication rate with 3 days of nitazoxanide (79%) than with 3 days of mebendazole plus quifamide (74%).[176] Another Mexican study has documented its *in vitro* effectiveness against trophozoites of *E. histolytica* and *Giardia*.[177] Nitazoxanide was best for eradication of *H. nana* (90–100%) and worst for giardiasis (56–74%). Comparative studies of Peruvian children with ascariasis, trichuriasis, hymenolepiasis and giardiasis reported cure rates for nitazoxanide of 89%, 89%, 82% and 85%, respectively, compared with 91%, 58%, 96% and 75–80% for albendazole, praziquantel (*H. nana*) or metronidazole (*Giardia*), respectively.[178,179] A recent Zambian trial of 3 days of nitazoxanide (vs. placebo) in 100 children with cryptosporidiosis showed clinical response rates of 56 vs. 23% and parasitological response rates of 52 vs. 14% in HIV-seronegative children, but no significant response in HIV-seropositive cases.[180]

Paromomycin

Paromomycin is a poorly absorbed aminoglycoside which reaches high concentrations in the intestine, but absorbed drug is excreted renally and is potentially ototoxic and nephrotoxic. It has been used for cryptosporidial diarrhea in AIDS patients, requiring continuous maintenance therapy, but appears now to be ineffective.[181,182]

Mass community anthelminthic treatment

UNICEF, the World Bank and WHO have promoted routine mass anthelminthic treatment programs as a cost-effective intervention, and school-based programs are popular.[183–185] Although most studies report prevalence, reducing the intensity of the worm burden is the major aim of control programs in children, who have the highest burden. Albendazole and praziquantel have broad-spectrum anthelminthic activity against ascariasis, trichuriasis, enterobiasis, hookworm, giardiasis, strongyloidiasis and schistosomiasis at relatively low cost and with low rates of resistance to these agents. Mass treatment protocols may reduce the risk of drug resistance by targeting school-age and preschool children, by only repeating treatment at intervals greater than the nematode generation time, by combining anthelminthic drugs in control programs to reduce or delay selection for resistance, and by monitoring drug resistance to benzimadoles using DNA probes.[2] Deworming programs were held back for young children because of concerns about their safety in children under 2 years of age (as well as in pregnancy and lactation). However, a recent WHO Informal Consultation that children over 12 months of age should be included in deworming campaigns using praziquantel and albendazole/mebendazole on the basis of improved safety data and risk–benefit analysis.[186]

The impact of helminth infections on growth and development is a controversial but important issue. A Cochrane systematic review of 30 randomized trials involving 15 000 children on the effects of antihelminthic treatment of endemic communities on growth and cognitive performance was reported in 2000.[187,188] It found only modest weight gain of 0.1 kg (0.04–0.17) after a year of follow-up and no differences in cognitive performance, so concluded that the evidence for routine anthelminthic treatment to improve growth and cognitive performance was unconvincing. Critics of the review pointed out that poorly designed trials may have failed to document an effect, that short-term treatment cannot assess the long-term benefits of regular treatment and that the review hid the greatest effect of anthelminthic treatment on growth and development in children with heavy parasitic burdens.

Since the Cochrane review, there has been a study of 614 children 12–48 months at baseline, in a community of high parasite intensity in Tanzania who were randomized to single-dose mebendazole 500 mg 3-monthly vs. placebo and followed for 12 months. It reported modest reductions in prevalence of *Trichuris* (75 vs. 58%), *Ascaris* (49 vs. 27%) and hookworm (66 vs. 60%), but the effect on worm intensity was more significant, reducing *Ascaris* from 126 to 12 eggs per gram of feces (epg), *Trichuris* from 511 to 88 epg and hookworm from 198 to 119 epg.[189] A large randomized mass treatment trial of school children with albendazole and praziquantel in China, Kenya and the Philippines documented significant reductions ($p < 0.0001$) in mean egg counts at 45 days for hookworm (97 to 27), *Ascaris* (5903 to 626) and *Trichuris* (233 to 161), but the effects were limited by rapid reinfection (*Ascaris*) and single-dose albendazole ineffectiveness (*Trichuris*).[190] The most important short-term benefits at 6 months from treatment were modest rises in hemoglobin level and reductions in hepatomegaly (Kenya only) in the children treated with praziquantel, but catch-up growth did not occur in treated children compared to controls.

Another study in the low-intensity setting of Bangladesh followed 123 children aged 2–5 years for 12 months with 2-monthly mebendazole and showed reduced prevalences of *Trichuris* (65 to 9%), *Ascaris* (78 to 8%) and hookworm (4 to 0%) while associated with an increase in giardiasis (19 to 49%), but failed to document improved growth or improvements in intermediate variables (intestinal permeability, plasma albumin, α_1-antichymotrypsin).[191] The increase in giardiasis with mebendazole was found in an earlier Bangladeshi study,[192] but could be prevented by substituting albendazole, which has anti-giardial activity. Confirmation of the limited effect of helminths on growth has come from indirect calorimetry, which showed no treatment effect on energy metabolism with low-level hookworm, *Ascaris*, *Trichuris* or *Strongyloides* infections.[193] A Malaysian study found that intestinal helminths did not contribute to poor school attendance.[194]

A 9-year cohort study of 119 children in a Brazilian shantytown showed that, in this setting, the burden of diarrheal disease and helminth infections in children under 2 years were independently associated with stunting by 2–7 years of age, even controlling for confounders.[195] Thus, early childhood helminth infections were associated with a 4.6-cm shortfall by age 7 years, compared to 3.6 cm attributed to the mean 9.1 episodes of diarrhea before the age of 2 years. There is also indirect evidence that intestinal nematodes affect productivity in adults through both disease-related morbidity and ill-health in childhood.[196] A Zairian study of 358 moderately malnourished preschool children randomized them to either vitamin A, mebendazole 500 mg 3-monthly or no treatment.[197] The vitamin A-deficient children showed significant catch-up growth on vitamin A treatment, but deworming did not improve growth, because only 12 of 123 in the mebendazole group had ascariasis of low intensity, making the claim in the title of the article misleading.

A South African randomized trial of 428 schoolchildren with a high prevalence of *Trichuris*, hookworm and schistosomiasis found that combination treatment with 3 days of albendazole and single-dose praziquantel 6-monthly and iron supplementation weekly for 10 weeks reduced worm prevalence and increased hemoglobin levels, but did not improve growth.[198] A Kenyan study showed that albendazole was more effective than mebendazole in reducing worm burdens in schoolchildren.[199] However, a Tanzanian study of 2294 schoolchildren from a very high prevalence setting showed that single-dose albendazole vs. mebendazole reduced the parasite burden of *Ascaris* by 97% vs. 97%, of *Trichuris* by 73% vs. 82%, and of hookworm by 98% vs. 82%, respectively.[200] Moreover, the high reinfection rate in this setting meant that the impact of chemotherapy was short-lived, so 4-monthly treatment would be necessary to reduce long-term morbidity.[64] In South African schoolchildren, a single dose of albendazole and praziquantel reduced prevalence rates of *Ascaris*, *Trichuris* and *S. haematobium* from 29.5 to 4.7%, 51.9 to 38.0% and 22.3 to 3.3%, respectively.

Invasive parasites which are known to cause malabsorption, weight loss or prolonged diarrhea, such as *Giardia*, *Cryptosporidium* and *Strongyloides*, are the most likely to affect growth, so specific studies have examined this in community settings. *Giardia* is the most prevalent intestinal protozoan parasite, and certainly can cause persistent diarrhea with malabsorption, weight loss and mucosal damage, but the key public health question is whether the high rates of infection without overt clinical symptoms contribute to poor growth of preschool children in the developing world. Lunn and colleagues examined this question in 60 infants in The Gambia where both giardiasis and poor growth are known to be highly prevalent.[201,202] *Giardia*-specific plasma immunoglobulins were used for diagnosis and did not explain the observed growth faltering. *Giardia* infection was not associated with diarrhea in this context, but mild infections may have caused minimal abnormalities in intestinal permeability and α_1-antichymotrypsin, an acute-phase reactant protein. They concluded that giardiasis was unlikely to be a major cause of the poor growth of rural Gambian infants. Rapid reinfection after treatment was also documented for giardiasis in Egypt and Peru, where 98% of children were reinfected within 6 months of tinidazole treatment and stool excretion lasted a mean of 3.2 months.[203,204]

Finally, studies have shown that control of intestinal parasitic infections is more than a question of mass chemotherapy, but is influenced by social and cultural factors that affect human behavior, such as treatment seeking and promiscuous defecation.[205,206]

Conclusion

The most prevalent intestinal parasites associated with morbidity in children are the protozoa *Cryptosporidium*, *Giardia* and *Entameoba histolytica*, and the helminths *Trichuris*, *Ascaris*, hookworm and *Strongyloides*. Although most infected children remain asymptomatic, some children with high intensity of infection have manifestations of severe and persistent enteropathy, particularly with strongyloidiasis, cryptosporidiosis, giardiasis and trichuriasis. In spite of reductions in overall child mortality rates over recent decades, intestinal parasites remain highly prevalent in children in the developing world with no evidence of decreases in either global prevalence or morbidity, despite effective treatment being available. Recent advances in molecular biology and immunology of parasites are improving diagnostic techniques and open the way for the development of vaccines to control them. New vaccines and mass chemotherapy programs appear to be more effective approaches in the control of intestinal parasites in the short-term than improvements in hygiene, sanitation and living standards.

REFERENCES

1. Booth M, Bundy DA, Albonico M et al. Associations among multiple geohelminth species infections in schoolchildren from Pemba Island. *Parasitology* 1998; **116**: 85–93.
2. Anonymous. *Prevention and Control of Schistosomiasis and Soil-Transmitted Helminthiasis. WHO Technical Report Series 912*. Geneva: World Health Organization. 2002: 1–57.
3. Yu SH, Xu LQ, Jiang ZX et al. Nationwide survey of human parasite in China. *Southeast Asian J Trop Med Public Health* 1994; **25**: 4–10.
4. Brooker S, Rowlands M, Haller L et al. Towards an atlas of human helminth infection in sub-Saharan Africa: the use of geographical information systems (GIS). *Parasitol Today* 2000; **16**: 303–307.
5. The Partnership for Child Development. The health and nutritional status of schoolchildren in Africa: evidence from school-based health programmes in Ghana and Tanzania. *Trans R Soc Trop Med Hyg* 1998; **92**: 254–261.
6. Amin OM. Seasonal prevalence of intestinal parasites in the United States during 2000. *Am J Trop Med Hyg* 2002; **66**: 799–803.
7. Booth M, Mayombana C, Machibya H et al. The use of morbidity questionnaires to identify communities with high prevalences of schistosome or geohelminth infections in Tanzania. *Trans R Soc Trop Med Hyg* 1998; **92**: 484–490.

8. Tshikuka JG, Gray DK, Scott M, Olela KN. Relationship of childhood protein–energy malnutrition and parasite infections in an urban African setting. *Trop Med Int Health* 1997; **2**: 374–382.
9. Genta RM. Diarrhea in helminthic infections. *Clin Infect Dis* 1993; **16(Suppl 2)**: S122–S129.
10. Kukuruzovic RH, Robins Browne RM, Anstey N, Brewster DR. Enteric pathogens, intestinal permeability and nitric oxide production in childhood diarrheal disease. *Pediatr Infect Dis J* 2002; **21**: 730–739.
11. Gillin FD, Reiner DS, Gault MJ et al. Encystation and expression of cyst antigens by *Giardia lamblia in vitro*. *Science* 1987; **235**: 1040–1043.
12. Lujan HD, Mowatt MR, Byrd LG, Nash TE. Cholesterol starvation induces differentiation of the intestinal parasite *Giardia lamblia*. *Proc Natl Acad Sci USA* 1996; **93**: 7628–7633.
13. Touz MC, Nores MJ, Slavin I et al. Membrane-associated dipeptidyl peptidase IV is involved in encystation-specific gene expression during *Giardia* differentiation. *Biochem J* 2002; **364**: 703–710.
14. Thompson SC. *Giardia lamblia* in children and the child care setting: a review of the literature. *J Paediatr Child Health* 1994; **30**: 202–209.
15. Nuchprayoon S, Siriyasatien P, Kraivichian K et al. Prevalence of parasitic infections among Thai patients at the King Chulalongkorn Memorial Hospital, Bangkok, Thailand. *J Med Assoc Thai* 2002; **85 (Suppl 1)**: S415–S423.
16. Molbak K, Wested N, Hojlyng N et al. The etiology of early childhood diarrhea: a community study from Guinea-Bissau. *J Infect Dis* 1994; **169**: 581–587.
17. Newman RD, Moore SR, Lima AA et al. A longitudinal study of *Giardia lamblia* infection in north-east Brazilian children. *Trop Med Int Health* 2001; **6**: 624–634.
18. Mahmud MA, Chappell CL, Hossain MM et al. Impact of breast-feeding on *Giardia lamblia* infections in Bilbeis, Egypt. *Am J Trop Med Hyg* 2001; **65**: 257–260.
19. Chunge RN, Nagelkerke N, Karumba PN et al. Longitudinal study of young children in Kenya: intestinal parasitic infection with special reference to *Giardia lamblia*, its prevalence, incidence and duration, and its association with diarrhoea and with other parasites. *Acta Trop Basel* 1991; **50**: 39–49.
20. Nain CK, Dutt P, Vinayak VK. Alterations in enzymatic activities of the intestinal mucosa during the course of *Giardia lamblia* infection in mice. *Ann Trop Med Parasitol* 1991; **85**: 515–522.
21. Buret AG, Mitchell K, Muench DG, Scott KG. *Giardia lamblia* disrupts tight junctional ZO-1 and increases permeability in non-transformed human small intestinal epithelial monolayers: effects of epidermal growth factor. *Parasitology* 2002; **125**: 11–19.
22. Hicks SJ, Theodoropoulos G, Carrington SD, Corfield AP. The role of mucins in host-parasite interactions. Part I. Protozoan parasites. *Parasitol Today* 2000; **16**: 476–481.
23. Pettoello MM, Guandalini S, Ecuba P et al. Lactose malabsorption in children with symptomatic *Giardia lamblia* infection: feasibility of yogurt supplementation. *J Pediatr Gastroenterol Nutr* 1989; **9**: 295–300.
24. Moya-Camarena SY, Sotelo N, Valencia ME. Effects of asymptomatic *Giardia intestinalis* infection on carbohydrate absorption in well-nourished Mexican children. *Am J Trop Med Hyg* 2002; **66**: 255–259.
25. Jove S, Fagundes-Neto U, Wehba J et al. Giardiasis in childhood and its effects on the small intestine. *J Pediatr Gastroenterol Nutr* 1983; **2**: 472–7.
26. Hjelt K, Paerregaard A, Krasilnikoff PA. Giardiasis: haematological status and the absorption of vitamin B12 and folic acid. *Acta Paediatr* 1992; **81**: 29–34.
27. Goto R, Panter-Brick C, Northrop-Clewes CA et al. Poor intestinal permeability in mildly stunted Nepali children: associations with weaning practices and *Giardia lamblia* infection. *Br J Nutr* 2002; **88**: 141–149.
28. Scott KG, Meddings JB, Kirk DR et al. Intestinal infection with *Giardia* spp. reduces epithelial barrier function in a myosin light chain kinase-dependent fashion. *Gastroenterology* 2002; **123**: 1179–1190.
29. Roberts Thomson IC, Mitchell GF, Anders RF et al. Genetic studies in human and murine giardiasis. *Gut* 1980; **21**: 397–401.
30. Char S, Cevallos AM, Yamson P et al. Impaired IgA response to *Giardia* heat shock antigen in children with persistent diarrhoea and giardiasis. *Gut* 1993; **34**: 38–40.
31. Walterspiel JN, Morrow AL, Lourdes Guerrero M et al. Secretory anti-*Giardia lamblia* antibodies in human milk: protective effect against diarrhea. *Pediatrics* 1994; **93**: 28–31.
32. Di Prisco MC, Hagel I, Lynch NR et al. Association between giardiasis and allergy. *Ann Allergy Asthma Immunol* 1998; **81**: 261–265.
33. Cevallos AM, Carnaby S, James M, Farthing MJ. Small intestinal injury in a neonatal rat model of giardiasis is strain dependent. *Gastroenterology* 2002; **109**: 766–773.
34. Jimenez JC, Rodriguez N, Di Prisco MC et al. Haemoglobin concentrations and infection by *Giardia intestinalis* in children: effect of treatment with secnidazole. *Ann Trop Med Parasitol* 1999; **93**: 823–827.
35. Lane S, Lloyd D. Current trends in research into the waterborne parasite *Giardia*. *Crit Rev Microbiol* 2002; **28**: 123–147.
36. Matsuyama W, Mizoguchi A, Iwami F et al. [A case of pulmonary infiltration with eosinophilia caused by *Ascaris suum*]. *Nihon Kokyuki Gakkai Zasshi* 1998; **36**: 208–12.
37. de Silva NR, Chan MS, Bundy DA. Morbidity and mortality due to ascariasis: re-estimation and sensitivity analysis of global numbers at risk. *Trop Med Int Health* 1997; **2**: 519–528.
38. Hall A, Holland C. Geographical variation in Ascaris lumbricoides fecundity and its implications for helminth control. *Parasitol Today* 2000; **16**: 540–544.
39. Geissler PW, Mwaniki D, Thiong F, Friis H. Geophagy as a risk factor for geohelminth infections: a longitudinal study of Kenyan primary schoolchildren. *Trans R Soc Trop Med Hyg* 1998; **92**: 7–11.
40. Saathoff E, Olsen A, Kvalsvig JD, Geissler PW. Geophagy and its associates with geohelminth infection in rural schoolchildren from northern KwaZulu-Natal, South Africa. *Trans R Soc Trop Med Hyg* 2002; **96**: 485–90.
41. Muller R. *Worms and Human Disease*. 2nd edn. Wallingford, UK: CABI Publishing, 2002.
42. Kennedy MW. The nematode polyprotein allergens/antigens. *Parasitol Today* 2000; **16**: 373–380.
43. Viney M. How do host immune responses affect nematode infections? *Trends Parasitol* 2002; **18**: 63–66.
44. Scott ME, Koski KG. Zinc deficiency impairs immune responses against parasitic nematode infections at intestinal and systemic sites. *J Nutr* 2000; **130**: 1412S–1420S.
45. Cooper PJ, Chico M, Sandoval C et al. Human infection with *Ascaris lumbricoides* is associated with suppression of the interleukin-2 response to recombinant cholera toxin B subunit following vaccination with the live oral cholera vaccine CVD 103-HgR. *Infect Immun* 2001; **69**: 1574–1580.

46. Cooper PJ, Chico ME, Losonsky G et al. Albendazole treatment of children with ascariasis enhances the vibriocidal antibody response to the live attenuated oral cholera vaccine CVD 103-HgR. *J Infect Dis* 2000; **182**: 1199–1206.
47. Wolday D, Mayaan S, Mariam ZG et al. Treatment of intestinal worms is associated with decreased HIV plasma viral load. *J Acquir Immune Defic Syndr* 2002; **31**: 56–62.
48. Cooper PJ, Chico ME, Sandoval C et al. Human infection with *Ascaris lumbricoides* is associated with a polarized cytokine response. *J Infect Dis* 2000; **182**: 1207–1213.
49. Behm CA,.Ovington KS. The role of eosinophils in parasitic helminth infections: insights from genetically modified mice. *Parasitol Today* 2000; **16**: 202–209.
50. Meeusen EN, Balic A. Do eosinophils have a role in the killing of helminth parasites? *Parasitol Today* 2000; **16**: 95–101.
51. Lynch NR, Hagel I, Perez M et al. Effect of anthelmintic treatment on the allergic reactivity of children in a tropical slum. *J Allergy Clin Immunol* 1993; **92**: 404–411.
52. Perzanowski MS, Ng'ang'a LW, Carter MC et al. Atopy, asthma, and antibodies to *Ascaris* among rural and urban children in Kenya. *J Pediatr* 2002; **140**: 582–588.
53. Lynch NR, Hagel IA, Palenque ME et al. Relationship between helminthic infection and IgE response in atopic and nonatopic children in a tropical environment. *J Allergy Clin Immunol* 1998; **101**: 217–221.
54. Gendrel D, Richard Lenoble D, Kombila M et al. Influence of intestinal parasitism on lactose absorption in well-nourished African children. *Am J Trop Med Hyg* 1992; **46**: 137–140.
55. Raj SM, Sein KT, Anuar AK, Mustaffa BE. Effect of intestinal helminthiasis on intestinal permeability of early primary schoolchildren. *Trans R Soc Trop Med Hyg* 1996; **90**: 666–669.
56. Chitkara RK, Sarinas PS. Dirofilaria, visceral larva migrans, and tropical pulmonary eosinophilia. *Semin Respir Infect* 1997; **12**: 138–148.
57. de Silva NR, Guyatt HL, Bundy DA. Morbidity and mortality due to *Ascaris*-induced intestinal obstruction. *Trans R Soc Trop Med Hyg* 1997; **91**: 31–36.
58. Carneiro FF, Cifuentes E, Tellez-Rojo MM, Romieu I. The risk of *Ascaris lumbricoides* infection in children as an environmental health indicator to guide preventative activities in Caparao and Alto Caparo, Brazil. *Bull World Health Organ* 2002; **80**: 40–46.
59. Olsen A, Samuelsen H, Onyango-Ouma W. A study of risk factors for intestinal helminth infections using epidemiological and anthropological approaches. *J Biosoc Sci* 2001; **33**: 569–584.
60. Adenusi AA. The distribution of *Necator americanus* and *Ancylostoma duodenale* among schoolchildren in Lagos, Nigeria. *Trans R Soc Trop Med Hyg* 1997; **91**: 270.
61. Walker NI, Croese J, Clouston AD et al. Eosinophilic enteritis in northeastern Australia. Pathology, association with *Ancylostoma caninum*, and implications. *Am J Surg Pathol* 1995; **19**: 328–37.
62. Sen L, Ghosh K, Bin Z et al. Hookworm burden reductions in BALB/c mice vaccinated with recombinant *Ancylostoma* secreted proteins (ASPs) from *Ancylostoma duodenale*, *Ancylostoma caninum* and *Necator americanus*. *Vaccine* 2000; **18**: 1096–1102.
63. Yu SH, Jiang ZX, Xu LQ. Infantile hookworm disease in China. A review. *Acta Trop* 1995; **59**: 265–270.
64. Albonico M, Smith PG, Ercole E et al. Rate of reinfection with intestinal nematodes after treatment of children with mebendazole or albendazole in a highly endemic area. *Trans R Soc Trop Med Hyg* 1995; **89**: 538–541.
65. Olsen A, Nawiri J, Friis H. The impact of iron supplementation on reinfection with intestinal helminths and *Schistosoma mansoni* in western Kenya. *Trans R Soc Trop Med Hyg* 2000; **94**: 493–499.
66. Guyatt HL, Brooker S, Kihamia CM et al. Evaluation of efficacy of school-based anthelmintic treatments against anemia in children in the United Republic of Tanzania. *Bull World Health Organ* 2001; **79**: 695–703.
67. Beasley NM, Tomkins AM, Hall A et al. The impact of population level deworming on the haemoglobin levels of schoolchildren in Tanga, Tanzania. *Trop Med Int Health* 1999; **4**: 744–750.
68. Stephenson LS, Holland CV, Cooper ES. The public health significance of *Trichuris trichiura*. *Parasitology* 2000; **121 (Suppl)**: S73–S95.
69. Brown CJ, McCloskey DJ, Bundy DA, Navarrete CV. Parasitic infection with *Trichuris trichiura* influences plasma levels of soluble HLA class I. *Hum Immunol* 1999; **60**: 1067–1071.
70. Needham C, Kim HT, Hoa NV *et al.* Epidemiology of soil-transmitted nematode infections in Ha Nam Province, Vietnam. *Trop Med Int Health* 1998; **3**: 904–912.
71. MacDonald TT, Choy MY, Spencer J et al. Histopathology and immunohistochemistry of the caecum in children with the *Trichuris* dysentery syndrome. *J Clin Pathol* 1991; **44**: 194–199.
72. Cooper ES, Whyte Alleng CA, Finzi Smith JS et al. Intestinal nematode infections in children: the pathophysiological price paid. *Parasitology* 1992; **104 (Suppl)**: S91–103.
73. Cooper ES, Ramdath DD, Whyte Alleng C et al. Plasma proteins in children with *Trichuris* dysentery syndrome. *J Clin Pathol* 1997; **50**: 236–240.
74. Duff EM, Anderson NM, Cooper ES. Plasma insulin-like growth factor-1, type 1 procollagen, and serum tumor necrosis factor alpha in children recovering from *Trichuris* dysentery syndrome. *Pediatrics* 1999; **103**: e69.
75. MacDonald TT, Spencer J, Murch SH et al. Immunoepidemiology of intestinal helminthic infections. 3. Mucosal macrophages and cytokine production in the colon of children with *Trichuris trichiura* dysentery. *Trans R Soc Trop Med Hyg* 1994; **88**: 265–268.
76. Cooper ES, Spencer J, Whyte-Alleng CA *et al.* Immediate hypersensitivity in colon of children with chronic *Trichuris trichiura* dysentery. *Lancet* 1991; **338**: 1104–1107.
77. Raj SM. Fecal occult blood testing on *Trichuris*-infected primary school children in northeastern peninsular Malaysia. *Am J Trop Med Hyg* 1999; **60**: 165–166.
78. Kaur G, Raj SM, Naing NN. Trichuriasis: localized inflammatory responses in the colon. *Southeast Asian J Trop Med Public Health* 2002; **33**: 224–228.
79. Kamath KR. Severe infection with *Trichuris trichiura* in Malaysian children. A clinical study of 30 cases treated with stilbazium iodine. *Am J Trop Med Hyg* 1973; **22**: 600–605.
80. Mathan VI,.Baker SJ. Whipworm disease. Intestinal structure and function of patients with severe *Trichuris trichuria* infestation. *Am J Dig Dis* 1970; **15**: 913–918.
81. Gilman RH, Davis C, Fitzgerald F. Heavy *Trichuris* infection and amoebic dysentery in Orang Asli children. A comparison of the two diseases. *Trans R Soc Trop Med Hyg* 1976; **70**: 313–316.
82. Noorizan AM, Mahendra RS. *Trichuris* dysentery syndrome: evidence that it may be underdiagnosed in Kelantan. *Med J Malaysia* 2001; **56**: 53–57.

83. Phillips AD, Thomas AG, Walker-Smith JA. *Cryptosporidium*, chronic diarrhea and the proximal small intestinal mucosa. *Gut* 1992; **33**: 1057–1061.
84. Bern C, Ortega Y, Checkley W et al. Epidemiologic differences between cyclosporiasis and cryptosporidiosis in Peruvian children. *Emerg Infect Dis* 2002; **8**: 581–585.
85. Nchito M, Kelly P, Sianongo S et al. Cryptosporidiosis in urban Zambian children: an analysis of risk factors. *Am J Trop Med Hyg* 1998; **59**: 435–437.
86. Molbak K, Hojlyng N, Ingholt L et al. An epidemic outbreak of cryptosporidiosis: a prospective community study from Guinea Bissau. *Pediatr Infect Dis J* 1990; **9**: 566–570.
87. Molbak K, Aaby P, Hojilyng N, Da Silva APJ. Risk factors for *Cryptosporidium* diarrhea in early childhood: a case–control study from Guinea-Bissau, West Africa. *Am J Epidemiol* 1994; **139**: 734–740.
88. Molbak K, Hojlyng N, Gottschau A *et al.* Cryptosporidiosis in infancy and childhood mortality in Guinea Bissau, west Africa. *Br Med J* 1993; **307**: 417–420.
89. Molbak K, Lisse IM, Hojlyng N, Aabÿ P. Severe cryptosporidiosis in children with normal T-cell subsets. *Parasite Immunol* 1994; **16**: 275–277.
90. Iqbal J, Hira PR, Al Ali F, Philip R. Cryptosporidiosis in Kuwaiti children: seasonality and endemicity. *Clin Microbiol Infect* 2001; **7**: 261–266.
91. Adegbola RA, Demba E, De Veer G, Todd J. *Cryptosporidium* infection in Gambian children less than 5 years of age. *J Trop Med Hyg* 1994; **97**: 103–107.
92. Javier Enriquez F, Avila CR, Ignacio Santos J et al. *Cryptosporidium* infections in Mexican children: clinical, nutritional, enteropathogenic, and diagnostic evaluations. *Am J Trop Med Hyg* 1997; **56**: 254–257.
93. Agnew DG, Lima AA, Newman RD et al. Cryptosporidiosis in northeastern Brazilian children: association with increased diarrhea morbidity. *J Infect Dis* 1998; **177**: 754–760.
94. McDonald AC, MacKenzie WR, Addiss DG et al. *Cryptosporidium parvum*-specific antibody responses among children residing in Milwaukee during the 1993 waterborne outbreak. *J Infect Dis* 2001; **183**: 1373–1379.
95. Cicirello HG, Kehl KS, Addiss DG et al. Cryptosporidiosis in children during a massive waterborne outbreak in Milwaukee, Wisconsin: clinical, laboratory and epidemiologic findings. *Epidemiol Infect* 1997; **119**: 53–60.
96. Cordell RL, Thor PM, Addiss DG et al. Impact of a massive waterborne cryptosporidiosis outbreak on child care facilities in metropolitan Milwaukee, Wisconsin. *Pediatr Infect Dis J* 1997; **16**: 639–644.
97. Moore R, Tzipori S, Griffiths JK et al. Temporal changes in permeability and structure of piglet ileum after site-specific infection by *Cryptosporidium parvum*. *Gastroenterology* 1995; **108**: 1030–1039.
98. Capet C, Kapel N, Huneau JF *et al. Cryptosporidium parvum* infection in suckling rats: impairment of mucosal permeability and Na(+)-glucose cotransport. *Exp Parasitol* 1999; **91**: 119–125.
99. Wyatt CR, Brackett EJ, Savidge J. Evidence for the emergence of a type-1-like immune response in intestinal mucosa of calves recovering from cryptosporidiosis. *J Parasitol* 2001; **87**: 90–95.
100. Pollok RC, Farthing MJ, Bajaj-Elliott M et al. Interferon gamma induces enterocyte resistance against infection by the intracellular pathogen *Cryptosporidium parvum*. *Gastroenterology* 2001; **120**: 99–107.
101. Hayward AR, Chmura K, Cosyns M. Interferon-gamma is required for innate immunity to *Cryptosporidium parvum* in mice. *J Infect Dis* 2000; **182**: 1001–1004.
102. Lawrence CE, Paterson JC, Higgins LM et al. IL-4-regulated enteropathy in an intestinal nematode infection. *Eur J Immunol* 1998; **28**: 2672–2684.
103. Garside P, Kennedy MW, Wakelin D, Lawrence CE. Immunopathology of intestinal helminth infection. *Parasite Immunol* 2000; **22**: 605–612.
104. Leitch GJ, He Q. Reactive nitrogen and oxygen species ameliorate experimental cryptosporidiosis in the neonatal BALB/c mouse model. *Infect Immun* 1999; **67**: 5885–5891.
105. Leitch GJ, He Q. Arginine-derived nitric oxide reduces fecal oocyst shedding in nude mice infected with *Cryptosporidium parvum*. *Infect Immun* 1994; **62**: 5173–5176.
106. Goodgame RW, Kimball K, Ou CN et al. Intestinal function and injury in acquired immunodeficiency syndrome-related cryptosporidiosis. *Gastroenterology* 1995; **108**: 1075–1082.
107. Checkley W, Epstein LD, Gilman RH et al. Effects of *Cryptosporidium parvum* infection in Peruvian children: growth faltering and subsequent catch-up growth. *Am J Epidemiol* 1998; **148**: 497–506.
108. Molbak K, Andersen M, Aaby P et al. *Cryptosporidium* infection in infancy as a cause of malnutrition: a community study from Guinea-Bissau, West Africa. *Am J Clin Nutr* 1997; **65**: 149–152.
109. Guarino A, Castaldo A, Russo S et al. Enteric cryptosporidiosis in pediatric HIV infection. *J Pediatr Gastroenterol Nutr* 1997; **25**: 182–187.
110. Sarabia Arce S, Salazar Lindo E, Gilman RH et al. Case–control study of *Cryptosporidium parvum* infection in Peruvian children hospitalized for diarrhea: possible association with malnutrition and nosocomial infection. *Pediatr Infect Dis J* 1990; **9**: 627–631.
111. Checkley W, Gilman RH, Epstein LD et al. Asymptomatic and symptomatic cryptosporidiosis: their acute effect on weight gain in Peruvian children. *Am J Epidemiol* 1997; **145**: 156–163.
112. Xiao L, Bern C, Limor J et al. Identification of 5 types of *Cryptosporidium* parasites in children in Lima, Peru. *J Infect Dis* 2001; **183**: 492–497.
113. Genta RM. Global prevalence of strongyloidiasis: critical review with epidemiologic insights into the prevention of disseminated disease. *Rev Infect Dis* 1989; **11**: 755–767.
114. Egido JM, De Diego JA, Penin P. The prevalence of enteropathy due to strongyloidiasis in Puerto Maldonado (Peruvian Amazon). *Braz J Infect Dis* 2001; **5**: 119–123.
115. Clyne M, Labigne A, Drumm B. *Helicobacter pylori* requires an acidic environment to survive in the presence of urea. *Infect Immun* 1995; **63**: 1669–1673.
116. Quiros A, Quiros E, Gonzalez I et al. *Helicobacter pylori* seroepidemiology in risk groups. *Eur J Epidemiol* 1994; **10**: 299–301.
117. Barnish G, Ashford RW. Strongyloides cf. fuelleborni and hookworm in Papua New Guinea: patterns of infection within the community. *Trans R Soc Trop Med Hyg* 1989; **83**: 684–688.
118. Milner PF, Irvine RA, Barton CJ et al. Intestinal malabsorption in *Strongyloides stercoralis* infestation. *Gut* 1965; **6**: 574–581.
119. Sipahi AM, Damiao AO, Simionato CS et al. Small bowel bacterial overgrowth in strongyloidiasis. *Digestion* 1991; **49**: 120–124.
120. Werneck-Silva AL, Sipahi AM, Damiao AO et al. Intestinal permeability in strongyloidiasis. *Braz J Med Biol Res* 2001; **34**: 353–357.
121. Sullivan PB, Lunn PG, Northrop Clewes CA, Farthing MJ. Parasitic infection of the gut and protein-losing

enteropathy. *J Pediatr Gastroenterol Nutr* 1992; **15**: 404–407.

122. Burke JA. Strongyloidiasis in childhood. *Am J Dis Child* 1978; **132**: 1130–1136.
123. Atkins NS, Conway DJ, Lindo JF et al. L3 antigen-specific antibody isotype responses in human strongyloidiasis: correlations with larval output. *Parasite Immunol* 1999; **21**: 517–526.
124. Walker AC, Blake G, Downing D. A syndrome of partial intestinal obstruction due to *Strongyloides stercoralis*. *Med J Aust* 1976; **1**: 47–48.
125. Walker-Smith JA, McMillan B, Middleton AW et al. Strongyloidiasis causing small-bowel obstruction in an Aboriginal infant. *Med J Aust* 1969; **2**: 1263–1265.
126. Vince JD, Ashford RW, Gratten MJ, Bana-Koiri J. *Strongyloides* species infestation in young infants of Papua, New Guinea: association with generalized oedema. *P N G Med J* 1979; **22**: 120–127.
127. Barnish G, Barker J. An intervention study using thiabendazole suspension against *Strongyloides fuelleborni*-like infections in Papua New Guinea. *Trans R Soc Trop Med Hyg* 1987; **81**: 60–63.
128. Robinson RD, Lindo JF, Neva FA et al. Immunoepidemiologic studies of *Strongyloides stercoralis* and human T lymphotropic virus type I infections in Jamaica. *J Infect Dis* 1994; **169**: 692–696.
129. Siddiqui AA, Berk SL. Diagnosis of *Strongyloides stercoralis* infection. *Clin Infect Dis* 2001; **33**: 1040–1047.
130. Sato Y, Kobayashi J, Shiroma Y. Serodiagnosis of strongyloidiasis. The application and significance. *Rev Inst Med Trop Sao Paulo* 1995; **37**: 35–41.
131. Gyorkos TW, Genta RM, Viens P, MacLean JD. Seroepidemiology of *Strongyloides* infection in the Southeast Asian refugee population in Canada. *Am J Epidemiol* 1990; **132**: 257–264.
132. Haque R, Faruque AS, Hahn P et al. *Entamoeba histolytica* and *Entamoeba dispar* infection in children in Bangladesh. *J Infect Dis* 1997; **175**: 734–736.
133. Heckendorn F, N'Goran EK, Felger I et al. Species-specific field testing of *Entamoeba* spp. On an area of high endemicy. *Trans R Soc Trop Med Hyg* 2002; **96**: 521–528.
134. Braga LL, Gomes ML, Da Silva MW et al. Household epidemiology of *Entamoeba histolytica* infection in an urban community in northeastern Brazil. *Am J Trop Med Hyg* 2001; **65**: 268–271.
135. Stanley SL. Pathophysiology of amoebiasis. *Trends Parasitol* 2001; **17**: 280–285.
136. Haque R, Duggal P, Ali IM et al. Innate and acquired resistance to amebiasis in Bangladeshi children. *J Infect Dis* 2002; **186**: 547–552.
137. Haque R, Ali IM, Petri WA Jr. Prevalence and immune response to *Entamoeba histolytica* infection in preschool children in Bangladesh. *Am J Trop Med Hyg* 1999; **60**: 1031–1034.
138. Ayeh-Kumi PF, Ali IM, Lockhart LA et al. *Entamoeba histolytica*: genetic diversity of clinical isolates from Bangladesh as demonstrated by polymorphisms in the serine-rich gene. *Exp Parasitol* 2001; **99**: 80–88.
139. Sirivichayakul C, Radomyos P, Praevanit R et al. *Hymenolepis nana* infection in Thai children. *J Med Assoc Thai* 2000; **83**: 1035–1038.
140. Liu LX, Chi J, Upton MP, Ash LR. Eosinophilic colitis associated with larvae of the pinworm *Enterobius vermicularis*. *Lancet* 1995; **346**: 410–412.
141. Sinniah B, Leopairut J, Neafie RC et al. Enterobiasis: a histopathological study of 259 patients. *Ann Trop Med Parasitol* 1991; **85**: 625–635.
142. Hoge CW, Shlim DR, Rajah R et al. Epidemiology of diarrheal illness associated with coccidian-like organism among travellers and foreign residents in Nepal. *Lancet* 1993; **341**: 1175–1179.
143. Ho AY, Lopez AS, Eberhart MG et al. Outbreak of cyclosporiasis associated with imported raspberries, Philadelphia, Pennsylvania, 2000. *Emerg Infect Dis* 2002; **8**: 783–788.
144. Katz D, Kumar S, Malecki J et al. Cyclosporiasis associated with imported raspberries, Florida, 1996. *Public Health Rep* 1999; **114**: 427–438.
145. Quintero-Betancourt W, Peele ER, Rose JB. *Cryptosporidium parvum* and *Cyclospora cayetanensis*: a review of laboratory methods for detection of these waterborne parasites. *J Microbiol Methods* 2002; **49**: 209–224.
146. Bern C, Hernandez B, Lopez MB et al. The contrasting epidemiology of *Cyclospora* and *Cryptosporidium* among outpatients in Guatemala. *Am J Trop Med Hyg* 2000; **63**: 231–235.
147. Eberhard ML, Nace EK, Freeman AR et al. *Cyclospora cayetanensis* infections in Haiti: a common occurrence in the absence of watery diarrhea. *Am J Trop Med Hyg* 1999; **60**: 584–586.
148. Chacin-Bonilla L, Estevez J, Monsalve F, Quijada L. *Cyclospora cayetanensis* infections among diarrheal patients from Venezuela. *Am J Trop Med Hyg* 2001; **65**: 351–354.
149. Pape JW, Verdier RI, Boncy M et al. *Cyclospora* infection in adults infected with HIV. Clinical manifestations, treatment, and prophylaxis. *Ann Intern Med* 1994; **121**: 654–657.
150. Connor BA, Shlim DR, Scholes JV et al. Pathologic changes in the small bowel in nine patients with diarrhea associated with a coccidia-like body. *Ann Intern Med* 1993; **119**: 377–382.
151. Rigo CR,.Franco RM. [Comparison between the modified Ziehl–Neelsen and acid-fast-trichrome methods for fecal screening of *Cryptosporidium parvum* and *Isospora belli*]. *Rev Soc Bras Med Trop* 2002; **35**: 209–214.
152. Sherchand JB,.Cross JH. Emerging pathogen *Cyclospora cayetanensis* infection in Nepal. *Southeast Asian J Trop Med Public Health* 2001; **32 (Suppl 2)**: 143–150.
153. Rizk H, Soliman M. Coccidiosis among malnourished children in Mansoura, Dakahlia Governorate, Egypt. *J Egypt Soc Parasitol* 2001; **31**: 877–886.
154. Madico G, McDonald J, Gilman RH et al. Epidemiology and treatment of *Cyclospora cayetanensis* infection in Peruvian children. *Clin Infect Dis* 1997; **24**: 977–981.
155. Hoge CW, Shlim DR, Ghimire M et al. Placebo-controlled trial of co-trimoxazole for *Cyclospora* infections among travellers and foreign residents in Nepal. *Lancet* 1995; **345**: 691–693.
156. Horton J. Albendazole: a review of anthelmintic efficacy and safety in humans. *Parasitology* 2000; **121 (Suppl)**: S113–S132.
157. Forrester JE, Bailar JC III, Esrey SA et al. Randomised trial of albendazole and pyrantel in symptomless trichuriasis in children. *Lancet* 1998; **352**: 1103–1108.
158. Montresor A, Stoltzfus RJ, Albonico M et al. Is the exclusion of children under 24 months from anthelmintic treatment justifiable? *Trans R Soc Trop Med Hyg* 2002; **96**: 197–199.
159. Zulu I, Veitch A, Sianongo S et al. Albendazole chemotherapy for AIDS-related diarrhea in Zambia – clinical, parasitological and mucosal responses. *Aliment Pharmacol Ther* 2002; **16**: 595–601.
160. Belizario VY, Amarillo ME, de Leon WU et al. A comparison of the efficacy of single doses of

albendazole, ivermectin, and diethylcarbamzine alone or in combinations against *Ascaris* and *Trichuris* spp. *Bull World Health Organ* 2003; **81**: 35–42.

161. Hall A, Nahar Q. Albendazole as a treatment for infections with *Giardia duodenalis* in children in Bangladesh. *Trans R Soc Trop Med Hyg* 1993; **87**: 84–86.
162. Ermis B, Aslan T, Beder L, Unalacak M. A randomized placebo-controlled trial of mebendazole for halitosis. *Arch Pediatr Adolesc Med* 2002; **156**: 995–998.
163. Marti H, Haji HJ, Savioli L et al. A comparative trial of a single-dose ivermectin versus three days of albendazole for treatment of *Strongyloides stercoralis* and other soil-transmitted helminth infections in children. *Am J Trop Med Hyg* 1996; **55**: 477–481.
164. Behnke JM, Pritchard DI, Wakelin D et al. Effect of ivermectin on infection with gastro-intestinal nematodes in Sierra Leone. *J Helminthol* 1994; **68**: 187–195.
165. Datry A, Hilmarsdottir I, Mayorga Sagastume R et al. Treatment of *Strongyloides stercoralis* infection with ivermectin compared with albendazole: results of an open study of 60 cases. *Trans R Soc Trop Med Hyg* 1994; **88**: 344–345.
166. Gann PH, Neva FA, Gam AA. A randomized trial of single- and two-dose ivermectin versus thiabendazole for treatment of strongyloidiasis. *J Infect Dis* 1994; **169**: 1076–1079.
167. Misra PK, Kumar A, Agarwal V, Jagota SC. A comparative clinical trial of albendazole versus metronidazole in children with giardiasis. *Indian Pediatr* 1995; **32**: 779–782.
168. Lares Asseff I, Cravioto J, Santiago P, Perez Ortiz B. A new dosing regimen for metronidazole in malnourished children. *Scand J Infect Dis* 1993; **25**: 115–121.
169. Addiss DG, Juranek DD, Spencer HC. Treatment of children with asymptomatic and nondiarrheal *Giardia* infection. *Pediatr Infect Dis J* 1991; **10**: 843–846.
170. Ish Horowicz M, Korman SH, Shapiro M et al. Asymptomatic giardiasis in children. *Pediatr Infect Dis J* 1989; **8**: 773–779.
171. Pickering LK, Engelkirk PG. *Giardia lamblia. Pediatr Clin North Am* 1988; **35**: 565–577.
172. Zaat JO, Mank T, Assendelft WJ. Drugs for treating giardiasis. *Cochrane Database Syst Rev* 2000; CD000217.
173. Gilles HM, Hoffman PS. Treatment of intestinal parasitic infections: a review of nitazoxanide. *Trends Parasitol* 2002; **18**: 95–97.
174. Rossignol JF, Ayoub A, Ayers MS. Treatment of diarrhea caused by *Giardia intestinalis* and *Entamoeba histolytica* or *E. dispar*: a randomized, double-blind, placebo-controlled study of nitazoxanide. *J Infect Dis* 2001; **184**: 381–384.
175. Rossignol JF, Ayoub A, Ayers MS. Treatment of diarrhea caused by *Cryptosporidium parvum*: a prospective randomized, double-blind, placebo-controlled study of Nitazoxanide. *J Infect Dis* 2001; **184**: 103–106.
176. Davila-Gutierrez CE, Vasquez C, Trujillo-Hernandez B, Huerta M. Nitazoxanide compared with quinfamide and mebendazole in the treatment of helminthic infections and intestinal protozoa in children. *Am J Trop Med Hyg* 2002; **66**: 251–254.
177. Cedillo-Rivera R, Chavez B, Gonzalez-Robles A et al. *In vitro* effect of nitazoxanide against *Entamoeba histolytica, Giardia intestinalis* and *Trichomonas vaginalis* trophozoites. *J Eukaryot Microbiol* 2002; **49**: 201–208.
178. Ortiz JJ, Chegne NL, Gargala G, Favennec L. Comparative clinical studies of nitazoxanide, albendazole and praziquantel in the treatment of ascariasis, trichuriasis and hymenolepiasis in children from Peru. *Trans R Soc Trop Med Hyg* 2002; **96**: 193–196.
179. Ortiz JJ, Ayoub A, Gargala G et al. Randomized clinical study of nitazoxanide compared to metronidazole in the treatment of symptomatic giardiasis in children from Northern Peru. *Aliment Pharmacol Ther* 2001; **15**: 1409–1415.
180. Amadi B, Mwiya M, Musuku J et al. Effect of nitazoxanide on morbidity and mortality in Zambian children with cryptosporidiosis: a randomised controlled trial. *Lancet* 2002; **360**: 1375–1380.
181. Bissuel F, Cotte L, Rabodonirina M et al. Paromomycin: an effective treatment for cryptosporidial diarrhea in patients with AIDS. *Clin Infect Dis* 1994; **18**: 447–449.
182. Hewitt RG, Yiannoutsos CT, Higgs ES et al. Paromomycin: no more effective than placebo for treatment of cryptosporidiosis in patients with advanced human immunodeficiency virus infection. AIDS Clinical Trial Group. *Clin Infect Dis* 2000; **31**: 1084–1092.
183. Anonymous. *World Development Report 1993: Investing in Health.* New York: Oxford University Press, 1993.
184. World Health Organization. *Guidelines for the Evaluation of Soil-transmitted Helminthiasis and Schistosomiasis at Community Level: a Guide for Managers of Control Programmes.* Geneva: WHO, 1998.
185. Brooker S, Marriot H, Hall A et al. Community perception of school-based delivery of anthelmintics in Ghana and Tanzania. *Trop Med Int Health* 2001; **6**: 1075–1083.
186. Allen HE, Crompton DW, de Silva N et al. New policies for using antihelmintics in high risk groups. *Trends Parasitol* 2002; **18**: 381–382.
187. Dickson R, Awasthi S, Williamson P et al. Effects of treatment for intestinal helminth infection on growth and cognitive performance in children: systematic review of randomised trials. *Br Med J* 2000; **320**: 1697–1701.
188. Dickson R, Awasthi S, Demellweek C, Williamson P. Anthelmintic drugs for treating worms in children: effects on growth and cognitive performance. *Cochrane Database Syst Rev* 2000; CD000371.
189. Stoltzfus RJ, Kvalsvig JD, Chwaya HM *et al.* Effects of iron supplementation and anthelmintic treatment on motor and language development of preschool children in Zanzibar: double blind, placebo controlled study. *Br Med J* 2001; **323**: 1389–1393.
190. Olds GR, King C, Hewlett J et al. Double-blind placebo-controlled study of concurrent administration of albendazole and praziquantel in schoolchildren with schistosomiasis and geoheminths. *J Infect Dis* 1999; **179**: 996–1003.
191. Northrop-Clewes CA, Rousham EK, Mascie-Taylor CN, Lunn PG. Anthelmintic treatment of rural Bangladeshi children: effect on host physiology, growth, and biochemical status. *Am J Clin Nutr* 2001; **73**: 53–60.
192. Rousham EK. An increase in *Giardia duodenalis* infection among children receiving periodic anthelmintic treatment in Bangladesh. *J Trop Pediatr* 1994; **40**: 329–333.
193. Stettler N, Schutz Y, Jequier E. Effect of low-level pathogenic helminth infection on energy metabolism in Gambian children. *Am J Trop Med Hyg* 1998; **58**: 476–479.
194. Raj SM, Sein KT, Anuar AK, Mustaffa BE. Effect of intestinal helminthiasis on school attendance by early primary schoolchildren. *Trans R Soc Trop Med Hyg* 1997; **91**: 131–132.
195. Moore SR, Lima AA, Conaway MR et al. Early childhood diarrhea and helminthiases associated with

long-term linear growth faltering. *Int J Epidemiol* 2001; **30**: 1457–1464.
196. Guyatt HL. Do intestinal nematodes affect productivity in adults? *Parasitol Today* 2000; **16**: 153–158.
197. Donnen P, Brasseur D, Dramaix M et al. Vitamin A supplementation but not deworming improves growth of malnourished preschool children in eastern Zaire. *J Nutr* 1998; **128**: 1320–1327.
198. Taylor M, Jinabhai CC, Couper I et al. The effect of different anthelmintic treatment regimens combined with iron supplementation on the nutritional status of schoolchildren in KwaZulu-Natal, South Africa: a randomized controlled trial. *Trans R Soc Trop Med Hyg* 2001; **95**: 211–216.
199. Muchiri EM, Thiong'o FW, Magnussen P, Ouma JH. A comparative study of different albendazole and mebendazole regimens for the treatment of intestinal infections in school children of Usigu Division, Western Kenya. *J Parasitol* 2001; **87**: 413–418.
200. Albonico M, Renganathan E, Bosman A et al. Efficacy of a single dose of mebendazole on prevalence and intensity of soil-transmitted nematodes in Zanzibar. *Trop Geogr Med* 1994; **46**: 142–146.
201. Lunn PG, Erinoso HO, Northrop-Clewes CA, Boyce SA. *Giardia intestinalis* is unlikely to be a major cause of the poor growth of rural Gambian infants. *J Nutr* 1999; **129**: 872–877.
202. Sullivan PB, Marsh MN, Phillips MB et al. Prevalence and treatment of giardiasis in chronic diarrhea and malnutrition. *Arch Dis Child* 1991; **66**: 304–306.
203. Sullivan PS, DuPont HL, Arafat RR et al. Illness and reservoirs associated with *Giardia lamblia* infection in rural Egypt: the case against treatment in developing world environments of high endemicity. *Am J Epidemiol* 1988; **127**: 1272–1281.
204. Gilman RH, Marquis GS, Miranda E et al. Rapid reinfection by *Giardia lamblia* after treatment in a hyperendemic Third World community. *Lancet* 1988; **1**: 343–345.
205. Rousham EK. Perceptions and treatment of intestinal worms in rural Bangladesh: local differences in knowledge and behaviour. *Soc Sci Med* 1994; **39**: 1063–1068.
206. Muller M, Sanchez RM, Suswillo RR. Evaluation of a sanitation programme using eggs of *Ascaris lumbricoides* in household yard soils as indicators. *J Trop Med Hyg* 1989; **92**: 10–16.
207. Albert MJ, Faruque AS, Faruque SM et al. Case–control study of enteropathogens associated with childhood diarrhea in Dhaka, Bangladesh. *J Clin Microbiol* 1999; **37**: 3458–3464.
208. Huilan S, Zhen LG, Mathan MM et al. Etiology of acute diarrhea among children in developing countries: a multicentre study in five countries. *Bull World Health Organ* 1991; **69**: 549–555.
209. Loening WE, Coovadia YM, van den Ende J. Aetiological factors of infantile diarrhea: a community-based study. *Ann Trop Paediatr* 1989; **9**: 248–255.

12 Post-infectious persistent diarrhea in developing countries

Zulfiqar A Bhutta

Global significance of diarrheal disorders and persistent diarrhea

Despite considerable advances in the understanding and management of diarrheal disorders in childhood, they are still responsible for a major burden of childhood deaths globally, with an estimated 2.5 million deaths.[1] In an estimate of the global burden of diarrheal disorders in 1980 the World Health Organization (WHO) calculated that there were over 700 million episodes of diarrhea annually in children under 5 years of age in developing countries (excluding China), with approximately 4.6 million deaths.[2] Reviews in the early 1990s suggested that diarrheal disorders still accounted for almost a third of all admissions to health facilities in developing countries,[3] with an estimated incidence of diarrheal disorders at around 2.6 episodes/child per year. More recent reviews of studies published in the past 10 years indicate that, while global mortality may have reduced, the incidence remained unchanged at about 3.2 episodes/child year.[4,5] These findings indicate the continuing need to focus on prevention and management of childhood diarrhea in developing countries.

It is recognized that most diarrheal disorders form a continuum, with the majority of cases resolving within the first week of the illness. However, a smaller proportion of diarrheal illnesses fail to resolve and may persist for longer than 2 weeks. Persistent diarrhea has been defined as an episode that begins acutely but lasts for 14 days or longer. It has been shown to identify children with a substantially increased diarrheal burden and leads to the majority of all diarrhea-related deaths.[6] In a prospective study of diarrheal disorders in north India, persistent diarrhea accounted for only 5% of all diarrheal episodes, but the case/fatality rate for persistent diarrhea was 14% in comparison with 0.7% for episodes of shorter duration.[7] In a similar prospective study of diarrheal episodes in the community in and around Lahore (Pakistan), persistent diarrhea accounted for 8–18% of all diarrheal episodes but 54% of all diarrheal deaths.[8] Figure 12.1 indicates the relative proportion of diarrheal episodes from several prospective community-based studies in developing countries.[7,9–11]

It is important to emphasize that the bulk of the epidemiological information on the relationship of acute diarrheal disorders to persistent diarrhea is derived from studies undertaken over 10–15 years ago, and that there is a paucity of recent data on this subject, especially from areas non-endemic for HIV.[5] However, it is evident from studies in HIV-endemic areas that chronic enteropathy and persistent diarrhea is a common manifestation of advancing HIV infection and AIDS.

Pathogenesis of persistent diarrhea

Although a close relationship between diarrheal disease and malnutrition has long been recognized,[12] this has been challenged.[13] The relationship of persistent diarrhea to malnutrition is less controversial, as the disorder is commonly seen in association with significant malnutrition. In a verbal autopsy study of diarrheal deaths in Bangladesh, Fauveau et al[14] found that almost half the deaths were in malnourished children with persistent diarrhea, and the relative risk of dying with persistent diarrhea and severe malnutrition was 17-fold higher than in children with lower degrees of malnutrition.

There are several reasons for malnutrition both to predispose to persistent diarrhea and to follow it.

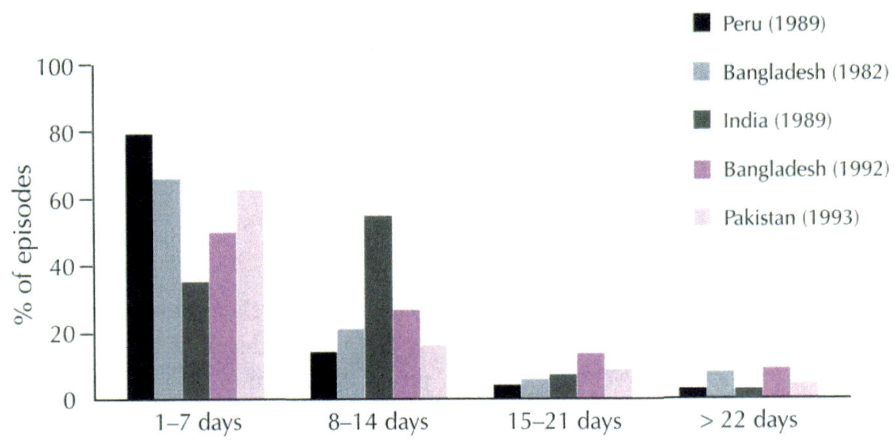

Figure 12.1 Distribution of diarrheal episodes in community-based studies. From references 7 and 9–11.

These range from achlorhydria with increased risk of small-bowel contamination, systemic immune deficiency, intestinal and pancreatic enzyme deficiency and altered intestinal mucosal repair mechanisms following an infectious insult. An independent relationship has also been demonstrated between cutaneous anergy and the subsequent risk of development of persistent diarrhea.[15] There has been much interest in the possibility that such transient immune deficiency may also be a marker of concomitant micronutrient deficiency.[16–18] The most striking example of the critical role that the immune system plays in the pathogenesis of persistent diarrhea is the relationship between HIV/AIDS and persistent diarrhea. This is exemplified by the host of studies linking persistent diarrhea with cryptosporidiosis[19] and other parasitic infections[20,21] in Africa and Asia.

A clear understanding of alterations in intestinal morphology and physiology is crucial towards the development of interventional strategies, but there has been little progress in our understanding of this problem in developing countries. This has been largely due to a paucity of studies formally evaluating intestinal biopsy findings in representative populations. A wide variety of pathological changes have been described after persistent diarrhea, ranging from near-normal appearance to mucosal flattening, crypt hypertrophy and lymphocytic infiltration of the mucosa.[22] Recent electron microscopic studies of the intestinal mucosa in persistent diarrhea have revealed patchy villous atrophy and intraepithelial lymphocytic infiltration[23] as well as severe mucosal damage and villous atrophy.[24]

Poor intestinal repair is regarded as a key component of the abnormal mucosal morphology. However, the exact factors underlying this ineffective repair process and continuing injury are poorly understood (Figure 12.2). The end result of this mucosal derangement is poor absorption of luminal nutrients, as well as increased permeability of the bowel to abnormal dietary or microbial antigens.[25–27] Alterations of intestinal permeability in early childhood may reflect changes in intestinal mucosal maturation[28] and may be affected by concomitant enteric infections.[29]

Risk factors for persistent diarrhea

It is important to recognize the major risk factors for development of persistent diarrhea, as appropriate case management of acute diarrhea is key to the prevention of prolonged episodes.

Specific pathogens

The association of specific bacterial and viral infections with persistent diarrhea has been the subject of considerable debate.[30,31] Evidence from

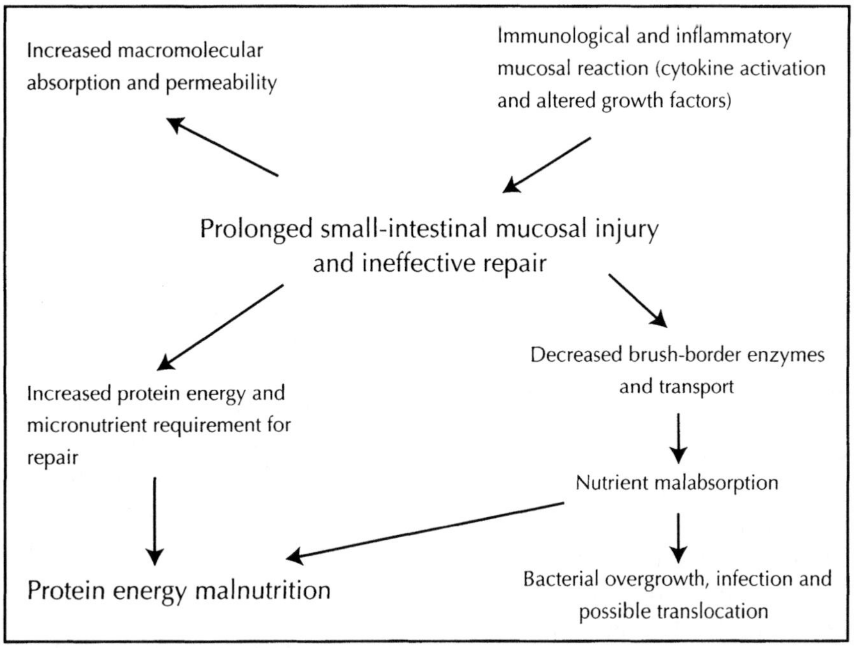

Figure 12.2 Mechanisms and effects of enteropathy of malnutrition and prolonged diarrhea.

Bangladesh suggests that recurrent bouts of infection with pathogens such as *Shigella* lead to prolongation of the duration of successive diarrheal episodes. Although several studies have identified an association between persistent diarrhea and enteroaggregative *Escherichia coli* in the small bowel, this is by no means pathognomonic,[32] nor is there a particular pattern of small-bowel microbial colonization or overgrowth seen in most cases. In parts of Africa endemic for HIV an association of persistent diarrhea with cryptosporidiosis and other pathogens[19–21,33] is well recognized, but may represent a manifestation of immunodeficiency.

Malnutrition

Persistent diarrhea is commonly seen in association with significant malnutrition, and the relationship may be bi-directional. It is widely recognized that diarrheal episodes, especially if invasive, may become prolonged in malnourished children. The recent evidence of micronutrient deficiencies, especially of zinc and vitamin A in malnourished children with persistent diarrhea, indicates impaired immunological mechanisms for clearing infections as well as ineffective mucosal repair mechanisms. From initial studies indicating the potential benefit of zinc supplementation on reducing the risk of prolonged diarrhea,[34] the evidence of the benefit of zinc supplements in children with persistent diarrhea was equivocal.[35,36] However, a recent meta-analysis of zinc supplementation in diarrheal illnesses indicated a significant reduction in duration and severity of diarrheal illnesses.[37] Thus, zinc deficiency may significantly contribute to the prolongation of mucosal injury and delayed intestinal repair mechanisms.

Dietary risk factors

While many children with persistent diarrhea are lactose-intolerant, the role of specific dietary allergies in inducing and perpetuating enteropathy of malnutrition is unclear. Several studies have highlighted the high risk of prolonged diarrhea with lactation failure and early introduction of artificial feeds in developing countries. In particular, the administration of unmodified cow's or buffalo's milk is associated with prolongation of diarrhea, suggesting the potential underlying role of milk protein enteropathy.[26,38]

Inappropriate management of acute diarrhea

The association of prolongation of diarrhea with starvation and inappropriately prolonged administration of parenteral fluids has been recognized for over half a century. Continued breast feeding is important; unnecessary food withdrawal, and replacement of luminal nutrients, especially breast milk, with non-nutritive agents is a major factor in prolonging mucosal injury after diarrhea. In particular, blanket administration of antibiotics and antimotility agents and semi-starvation diets should be avoided in cases of prolonged diarrhea.[39,40] While parenteral nutrition has been occasionally life saving in selected cases in developing countries,[41] it is clearly an impractical option for most of the developing world. There is now clear evidence supporting the enteral route for nutritional rehabilitation of malnourished children with persistent diarrhea.[12] Starvation has been shown to have deleterious effects on the intestinal mucosa,[42] with a reduction in the nutritive transporters for glutamine and arginine.[43] It is therefore imperative that malnourished children with persistent diarrhea should receive enteral nutrition during their period of rehabilitation.

The aforementioned risk factors highlight the importance of recognizing that optimal management of diarrheal episodes is key to the prevention of persistent diarrhea. It is thus necessary that, given the close relationship between diarrheal disorders and malnutrition, persistent diarrhea be widely recognized as a nutritional disorder,[44,45] and optimal nutritional rehabilitation be considered as the cornerstone of its management.[12]

Principles of management of persistent diarrhea

In general the management of persistent diarrhea in malnourished children represents a blend of the principles of management of diarrhea and malnutrition. Associated malnutrition may be quite severe in affected children, necessitating rapid nutritional rehabilitation, often in hospital. Given the chronicity of the disorder, prolonged hospitalization may be problematic in developing countries and, whenever possible, ambulatory or home-based therapy must be supported.

The following represent the basic principles of management of persistent diarrhea. A suggested therapeutic approach is indicated in Figure 12.3.

Rapid resuscitation, antibiotic therapy and stabilization

Most children with persistent diarrhea and associated malnutrition are not severely dehydrated, and oral rehydration may be adequate. However, acute exacerbations and associated vomiting may require brief periods of intravenous rehydration with Ringer's lactate. Acute electrolyte imbalance such as hypokalemia and severe acidosis may require correction. More importantly, associated systemic infections (bacteremia, pneumonia and urinary tract infection) are well recognized in severely malnourished children with persistent diarrhea and a frequent cause of early mortality. Children must be screened for these at admission. Almost 30–50% of malnourished children with persistent diarrhea may have an associated systemic infection requiring resuscitation and antimicrobial therapy.[46,47] In severely ill children requiring hospitalization, it may be best to cover with parenteral antibiotics at admission (usually ampicillin and gentamicin) while awaiting the results of cultures. It should be emphasized that there is little role for oral antibiotics in persistent diarrhea, as in most cases the original bacterial infection triggering the prolonged diarrhea has disappeared by the time the child presents. One possible exception may be adjunctive therapy for cryptosporidiosis in children with HIV and persistent diarrhea.[48]

Oral rehydration therapy

This is the preferred mode of rehydration and replacement of on-going losses. While in general the standard WHO oral rehydration solution (ORS) is adequate, recent evidence indicates that hypo-osmolar rehydration fluids[49,50] as well as cereal-based oral rehydration fluids may be advantageous in malnourished children. In general replacing each stool with about 50–100 ml ORS is safe.

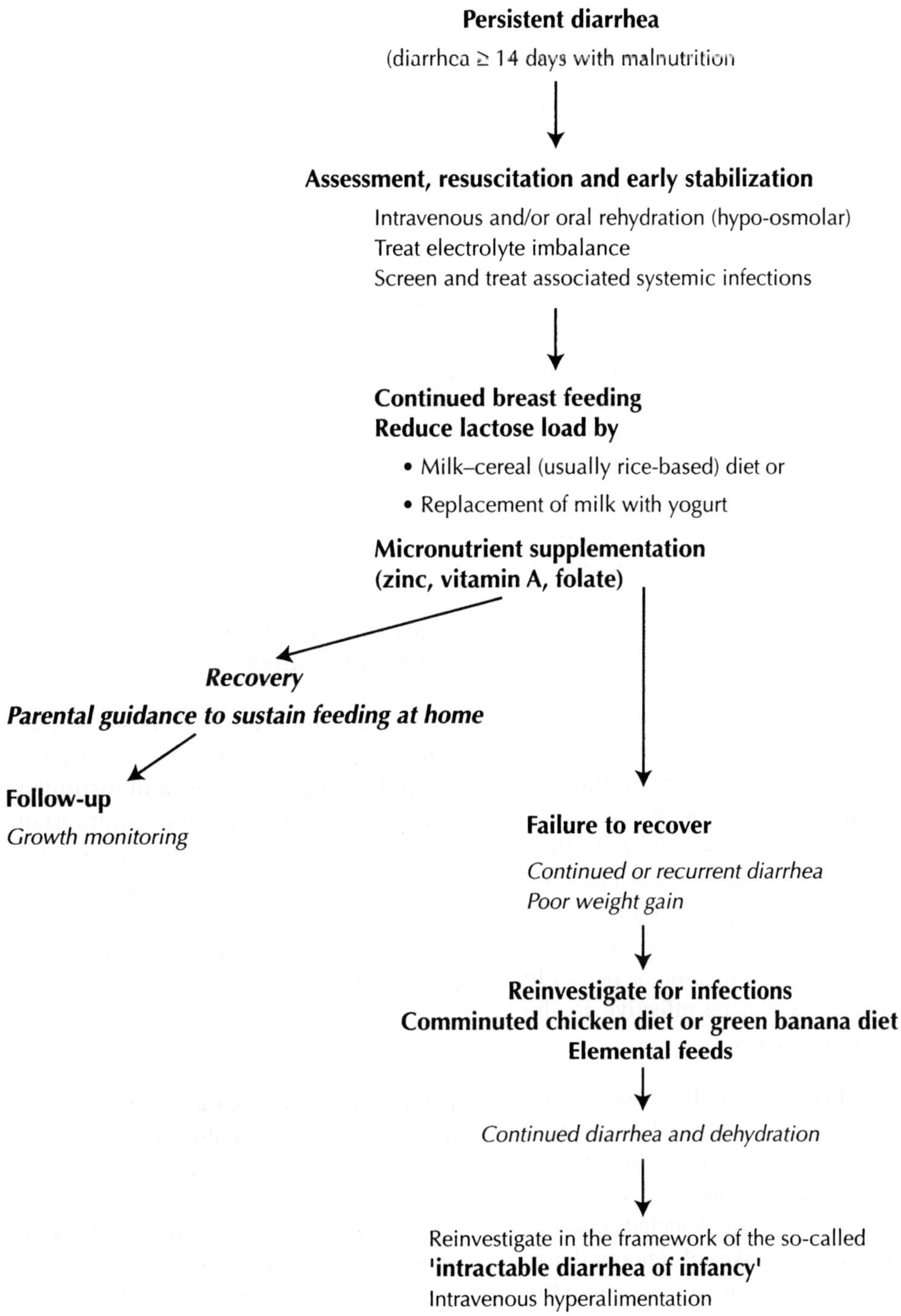

Figure 12.3 Therapeutic approach to the management of persistent diarrhea.

Enteral feeding and diet selection

Irrespective of the cellular mechanisms and structural alterations in malnourished children with persistent diarrhea, the end result is one of altered brush-border and luminal enzymes, with consequent malabsorption. Despite the aforementioned alterations in digestive and absorptive mechanisms, analysis of studies of metabolic balance in children with persistent diarrhea indicates that satisfactory carbohydrate, protein and fat absorption can take place on a variety of diets.[12,38]

It is exceedingly rare to find persistent diarrhea in exclusively breast-fed infants, and with the exception of situations where persistent diarrhea accompanies perinatally acquired HIV infection, breast feeding must be continued. Most children with persistent diarrhea are not lactose intolerant, although administration of a lactose load exceeding 5 g/kg per day is associated with higher purging rates and treatment failure. In general therefore withdrawal of milk and replacement with specialized (and expensive) lactose-free formulations is unnecessary. Alternative strategies for reducing the lactose load in malnourished children with persistent diarrhea include the addition of milk to cereals as well as replacement of milk with fermented milk products such as yogurt. These dietary interventions have now been extensively evaluated in several studies in South Asia, and found to be of equivalent efficacy to expensive formulations.[51,52]

Rarely, when dietary intolerance precludes the administration of cow's milk-based formulations or milk, it may be necessary to administer specialized milk-free diets such as a comminuted or blenderized chicken-based diet or an elemental formulation.[53] It must be pointed out that, although effective in some settings,[54] the latter are unaffordable in most developing countries. In addition to rice–lentil formulations such as *khitchri*, the addition of green banana or pectin to the diet[55] has been shown to be effective in the treatment of persistent diarrhea.

The usual energy density of any diet used for the therapy of persistent diarrhea should be around 1 kcal/g, aiming to provide an energy intake of a minimum of 100 kcal/kg per day, and a protein intake of 2–3 g/kg per day. In selected circumstances when adequate intake of energy-dense food is problematic, the addition of amylase to the diet through germination techniques may also be helpful.

Micronutrient supplementation

It is now widely recognized that most malnourished children with persistent diarrhea have associated deficiencies of micronutrients including zinc, iron and vitamin A. This may be a consequence of poor intake and continued enteral losses, and requires replenishment during therapy.[56] While the evidence supporting zinc administration in children with persistent diarrhea is persuasive, it is likely that these children have multiple micronutrient deficiencies. Concomitant vitamin A administration to children with persistent diarrhea has been shown to improve outcome[57,58] especially in HIV-endemic areas.[59] It is therefore important to ensure that all children with persistent diarrhea and malnutrition receive an initial dose of 100 000 U of vitamin A and a daily intake of at least 3–5 mg/kg per day of elemental zinc. While the association of significant anemia with persistent diarrhea is well recognized, iron replacement therapy is best initiated only after recovery from diarrhea has started and the diet is well tolerated.

Follow-up and nutritional rehabilitation in community settings

Given the high rates of relapse in most children with persistent diarrhea, it is important to address the underlying risk factors and institute preventive measures. These include appropriate feeding (breast feeding, complementary feeding) and close attention to environmental hygiene and sanitation. This poses a considerable challenge in communities deprived of basic necessities such as clean water and sewage disposal.

In addition to the preventive aspects, the challenge in most settings is to develop and sustain a form of dietary therapy using inexpensive, home-available and culturally acceptable ingredients that can be used to manage children with persistent diarrhea. Given that the majority of cases of persistent diarrhea occur in the community and that parents are frequently hesitant to seek institutional help, there is a need to develop and implement inexpensive and practical home-based therapeutic measures.[12] Recent data indicate that it may be entirely feasible to do so in community settings.[60,61]

Conclusion

Most of the knowledge and tools needed to prevent diarrhea-associated mortality in developing countries and especially persistent diarrhea are available. These require concerted and sustained implementation in public health programs.[62] Given the emerging evidence of the long-term impact of childhood diarrhea on developmental outcomes,[63] it is imperative that due emphasis is placed on prompt recognition and appropriate management of persistent diarrhea.

REFERENCES

1. Black RE, Morris SS, Bryce J. Where and why are 10 million children dying every year? *Lancet* 2003; **361**: 2226–2234.
2. Snyder JD, Merson MH. The magnitude of the global problem of acute diarrheal disease: a review of active surveillance data. *Bull World Heath Organ* 1982; **60**: 605–613.
3. Bern C, Martines J, Zoysa ID, Glass RI. The magnitude of the global problem of diarrheal disease: a ten year update. *Bull World Health Organ* 1992; **70**: 705–714.
4. Yusufzai M, Bhutta ZA. In Bhutta ZA, ed. *Contemporary Issues in Childhood Diarrhea and Malnutrition*. Oxford: Karachi, 1997.
5. Kosek M, Bern C, Guerrant RL. The global burden of diarrheal disease as estimated from studies published between 1990 and 2000. *Bull World Health Organ* 2003; **81**; 197–204.
6. Moore SR, Lima AA, Schorling JB et al. Changes over time in the epidemiology of diarrhea and malnutrition among children in an urban Brazilian shantytown, 1989 to 1996. *Int J Infect Dis* 2000; **4**: 179–186.
7. Bhan MK, Bhandari N, Sazawal S et al. Descriptive epidemiology of persistent diarrhea among young children in rural north India. *Bull World Health Organ* 1989; **67**: 281–288.
8. Khan SR, Jalil F, Zaman S et al. Early child health in Lahore, Pakistan: X. Mortality. *Acta Paediatr Suppl* 1993; **390**: 109–117.
9. Black RE, Brown KH, Becker S, Yunus M. Longitudinal studies of infectious diseases and physical growth of children in rural Bangladesh. I. Patterns of morbidity. *Am J Epidemiol* 1982; **115**: 305–314.
10. Lanata CF, Black RE, Gilman RH et al. Epidemiologic, clinical, and laboratory characteristics of acute vs persistent diarrhea in periurban Lima, Peru. *J Pediatr Gastroenterol Nutr* 1991; **12**: 82–88.
11. Mahmud A, Jalil F, Karlberg J, Lindblad BS. Early child health in Lahore, Pakistan: VII. Diarrhea. *Acta Paediatr Suppl* 1993; **390**: 79–85.
12. Bhutta ZA, Hendricks KM. Nutritional management of persistent diarrhea in childhood: a perspective from the developing world. *J Pediatr Gastroenterol Nutr* 1996; **22**: 17–37.
13. Briend A. Is diarrhea a major cause of malnutrition among under-fives in developing countries? A review of available evidence. *Eur J Clin Nutr* 1990; **44**: 611–628.
14. Fauveau V, Henry FJ, Briend A et al. Persistent diarrhea as a cause of childhood mortality in rural Bangladesh. *Acta Paediatr Suppl* 1992; **381**: 12–14.
15. Baqui AH, Black RE, Sack RB et al. Malnutrition, cell-mediated immune deficiency and diarrhea: a community-based longitudinal study in rural Bangladeshi children. *Am J Epidemiol* 1993; **137**: 355–365.
16. Azim T, Ahmad SM, Sefat-E-Khuda et al. Immune response of children who develop persistent diarrhea following rotavirus infection. *Clin Diagn Lab Immunol* 1999; **6**: 690–695.
17. Raqib R, Mia SM, Qadri F et al. Innate immune responses in children and adults with Shigellosis. *Infect Immun* 2000; **68**: 3620–3629.
18. Taniguchi K, Rikimaru T, Yartey JE et al. Immunological background in children with persistent diarrhea in Ghana. *Pediatr Int* 1999; **41**: 162–167.
19. Amadi B, Kelly P, Mwiya M et al. Intestinal and systemic infection, HIV, and mortality in Zambian children with persistent diarrhea and malnutrition. *J Pediatr Gastroenterol Nutr* 2001; **32**: 550–554.
20. Tumwine JK, Kekitiinwa A, Nabukeera N et al. *Enterocytozoon bieneusi* among children with diarrhea attending Mulago Hospital in Uganda. *Am J Trop Med Hyg* 2002; **67**: 299–303.
21. Chokephaibulkit K, Wanachiwanawin D, Tosasuk K et al. Intestinal parasitic infections among human immunodeficiency virus-infected and -uninfected children hospitalized with diarrhea in Bangkok, Thailand. *Southeast Asian J Trop Med Public Health* 2001; **32**: 770–775.
22. Sullivan PB, Marsh MN, Mirakian R et al. Chronic diarrhea and malnutrition – histology of the small intestinal lesion. *J Pediatr Gastroenterol Nutr* 1991; **12**: 195–203.
23. Shiner M, Nichols VN, Barrish JP, Nichols BL. Pathogenesis of small-intestinal mucosal lesions in chronic diarrhea of infancy: II. An electron microscopic study. *J Pediatr Gastroenterol Nutr* 1990; **11**: 464–480.
24. Fagundes-Neto U, De Martini-Costa S, Pedroso MZ, Scaletsky IC. Studies of the small bowel surface by scanning electron microscopy in infants with persistent diarrhea. *Braz J Med Biol Res* 2000; **33**: 1437–1442.
25. Manuel PD. The role of cow's milk protein intolerance in chronic diarrhea in a developing community. In Walker-Smith JA, McNeish AS, eds. *Diarrhea and Malnutrition in Childhood*. London: Butterworth, 1986: 193–199.
26. Lunn PG, Northrop-Clewes CA, Downes RM. Chronic diarrhea and malnutrition in the Gambia: studies on intestinal permeability. *Trans R Soc Trop Med Hyg* 1991; **85**: 8–11.
27. Sullivan PB, Lunn PG, Northrop-Clewes C et al. Persistent diarrhea and malnutrition – the impact of treatment on small bowel structure and permeability. *J Pediatr Gastroenterol Nutr* 1992; **14**: 208–215.
28. Jakobsson I. Intestinal permeability in children of different ages and with different gastrointestinal diseases. *Pediatr Allergy Immunol* 1993; **4**(Suppl 3): 33–39.

29. Holm S, Lindberg T, Gothefors L. Macromolecular absorption during and after gastroenteritis in children. *Acta Pediatr Scand* 1992; **81**: 585–588.
30. Okeke IN, Nataro JP. Enteroaggregative *Escherichia coli*. *Lancet Infect Dis* 2001; **1**: 304–313.
31. Unicomb LE, Banu NN, Azim T et al. Astrovirus infection in association with acute, persistent and nosocomial diarrhea in Bangladesh. *Pediatr Infect Dis J* 1998; **17**: 611–614.
32. Fraser D, Dagan R, Porat N et al. Persistent diarrhea in a cohort of Israeli Bedouin infants: role of enteric pathogens and family and environmental factors. *J Infect Dis* 1998; **178**: 1081–1088.
33. Germani Y, Minssart P, Vohito M et al. Etiologies of acute, persistent, and dysenteric diarrheas in adults in Bangui, Central African Republic, in relation to human immunodeficiency virus serostatus. *Am J Trop Med Hyg* 1998; **59**: 1008–1014.
34. Sazawal S, Black RE, Bhan MK et al. Zinc supplementation in young children with acute diarrhea in India. *N Engl J Med* 1995; **333**: 839–844.
35. Bhutta ZA, Nizami SQ, Isani Z. Zinc supplementation during persistent diarrhoea of childhood in Pakistan. *Pediatrics* 1999; **103**: e42.
36. Roy SK, Tomkins AM, Mahalanabis D et al. Impact of zinc supplementation on persistent diarrhoea in malnourished Bangladeshi children. *Acta Paediatr* 1998; **87**: 1235–1239.
37. Bhutta ZA, Bird SM, Black RE et al. Therapeutic effects of oral zinc in acute and persistent diarrhea in children in developing countries: pooled analysis of randomized controlled trials. *Am J Clin Nutr* 2000; **72**: 1516–1522.
38. Bhutta ZA, Molla AM, Isani Z et al. Nutrient absorption and weight gain in persistent diarrhoea: comparison of a traditional rice–lentil–yogurt–milk diet with soy formula. *J Pediatr Gastroenterol Nutr* 1994; **18**: 45–52.
39. Sodemann M, Jakobsen MS, Molbak K et al. Episode-specific risk factors for progression of acute diarrhoea to persistent diarrhoea in west African children. *Trans R Soc Trop Med Hyg* 1999; **93**: 65–68.
40. Mahmud MA, Hossain MM, Huang DB et al. Sociodemographic, environmental and clinical risk factors for developing persistent diarrhoea among infants in a rural community of Egypt. *J Health Popul Nutr* 2001; **19**: 313–319.
41. Vaidya U, Bhave S, Pandit A. Parenteral nutrition in the management of severe protracted diarrhea. *Indian J Pediatr* 1993; **60**: 19–24.
42. Illig KA, Ryan CK, Hardy DJ et al. Total parenteral nutrition-induced changes in gut mucosal function: atrophy alone is not the issue. *Surgery* 1992; **112**: 631–637.
43. Sarac TP, Souba WW, Miller JH et al. Starvation induces differential small bowel luminal amino acid transport. *Surgery* 1994; **116**: 679–686.
44. Lo CW, Walker WA. Chronic protracted diarrhea in infancy: a nutritional disease. *Pediatrics* 1983; **72**: 786–800.
45. Lima AA, Moore SR, Barboza MS Jr et al. Persistent diarrhea signals a critical period of increased diarrhea burdens and nutritional shortfalls: a prospective cohort study among children in northeastern Brazil. *J Infect Dis* 2000; **181**: 1643–1651.
46. Bhutta ZA, Nizami SQ, Thobani S. Factors determining recovery during nutritional therapy of persistent diarrhoea: the impact of diarrhoea severity and intercurrent infections. *Acta Paediatrica* 1997; **86**: 796–802.
47. Alam NH, Faruque AS, Dewan N et al. Characteristics of children hospitalized with severe dehydration and persistent diarrhoea in Bangladesh. *J Health Popul Nutr* 2001; **19**: 18–24.
48. Amadi B, Mwiya M, Musuku J et al. Effect of nitazoxanide on morbidity and mortality in Zambian children with cryptosporidiosis: a randomised controlled trial. *Lancet* 2002; **360**: 1375–1380.
49. Sarker SA, Mahalanabis D, Alam NH et al. Reduced osmolarity oral rehydration solution for persistent diarrhea in infants: a randomized controlled clinical trial. *J Pediatr* 2001; **138**: 532–538.
50. Dutta P, Mitra U, Dutta S et al. Hypo-osmolar oral rehydration salts solution in dehydrating persistent diarrhoea in children: double-blind, randomized, controlled clinical trial. *Acta Paediatr* 2000; **89**: 411–416.
51. Bhutta ZA, Molla AM, Isani Z et al. Dietary management of persistent diarrhoea: comparison of a traditional rice–lentil based diet with soy formula. *Pediatrics* 1991; **88**: 1010–1018.
52. Ashraf H, Ahmed S, Fuchs GJ, Mahalanabis D. Persistent diarrhoea: associated infection and response to a low lactose diet. *J Trop Pediatr* 2002; **48**: 142–148.
53. International Working Group on Persistent Diarrhea. Evaluation of the efficacy of an algorithm for the treatment of persistent diarrhea: a multicentre study. *Bull World Health Organ* 1996; **74**: 479–489.
54. Amadi B. Role of food antigen elimination in treating children with persistent diarrhea and malnutrition in Zambia. *J Pediatr Gastroenterol Nutr* 2002; **34** (Suppl 1): S54–S56.
55. Rabbani GH, Teka T, Zaman B et al. Clinical studies in persistent diarrhea: dietary management with green banana or pectin in Bangladeshi children. *Gastroenterology* 2001; **121**: 554–560.
56. Mahalanabis D, Bhan MK. Micronutrients as adjunct therapy of acute illness in children: impact on the episode outcome and policy implications of current findings. *Br J Nutr* 2001; **85** (Suppl 2): S151–S158.
57. Rahman MM, Vermund SH, Wahed MA et al. Simultaneous zinc and vitamin A supplementation in Bangladeshi children: randomised double blind controlled trial. *BMJ* 2001; **323**: 314–318.
58. Khatun UH, Malek MA, Black RE et al. A randomized controlled clinical trial of zinc, vitamin A or both in undernourished children with persistent diarrhea in Bangladesh. *Acta Paediatr* 2001; **90**: 376–380.
59. Villamor E, Mbise R, Spiegelman D et al. Vitamin A supplements ameliorate the adverse effect of HIV-1, malaria, and diarrheal infections on child growth. *Pediatrics* 2002; **109**: E6.
60. Bhandari N, Bahl R, Saxena M et al. Prognostic factors for persistent diarrhoea managed in a community setting. *Indian J Pediatr* 2000; **67**: 739–745.
61. Valentiner-Branth P, Steinsland H, Santos G et al. Community-based controlled trial of dietary management of children with persistent diarrhea: sustained beneficial effect on ponderal and linear growth. *Am J Clin Nutr* 2001; **73**: 968–974.
62. Jones GR, Steketee RW, Black RE, Bhutta ZA, Morris SS and the Bellagio Child Survival Study Group. How many child deaths can we prevent this year? *Lancet* 2003; **362**: 65–71.
63. Niehaus MD, Moore SR, Patrick PD et al. Early childhood diarrhea is associated with diminished cognitive function 4 to 7 years later in children in a northeast Brazilian shantytown. *Am J Trop Med Hyg* 2002; **66**: 590–593.

13 Small-bowel bacterial overgrowth

Mauro Batista de Morais and Ulysses Fagundes-Neto

Introduction

Small-bowel bacterial overgrowth (SBBO) is characterized by the colonization of the small intestine by bacteria that are normally found only in the colonic microbiota.

In the literature, SBBO has received many names such as 'the blind loop syndrome',[1] 'stagnant loop syndrome',[2] 'small intestinal stasis syndrome',[3] and the 'contaminated small bowel syndrome'.[4]

Initially, SBBO descriptions predominated in patients with surgical or anatomical abnormalities, and later SBBO was recognized in children who did not present anatomical abnormalities, in situations such as protein–energy malnutrition, acute diarrhea, persistent diarrhea and environmental enteropathy. These findings characterize SBBO as an important public health problem, occurring especially in the pediatric population in less-developed countries. SBBO can cause asymptomatic intestinal malabsorption and/or chronic diarrhea and may be associated with protein–energy malnutrition and stunting.

Etiology

SBBO is a syndrome that can cause functional and morphological abnormalities of the digestive tract, resulting in a disturbance in the homeostasis of the bacterial flora in the small intestine and a consequent imbalance of the mechanisms that control the flora.[5,6] Therefore, for better understanding of the development of SBBO, the microflora that is normally found in the digestive tract and its regulatory mechanisms are briefly described.

It is generally accepted that the upper digestive tract (stomach, duodenum, jejunum) is sterile, as found in 70% of the population, or may present a scarce microflora made up of facultative microorganisms, predominantly Gram-positive bacteria. The concentration of bacteria (*Streptococcus, Lactobacillus,* aerobes and diphtheroids) and yeast is normally no greater than 10^4 colonies/ml in the fluid of the small bowel. These micro-organisms come from the oral cavity, colonizing the upper small intestine after surviving the gastric juice. The terminal portion of the ileum comprises a transition zone and the microbiota begins to change with the appearance of Gram-negative bacteria, such as coliforms and bacteroids. The ileocecal valve acts as a true barrier, separating the Gram-positive species, which predominate in the upper small intestine, from the Gram-negative species, which inhabit the colon, where the anaerobic bacterial population represents the main portion of colonic microflora. Bacteroids, anaerobic *Lactobacilli* and *Clostridium* spp are the main components of the colonic flora and exist in concentrations ranging between 10^8 and 10^{11} colonies/ml, surpassing the facultative or aerobic microflora in a proportion of 1000–10 000 : 1. Table 13.1 shows the microflora of various segments of the digestive tract.[5–7]

The maintenance of the intestinal microbiota with the characteristics mentioned above depends upon the action of various regulatory mechanisms, such as diet, digestive tube motility, gastric acidity, the intestinal immunological system and the integrity of the ileocecal valve.[5,6]

Diet type

Animals raised in sterile environmental conditions, including feed, are different from animals raised under normal conditions that present digestive tract colonization. Animals free of bacteria

Table 13.1 Microflora of the digestive tract

Site	Concentration of micro-organisms/ml	Description
Stomach, duodenum, jejunum, proximal ileum	$<10^4$	mostly Gram-positive, *Streptococcus, Lactobacillus,* diphtheroids and yeast
Distal ileum	$10^5 - 10^8$	besides organisms of the proximal digestive tract, Gram-negative, *Bacteroides* and coliforms
Colon	$10^9 - 10^{11}$	mostly anaerobic bacteria, 95% *Bacteroides, Clostridium* and bifidobacteria
Stool	10^{12}	same as the colon

present a dilated cecum, underdeveloped lymphatic tissue and reduced levels of immunoglobulins in the serum. The intestinal wall of these animals is thinner, and lymphoplasmocytic infiltration is not observed in the lamina propria as in animals raised in normal environments, which present digestive tube colonization.[1,5] In the human being, during gestation, the intestine of the fetus is sterile. Shortly after birth, the intestine of the newborn is rapidly colonized by bacteria from the vaginal canal of the mother and from the environment. However, the bacterial flora also depends on the type of milk used in the diet. In infants who receive breast milk, *Lactobacillus bifidus* predominates and represents from 95% to 99% of the bacteria in the intestinal lumen. When an unweaned infant is fed with milk-based formulas, in addition to the bifidobacteria, bacteroids and anaerobes also appear.[5,7]

It is noteworthy that coprophagous animals present a greater number of bacteria in the proximal small intestine than do humans, but in the colon the number of bacteria is similar.[6] Under suitable environmental conditions, especially when climatic conditions are favorable, humans may ingest food with higher quantities of bacteria that are able to defeat the antibacterial barriers of the digestive tube.[6] Bacterial contamination of the lacteal contents of feeding bottles prepared in households for infants is observed frequently in developing countries, and is more frequent in families of low socioeconomic status.[8]

Gastric acid secretion

Gastric acid secretion is considered one of the most important factors for the regulation of small-intestine microflora, because it destroys a large amount of the bacteria that come from the oral cavity or from ingested food. In patients with hypochlorhydria or achlorhydria, secondary to gastrectomy or the use of antacids, an increase in the number of proximal small-intestine bacteria can be observed. In the small intestine, the digestive pancreatic and biliary secretions work together to control the intestinal microbiota.[5,6]

Digestive tract motility

Propelling peristaltic movements in the craniocaudal direction plays an important role in the maintenance of intestinal microbiota. Dixon's classic study[9] demonstrated, by inoculating the intestinal lumen with a mixture of erythrocytes marked with radioactive chromium and bacteria, that peristaltic movements are fundamental in the elimination of these elements. The integrity of the autonomic nervous system and the intestinal musculature are fundamental for the maintenance of intestinal motility. For example, in intestinal pseudo-obstruction syndrome, which is associated with profound abnormalities of intestinal motility, SBBO is frequent.[10]

Intestinal mucosal immunity

Intestinal mucosal immune responses are different from those that occur systemically. One of the fundamental differences is the production of immunoglobulin A (IgA), which is secreted in the intestine. IgA is the main class of antibodies produced in the intestine, as illustrated by the larger number of IgA-producing cells: a proportion of 20 for each IgG-producing cell and three for each producing IgM. Secretory IgA differs from serum IgA, as it is in dimeric form, created by the secretory piece, which confers resistance against proteolysis in the intestinal lumen. Secretory IgA can impede the adherence of micro-organisms to the surface of enterocytes, an important control mechanism to prevent SBBO. It is important to emphasize that newborns have a smaller population of plasma cells in the lamina propria, which explains their reduced ability to respond to local antigenic stimuli. At this stage of life, the colostrum and mother's milk are rich in secretory IgA and play an important role in the newborn's defense mechanism.[5,7,11]

Ileocecal valve

This valve acts as a barrier separating Gram-positive bacteria that inhabit the proximal small intestine from the Gram-negative bacteria and anaerobes that comprise the colonic bacterial flora. In the absence of the ileocecal valve due to intestinal resection, a retrograde colonization of the small intestine with bacteria that are normally found only in the colon is observed.[6]

SBBO develops when an alteration of one or more of the intestinal mucosa regulatory mechanisms occurs. Theoretically, bacteria responsible for SBBO may come either from the environment, by the ingestion of contaminated food or water, or from the colonic microflora itself, as a result of proximal colonization due to intestinal motility disturbances or ileocecal valve functional insufficiency.

Pathophysiology

In patients with SBBO, functional and/or morphological alterations can be observed, owing to the capacity of these bacteria to promote deconjugation of bile salts, such as 7α-dehydroxylation, which transforms them into secondary bile salts. The deconjugation of bile salts causes a reduction in the capacity to form mixed micelle, which is important in the process of lipid digestion and absorption, because the concentration in the intestinal lumen does not achieve a critical micellar concentration. Therefore, lower solubility of fats in the diet causing steatorrhea is observed. On the other hand, the secondary bile acids (deoxycholic and lithocholic) have a large capacity to provoke lesions in the intestinal mucosa, causing partial villous atrophy that may be associated with the secretion of electrolytes and malabsorption of glucose.[5,12,13]

Patients with SBBO also present reduced absorption of carbohydrates from the diet by:

(1) Metabolism of carbohydrates by the SBBO bacteria, which generates short-chain fatty acids (acetic, propionic and butyric acids) and gases, such as hydrogen, which, after diffusion through the intestinal mucosa, pass through to the circulatory system and reach the lungs, where they are eliminated in respiration.

(2) Reduction in the activity of disaccharidases due to alterations in the ultrastructure of the small intestine.

Consequently, the unabsorbed carbohydrates remain in the intestinal lumen in their original form or in the form of short-chain fatty acids as a result of bacterial fermentation, generating osmotic pressure that promotes the secretion of water into the intestinal lumen.[5,11]

Evidence also exists of a reduction in protein digestion and absorption from the diet due to intraluminal protein catabolism as well as a reduction in the transport and uptake of amino acids by the intestinal mucosa.[5,11]

SBBO may also cause malabsorption of liposoluble vitamins A and D accompanied by steatorrhea. Reduction in the absorption of vitamin B_{12} may

Table 13.2 Probable effects of bacterial overgrowth

Intraluminal	Mucosal	Systemic
Bile salt deconjugation	Deficiency of disaccharidases	Absorption of bacterial toxins and antigens
Decrease of the biliary salt 'pool'	Enterocyte damage	Hepatic inflammation
Steatorrhea	Inflammation	Immune complex formation
Vitamin B_{12} malabsorption	Protein loss	Vasculitis
Production of short-chain fatty acids	Bleeding	Polyarthritis

occur, owing to the consumption of vitamins by bacteria present in the intestinal lumen, especially *Bacteroides*.[5,11]

Systemic effects of SBBO are associated with the absorption of antigens and bacterial products through the injured intestinal mucosa.[6] Table 13.2 lists the effects of an overgrowth of bacteria on its host.

Diagnosis

Research to characterize the digestive tract microflora has developed mainly from the 1960s onward. The micro-organisms of the digestive tube flora, made up of aerobic and anaerobic bacteria, protozoa and even some viruses, form a complex ecosystem. The terms 'indigenous flora' and 'microbiota' are used as synonyms for normal flora and refer to micro-organisms that can be found in normal individuals. Therefore, in order to establish a diagnosis for SBBO, it is necessary to define the location, the count and the type of bacteria found. In general, studies regarding normal flora have been carried out by analyzing fluid collected by intubation of the Treitz angle region. Dickman et al[14] studied the intestinal fluid of 22 healthy individuals, finding 10^3 bacteria/ml in 16 of them and 10^4 bacteria/ml in two individuals. In another study, Thadepalli et al[15] found up to 10^4 bacteria/ml in six of 28 individuals. Fagundes-Neto et al[16] evaluated the small-bowel microflora in children who were not undernourished or presenting diarrhea, and found similar numbers of bacteria.

Many authors[17–27] characterize SBBO based on bacterial count, without taking into consideration the family or genus of these micro-organisms. According to this quantitative principle, various cut-off points can be found in the literature:

(1) $\geq 10^4$ bacteria/ml;[17–21]

(2) $\geq 10^5$ bacteria/ml;[22–25]

(3) $\geq 10^6$ bacteria/ml.[26,27]

Other authors[28,29] have used criteria that take into consideration the family as well as the number of the bacteria, characterizing SBBO when $\geq 10^3$ coliforms and aerobic or anaerobic enterobacteria/ml are found in the intestinal fluid.

Finally, there is a group of authors that considers SBBO to be the presence, in any concentration, of aerobic or anaerobic bacteria of the colonic microflora.[16,30–33]

In spite of the lack of consensus on the interpretation of results, the intestinal fluid culture is considered the gold standard test for the diagnosis of SBBO.[6,22,28] However, the invasive character of duodenal intubation and the high cost of aerobic and anaerobic microbiological study have driven research into lower cost, non-invasive methods, of which the hydrogen breath test has shown itself to be the most important.

The basic principle of the hydrogen breath test is the fermentation of carbohydrates by bacteria present in the intestinal lumen, which generates, among other products, hydrogen. After it diffuses through the intestinal mucosa and reaches the lungs through the circulatory system, the hydrogen is eliminated in exhaled air. Normally, fermenting bacteria are found only in the colon: so, when an unabsorbed carbohydrate reaches the colon, it is fermented and the elimination of hydrogen through the breath occurs about 10 min after it reaches the large intestine. Under these circumstances, the carbohydrate must travel the entirety of the small intestine for it to begin to produce hydrogen. This orocecal transit time varies according to the type of carbohydrate and its concentration in the administered solution. The lactulose solution employed in the hydrogen breath test for SBBO diagnosis presents a mean orocecal transit time of approximately 90 min. When SBBO is present, bacterial fermentation occurs prematurely, while still in the small intestine, elevating the concentration of hydrogen in the breath in the samples collected in the 60 min following the ingestion of the carbohydrate. Ideally, when the unabsorbed carbohydrate reaches the colon, it will produce a second peak of hydrogen corresponding to its fermentation by the colonic flora. Thus, after the ingestion of a carbohydrate that is not absorbed, such as lactulose, in individuals with bacterial overgrowth, two peaks in hydrogen production are expected: the first is an early peak, generated by the bacteria of the SBBO, while the second is a late peak, due to the normal production of hydrogen in the colon, as illustrated in Figure 13.1. The other carbohydrate used in the hydrogen breath test is glucose. As glucose is, in ordinary circumstances, completely absorbed by the small intestine, there should be no delayed peak, except if the patient presents intestinal malabsorption of glucose associated with SBBO.[19,34–36]

Most studies relating the hydrogen breath test to the culture of intestinal fluid have been carried out in adults. However, common criteria were not used for the interpretation of intestinal fluid cultures, which is considered the gold standard for the characterization of SBBO. The main points of these studies are summarized in Table 13.3.[22,26,35,37–39]

To our knowledge, only six studies have been carried out in children. Davidson et al[40] studied nine children aged 2–34 months, and characterized SBBO as the presence of more than 10^4 bacteria/ml in duodenal fluid. Lactose, sucrose and lactulose were used as substrates. SBBO was deter-

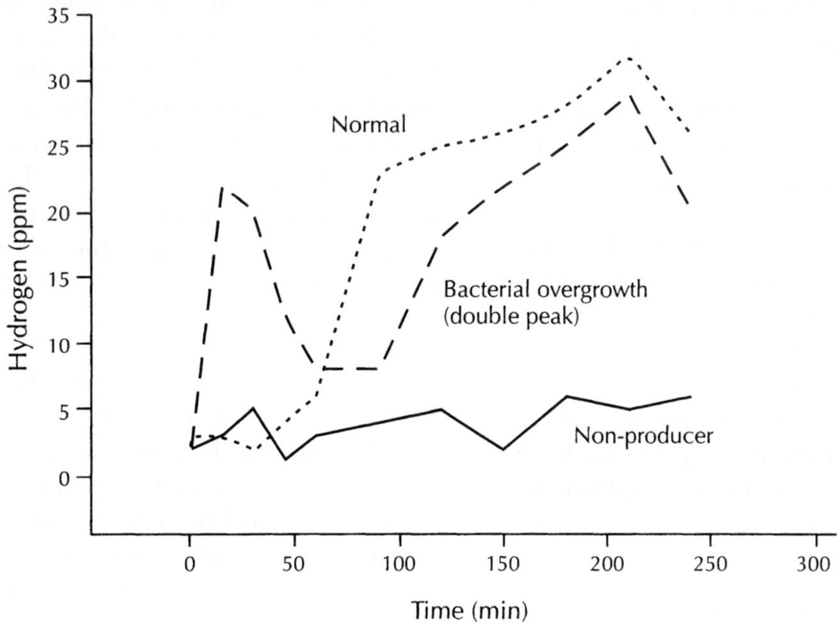

Figure 13.1 Schematic representation of possible results of the hydrogen breath test with lactulose.

Table 13.3 Studies in adults evaluating the diagnostic performance of the hydrogen breath test for the diagnosis of small-bowel bacterial overgrowth

Authors and reference	Number of patients	Probe	Criteria for bacterial overgrowth*	Sensitivity (%)	Specificity (%)
King and Toskes[26]	20	lactulose 10g	>10ppm	61	41
Kerlin and Wong[37]	45	glucose 50g	>12ppm	93	78
Corazza *et al*[35]	77	lactulose 12g	>10ppm	68	44
Riordan *et al*[38]	42	lactulose 10g	>16ppm	20	75
Riordan *et al*[22]	28	lactulose 10g	>10ppm	16	70
MacMahon *et al*[39]	30	glucose 50g	>10ppm	75	30

*Increment of breath hydrogen concentration before colonic peak

mined by the presence of a double peak. Boissieu et al[41] studied cultures of intestinal fluid and the hydrogen breath test after administering glucose to five children. A study carried out by Khin-Maung et al,[27] with 19 children aged from 3 to 5 years, considered SBBO to be a concentration of more than 10^6 bacteria/ml in the enteral fluid. After ingestion of 10g of lactulose, an increase of more than 10ppm in samples collected after 20, 40 and 60min was considered indicative of SBBO. Only two of the children with positive cultures presented a hydrogen breath test indicative of SBBO. Furthermore, three of the nine children with positive cultures did not present a positive hydrogen breath test indicative of SBBO.

Marcelino[42] carried out a study in our institution and observed that only three of 18 unweaned infants, with acute or persistent diarrhea and SBBO, according to an intestinal fluid culture of the small intestine, presented a rise in breath hydrogen of more than 20ppm after the ingestion of 10g of lactulose. It should be pointed out that almost 80% of the unweaned infants studied were not hydrogen producers and many presented secondary lactose malabsorption.

Guno et al[43] studied SBBO in 31 infants with ages ranging from 2 to 24 months suffering from protein–energy malnutrition. The culture of the small-bowel fluid revealed that SBBO was present in ten of the 31 patients. The sensitivity and specificity of the hydrogen breath test using lactulose was 72% and 90%, respectively, while the scores for the hydrogen breath test using glucose were 55% and 90%, respectively. The authors did not include criteria for interpretation of the breath test.

Silva[33] compared the results of the culture of aerobic and anaerobic organisms in the intestinal fluid of 31 children, with ages ranging from 6 months to 16 years, with the increase in breath hydrogen after the ingestion of 10g of lactulose. SBBO was characterized by the presence of any bacterium from the colonic flora in the duodenum, and was found in 16 (51.6%) of the 31 children. Given the minimum increase of 10ppm in breath hydrogen concentration in the samples collected up to 60min, the sensitivity of the hydrogen test was 75% and specificity 60%.

Analysis of the available information shows that both in adults and in children, irrespective of the carbohydrate that is used – lactulose or glucose – the occurrence of false-positive and false-negative results in the hydrogen breath test in relation to culture requires cautious application of this test in researching SBBO in a individual patient.

Another utilization of the hydrogen breath test is the analysis of groups of individuals in order to obtain information about the bacterial flora of the

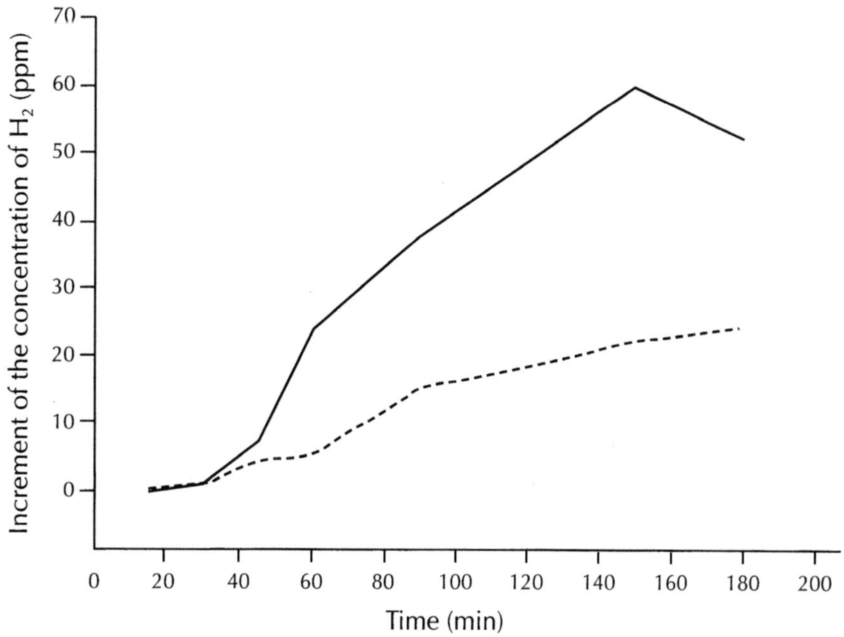

Figure 13.2 Median of the increment of the concentration of hydrogen in the expired air of 16 patients with bacterial overgrowth (unbroken line) and in 15 patients without bacterial overgrowth (dotted line) according to culture of the intestinal fluid. Differences at 15 min, $p = 0.98$; 30 min, $p = 0.90$; 45 min, $p = 0.58$; 60 min, $p = 0.26$; 90 min, $p = 0.075$; 120 min, $p = 0.028$; 150 min, $p = 0.031$; 180 min, $p = 0.007$.

digestive tract in varying environmental conditions. The results obtained by Silva,[33] with two groups of children (15 with SBBO and 16 without SBBO) can, in this light, be reanalyzed differently. Figure 13.2 presents the median values of increases in hydrogen on expiration. It can be seen that the SBBO groups produced a greater amount of hydrogen after 60 min, and that there was a statistically significant difference in hydrogen increases at 120, 150 and 180 min of the test. The data suggest two possibilities: that individuals with SBBO may not present a double peak of hydrogen; or that the colonic flora of children with SBBO has a greater hydrogen-producing capacity. This is based on the observation that, at the beginning of the test, the difference in hydrogen production in expired breath in SBBO patients was lower than after 60 min of the test. This second aspect was further analyzed using the area under the curve as the basis for calculation. In the fasting sample until 60 min, the 16 patients with SBBO presented a median hydrogen production rate (720 ppm/min) not statistically different from the 15 patients without SBBO (923 ppm/min). In turn, from 60 to 180 min this parameter was significantly higher ($p = 0.017$) in SBBO patients (6943 ppm/min) compared to patients without SBBO (3074 ppm/min).

Clinical presentation

SBBO may be asymptomatic or may present with chronic diarrhea associated with malabsorption of macronutrients. SBBO may thus lead to or aggravate protein–energy malnutrition.[5,6] In children, SBBO has also been linked to recurrent abdominal pain that responded to antimicrobial treatment.[41]

Several disorders may predispose to the development of SBBO (Table 13.4). It is therefore crucial that in every child diagnosed with SBBO a careful work-up be performed, aimed at ruling out these underlying conditions.

We will focus here on SBBO associated with acute or persistent diarrhea and with environmental factors, given their high incidence and prevalence, particularly in young infants and in children living in unfavorable environments.

Table 13.4 Clinical conditions associated with small-bowel bacterial overgrowth

Anatomic abnormalities
Congenital intestinal obstruction
Acquired strictures and stenosis (e.g. Crohn's disease)
Intestinal fistula
Abnormalities of intestinal motility
Pseudo-obstruction syndrome
Scleroderma
Damage of the myenteric plexus
Post-surgery complications
Stasis of the afferent loop
Gastroenterostomy
Enteroenterostomy
Colectomy or jejunoileal anastomosis
Without anatomic abnormalities
Carbohydrate malabsorption
Immunological deficiency
Giardia infection
Acute and persistent diarrhea
Environmental enteropathy

Small-bowel bacterial overgrowth in acute and persistent diarrhea

In developing countries, these two conditions account for a major proportion of deaths in the early years of life, and it should be emphasized that mortality due to persistent infectious diarrhea is much greater than that due to its acute phase.[44,45] SBBO does occur in children with acute diarrhea and is considered one of the factors leading to its perpetuation. In the 1970s, Fagundes-Neto et al[46] and Albert et al[47] showed a raised incidence of SBBO in children with acute diarrhea. A later study by Penny et al[48] showed that SBBO was more frequent in children with persistent diarrhea (80%) than in acute diarrhea (40%). In a study carried out in Cuba, Cristia et al[49] observed a similar frequency of SBBO in unweaned infants who had been hospitalized with acute and persistent diarrhea. From a functional point of view, Coello Ramirez and Lifschitz[50] found a correlation between SBBO and malabsorption of carbohydrates.

Studies in Brazil[31,32,42] and in other countries[48] have shown an association between SBBO and severe acute diarrhea or persistent diarrhea caused by classic enteropathogenic *Escherichia coli*.

SBBO can thus be present in both acute and persistent diarrhea, aggravating the clinical manifestations of patients, and, in conjunction with other factors, prolonging its course. Being aware of this possibility is obviously necessary for proper and timely diagnostic and therapeutic interventions.

Small-bowel bacterial overgrowth in environmental enteropathy

In the 1960s, several studies in tropical countries showed that adults without clinical gastrointestinal manifestations presented histological changes in the small intestine and reduction of D-xylose absorption capacity, compared to healthy adults living in developed countries.[51,52] With regard to morphology, the abnormalities observed in the small intestine were reduced height of the intestinal villi and increased lymphoplasmocytic infiltrate in the lamina propria. The disorder was initially named tropical enteropathy. However, the possibility of a spontaneous normalization of the defect in D-xylose absorption after a change of environment, as observed in Indians and Pakistanis who moved to New York,[53] its close link with unfavorable environmental conditions, as well as the occurrence of this disorder in nontropical regions, led in the 1980s to a redefinition of this clinical condition as 'environmental enteropathy' by Fagundes-Neto et al.[54,55] Environmental enteropathy can thus be defined as a set of unspecific morphological and functional abnormalities of the small intestine that are potentially reversible with a change in environmental conditions. From the clinical standpoint, it may be asymptomatic or associated with chronic diarrhea or with recurrent bouts of diarrhea. Stunted growth and protein–energy malnutrition often occur, as a result of the combination of malabsorption and inadequate nutrition, related to underprivileged socioeconomic conditions. Environmental enteropathy may be associated with. SBBO. The high prevalence of SBBO in this disorder was confirmed by studies on slum-dwelling infants in the city of São Paulo,[56,57] including 40 unweaned infants without diarrhea but presenting blunted D-xylose absorption and histological abnormalities of the small intestinal mucosa. SBBO was found in 61.2% of such infants. Study of the intestinal ultrastructure in these patients showed several abnormalities, such as decreased number and fusion of microvilli, cytoplasmic vacuolization and derangement of the mitochondria and endoplasmic reticulum. Taken together, these data[56,57] showed that exposure to unsuitable environmental conditions can damage the intestinal digestive–absorptive functions.

Use of the hydrogen breath test with lactulose to characterize SBBO has enabled research into environmental enteropathy in larger numbers of children, leading to a social vision of the threat that SBBO represents to the infant population. Pereira et al[58] studied 340 children under 5 years of age and found SBBO in 27.2% of this population in a town in Australia.

In Brazil, several studies have been performed using the hydrogen breath test with lactulose to characterize SBBO associated with environmental enteropathy. One such study[59] involved 83 schoolchildren who lived in a rural area, an urban area and a slum (favela) area of a city in the interior of São Paulo State, south-east Brazil. SBBO was detected in 7.2% of the children investigated. In the same study, the proportion of SBBO in the slum-dwelling children (18.2%) was statistically higher than that of the non-slum-dwelling children, in whom SBBO was not identified. These data thus demonstrated an association between unsuitable environmental conditions and SBBO.[39]

Two studies performed in 5–10-year-old children are also of interest. The first[60] was carried out in Indian children living in a reservation in Mato Grosso do Sul and found SBBO in 11.5% of the 252 children studied. The second[61] compared 50 slum-dwelling children with 50 control children who lived in domiciles with adequate food and environmental conditions and came from families with a solid socioeconomic background. SBBO was investigated by means of the hydrogen breath test with lactulose (10 g) on one day and then with glucose (50 g) on the next. After excluding non-hydrogen-producing children, SBBO (increase of 20 ppm in hydrogen concentration in the first hour after ingestion of lactulose) was observed in 50.0% (23/46) of slum-dwelling children and in 2.2% (1/46) of control children. The hydrogen test with glucose did not enable characterization of greater frequency of SBBO in slum-dwelling children. Figure 13.3 displays the curves based on the average concentrations of hydrogen in exhaled air, showing that production of hydrogen in slum-dwelling children was greater than in the control group, indirectly indicating a greater quantity of lactulose-fermenting bacteria. On the other hand, the glucose test did not draw a distinction between the groups. The average (±SD) of the z-scores of weight for age (-0.45±0.95) and height for age (-0.66±1.05) of the slum-dwelling children were lower than those of the control group (+0.39 ±0.97 and +0.18±0.84, respectively); the difference was statistically significant and showed an association between SBBO and protein–energy malnutrition.[61]

The evidence presented shows that unfavorable environmental conditions with lack of basic sanitation or inadequate supply of treated water can prompt the consumption of contaminated water and food that cause episodes of acute infectious diarrhea. This chronic state of environmental aggression may then cause long-lasting abnormalities of intestinal function that by inducing environmental enteropathy, ends up by negatively impacting the health of a large portion of the world population.

Treatment

Treatment of SBBO depends fundamentally on the patient's general characteristics, especially on the presence of those clinical conditions listed in Table 13.3. Obviously, when possible, one should treat the predisposing conditions, improving factors to control bacterial flora.

In patients with clinical conditions associated with SBBO in whom treatment of the underlying disease does not always produce satisfactory results, such as in intestinal pseudo-obstruction syndrome and ileocecal valve resection, use of antibiotics is indicated.

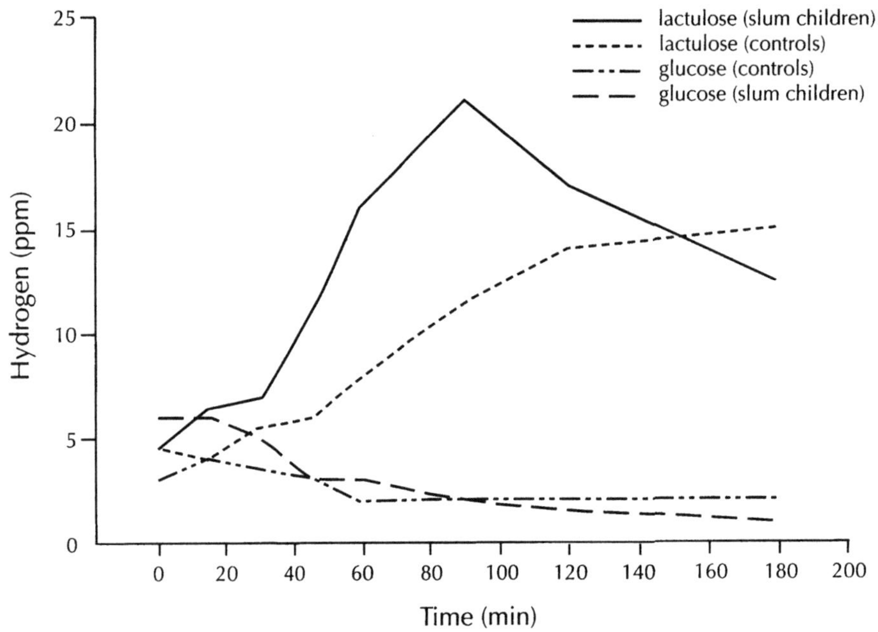

Figure 13.3 Median of the concentration of hydrogen in the expired air in the children living in a slum ($n = 50$) and controls ($n = 50$) after the administration of 10 g of lactulose and 50 g of glucose on different days.

Boissieu et al[41] observed the disappearance of symptoms attributed to SBBO, such as chronic abdominal pain and chronic diarrhea, after antibiotic therapy.

Lichtman[6] reviewed the literature in 2000 on the use of antibiotics in the treatment of SBBO. Most reports dealt with small groups of patients, with different underlying diseases predisposing towards SBBO; there were no controlled studies or series with a sufficient number of patients. Therefore, based on his own experience and in view of the scanty evidence from the literature, this author recommended the use of antibiotics effective against bacteroids, such as metronidazole, chloramphenicol and tetracycline. In children, an initial course of metronidazole for 2–4 weeks is considered the first choice.

In our practice, we normally prescribe courses of metronidazole and trimethoprim–sulfamethoxazole.

In the case of SBBO associated with severe acute diarrhea and with persistent diarrhea, a double-blind placebo-controlled study was carried out by our group to assess the effect of oral polymyxin for 7 days on the clinical course and on the proximal small-intestine fluid culture in 25 hospitalized infants.[32] Both groups were on the same basic and dietary treatments; pre-treatment rates of SBBO were 61.5% in the polymyxin group and 71.4% in the placebo group. Both groups had a satisfactory clinical course. SBBO, however, persisted after treatment in a high proportion of patients: 76.9% of those given polymyxin and 57.1% on the placebo (NS). However, in the group treated with polymyxin a reduced need for other antibiotics for suspected systemic infections was found ($p = 0.08$).

Recently, growing attention has been given to the possible use of probiotics in a variety of gastrointestinal disorders, including SBBO, and some preliminary evidence of possible efficacy is beginning to emerge. In fact, the risk of bacterial translocation in experimental short-bowel syndrome, a condition characterized by frequent episodes of SBBO, has been found to be reduced by the administration of *Bifidobacterium lactis* in rats.[62] Furthermore, two strains of lactobacilli (*Lactobacillus casei* and *L. acidophilus* strains cerela) have been found useful in the treatment of SBBO-related chronic diarrhea.[63]

When SBBO is associated with environmental enteropathy, there is no evidence that antibiotics can help control it; in addition, the chronic nature of the process with possible recurrences clearly discourages this type of treatment. However, environmental enteropathy shows spontaneous regression once appropriate environmental conditions are restored. It is obvious, therefore, that the mainstay for the approach to this socially relevant problem has to be through creating suitable living conditions for such a wide proportion of the world's children.

REFERENCES

1. Ellis H, Smith ADM. The blind loop syndrome. *Monogr Surg Sci* 1977; **4**: 193–197.
2. Gorbach SL, Tabaqchali S. Bacteria, bile and small bowel. *Gut* 1969; **10**: 963–972.
3. Ament MF, Shimoda SS, Sanders DP. Phatogenesis of steatorrhea in three cases of small intestinal stasis syndrome. *Gastroenterology* 1972; **63**: 728.
4. Gracey M. The contaminated small bowel symdrome: pathogenesis, diagnosis, and treatment. *Am J Clin Nutr* 1979; **32**: 234–243.
5. Fagundes Neto U. *Enteropatia Ambiental uma Conseqüência do Fracasso das Políticas de Saúde Pública.* Rio de Janeiro: Livraria e Editora Revinter Ltda; 1996.
6. Lichtman SN. Bacterial overgrowth. In Walker WA, Durie PT, Hamilton JR et al. *Pediatric Gastrointestinal Disease*, 3rd edn. Ontario: BC Decker, 2000: 569–581.
7. Araya M, Figueroa G. Flora residente intestinal. Funciones fisiológicas y alterações. *Rev Chil Pediatr* 1985; **56**: 490–496.
8. Morais TB, Morais MB, Sigulem DM. Bacterial contamination of the lacteal contents of feeding bottles in metropolitan. *Bull World Health Organ* 1998; **76**: 173–181.
9. Dixon JM. The fate of bacteria in the small intestine. *J Path Bact* 1960; **79**: 131–139.
10. Ament EM, Vargas J. Diagnóstico e tratamento da síndrome da pseudo-obstrução intestinal crônica na criança. In Fagundes Neto U, Wehba J, Pena FJ, eds. *Gastrenterologia Pediátrica*, 2nd edn. Rio de Janeiro: MEDSI, 1991: 349–368.
11. King CE, Tokes PP. Small intestine bacterial overgrowth. *Gastroenterology* 1979; **76**: 1035–1055.
12. Simon GL, Gorbach SL. Intestinal flora in health and disease. *Gastroenterology* 1984; **86**: 174–193.
13. Kocoshis AS, Scheletewitz K, Lovelace G, Laine AR. Duodenal bile acids among children: keto derivatives and aerobic small bowel bacterial overgrowth. *J Pediatr Gastroenterol Nutr* 1987; **6**: 686–696.
14. Dickman MD, Chappelka AR, Schaelder RW. The microbial ecology of the upper small bowel. *AJG* 1976; **65**: 57–62.
15. Thadepalli H, Ann Lou SM, Bach VT et al. Microflora of the human small intestine. *A J Surge* 1979; **138**: 845–850.
16. Fagundes Neto U, Reis MHL, Webha J et al. Small bowel bacterial flora in normal and in children with acute diarrhea. *Arq Gastroenterol São Paulo* 1980; **17**: 103–108.
17. Drasar BS, Shiner M. Studies on the intestinal flora: part II. Bacterial flora of the small intestine in patients with gastrointestinal disorders. *Gut* 1969; **10**: 812–819.
18. Isaacs PET, Kim YS. The contaminated small bowel syndrome. *Am J Med* 1979; **67**: 1049–1057.
19. Davidson GP, Butler RN. Breath analysis. In Walker WA, Durie PD, Hamilton JR et al., eds. *Pediatric Gastrointestinal Disease,* 3rd edn. Ontario: BC Decker, 2000: 1529–1537.
20. Kirsch M. Bacterial overgrowth. *Am J Clin Nutr* 1990; **85**: 231–237.
21. Suarez L, Perdomo M, Escobar H. Microflora bacteriana y ecosistema intestinal isiopatologia del intestino delgado contaminado. Diarréia aguda. Meio ambiente en Espana. *GEN* 1994; **48**: 61–64.
22. Riordan SM, Mciver CJ, Walker BM et al. The lactulose breath hydrogen test and small intestinal bacterial overgrowth. *Am J Gastroenterol* 1996; **91**: 1795–1803.
23. Bouhnik Y, Alain S, Attar A et al. Bacterial populations contaminating the upper gut in patients with small intestinal bacterial overgrowth syndrome. *Am J Gastroenterol* 1999; **94**: 1328–1331.
24. Attar A, Flourié B, Rambaud JC et al. Antibiotic efficacy in small intestinal bacterial overgrowth-related chronic diarrhea: a crossover, randomized trial. *Gastroenterology* 1999; **117**: 794–797.
25. Bardhan PK, Feger A, Kogon M et al. Urinary choloyl-PABA excretion in diagnosing small intestinal bacterial overgrowth. *Dig Dis Sci* 2000; **45**: 474–479.
26. King CE, Toskes PP. Comparison of the 1-Gram [^{14}C] xylose, 10-Gram lactulose-H_2, and 80-Gram glucose-H_2 breath test in patients with small intestine bacterial overgrowth. *Gastroenterology* 1986; **91**: 1447–1451.
27. Khin-Maung U, Tin-Ay, Ku-Tin M et al. *In vitro* hydrogen production by enteric bacteria cultured from children with small bowel bacterial overgrowth. *J Pediatr Gastroenterol Nutr* 1992; **14**: 192–197.
28. Rumessen JJ, Gudmand-Hoyer E, Bachmann E, Justesen T. Diagnosis of bacterial overgrowth of small intestine: comparison of the ^{14}C D-xylose breath test and jejunal cultures in 60 patients. *Scand J Gastroenterol* 1985; **20**: 1267–1275.
29. Farfán GF, Augusto CY, Raúl RL, Tello RC. Sobrepoblacion bacteriana del intestino delgado y diarrea cronica: estudo clínico y bacteriológico de 40 casos. *Diagnostico* 1991; **28**: 41–47.
30. Challacombe DN, Richardson MJ, Andersoon CM. Bacterial microflora of the upper gastrointestinal tract in infants without diarrhoea. *Arch Dis Child* 1974; **49**: 264–269.
31. Cruz AS, Fagundes Neto U. Influência da *Escherichia coli* enteropatogênica clássica sobre a proliferação bacteriana no intestino delgado na diarréia aguda e persistente do lactente. *Rev Ass Med Brasil* 1996; **42**: 89–94.

32. Tahan S. *O efeito de um antimicrobiano na microbiota duodenal e na evolução clínica de lactentes hospitalizados por diarréia aguda e persistente: um ensaio clínico duplo-cego randomizado.* Thesis, Universidade Federal de São Paulo, 2000.
33. Silva NS. *Cultura de bactérias aeróbias e anaeróbias e teste do hidrogênio no ar expirado no diagnóstico de sobrecrescimento bacteriano no intestino delgado.* Thesis, Universidade Federal de São Paulo, 2001.
34. Levitt MD, Bond JH. Volume, composition, and source of intestinal gas. *Gastroenterology* 1970; **59**: 921–929.
35. Corazza G, Menozzi GM, Strocchi A et al. The diagnosis of small bowel bacterial overgrowth. *Gastroenterology* 1990; **98**: 302–309.
36. Perman JA. Clinical application of breath hydrogen measurements. *Can J Physiol Phamacol* 1991; **69**: 111–115.
37. Kerlin P, Wong L. Breath hydrogen testing in bacterial overgrowth of the small intestine. *Gastroenterology* 1988; **95**: 982–988.
38. Riordan SM, Mciver CJ, Bolin TD, Duncombe VM. Fasting breath hydrogen concentrations in gastric and small-intestinal bacterial overgrowth. *Scand J Gastroenterol* 1995; **30**: 252–257.
39. MacMahon M, Gibbons N, Mullins E et al. Are hydrogen breath tests valid in the elderly? *Gerontology* 1996; **42**: 40–45.
40. Davidson GP, Robb TA, Kirubakaran CP. Bacterial contamination of the small intestine as an important cause of chronic diarrhea and abdominal pain: diagnosis by breath hydrogen test. *Pediatrics* 1984; **74**: 229–235.
41. Boissieu D, Chaussain M, Badoual J et al. Small-bowel bacterial overgrowth in children with chronic diarrhea, abdominal pain, or both. *J Pediatr* 1996; **128**: 203–207.
42. Marcelino RT. *Teste do hidrogênio no ar expirado no diagnóstico do sobrecrescimento bacteriano do intestino delgado.* Thesis, Universidade Federal de São Paulo, 1995.
43. Guno MJV, Nolasco ET, Rogacion JM et al. Small bowel bacterial overgrowth in severely malnourished filipino children using breath hydrogen tests. *J Pediatr Gastrentrol Nutr* 2000; **31**(Suppl 2): 240.
44. World Health Organization. Persistent diarrhoea in children in developing countries. Report of a WHO Meeting. *Bull World Health Organ* 1988; **66**: 709–717.
45. World Health Organization. Evalution of an algorithm for the treatment of persistent diarrhea: a multicentre study. *Bull World Health Organ* 1996; **74**: 479–489.
46. Fagundes Neto U, Toccalino H, Dujovney F. Stool bacterial aerobic overgrowth in the small intestine of children with acute diarrhoea. *Acta Paediatr Scand* 1976; **65**: 609–615.
47. Albert MJ, Bhat P, Rojand D et al. Jejunal microbial flora of Southern India infants in health and with acute gastroenteritis. *J Med Microbiol* 1978; **11**: 43–44.
48. Penny ME, Silva DGH, Mcneish AS. Bacterial contamination of the small intestine of infants with enteropathogenic *Escherichia coli* and other enteric infections: a factor in the aetiology of persistent diarrhoea? *Br Med J* 1986; **292**: 1223–1225.
49. Cristia YG, Arbelo TF, Vivanca MVP et al. Estudos de la microflora intestinal in niños com diarreia aguda y persistent. *GEN* 1994; **48**: 236–244.
50. Coello-Ramirez P, Lifschitz F. Enteric microflora and carbohydrate intolerance in infants with diarrhea. *Pediatrics* 1972; **49**: 233–242.
51. Sprinz H, Sribhibhadh R, Gangarosa et al. Biopsy of small bowel of Thai people. *Am J Clin Pathol* 1962; **38**: 43–51.
52. Klipstein FA. Recent advances in tropical malabsorption. *Scand J Gastroenterol Suppl* 1970; **6**: 93–114.
53. Gerson CD, Kent TH, Saha JR et al. Recovery of small-intestinal structure and function after residence in the tropics. II. Studies in Indians and Pakistanis living in New York City. *Ann Intern Med* 1971; **75**: 41–48.
54. Fagundes-Neto U, Viaro T, Wehba J et al. Enteropatia tropical: na infância: uma síndrome decorrente da contaminação ambiental (enteropatia ambiental). *J Pediatr (Rio de J)* 1983; **54**: 313–319.
55. Fagundes-Neto U, Viaro T, Wehba J et al. Tropical enteropathy (environmental enteropathy) in early childhood: a syndrome caused by contaminated environment. *J Trop Pediatr* 1984; **30**: 204–209.
56. Fagundes Neto U, Martins MCV, Lima FMLS et al. Symptomatic environmental enteropathy in infancy: bacterial proliferation, functional and morphological alterations of the small bowel. *Rev Hosp São Paulo Esc Paul Med* 1992; **4**: 64–70.
57. Gusmão RHP, Martins MCV, Gusmão SRB, Fagundes Neto U. Enteropatia ambiental: estudo ultra-estrutural da mucosa jejunal de criancas assintomaticas [Ambiental intestinal diseases: ultrastructure of the jejunum mucosa of asymptomatic children]. *J Pediatr (Rio de J)* 1993; **69**: 21–26.
58. Pereira SP, Khin-Maung U, Bolin TD et al. A pattern of breath hydrogen excretion suggesting small bowel bacterial overgrowth in Burmese village children. *J Pediatr Gastroenterol Nutr* 1991; **13**: 32–38.
59. Reis JC, Morais MB, Fagundes-Neto U. Teste do H_2 no ar expirado na avaliação de absorção de lactose e sobrecrescimento bacteriano no intestino delgado de escolares. *Arq Gastroenterol* 1999; **36**: 169–176.
60. Alves GMS, Morais MB, Fagundes-Neto U. Estado nutricional e teste do hidrogênio no ar expirado com lactose e lactulose em crianças indígenas terenas. *J Pediatr (Rio de J)* 2002; **78**: 113–119.
61. Reis JC. *Utilização da glicose e lactulose no diagnóstico de sobrecrescimento bacteriano no intestino delgado por meio do teste do hidrogênio no ar expirado.* Thesis, Universidade Federal de São Paulo, 2002.
62. Eizaguirre I, Urkia NG, Asensio AB et al. Probiotic supplementation reduces the risk of bacterial translocation in experimental short bowel syndrome. *J Pediatr Surg* 2002; **37**: 699–702.
63. Gaon D, Garmendia C, Murrielo NO et al. Effect of *Lactobacillus* strains (*L. casei* and *L. acidophillus* strains cerela) on bacterial overgrowth-related chronic diarrhea. *Med (Buenos Aires)* 2002; **62**: 159–163.

14 Functional abdominal pain and other functional bowel disorders

Miguel Saps and Carlo Di Lorenzo

Introduction

The classic definition of recurrent abdominal pain has been based on the work of Apley and Naish,[1] who described children who presented with intermittent episodes of abdominal pain occurring for at least 3 months without any identifiable cause and interfering with daily activities. The term 'chronic abdominal pain' is often used interchangeably with 'recurrent abdominal pain'. Chronic abdominal pain is abdominal pain that is continuous, persistent, or intermittent over a period of a few months. The pain may wax and wane, with some days being better than others.[2] On occasions, relatively short asymptomatic periods may be interposed with 'painful periods', but the episodes of wellness rarely last long, generating a condition that profoundly distresses the daily life of children and their families. It is important to emphasize that recurrent abdominal pain represents a description and not a diagnosis. Many conditions can cause abdominal pain that is recurrent, but in clinical practice most children and adolescents presenting with this symptom have a functional disorder without any evidence of organic disease. They are considered to have 'functional abdominal pain'. In this chapter we discuss conditions associated with functional alterations of the gastrointestinal (GI) system, called functional bowel disorders, and we only briefly describe those organic diseases causing abdominal pain (in the section dedicated to the differential diagnosis).

Epidemiology

Chronic abdominal pain is one of the most common pediatric complaints,[3] accounting for 2–4% all of pediatric office visits.[4] Symptoms consistent with irritable bowel syndrome (IBS), one of the most common functional bowel disorders, occur in 14% of all high-school students and 6% of all middle-school students.[5] IBS is more prevalent than other medical conditions such as hypertension, asthma and diabetes that tend to receive greater medical attention.[6] As many patients with IBS do not seek medical attention, assessing the prevalence of IBS is often difficult. Current estimates suggest that only one in four patients with symptoms of IBS seek medical care for their symptoms.[7] Population-based studies of adults have shown IBS-type symptoms in 13–15% of adult females, with abdominal pain reported as the most common complaint.[8] Reports from Kenya, Poland, Russia, India and Pakistan reveal that, although the relative frequency of an organic etiology for chronic pain may differ in various regions of the world, functional abdominal pain is probably a universal problem.[9–12] A Malaysian study in 1500 schoolchildren found evidence of chronic abdominal pain in 10% of children, concluding that, in spite of differences in diet, customs and culture, the overall prevalence of this entity was similar across regions.[13] A Danish study also demonstrated that 15% of children aged 9–12 years had recurrent abdominal pain.[14]

Quality of life in patients with IBS is substantially poorer than in the general population or in those suffering from asthma or migraine.[15] Costs related to functional bowel disorders are also enormous, with direct and indirect medical expenses associated with IBS being estimated as up to US$ 30 billion a year, comparable to those of asthma, stroke, hypertensive disease, migraine and arthritis.[16–18] IBS also has a high impact on a patient's productivity, as a result of missed working days.[19] A recent survey of adult patients suffering from

IBS showed that 15% believed that IBS would stop them from finding a long-term partner, 16% had turned down a date in fear of the embarrassment that may result from intimacy, and 17% stated that they had a relationship ending as a consequence of IBS.[20] The survey also revealed that 12% of respondents had to give up working, while 35% of employed respondents reported having lost work time due to IBS. In addition to the direct and indirect costs, IBS patients are affected by intangible costs and social stigma. In 14% of cases, IBS symptoms were not accepted as a valid reason for absence by their employers. One-third of the patients with IBS had refrained from applying for promotions for positions involving multiple meetings and presentations.[20]

Physiology of the gastrointestinal pain response

Visceral pain perception involves a complex pathway of peripheral and central nervous structures that encode, relay and modify the afferent stimulus.

The enteric nervous system (ENS) is organized into two major plexuses providing the intrinsic innervation of the gut. The plexuses and the nerves connecting them constitute a continuous network around the circumference of the GI tract and along its length. The myenteric plexus, also known as Auerbach's plexus, is situated between the external longitudinal and internal circular muscle layers, and the submucosal plexus (Meissner's plexus) lies between the circular muscle layer and the mucosa. The myenteric plexus is larger and projects fibers primarily to the smooth muscle of the gut controlling motility. Meanwhile, the submucosal plexus projects into the mucosa and submucosa and includes more sensory cells and the neurons that control gland secretion. Although the two intestinal plexuses are separated spatially, interconnections bind the two networks into a functionally unified nervous system. The characteristics of this mesh of sensory fibers, interneurons and motor neurons, enables this mini-brain or 'gut brain' to integrate the sensory information, organize the motor and secretory responses and influence the luminal absorption, producing a functional state that is adapted to the well-being of the individual. Although the ENS receives input from the central and autonomic nervous systems, it can function independently. The ENS performs most of its functions in the absence of central nervous system (CNS) control, locally integrating the information of intrinsic afferent fibers (for example, luminal distension and chemical stimuli) with efferent axons, resulting in motor reflexes or secretory or absorptive responses.

The extrinsic nervous system consists of afferent and efferent fibers connecting the ENS with the CNS. This communication allows the CNS continuously to integrate the information from the gastrointestinal tract with incoming information from other organs and from the environment, in order to initiate an adequate response. Under physiological conditions, most of these processes do not reach the level of conscious perception.[21] However, sensations that trigger a particular behavior, including hunger, satiety and need to defecate, reach the cortex. The constant influence of the CNS on the ENS through activation of a subset of vagal and sacral parasympathetic fibers is exemplified by the relation between psychological stress and gastrointestinal response, manifested clinically by the occurrence of vomiting or diarrhea in patients experiencing a stressful event.

The ENS and the brain use multiple neurotransmitters for chemical signaling and exchanging of inhibitory or excitatory information. They include excitatory neurotransmitters such as acetylcholine and substance P, and gut inhibitory neurotransmitters such as nitric oxide, ATP, vasoactive intestinal peptide (VIP), cholecystokinin, enkephalins, calcitonin gene-related peptide (CGRP), norepinephrine (noradrenaline), epinephrine (adrenaline) and others. Other neurotransmitters such as serotonin (5-hydroxytryptamine; 5-HT) and histamine have more complex effects. Ninety-five per cent of the total body 5-HT lies within the gut. Of the total gut 5-HT, 90% is found in the granules of the enteroendocrine cells, and 10% in the neurons of the myenteric plexus.[22,23] 5-HT plays a role in regulating GI motility and intestinal secretion.[22] 5-HT receptors appear to participate in mucosal sensory processing within the gut. Distension and stroking of mechanosensitive receptors in the enteroendocrine cells triggers the release of 5-HT.[24] There are at least seven main classes of 5-HT receptor and 22 subclasses that can be differentiated on the basis of structure and function. Four classes have been reported in the human GI tract (5-HT_1, 5-HT_2, 5-HT_3 and 5-HT_4).[25] Serotonin action is complex, with mixed effects ranging from smooth muscle contraction via cholinergic nerves, to relaxation through stimulation of inhibitory nitric oxide-releasing neurons. Higher levels of serotonin are present in diarrhea-predominant IBS.[26] The ENS has the ability to modulate signal transduction by enhancing or inhibiting the activation of nociceptors through alteration in smooth muscle tone and contractile activity. Visceral pain may be modulated also at the CNS level by emotional or cognitive factors, providing a rationale for the use of centrally acting agents or cognitive behavioral treatments in functional bowel disorders. Neuroimaging studies have provided information on differences in brain processing of visceral stimuli between normal individuals and those suffering from IBS, revealing an increased activity at the level of the anterior cingulated cortex, prefrontal cortex, insular cortex and thalamus (the areas associated with emotional responses) in patients with IBS compared to asymptomatic individuals.[27–29]

Pathophysiology

Several hypotheses have been put forward to explain the cause of functional recurrent abdominal pain. We examine them in the following sections.

Visceral hyperalgesia

The visceral hyperalgesia hypothesis proposes that greater sensitivity of visceral afferent pathways or central amplification of visceral input lead to an enhanced perception of visceral stimuli. There is evidence that the pain and discomfort of IBS might be due to hyperalgesia and allodynia of the gut. While in hyperalgesia a painful stimulus is perceived as even more painful, in allodynia a non-painful stimulus becomes painful.[30] A noxious stimulus applied to a particular area of the gut may sensitize primary afferent fibers and nociceptors of adjacent areas, causing painful sensations with a low-intensity stimulus, resulting in primary hyperalgesia.

Most IBS patients experience rectal discomfort at lower intraluminal volumes or pressures[31,32] and have diminished tolerance to intestinal gas.[33] Trimble et al[31] found that patients presenting with one functional bowel disorder frequently had additional symptoms referable to other parts of the digestive system, suggesting that enhanced visceral nociception may be a pan-intestinal phenomenon. For example, it has been reported that in addition to the features of rectal hyperalgesia, IBS patients have a decreased sensory threshold to balloon distension of the esophagus. Children with functional abdominal pain exhibited generalized visceral hyperalgesia, whereas IBS patients had rectal but not gastric hyperalgesia.[32] Different GI symptoms were reproduced by stimulation of the predominant site of hyperalgesia, providing a physiological explanation of symptoms in children who have distinct phenotypic presentations.

Dysmotility

In addition to a greater intestinal sensitivity, patients with functional bowel disorders may display abnormal motility. Various types of motor disturbances have been documented in IBS, apparently reflecting dysfunction at one or more levels of the brain–gut axis.[34] Although the pathophysiology of IBS is commonly attributed to dysfunction of the large intestine, evidence exists to incriminate the small bowel as well.[35] Postprandial motor dysfunction in the small bowel appears to be more prevalent among IBS patients who exhibit underlying visceral hypersensitivity in the fasting state. Abdominal cramping has been associated with the passage of high-amplitude contractions through the ileocecal region.[36] Bloating has been explained by an abnormal transit and pooling of gas in conjunction with gut hypersensitivity.[33] Manometric studies have demonstrated postprandial antral hypomotility in children and adults with functional dyspepsia.[37] However, not all studies have demonstrated differences between patients and control subjects.[38,39] Motility changes in IBS are neither specific nor predictable and do not serve as a diagnostic marker or as an aid to the selection of treatment.[40] It has been suggested than, rather than having a persistent motility abnormality, patients with functional bowel disorders exhibit an abnormal motor response to a variety of physiological stimuli.[41]

Brain–gut interaction

The shortcomings of isolated experimental or observational models in explaining the complex nature of functional bowel disorders have led research to focus on the alterations in the communications between the CNS and the GI tract, hence the term 'brain–gut' interaction.[6,42] There are multiple examples of brain–gut interaction, the most common being the subjects who, under emotionally stressful situations, develop diarrhea, nausea or vomiting. Anger and aggression increase colonic motility, while hopelessness results in decreased motility.[43] The brain–gut model links alterations in peripheral sensory afferent communication from the gut (e.g. visceral hyperalgesia) to CNS processing of the sensory stimuli and its efferent signaling to the gut. In IBS patients multiple studies have shown that both gut and brain show an exaggerated responsiveness to different stimuli. Patients with IBS have significantly greater electroencephalogram (EEG) abnormalities than controls.[44] Dynamic brain imaging technologies such as positron emission tomography (PET) and functional magnetic resonance imaging (fMRI) have recently been applied to the study of the gut–brain axis in order to identify the areas of the brain activated by visceral sensations. Studies with these techniques have suggested an abnormal cerebral processing of visceral stimuli in patients with functional bowel disorders.[27,28]

Inflammation

There is evidence that IBS can occur following a gastrointestinal infection resulting in transient inflammation. Gwee et al reported that 20–25% of patients admitted to the hospital for bacterial gastroenteritis developed symptoms consistent with IBS in the first 3 months.[45] Rectal biopsies prospectively obtained during and after acute gastroenteritis from patients who developed post-infectious IBS and a control group, showed that the former group exhibited significantly greater expression of interleukin (IL)-1β mRNA.[46] A recent study examining full-thickness biopsies from the jejunum of patients with severe IBS revealed inflammation and neuronal degeneration in the myenteric plexus, suggesting a possible pathogenetic role of inflammation.[47] Animal studies also seem to indicate that inflammation may produce persistent neuromuscular gut dysfunction.[48] Mild mucosal inflammation may perturb neuromuscular function also at remote non-inflamed sites. The gut dysfunction may persist even after reduction of the mucosal inflammation. Substances that mediate these changes are not fully understood, but there is growing recognition of the role of serotonin as a sensitizing agent.

Immunity

The mucosal immune system mediates the clinical impact of stress and other psychological factors on the gut. Vagal afferents can be activated by products of mast cell degranulation, resulting in sensitization of silent nociceptors. Mast cell mediators may be released in response to luminal macromolecules, a phenomenon that could explain brain–immune system interactions within the gut. A descending input by the vagus nerve may also reciprocally affect mast cell degranulation, resulting in local effects on secretomotor activity.

Stressors

Stressful events have long been believed to be important in the development of symptoms in functional bowel disorders.[49] Physiological reactions to stressors should be considered as attempts by the body to adapt – a natural coping mechanism, in which, if stressors are not too extreme or long standing, the subject is usually successful in reaching a homeostatic state. However, at times the body loses the capacity to adapt and deleterious behavioral responses may arise. Chronic exposure to threat is associated with alterations in the autonomic outflow, resulting in activation of the hypothalamic–hypopituitary–adrenal axis with alteration in pain modulation. Corticotropin releasing hormone seems to be the hormonal mediator of the stress response. Intracerebroventricular injection of corticotropin releasing factor, which mimics the responses to stress in animals, exacerbates nociceptive responses associated with increased release of histamine.[50] In humans, possibly as a primitive response to danger, stress induces delayed gastric emptying, slower small-bowel activity and accelerated colonic transit.[51–54]

These alterations may presumably cause diarrhea, constipation or abdominal distension depending on the predominant abnormality.

Genetics

A recent study showed a significant association between subjects with abdominal pain or bowel disturbances and first-degree relatives with IBS and dyspepsia.[55] Twin studies have shown a 17% concordance for IBS in monozygotic patients with only 8% concordance in dizygotic twins. Although these data suggest a specific role for heredity in the development of IBS, the same study showed a higher correlation of IBS with parental symptoms, suggesting that social learning from the patient's environment has an equal or greater influence.[56]

Biopsychosocial model

The biopsychosocial model[57] provides a framework to integrate the biological and psychosocial processes, in an attempt to understand the underlying pathophysiological mechanisms determining disease susceptibility, and to explain the clinical variability and outcome among individuals.

The biopsychosocial model, proposed as an alternative to the traditional biomedical model, conceptualizes the general state of health as resulting from the integration of medical and psychosocial factors. To understand this model, one should differentiate between *disease*, which is the abnormality of the structure and/or function of organs and tissues (physical component), and *illness*, defined as the patient's perception of health and bodily dysfunction (psychological component). In Engel's model,[57] illness and disease result from interactions at the cellular, tissue, interpersonal and environmental levels resulting in a clinical outcome. The biopsychosocial model assumes that genetic influences on disease susceptibility and behavior result in a biological and psychosocial predisposition that will influence later psychosocial experiences, physiological functioning, or susceptibility to a pathological condition. This particular background is affected by physical and environmental exposures such as infection, food intolerance and social exposures including friends, family and community to influence the patient's attitude towards illness.[58] Stress acting on a vulnerable GI tract leads to an imbalance in the system, resulting in an alteration of the brain–gut axis. Multiplicity of stressors reinforces and up-regulates the response. It is well recognized that some IBS patients report initiation or exacerbation of symptoms at times of stress, trauma and major loss.[59] Traumatic *early life events* such as child abuse may predispose to functional bowel disorders.[60] There have been reports of a greater prevalence of sexually and physically abusive experiences in individuals with IBS than in patients with organic gastrointestinal disorders and non-patient populations.[61] The interaction of the previously described subsystems with psychosocial modifiers (concurrent psychiatric diagnosis, life stress, social support, coping mechanisms) affects the behavior of the individual, the biological nature of the condition and, ultimately, the clinical outcome. New or uncontrollable threatening situations may result in emotional and physiological arousal. Psychosocial factors may affect the end result (clinical presentation and outcome) acting on gut physiology, modulating symptoms experience, and influencing health behavior and therapeutic interventions (Figure 14.1). The relative contribution of the medical and psychosocial factors varies among patients. This model should be considered when

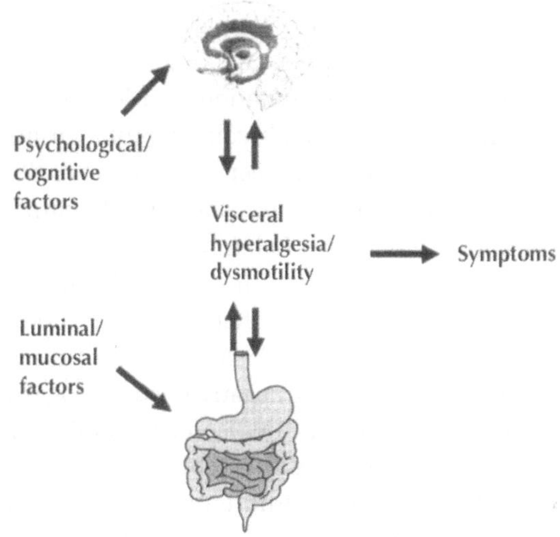

Figure 14.1 Proposed pathophysiological model for functional bowel disorders.

planning therapy, as failure to link the disease and illness components will reduce the likelihood of an effective treatment.

Functional bowel disorders presenting with abdominal pain

Irritable bowel syndrome

IBS is the most common painful functional gastrointestinal disorder in children, with symptoms arising with similar incidence in both genders.[5,62] Because there are no known biochemical or structural markers for IBS, the diagnosis is based on typical symptoms with the aid of negative results of a limited diagnostic evaluation. Despite their limited validation, the most widely accepted criteria for definition of all functional bowel disorders in children are the Rome II criteria (Table 14.1). The criteria for IBS require abdominal pain associated with bowel movements or with change in stool frequency or stool characteristics.[63,64] Patients with IBS may be classified into those with a predominance of diarrhea, those who tend to have constipation, and those whose symptoms alternate from diarrhea to constipation.

Functional dyspepsia

According to Rome II criteria, functional dyspepsia is persistent or recurrent pain or discomfort centered in the upper abdomen. Functional dyspepsia has two presentations – ulcer-like and dysmotility-like – although considerable variation and overlap occur between the two entities. Symptoms include upper abdominal pain or discomfort, bloating, belching, early satiety, nausea, retching, or vomiting. The diagnosis is based on symptoms, as there are no biologic markers for this condition.[65] A controversial issue is the requirement for a negative esophagogastroduodenoscopy to reach the diagnosis (Table 14.1). Dyspeptic symptoms are frequent in children. An Italian school study in children 6–19 years of age revealed symptoms of dyspepsia in 45% of children.[66] Although the link between *Helicobacter pylori* infection and the development of chronic abdominal pain is controversial, there seems to be evidence of an increased risk of dyspepsia in adult patients infected with *H. pylori*.[67] This link has not been clearly defined in children, where it remains unknown whether *H. pylori*-induced gastritis (when not associated with peptic ulcer) is responsible for clinical symptoms.[68]

Functional abdominal pain

Although the terminology seems confusing, it should be noted that the term 'functional abdominal pain' has been considered by the Rome II committee members as one of the categories of abdominal pain, being an entity by itself (Table 14.1). This group comprises patients with pain that is usually located in the periumbilical region and is not consistently related to eating, defecation, menses, or exercise. Patients may have associated headache, dizziness, light-headedness, nausea and vomiting. As with other forms of pain of functional origin, the diagnosis is clinical.

Abdominal migraine

In some children with a personal and family history of migrainous headache, the abdominal pain may be acute, severe and non-colicky, and often associated with pallor and anorexia. This is sometimes referred to as abdominal migraine. Children with abdominal migraine are completely healthy between attacks, but suffer a feeling of intense misery during attacks, interrupting their activities, and seeking out a quiet, dark room. Pain is usually periumbilical, incapacitating and poorly defined. Bouts of pain can last from a few hours up to 2–3 days. Peak prevalence is at 10 years of age, declining rapidly thereafter, although occasionally it may persist into adulthood.[69]

In contrast to children, adults with migraine headaches usually do not have abdominal pain.[70] Follow-up studies have shown an evolution of children with abdominal migraine into adults with migraine headaches,[71] and the episodes of abdominal pain have been considered a prodrome to migraine headaches. The clinical features of abdominal migraine and cyclic vomiting syndrome (recurrent, sudden, self-limiting episodes of nausea, vomiting and lethargy) show considerable similarity; treatment of the two conditions often utilizes similar pharmacological agents.[72]

Table 14.1 Rome II criteria for functional bowel disorders associated with abdominal pain or discomfort (from reference 74)

Functional dyspepsia

In children mature enough to provide an accurate pain history, at least 12 weeks, which need not be consecutive, within the preceding 12 months of:

(1) Persistent or recurrent pain or discomfort centered in the upper abdomen (above the umbilicus); and
(2) No evidence (including upper endoscopy) that organic disease is likely to explain the symptoms; and
(3) No evidence that dyspepsia is exclusively relieved by defecation or associated with the onset of a change in stool frequency or stool form.

Irritable bowel syndrome

In children old enough to provide an accurate pain history, at least 12 weeks, which need not be consecutive, in the preceding 12 months of:

(1) Abdominal discomfort or pain that has two out of three features:
  (a) Relieved with defecation; and/or
  (b) Onset associated with a change in frequency of stool; and/or
  (c) Onset associated with a change in form (appearance) of stool; and
(2) There are no structural or metabolic abnormalities to explain the symptoms.

The following symptoms also support a diagnosis of irritable bowel syndrome:

  (a) Abnormal stool frequency defined as more than three bowel movements per day or fewer than three bowel movements per week;
  (b) Abnormal stool form (lumpy/hard or loose/watery);
  (c) Abnormal stool passage (straining, urgency, or feeling of incomplete evacuation);
  (d) Passage of mucus with stool;
  (e) Bloating or feeling of abdominal distension.

Functional abdominal pain:

At least 12 weeks of:

(1) Nearly continuous abdominal pain in a school-aged child or adolescent; and
(2) No or only occasional relation of pain with physiological events (e.g. eating, menses, or defecation); and
(3) Some loss of daily functioning; and
(4) The pain is not feigned (e.g. malingering); and
(5) The patient has insufficient criteria for other functional gastrointestinal disorders that would explain the abdominal pain.

Abdominal migraine:

In the preceding 12 months:

(1) Three or more paroxysmal episodes of intense, acute midline, abdominal pain lasting 2 h to several days, with intervening symptom-free intervals lasting weeks to months; and
(2) No evidence of absence of metabolic, gastrointestinal and central nervous system structural or biochemical diseases; and
(3) Two of the following features:
  (a) Headache during episodes;
  (b) Photophobia during episodes;
  (c) Family history of migraines;
  (d) Headache confined to one side only;
  (e) An aura or warning period consisting of either visual disturbances, sensory symptoms, or motor abnormalities.

Differential diagnosis

A number of clinical features ('red flags') are commonly considered as orienting towards an organic etiology, although definitive proof for their predictive value is scant. Elements that have been classically associated with a greater likelihood of an organic condition are listed in Table 14.2. The presence of an isolated symptom (such as isolated abdominal pain) is usually thought to be consistent with a functional disorder, while multiple symptoms (such as abdominal pain with weight loss, or vomiting, or diarrhea) are more likely to be due to an organic condition. There are almost endless causes of chronic organic abdominal pain in children. The most common are listed in Table 14.3.

Peptic disease

Pain related to peptic ulcer disease is usually epigastric and non-radiating, but may also be generalized or periumbilical. It occasionally awakens the patient from sleep. It may occur at any time of the day and frequently children experience exacerbation rather than relief with meals. A review of 160 children concluded that epigastric pain, food-related pain, vomiting, bleeding and family history were important factors in the diagnosis of peptic ulcer in childhood.[73] However, the clinical presentation of ulcer may have symptoms that overlap with some functional bowel disorders such as functional dyspepsia. A favorable response to antacids or H_2 blockers may orient towards a peptic disease, but there is evidence that anti-secretory therapy may also be effective in dyspepsia. Therefore, as symptoms and therapeutic response may be indistinguishable, the definitive diagnosis of peptic disease requires esophagogastroduodenoscopy.[74]

Table 14.2 Chronic abdominal pain 'red flags': signs and symptoms suggesting an organic etiology

Age <5 years
Pain further away from the umbilicus
Fever
Emesis
Weight loss
Growth deceleration
Pain awakening the child at night
Blood in stools
Perianal disease
Elevated erythrocyte sedimentation rate
Elevated white cell count
Hypoalbuminemia
Anemia
Dysuria, hematuria
Joint involvement
Family history of inflammatory bowel disease

While it is accepted that *H. pylori* infection causes both gastritis and duodenal ulcer disease, its etiologic role in functional dyspepsia is still controversial. Dyspepsia associated with epigastric pain was frequently found in preschool and school children infected by *H. pylori*.[66,75] These findings are contradicted by other reports. A German study concluded that *H. pylori* infection in children was mostly asymptomatic and not associated with specific gastrointestinal symptoms.[76] A review of 2715 children with *H. pylori* infection found abdominal pain in 5–17% of cases. However, abdominal pain was also found in 5–29% of patients without *H. pylori* infection.[77] Universal testing or treatment of *H. pylori* infection in children with either recurrent pain referable to the epigastrium or recurrent periumbilical abdominal pain is currently not recommended.

Pancreatitis

Pain resulting from pancreatic inflammation is usually epigastric, radiating to the sides or back, with pain episodes frequently triggered or aggravated by meals. Nausea and vomiting are often present. Severe abdominal tenderness in the epigastric area and decreased bowel sounds are characteristic. Chronic pancreatitis is an inflammatory disease characterized by recurrent episodes of abdominal pain that in certain individuals may result in progressive structural changes and permanent impairment of exocrine and endocrine functions.[78]

Table 14.3 Causes of chronic abdominal pain

Functional	**Respiratory**
Irritable bowel syndrome	infection, tumor or inflammation vicinity of diaphragm
Functional abdominal pain syndrome	
Dyspepsia	**Genital**
Abdominal migraine	hematocolpos
Constipation	endometriosis
	mittelschmertz
Organic	tumor
Gastrointestinal	
esophagitis	**Urinary**
gastritis	ureteropelvic junction obstruction
duodenitis	recurrent pyelonephritis
peptic ulcer	recurrent cystitis
eosinophilic gastroenteritis	hydronephrosis
malrotation	nephrolithiasis
cysts (duplication or mesenteric)	
celiac disease	**Metabolic**
parasites	porphyria
hernias	diabetes
tumors	lead poisoning
foreign body	
intussusception	**Hematological**
inflammatory bowel disease	angioedema
	collagen vascular disease
Hepatobiliary	sickle cell disease
chronic hepatitis	
cholelithiasis	**Musculoskeletal**
cholecystitis	trauma
choledochal cyst	inflammation
sphincter of Oddi dysfunction	infection
	tumor
Pancreatic	
pancreatitis	**Psychiatric**
pseudocyst	conversion reaction

Carbohydrate intolerance

In children with chronic abdominal pain, increased flatulence and bloating, the diagnosis of carbohydrate intolerance should be considered. The breath hydrogen test following a lactose or fructose load will confirm the diagnosis. Exclusion of these offending agents may improve the symptoms. On the other hand, lactose intolerance has a very high prevalence in the general population and symptoms after a lactose load develop in only a few of the self-reported milk-intolerant subjects.[79] In a large sample of American patients, lactose malabsorption was found in 21–25% of IBS patients,[81] a prevalence considered comparable to that in the general American population. Lebenthal et al[84] found a similar prevalence of lactase deficiency in children with recurrent abdominal pain and in children of a control group of similar ethnic background. Moreover, a lactose-free elimination diet resolved symptoms in a similar percentage of patients in the lactose absorbers and in the lactose malabsorbers. As a result of the high independent prevalence of both conditions in the general population, the presence of chronic abdominal pain and lactose intolerance in one patient may be merely coincidental. Thus, the recommendation of an exclusion diet should be made with reasonable expectations, as it may be helpful in the resolution of symptoms in only a limited number of patients.

Inflammatory bowel disease

Occult IBD was found in 1% of adult patients[80] and in 3–4% of pediatric patients[62] evaluated for IBS. Some patients may complain for months or years of vague abdominal pain and intermittent diarrhea before being diagnosed as having IBD. The presentation of the abdominal pain is variable, depending on the site of bowel involvement. Terminal ileum and cecal disease in the setting of Crohn's disease is often associated with right lower quadrant discomfort and tenderness. Diagnosis is frequently delayed, with an average lag in diagnosis of approximately 7 months.[82] A decrease in growth preceded the onset of any symptoms by at least 1 year in 24 of 50 patients with Crohn's disease.[83]

Chronic constipation

IBS with constipation predominance and chronic constipation present many descriptive similarities.[65] However, constipation in combination with abdominal pain has a wide differential diagnosis and constipation should not be judged as causing abdominal pain without consideration of alternative diagnoses. In chronic constipation physical examination may reveal a fecal mass in the left lower quadrant and suprapubic region. Examination of the perineum should include assessment of the lower back, sacrum and site of the anus. Anal examination may reveal the presence of a fissure or a sentinel skin tag indicative of a fissure. Rectal examination may reveal the presence of a dilated rectum containing a hard fecal mass. A flat plate radiograph may help in the diagnosis in cases where obesity precludes an appropriate abdominal examination.

Gallstones

Cholelithiasis is considered uncommon in infancy, childhood and adolescence, with a prevalence ranging from 0.2 to 0.5%.[84] In older children, obesity, ileal disease and a family history of childhood gallstones have been associated with cholelithiasis.[85] Children with gallstones may have colicky or unspecific pain or remain asymptomatic. The pain is mostly located in the right upper quadrant or in the epigastrium, and may radiate to the back or right shoulder. Nausea and vomiting are present in more than 50% of cases. Fatty food intolerance is not commonly reported in children. Other biliary tree pathologies such as choledochal cyst may present with abdominal pain. Presentation is age dependent, with jaundice prevailing in children and abdominal pain in adults.[86]

Parasitic infections

Positive fecal ova and parasite tests were found in only 2% of adult patients with IBS.[80] *Giardia lamblia, Dientamoeba fragilis, Cryptosporidium* and *Blastocystis hominis* may be found in patients presenting with abdominal pain, often accompanied by anorexia, abdominal distension and diarrhea. *Blastocystis hominis* is most likely to be non-pathogenic in the immunocompetent human host.[87]

Small-bowel bacterial overgrowth

Symptoms of IBS may overlap with those of small-intestinal bacterial overgrowth (SBBO). Pimentel et al,[88] in a prospective study, showed that 78% of IBS patients had SBBO diagnosed by a lactulose hydrogen breath test, and that the eradication of the overgrowth improved diarrhea and abdominal pain. A study of IBS patients with SBBO demonstrated significant motility abnormalities,[89] leading the authors to conclude that dysmotility was the pathogenic mechanism linking SBBO to IBS. Another controlled study looking at the effects of antibiotics on IBS patients with alterations of the duodenal and colonic flora has also shown a significant improvement of symptoms in the group of patients receiving antibiotics.[90]

Celiac disease

Patients with celiac disease may present with symptoms mimicking other conditions.[91] A recent study has shown that celiac disease patients were initially diagnosed as having IBS in 37% of cases.[92] In this study, only 32% of adults with celiac disease were underweight, and only 50% reported frequent diarrhea and weight loss. Anemia was present in 67% of the cases. Patients frequently presented with abdominal pain and bloating or gas which are common clinical manifestations of functional bowel disorder. The Dutch College of General Practitioners states that celiac disease should be added to the differential diagnosis of IBS.[93] A Canadian study revealed that, prior to being diagnosed as celiac disease, 37% of respondents consulted four or more family doctors.[94] An Israeli study in 270 consecutive patients who underwent endoscopy for abdominal pain demonstrated celiac disease in one out of 23 of the patients.[95]

Genitourinary disorders

Pyelonephritis and obstructive conditions such as ureteral or pelviureteric junction obstruction may present with recurrent cramping abdominal pain, despite normal physical examination and urinalysis.[96] Hematuria can be present in the setting of urinary tract infections, abuse, trauma, Henoch–Schönlein purpura, or renal stones. Dysuria associated with abdominal pain can represent a sign of pyelonephritis, abuse, trauma, or a sexually transmitted disease.[97] In adolescent girls, a history of mid-lower abdominal pain was found to have low sensitivity but high specificity for gynecological diseases.[98] Gynecological pathology such as ovarian cysts, congenital uterine abnormalities and endometriosis should also be considered in the differential diagnosis of abdominal pain. Hematocolpos[99] due to imperforate hymen may present with periodic lower abdominal pain and urinary retention. Endometriosis may begin 3–4 years after menarche. Clinically it may manifest as cyclic abdominal pain, nausea, vomiting, constipation or diarrhea.[100]

Congenital anomalies

Malrotation presents usually early in life, with 85% of all cases of midgut volvulus occurring in the first year. In neonates, symptoms are usually dramatic with sudden onset of bilious vomiting and a visibly seriously ill patient. Older infants may present with episodes of colicky abdominal pain. In one series, 20% of cases of malrotation in patients over 1 year of age presented with chronic abdominal pain.[101] These patients often have vague, long-standing abdominal complaints with or without emesis. The pain is often postprandial and may be accompanied by bilious emesis and diarrhea or evidence of malabsorption or protein-losing enteropathy associated with bacterial overgrowth. Duplications of the alimentary tract are uncommon congenital abnormalities. The clinical presentations may be vague and diverse, depending on the location of the duplication.[102] Presenting signs and symptoms include abdominal mass, vomiting, decreased oral intake, gastrointestinal bleeding, periumbilical tenderness and abdominal distension.

Musculoskeletal pain

Pain related to trauma is usually well localized and sharp in nature, and may be exacerbated by movement. Patients usually are able to recall a history of trauma or strain, but occasionally that history cannot be elicited. The diagnosis of costochondritis should be considered in adolescent patients complaining of chest or upper abdominal pain. Costochondritis pain originates in the anterior chest wall, from where it may radiate into the chest, back, or abdomen. Pain is reproducible by palpating the affected costal cartilage.[103]

Miscellaneous

Familial Mediterranean Fever (FMF) is a hereditary disease with an autosomal recessive transmission that primarily affects populations of non-Ashkenazi Jews, Armenians, Arabs and Turks.[104] A typical attack consists of fever and inflammation of serous membranes lasting from 1 to 4 days. Between attacks, FMF patients are asymptomatic and appear healthy. The frequency of the attacks varies from weekly to one every 3–4 months or less. Severe abdominal pain similar to acute peritonitis is present in 95% of patients. Other symptoms may include chest pain, arthritis and rash. Attacks may be triggered by physical and emotional stress, menstruation and a high-fat diet. There are no specific laboratory tests for FMF, although a genetic diagnosis might become available in the foreseeable future. During attacks, acute-phase reactants may be elevated.

Diagnostic testing

In patients with no alarm symptoms, the Rome criteria have a positive predictive value of approximately 98%, with additional diagnostic tests providing a yield of 2% or less.[105] When needed, the exclusion of an organic condition can be accomplished by utilizing inexpensive, non-invasive and easily available diagnostic tests such as complete blood cell count, erythrocyte sedimentation rate, chemistry panel, liver and thyroid function studies, urine analysis and stool examination for blood, ova and parasites. Need for other diagnostic tests should be based on history and physical examination findings. The physician should avoid the lure of having to 'rule out' an organic disease at all cost. Performing multiple tests may provide results that often are unrelated to the presenting symptom or have no clinical relevance (such as a mildly elevated sedimentation rate). Repeating tests to confirm the serendipitous findings may further increase anxiety and undermine the clinical diagnosis of functional bowel disorder. One could use time as the *physician's ally*, assuring the patient that no test is necessary at this point but if further symptoms present or the current symptom worsens the physician will not hesitate to proceed with further work-up.

Blood and stool studies

Hamm et al[80] studied 1452 patients with an established diagnosis of IBS and found that screening tests showed a low incidence of thyroid dysfunction, ova and parasite infestation, or colonic pathology. The authors concluded that limited detection rates, added costs and the inconvenience of these tests made the routine use of endoscopy, radiography, thyroid function tests, fecal ova and parasite determination and the lactose hydrogen breath test questionable in the diagnostic evaluation of established IBS patients. In accordance with these results, Tolliver et al[106] performed fecal ova and parasite determinations in 196 patients with a possible diagnosis of IBS, and found no evidence of infection in any of them. In the same study, complete blood cell count, sedimentation rate, serum chemistries, thyroid profile and urinalysis were normal or yielded no useful clinical information.

A study designed to investigate the prevalence of elevated antiendomysial antibody titers in children with recurrent abdominal pain compared with healthy children found no association between abdominal pain and celiac disease.[107] The study showed that 1% of patients in each group had positive celiac disease antibodies. An adult investigation studied serum antibody testing for celiac disease in patients with IBS symptoms and a control group, followed by upper endoscopy in positive cases. The study revealed that 4.6% of patients in the group with possible IBS had positive antibodies in comparison with 0.67% in the control group, suggesting that testing for celiac disease may be one of the few cost-effective evaluations in patients with IBS.[108]

Endoscopic studies

A study investigating the presence of gastroesophageal reflux in children with recurrent abdominal pain concluded that pathological gastroesophageal reflux is a frequent finding in such children.[109] Treatment of gastroesophageal reflux in this group of patients resulted in resolution or improvement of abdominal pain in 71% of cases. Another study evaluating findings on endoscopic examinations in 62 Indonesian children with recurrent abdominal pain revealed pathological abnormalities including esophagitis, erosions and duodenitis in 50% of the patients.[110] In the absence of peptic ulcers, it is unclear how much these pathological findings contribute to the patients' symptoms. Endoscopy and biopsy performed in children evaluated for dyspepsia demonstrated that most children did not have significant mucosal disease. Inflammation without evidence of peptic ulceration was found in 38% of the patients with *H. pylori* being identified in only five cases.[111] Follow-up at 6 months to 2 years revealed that most subjects improved, regardless of the cause of dyspepsia.

Ultrasound

The diagnostic yield of a sonographic examination of the abdomen in children presenting with functional bowel disorders seems to be extremely low. Yip et al, in a retrospective evaluation of 644 ultrasound studies performed in children with the diagnosis of recurrent abdominal pain found abnormalities in only ten children, concluding that only children who have abdominal pain with atypical clinical features should receive sonographic screening.[112] In another study, the evaluation of 57 patients with chronic abdominal pain by abdominal and/or pelvic sonography revealed only one case of ovarian cyst that later resolved spontaneously.[113] Stordal et al[114] studied 44 children with recurrent abdominal pain without finding any abnormalities on ultrasound that could be related to the symptoms.

Intraesophageal pH monitoring

The diagnostic yield of esophageal pH monitoring in children presenting with chronic abdominal pain is controversial. A study of 44 children presenting with recurrent abdominal pain demonstrated gastroesophageal reflux in 25% of cases.[114] No studies have compared outcomes between children who had pH monitoring studies and those who did not. The inconvenience associated with this test and its cost preclude its use at least in the initial evaluation of chronic abdominal pain.

Lactose hydrogen breath test

This test is often used to diagnose lactose intolerance in patients with functional bowel disorders, but the cause–effect relationship between lactose intolerance and symptoms has been questioned.[81] Lactose intolerance is discussed in more detail in a previous section of this chapter.

Treatment

There is no uniformly successful treatment or cure for functional bowel disorders. Once the diagnosis has been made, it is essential to emphasize the benign aspects of the history, physical examination and laboratory tests in order effectively to reassure the patient and the family of their significance. Initial treatment of functional pain is based on reassurance and establishing an effective physician–patient–family relationship. Alleviating symptoms is one of the main goals of caring for patients with functional bowel disorders, but a rational management of these disorders is often challenging, owing to the lack of objective diagnostic criteria and unclear pathogenesis. As a consequence, there are no specific, universally effective therapies.[115]

Reassurance

It is of great importance to assure the family and the patient that the physician believes that the symptoms are 'real' and that an organic or progressive disease is not present. An extensive explanation of the nature of the disorder should be given, discussing the problem as a common diagnosis and not just an exclusion of an organic disease. A comprehensive but easily understandable description of the nature of this group of disorders should be attempted. Comparisons with other common and benign entities such as headaches or muscle cramps may help. The family and the patient should be encouraged to ask questions and share their concerns, which should be addressed in depth to avoid fears and misconceptions.

The main goal of the therapy is to re-establish a normal daily life for the patient and the family. The family should be discouraged from reinforcing the symptoms by allowing the child to miss school and leisure activities. Patients with perceived low self-worth and academic competence may find the relief of responsibility as a benefit of the pain experience;[116] meanwhile, patients with adequate perception of their self-worth may find it discouraging. Fordyce and others have suggested that positive attention from others may serve as a secondary gain, transforming the painful experience into a rewarded activity that in turn could reinforce symptoms, leading to further disability.[117,118] However, negative attention to pain in children with low self-esteem has been associated with increased pain behavior, possibly by creating affective distress that may further contribute to somatic symptoms.[116] Thus, the parents' attitude towards the pain experience should be balanced, showing support and understanding, but being aware that excessive attention to the painful experience and missing activities may allow some patients (especially those with low self-worth) to develop a sick role, perpetuating the symptoms.

Behavior alternative to assuming the sick role should be encouraged and rewarded. Patients should be encouraged to discuss perceived triggering factors. Psychosocial stressors at home or school should be addressed. At school, strict toilet times or issues relating to social embarrassment to attend the restrooms should be discussed. It is often useful to communicate with the school nurse or teacher in order to address these issues.

Owing to the high index of symptomatic success with reassurance, medications are not necessary for every patient with functional abdominal pain. Drug therapy should be recommended only for patients with symptoms interfering with satisfactory quality of life.

Diet

A detailed dietary history may identify factors that patients may feel as aggravating or provoking the symptoms. Food intolerance was perceived as a problem by 20% in an unselected UK population who responded to a questionnaire, but with controlled challenge the prevalence was slightly higher than 1%.[119] Food-induced symptoms are common reports among IBS patients, with 20–65% attributing their symptoms to adverse food reactions.[120,121] In a study of 200 IBS patients,[120] the effect of an exclusion diet was evaluated, with a symptomatic improvement in almost 50% of patients, indicating that a significant proportion of IBS patients could benefit from therapeutic dietary manipulation. However, such intervention is still controversial because the observed response rate replicates the average placebo response rate in IBS trials.[40] Within IBS patients the subgroup of patients with diarrhea-predominant symptoms seems to benefit the most by a trial of exclusion diet. Among those with abdominal pain with or without diarrhea, lactose, or excessive fructose or sorbitol intake may induce symptoms. The avoidance of gas-forming foods such as legumes, complex carbohydrates, lactose and fructose may provide symptomatic relief in some patients.

High-fiber diets have long been used in adult IBS patients but the data in children are still preliminary and accomplishing a substantial increase in fiber consumption may be difficult.[122,123] As fibers decrease the whole-gut transit time, fiber-enriched diets may be more useful in the subgroup of patients with constipation.[124,125] Fiber may also decrease intraluminal pressures, reducing wall tension and pain.[126] In committed families wishing to increase dietary fibers, the change should be attempted gradually, as the excess of undigested carbohydrates in the colon results in fermentation with consequent increase of gas, aggravating IBS symptoms.[127] Frequently, non-pharmacological strategies alone fail to bring complete relief to IBS patients, necessitating pharmacotherapy (Table 14.4).

Laxatives

Patients with severe constipation may find relief by combining fiber with a laxative. It is our preference to use polyethylene glycol or a senna derivative, but other laxatives may be used according to the practitioner's preference. Lactulose should be avoided, as the increase of gas production derived from its use may trigger pain.

Anticholinergic and antidiarrheal medications

Some patients with diarrhea seem to benefit from an antidiarrheal preparation such as loperamide or diphenoxylate. Studies in adults[6] and anecdotal experience seem to demonstrate that some patients find relief by using anticholinergics such as hyoscyamine,[128] dicyclomine or others that may modify intestinal tone and motility. These agents are best used on a sporadic basis, whenever the symptoms are present much like analgesics are used for headaches. When giving medications for pain, the high placebo response rate should be considered, as several preparations may work in the short term, only to relapse after a variable period of time.[129]

Tricyclic antidepressants

An additional option for treating chronic abdominal pain is the use of tricyclic antidepressants (TCA). TCA are used at smaller doses (0.2–0.4 mg/kg per day, 5–50 mg/day) than needed for treatment of clinical depression. The analgesic effects of TCA and other antidepressants are independent of their effects on depression, and this information should be shared with the family and the patient. The beneficial effect of the TCA starts

Table 14.4 Drugs approved for treatment of IBS and scientific evidence

	USA	Canada	Scientific evidence
Dicyclomine	yes	yes	
Propantheline		yes	
Hyoscymine	yes	yes	
Hyoscine/atropine	yes	yes	
Peppermint oil		yes	yes
Tegaserod	yes	yes	yes
Alosetron	yes (restricted)		yes

Source: physicians' desk reference 2001 (USA)
Compendium of Pharmaceuticals and Specialties (Canada)

3–7 days after the beginning of the treatment, while it takes 2–3 weeks for the onset of the antidepressant effects.[130] Relief of chronic pain with the use of antidepressants has been documented in the absence of any measurable antidepressant response, both in depressed patients[131] and in patients without clinical depression. In addition to its action on noradrenergic and serotoninergic receptors, the TCA have antimuscarinic and antihistaminic effects. Thus, these agents are especially effective in diarrhea-predominant patients[132] and those with disturbed sleep, when slowing intestinal transit and the side-effects of sleepiness may be of therapeutic value. The medication is best administered at bedtime. Other side-effects such as undesirable weight gain and the possibility of cardiac arrhythmias, although rare at such low doses, demand caution when prescribing these drugs. Electrocardiogram (EKG) monitoring can be performed at the practitioner's discretion. Amitriptyline, although probably more effective, has greater sedative and anticholinergic effects than imipramine.[133] It is recommended that the medication be started at low doses, increasing the dose progressively as needed to achieve a full dose in weeks.[134] Other antidepressant drugs, such as selective serotonin reuptake inhibitors (SSRIs) are also being used in the relief of chronic pain.[135]

Selective serotonin re-uptake inhibitors

SSRIs, such as paroxetine, fluoxetine, or sertraline, also seem to have therapeutic value in relieving symptoms in adult patients with functional bowel disorders.[128] SSRIs have become the most frequently prescribed antidepressant medications, owing to their favorable side-effect profile.[136] Despite the growing popularity of SSRIs, there are few controlled studies of their efficacy in managing chronic pain syndromes. The effects of TCAs and SSRIs in the GI tract are different, with the TCAs slowing intestinal transit and SSRIs increasing motility in the small intestine.[39,137] Thus, a patient in whom the main symptom is constipation may benefit most from an initial trial of an SSRI, whereas a patient with increased bowel frequency may benefit from an antidepressant with anticholinergic properties. Recent reviews concluded that, although SSRIs may be effective, in most circumstances TCAs should remain the first-line antidepressant agents for chronic pain.[131]

Serotonin receptor antagonists

There has been much recent interest in clinical gastrointestinal pharmacology focused on 5-HT_3 and 5-HT_4 receptors. Such receptors have been shown to be involved in diverse sensory and motor regulatory processes in the GI tract. The 5-HT_3 receptor has a role in modulating colonic motility and visceral pain, increasing the threshold for sensation and discomfort, slowing colonic transit and improving stool consistency.[138] A number of selective 5-HT_3 antagonists have been developed including ondansetron, granisetron, tropisetron renzapride and zacopride. Ondansetron was the first 5-HT_3 to be evaluated for its effects on the gut. It demonstrated some benefits in diarrhea-predominant IBS, but no improvement in abdominal pain. Similarly, no reduction in pain was seen with granisetron. This modest efficacy led to the search for a 5-HT_3 with greater potency. Alosetron, a newer 5-HT_3 receptor antagonist, has greater potency than ondansetron, and good bioavailability.[139] Treatment with alosetron has led to significant relief of abdominal pain and discomfort in women with diarrhea-predominant IBS. Though generally safe, its use has been associated with severe constipation and ischemic colitis. It is currently available in the USA as part of a limited access program.

5-HT_4 agonists such as tegaserod and prucalopride, have been developed for patients with IBS and constipation. Tegaserod has demonstrated efficacy in the short-term relief of abdominal pain and discomfort in adult women with constipation-predominant IBS[140] and is commercially available for this indication. Adverse events, particularly loose stools, are compatible with an exaggerated pharmacological response to tegaserod and are most common during the first 2 days of therapy.

Alternative and complementary therapy

Despite the interventions described above, some patients will continue to experience symptoms, suggesting that current treatments that target the predominant symptom are only partially effective, presumably because they do not resolve the underlying cause of functional bowel disorder.[6] The large number of patients in whom these therapies fail has prompted an interest in alternative therapies such as diet supplements, probiotics and ancient therapeutic modalities such as Chinese medicine.

Peppermint oil (*Mentha piperita*), which is commonly found in many over-the-counter preparations for IBS, has long been recognized as a spasmolytic agent that relaxes GI smooth muscle, relieving pain. Placebo-controlled studies have shown an overall improvement in IBS patients who used peppermint oil.[141,142] A double-blind clinical trial in Chinese medicine demonstrated that herbal therapy was effective in the management of symptoms related to IBS.[143] Natural and herbal medications are not without adverse effects, and patients should not take these products without medical supervision. A variety of other herbal preparations have been studied with different methodologies, resulting in mixed results. More well-designed, controlled trials must be performed to identify other complementary therapies, with validation of the safety and efficacy of their use.[73]

Another alternative therapeutic strategy for patients with significant pain is to use hypnotherapy or psychotherapy.[144–146] Hypnotherapy has been shown to be effective in the treatment not only of gastrointestinal symptoms but also of urological, sexual and psychological symptoms that are often associated features of IBS in adults.[147] Effective psychological treatments include cognitive–behavioral interventions, dynamic or interpersonal psychotherapy and stress management. In a review of published psychological trials, Talley et al found methodological problems in all the studies, concluding that the efficacy of psychological treatment for IBS could not yet be established.[148]

Despite the fact that alterations of enteric flora may play a role in IBS, convincing evidence for a pathogenic role of bacterial overgrowth or for a beneficial effect of probiotic therapy is still scant. A review of the therapeutic role of probiotics concluded that further studies are needed to identify particular subgroups of patients with IBS who could benefit from their use.[149] More recently, however, a very encouraging randomized, double-blind and placebo-controlled study in adults with diarrhea-predominant IBS showed efficacy for the probiotic preparation 'VSL#3'.[150] These findings will of course have to be reproduced in children.

In chronic cases of refractory pain, referral to specialized treatment centers for an interdisciplinary pain management approach may be the most efficient method of treating disability.

Natural history

Functional abdominal pain is not always a benign condition with a satisfactory outcome. Long-term psychiatric disorders have been identified in patients suffering from functional abdominal pain in childhood.[151] Children with abdominal pain do not necessarily continue to experience physical symptoms in adulthood but may have an increased risk of adult psychiatric disorders.[152]

Future trends

The key to revealing the mechanisms and improving therapy of functional bowel disorders lies in the collaborative efforts among basic scientists, clinical investigators, physicians and behavioralists. Progress in better understanding of the sensory mediators and the causes of visceral afferent dysfunction should lead to treatments that reduce the visceral perception or reflex motor responses that lead to symptoms. We should continue to pursue investigations looking for biological markers of this group of disorders. Education of patients and physicians on the nature and therapy of this group of conditions, in conjunction with early identification of psychosocial variables and development of better therapies, are fundamental strategies in order to reduce patient suffering and the elevated costs to society associated with functional bowel disorders.

REFERENCES

1. Apley J, Naish N. Recurrent abdominal pain: a field survey of 1000 school children. *Arch Dis Child* 1958; **33**: 165–170.
2. Russell, G, Abu-Arafeh, Ishaq S et al. Abdominal migraine: evidence for existence and treatment options. *Paediatric Drugs.* 2002; **4**: 1–8.
3. Alfven G. The covariation of common psychosomatic symptoms among children from socioeconomically differing residential areas: an epidemiologic study. *Acta Paediatr* 1993; **82**: 484–487.
4. Starfield B, Hoekelman RA, McCormick M et al. Who provides health care to children and adolescents in the United States? *Pediatrics* 1984; **74**: 991–997.
5. Hyams JS, Burke G, Davis PM et al. Abdominal pain and irritable bowel syndrome in adolescents: a community-based study. *J Pediatr* 1996; **129**: 220–226.
6. Camilleri M, Choi M. Review article: irritable bowel syndrome *Aliment Pharmacol Ther* 1997; **11**: 3–15.
7. Drossman DA, Thompson WG. The irritable bowel syndrome: review and a graduated multicomponent treatment approach. *Ann Intern Med* 1992; **116**: 1009–1016.
8. Heaton KW, O'Donnell LJD, Braddon FEM et al. Symptoms of irritable bowel syndrome in a British urban community: consulters and nonconsulters. *Gastroenterology* 1992; **102**: 1962–1967.
9. Cross AW. Recurrent abdominal pain and duodenal ulcers in Kenyan children. *East Afr Med J* 1977; **54**: 548–551.
10. Skorochodzki J, Oldak E, Taraszkiewicz F et al. Frequency of giardiasis in children with chronic abdominal pain coming from North-East Poland. *Przegl Epidemiol* 1998; **52**: 309–315.
11. Dutta S, Mehta M, Verma IC. Recurrent abdôminal pain in Indian children and its relation with school and family environment. *Indian Pediatr* 1999; **36**: 917–920.
12. Hafeez A, Ali S, Hassan M. Recurrent abdominal pain and *Helicobacter pylori* infection in children. *J Pak Med Assoc* 1999; **49**: 112–114.
13. Boey C, Yap S, Goh KL. The prevalence of recurrent abdominal pain in 11- to 16-year-old Malaysian schoolchildren. *J Paediatr Child Health* 2000; **36**: 114–116.
14. Lundby L, Sandbaek A, Juul S. Recurrent abdominal pain in schoolchildren 9–12 years of age. *Ugeskr Laeger* 1990; **152**: 2851–2854.
15. Frank L, Kleinman L, Rentz A et al. Health-related quality of life associated with irritable bowel syndrome: comparison with other chronic diseases. *Clin Ther* 2002; **24**: 675–689.
16. Drossman DA, Li Z, Andruzzi E et al. US householder survey of functional gastrointestinal disorders. *Dig Dis Sci* 1993; **38**: 1569–1580.
17. Talley NJ, Gabriel SE, Harmsen WS et al. Medical costs in community subjects with irritable bowel syndrome. *Gastroenterology* 1995; **109**: 1736–1741.
18. Martin R, Barron JJ, Zacker C. Irritable bowel syndrome: toward a cost-effective management approach. *Am J Manag Care* 2001; **7**: S268–S275.
19. Hahn BA, Yan S, Strassels S. Impact of irritable bowel syndrome on quality of life and resource use in the United States and United Kingdom. *Digestion* 1999; **60**: 77–81.
20. Silk DB. Impact of irritable bowel syndrome on personal relationships and working practices. *Eur J Gastroenterol Hepatol* 2001; **13**: 1327–1332.
21. Andrews PLR. Modulation of visceral afferent activity as a therapeutic possibility for gastro-intestinal disorders. In Read NW, ed. *Irritable Bowel Syndrome.* London: Blackwell Scientific, 1991: 91–121.
22. Talley NJ. Serotoninergic neuroenteric modulators. *Lancet* 2001; **358**: 2061–2068.
23. Spiller RC. Effects of serotonin on intestinal secretion and motility. *Curr Opin Gastroenterol* 2001; **17**: 99–103.
24. Kellum JM, Albuquerque FC, Stoner MC et al. Stroking human jejunal mucosa induces 5-HT release and Cl- secretion via afferent neurons and 5-HT_4 receptors. *Am J Physiol* 1999; **277**: G515–G520.
25. De Ponti F, Tonini M. Irritable bowel syndrome: new agents targeting serotonin receptor subtypes. *Drugs* 2001; **61**: 317–332.
26. Bearcroft CP, Perrett D, Farthing MJG. Postprandial plasma 5-hydroxytryptamine in diarrhea predominant irritable bowel syndrome: a pilot study. *Gut* 1998; **42**: 42–46.

27. Silverman DHS, Munakata JH, Ennes H et al. Regional cerebral activity in normal and pathological perception of visceral pain. *Gastroenterology* 1997; **112**: 64–72.
28. Mertz M, Morgan V, Tanner G et al. Regional cerebral activation in irritable bowel syndrome and control subjects with painful and non-painful rectal distention. *Gastroenterology* 2000; **118**: 842–848.
29. Read NW. Rectal distention: from sensation to feeling. An up-to-date evaluation of brain-imaging in IBS patients and interpretation in terms of psychophysical factors of higher brain function. *Gastroenterology* 2000; **118**: 972–974.
30. Merskey H, Bogduk N. *Classification of Chronic Pain*, 2nd edn. Seattle: IASP Press, 1994.
31. Trimble KC, Farouk R, Pryde A et al. Heightened visceral sensation in functional gastrointestinal disease is not site-specific. Evidence for a generalized disorder of gut sensitivity. *Dig Dis Sci* 1995; **40**: 1607–1613.
32. Di Lorenzo C, Youssef NN, Sigurdsson L et al. Visceral hyperalgesia in children with functional abdominal pain. *J Pediatr* 2001; **138**: 838–843.
33. Serra J, Azpiroz F, Malagelada JR. Impaired transit and tolerance of intestinal gas in the irritable bowel syndrome. *Gut* 2001; **48**: 14–19.
34. Kellow JE, Phillips SF, Miller LJ et al. Dysmotility of the small intestine in irritable bowel syndrome. *Gut* 1988; **29**: 1236–1243.
35. Kellow JE, Phillips SF. Altered small bowel motility in irritable bowel syndrome is correlated with symptoms. *Gastroenterology* 1987; **92**: 1885–1893.
36. Kellow JE, Delvaux M, Azpiroz F et al. Principles of applied neurogastroenterology: physiology/motility-sensation. *Gut* 1999; **45** (Suppl): 17–24.
37. Di Lorenzo C, Hyman PE, Flores AF et al Antroduodenal manometry in children and adults with severe non-ulcer dyspepsia. *Scand J Gastroenterol* 1994; **29**: 799–806.
38. Latimer P, Sarna S, Campbell D et al. Colonic motor and myoelectrical activity: a comparative study of normal subjects, psychoneurotic patients, and patients with irritable bowel syndrome. *Gastroenterology* 1981; **80**: 893–901.
39. Gorard DA, Libby GW, Farthing MJ. Ambulatory small intestinal motility in diarrhoea predominant irritable bowel syndrome. *Gut* 1994; **35**: 203–210.
40. Camilleri M, Heading RC, Thompson WG. Clinical perspectives, mechanisms, diagnosis and management of irritable bowel syndrome. *Aliment Pharmacol Ther* 2002; **16**: 1407–1430.
41. Van Ginkel R, Voskuijl WP, Benninga MA et al. Alterations in rectal sensitivity and motility in childhood irritable bowel syndrome. *Gastroenterology* 2001; **120**: 31–38.
42. Mayer EA, Gebhart GF. Basic and clinical aspects of visceral hyperalgesia. *Gastroenterology* 1994; **107**: 271–293.
43. Welgan P, Meshkinpour H, Beeler M. Effect of anger on colon motor and myoelectric activity in irritable bowel syndrome. *Gastroenterology* 1988; **94**: 1150–1156.
44. Nomura T, Fukudo S, Matsuoka H et al. Abnormal electroencephalogram in irritable bowel syndrome. *Scand J Gastroenterol* 1999; **34**: 478–484.
45. Gwee KA, Graham JC, McKendrick MW et al. Psychometric scores and persistence of irritable bowel after infectious diarrhea. *Lancet* 1996; **20**: 150–153.
46. Gwee KA, Collins SM, Read NW et al. Increased rectal mucosal expression of interleukin 1beta in recently acquired post-infectious irritable bowel syndrome. *Gut* 2003; **52**: 523–526.
47. Tornblom H, Lindberg G, Nyberg B et al. Full-thickness biopsy of the jejunum reveals inflammation and enteric neuropathy in irritable bowel syndrome. *Gastroenterology* 2002; **123**: 1972–1979.
48. Barbara G, Vallance BA, Collins SM et al. Persistent intestinal neuromuscular dysfunction after acute nematode infection in mice. *Gastroenterology* 1997; **113**: 1224–1232.
49. Boey CC, Goh KL. Psychosocial factors and childhood recurrent abdominal pain. *J Gastroenterol Hepatol* 2002; **17**: 1250–1253.
50. Gue M, Del Rio-Lacheze C, Eutamene H et al. Stress-induced visceral hypersensitivity to rectal distension in rats: role of CRF and mast cells. *Neurogastroenterol Motil* 1997; **9**: 271–279.
51. Beglinger C, Degen L. Role of thyrotrophin releasing hormone and corticotrophin releasing factor in stress related alterations of gastrointestinal motor function. *Gut* 2002; **51** (Suppl): 145–149.
52. Whitehead WE, Crowell MD, Robinson JC et al. Effects of stressful life events on bowel symptoms: subjects with irritable bowel syndrome compared with subjects without bowel dysfunction. *Gut* 1992; **33**: 825–30.
53. Drossman DA, Sandler RS, McKee DC et al. Bowel patterns among subjects not seeking health care. Use of a questionnaire to identify a population with bowel dysfunction. *Gastroenterology* 1982; **83**: 529–534.
54. Kumar D, Wingate DL. The irritable bowel syndrome: a paroxysmal motor disorder. *Lancet* 1985; **2**: 973–977.
55. Locke GR 3rd, Zinsmeister AR, Talley NJ et al. Familial association in adults with functional gastrointestinal disorders. *Mayo Clin Proc* 2000; **75**: 907–912.
56. Levy RL, Jones KR, Whitehead WE et al. Irritable bowel syndrome in twins: heredity and social learning both contribute to etiology. *Gastroenterology* 2001; **121**: 799–804.
57. Engel GL. The need for a new medical model: a challenge for biomedicine. *Science* 1977; **196**: 129–136.
58. Drossman DA. Gastrointestinal illness and the biopsychosocial model. *Psychosom Med* 1998; **60**: 258–267.
59. Leserman J, Li Z, Hu Y et al. How multiple types of stressors impact on health. *Psychosom Med* 1998; **60**: 175–181.
60. Drossman DA, Talley NJ, Leserman J et al. Sexual and physical abuse and gastrointestinal illness. *Ann Intern Med* 1995; **123**: 782–794.
61. Delvaux M, Denis P, Allemand H. Sexual abuse is more frequently reported by IBS patients than by patients with organic digestive diseases or controls. Results of a multicentre inquiry, French Club of Digestive Motility. *Eur J Gastroenterol Hepatol* 1997; **9**: 345–352.
62. Hyams JS, Treem WR, Justinich CJ et al. Characterization of symptoms in children with recurrent abdominal pain: resemblance to irritable bowel syndrome. *J Pediatr Gastroenterol Nutr* 1995; **20**: 209–214.
63. Drossman DA. The functional gastrointestinal disorders and the Rome II process. *Gut* 1999; **45**: II1–II5.
64. Thompson WG, Longstreth GF, Drossman DA et al. Functional bowel disorders and functional abdominal pain. *Gut* 1999; **45**: II43–II47.
65. Hyams J, Colletti R, Faure C et al. Functional gastrointestinal disorders: Working Group Report of the First World Congress of Pediatric Gastroenterology, Hepatology, and Nutrition. *J Pediatr Gastroenterol Nutr* 2002; **35**: S110–S117.
66. De Giacomo C, Valdambrini V, Lizzoli F et al. A population-based survey on gastrointestinal tract symptoms and *Helicobacter pylori* infection in children and adolescents. *Helicobacter* 2002; **7**: 356–363.

67. Jaakkimainen RL, Boyle E, Tudiver F. Is *Helicobacter pylori* associated with non-ulcer dyspepsia and will eradication improve symptoms? A meta-analysis. *BMJ* 1999; **319**: 1040–1044.
68. Hyams J, Hyman PE. Recurrent abdominal pain. *J Pediatr* 1999; **135**: 401–402.
69. Dignan F, Abu-Arafeh I, Russell G. The prognosis of childhood abdominal migraine. *Arch Dis Child* 2001; **84**: 415–418.
70. Lanzi G, Zambrino CA, Balottin U et al. Periodic syndrome and migraine in children and adolescents. *Ital J Neurol Sci* 1997; **18**: 283–288.
71. Blau JN, MacGregor EA. Is abdominal pain a feature of adult migraine? *Headache* 1995; **35**: 207–209.
72. Abu-Arafeh I, Russell G. Cyclical vomiting syndrome in children: a population-based study. *J Pediatr Gastroenterol Nutr* 1995; **21**: 454–458.
73. Haas L, McClain C, Varilek G et al. Complementary and alternative medicine and gastrointestinal diseases. *Curr Opin Gastroenterol* 2000; **16**: 188–196.
74. Rasquin-Weber A, Hyman PE, Cucchiara S et al. Childhood functional gastrointestinal disorders. *Gut* 1999; **45**: II60–II68.
75. Frank F, Stricker T, Stallmach T et al. *Helicobacter pylori* infection in recurrent abdominal pain. *J Pediatr Gastroenterol Nutr* 2000; **31**: 424–427.
76. Bode G, Rothenbacher D, Brenner H et al. *Helicobacter pylori* and abdominal symptoms: a population-based study among preschool children in southern Germany. *Pediatrics* 1998; **101**: 634–637.
77. Splawski JB. *Helicobacter pylori* and nonulcer dyspepsia: is there a relation? *J Pediatr Gastroenterol Nutr* 2002; **34**: 274–277.
78. Mergener K, Baillie J. Chronic pancreatitis. *Lancet* 1997; **350**: 1379–1385.
79. Carroccio A, Montalto G, Cavera G et al. Lactose intolerance and self-reported milk intolerance: relationship with lactose maldigestion and nutrient intake. Lactase Deficiency Study Group. *J Am Coll Nutr* 1998; **17**: 631–636.
80. Hamm LR, Sorrells SC, Harding JP et al. Additional investigations fail to alter the diagnosis of irritable bowel syndrome in subjects fulfilling the Rome criteria. *Am J Gastroenterol* 1999; **94**: 1279–1282.
81. Lebenthal E, Rossi TM, Nord KS et al. Recurrent abdominal pain and lactose absorption in children. *Pediatrics* 1981; **67**: 828–832.
82. Heikenen JB, Werlin SL, Brown CW et al. Presenting symptoms and diagnostic lag in children with inflammatory bowel disease. *Inflamm Bowel Dis* 1999; **5**: 158–160.
83. Kanof ME, Lake AM, Bayless TM. Decreased height velocity in children and adolescents before the diagnosis of Crohn's disease. *Gastroenterology* 1988; **95**: 1523–1527.
84. Toscano E, Trivellini V, Andria G. Cholelithiasis in Down syndrome. *J Arch Dis Child* 2001; **85**: 242–243.
85. Wesdorp I, Bosman D, de Graaff A et al. Clinical presentations and predisposing factors of cholelithiasis and Sludge in Children. *J Pediatr Gastroenterol Nutr* 2000; **31**: 411–417.
86. de Vries JS, de Vries S, Aronson DC et al. Choledochal cysts: age of presentation, symptoms, and late complications related to Todani's classification. *J Pediatr Surg* 2002; **37**: 1568–1573.
87. Herwaldt BL, de Arroyave KR, Wahlquist SP et al. Multiyear prospective study of intestinal parasitism in a cohort of Peace Corps volunteers in Guatemala. *J Clin Microbiol* 2001; **39**: 34–42.
88. Pimentel M, Chow EJ, Lin HC. Eradication of small intestinal bacterial overgrowth reduces symptoms of irritable bowel syndrome. *Am J Gastroenterol* 2000; **95**: 3503–3506.
89. Pimentel M, Soffer EE, Chow EJ et al. Lower frequency of MMC is found in IBS subjects with abnormal lactulose breath test, suggesting bacterial overgrowth. *Dig Dis Sci* 2002; **47**: 2639–2643.
90. Yakovenko E, Grigoriev P, Tcherenchimediin S et al. Is irritable bowel syndrome (IBS) related to altered gut flora? *Gut* 1997; **41**: 123A.
91. Guandalini S. Celiac disease. *School Nurse News* 2003; **20**: 24–27.
92. Zipser RD, Patel S, Yahya KZ et al. Presentations of adult celiac disease in a nationwide patient support group. *Dig Dis Sci* 2003; **48**: 761–764.
93. Kleibeuker JH. The Dutch College of General Practitioners' 'Irritable bowel syndrome' standard; reaction from the field of gastroenterology. *Ned Tijdschr Geneeskd* 2002; **146**: 790–791.
94. Cranney AB, Zarkadas M, Graham ID et al. The Canadian celiac health survey – The Ottawa chapter pilot. *BMC Gastroenterol* 2003; **3**: 8.
95. Yassin K, Lachter J, Suissa A et al. Undiagnosed celiac disease in adults unmasked by endoscopy. *Harefuah* 2003; **142**: 14–16.
96. Byrne WJ, Arnold WC, Stannard MW et al. Ureteropelvic junction obstruction presenting with recurrent abdominal pain: diagnosis by ultrasound. *Pediatrics* 1985; **76**: 934–937.
97. McDonald JA. Abdominal pain in the adolescent female. *CPEM* 2002; **3**: 33–44.
98. Yamamoto W. The relationship between abdominal pain regions and specific diseases: an epidemiologic approach to clinical practice. *J Epidemiol* 1997; **7**: 27–32.
99. Kumar A, Mittal M, Prasad S et al. Haematocolpos – an uncommon cause of lower abdominal pain in adolescent girls. *J Indian Med Assoc* 2002; **100**: 240–241.
100. Tsenov D. Endometriosis in adolescence – characteristic features. *Akush Ginekol* 2000; **40**: 24–26.
101. Sprigland N, Brandt ML, Yazbeck S. Malrotation presenting beyond the neonatal period. *J Pediatr Surg* 1990; **25**: 1139–1142.
102. Otter ML, Marks CG, Cook MG. An unusual presentation of intestinal duplication with a literature review. *Dig Dis Sci* 1996; **41**: 627–629.
103. Brown RT. Costochondritis in adolescents. *J Adolesc Health Care* 1981; **1**: 198–201.
104. Ben-Chetrit E, Levy M. Familial mediterranean fever. *Lancet* 1998; **351**: 659–664.
105. Olden KW. Diagnosis of irritable bowel syndrome. *Gastroenterology* 2002; **122**: 1701–1141.
106. Tolliver BA, Herrera JL, DiPalma JA. Evaluation of patients who meet clinical criteria for irritable bowel syndrome. *Am J Gastroenterol* 1994; **89**: 176–178.
107. Fitzpatrick KP, Sherman PM, Ipp M et al. Screening for celiac disease in children with recurrent abdominal pain. *J Pediatr Gastroenterol Nutr* 2001; **33**: 250–252.
108. Wahnschaffe U, Ullrich R, Riecken EO et al. Celiac disease-like abnormalities in a subgroup of patients with irritable bowel syndrome. *Gastroenterology* 2001; **121**: 1329–1338.
109. van der Meer SB, Forget PP, Kuijten RH et al. Gastroesophageal reflux in children with recurrent abdominal pain. *Acta Paediatr* 1992; **81**: 137–140.
110. Soeparto P. Endoscopic examinations in children with recurrent abdominal pain. *Paediatr Indones* 1989; **29**: 221–227.

111. Hyams JS, Davis P, Sylvester FA et al. Dyspepsia in children and adolescents: a prospective study. *J Pediatr Gastroenterol Nutr* 2000; **30**: 413–418.
112. Yip WC, Ho TF, Yip YY et al. Value of abdominal sonography in the assessment of children with abdominal pain. *J Clin Ultrasound* 1998; **26**: 397–400.
113. Schmidt RE, Babcock DS, Farrell MK. Use of abdominal and pelvic ultrasound in the evaluation of chronic abdominal pain. *Clin Pediatr (Phila)* 1993; **32**: 147–150.
114. Stordal K, Nygaard EA, Bentsen B. Organic abnormalities in recurrent abdominal pain in children. *Acta Paediatr* 2001; **90**: 638–642.
115. Sperling MS, McQuaid KR. Rational medical therapy of functional GI disorders. In KW Olden, ed. *Handbook of Functional Gastrointestinal Disorders.* New York: Marcel Dekker, 1996: 269–328.
116. Walker LS, Claar RL, Garber J. Social consequences of children's pain: when do they encourage symptom maintenance? *J Pediatr Psychol* 2002; **27**: 689–698.
117. Fordyce WE. The cognitive/behavioral perspective on clinical pain. In JD Loeser, KJ Egan, eds. *Managing the Chronic Pain Patient.* New York: Raven Press, 1989: 51–64.
118. Fishbain DA, Rosomoff HL, Cutler RB et al. Secondary gain concept: a review of the scientific evidence. *Clin J Pain* 1995; **11**: 6–21.
119. Young E, Stoneham MD, Petruckevitch A et al. A population study of food intolerance. *Lancet* 1994; **343**: 1127–1130.
120. Nanda R, James R, Smith H et al. Food intolerance and the irritable bowel syndrome. *Gut* 1989; **30**: 1099–1104.
121. Dainese R, De Galliani EA, Lazzari F et al. Discrepancies between reported food intolerance and sensitization test findings in irritable bowel syndrome patients. *Am J Gastroenterol* 1999; **94**: 1892–1897.
122. Aggett PJ, Agostoni C, Axelsson I et al. Nondigestible carbohydrates in the diets of infants and young children: a commentary by the ESPGHAN committee on nutrition. *J Pediatr Gastroenterol Nutr* 2003; **36**: 329–337.
123. Saldanha LG. Fiber in the diet of US children: results of national surveys. *Pediatrics* 1995; **96**: 994–997.
124. Hillemeier C. An overview of the effects of dietary fiber on the gastrointestinal transit. *Pediatrics* 1995; **96**: 997–999.
125. Roma E, Adamidis D, Nikolava R et al. Diet and chronic constipation in children: the role of fiber. *J Pediatr Gastroenterol Nutr* 1999; **28**: 169–174.
126. Malcolm A, Phillips SP, Camilleri M et al. Pharmacological modulation of rectal tone alters perception of distention in humans. *Am J Gastroenterology* 1997; **92**: 2073–2079.
127. Anderson JW, Smith BM, Gustafson NJ. Health benefits and practical aspects of high fiber diets. *Am J Clin Nutr* 1994; **59**: 1242S–1247S.
128. Wald A. Irritable bowel syndrome. *Curr Treat Options Gastroenterol* 1999; **2**: 13–19.
129. Spiller RC. Problems and challenges in the design of irritable bowel syndrome clinical trials: experience from published trials. *Am J Med* 1999; **107**: 91S–97S.
130. Hameroff SR, Weiss JL, Lerman JC et al. Doxepin effects on chronic pain and depression: a controlled study. *J Clin Psychiatry* 1984; **45**: 45–52.
131. Fishbain D. Evidence-based data on pain relief with antidepressants. *Ann Med* 2000; **32**: 305–316.
132. Greenbaum DS, Mayle JE, Vanegeren LE et al. Effects of desipramine on irritable bowel syndrome compared with atropine and placebo. *Dig Dis Sci* 1987; **32**: 257–266.
133. Tura B, Tura SM. The analgesic effect of tricyclic antidepressants. *Brain Res* 1990; **518**: 19–22.
134. Hyams JS, Hyman PE. Recurrent abdominal pain and the biopsychosocial model of medical practice. *J Pediatr* 1998; **133**: 473–478.
135. Jung, AC, Staiger T, Sullivan M. The efficacy of selective serotonin reuptake inhibitors for the management of chronic pain. *J Gen Int Med* 1997; **12**: 384–389.
136. Olfson M, Klerman G. Trends in prescription of antidepressants by office-based psychiatrists. *Am J Psychiatry* 1993; **150**: 571–577.
137. Gorard DA, Libby GW, Farthing MJ. Effect of a tricyclic antidepressant on small intestinal motility in health and diarrhea-predominant irritable bowel syndrome. *Dig Dis Sci* 1995; **40**: 86–95.
138. Camilleri M, Chey WY, Mayer EA. A randomized controlled clinical trial of the serotonin type 3 receptor antagonist alosetron in women with diarrhea-predominant irritable bowel syndrome. *Arch Intern Med* 2001; **161**: 1733–1740.
139. Gunput MD. Review article: clinical pharmacology of alosetron. *Aliment Pharmacol Ther* 1999; **13** (Suppl 2): 70–76.
140. Wagstaff A, Frampton J, Croom K. Tegaserod: a review of its use in the management of irritable bowel syndrome with constipation in women. *Drugs* 2003; **63**: 1101–1120.
141. Pittler MH, Ernst E. Peppermint oil for irritable bowel syndrome: a critical review and meta-analysis. *Am J Gastroenterol* 1998; **93**: 1131–1135.
142. Kline RM, Kline JJ, Di Palma J et al. Enteric-coated, pH-dependent peppermint oil capsules for the treatment of irritable bowel syndrome in children. *J Pediatr* 2001; **138**: 125–128.
143. Bensoussan A, Talley NJ, Hing M et al. Treatment of irritable bowel syndrome with Chinese herbal medicine: a randomized controlled trial. *JAMA* 1998; **280**: 1585–1989.
144. Whorwell PJ, Prior A, Faragher EB. Controlled trial of hypnotherapy in the treatment of severe refractory irritable-bowel syndrome. *Lancet* 1984; **2**: 1232–1234.
145. Lea R, Houghton LA, Calvert EL et al. Gut-focused hypnotherapy normalizes disordered rectal sensitivity in patients with irritable bowel syndrome. *Aliment Pharmacol Ther* 2003; **17**: 635–642.
146. Whitehead WE, Crowell MD. Psychologic considerations in the irritable bowel syndrome. *Gastroenterol Clin North Am* 1991; **20**: 249–267.
147. Houghton LA, Whorwell PJ. Symptomatology, quality of life and economic features of irritable bowel syndrome – the effect of hypnotherapy. *Aliment Pharmacol Ther* 1996; **10**: 91–95.
148. Talley NJ, Owen BK, Boyce P et al. Psychological treatments for irritable bowel syndrome: a critique of controlled clinical trials. *Am J Gastroenterol* 1996; **91**: 277–286.
149. Gionchetti P, Rizzello F, Campieri M. Probiotics in gastroenterology. *Curr Opin Gastroenterol* 2002; **18**: 235–239.
150. Kim HJ, Camiller M, McKinzie S et al. A randomized controlled trial of a probiotic, VSL#3, on gut transit and symptoms in diarrhoea-predominant irritable bowel syndrome. *Aliment Pharmacol Ther* 2003; **17**: 895–904.
151. Campo JV, Di Lorenzo C, Chiappetta L et al. Adult outcomes of pediatric recurrent abdominal pain: do they just grow out of it? *Pediatrics* 2001; **108**: E1.
152. Hotopf M, Carr S, Mayou R et al. Why do children have chronic abdominal pain, and what happens to them when they grow up? Population based cohort study. *BMJ* 1998; **316**: 1196–1200.

15 Disorders of sucking and swallowing

Erasmo Miele and Annamaria Staiano

Introduction

The development of feeding skills is an extremely complex process influenced by multiple anatomic, neurophysiological, environmental, social and cultural factors. This entire process is dynamic because of ongoing growth and development. Functional feeding skills, which depend on the integrity of anatomic structures, undergo change based on neurological maturation and experimental learning.

There are a variety of neurological, neuromuscular conditions in children and in infants that can impair the physiological phases of sucking and swallowing and cause disorders of feeding and dysphagia.

In recent years, there has been an increase in infant swallowing disorders as a result of improved survival rates for infants born prematurely or with life-threatening medical disorders. Disorders of feeding and swallowing in children are serious and potentially fatal problems. Aspiration due to dysphagia may lead to severe pulmonary disease, and impaired oral and pharyngeal function may rapidly result in failure to thrive. Prompt evaluation of swallowing disorders is therefore critical.

The differential diagnosis of dysphagia in children is widespread. The diagnostic work-up can be extremely difficult and exhaustive in many cases. Because of this complexity, multidisciplinary team evaluations should be conducted.

Successful rehabilitation of children with swallowing disorders requires knowledge of the parameters of normal and abnormal swallowing plus skill in the integration of a variety of essential therapeutic techniques.

Epidemiology and etiology

Data on the incidence of swallowing disorders are lacking, because in clinical practice, disorders of swallowing are often considered in the general context of a feeding disorder. Feeding is a complex process that involves a number of phases in addition to the act of swallowing, including the recognition of hunger (appetite), the acquisition of food and the ability to bring the food to the mouth.[1] The estimated prevalence of feeding problems in the pediatric population ranges from 25 to 35% in normally developing children, and from 40 to 93% in children with developmental delay.[2,3]

Disorders of sucking and swallowing may be caused by multiple etiological factors that may interfere with the child's ability to coordinate swallowing and breathing maneuvers and may be manifested as a unique set of symptoms. Potential causes are in three broad categories: immaturity, delay, or a defect in neuromuscular control; an anatomic abnormality of the aerodigestive tract; and/or systemic illness. The magnitude of the dysfunction depends on the balance between the extent of the structural or functional abnormality and the child's compensatory adaptations.[4] Disorders associated with sucking and swallowing difficulties are listed in Table 15.1.[5]

Pathophysiology

The fetus is capable of swallowing amniotic fluid *in utero*, indicating that the motor program for swallowing functions before gestation is complete.

However, oral feeding is not initiated in preterm infants before 32 weeks of postconceptional age, partly because the coordination of sucking,

Table 15.1 Differential diagnosis in dysphagia (adapted from reference 5)

Prematurity

Upper airway obstruction
Nasal and nasopharyngeal
- cohanal atresia, stenosis, septal deflections and abscess, infections, tumors, sinusitis

Oropharynx
- defects of lips and alveolar processes, cleft lip or palate, hypopharyngeal stenosis, craniofacial syndromes or sequences (e.g. Cruzon, Treacher–Collins syndrome, Pierre Robin sequence)

Laryngeal
- laryngeal cleft and cyst, laryngomalacia, subglottic stenosis and paralysis

Congenital defects of the larynx, trachea and esophagus
Laryngotracheoesophageal cleft
Tracheoesophageal fistula with associated esophageal atresia
Esophageal anomalies (e.g. strictures, webs)
Vascular anomalies
- aberrant right subclavian artery
- double aortic arch
- right aortic arch with left ligamentum

Acquired anatomic defects
Trauma
- external trauma, intubation, endoscopic, foreign body

Chemical ingestion

Neurological disorders
Central nervous system
- trauma
- hypoxia and anoxia
- cortical atrophy, hypoplasia, agenesis
- infections (meningitis, brain abscess)

Peripheral nervous system disease
Trauma
Congenital defects

Neuromuscular disorders
Guillain–Barré syndrome
Poliomyelitis (bulbar paralysis)
Myasthenia gravis
Myotonic muscular dystrophy

Anatomic and functional defects
Crycopharyngeal dysfunction
Esophageal achalasia
Esophageal spasm
Paralysis of the esophagus
Associated atresia-tracheoesophageal fistula, nerve defect
Peptic and eosinophilic esophagitis
Riley-Day syndrome (Dysautonomia)
Brain stem compression (e.g. Chiari malfomation, tumor)

swallowing and respiration is not established.[6] Even at 34 weeks, the minute ventilation during sucking decreases more than that of infants at 36–38 weeks. Therefore, the co-ordination between swallowing and breathing is not yet fully organized at 34 weeks of postconceptional age.[7,8]

Anatomic structures, which are essential to competent feeding skills, undergo growth that changes their physical relationship to one another and consequently affects their function. The swallowing mechanism, by which food is transmitted to the stomach and digestive organs, is a complex action involving 26 muscles and five cranial nerves. The neurophysiological control involves sensory afferent nerve fibers, motor efferent fibers, paired brainstem swallowing centers, and suprabulbar neural input. Structural integrity is essential to the development of normal feeding and swallowing skills.[9]

Deglutition is generally divided into phases of swallowing, based on anatomic and functional characteristics: pre-oral, pharyngeal and esophageal.[10,11]

Anatomic considerations

An understanding of the anatomy of the pharynx is essential to a thorough understanding of the swallowing process. The anatomy changes during development. The tongue, the soft palate and the arytenoid mass (arytonoid cartilage, false vocal cords and true vocal cords) are larger relative to their surrounding chambers when compared with the adult.[12] In the infant, the tongue lies entirely within the oral cavity, resulting in a small oropharynx.[12,13] In addition, a sucking pad, composed of densely compacted fatty tissue that further reduces the size of the oral cavity, stabilizes the lateral walls of the oral cavity. The larynx lies high in the infant, and the tip of the epiglottis extends to and may overlap the soft palate. These anatomic relationships are ideal for the normal infant feeding pattern of sucking or suckling feeding a breast or a bottle in a recumbent position.[14] In the infant, the larynx sits high in the neck at the level of vertebrae C1 to C3, allowing for the velum, tongue and epiglottis to approximate, thereby functionally separating the respiratory and digestive tracts. This separation allows the infant to breathe and feed safely. By age of 2–3 years, the larynx descends, decreasing the separation of the swallowing and digestive tracts[2,15] (Figure 15.1).

Development and normal swallowing function

The newborn infant is reflex bound and automatically makes certain oral motor movements. For example, the newborn's automatic-phasic bite

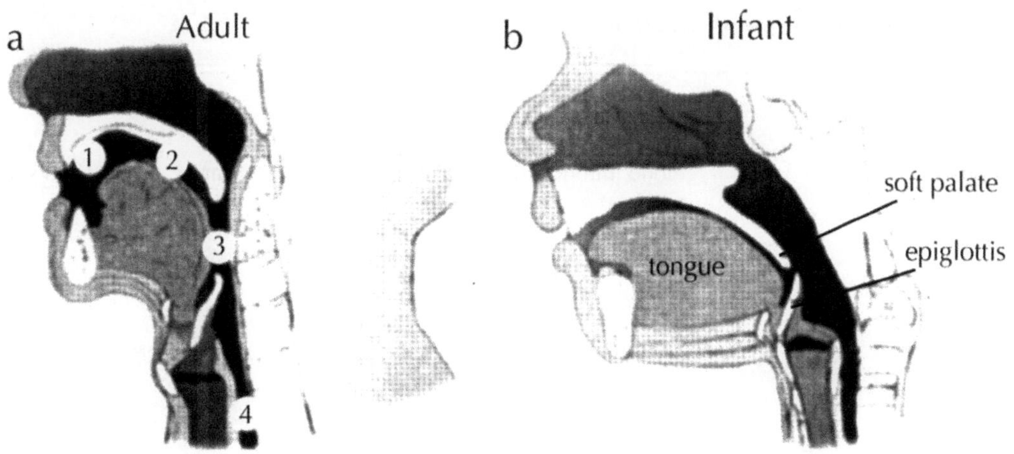

Figure 15.1 (a) The adult oropharynx. The phases of swallowing are labeled. 1, preparatory phase; 2, oral phase; 3, pharyngeal phase; 4, esophageal phase. (b) The infant oropharynx. Note that the infant oral cavity providing little space for manipulation of the food bolus. The larynx is elevated so that the epiglottis almost touches the soft palate. The tongue is entirely within the oral cavity, with no oral pharynx. Reproduced with permission from reference 15.

pattern, although it may look like chewing, actually starts liquid flowing into the mouth with its pump-like action. The rooting reflex elicited by stroking the side of the mouth and resulting in the head turning towards the source of stimulation, is a food-seeking response. Over time, these reflexive movements of the newborn are gradually refined and incorporated into more voluntary feeding patterns.[14]

Therefore, by increasing the intraoral space, the infant begins to suppress reflexive suckling patterns and starts to use voluntary sucking patterns. In contrast to suckling, true sucking involves a raising and lowering of the body of the tongue with increased use of intrinsic musculature. Most infants complete the gradual transition from suckling to true sucking by 9 months of age. This is considered a critical step in the development of oral skills that will permit handling of thicker textures and spoon-feeding.[16]

As with sucking, chewing patterns emerge gradually during infancy. Between birth and 5 months of age, a phasic bite-release pattern develops. Jaw opening and closing begins as a reflex and evolves into a volitionally controlled bite. True chewing develops as activity of the tongue, cheeks and jaws co-ordinate to participate in the breakdown of solid food. The eruption of the deciduous teeth between the ages of 6 and 24 months provides a chewing surface and increased sensory input to facilitate the development of chewing.[16]

The concept of a 'critical period' is relevant to feeding development. A critical period is a fairly well-delineated period of the time during which a specific stimulus must be applied in order to produce a particular action. After such a critical period a particular behavior pattern can no longer be learned. The 'sensitive period' is the optimal time for the application of a stimulus. After the sensitive period, it is more difficult to learn a specific pattern of behavior.[17]

Current knowledge of the swallowing mechanism is derived mainly from radiographic studies, which have been in use since the early 1900s. Plain films of the pharynx were replaced in the 1930s by cineradiography, which, in the 1970s, was subsequently replaced by videofluoroscopy. Videofluoroscopy permits instant analysis of bolus transport, aspiration and pharyngeal function.[18] Using this descriptive method deglutition can be divided into four phases: the oral preparatory phase, oral voluntary phase, pharyngeal phase, and esophageal phase (Table 15.2).[19]

The oral preparatory phase occurs after food is placed into the mouth. The food is prepared for pharyngeal delivery by mastication and mixing with saliva. This is a highly co-ordinated activity

Table 15.2 Phases of normal deglutition

Phase	Activities	Time
Pre-oral phase (voluntary)	food introduced into the oral cavity	varies; depends on substance
Oral phase (voluntary/involuntary)	bolus formation and passage to the pharynx	Less than 1 s
Pharyngeal phase (involuntary)	respiration ceases; pharyngeal peristalsis; epiglottis closes; larynx closes, elevates and draws forward. UES relaxes	1 s or less
Esophageal phase (involuntary)	esophageal peristalsis; opening of lower esophageal sphincter	8–20 s

UES, upper esophageal sphincter

that is rhythmic and controlled to prevent injury to the tongue. The tongue is elevated towards the palate by the combined actions of the digastric, genioglossus, geniohyoid and mylohyoid muscles. Intrinsic tongue muscles produce both the initial depression in the dorsum that receives the food and the spreading action that distributes the food throughout the oral cavity. The buccinator muscles hold food between the teeth in dentulous infants and help to generate suction in neonates. In this phase, the soft palate is against the tongue base secondary to contraction of the palatoglossus muscles, which allows nasal breathing to continue.[2,20]

During, the oral propulsive phase, the bolus is propelled into the oropharynx. The oral phase is characterized by elevation of the tongue and a posterior sweeping or stripping action produced mainly by the action of styloglossus muscles. This propels the bolus into the pharynx and triggers the 'reflex swallow'. The receptors for this reflex are thought to be at the base of the anterior pillars, but there is evidence that others exist in the tongue base, epiglottis and pyriform fossae. Sensory impulses for the reflex are conducted through the afferent limbs of cranial nerves V, IX and X to the swallowing center. Oral transit time is less than 1 s.[2,21]

The pharyngeal phase of deglutition is the most complex and critical. The major component of the pharyngeal phase is the reflex swallow. This results from motor activity stimulated by cranial nerves IX and X. The reflex swallow may be triggered by a voluntary oral phase component or any stimulation of the afferent receptor in and around the anterior pillar.[2] Bolus passage through the pharynx is accompanied by soft palate elevation, lingual thrust, laryngeal elevation and descent upper esophageal sphincter (UES) relaxation and pharyngeal constrictor peristalsis. The pharyngeal phase commences as the bolus head is propelled past the tongue pillars and finishes as the bolus tail passes into the esophagus.[21] Once it begins, the pharyngeal phase is very quick, (1 s or less).[2] It is characterized biomechanically by the operation of three valves and several propulsive mechanisms. The larynx closes and the palate elevates to disconnect the respiratory tract. The UES opens to expose the esophagus. At the completion of the pharyngeal phase, the airway valves (larynx, palate) open, and the UES closes so that respiration can resume.[21]

Pharyngeal bolus transit occurs in two phases: an initial thrust phase and a mucosal clearance phase.[22] Bolus thrust, which propels most of the bolus into the esophagus, is provided by lingual propulsion, laryngeal elevation and gravity. The tongue has been linked to a piston, pumping the bolus though the pharynx.[23] Patients with tongue impairment cannot generate large bolus driving forces despite an intact pharyngeal constrictor mechanism.[24] Laryngeal elevation creates a negative post-crycoid pressure to suck the oncoming bolus towards the esophagus, and the elevated larynx holds the pharyngeal lumen open to minimize pharyngeal resistance.[23]

As the bolus enters the pharynx and is stripped inferiorly by the combined effects of gravity, the negative pressure mentioned above and the sequential contractions of the pharyngeal constrictors, the soft palate moves against the posterior pharyngeal wall to close off the nasopharyngeal port. The bolus divides around the epiglottis, combines and passes through the crycopharyngeal muscle, or upper esophageal sphincter.[2]

The UES is the high-pressure zone located between the pharynx and the cervical esophagus. The physiological role of this sphincter is to protect against reflux of food into the airways as well as to prevent entry of air into the digestive tract.[25] Posteriorly and laterally the cricopharyngeus muscle is a definitive component of the UES. The crycopharyngeus has many unique characteristics: it is tonically active, has a high degree of elasticity, does not develop maximal tension at basal length and is composed of a mixture of slow- and fast-twitch fibers, with the former predominating. These features enable the crycopharyngeus to maintain a resting tone and yet be able to stretch open by distracting forces, such as a swallowed bolus and hyoid and laryngeal excursion. The crycopharyngeus muscle, however, constitutes only the lower one-third of the entire high-pressure zone. The thyropharyngeus muscle accounts for the remaining upper two-thirds of the UES.

The UES function is controlled by a variety of reflexes that involve afferent inputs to the motorneurons innervating the sphincter.[25] Based, on functional studies, it is believed that the major motor nerve of the crycopharyngeus muscle is the pharyngoesophageal nerve. Vagal efferents probably reach the muscle by the pharyngeal plexus, using the pharyngeal branch of the vagus.[26] The superior laryngeal nerve may also contribute to motor control of the crycopharyngeus muscle.[1] Sensory information from the UES is probably provided by the glossopharyngeal nerve and the sympathetic nervous system. There is probably little or no contribution by the sympathetic nervous system to crycopharyngeal control.[26]

The relaxation phase begins as the genioglossus and suspensory muscles pulls the larynx anteriorly and superiorly. The bolus is carried into the esophagus by a series of contraction waves that are a continuation of the pharyngeal stripping action.[2] Proposed functions of the UES include prevention of esophageal distension during normal breathing and protection of the airway against aspiration following an episode of acid reflux.[1,26] Qualitative abnormalities of the UES have been documented in infants with reflux disease.[27]

The esophageal phase occurs as the bolus is pushed through the esophagus to the stomach by esophageal peristalsis. Esophageal transit time varies from 8 to 20 s.[14]

Dysphagia

Dysphagia is an impairment of swallowing involving any structures of the upper gastrointestinal tract from the lips to the lower esophageal sphincter.[28] Dysphagia in children is generally classified as either oral dysphagia (abnormal preparatory or oral phase) or pharyngeal dysphagia (abnormal pharyngeal phase).

Oral dysphagia is seen most commonly in children with neurodevelopmental disorders. Infants with oral dysphagia often have an impaired oral preparatory phase. These children typically demonstrate poor lingual and labial co-ordination, resulting in anterior substance loss and a poor labial seal for sucking or removing food from a spoon. Other abnormal patterns include jaw thrust and tongue thrust on presentation of food. Oral dysphagia may also involve the oral phase of swallowing. Children with impaired oral phase function often have difficulty in co-ordinating the 'suck, swallow, breathe' pattern of early oral intake, resulting in diminished endurance during oral feeds. Apraxia of the oral swallow as well as reduction of oral sensation are also common. Other deficits include reduced bolus formation and transport, abnormal holding patterns, incomplete tongue-to-palate contact and repetitive lingual pumping.[14]

Oropharyngeal dysphagia results from either oropharyngeal swallowing dysfunction or perceived difficulty in the process of swallowing. Major categories of dysfunction are: an inability or excessive delay in initiation of pharyngeal swallowing; aspiration of ingestate; nasopharyngeal regurgitation; and residue of ingestate within the pharyngeal cavity after swallowing. Each of these categories of dysfunction can be mechanically subcategorized using fluoroscopic and/or manometric data.[18]

Clinical signs and symptoms

Clinical signs and symptoms of sucking and swallowing disorders in infants and in children are listed in Table 15.3.

Complications

Malnutrition

In the severely affected child with impaired swallowing, poor oral and/or pharyngeal function may lead to decreased energy intake as a consequence of prolonged feeding time and the inability to ingest adequate volumes, and malnutrition may result.[1] Malnutrition has many adverse effects. The most significant effects are on behavior and immune status. Malnutrition negatively influences immune status. This leads to recurrent infections that increase caloric requirements but decrease intake, leading to a worsening nutritional status. In addition, malnutrition causes behavioral apathy, weakness and anorexia, which can all profoundly affect feeding and secondarily, nutritional status. Thus, although malnutrition is often a direct result of poor feeding skills, it can also have a compounding, and even perpetuating, effect on feeding problems in children.[14]

Table 15.3 Clinical signs and symptoms of dysfunctional sucking and swallowing

Clinical signs	Odynophagia
Failure to thrive	Atypical chest pain
Meal-time distress	*Respiratory manifestations*
Refusing food	Coughing
Nasal regurgitation	Choking
Wet or hoarse voice	Stridor
Drooling	Change in respiration pattern after swallowing
Spitting	Apnea and bradycardia (predominantly in infants)
Vomiting	Noisy breathing after feeding
Gastroesophageal or pharyngeal reflux	Chronic recurrent wheezing
Symptoms	Chronic recurrent bronchitis, pneumonia and atelectasis
Oral–tactile hypersensitivity	
Feeling of obstruction	

Sialorrea

Sialorrea (excessive drooling) is defined as the unintentional loss of saliva and other oral contents from the mouth. Drooling usually occurs in patients with neurological disease complicated by abnormalities of the oral phase of deglutition. Clinical complications of drooling include soaking of clothes, offensive odors, macerated skin and, if 'posterior' drooling occurs, aspiration.[29]

Respiratory complications

Respiratory complications of swallowing disorders include apnea and bradycardia, choking episodes, chronic or recurrent pneumonia, bronchitis and atelectasis.[30]

Apnea and bradycardia may result from stimulation of laryngeal chemoreceptors without evidence of aspiration or as a consequence of hypoxemia. Hypoxemia may result from the effects of direct aspiration on gas exchange, from apnea triggered by laryngeal and nasopharyngeal chemoreceptors, or in patients with compromised lung function as a result of a normal decrease in minute ventilation that occurs with suckle feeding.[31–33] Symptoms such as chronic recurrent coughing, choking and postprandial congestion or wheezing generally indicate the occurrence of aspiration. Infants, especially premature infants, appear to be at increased risk of respiratory disease from dysfunctional swallowing.[4] Clinical manifestations of dysfunctional sucking and swallowing in infants are primarily apnea and bradycardia during feeding, although chronic or recurrent respiratory problems (congestion, cough, wheezing) are also seen.[30] Congested or noisy breathing during and following feeding is also a common complaint of parents of infants with dysfunctional swallowing. Dysphagia can also be an important but under-recognized cause of chronic or recurrent bronchitis, asthma and pneumonia in infants.[4]

Respiratory disease secondary to dysphagia in an older child is typically seen in a neurologically impaired host.[34,35] Apnea and bradycardia are uncommon in an older child. Bronchitis, pneumonia, atelectasis and recurrent wheezing are more likely to be seen in this population. Feeding and swallowing evaluation should be considered in those with central nervous system (CNS) injury affecting cranial nerve function and difficult-to-control chronic or recurrent bronchitis, wheezing, pneumonia, or asthma. Tracheobronchomalacia, a complication of chronic inflammation of the major airways, occurs commonly. Dysfunctional swallowing is also encountered in children with a tracheostomy. The tracheostomy may interfere with normal laryngeal function during swallowing and predispose to aspiration.[28]

Aspiration may also occur in children with disorders of swallowing after an episode of gastroesophageal reflux; also acid reflux may result in bronchospasm, pneumonia or apnea.[36,37] The most obvious sign that a person may have aspirated is the post-swallow cough, but in the swallowing-impaired child other more insidious indicators may be present. 'Silent aspiration' with no clinical signs can account for over half of all cases of radiologically defined aspiration.[28,38]

Diagnosis

Feeding disorders and dysphagia in infants and in children can be both physiological and behavioral in nature.[39] The evaluation of feeding and swallowing dysfunction is best performed as a multidisciplinary process with co-ordinated input from a variety of team members, including pediatricians, pediatric gastroenterologists, developmental pediatricians, speech–language pathologists, occupational therapists, and pediatric dietitians.[40] The goals of this evaluation include the following: ascertaining whether oropharyngeal dysphagia is likely, and identifying the etiology; identifying structural etiologies of oropharyngeal dysfunction; ascertaining the functional integrity of the oropharyngeal swallow; evaluating the risk of aspiration pneumonitis; and determining whether the pattern of dysphagia is amenable to therapy.[41] The investigation and management of swallowing disorders are summarized in the Figure 15.2.

History

A comprehensive history, obtained from individuals directly involved in caring for the child (e.g. parents, feeding specialist) is essential in evaluating children with swallowing disorders. The evaluation begins with a focused feeding history, including current diet, textures, route and time of administration, modifications and feeding position. Medical co-morbidites that may affect swallowing need to be investigated.

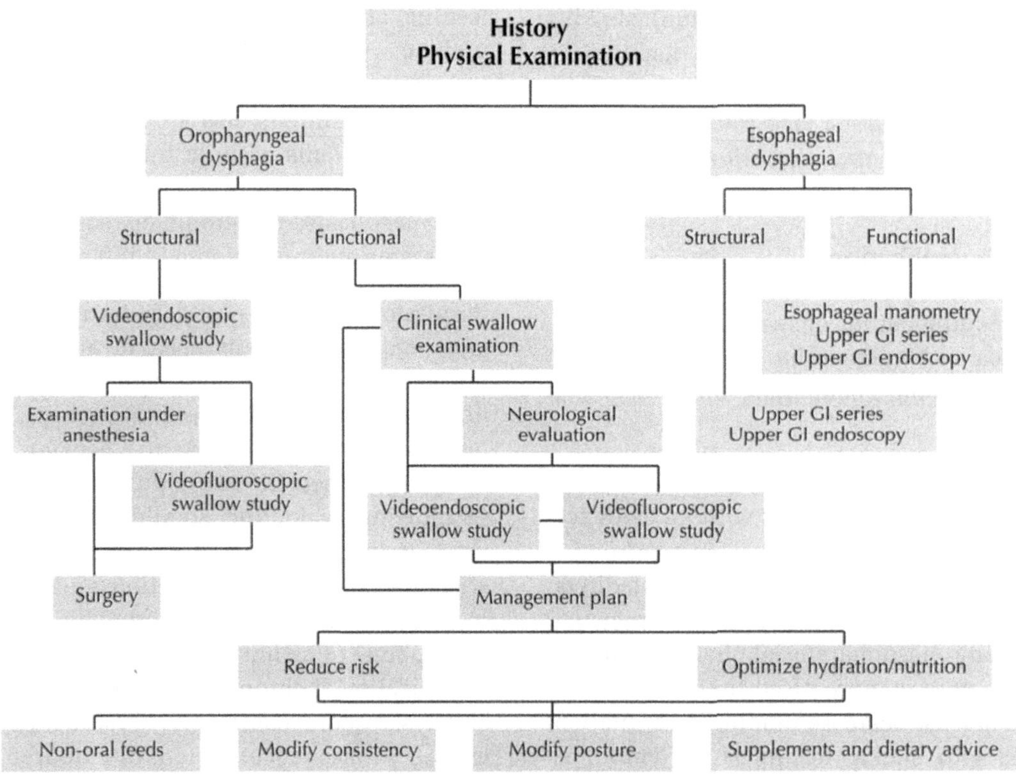

Figure 15.2 Flow chart for the investigation and management of dysphagia in children. Adapted from reference 28. GI, gastrointestinal.

The child's caregivers should also be questioned regarding associated symptoms such as oral aversion, weak sucking, irritable behavior, gagging and choking, and disruptions in breathing or apnea. Postural or positional change during feeding may be reported in children with dysphagia. Odynophagia and emesis may be related to pharyngeal and/or esophageal disorders. A history of recurrent pneumonia may indicate chronic aspiration; a history of stridor in relation to feeding may indicate a glottic or subglottic abnormality contributing to feeding disorders. Determining whether these symptoms occur before, during or after the swallow helps localize the affected phase.[16,17]

In addition, nutritional and psychological assessment should be evaluated. Many patients with swallowing disorders have a concurrent illness that may increase metabolic needs. Psychological assessments help to identify behavioral and parental factors that may be contributing to a feeding disorder. Psychosomatic causes of dysphagia should be considered in adolescents with dysphagia.[2,42,43]

Physical and clinical evaluation

The aims of physical examination in dysphagic patients are: to identify underlying systemic or metabolic disease when present; to localize the neuroanatomic level and severity of a causative neurological lesion when present; and to detect adverse sequelae such as aspiration pneumonia or nutritional deficiency.[18]

The physical examination views the whole child and specifically focuses on the upper aerodigestive tract, beginning with an examination for structural and functional abnormalities. Oral cavity anatomic abnormalities, such as ankyloglossia, cleft lip or palate, or macroglossia, need to be excluded.[2] The palatal gag is perhaps the most commonly assessed reflex and should be evaluated.[29] A hyperactive gag can result in significant feeding difficulties; in the past an absent gag reflex was viewed as an indication to stop oral feeding.[4,34]

It is critical that observation of the feeding process be included.[40] This part of the examination is best performed in conjunction with a feeding and swallowing specialist, such as a speech–language pathologist or an occupational therapist. This examination includes assessments of posture, positioning, patient motivation, oral function, efficiency of oral intake and clinical signs of safety. During the feeding trial, the presence of abnormal movements such as jaw thrust, tongue thrust, tonic bite reflex and jaw clenching are noted. A variety of therapeutic positions, techniques and adaptive feeding utensils may be used.[1,16]

A variety of assessment scales may be used to detail and quantitate results of the swallowing evaluation. However, all assessments are based on similar observation of feeding structure and function.[44]

Usually, a careful developmental, medical and feeding history provides clues to the diagnosis that guide the selection of further diagnostic tests. Only after all reasonable physical causes have been ruled out should a feeding or swallowing disorder be attributed to a purely behavioral cause.[2]

Diagnostic tests

Radiographic assessment

Videofluoroscopy represents the gold standard for evaluation of children with swallowing disorders. A videofluoroscopic swallow study is ideally performed by a consultant radiologist and specialist speech and language therapist.[45] A series of swallows of varied volumes and consistencies of contrast material are imaged in a lateral projection, and framed to include the oropharynx, palate, proximal esophagus and proximal airway. Studies are recorded on videotape to permit instant replay, in slow motion if necessary, and examination of both the presence and mechanism of the swallowing dysfunction. The videofluoroscopic study provides evidence of all four categories of oropharyngeal swallowing disorders: inability or excessive delay in initiation of pharyngeal swallowing; aspiration of ingestate; nasopharyngeal regurgitation; and residue of ingestate within the pharyngeal cavity after swallowing. Furthermore, the procedure allows for testing of the efficacy of compensatory dietary modifications, postures, swallowing maneuvers and facilatory techniques in correction of observed dysfunction. Generally, the videofluoroscopic evaluation is completed by esophagography to evaluate the esophageal phase of deglutition (Figure 15.3).[18]

Ultrasonography

Ultrasound imaging has been used to a limited extent in the assessment of oral phase dysphagia.

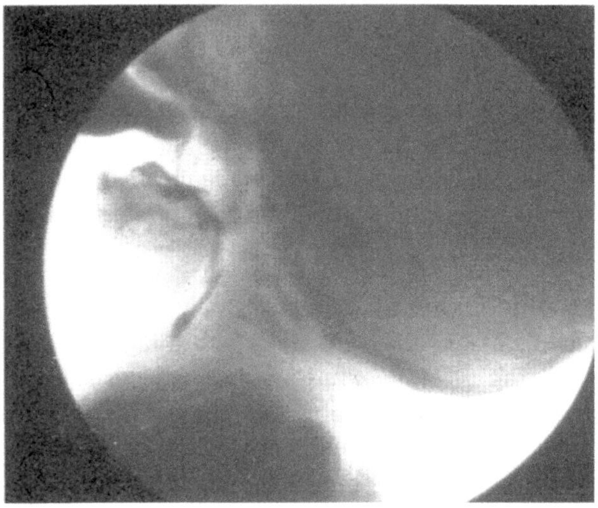

Figure 15.3 Lateral fluoroscopic projection of an infant showing contrast material in the valleculas, pyriform sinuses, laryngeal vestibule and esophagus.

Using a transducer positioned in the submental region, ultrasonography allows observation of the motion of structures in the oral cavity such as the tongue and floor of the mouth during feeding and deglutition, but lacks sensitivity in visualizing pharyngeal motion and for determining whether aspiration has occurred. Ultrasonography represents the only method of imaging that can study infants during breast feeding, and may be particularly useful in distinguishing an infant's inability to attach from maternal factors contributing to feeding difficulties.[16] Unfortunately, laryngeal penetration and aspiration are not easily detected, because of the shadows cast by the laryngeal structures (Figure 15.4).[4,46,47]

Pharyngeal manometry

Intraluminal manometry, performed using a transnasally positioned manometric assembly, can quantify the strength of pharyngeal contraction, the completeness of UES relaxation and the relative time of these two events. Most studies have indicated that manometry of the UES and pharynx provides useful information, primarily in patients who have symptoms of oropharyngeal dysfunction.

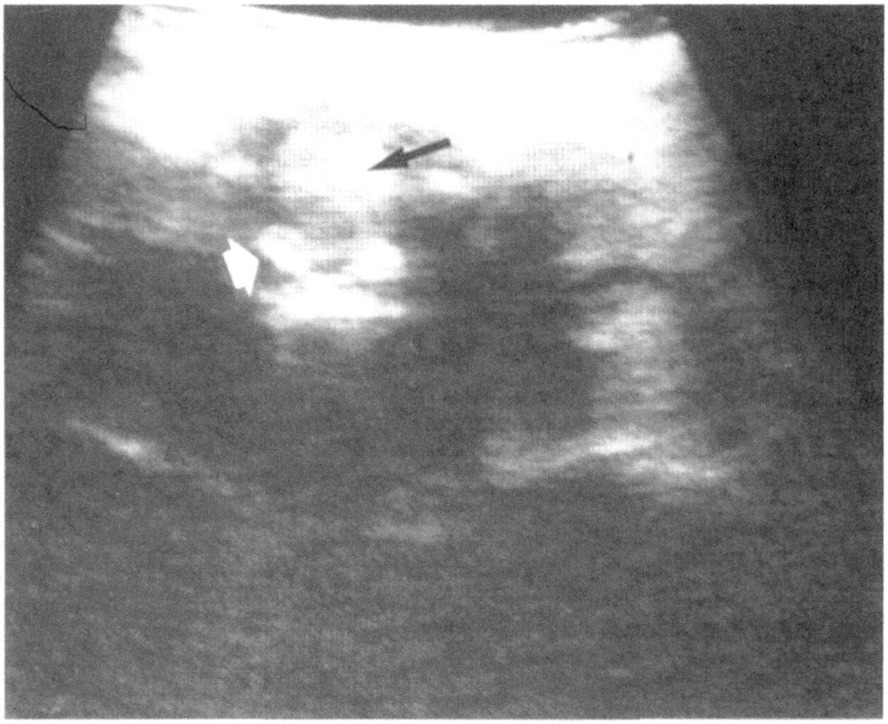

Figure 15.4 Transverse ultrasound scan of the larynx at the level of the vocal cords. During swallowing the vocal cords (white arrow) adduct and the glottis closes (black arrow).

The co-ordination of muscle activity at various levels can be obtained by simultaneous recording of pressure in the pharynx, at the level of the crycopharyngeus, and in the esophagus. Anatomical references are not avalaible with this technique (Figure 15.5).[27,48]

Fiberoptic endoscopic examination

Pediatric fiberoptic endoscopic examination is a relatively new diagnostic method to complement the current armamentarium of techniques for evaluating dysphagia and/or aspiration. The procedure is performed by passing a flexible laryngoscope into the oropharynx after anesthetizing the nares and nasopharynx.[49] It provides the ability to diagnose many of the laryngeal disorders that may affect the child, while at the same time evaluating the swallowing mechanism itself. The procedure involves five components: assessment of the anatomy as it affects swallowing; evaluation of movement and sensation of critical structures; assessment of secretion management; direct assessment of swallowing function for food and for liquid; and the patient's response to therapeutic maneuvers. In experienced hands, this test can be performed in children with minimal discomfort.[50,51]

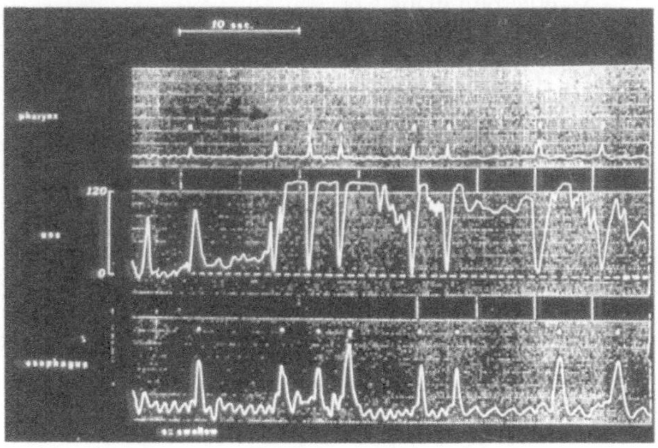

Figure 15.5 Upper esophageal sphincter (UES) motility in a control child. The pressure is recorded in the pharynx, in the UES, and in the cervical esophagus. Note that the onset of UES relaxation precedes pharyngeal contraction, which is terminated before the return of UES pressure to resting values. UES relaxation is complete to the level of the esophageal resting pressure (dashed line). Contraction of the UES continues into the cervical esophagus as the primary wave (dots) of swallowing. From reference 27.

Scintigraphy

Scintigraphy is a radionuclide evaluation using technetium-99m-labeled sulfur colloid mixed in the infant's formula. It has been proposed as an alternative and perhaps more sensitive way of quantifying aspiration, transit times, gastroesophageal reflux and pharyngeal residue. Based on a case report, the radionuclide salivagram has also been used to document aspiration of saliva. The major limitations of this technique are the poor definition of the anatomy and the poor sensitivity for detecting aspiration during swallowing in known aspirators. At present, the use of this technique in pediatric patients is limited.[51,52]

Treatment options

Optimal management strategies are critical for infants and children with feeding and swallowing problems. The management of swallowing dysfunction involves a team approach. Individuals involved in addition to the medical team include a swallowing expert (speech–language pathologist or occupational therapist), a nutritionist and the family. Since swallowing abnormalities arise from a diverse group of underlying disorders, management techniques must be individualized. This heterogeneity is also reflected in the fact that patients have different potentials for recovery.[1]

Although total oral feeding may not be a realistic goal, it is the universal hope of caregivers. Professionals are obliged to point out prerequisites for oral feeding and to discuss the probability that an individual child may reach the goal. These management decisions are typically made on the basis of clinical observations and assessments. In addition, important information is obtained through an instrumental assessment by videofluoroscopic swallow study. A methodical videofluoroscopic swallowing study defines the anatomy of the oropahrynx; detects dysfunction as evident by aspiration, poor clearance, or poor control of the bolus; determines the mechanism responsible for the dysfunction; and examines the short-term effects of the therapeutic strategies designed to eliminate or compensate for that dysfunction.[53] Management decisions may incorporate nutritive recommendations, medical and surgical decisions, position guidelines, oral–motor swallowing practice and behavioral intervention.[54]

The clinical and instrumental evaluation of children with sucking and swallowing disorders should allow for the recognition of treatable anatomic or inflammatory lesions.

A child may refuse to eat even if his anatomic abnormality has been corrected, because of learned aversion to feeding. Behavior therapy can often overcome this type of conditioned food refusal.[2,55]

Various therapeutic approaches may improve the efficiency and safety of feeding. Management techniques involve devising compensatory strategies to minimize swallowing-related complications.[56] These include changing the textures of foods; pacing of feeding; changing the bottle or utensils; and changing the alignment of the head, neck and body when feeding (Table 15.4).[49]

Frequently, children with severe anatomic disorders but normal neurological function develop their own adaptive strategies to allow for safe oral feeding. Unfortunately, many children with feeding disorders have non-correctable neurological or anatomic abnormalities that make oral feeding difficult or unsafe. Some patients cannot obtain adequate nutrition by mouth because of a risk for aspiration. Thus, supplying a portion of the patient's nutrition by nasogastric or gastrostomy feeding may be beneficial.[2] For those children who have been intubated, management includes teaching techniques that will facilitate the transition from non-oral to oral feeding. However, there is little evidence that non-oral feeding reduces or eliminates the risk of aspiration.[57–59]

The strongest evidence-based recommendation that can be made pertains to diet modification. Furthermore, the literature provides reasonable evidence of the plausibility of swallowing therapy but minimal evidence of efficacy. Nonetheless, although no hard evidence supports its efficacy, the available data are inconclusive and swallowing therapy has not been proved to be ineffective. Thus, the current weight of opinion, combined with the convincing demonstration of biological plausibility for specific techniques and the consistency of low-grade evidence, is the basis for recommending that swallowing therapy should be used. Large-scale randomized, controlled trials are needed to clarify the current recommendations.[18]

Prognosis

The prognosis depends on underlying conditions that predispose to impaired sucking and swallowing. However, the early recognition of feeding problems, the diagnosis of underlying disorders and appropriate intervention improve outcomes for the child and the family.

Table 15.4 Swallowing strategies for pediatric dysphagia
Behavioral training
Dietary modification
thickened liquids
thin liquids
Proper intrabolus placement
modification of feeding utensils and bolus presentation
Swallowing exercises
supraglottic swallow
supersupraglottic swallow
effortful swallow
Mendelsohn maneuver
Modification of body tone, posture, seating and positioning
head tilt
chin tuck
head rotation
lying on the side, elevation
Suckle-feeding-valved feeding bottle
Crycopharyngeal myotomy
Facilitatory techniques
biofeedback
thermal stimulation
gustatory stimulation
Provision of alternative means of enteral nutrition
nasogastric feeding
gastrostomy tube (surgical or endoscopic)

REFERENCES

1. Tuchman DN. Disorders of deglutition. In Walker WA, Durie PR, Walker-Smith JA, Watkins JB, eds. *Pediatric Gastrointestinal Disease*, 3rd edn. Hamilton, Ontario, Canada: BC Decker, 2000: 277–288.
2. Rudolph CD, Link DT. Feeding disorders in infants and children. *Pediatr Clin North Am* 2002; **49**: 97–112.
3. Del Giudice E, Staiano A, Capano G et al. Gastrointestinal manifestations in children with cerebral palsy. *Brain Dev* 1999; **21**: 307–311.
4. Loughlin GM, Lefton-Greif MA. Dysfunctional swallowing and respiratory disease in children. *Adv Pediatr* 1994; **41**: 135–162.
5. Cohen SR. Difficulty with swallowing. In Bluestone CD, Stool SE, Arjona SK, eds. *Pediatric Otolaryngology*. Philadelphia: WB Saunders, 1983.
6. Wolff Ph. The serial organization of sucking in the young infant. *Pediatrics* 1968; **42**: 943–956.
7. Mizuno K, Ueda A. The maturation and coordination of sucking, swallowing, and respiration in preterm infants. *J Pediatr* 2003; **142**: 36–40.
8. Mathew OP. Science of bottle-feeding. *J Pediatr* 1991; **119**: 511–519.
9. Derkay CS, Schecter GL. Anatomy and physiology of pediatric swallowing disorders. *Otolaryngol Clin North Am* 1998; **31**: 397–404.
10. Miller AJ. Deglutition. *Physiol Rev* 1982; **62**: 129–184.
11. Morrell RM. The neurology of swallowing. In Groher ME, ed. *Dysphagia and Management*. Boston: Butterworth, 1984: 3.
12. Bosma JF. Postnatal ontogeny of performances of the pharynx, larynx, and mouth. *Am Rev Respir Dis* 1985; **131**: S10–S15.
13. Tuchman DN. Dysfunctional swallowing in the pediatric patient: clinical considerations. *Dysphagia* 1988; **2**: 203–208.
14. Stevenson RD, Allaire JH. The development of normal feeding and swallowing. *Pediatr Clin North Am* 1991; **38**: 1439–1453.
15. Rudolph CD. Diagnosis and management of children with feeding disorders. In Hyman P, Di Lorenzo C, eds. *Gastrointestinal Motility Disorders in Children*. New York: Academy Professional Information Services, 1994: 33–54.
16. Darrow DH, Harley CM. Evaluation of swallowing disorders in children. *Otolaryngol Clin North Am* 1998; **31**: 405–418.
17. Illingworth RS, Lister J. The critical or sensitive period, with special reference to certain feeding problems in infants and in children. *J Pediatr* 1964; **65**: 839–843.
18. Cook IJ, Kahrilas PJ. AGA technical review on management of oropharyngeal dysphagia. *Gastroenterology* 1999; **116**: 455–478.
19. Logemann JA. *Evaluation and Treatment of Swallowing Disorders*. San Diego, CA: College Hill, 1983.
20. Dodds WJ, Stewart ET, Logemann JA. Physiology and radiology of the normal oral and pharyngeal phases of swallowing. *Am J Roentgenol* 1990; **154**: 953–963.
21. Mendelsohn M. New concepts in dysphagia management. *J Otolaryngol* 1993; **22** (Suppl 1): 1–24.
22. McConnel FMS. Analisys of pressure generation and bolus transit during pharyngeal swallowing. *Laryngoscope* 1988; **98**: 71–78.
23. McConnel FM, Cerenko D, Mendelsohn MS. Dysphagia after total laryngectomy. *Otolaryngol Clin North* Am 1988; **21**: 721–726.
24. Curtis DJ, Cruess DF, Dachman AH. Normal erect swallowing. Normal function and incidence of variations. *Invest Radiol* 1985; **20**: 717–726.
25. Sivarao DV, Goyal RK. Functional anatomy and physiology of the upper esophageal sphincter. *Am J Med* 2000; **108** (Suppl 4a): 27S–37S.
26. Palmer ED. Disorders of the cricopharyngeus muscle: a review. *Gastroenterology* 1976; **71**: 510–519.
27. Staiano A, Cucchiara S, De Vizia B et al. Disorders of upper esophageal sphincter motility in children. *J Pediatr Gastroenterol Nutr* 1987; **6**: 892–898.
28. Leslie P, Carding PN, Wilson JA. Investigation and management of chronic dysphagia. *BMJ* 2003; **326**: 433–436.
29. Myer CM. Sialorrea. *Pediatr Clin North Am* 1989; **36**: 1495–1500.
30. Loughlin GM. Respiratory consequences of dysfunctional swallowing and aspiration. *Dysphagia* 1989; **3**: 126–310.
31. Durand M, Leahy FN, MacCallum M et al. Effect of feeding on the chemical control of breathing in the newborn infant. *Pediatr Res* 1981; **15**: 1509–1512.
32. Thach BT. Maturation and transformation of reflexes that protect the laryngeal airway from liquid aspiration from fetal to adult life. *Am J Med* 2001; **111** (Suppl 8A): 69S–77S.
33. Hoekstra RE, Perkett EA, Dugan M, Knox GE. Follow-up of the very low birth weight infant (less than 1251 grams). *Minn Med* 1983; **66**: 611–613.
34. Tuchman DN. Cough, choke, spitter: the evaluation of the child with dysfunctional swallowing. *Dysphagia* 1989; **3**: 111–116.
35. Rogers BT, Arvedson J, Msall M, Demerath RR. Hypoxemia during oral feeding of children with severe cerebral palsy. *Dev Med Child Neurol* 1993; **35**: 3–10.
36. Berquist WE, Ament ME. Upper GI function in sleeping infants. *Am Rev Respir Dis* 1985; **131**: S26–S29.
37. Boyle JT, Tuchman DN, Altschuler SM et al. Mechanisms for the association of gastroesophageal reflux and bronchospasm. *Am Rev Respir Dis* 1985; **131**: S16–S20.
38. Smith CH, Logemann JA, Colangelo LA et al. Incidence and patient characteristics associated with silent aspiration in the acute care setting. *Dysphagia* 1999; **14**: 1–7.
39. Sonies BC. Swallowing disorders and rehabilitation techniques. *J Pediatr Gastroenterol Nutr* 1997; **25** (Suppl 1): S32–S33.
40. Kramer SS, Eicher PM. The evaluation of pediatric feeding abnormalities. *Dysphagia* 1993; **8**: 215–224.
41. American Gastroenterological Association. American Gastroenterological Association Medical Position Statement on Management of Oropharyngeal Dysphagia. *Gastroenterology* 1999; **116**: 452–454.
42. Kovar AJ. Nutrition assessment and management in pediatric dysphagia. *Semin Speech Lang* 1997; **18**: 39–49.
43. Babbitt RL, Hoch TA, Coe DA et al. Behavioral assessment and treatment of pediatric feeding disorders. *J Dev Behav Pediatr* 1994; **15**: 278–291.
44. Gisel EG, Alphonce E, Ramsay M. Assessment of ingestive and oral praxis skills: children with cerebral palsy vs. controls. *Dysphagia* 2000; **15**: 236–244.
45. Ekberg O, Olsson R, Bulow M. Radiologic evaluation of dysphagia. *Abdom Imag* 1999; **24**: 444.

46. Bu'Lock F, Woolridge MW, Baum JD. Development of co-ordination of sucking, swallowing and breathing: ultrasound study of term and preterm infants. *Dev Med Child Neurol* 1990; **32**: 669–678.
47. Rudolph CD. Feeding disorders in infants and children. *Pediatrics* 1994; **125**: S116–S124.
48. Hila A, Castell JA, Castell DO. Pharyngeal and upper esophageal sphincter manometry in the evaluation of dysphagia. *J Clin Gastroenterol* 2001; **33**: 355–361.
49. Broniatowski M, Sonies BC, Rubin JS et al. Current evaluation and treatment of patients with swallowing disorders. *Otolaryngol Head Neck Surg* 1999; **120**: 464–473.
50. Langmore SE, Schatz K, Olsen N. Fiberoptic endoscopic examination of swallowing safety: a new procedure. *Dysphagia* 1988; **2**: 216-219.
51. Hamlet SL, Mutz J, Patterson, R, Jones L. Pharyngeal transit time: assessment with videofluoroscopic and scintigraphic techniques. *Dysphagia* 1989; **4**: 4–7.
52. Silver KH, Nostrand DV. Scintigraphic detection of salivary aspiration: description of a new diagnostic technique and case reports. *Dysphagia* 1992; **7**: 45–49.
53. Logemann JA. Role of the modified barium swallow in management of patients with dysphagia. *Otolaryngol Head Neck Surg* 1997; **116**: 335–338.
54. Arvedson JC. Management of pediatrics dysphagia. *Otolaryngol Clin North Am* 1998; **31**: 453–476.
55. Babbitt RL, Hoch TA, Coe DA et al. Behavioral assessment and treatment of pediatric feeding disorders. *J Dev Behav Pediatr* 1994; **15**: 278–291.
56. Helfrich-Miller KR, Rector KL, Straka JA. Dysphagia: its treatment in the profoundly retarded patient with cerebral palsy. *Arch Phys Rehabil* 1986; **67**: 520–525.
57. Croghan JE, Burke EM, Caplan S, Denman S. Pilot study of 12-month outcomes of nursing home patients with aspiration on videofluoroscopy. *Dysphagia* 1994; **9**: 141–146.
58. Groher ME. Bolus Management and aspiration pneumonia in patient with pseudobulbar dysphagia. *Dysphagia* 1987; **1**: 215–216.
59. Shaker R, Easterling C, Kern M et al. Rehabilitation of swallowing by exercise in tube-fed patients with pharyngeal dysphagia secondary to abnormal UES opening. *Gastroenterology* 2002; **122**: 1314–1321.

Additional educational resource

Resource center: resources for normal swallowing and swallowing disorders (www.dysphagia.com). This multi-disciplinary website has a wealth of information on dysphagia, references to texts, archives and links to other related sites; it is user-friendly and comprehensive.

16 Constipation and encopresis in childhood

Jan Taminiau and Marc Benninga

Epidemiology

Constipation is a common disorder in Western societies. Survey estimates of the prevalence of constipation in childhood vary between 2 and 15%. The average prevalence of constipation increases from childhood (2%) exponentially to 15% in adults. It is estimated that a general practitioner will see 20–30 children with constipation per year in an average practice of 2500 patients. Around 3% of a pediatrician's practice consists of children with chronic constipation. For the pediatric gastroenterologist, consultation rates vary between 10 and 20%. Thus, a substantial number of children have constipation,[1] and this problem is of paramount practical importance for physicians.

Normal physiology

The Rome II criteria are currently used to define childhood constipation based on the presenting symptom profile. Two subgroups, namely functional constipation and functional fecal retention, are distinguished. Functional constipation is defined as follows: in infants and children at least 2 weeks of scybalous, pebble-like hard stools for a majority of stools; or firm stools two or fewer times/week; and no evidence of structural or metabolic disease.[2]

Functional fecal retention in contrast, is defined as follows: from infancy to 16 years old, a history of at least 12 weeks of passage of large-diameter stools at intervals, fewer than two times/week; and retentive posturing, avoiding defecation by purposefully contracting the pelvic floor. As pelvic floor muscles fatigue, the child uses the gluteal muscles, squeezing the buttocks together. The main difference between functional constipation and functional fecal retention is the occurrence of retentive posturing in the latter. Retentive posturing is the behavioral withholding of stool during the sensation of urge, which, according to the authors of the Rome II criteria, mostly results from painful defecation.

However, the Rome II criteria exclude a very common and major symptom of constipation, namely fecal soiling (if substantial called encopresis), which is not included in the definition. Therefore, to study constipation in children and define suitable end-points in pediatric research, a different definition of constipation has been used in children over 4 years of age. Pediatric constipation is thus diagnosed if at least two out of the four following criteria are fulfilled two or fewer bowel movements/week without laxatives; two or more soiling episodes/week; periodic passage of a very large amount of stool once every 7–30 days; or palpable abdominal or rectal mass on physical examination. Using this last definition, a small group of children (between 10 and 20%) do not fulfill these criteria, but still appear constipated, having a low frequency of defecation with production of firm hard stools with retentive posturing or painful experience. This last group is difficult to study, but will usually be included by the consulting physician for treatment efforts.[3]

Functional non-retentive fecal soiling

The Rome II group defined functional non-retentive fecal soiling as follows: once a week, or more, for the preceding 12 weeks, in a child older than 4 years (who failed to be toilet trained), a history of defecation into places and at times inappropriate to the social contacts; in the absence of structural or inflammatory disease; and in the absence of signs of fecal retention. Many studies performed in encopretic children assumed that these children were constipated. Therefore, the new definition of encopresis or functional non-retentive fecal soiling states that this is a separate entity. Although in the current literature sometimes a difference is made between soiling (loss of small amounts of feces due to overflow) and encopresis (normal bowel movement) the terms are used interchangeably. Sometimes the term solitary encopresis is used in a research environment; the children who presented for constipation with soiling and encopresis (around one in three) proved to have solitary encopresis or functional non-retentive fecal soiling without any sign of constipation, and needed a different treatment strategy.[4]

Clinical presentation

The functional diagnosis of constipation

Constipation, in approximately 5–10% of the patients, is a symptom of an underlying disorder. In the remaining 90–95% of the patients constipation is idiopathic. This label implies that no clear underlying mechanism explains the defecation problem. The differential diagnosis is large, but it is highly unlikely that one of these diagnoses is missed on clinical grounds, and therefore investigations should be limited and approached cautiously. The main presenting symptoms of constipation in children are a combination of a low defecation frequency and soiling or encopresis. The latter occurs several times a day and, in severe fecal retention, also at night. If specifically asked, most children will report production of a large amount of stools, which might clog the toilet with the frequency of once a week or once a month. Often, the evacuation of such large amounts of stool is preceded by an increase of soiling frequency. At physical examination in constipated children, the rectal fecal impaction might be palpated with firm abdominal scybala, but usually manual palpation of a rectal examination with abdominal palpation as well identifies the large fecal mass.[5] Table 16.1 reports the prevalence of symptoms associated with constipation.

Table 16.1 The reported symptomatology of childhood constipation

Clinical features	Percentages
Bowel history	
Infrequent defecation	80–100
Abdominal pain	10–64
Vomiting	8–10
Anorexia or poor appetite	10–47
Abdominal distension	0–61
Passage of large stool	45–75
Passage of hard stool	58–100
Painful defecation	50–90
Psychological problems	20–62
Urinary problems	5–43
Fecal incontinence	35–96
Positive family history	9–49
Physical examination	
Fissures and rectal bleeding	5–55
Rectal prolapse	0–3
Abdominal mass	30–71
Rectal mass	28–100

Percentages are adapted from references

Defecation frequency

The average neonate has a defecation frequency of between one and four times daily. Ninety-nine per cent of newborns pass the first stool within 48 h. However, newborns with low birth weights or premature infants might have a delayed passage of the first stool. Eighty per cent of infants weighing less than 2500 g pass meconium within the first 24 h of life. If birth weight declines to 1000–1500 g, the first stool will be passed after 48 h in 22–60% of children. This is still within the physiological range. In large cohort studies in normal children, the stool frequency varied greatly from once daily to once every other day. Therefore, a frequency of less than three times a week is considered abnormal, but other signs of constipation are necessary to decide on the clinical symptomatology of constipation.[6]

Normal anatomy and physiology of anorectal function

The most distal part of the gastrointestinal tube is formed by the anal sphincter complex, and is responsible for maintaining fecal continence. This sphincter complex is embedded in the striated pelvic floor, where the puborectalis muscle joins the upper end of the external anal sphincter with a sling. The anal sphincter complex therefore consists of a smooth muscle component of the internal anal sphincter and a striated muscle component of the external anal sphincter and the puborectalis muscle. The internal anal sphincter is tonically contracted and generates 85% of the anal resting pressure, keeping the anal canal closed at rest. It is not under voluntary control, and is innervated by the enteric nervous system. Stimulation of mechanoreceptors in the rectal wall and the sigmoid activates intramural inhibitory neurons, leading to relaxation of the internal anal sphincter, called the anorectal inhibition reflex.[7] This occurs after presentation of stool or gas to the anal canal. The external anal sphincter is innervated by the pudendal nerve and is under voluntary control. This muscle is to some degree contracted, but on demand it might be contracted or relaxed upon the decision to defecate or to have it postponed. The puborectalis muscle ends from the pubic bone, loops around the caudal part of the rectum at the junction with the anal canal and ends at the os pubis. This muscle is tonically contracted, maintains and forms the anorectal angle and keeps the rectum and anus closed during episodes of increased abdominal pressure. The pelvic floor and gluteus muscles can assist the anal sphincter complex in contraction. Sensation arising from the anorectal area is crucial for detecting the presence, volume and consistency of feces and gas in the rectum. Mucosal and intramuscular receptors are involved. These nerve endings detect the nature of the anal contents, discriminating between gas, liquids and solid feces. Intramural stretch and/or pressure receptors detect the degree of rectal filling and produce sensations of desire to defecate and urgency. Receptors located in the pelvic floor and/or the pelvis detect increases in intra-abdominal pressure, causing changes in the anal sphincter complex, leading to expulsion of rectal contents. These receptors also activate compensatory reflexes to increase anal sphincter pressure and ensure fecal continence. Sensations arising from the anorectal area are transported by afferent neural pathways to the spine via ascending nerves in the spinal cord (the spinal thalamic tract). The information is transported to the thalamus. This sensory information is transferred to the limbic and somatosensory areas of the cerebellum, where sensations such as flatus and the desire to defecate will be perceived.[8]

Normal anorectal function depends on the complex interplay between the different anorectal and pelvic anatomic structures. The main task of the anorectum is to assure continuous fecal continence.

Defecation might be considered as a controlled episode of incontinence at a socially acceptable moment. Normal defecation is a complex mechanism depending on normal sensation and motility of the anorectal area, pelvic floor, sigmoid and descending colon, and also involving the abdominal and respiratory musculature. Psychological factors have a major impact on these pathways.

Fecal continence is produced by different mechanisms.[9] First, the caudal end of the rectum is closed by the anal sphincter complex, creating an anal sphincter resting pressure of around 40 mmHg, to which the internal sphincter contributes 85%, and the external anal sphincter 15%. A reflex of the external anal sphincter increases this pressure when the intra-abdominal pressure increases acutely and counteracts imminent loss of feces. This is probably an important mechanism in normal daily life, since coughing, laughing, bending, sneezing, etc. instantly increase intra-abdominal pressure. This function of the anal sphincter for keeping the gate closed is supported by rectal motility, which is directed antegrade, to keep the rectum empty, transporting the feces back to the sigmoid and away from the anal canal. A third mechanism takes care of continence by a sensation in the cranial part of the anal sphincter. These receptors are located in the area of the skin close to the surface of the anus.

Transsection studies have shown that sensation is not lost, emphasizing the distal location of this sensation. Triggering of these receptors in the anal canal by feces or gas will result in the sensation of imminent loss, and gives the person the ability to prevent this loss of feces and gas by contracting the pelvic floor muscles. When defecation is not desired, the external sphincter complex and the pelvic floor muscles remain contracted until the rectal wall has adapted to the increased rectal volume; when the intrarectal pressure decreases, the sensation of urge will disappear. In addition, retrograde contraction of the caudal part of the rectum starts to occur, and transports the feces back into the sigmoid colon. The interplay of all these mechanisms starts when feces or gas enters the rectum, owing to increased propulsive activity of the colon after ingestion of a meal. Filling the rectal vault, these feces lead to an increase of intrarectal pressure and triggering of receptors located in the rectal wall. This induces the inhibition reflex, leading to a decrease of anal sphincter pressure (internal sphincter), which is more pronounced when rectal filling increases. Above a certain threshold in rectal pressure, the perception of urge occurs. At that time, due to a reflex triggered by this sensation of urge, the external anal sphincter complex contracts for a short time, preventing immediate loss of feces, thus creating time to consider whether the pelvic floor has to be contracted to stop imminent defecation or to permit the defecation process to continue. Defecation occurs when there is a difference in pressure in the rectum on the one hand (rectal contractions and straining), and the pelvic floor on the other hand (relaxation of the anal sphincter complex and pelvic floor, and flattening of the anorectal angle).[10]

Training is essential when a child tries to defecate without a sensation of urge (e.g. during toilet training). During the process of toilet training the child starts to obtain control of these complex mechanisms in the defecation process. The will of the child seems to be a crucial factor in this process. Aberrations in these complex interacting mechanisms might lead to clinical signs and symptoms of constipation and fecal incontinence. The pathophysiological mechanisms of these clinical entities are largely unknown. In the past decades, only little progress has been made in resolving these mechanisms.[11]

Colonic propagated contractions are tonic and phasic and propel the luminal contents to the distal colon and rectum. Non-propagated contractions move fecal material antegrade and retrograde and mix a shift of the fecal contents over short distances. High-amplitude propagated contractions (HAPCs) are a pattern of colonic motility originating in the proximal colon and proceeding to the distal sigmoid colon, and are associated with mass movements. They have an amplitude of at least 100 mmHg, duration of <10 s, and an unequivocal propagation of at least 30 cm. Children have more frequent HAPCs than adults, and HAPCs are more often associated with an urge to defecate or tenesmus in children than in adults. The number of HAPCs is increased after meals and upon awakening. The rectal motor complex is a cluster of contractions at a rate of 7–9/min found only in the rectum, and not related to feeding and awakening. They might have a role in keeping the rectum empty, especially at night, but their function is not yet well understood. The migrating motor complex (MMC) is the beginning of phase III motility. The MMC migrates slowly to the distal bowel, interrupted by feeding, and is probably necessary to prevent bacterial overgrowth during the interdigestive periods.

Pathophysiology of functional constipation

The pathophysiology underlying functional constipation might be multifactorial and is certainly not well understood. Functional constipation results from abnormal function of the colon, rectum and sphincter complex, and conscious and subconscious factors in the child. Two main subgroups are described: slow-transit constipation; and outlet obstruction, leading to retention of feces in the rectum and extending to the whole colon. It is unclear whether different pathophysiological mechanisms are involved in each of these forms of constipation.

Slow-transit constipation

This can be diagnosed by colonic transit time measurements, showing an overall delay in colonic transit time over the whole colon. Both muscular (impaired contractility) and neural (uncoordinated activity) mechanisms may lead to impairment of propulsion of fecal contents leading to slow-transit constipation.[12] Mechanisms underlying these entities might be an impairment of neural transmitter function, such as nitric oxide (NO) or substance P, or aberrations in the interstitial cells of Cajal. However, this entity remains extremely difficult to explain and might be secondary to the effect of stasis.

In addition to neuromuscular dysfunction, constipation can also result from massive fecal retention in the rectum. It has been shown that voluntary retention of feces can cause a delay in colonic transit in healthy volunteers. Similarly, massive fecal retention in children can also inhibit colonic transit and thus indirectly leads to prolonged transit time. In several children, slow-transit constipation after treatment changes to outlet obstruction with only a delay in the rectosigmoid region.

An alternative mechanism leading to constipation is the so-called outlet obstruction or abnormalities in the dynamics underlying defecation. In these children, the delay in colonic transit involves the rectum. This mechanism is found in approximately 40–60% of constipated children. It should be noted that 50% of constipated children, all presenting with the same symptomatology, have normal colonic transit time.[13–15] This observation strongly suggests that abnormal transit times are secondary events in children with constipation. It is also supported by normalization of transit time in slow-transit constipation after successful treatment.

Another alternative mechanism might be abnormal sphincter function.[16,17] Under normal circumstances, the pressure generated by the anal sphincter complex should drop during an attempt to defecate, allowing expulsion of fecal contents. As stated above, in 40% of children with constipation, colonic transit is delayed in the rectum, and it was suggested that this abnormal obstruction is the result of abnormal defecation dynamics. However, using anorectal manometry, a paradox for contraction in the anal sphincter complex is observed in more than 50% of constipated children. This contraction of the anal sphincter complex might lead to fecal accumulation and constipation. This abnormality might be the underlying pathophysiological mechanism of childhood constipation, reflecting the observed stool withholding behavior/retentive posturing. Possible suggested causes leading to this behavior might be pain, resulting from the previous production of a large, hard stool; anal fissures; primary behavioral mechanisms; not taking time to visit the toilet; and avoiding other toilets, mainly at school. However, abnormal defecation dynamics have not only been observed in fecal retention and constipation, but similarly in children with functional non-retentive fecal soiling. In addition, a large study, comparing conventional treatment with additional biofeedback training in constipated children, showed that biofeedback training could normalize the aberrant sphincter contraction, but, it did not lead to a larger success rate in children receiving additional biofeedback training.[1] These observations argue against a major contribution of abnormal defecation dynamics to the development of constipation in children.

As explained previously, different types of nerve endings, giving rise to sensations of flatus, urge to defecate and pain, sense the arrival of fecal material into the rectum. This sensory information is important for initiating the defecation process. Abnormalities in rectal sensation are believed to play an important role in the pathogenesis of constipation. Children usually report that they do not feel the sensation or urge to defecate. Several studies have investigated rectal sensitivity in children with constipation. In these studies, rectal sensation is determined by inflation of a rectal balloon, measuring the volume at which the sensation of urge is perceived. These studies showed impaired rectal sensation in a subgroup of patients with constipation. In the majority of children, however, rectal sensation was normal and present after insufflation of only 20 ml of air in the balloon. Rectal volumes are obviously age-dependent, with a barostat (an insufflatable rectal balloon that can keep the volume constant while varying the pressure, or vice versa) showing that one subgroup needs higher pressures with a normal volume to feel urge, but children in another subgroup need higher volumes with a normal pressure to feel urge.

Abnormal rectal sensation does not seem to be an important pathophysiological entity. In fact, a number of studies in children with constipation have documented a normal anal resting pressure, as well as a normal maximal rectal squeeze pressure.

To date, no consistent abnormalities in motility testing have been recorded in children with constipation. There were no differences in motility parameters between children with long-standing constipation and those who have had constipation for only a short period. Furthermore, there were no indications of neuromuscular damage due to abnormalities caused by constipation or its therapy.

Therefore, it is fair to conclude that, there is no current explanation of the cause(s) of constipation or suggested pathophysiological mechanisms. All assumed mechanisms have been found to be normal in the majority of children with constipation with a mainly uniform clinical presentation.

Children with functional non-retentive fecal soiling, in studies on its pathophysiology, show normal anal sphincter resting pressure, normal maximal squeeze pressure and normal rectal sensation. Also, colonic transit time measurements were normal in all children with this entity.[18–20]

Medical history

Symptoms of constipation in most children start in more than 38–65% before the age of 6 months, and some have even described bowel problems in 40% of children in the first months of life. Stool habits might change, owing to stress factors and change in nutrition, for instance change from breast feeding to formula feeding. Specific questions regarding the presence of soiling and encopresis should be asked, and also regarding the frequency and whether it is present at night-time. These children produce an enormous amount of stool once every 7–30 days, which is almost never spontaneously presented as a symptom during a first doctor's visit. It must also be asked whether this enormous amount of stool has been produced just before the visit to the doctor (the rectum might then be empty for rectal examination). Questions about retentive posturing should be asked, but might be difficult to answer; nevertheless, the parents might notice whether stools are produced with pain and also if any of these symptoms started after a period in which defecation and stools were completely normal. When the frequency is less than three times a week, soiling and encopresis are present, and large amounts of stool are occasionally produced, the diagnosis of functional constipation is likely. When a child has a painful stressful production of hard stools without soiling and encopresis and retentive posturing, even at an almost normal frequency, constipation will still be considered probable by the physician, and a therapeutic attempt should be initiated.[21–23]

In developed societies most children are toilet trained by the age of 2–3 years. There is no relation between failed toilet training and the development of constipation or functional non-retentive fecal soiling. Before the age of 4 years, the diagnosis of constipation can be made only on low or decreased frequency of defecation, production of occasional voluminous stools, production of hard stools with discomfort, pain and/or retentive posturing. In infants, the diagnosis of constipation can be inferred when they cry before, during and after defecation, and this consists of firm, hard stools. Behavioral problems occur often, but they are almost invariably secondary to the social consequences and depend on individual styles of coping. Such problems typically improve considerably once the defecation difficulties are successfully treated. However, poor social behavior, or an inadequate parent–child relationship may be associated with the continuation of defecation problems. Urinary problems, diurnal and also nocturnal enuresis, are secondary to the defecation problems and usually improve after successful treatment.

Physical examination

Abdominal masses should be gently looked for by palpation in the lower abdominal quadrants and suprapubic area. The stool mass might be palpable extending from the pelvis, but smaller scybala might also be detected. Usually, a bimanual palpation through a rectal examination with one hand combined with abdominal palpation with the other hand, clearly defines the rectal mass of stool the best. At the first visit a rectal examination should be attempted in all children who present with constipation or non-functional fecal retention. Only in 10–15% of children is the fear of examination too high, when this procedure has to be omitted. Otherwise, it is well perceived and gives the essential information about the rectal fecal mass. Anal fissures can be clearly visualized by spreading the anus, and during the examination anatomical abnormalities should be inspected, checking the anal position in the perineum and its asymmetry: an ectopic anus can in fact be the cause of constipation. The inspection of the lower lumbar and sacral spine areas should be focused on dimpling, surgical scars and hair tufting. Also, tendon reflexes should be evoked. Usually, the school-aged child has stools or soiling in his underpants and one should be aware of the production of a large amount of stool just prior to the visit to the physician. That might interfere with the examination results. Fissures are considered to be related to the initiation of constipation only in very young infants; an abdominal and/or rectal mass is found in 30–100%, depending on the investigator.[24]

Differential diagnosis

Over 90% of pediatric patients with constipation have functional constipation or non-retentive functional fecal soiling. Only in a very small number of children is a distinct etiology established, and these cases are not easily overlooked.

Changed dietary habits might decrease the intake of fluids and food. The change from breast milk to formula feeding as an initiating point is highly suggestive of constipation.

A careful perianal examination will disclose an imperforate anus, or an abnormal anteriorly displaced anus, as well as other congenital anatomic and structural defects.

Spinal abnormalities are indicated by abnormalities of the skin, and also growth impairment and a combination of fecal and urinary incontinence or constipation.

Metabolic disturbances are related to severe dehydration, as is seen in diabetes insipidus, hypocalcemia and renal tubular acidosis, and are not easily overlooked.

Hypothyroidism is screened for in the neonatal period and might still occur later, but is not easily overlooked as a symptom complex in a child.

Hirschsprung's disease is suspected after a delayed production of meconium beyond 48 h after birth, and continuing defecation problems usually with distended abdomen and poor appetite, failure to gain weight and vomiting. Also, the history would often document episodes of acute, severe enterocolitis with explosive diarrhea. Clinically, the diagnosis is made by insertion of a catheter through the anus in the distended part, after which decompression follows (see Chapter 17).

Also, Hirschsprung's disease might involve a very small segment of the anorectum and present as constipation. In practice, this is seen only on extremely rare occasions. We have not made this diagnosis in our practice for decades.

Recently, magnetic resonance imaging (MRI) of the pelvis and distal colon has been proposed in order to detect small abnormalities, cysts, tumors or tethered cord which may be the basis of constipation without any other neurological symptom. This approach, however, has not been performed in a large population, and is currently awaiting some protocol definitions.[25]

Examinations

Plain abdominal X-ray

On a plain abdominal radiograph some amount of stool is always visible. The simple report of 'stools in the colon' should therefore not be regarded as indicative of constipation. Barr et al tried to develop a scoring system to define constipation. Although this scoring system is used to diagnose constipation in children with chronic abdominal pain as the only symptom, the method is subject to large intra- and interobserver variability.[26,27]

Colonic transit times are measured by the Metcalf method. Swallowed radio-opaque tiny rings allow the intestinal transit to be measured. This test shows normal transit times in half of the constipated children and is therefore only useful to diagnose slow-transit constipation, a clinical entity usually apparent with night-time soiling and resistance to treatment. The upper limit of colonic transit is 63h. A colonic transit time delayed to more than 100h is defined as slow-transit constipation. A palpable rectal mass is always found. The method can also be used to support the diagnosis of functional non-retentive fecal soiling, but it has no place in the general management of children with constipation.

Barium enema

A barium enema performed in the unprepared colon might delineate the transition zone in Hirschsprung's disease in young infants, but is of limited value, as the transition zone is often difficult to see and might only be of value to the operating surgeon preoperatively after the diagnosis has been made.

Defecography

Defecography uses a relatively high radiation exposure and is difficult and unreliable in children.

Anorectal manometry

Anorectal manometry is a relatively safe, minor invasive technique. With an open perfusion system, pressures may be assessed in anal sphincter muscles at rest, at squeezing and during straining. During defecation, the pelvic pressure or rectal pressure increases, owing to abdominal muscle contraction, and the anal canal pressure decreases, creating a difference to allow defecation. A rectal balloon might be inflated to assess the rectal anal inhibitory reflex against relaxation of the internal anal sphincter. In the clinical setting, except for Hirschsprung's disease, the majority of children have normal anorectal pressures.

Rectal sensitivity after inflation of a balloon is normal. Children who have abnormal defecation dynamics, in an attempt to defecate the balloon, will contract the anal sphincters at the same time that they contract the abdominal musculature. This can be shown on a screen and children can learn to relax instead of having this paradoxical contraction during defecation of the anal musculature. The training by reinforcement is called biofeedback training.

Anorectal manometry is normal in children with functional constipation or functional non-fecal retention, and therefore this should not be used.[1]

Colonic manometry

Colonic manometry[28] requires colonoscopic placement of the catheter with motility recordings, which are measured the day after placement. Colonic motility can be tested over hours, possibly with bisacodyl administration to enable propagated contractions to be endured. This test is reserved for children with intractable constipation. Some investigators can differentiate children with functional fecal retention from those with no neuropathy or myopathy of the colon with this technique. The technique is still used in a few centers; however, its value in the diagnostic process of constipation has to be assessed.

Treatment

Only a few studies, most of them with small patient numbers, have been performed to evaluate treatment for children with defecation disorders. Treatment of constipation is mainly based on empirical experience, rather than on placebo-controlled, randomized studies. The main reason for a consultation is interference with social activities of the child and its family because of the defecation problems (soiling and encopresis). They should be educated and the problem should be demystified.[29] It should be stressed that the prevalence of constipation and soiling is quite common. The relationship between fecal impaction and overflow diarrhea should be explained with the help of drawings, and the involuntary nature of the loss of feces in the underwear made clear. The objective of this is to make parents start to feel more comfortable and decrease the feeling of shame in the child. The child and parents almost invariably accept a positive non-accusatory approach with relief. Organic versus functional disease should be explained clearly, once the history and physical examination have been evaluated and the diagnosis is made with confidence. It should be stressed that there is no need for further investigation. The therapy is stressful and might be long lasting. The child is the only one who is responsible for completing the treatment. Behavioral therapy (see below) is not generally recommended; if the treatment is successful, the behavior abnormalities usually normalize too. It is helpful to advise that a diary is kept to follow and gain insight into the therapeutic progress; it might also motivate the child. The child has to fill in the diary himself, and that enhances responsibility. It might also be linked to a reward system.[30–33]

Another simple general measure is toilet training to normalize defecation. It should be explained that the sensation of defecation must be felt by the child and, usually from the age of 4, will be admitted by the child when it is explained well. The treatment of the child should involve an instruction to attempt to defecate three times a day for 5 min after each meal. This should stimulate straining actively and the child should be able to place his feet on a footrest or on the ground (the younger ones usually need a footrest). This is important, to flatten the anorectal angle, facilitating fecal expulsion. Using this approach, the child will be forced to focus on its bowel function. The emptying of the rectum will reduce the risk of fecal soiling during the rest of the day. This approach is only successful in 50% of children with severe constipation referred to a tertiary hospital, without any added pharmacological treatment.

Fluid intake

Fluid intake of children with constipation has been found to be slightly lower than normal,[33] and so is energy intake, estimated in a prospective study to be around 100 kcal/day lower. Fiber intake of children with constipation was also slightly lower than controls, but in 6 months after reinforcement we found that it could be increased in some by only around 9 g while it was actually decreased in others up to 16 g. The total amount remained less than 20 g and no child achieved 30 g/day. There was no relation between fiber intake, colonic transit times and success in treatment. Therefore, while we would still recommend increasing fiber intake in constipated children, one might not expect much success in children from this intervention alone.[34]

Pharmacotherapy

No double-blind randomized study on oral or rectal laxatives has been performed in children with constipation, except for the use of cisapride.[35] The effect of lactulose, one of the most widely used stool softeners, has not been investigated. An evidence-based treatment cannot be constructed. Almost all advice concerning the use of oral or rectal laxatives is currently based on clinical empirical experience.

The major aim of medical therapy is two-fold: to remove fecal impaction; and to prevent its recurrence by avoiding prolonged rectal distension.

Removing fecal impaction

The most convenient approach in the majority of cases is by daily enemas, better administered after returning from school, as it might take some time to induce defecation.[36] The effect is mainly due to a sudden increase in rectal filling, which leads to a strong rectal contraction and reflex relaxation of the internal anal sphincter, often followed by a bowel movement. The advantage of an enema strategy is a direct effect on overflow incontinence and relief for the child and parents. Enemas have the effect of hyperosmosis and increased fluids in the colon; furthermore, they lubricate the feces and distend the colon. Enemas used in children may contain dioctyl sodium sulfosuccinate and sorbitol or phosphate. Also, oil enemas and tap water enemas can be used. Hyperphosphate enemas in children have some risk when the enema administration is not followed by defecation and might lead, through retention, to hyperphosphatemia, subsequent hypocalcemia, hypokalemia and dehydration.[37,38] Also, hypocalcemia might lead to tetany and cardiac abnormalities in children, which in practice it is mainly seen in treatment of Hirschsprung's disease prior to surgery. Enemas should contain a sufficient amount of fluid: under 2 years of age around 60 ml and above 2 years of age 120 ml. Usually, evacuation is achieved within 3 days with consecutive daily enemas. Otherwise, it should be continued until the fecal mass has been removed successfully. When soiling relapses or the defecation frequency does not normalize with adequate treatment with oral laxatives, enemas are added to long-term treatment on an individual basis, usually 2–3 times weekly. When this procedure for severe fecal impaction is unsuccessful, and also in children who are treated for constipation and have recurrent large impaction, intermittent nasogastric lavage treatment might be tried. A safe and efficient method to clean the intestine is the balanced electrolyte solution of non-resorbable polyethylene glycol. This solution is often well taken by the child and, if he cannot swallow the required quantity, nasogastric tubes might be used. The recommended volume varies between 14 and 40 ml/kg per h, not to exceed 1litre/h, and treatment should be continued until clear fluid is excreted through the rectum, an effect usually reached within 24 h. This treatment gives some temporary relief, but is not a substitute for other treatment protocols.

Preventing recurrence of fecal impaction

The remaining initial treatment after desimpaction is achieved involves osmotic laxatives (lactulose, lactitol) at a dose of 1–6 g/kg body weight per day. The main function is to loosen stool consistency, and enhance the rectal sensation and urge of the child to defecate. The dose might be increased without any danger up to 20–40 g daily. Side-effects are initially bloating, flatulence and increase of abdominal pain, but these symptoms usually disappear after the first 1–2 weeks. Therapy should be continued for at least 3–6 months until constipation has disappeared; the dose should be titrated individually. If this treatment is insufficient, recently polyethylene glycol has been shown to be effective in treating constipation in children at a dose of 0.8 g/kg per day. It also functions as an osmotic laxative.[39,40] It has fewer side-effects in terms of flatulence and abdominal pain, and its tasteless nature increases compliance. The effects are comparable to those of lactulose.

Another laxative is mineral oil, an emollient agent, at a dose of 1–3 ml/kg per day, whose main function is to keep the rectal walls lubricated. Disadvantages are anal oil seepage with coloring of the underwear, which is not removable with washing, and the risk of aspiration and chemical pneumonia in very young children, and in children with cerebral palsy or other causes of mental retardation. Milk of magnesia is a relatively non-absorbable laxative, and can be given at a dose of 1 ml/kg per day. The treatment might be started at a higher dose, up to 3 ml/kg per day. Prokinetic agents, such as cisapride at a dose of 0.2 mg/kg body weight three times daily, have some transient effect on constipation, but this drug is no longer available.

Stimulant laxatives such as bisacodyl, sodium picosulfate and senna alkaloids should be used with caution and have no advantage over osmotic laxatives. Biofeedback training has been shown to normalize defecation dynamics, but has no place in management, because it does not influence therapeutic outcome. Surgical colostomies for antegrade enemas have been successfully tried, but also have their complications; at present, indications are difficult to establish.

In functional non-retentive fecal soiling, biofeedback training showed a minor effect on treatment outcome.[41] In this form of constipation, the main treatment is laxatives. Daily enemas in the morning might help to have a clean day, which might stimulate the defecation behavior. Oral laxatives usually worsen soiling and encopresis and should be avoided in these children with functional non-retentive fecal soiling.

Biofeedback training compared to conventional treatment

In a large cohort of 200 children who had conventional treatment and one arm of biofeedback training added, they did learn to normalize their defecation dynamics, but this normalization had no influence on outcome of treatment. Only in functional non-retentive fecal soiling did biofeedback have a modest effect in a sample of 100 tested children.

Prognosis

In a cohort of more than 400 constipated children, follow-up was obtained by annual telephone contact in more than 95% of children. Mean follow-up was 5 years (range 1–8). The cumulative percentage of children who were successfully treated during follow-up was 60% in 1 year, increasing to 80% in 8 years (Figure 16.1). Interestingly, successful treatment was more

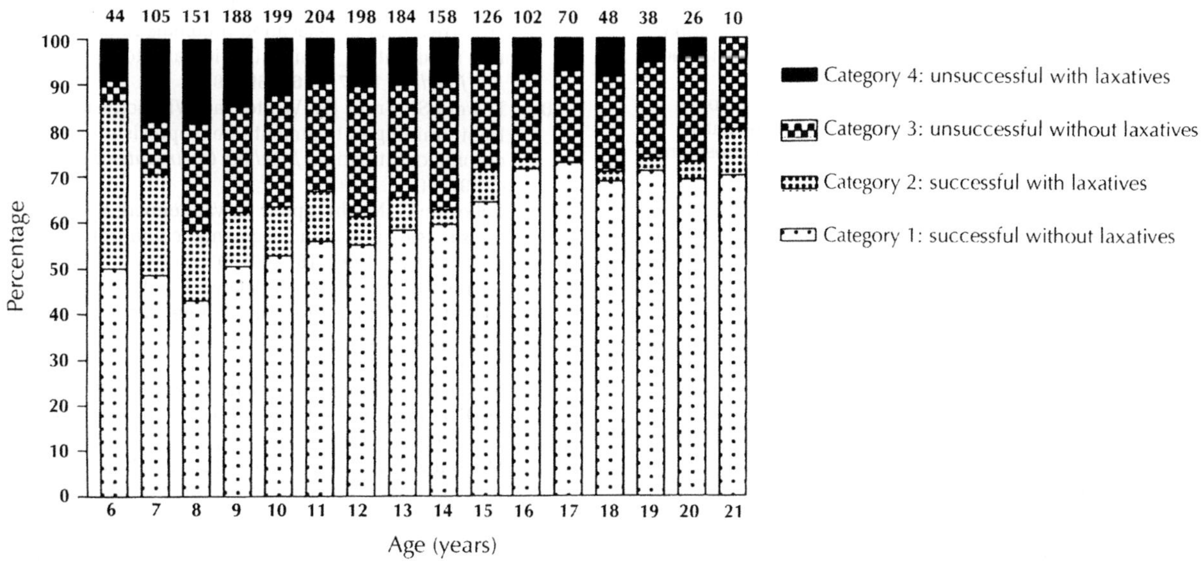

Figure 16.1 Outcome with and without laxatives.

frequent in children without encopresis, and in children with an age at onset of defecation difficulty older than 4 years. In the group of successfully treated children, approximately 50% remained symptom free during the follow-up period, while the other half experienced at least one period of relapse. The relapses occurred more frequently in boys than in girls. In a subset of children aged 16 years and older, constipation was still present in around 30%, thus continuing into adulthood.[42]

REFERENCES

1. van der Plas RN, Benninga MA, Büller HA et al. Biofeedback training in treatment of childhood constipation: a randomized, controlled study. *Lancet* 1996; **348**: 776–780.
2. Rasquin-Weber A, Human PE, Cuccchiara S et al. Childhood functional gastrointestinal disorders. *Gut* 1999; **45**(Suppl 2): 60–68.
3. Loening-Baucke V. Constipation in children. *Gastroenterology* 1993; **105**: 1557–1564.
4. Benninga MA, Buller HA, Heymans HS et al. Is encopresis always the result of constipation? *Arch Dis Child* 1994; **71**: 186–193.
5. Loening-Baucke V. Factors determining outcome in children with chronic constipation and fecal soiling. *Gut* 1989; **30**: 999–1006.
6. Weaver LT, Lucas A. Development of bowel habit in preterm infants. *Arch Dis Child* 1993; **68**: 317–320.
7. Wald A. Colonic and anorectal motility testing in clinical practice. *Am J Gastroenterol* 1994; **89**: 2109–2115.
8. Carlstedt A, Nordgren S, Fasth S et al. Sympathetic nervous influence on the internal anal sphincter and rectum in man. *Int J Colorect Dis* 1988; **3**: 90–95.
9. Sarna SK. Physiology and pathophysiology of colonic motor activity (1). *Dig Dis Sci* 1991; **36**: 827–862.
10. Benninga MA, Wijers OB, Hoeven van der CW et al. Manometry, profilometry, and endosonography: normal physiology and anatomy of the anal canal in healthy children. *J Pediatr Gastroenterol Nutr* 1994; **18**: 68–77.
11. Di Lorenzo C, Flores AF, Hyman PE. Age-related changes in colon motility. *J Pediatr* 1995; **127**: 593–596.
12. Wheatly JM, Hutson JM, Chow CW et al. Slow-transit constipation in childhood. *J Pediatr Surg* 1999; **34**: 829–832.

13. Corazziari E, Cucchiara S, Staiano A et al. Gastrointestinal transit time, frequency of defecation, and anorectal manometry in healthy and constipated children. *J Pediatr* 1985; **106**: 379–382.
14. Benninga MA, Büller HA, Tytgat GNJ et al. Colonic transit time in constipated children: does pediatric slow-transit constipation exist? *J Pediatr Gastroenterol Nutr* 1996; **23**: 241–251.
15. Metcalf AM, Phillips SF, Zinsmeister AR et al. Simplified assessment of segmental colonic transit. *Gastroenterology* 1987; **92**: 40–47.
16. Loening-Baucke VA, Younoszai MK. Abnormal anal sphincter response in chronically constipated children. *J Pediatr* 1982; **100**: 213–218.
17. Read NW, Timms JM. Pathophysiology of constipation. *Acta Gastroenterol Belg* 1987; **50**: 393–404.
18. Steffen R, Loening-Baucke V. Constipation and encopresis. In Wycki R, Hyams JS, eds. *Pediatric Gastrointestinal Disease*, 2nd edn. Philadelphia: WB Saunders, 1999: 43–50.
19. Cucchiara S, Coremans G, Staiano A et al. Gastrointestinal transit time and anorectal manometry in children with fecal soiling. *J Peditar Gastroenterol Nutr* 1984; **3**: 545–550.
20. Borowitz SM, Sutphen J, Ling W, Cox DJ. Lack of correlation of anorectal manometry with symptoms of chronic childhood constipation and encopresis. *Dis Colon Rectum* 1996; **39**: 400–405.
21. van der Plas RN, Benninga MA, Redekop WK et al. How accurate is the recall of bowel habits in children with defecation disorders? *Eur J Pediatr* 1997; **156**: 178–181.
22. Loening-Baucke V. Constipation in early childhood: patient characteristics, treatment, and longterm follow up. *Gut* 1993; **34**: 1400–1404.
23. Loening-Baucke V. Urinary incontinence and urinary tract infection and their resolution with treatment of chronic constipation of childhood. *Pediatrics* 1997; **100**: 228–232.
24. Meunier P, Mollard P, Marechal JM. Physiopathology of megarectum: the association of megarectum with encopresis. *Gut* 1976; **17**: 224–227.
25. Andrade R, Fortunato C, Nurko S. Spinal cord abnormalities in children with constipation. *Gastroenterology* 2002; **122**: A315.
26. Benninga MA, Büller HA, Staalman CR et al. Defecation disorders in children, colonic transit time versus the Barr-score. *Eur J Pediatr* 1995; **154**: 277–284.
27. Barr RG, Levine MD, Wilkinson RH, Mulvihill D. Chronic and occult stool retention: a clinical tool for its evaluation in school-aged children. *Clin Pediatr (Phila)* 1979; **18**: 674, 676.
28. Di Lorenzo C, Flores AF, Reddy SN, Hyman PE. Use of colonic manometry to differentiate causes of intractable constipation in children. *J Pediatr* 1992; **120**: 690–695.
29. van der Plas RN, Benninga MA, Taminiau JA, Büller HA. Treatment of defecation problems in children: the role of education, demystification and toilet training. *Eur J Pediatr* 1997; **156**: 689–692.
30. Lowery SP, Srour JW, Whitehead WE, Schuster MM. Habit training as treatment of encopresis secondary to chronic constipation. *J Pediatr Gastroenterol Nutr* 1985; **4**: 397–401.
31. Roberson G, Meshkinpour H, Vandenberg K et al. Effects of exercise on total and segmental colon transit. *J Clin Gastroenterol* 1993; **16**: 300–303.
32. Levine MD, Mazonson P, Bakow H. Behavioral symptom substitution in children cured of encopresis. *Am J Dis Child* 1980; **134**: 663–667.
33. Stark LJ, Spirito A, Lewis AV, Hart KJ. Encopresis: behavioral parameters associated with children who fail medical management. *Child Psychiatry Hum Dev* 1990; **20**: 169–179.
34. Mooren GC, van der Plas RN, Bossuyt PM et al. Het verband tussen inname van voedingsvezels en chronische obstipatie bij kinderen. *Ned Tijdschr Geneesk* 1996; **140**: 2036–2039.
35. Nurko S, Garcia-Arnada JA, Guerrero VY, Worona LB. Treatment of intractable constipation in children: experience with cisapride. *J Pediatr Gastroenterol Nutr* 1996; **22**: 38–44.
36. Price KJ, Elliott TM. What is the rule of stimulant laxatives in the management of childhood constipation and soiling? (Cochrane Review). *Cochrane Database Syst Rev* 2001; **3**: CD002040.
37. Martin RR, Lisehora GR, Braxton M Jr, Barcia PJ. Fatal poisoning from sodium phosphate enema: case report and experimental study. *JAMA* 1987; **257**: 2190–2192.
38. Sotos JF, Cutler EA, Finkel MA, Doody D. Hypocalcemic coma following two pediatric phosphate enemas. *Pediatrics* 1977; **60**: 305–307.
39. Loening-Baucke V. Polyethylene glycol without electrolytes for children with constipation and encopresis. *J Ped Gastroent Nutr* 2002; **34**: 372–377.
40. Youssef NN, Peters JM, Hnederson W et al. Dose response of PEG 3350 for the treatment of childhood fecal impaction. *J Pediatr* 2002; **141**: 410–415.
41. van Ginkel R, Benninga MA, Blommaart PJ et al. Lack of benefit of laxatives as adjunctive therapy for functional nonretentive fecal soiling in children. *J Pediatr* 2000; **137**: 808–813.
42. van Ginkel R, Reitsma JB, Buller HA et al. Childhood constipation: longitudinal follow-up beyond puberty. *Gastroenterology* 2003; **125**: 357–363.

17 Hirschsprung's disease and intestinal neuronal dysplasias

Annamaria Staiano, Lucia Quaglietta and Renata Auricchio

Introduction

Hirschsprung's disease is a heterogeneous genetic disorder, resulting from an anomaly of the enteric nervous system of neural crest cell origin, characterized by the absence of parasympathetic intrinsic ganglionic cells in the submucosal and myenteric plexuses. It is regarded as the consequence of the premature arrest of the craniocaudal migration of vagal neural crest cells in the hindgut, between the 5th and 12th weeks of gestation, to form the enteric nervous system, and is therefore considered a neurocristopathy.[1]

Epidemiology

Hirschsprung's disease occurs in approximately 1 of 5000 live births, and with a male predominance of 4 : 1. It is generally sporadic, although in 3–7% of cases a genetic transmission has been reported.[1] The risk for short-segment disease is 5% in brothers and 1% in sisters of index cases; for long-segment disease the risk is 10%, regardless of sex.[2]

Etiology

Hirschsprung's disease is characterized by the congenital absence of ganglionic cells in the submucosal and myenteric plexuses in the distal bowel, and variable proportion of the colon proximally. The embryonic disorder is a lack of the craniocaudal migration, differentiation and maturation of neuroblasts from the neural crests. The earlier the migration ceases, the longer the aganglionic segment will be. The aganglionic segment is permanently contracted, causing dilatation of its proximal tract.[3]

Hirschsprung's disease may be classified according to the length of the aganglionic segment: the classic form (short segment in 70–75% of cases) is limited to the rectum and sigmoid colon; the long segment, or subtotal colonic disease (10–15%), generally involves the bowel up to the splenic flexure; total colonic aganglionosis (TCA; 3–6%) may extend to involve a variable amount of the short bowel; and total intestinal aganglionosis is sometimes associated with intestinal malrotation or volvulus.[4] Ultrashort-segment aganglionosis is considered a functional alteration, without any detectable histological finding. Although longer aganglionic segments tend to produce more dramatic symptoms, some patients with even short-segment disease deteriorate rapidly.[5]

Pathophysiology

The hallmark of diagnosis is the absence of ganglionic cells from the myenteric and submucosal plexuses, as seen on a full-thickness or suction (mucosal–submucosal) biopsy of the rectum. Proximal contents fail to enter the unrelaxed, aganglionic segment. The lack of non-adrenergic–non cholinergic (NANC) inhibitory innervation is responsible for a tonic contraction of the affected segment, with absence of peristalsis and proximal dilatation of the gut.[6]

Morphologically, ganglionic cells are absent from the narrowed segment and for some distance (usually 1–5 cm) into the dilated segment. The pattern of nerve fibers is also abnormal; they are hypertrophic with abundant, thickened bundles. Specific stains for acetylcholinesterase are used to highlight the abnormal morphology.[7,8]

In recent years, new insights into the pathophysiology of Hirschsprung's disease have been gained. There is growing evidence suggesting that the disease might be the expression of a genetic alteration, as reported in the genetic section of this chapter.

It has also been suggested that abnormal expression of the muscular neural cell adhesion molecule is likely to be associated with an arrest in the craniocaudal migration of neural cells to their most distal location.[9] Furthermore, the lack of nitric oxide (NO)-producing nerve fibers in the aganglionic intestine probably contributes to the inability of the smooth muscle to relax, thereby causing lack of peristalsis.[10] In addition, in the aganglionic segments, interstitial cells of Cajal are scarce and their network appears to be disrupted.[11]

Clinical signs/symptoms

In the newborn, symptoms may appear during the first hours of life with failure to pass meconium, or in the first week with a picture of intestinal obstruction. However, the delay in passage of meconium is not constant, and a percentage of children still presents late or with complications despite a history of problems since birth. Enterocolitis, the most common complication, is always severe and is an important cause of mortality in these young patients.

In infants and children, the presentation is often less dramatic and may not mimic acute intestinal obstruction (Figure 17.1). Severe constipation and recurrent fecal impaction are more common. Physical examination reveals a distended abdomen and a contracted anal sphincter and rectum in most children. The rectum is devoid of stools, except in cases of short-segment aganglionosis. As the finger is withdrawn, there may be an explosive discharge of foul-smelling liquid stools, with decompression of the proximal normal bowel.

Complications

Over the past four decades, enterocolitis has been a major cause of morbidity and mortality in infants and children with Hirschsprung's disease. The mean incidence is 25%, but the range is great (from 17 to 50%) and may be differently estimated, depending on the manner in which it is diagnosed. Mortality rates range from 0 to 33%, probably reflecting differences in the diagnostic criteria.[12] Mortality also appears to be associated with other factors, such as trisomy 21. The classic clinical manifestations described for enterocolitis include abdominal distension, explosive diarrhea, vomiting, fever, lethargy, rectal bleeding and shock.[13]

Abdominal radiographs show the intestinal 'cut-off' sign in the rectosigmoidal region with absence of air distally. Other common findings are small-bowel dilatation in 74% of patients and multiple air–fluid levels.[14] Because of the risk of perforation, contrast enema should not be performed in the presence of clinical enterocolitis.

Postoperative enterocolitis has been associated with a fairly high rate of mortality in several series. In fact, when examining the deaths related to

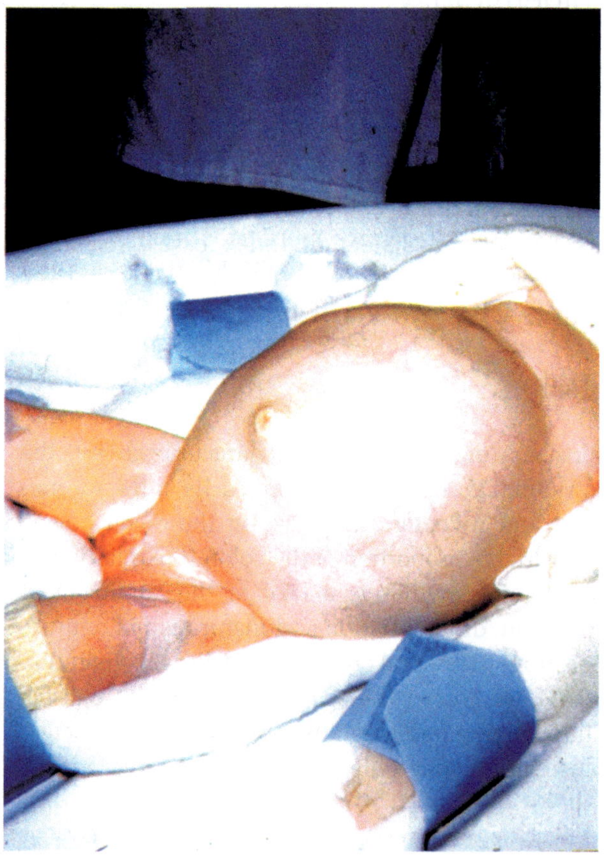

Figure 17.1 Severe abdominal distension in an infant with Hirschsprung's disease.

Hirschsprung's disease, several groups found that approximately 50% of deaths resulted from complications directly related to an enterocolitis episode.[15,16]

Rectal washouts should be the initial approach in the care of a child, regardless of age, who presents with enterocolitis. Along with washouts, intravenous antibiotics or oral metronidazole (in mild cases) should be used. Should the disease process fail to improve, or the infant's condition deteriorate, the performance of a leveling colostomy should be considered.[15,16]

Diagnosis with differential

For the diagnosis of Hirschsprung's disease, the subject's history is very important. The crucial elements to obtain are: the age of the appearance of symptoms; whether the passage of meconium has been normal or delayed; and whether the child presented with episodes of functional intestinal obstruction. In addition, a functional (idiopathic) megacolon must be ruled out. A clinical comparison between functional and congenital megacolon is shown in Table 17.1. When the history (early onset of constipation, absence of fecal soiling) and/or the physical examination (empty rectal ampulla) suggests an organic cause, anorectal manometry should be performed.

Anorectal manometry evaluates the response of the internal anal sphincter to inflation of a balloon in the rectal ampulla.[17] When the rectal balloon is inflated, there is normally a reflex relaxation of the sphincter. The rectoanal inhibitory reflex is absent in patients with Hirschsprung's disease; there is no relaxation, or there may even be paradoxical contraction of the internal anal sphincter (Figure 17.2). Anorectal manometry is particularly useful when the aganglionic segment is short and the results of radiological or pathological studies are equivocal.

Barium enema is helpful in the assessment of a transition zone between aganglionic and ganglionic bowel, and in giving an estimation of the length of an aganglionic segment. Demonstration of the transition zone is easier if no effort is made to cleanse the bowel (Figure 17.3). In the newborn, dilatation of the proximal ganglionic bowel may not have developed and radiological diagnosis may be more difficult. The sensitivity and specificity for recognition of a transition zone have been reported to be 80% and 76%, respectively.[18] The barium enema may not show a transition zone in cases of total colonic Hirschsprung's disease, or may be indistinguishable from cases of functional constipation when ultrashort-segment Hirschsprung's disease is present.

Nevertheless, the diagnosis is based on histological evidence. Since the mid-1970s,

Table 17.1 Differentiating types of megacolon in children

Signs and symptoms	Functional fecal retention	Colonic neuromuscular disorders
Soiling	common	rare
Obstructive symptoms	rare	common
Large-caliber stools	common	rare
Stool-withholding behavior	common	rare
Enterocolitis	never	possible
Associated upper-gastrointestinal symptoms	never	common
Symptoms from birth	rare	common
Localization of stools	rectum	rectal and extrarectal

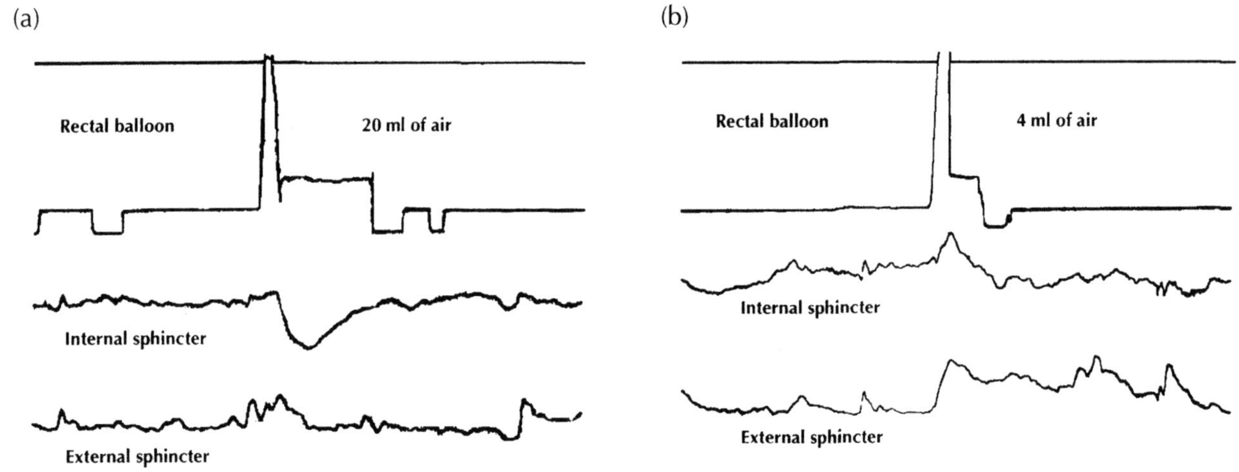

Figure 17.2 Anorectal manometry in a 2-month-old boy with functional constipation (a). Note that the distension of a rectal balloon with air for 1 s produces a decrease of anal pressure (rectosphincter reflex). (b) Anorectal manometry in a 3-month-old boy with Hirschsprung's disease. Distension of a rectal balloon with air for 1 s produces no decrease of anal pressure.

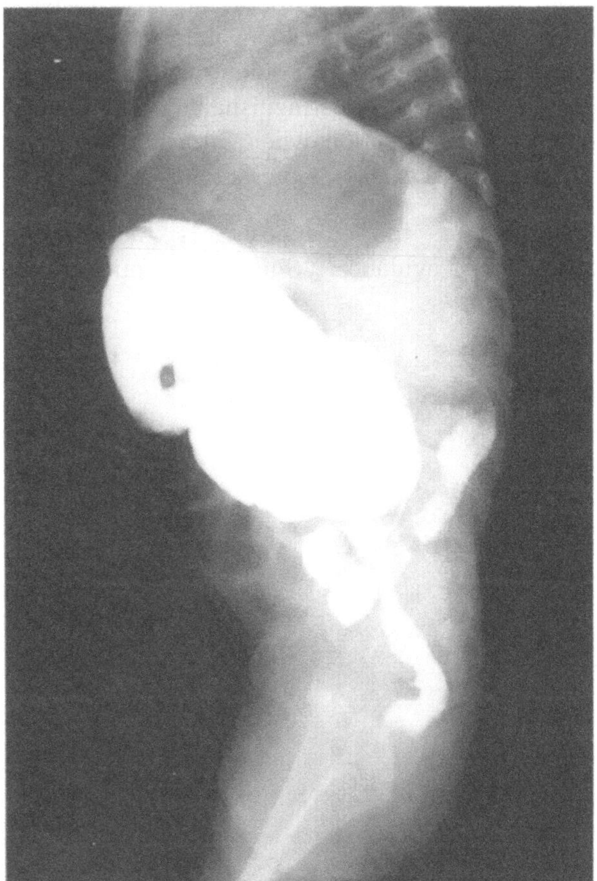

Figure 17.3 Barium enema showing a long, narrowed segment in a child with Hirschsprung's disease.

demonstration of acetylcholinesterase activity in mucosal biopsies has allowed the non-invasive suction rectal biopsy technique to become the most reliable diagnostic method for aganglionosis.[7,8] The histological diagnosis is based on the demonstration of the total absence of ganglionic cells in the affected segment of the intestine, with an overgrowth of large nerve trunks in the intermuscular and submucosal zones (Figures 17.4 and 17.5).[19] Two small samples of rectal mucosa and submucosa, taken using the suction rectal biopsy technique, are sufficient for diagnosis. The two pieces must be taken not less than 2 cm above the dentate line, to avoid the physiological hypoganglionic zone, and not more than 5 cm above the dentate line, to avoid missing the diagnosis of a short-segment disease. Acetylcholinesterase activity in the normal colon shows only a few fibers in the lamina propria and muscularis mucosae; in Hirschsprung's disease there is an increase in thick, knotted acetylcholinesterase-positive nerve fibers in the muscularis mucosae and lamina propria, and hypertrophied nerve trunks in the submucosa.

The hyperplastic nerve trunks in the lamina propria, submucosa and muscularis propria are both adrenergic and cholinergic. Thus, these are extrinsic nerve fibers that are hyperplastic, owing

cholinesterase technique has been found to be of great value in determining the extent of IND intraoperatively.[42]

Genetic aspects

Hirschsprung's disease

HSCR occurs as an isolated trait in 70% of patients, and is associated with chromosomal abnormality in 12% of cases, trisomy 21 being by far the most frequent (> 90%). Additional congenital anomalies are found in 18% of cases, and include gastrointestinal malformation, cleft palate, polydactyly, cardiac septal defects and craniofacial anomalies. The higher rate of associated anomalies in familial cases than in isolated cases (39% vs. 21%) strongly suggests syndromes with Mendelian inheritance.[43] Isolated HSCR appears to be a multifactorial malformation with low, sex-dependent penetrance, variable expression according to the length of the aganglionic segment, and a suggestion of involvement of one or more gene(s) with low penetrance.[44] These parameters must be taken into account for accurate evaluation of the recurrence risk in relatives. Segregation analyses suggested an oligogenic mode of inheritance in isolated HSCR. With a relative risk as high as 200, HSCR is an excellent model for the approach to common multifactorial diseases.

A large number of chromosomal anomalies have been described in HSCR patients. Free trisomy 21 (Down's syndrome) is by far the most frequent, involving 2–10% of ascertained HSCR cases. Syndromes associated with HSCR can be classified as: pleiotropic neurocristopathies; syndromes with HSCR as a mandatory feature; and occasional association with recognizable syndromes. The neural crest is a transient and multipotent embryonic structure that gives rise to neuronal, endocrine and paraendocrine, craniofacial, conotruncal heart and pigmentary tissues. Neurocristopathies encompass tumors, malformations and single or multifocal abnormalities of the tissues mentioned above in various combinations. Multiple endocrine neoplasia type 2 (MEN 2) and Waardenburg syndrome are the most frequent neurocristopathies associated with HSCR.[45]

Waardenburg syndrome, an autosomal dominant condition, is by far the most frequent condition combining pigmentary anomalies and sensorineural deafness, resulting from the absence of melanocytes of the skin and the stria vascularis of the cochlea. The combination of HSCR with Waardenburg syndrome defines the WS4 type (Shah–Waardenburg syndrome). Indeed, homozygous mutations of the endothelin pathway and heterozygous *SOX10* mutations have been identified in WS4 patients with central nervous system involvement including seizures, ataxia and demyelinating peripheral and central neuropathies.[46]

A wide spectrum of additional isolated anomalies have been described among HSCR cases with an incidence of sporadic types varying from 5 to 30%.[47,48] No constant pattern is observed. These anomalies include distal limb, sensorineural, skin, gastrointestinal, central nervous system, genital, kidney and cardiac malformations, and facial dysmorphic features.

These data highlight the importance of a careful assessment by a clinician trained in dysmorphology for all newborns diagnosed with HSCR. Skeletal X-ray and cardiac and urogenital echographic survey should be systematically performed. The observation of one additional anomaly to HSCR should prompt chromosomal studies.

Molecular genetics

Eight genes are known to be involved in HSCR in humans, namely the proto-oncogene *RET* (*RET*), glial cell line-derived neurotrophic factor (*GDNF*), neurturin (*NTN*), endothelin B receptor (*EDNRB*), endothelin 3 (*EDN3*), endothelin converting enzyme 1 (*ECE1*), *SOX10* and *SIP1* genes. RET and EDNRB signaling pathways were considered biochemically independent. However, an HSCR patient heterozygous for weak hypomorphic mutations in both *RET* and *EDNRB* has recently been reported.[49] Each mutation was inherited from a healthy parent. Sox10, otherwise, is involved in cell lineage determination and could be responsible of the reduced expression of EDNRB in the *dom* mouse.

The RET signaling pathway

The first observation was about an interstitial deletion of chromosome 10q11.2 in patients with TCA and mental retardation.[50] The proto-oncogene *RET*, identified as disease-causing in MEN 2 and mapping to 10q11.2, was regarded as a good candidate gene, owing to the concurrence of MEN 2A and HSCR in some families and the expression in neural crest-derived cells. Consequently, *RET* gene mutations were identified in HSCR patients.[51] Expression and penetrance of a *RET* mutation is variable and sex dependent within HSCR families (72% males and 51% females). Over 80 mutations have been identified including large deletions encompassing the *RET* gene, microdeletions and insertions, nonsense, missense and splicing mutations.[52,53] Haploinsufficiency is the most likely mechanism for HSCR mutations. Biochemical studies showed variable consequences of some HSCR mutations (misfolding, failure to transport the protein to the cell surface, abolished biological activity).

Despite extensive mutation screening, a *RET* mutation is identified in only 50% of familial and 15–20% of sporadic HSCR cases.[54] However, most families, with a few exceptions, are compatible with linkage at the *RET* locus.[55]

Mutations in the *RET* ligand, such as *GDNF*, *GFRA1-4*, *NTN*, persephin (*PSPN*) and artemin (*ARTN*), may occur, but are not sufficient to lead to HSCR.

The endothelin signaling pathway

A susceptibility locus for HSCR in 13q22 was suggested for three main reasons: a significant lod score at 13q22 in a large inbred Old Order Mennonite community with multiple cases of HSCR; *de novo* interstitial deletion of 13q22 in several patients with HSCR; and synteny between the murine locus for *piebald-lethal*, a model of aganglionosis, and 13q22 in humans. Subsequently, an *EDNRB* missense mutation was identified in the Mennonite kindred.[56,57] Both *EDNRB* and *EDN3* were screened in a large series of isolated HSCR patients, and *EDNRB* mutations were identified in approximately 5% of the patients. It is worth mentioning that the penetrance of *EDN3* and *EDNRB* heterozygous mutations was incomplete in those HSCR patients, *de novo* mutations have not hitherto been observed and short HSCR (S-HSCR) is largely predominant.[58]

SOX10

The last *de novo* mouse model for WS4 in humans is *dominant megalon* (*Dom*). The *Dom* gene is *SOX10*, a member of the sex-determining factor (SRY)-like, high mobility group (HMG) DNA binding proteins. Subsequently, heterozygous *SOX10* mutations have been identified in familial and isolated patients with WS4 (including *de novo* mutation) with high penetrance.[59]

Intestinal neuronal dysplasia

Studies have been performed to investigate the potential role of HSCR-associated *RET*, *GDNF*, *EDNRB* and *EDN*3 genes in the development of IND. They demonstrated that only three RET mutation were detected in patients with HSCR, no mutation in this gene was observed in IND and mixed HSCR/IND patients, HSCR and HSCR/IND patients showed over-representation of a specific *RET* polymorphism in exon 2, while IND patients exhibited a significantly lower frequency of the same polymorphism comparable with that of controls. These findings may suggest that IND is genetically different from HSCR.

A homozygous mutation of the *EDNRB* gene in spotting lethal (sl/sl) rats leads to the HSCR phenotype with long segmented aganglionosis. The heterozygous (+/sl) *EDNRB*-deficient rats revealed more subtle abnormalities of the enteric nervous system: the submucous plexus was characterized by a significantly increased ganglionic size and density, and the presence of hypertrophied nerve fiber strands, resembling the histopathological criteria for IND. Other animal models, such as *Ncx*/*Hox*11L.1-deficient mice, suggest that many other genes could be involved in the pathogenesis of IND.[60]

REFERENCES

1. Taviras S, Pachinis V. Development of the mammalian enteric system. *Curr Opin Genet Dev* 1999; **9**: 321.
2. Lyonnet S, Bolino A, Pelet A et al. A gene for Hirschsprung disease maps to the proximal long arm of chromosome 10. *Nat Genet* 1993; **4**: 346–350.
3. Gershon MD, Chalazonitis A, Rothman TP. From neural crest to bowel: development of the enteric nervous system. *J Neurobiol* 1993; **24**: 199–214.
4. Badner JA, Sieber Wk, Garver KL et al. A genetic study of Hirschsprung's disease. *Am J Hum Genet* 1990; **46**: 568–580.
5. Staiano A, Corazziari E, Andreotti MR, Clouse RE. Esophageal motility in children with Hirschsprung's disease. *Am J Dis Child* 1991; **145**: 310–313.
6. Larsson LT, Shen Z, Ekbland E et al. Lack of neuronal nitric oxide synthase in nerve fibers of aganglionic intestine: a clue to Hirschsprung's disease. *J Pediatr Gastroenterol Nutr* 1995; **20**: 49–53.
7. Meier-Ruge W. Uber Ein Erkrankungsbild des colon mit Hirschsprung-Symptomatik. *Vehr Dtsch Ges Pathol* 1971; **55**: 506–510.
8. Lake BD, Puri P, Nixon HH, Claireaux AE. Hirschsprung's disease. An appraisal of histochemically demonstrated acetylcholinesterase activity in suction rectal biopsy specimens as an aid to diagnosis. *Arch Path Lab Med* 1978; **26**: 288–291.
9. Romanska HM, Bishop AE, Brereton RJ et al. Increased expression of muscular neural cell adhesion molecule in congenital aganglionosis. *Gastroenterology* 1993; **105**: 1104–1109.
10. Vanderwinden JM, De Laet MH, Schiffmann SN et al. Nitric oxide synthase distribution in the enteric nervous system of Hirschsprung's disease. *Gastroenterology* 1993; **105**: 969–973.
11. Vanderwinden JM, Rumessen JJ, Liu H et al. Interstitial cells of cajal in human colon and in Hirschsprung's disease. *Gastroenterology* 1996; **111**: 901–910.
12. Coran AG, Teitelbaum DH. Recent advances in management of Hirschsprung's disease. *Am J Surg* 2000; **180**: 382–387.
13. Bill JAH, Chapman ND. The enterocolitis of Hirschsprung's disease: its natural history and treatment. *Am J Surg* 1962; **103**: 70–74.
14. Elhalaby EA, Coran AG, Blane CE et al. Enterocolitis associated with Hirschsprung's disease: a clinical–radiological characterization based on 168 patients. *J Pediatr Surg* 1995; **30**: 1023–1027.
15. Swenson O, Fisher JH. Hirschsprung's disease during infancy. *Surg Clin North Am* 1956; **36**: 115–122.
16. Marty TL, Matlak ME, Hendrickson M et al. Unexpected death from enterocolitis after surgery for Hirschsprung's disease. *Pediatrics* 1995; **96**: 118–121.
17. Loening-Baucke V. Modulation of abnormal defecation dynamics by biofeedback treatment in chronically constipated children with encopresis. *J Pediatr* 1990; **116**: 214–222.
18. Taxman TI, Yulish BS, Rothstein FC. How useful is barium enema in diagnosis of infantile Hirschsprung's disease? *Am J Dis Child* 1986; **140**: 881–884.
19. Aldridge RT, Campbell PE. Ganglion cells distribution in the normal rectum and anal canal: a basis for diagnosis of Hirschsprung's disease by anorectal biopsy. *J Pediatr Surg* 1968; **3**: 475–489.
20. Milla PJ. Regulatory gut peptides in intestinal neuronal dysplasia and Hirschsprung's disease. In Hadziselimovic F, Herzog B, eds. *Falk Symposium 65. Inflammatory Bowel Disease and Morbus Hirschsprung*. Dordrecht: Kluwer Academic Publishers, 1992: 239–250.
21. Hellstrom PM, Lundberg JM, Holfelt T, Goldstein M. Neuropeptide Y, peptide YY and sympathetic control of rectal tone and anal canal pressure in the cat. *Scand J Gastroenterol* 1989; **24**: 231–243.
22. Langer JC, Fitzgerald PG, Winthrop AL et al. One vs two stage Soave pull-through for Hirschsprung's disease in the first year of life. *J Pediatr Surg* 1996; **31**: 33–37.
23. Pierro A, Fasoli L, Kiely EM et al. Staged pull-through for rectosigmoid Hirschsprung's disease is not safer than primary pull-through. *J Pediatr Surg* 1997; **32**: 505–509.
24. Hackam DJ, Superina RA, Pearl RH. Single stage repair of Hirschsprung's disease: a comparison of 109 patients over 5 years. *J Pediatr Surg* 1997; **32**: 1028–1031.
25. Jona JZ, Cohen RD, Georgeson KE et al. Laparoscopic pull-through procedure for Hirschsprung's disease. *Semin Pediatr Surg* 1998; **7**: 228–231.
26. Smith BM, Stainer RB, Lobe TE. Laparoscopic Duhamel pull-through procedure for Hirschsprung's disease in Childhood. *J Laparoendosc Surg* 1994; **4**: 273–276.
27. Curran TJ, Raffensperger JG. Laparoscopic Swenson pull-through: a comparison with the open procedure. *J Pediatr Surg* 1996; **31**: 1155–1156.
28. De La Torre- Mondragon L, Ortega-Salgado JA. Transanal endorectal pull-through for Hirschsprung's disease. *J Pediatr Surg* 1998; **33**: 1283–1286.
29. Langer JC, Minkes RK, Mazziotti MV et al. Transanal one-stage Soave procedure for infants with Hirschsprung's disease. *J Pediatr Surg* 1999; **34**: 148–152.
30. Albanese CT, Jennings RW, Smith B et al. Perineal one-stage pull-through for Hirschsprung's disease. *J Pediatr Surg* 1999; **34**: 377–380.
31. Langer JC, Scifert M, Mikes RK. One stage Soave pull-through for Hirschsprung's disease. A comparison of the transanal and open approach. *J Pediatr Surg* 2000; **35**: 820–822.
32. Teeraratkul S. Transanal one stage endorectal pull-through for Hirschsprung's disease in infants and children. *J Pediatr Surg* 2003; **38**: 184–187.
33. Miele E, Tozzi A, Staiano A et al. Persistence of abnormal gastrointestinal motility operation for Hirschsprung's disease. *Am J Gastroenterol* 2000; **95**: 1226–1230.
34. Di Lorenzo C, Flores AF, Reddy SN et al. Small bowel neuropathy in symptomatic children after surgery for Hirschsprung's disease. *Gastroenterology* 1997; **112**: 783A.
35. Fadda B, Meier WA, Meier-Ruge W et al. Neuronale intestinale Dysplasie: Eine Kritische 10-Jahres-Analyse Klinischer und Bioptischer Diagnostik. *Z Kinderchir* 1983; **38**: 305–311.
36. Smith VV. Isolated intestinal neuronal dysplasia: a descriptive pattern or a distinct clinicopathological entity? In Hadziselimomic F, Herzog B, eds. *Inflammatory Bowel Disease and Morbus Hirschsprung*. Dordrecht, The Netherlands: Kluwer Academic, 1992: 203–214.
37. Kobayashi H, Hirakawa H, Surana R et al. Intestinal neuronal dysplasia is a possible cause of persistant bowel symptoms after pull-through operation for Hirschsprung's disease. *J Pediatr Surg* 1995; **30**: 253–259.

38. Fadda B, Pistor G, Meier-Ruge W et al. Symptoms, diagnosis and therapy of neuronal intestinal dysplasia masked by Hirschsprung's disease. *J Pediatr Surg* 1987; **2**: 76–80.
39. Borchard F, Meier-Ruge W, Wiebecke B et al. Innervationsstrunger des Dickdarms – Klassifikation und Diagnostik. *Pathologe* 1991; **12**: 171–174.
40. Cord-Udy CL, Smith VV, Ahmed S et al. An evaluation of the role of suction rectal biopsy in the diagnosis of intestinal neuronal dysplasia. *J Pediatr Gastroenterol Nutr* 1997; **24**: 1–6.
41. Koletzko S, Jesh I, Faus- Kebler T et al. Rectal biopsy for diagnosis of intestinal neuronal dysplasia in children: a prospective study on interobserver variation and clinical outcome. *Gut* 1999; **44**: 856–861.
42. Kobayashi H, O'Briain S, Hirakawa H et al. A rapid tecnique for acetylcholinesterase staining. *Arch Pathol Lab Med* 1994; **118**: 1127–1129.
43. Brooks AS, Breuning MH, Meijers C. Spectrum of phenotypes associated with Hirschsprung disease: an evaluation of 239 patients from a single institution. *The Third International Meeting: Hirschsprung Disease and the Correlated Neurocristopathies.* France: Evian, 1998
44. Puffenberger EG, Kauffman ER, Bolk S et al. Identity-by-descent and association mapping of a recessive gene for Hirschsprung disease on human chromosome 13q22. *Hum Mol Genet* 1994; **3**: 1217–1225.
45. Decker RA, Peacock ML, Watson P. Hirschsprung disease in MEN 2A: increased spectrum of RET exon 10 genotypes and strong genotype–phenotype correlation. *Hum Mol Genet* 1998; **7**: 129–134.
46. Edery P, Attie T, Amiel J et al. Mutation of the endothelin-3 gene in the Waardenburg–Hirschsprung disease (Shah–Waardenburg syndrome). *Nat Genet* 1996; **12**: 442–444.
47. Sarioglu A, Tanyel FC, Buyukpamukcu N, Hicsonmez A. Hirschsprung-associated congenital anomalies. *Eur J Pediatr Surg* 1997; **7**: 331–337.
48 Auricchio A, Griseri P, Carpentieri ML et al. Double heterozygosity for a RET substitution interfering with splicing and an EDNRB missense mutation in Hirschsprung disease. *Am J Hum Genet* 1999; **64**: 1216–1221.
49. Martucciello G, Biocchini M, Dodero P et al. Total colonic aganglionosis associated with interstitial deletion of the long arm of chromosome 10. *Pediatr Surg Int* 1992; **7**: 308.
50. Edery P, Lyonnet S, Mulligan LM et al. Mutations of the RET proto-oncogene in Hirschsprung's disease. *Nature* 1994; **367**: 378–380.
51. Angrist M, Bolk S, Thiel B et al. Mutation analysis of the RET receptor tyrosine kinase in Hirschsprung disease. *Hum Mol Genet* 1995; **4**: 821–830.
52. Seri M, Yin L, Barone V et al. Frequency of RET mutations in long- and short-segment Hirschsprung disease. *Hum Mutat* 1997; **9**: 243–249.
53. Attie T, Pelet A, Edery P et al. Diversity of RET proto-oncogene mutations in familial and sporadic Hirschsprung disease. *Hum Mol Genet* 1995; **4**: 1381–1386.
54. Bolk S, Pelet A, Hofstra RM et al. A human model for multigenic inheritance: phenotypic expression in Hirschsprung disease requires both the RET gene and a new 9q31 locus. *Proc Natl Acad Sci USA* 2000; **97**: 268–273.
55. Borrego S, Ruiz A, Saez ME et al. RET genotypes comprising specific haplotypes of polymorphic variants predispose to isolated Hirschsprung disease. *J Med Genet* 2000; **37**: 572–578.
56. Kiss P, Orsztovics M. Association of 13q deletion and Hirschsprung's disease. *J Med Genet* 1989; **26**: 793–794.
57. Puffenberger EG, Hosoda K, Washington SS et al. A missense mutation of endothelin-B receptor gene in multigenic Hirschsprung's disease. *Cell* 1994; **30**: 1257–1266.
58. Auricchio A, Casari G, Staiano A, Ballabio A. Endothelin-B receptor mutations in patients with isolated Hirschsprung disease from a non-inbred population. *Hum Mol Genet* 1996; **5**: 351–354.
59. Southard-Smith EM, Angrist M, Eleison JS et al. The Sox10 (Dom) mouse: modeling the genetic variation of Waardenburg–Shah (WS4) syndrome. *Genom Res* 1999; **9**: 215–225.
60. Yamataka A, Datano M, Kobayashi H et al. Intestinal neuronal displasia-like pathology in Ncx/Hox11L.1 deficient mice. *J Pediatr Surg* 2001; **36**: 1293–1296.

Additional educational resources

www.1uphealth.com/health/hirschsprung_disease_info.htm
www.bdid.com/cam.htm
www.anatomy.med.unsw.edu.au/ebl/embryo/OMIM

18 Chronic intestinal pseudo-obstruction in childhood

Peter J Milla

Introduction

Chronic intestinal pseudo-obstruction (CIP) is a clinical syndrome characterized by signs of intestinal obstruction without mechanical occlusion of the gut. A number of other names have been used to described the disorder, including adynamic bowel, Hirschsprung's disease, megacystis, microcolon hypoperistalsis syndrome, visceral neuropathies and visceral myopathies. Initially, it was thought that CIP was a single disease entity without clearly defined pathology. Over the past 20 years, however, numerous reports have appeared which show that this is not the case.[1–4] CIP is a heterogeneous disorder associated with a wide variety of pathologies, some intrinsic to the gut, others multisystem disorders involving the gut or altering the environment within which the gut operates. The conditions cause disordered intestinal motor activity and may present acutely or chronically. The most common forms of pseudo-obstruction are acute in nature and occur as postoperative ileus or the ileus that is associated with electrolyte imbalance and metabolic disorder. Acute pseudo-obstruction episodes have also been reported in association with food-sensitive intestinal disease such as celiac disease and cow's milk protein intolerance, together with drugs such as vincristine. CIP was originally thought to involve only the small intestine, but it is now realized that it may be restricted to one region of the gut, such as in achalasia or Hirschsprung's disease, or it may be present diffusely throughout the gastrointestinal tract.

Clinical presentation

A child may present with either the primary or the secondary effects of the underlying disease. However, the clinical symptoms are variable and often non-specific. The location of the affected bowel, diffuse or regional, seems a more important determinant of the clinical presentation than the underlying disease. A child may be obstructed or complain of severe constipation depending upon whether the small intestine and colon or just the colon is affected. In addition, those with urinary tract involvement may initially present with acute or chronic urinary retention. These effects quite clearly are the result of the ability of the underlying disease of the neuromusculature of the gut to produce ordered motor activity. However, the effects of the underlying disease may also be secondary, such as the consequences of bacterial overgrowth, fecal impaction or adhesional obstruction associated with previous surgery. In neuropathic disorders the consequences of denervation may not only be on motor activity but also on secretomotor control and sensation. These effects may result in diarrhea or visceral hyperalgesia.

Although initial reports of CIP were in adults, it is now apparent that it probably occurs more commonly in infants. Indeed, when the presentation and mortality of cases published in the literature are considered, it is found to occur most commonly in children, with high morbidity and mortality. Considering these data[5] together with a large series from one center,[1] the conditions in childhood present most commonly during infancy, either in the neonatal period, or under the age of 1 year, during which time the highest mortality rates are suffered. In most cases an underlying abnormality of either smooth muscle or of enteric nerves is found when adequately sought. The clinical manifestation at presentation depends on both age and the type and extent of the condition affecting the neuromusculature of the gut.

Before birth

CIP may first be recognized before birth, either as part of a routine antenatal ultrasound scan or in the investigation of a mother with polyhydramnios. On abdominal ultrasound examination the fetus may have either dilated loops of bowel or a distended bladder, or both.

Birth and the neonatal period

The majority of children with CIP present either at birth or in the neonatal period.[1] In all series approximately half the infants have symptoms at birth or within the first few days of life. In those who present at birth, the labor and delivery are frequently difficult, owing to an already distended abdomen. After birth there is abdominal distension, failure to pass meconium and bilious vomiting. The abdominal distension is due to swallowed air, which distends and dilates the small bowel, but is not passed further through the gut. Contrast studies may show the presence of a microcolon or a short small intestine or, in approximately 34%, a malrotation. In some there may be a specific clinical syndrome of a congenitally short small intestine, pyloric stenosis and a malrotation.[6,7] In addition to gastrointestinal symptoms, there may also be failure to pass urine, megacystis and hydroureter or hydronephrosis. Incomplete bladder emptying often results in recurrent urinary tract infection, and this may completely overshadow the gastrointestinal symptoms.

Later infancy

After the neonatal period, although infants may present with an acute obstruction, the symptoms are often intermittent or slowly progressive. Initially some infants may appear completely healthy, taking breast feeds normally, but then suddenly develop an episode of obstruction following what appears to be an intercurrent enteric infection. In these infants persistence of vomiting for more than 7 days warrants further investigation in a patient who has been thought to have had acute gastroenteritis, as they may have developed an acute myositis, which is potentially treatable.[8] In other such infants, who have fed normally from birth, episodes of obstruction begin only when more complex foods are introduced into the diet and attempts are made at weaning. Urinary symptoms due to involvement of the urinary tract may continue to present for the first time during infancy.

Childhood

In later childhood the initial presentation may continue to indicate obstruction, but may simply be constipation, which becomes intractable. Severe abdominal pain may also occur, owing to distension of the bowel or as part of visceral hyperalgesia. In those with a distended abdomen, bowel sounds may be totally absent or very markedly reduced. If high-pitched bowel sounds are present, or if there is visible peristalsis, the distension of the gut is more likely to be secondary to a mechanical rather than a functional obstruction.

Investigation

In order to understand the pseudo-obstructive disorder and plan rational treatment, there are three steps in diagnosis: definition of the presence of functional obstruction. definition of the areas involved and the physiology of the affected areas; and delineating the disease process causing the functional obstruction.

CIP is due to disordered motor activity, and this results from disturbance of the control mechanisms of motor activity and disease of the smooth muscle coats. This may occur as a consequence of primary disease of the gut motor apparatus or because of involvement of the neuromusculature of the gut secondary to disease, which either affects the gut as part of a multisystem disease or is primarily elsewhere. It is useful to consider that the obstruction may be caused at different levels of control of gut motor activity: the end-organ smooth muscle; the enteric nervous system; the humoral environment provided by gut endocrine cells or immunocytes; or the extrinsic innervation. Disruption at one or all of these levels results in the lack of effective co-ordinated propulsive movement. Initial investigations were designed to demonstrate this.

Radiology and transit studies

Plain abdominal X-rays and abdominal ultrasound examinations may show the presence of large distended loops of gut, but it is difficult using such studies to define the area of the gut involved. Conventional contrast radiography will delineate anatomical abnormalities and together with studies by radioisotope and computed tomography (CT) scanning, may provide a measure of transit time and/or demonstrate disordered peristalsis. Limited descriptions of transit can be obtained using breath hydrogen or radio-opaque pellets and plain abdominal X-ray for whole bowel transit times. All of these methods provide a limited description of the disease but no clues to the nature of the disorder.

Surface electrogastrography

Electrogastrography (EGG) is defined as the recording of myoelectric activity of the smooth muscle of the stomach by means of electrodes attached to the abdominal skin surface. EGG was first devised by Alvarez in the 1920s using mechanical means of recording from a string galvanometer. The advent of powerful personal computers and the development of signal processing algorithms has allowed such data to be objectively analyzed. A great advantage of the methodology is that it is non-invasive and readily detects disturbance of gastric antral slow waves and, by suitable positioning, duodenal slow waves. This method has been used in patients with diffuse CIP to detect abnormal myoelectric activity. Persistent entral dysrhythmias have been found in the fasting state in both myopathic and neuropathic disorders.[9]

Manometry

Motor activity may be studied by measurement of intraluminal pressure changes and known manometry. This is helpful in delineating both the extent of the disordered motility and possibly the disease processes causing the disorder. In patients with suspected functional obstruction at least three areas of the gastrointestinal tract should be studied: the esophagus, the upper small intestine and the left colon, as the disease process may not be restricted to any one of these areas. In these areas swallow-induced peristalsis, fasting small intestinal motor activity and the gastrocolonic response to food or the induction of high-amplitude propagated contraction by bisacodyl can be used as tests of the integrity of the enteric nervous system and of the contractile activity of the smooth muscle.

Esophagus

Swallow-induced peristalsis and the associated relaxation of the lower esophageal sphincter can be studied using a Dent sleeve assembly modified for use in infants or young children.[10] Particular attention should be paid to the nature of the primary peristaltic sequence and whether secondary peristalsis occurs in response to reflux. The presence of tertiary contractions and the amplitude and form of the contractile waves should also be noted, as should the behavior of the lower esophageal sphincter.

Small intestine

Most studies of intestinal motor activity in children with CIP have utilized small intestinal manometry. The cyclical nature of fasting small intestinal motor activity is determined by the inherent activity of the enteric nervous system. This intrinsic property can be used to test the integrity of the enteric nervous system and whether extrinsic nervous modulation is present. Disruption of fasting activity and the establishment of postprandial activity results from the humorally mediated responses to food and clarifies whether enteroenteric responses are intact. In addition, these responses can be further tested by utilizing the motilin agonists erythromycin and somatostatin. The algorithm that the author uses to test motor functioning in pseudo-obstruction is shown in Figure 18.1. Some studies have shown that myopathic processes produce low-amplitude poorly propagated contractions[5,11] whereas neuropathic processes are associated with contractions of normal amplitude which are bizarre in wave form, abnormally propagated and, in phase 3 activity ill formed.[11,12] In addition, clustered phasic activity in phase 2 is often present. Disturbance of the neuroendocrine environment can also be shown where there are changes in frequency of

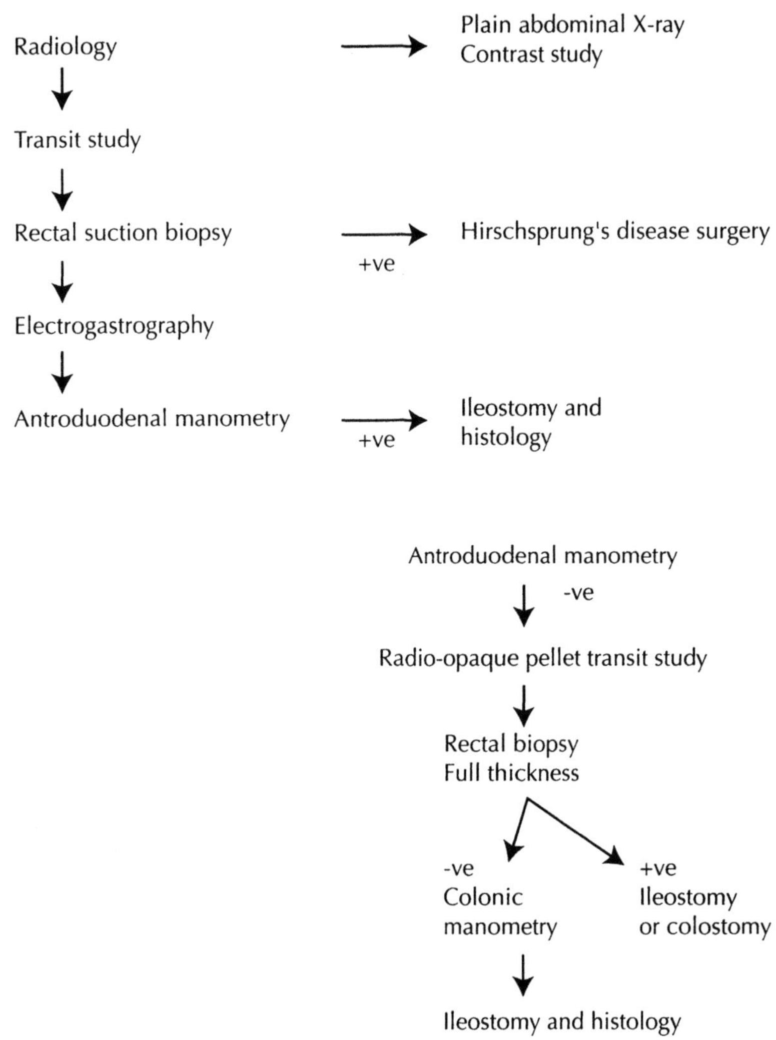

Figure 18.1 Investigation of intestinal pseudo-obstruction.

slow-wave activity and in frequency of phase 3 contractions. In conditions where there is increased secretion of catecholamines such as hyperthyroidism, ganglioneuroma and pheochromocytoma there is increased frequency of slow-wave rhythm; in preterm infants and hypothyroidism, there is decreased slow-wave frequency.

Colon

It is often useful to record simultaneously left-sided colonic motor activity and post-prandial small intestinal motility as a feed will also induce increased rectosigmoid contractions. In addition, the response of the descending colon to bisacodyl in inducing a high-amplitude propagated contraction can be demonstrated, and also whether this propagated contraction halts in the sigmoid colon. Thus, information regarding smooth muscle, local enteric nerves and those involved in the gastrocolonic response and colocolonic reflexes can be obtained.[13]

Etiology

The disease processes, which result in CIP, affect the control mechanisms of intestinal motility. The disorders and disease may primarily be of the intrinsic enteric nerves with or without involvement of the extrinsic autonomic nerves, the smooth muscle cells themselves or of the tumoral and endocrine environment. Good examples of the effect of disturbance of the endocrine environment are the ileus associated with vasoactive intestinal polypeptide-secreting tumors such as ganglioneuromas, and the constipation caused by hypothyroidism. These conditions will not be considered further here. A variety of diseases and drugs, which are listed in Table 18.1, may secondarily cause CIP. Such secondary disorders are much more common in adult life than in childhood. Primary disease of the gut neuromusculature may be due to disease of the enteric nerves or the smooth muscle cells or, at least theoretically, of the interstitial cells of Cajal. Surprisingly, there are virtually no descriptions of the primary pathology of interstitial cells of Cajal, which is said to occur in piebaldism, but there have been descriptions of alterations of these cells in hypertrophic pyloric stenosis and Hirschsprung's disease.[14,15] Definite diagnosis of neuromuscular disease requires careful study of the full thickness of the gastrointestinal wall in optimally orientated pieces of gut.

Table 18.1 Miscellaneous conditions causing intestinal pseudo-obstruction

Endocrine disorders
Hypothyroidism
Hypoparathyroidism
Pheochromocytoma
Carcinoid
Ganglioneuroblastoma/neuroma
Metabolic disorders
Uremia
Porphyria
Amyloidosis
Drugs
Antidepressants and anti-anxiety drugs
Anticholinergic agents
Opiates
Anticonvulsive cytotoxic drugs
Toxic agents
Alcohol in fetal alcohol syndrome
Irradiation

It is best carried out in centers that have experience of both the disease and the histopathological techniques required.

Primary visceral myopathies

Primary disorders of the intestinal smooth muscle coats may represent abnormalities in morphogenesis or intrinsic myocyte defects.[4] Abnormalities of morphogenesis of the muscle coats may result in the presence of an additional muscle coat or the absence of a muscle layer. This may occur diffusely throughout the gut or may only involve only a segment of the gut. Clinically, primary visceral myopathies occur as either familial genetic diseases with a defined mode of inheritance or, more often, as sporadic cases. Three types of familial visceral myopathy have been described in adults, which all initially presented in the second decade and should therefore be considered when symptoms begin during adolescence.

Familial visceral myopathy with diffuse abnormal muscle layering

This condition usually presents at birth, or shortly after, with functional obstruction. Investigation shows the presence of a short gut and a mid-gut malrotation. Three related males have been described with this condition (the index case, his half brother from the same mother, and his maternal uncle), suggesting an X-linked mode of inheritance.[4,6] The most striking histological finding was an extra circular muscle layer with the myenteric enteric plexus embedded within it. None of the patients tolerated enteral feeding, all required long-term parenteral nutrition and all died with septic complications of parenteral nutrition. One further sporadic case has since been described, also in a male child, aged 5 years, who has done well since birth with a decompression ileostomy and mixed enteral and parenteral nutrition.

Infantile visceral myopathy

Most cases occur sporadically but some families have been described with either a dominant gene with variable expressivity or autosomal recessive mode of inheritance. Most affected children develop symptoms at birth or within the first year of life often with severe constipation and abdominal distension. Failure to thrive and malnutrition are common. When recurrent episodes of functional obstruction occur, long-term parenteral nutrition is necessary. Usually the entire gastrointestinal tract is affected, and almost all patients have involvement of the urinary tract with megaureter and megacystis.

Smith and Milla,[4] studying 27 patients with smooth muscle disease, identified five histological phenotypes in full-thickness biopsies from such children using routine microscopy, histochemistry, immunocytochemistry (with monoclonal antibodies against different neural and smooth muscle markers) and electron microscopy. In two of the 27 patients, a severe myositis was found. This is considered separately. Twenty-five had a primary myopathic disorder which, on routine microscopy of paraffin sections of the smooth muscle, was abnormal in only 15. In the remaining patients myopathic changes would have been missed without application of other techniques, particularly electron microscopy.

These authors, like others, found the presence of gross fibrosis of the muscle layers and profound atrophy of the smooth muscle cells similar to that seen in adults with familial and sporadic forms of visceral myopathy. They were able to relate these changes to intrinsic myocyte defects or changes in the extracellular matrix. A myopathy with increased autophagic activity could sometimes be detected using histochemistry with increased acid phosphatase activity in the smooth muscle cells due to active lysozymes. However, but often electron microscopy was required, as the condition appeared to be active only in the central portions of the smooth muscle cells. A further and distinct myopathic subtype was found where there was a so-called pink blush in the circular muscle layer with nuclear crowding, possibly due to a disorganization of the muscle cells. On electron microscopy, the smooth muscle cells appeared to be separated from each other by material secreted either by the muscle cells themselves or the extracellular matrix. In patients with diffuse disease the prognosis is poor, with about 40% of them dying during childhood from the complications of malnutrition or long-term parenteral nutrition.[1] Those who tolerate some oral feeding generally survive into adult life.

Megacystis microcolon hypoperistalsis syndrome

This condition causes severe CIP and affects predominantly female infants.[5,16] Most cases present antenatally. Ultrasound scans show the presence of megacystis hydronephrosis and distended bowel. In addition, the proximal small bowel is often short and there is a malrotated midgut with microcolon located entirely on the left side of the abdomen. The myopathy causing the problem appears to be a degenerative condition of smooth muscle cells. Whilst most cases are sporadic, others appear to have been inherited in an autosomal recessive mode.

After birth, the affected infants develop massive abdominal distension, which is partly due to distended bowel and partly due to a distended bladder. Patients require a decompression ileostomy and either a vesicostomy or frequent catheterization to ensure that the urinary tract is decompressed. Almost all children require long-term parenteral nutrition for survival and, if this becomes problematic, small intestinal transplantation. Megacystis microcolon hypoperistalsis syndrome must be differentiated from prune belly syndrome, which is due to early intrauterine urethral obstruction and affects predominantly male infants. They present with a dilated abdomen, constipation, megacystis and hydronephrosis. Sometimes there is an intestinal malrotation present, but there is no hypoperistalsis and no microcolon.

Familial visceral myopathies types 1, 2 and 3

These conditions usually present in later childhood and have a number of distinctive features.

Familial visceral myopathy type 1 presents as a megaduodenum and is inherited as an autosomal dominant trait with a female predominance in frequency and severity.[17] The disease is characterized by foregut functional obstruction, although gastric emptying is often normal, and an elongated, redundant, usually dilated colon. Barium studies show an aperistaltic esophagus, sometimes normal gastric emptying but a flaccid and dilated duodenum with prolonged retention of barium. The bladder is affected in about half the cases, but is often asymptomatic.[17] Schuffler and Pope showed that there was marked thinning of muscle coats and degeneration with vacuolation of smooth muscle cells and replacement by fibrous tissue.[18] Some patients appear to be more mildly affected than others, and merely require dietary modification with either a low-fat, low-fiber, low-lactose diet or enteral feeding, together with the intermittent use of antibiotics to treat bacterial overgrowth. In patients with more severe disease surgical decompression of the foregut into the normal jejunum appears to be effective.[19]

Familial visceral myopathy type 2 is quite distinct and was first reported as oculogastrointestinal muscular dystrophy. Recently the mitochondrial-disease nature of the condition has resulted in it being renamed mitochondrial neurogastrointestinal encephalomyopathy.[20] It is inherited as an autosomal recessive trait and presents with external ophthalmoplegia with ptosis and diplopia, a cardiac conduction defect, mild muscular atrophy and dilatation of the entire gastrointestinal tract with scattered small-bowel diverticulae. Gastrointestinal symptoms with dyspepsia, retrosternal chest pain and weight loss may start during teenage years. In skeletal muscle biopsies a deficiency of cytochrome C oxidase has been demonstrated which results in the ragged red fibers typical of mitochondrial myopathies. Examination of the smooth muscle of the gut shows the presence of fibrosis and degeneration with vacuolation of the smooth muscle cells. Most patients have eventually required total parenteral nutrition.

Familial visceral myopathy type 3 is much less well understood. The data are from of one family in which there were four siblings who presented with dilatation of the entire gastrointestinal tract. The condition appeared to be inherited in an autosomal recessive fashion.[21]

Systemic disorders involving intestinal smooth muscle

Until recently the majority of myopathies involving multisystem disorders have been described in adults, but in whom the disease process has been in place for a number of years resulting in obvious damage to the intestinal smooth muscle coats, mostly with increased fibrosis. With modern physiological recording methods and histological techniques available in young children, myopathies associated with systemic disorders have been increasingly recognized. It is important to identify these conditions, as medical treatment may be available for them which can result in symptomatic improvement and even prevention of progression of the disease process, if it is put in place before fibrosis of the muscle coat has occurred.

Connective tissues disorders

Scleroderma, systemic lupus erythematosus and even dermatomyositis may all affect the muscle coats of the bowel. However, the best understood of these is scleroderma, a systemic disease characterized by the excessive deposition of collagen by fibroblasts in the skin and in many internal organs. It is associated with prominent and often severe alteration of the microvasculature, the autonomic nervous system and the immune system.[22] Gastrointestinal involvement with symptoms of clinical relevance occur in approximately 50% of patients with the systemic form of scleroderma. The esophagus is the most commonly affected part of the gastrointestinal tract, followed by the rectum and then the small intestine. The lesions of the muscle coat are similar throughout the gut with atrophy and fragmentation of the muscle coats, collagen infiltration and fibrosis in a later stage of the disease.

Enteric myositis

In Crohn's disease, infiltration of the smooth muscle layer with lymphocytes has been found, but no clue as to whether this is part of the Crohn's disease or an autoimmune phenomenon. Acquired myositis has been described in children in a number of reports. Two have presented with functional intestinal obstruction at 1 and 2.5 years of age. In these patients a dense lymphocyte infiltrate mainly of T cells was found along the large and small intestine. Both responded to immunosuppressive treatment. A further child with similar histological findings but in whom there was clear evidence of an autoimmune process has more recently been described.[8] In this patient features were noted that suggested that the intestinal muscle cells themselves were taking part in the inflammatory response. The patient responded to prednisolone, azathioprine and cyclophosphamide, but was dependent upon steroids.

A similar inflammatory cell infiltrate was described in 12 of 27 Bantu children from South Africa who had some sporadic form of an acquired degenerative enteric myopathy (V.V. Smith, personal communication). However, no information was given as to whether the children suffered from other autoimmune diseases or had autoantibodies present. Nor was there information about response to immunosuppressive treatment.

Muscular dystrophy

Gastrointestinal involvement may occur in a number of forms of muscular dystrophy including myotome muscular dystrophy and the dystrophinopathies Duchenne and Becker muscular dystrophy. Involvement of the smooth muscle of the gastrointestinal tract and bladder is well described in myotonic muscular dystrophy, and seemingly motor abnormalities can be found throughout the whole gastrointestinal tract.[23] Duchenne and the milder variety Becker muscular dystrophy are due to abnormalities of dysrophin.[24] The predominant effects are on skeletal and cardiac muscle. Abnormality of particularly the smooth muscle of the foregut also occurs, with impairment of gastric emptying and disordered proximal small intestinal motor activity demonstrable on manometry. Histological studies show that the intestinal smooth muscle cells become swollen, then destroyed, and progressively replaced by fat.[25]

Disorders of the enteric nervous system

The enteric nervous system is arranged in the form of two major plexuses: the myenteric plexus, which is located between the longitudinal and circular muscle layers and primarily provides motor innervation to the muscle coats; and the submucous plexus, which lies in the submucosa between the circular muscle layer and the muscularis mucosae.[26] The submucous plexus is important in regulating secretion by the mucosa and providing sensory innervation of the mucosa. As a whole it is a collection of neurons derived from neural crest cells and has been referred to as the 'brain of the gut' or the 'little brain'. Whilst there is a two-way flow of information between the central nervous system and the enteric nervous system, often referred to as the 'big brain' and 'little brain', respectively, the little brain can function independently of the big brain.[27] The neurons of the enteric nervous system are grouped into small ganglia that are connected by bundles of nerve processes forming the two major nerve plexuses. Ganglia consist of tightly packed neurons, terminal bundles of nerve fibers and glial cells, which usually outnumber the enteric neurons.[26] Normally, there are between five and seven neurons in a ganglion. There are numerous interneurons between the two plexuses and within the plexuses. Both are connected to the central autonomic neural network by parasympathetic and sympathetic nerves. Throughout the gastrointestinal tract there are also non-neural cells derived from the mesenchyme, the interstitial cells of Cajal, that generate and propagate slow waves.[28] The interstitial cells are important modulators of communication between nerves and muscle. The enteric nervous system is particularly concerned with the propulsion of the gut contents in an ordered physiologically effective fashion, and the control of secretion by the gut. Both quantitative and qualitative changes in the enteric nervous system have been identified and these are described below.

Primary visceral neuropathies

Primary visceral neuropathies can be subdivided into familial neuropathies, where a distinct pattern of inheritance is known, and sporadic cases, in which there are distinctive clinical and morphological findings. In this chapter, Hirschsprung's disease, which is clearly a primary visceral neuropathy, will not be discussed. A number of neuropathic motility disorders, including those that present with slow-transit constipation, remain unclassified, although most frequently degenerative changes are found in the enteric neurons.

Familial visceral neuropathy without extraintestinal manifestations

In this disorder it is mainly the colon and distal small intestine that are affected, and it is inherited as an autosomal dominant trait.[39] The age of onset may differ within the same family, but in general symptoms develop after infancy. Most patients present with severe slow-transit constipation associated with abdominal distension and colicky pain. In about half of the patients severe episodes of functional obstruction have occurred which have required decompression. To date, there have been no descriptions of any associated abnormalities, such as extrinsic autonomic dysfunction. Full-thickness biopsies of the affected parts of the bowel have shown evidence of degeneration, both on silver staining and on routine hematoxylin-and-eosin staining. No other abnormalities have been observed.

Familial visceral neuropathy with pyloric stenosis, a short small intestine and malrotation

This syndrome has been described in several families. An extended kindred from Sicily and Southern Italy has shown that it is inherited as an X-linked recessive trait through four generations. Linkage analysis assigns the genetic defect to a locus at XQ28. To date, the gene involved has not been identified. Affected infant boys usually present with functional obstruction in the neonatal period and most have died during the first year of life. Histology of the nerve plexuses has shown the presence of shrunken neurons with particular loss of argyrophilic neurons. However, apparent loss of argyrophilic neurons may be a normal finding at this age, as the acquisition of argyrophilia is associated with changes in the neurofilamentous content of the neuron and this occurs progressively during the first year of life.

Familial visceral neuropathy with neuronal intranuclear inclusions

This condition may be inherited as an autosomal dominant trait, as it was described in three siblings (two female, one male) and their father.[30] The patients developed symptoms during childhood and, in addition to pseud-obstruction, suffered from dysphagia, diarrhea and constipation. They became developmentally delayed, had autonomic dysfunction and ataxia, and developed dementia. A characteristic feature of the condition is the presence of eosinophilic intranuclear inclusions in the neurons of the myenteric plexus and in the central nervous system.[3] In some of the patients the intranuclear inclusions could be seen within the ganglion cells of the submucous plexus on suction rectal biopsy. This appears to be a progressive degenerative condition affecting a widespread class of neurons in both the enteric and the central nervous systems.

Familial visceral neuropathy with neurological involvement

A number of families have been described in which there are least two affected siblings. The condition is probably inherited as an autosomal recessive disorder. The symptoms start in early childhood, with neuropathic dysmotility of the gut and involvement of the central nervous system. The central nervous system disorder appears to consist of progressive sensory and motor peripheral neuropathies, ophthalmoplegia and hearing loss.[31] It seems highly likely that this is a mitochondrial disorder. On full-thickness biopsy, neurons in the myenteric plexus appear normal on conventional staining, but there is evidence of degeneration of argyrophobic C cells.

Familial visceral neuropathy associated with multiple endocrine neoplasia

The multiple endocrine neoplasia type 2 syndromes may be associated with involvement of the gastrointestinal tract. These include multiple endocrine neoplasia (MEN) 2A, MEN 2B and isolated medullary thyroid carcinoma. These conditions are inherited as autosomal dominant traits and are as a consequence of mutation of the gene encoding the RET tyrosine kinase receptor. It is extremely important in the development of the enteric nervous system as *RET* null knockout mice do not develop neurons within the gut.[32] There is now good evidence to show that *RET* is important not only for colonization of the primitive gastrointestinal tract by neural crest cells but also for their migration down the length of the gut and their further differentiation. In MEN 2A and isolated medullary thyroid carcinoma, there is an abnormality of the *RET* gene between codons 619 and 638, the cysteine-rich region of the gene, which results in the development of medullary thyroid carcinoma with or without pheochromocytoma. In about 5% of patients with MEN 2A, Hirschsprung's disease is also present with pheochromocytoma.[33]

In MEN 2B there is always involvement of the gastrointestinal tract, with transmural intestinal ganglioneuromatosis. In most patients, disorders of gastrointestinal motility are the first manifestations of the disease, but the presentation is variable both in severity and in time. Some patients present in early infancy, similarly to Hirschsprung's disease, but others not until adult life.[34] There is nearly always colonic dysfunction present and the most usual presentations are either with chronic constipation, episodes of functional obstruction or as if this were Hirschsprung's disease. In all the patients that the author has studied, evidence of medullary thyroid carcinoma has been present from very early on, either as clumps of malignant cells *in situ* within the thyroid gland or as an overt tumor. Frequently in those patients in whom there are only collections of cells *in situ* within the gland, screening investigations such as CT scanning of the thyroid and calcitonin determinations have not been helpful. It is only when there is a considerable mass of C cells present that the normal screening investigations become positive. It is for this reason, together with the fact that there is no satisfactory radiotherapeutic or chemotherapeutic treatment available, that prophylactic thyroidectomy is recommended.[35]

The characteristic histopathological findings are an increased density of nerve fibers and possibly ganglion cells in the submucosa and myenteric plexus with penetration of the hyperplastic nerve fibers into the mucosal area. The hyperplastic nerve fibers are accompanied by large ganglionic nodes containing numerous glial cells, with a normal to increased quantity of neurons. This abnormality of the enteric nervous system is present along the entire gastrointestinal tract and the hyperplastic neurons may be seen within the mouth or anal canal.[35]

Sporadic visceral neuropathies

Neuropathic dysmotility may also be produced by having too few neurons within the enteric nervous systems (hypoganglionosis) as well too many (hyperganglionosis) or none at all (aganglionosis). The conditions that cause these states are nearly always congenital, although both hypoganglionosis and aganglionosis may result from acquired disorders in which there is destruction of neurons. As these conditions are defined by the numbers of neurons present, it is clear that a reliable means of assessing neuronal density is required.[36] Neuronal density is affected by the age of the patient, tissue freshness and intestinal dilatation as well as by the disease process. It is therefore important that a standardized technique for assessing neuronal density be used. A full-thickness sample of intestine at an appropriate site, needing to be greater than 1 cm in length, is required. Preferably neurons should be counted in sections cut longitudinally along the long axis of the bowel rather than transversely.[36] If sections are cut transversely they should be at least 30 μm apart to avoid counting each neuron more than once. There are few published studies, especially in children, but Smith reported a mean neuronal density of 3.6 neurons/mm for the jejunum, 4.3/mm for the ileum and 7.7/mm for the colon, with no significant difference between transverse and longitudinal sections.[36]

Hypoganglionosis

A reduced number of neurons in the myenteric plexus, so-called hypoganglionosis, is perhaps the most frequent diagnosis in children who present with functional obstruction due to a visceral neuropathy. Hypoganglionosis also occurs commonly in children with severe slow-transit constipation. Navarro et al[3] reported hypoganglionosis of the myenteric plexus in 13 of 26 patients who presented with functional obstruction. Most commonly the hypoganglionosis was confined to the distal segment of the colon, and diffuse disease was uncommon. Histologically the ganglia were smaller than normal, often infiltrated with collagen, and there was a paucity of neurons within the ganglia. Between the ganglia there were numerous thickened nerve fibers that stained strongly with acetylcholinesterase. Krishnamurthy et al described a further series of patients with hypoganglionosis[37] in four of 26 children, but unlike those described by Navarro et al the nerve tracts did not strongly stain with cholinesterase. As in both of these series the majority of the children presented as infants, care must be taken in the interpretation of silver staining as during the first year of life there may be absence of silver staining. In the Krishnamurthy group[37] there were 19 children with a deficiency of argyrophilic neurons. When argyrophilic neurons were present, they were small and had few processes. It was suggested that these patients suffered from a defect in differentiation and maturation of neurons from primitive neuroblasts. As these processes continue after birth, this would explain why some infants during the first year of life may have apparent abnormalities of the myenteric plexus which are not the case.[38]

The problem of the diagnosis of hypoganglionosis is emphasized by the marked variability of the clinical course of such patients. Most will present in the newborn period with symptoms suggestive of Hirschsprung's disease, but others become symptomatic only during their preschool years. In those in which the disorder is restricted to the colon, ileostomy or colonic resection and the pull-through procedure relieves their symptoms, but those in whom the disease is diffuse remain dependent on parenteral nutrition for their survival.

Hyperganglionosis

Hyperganglionosis is characterized by an excess of intestinal neurons in the myenteric plexus with or without hyperplasia of nerve fibers. The condition may also affect the submucous plexus, but in some, the submucous plexus will be normal. Hyperganglionosis requires the presence of large ganglia containing more than seven ganglion cells at a greater density than the normal range for the region. There is also some evidence that infants, especially those during the neonatal period, have a higher neuronal density than that in older children.[38,39] Therefore, the finding of hyperganglionosis in a very small infant with dysmotility requires caution in its interpretation.

Marked hyperganglionosis is the hallmark of intestinal ganglioneuromatosis and MEN 2B. This is dealt with above and will not be considered further here. In view of the implications of MEN 2B in those with severe hyperganglionosis and ganglioneuromatosis, mutations of the *RET* gene should be sought in all patients who have severe hyperganglionosis even if only the submucous plexus is involved.

Intestinal neuronal dysplasia

Those with mild submucous hyperganglionosis have sometimes been reported to suffer from intestinal neuronal dysplasia, a term that has been used over the past 30 years to describe quantitative and qualitative abnormalities of enteric ganglia. The term was originally used to describe abnormalities of both the myenteric and submucous plexus.[40] However, over the past 20 years, diagnosis has largely been dependent on suction rectal biopsy and thus on changes in the submucous plexus and the mucosal innervation. The term has raised confusion and controversy among clinicians and pathologists. It appears to affect all age groups, although it is mostly seen in infants with chronic constipation and was first considered to be a developmental defect of the submucous plexus.[41] Part of the problem has been the lack of agreed criteria, and the confusion has been further compounded by the use of the histological description as a clinical diagnosis. No studies have shown a correlation between morphological features of intestinal neuronal dysplasia and symptoms or long-term outcome.[42,43] Nevertheless, surgical procedures have been recommended on the basis of the histological diagnosis. In one prospective study of rectal biopsies, the interobserver variation between centers was enormous and close to that which that might occur by chance. In this study,[43] 377 biopsies from 108 children aged 4–15 years were assessed by three experienced pathologists for a number of agreed histological features and a final diagnosis. Complete concordance was obtained for the diagnosis of Hirschsprung's disease, but in only 14% of the remainder was there concordance. Assessment of the clinical symptoms 1 year after biopsy, demonstrated that the diagnosis of intestinal neuronal dysplasia had no prognostic value for the outcome in these individuals. It seems, therefore, that intestinal neuronal dysplasia describes neither a specific histological nor a clinical entity, and remains controversial. This author can see very little use for the term until it is better defined. It should at the present time be avoided and certainly not used as a criterion for individual treatments.

Acquired visceral neuropathies

Damage to the enteric nervous system may occur from a variety of agents as well as being secondary to a systemic disease. Secondary visceral neuropathies may occur at any age, before or after birth, but most often occur in adults compared to children.

Infectious agents

Infectious agents may damage enteric neurons either by direct invasion of the neuron or by involvement in an inflammatory process, often autoimmune, that the infectious agent provokes. The best example of this is Chagas' disease, caused by infection with *Trypanosoma cruzi,* in which the inflammatory response to the parasite results in an autoimmune response in which antibodies to the muscarinic receptors on neurons is produced. Whilst the most common clinical presentation following such an infection is achalasia, other areas of the bowel may be affected, including the small and large intestines.

Functional obstructive episodes have also been observed with a variety of other infectious agents, including acute Lyme disease and the neurotrophic viruses from the herpes virus family, including cytomegalovirus, varicella zoster virus, Epstein–Barr virus and herpes simplex virus type 1.[44–46]

Chronic inflammation and autoimmune disease

A number of patients have been reported with different non-infectious inflammatory diseases. Clearly, classical mucosal inflammatory conditions such as Crohn's disease and necrotizing enterocolitis may result in damage to both enteric nerves and muscular structures of the bowel. However, other autoimmune diseases affecting the gut, such as celiac disease and ulcerative colitis, may also result in severe dysmotility. It is becoming apparent that the neuromusculature of the bowel may become involved in the inflammatory process.

Lymphocytic ganglionitis associated with the presence of circulating enteric neuronal antibodies has been described both in association with small round cell carcinoma as a paraneoplastic syndrome and in isolation.[47] In both settings acquired progressive aganglionosis occurs as a result of a severe T-cell-mediated inflammatory ganglionitis of both enteric plexuses. In the isolated form of the disease the antibody produced is similar to the Hu-protein antibody found in the paraneoplastic syndrome, but instead of antibody staining being restricted to the nucleus, it is present in the cytoplasm. In both forms of the disease, episodes of functional obstruction are responsive to immunosuppressive treatment, with a consequent fall in the titers of antibodies produced.

The enteric neuromusculature may also become involved in a variety of connective tissues disorders including systemic sclerosis, systemic lupus erythematosus and dermatomyositis.

Miscellaneous conditions

The enteric neuromusculature can be affected by a wide variety of other conditions or affected by toxic agents, drugs and irradiation. These are listed in Table 18.1.

Treatment

In all the primary and many of the secondary causes of functional obstruction, treatment is symptomatic and supportive unless the underlying disease process can be corrected by specific therapy. For example, celiac disease presenting with functional obstruction can be treated acutely with immunosuppression and then by a gluten-free diet. The slow-transit constipation that occurs with hypothyroidism will respond to thyroxin replacement therapy. Similarly, other forms of autoimmune disease which affect specifically the nerves and muscle of the bowel can be treated by appropriate immunosuppressive treatment. Where an isolated obstructing segment of gut can be discerned, surgery may bring very real benefit. This will be discussed further below.

Nutritional therapy plays an important role, as the majority of children die either as a consequence of malnutrition or of sepsis associated with parenteral nutrition. Wherever possible the enteral route should be used in preference to parenteral nutrition, and even if parenteral nutrition is required it is beneficial if small volumes of enteral feed can be maintained. In small infants, human milk is the preferred milk source, but if this is not available a whey protein hydrolysate formula should be used in preference to whole-protein-based cow's milk formula, as this empties faster from the stomach. In older children episodes of functional obstruction can often be managed with enteral feeding of protein hydrolysates where they have previously tolerated a low-fiber diet. If enteral feeding cannot provide sufficient nutrients for normal growth and development, then parenteral nutrition should be initiated before malnutrition develops. Experience of over 40 patients with severe recurrent episodes of pseudo-obstruction has shown that approximately half will require parenteral nutrition at some time during the course of their illness and, in a proportion, home parenteral nutrition may be required.

As a consequence of bowel dilatation and the development of blind loop syndromes, bacterial overgrowth frequently develops and will further enhance malabsorption due to fermentation of nutrients. Intermittent treatment with appropriate antibiotics is the recommended course of action, and this often improves symptoms.

The use of pharmaceutical agents to improve intestinal motility can be expected to be successful only if there is remaining function of enteric nerves and muscles for the drugs to have a beneficial effect. In general, in those with severe and recurrent episodes of functional obstruction, pharmaceutical agents play little role. Agents that have been tried include cisapride, domperidone, metoclopramide, erythromycin and octreotide. Ondansetron, a 5-hydroxytryptamine$_3$ antagonist, may be helpful in those cases in which the emetic reflex is activated, but it does not appear to affect episodes of obstruction.

Surgical intervention should be limited to the placement of decompression stomas, feeding gastrostomies and the provision of full-thickness intestinal biopsies for a specific diagnosis. Bowel resection may help in patients where the disease is limited to a specific segment of the gut such as the colon, but for those children with diffuse disease other than the placement of a decompression ileostomy, resection does not play a part. Similarly in those in whom a decompression ileostomy has produced relief, but there is diffuse disease, the urge to re-establish connection with the defunctioned limb of the bowel should be resisted as this will only result in further episodes of obstruction.[1] Wherever possible, unnecessary surgery should be avoided as it will only create adhesion and complications. A most difficult surgical decision is in an individual case defining whether an episode of obstruction is functional or is a consequence of mechanical obstruction caused by the presence of adhesions. Signs of peritonism, extreme dilatation and pain in association with a specific episode of obstruction points more towards a mechanical obstruction, than a functional obstruction and laparotomy may be necessary to relieve it.

For those infants born with primary neuromuscular disease and totally dependent on parenteral nutrition, the only therapeutic options are home parenteral nutrition or small-intestinal transplantation. Small-intestinal transplantation should be reserved for those who have severe parenteral nutrition-related liver disease or those whose intravenous access has become unreliable and precarious.

REFERENCES

1. Heney KES, Smith VV, Spitz L, Milla PJ. Chronic intestinal pseudo obstruction: treatment and long term follow up of 44 patients. *Arch Dis Child* 1999; **81**: 21–27.
2. Vargos J, Sachs P, Ament ME. Chronic intestinal pseudo obstruction in paediatrics. *J Paediatr Gastroenterol Nutr* 1998; **7**: 323–332.
3. Navarro J, Sonsino E, Boige N et al. Visceral neuropathies responsible for chronic intestinal pseudo obstruction syndrome in pediatric practice: analysis of 26 cases. *J Pediatr Gastronenterol Nutr* 1990; **11**: 179–195.
4. Smith VV, Milla PJ. Histological phenotypes of enteric smooth muscle disease causing functional intestinal obstruction in childhood. *Histopathology* 1997; **31**: 112–122.
5. Milla PJ. Clinical features of intestinal pseudo obstruction in Children. In Kamm MA, Lennard Jones JE, eds. *Constipation*. Petersfield, UK: Wrightson Bio Medical Publishing, 1994: 251–258.
6. Tanner MS, Smith V, Lloyd JK. Functional intestinal obstruction due to deficiency of argyrophil neurons in the myenteric plexus. Familial syndrome presenting

with short small bowel, malrotation and pyloric hypertrophy. *Arch Dis Child* 1976; **51**: 837–841.
7. Auricchio A, Brancholini V, Casari G et al. the locus for a novel syndromic form of intestinal pseudo obstruction maps to XQ28. *Am J Hum Genet* 1996; **58**: 743–749.
8. Ruuska TH, Karikoski R, Smith VV, Milla PJ. Acquired myopathic pseudo-obstruction may be due to autoimmune enteric leiomyositis. *Gastroenterology* 2002; **122**: 1133–1139.
9. Devane SP, Ravelli AM, Bisset WM et al. Gastric enteral dysrhythmias in children with chronic idiopathic intestinal pseudoobstruction. *Gut* 1992; **33**: 1477–1481.
10. Omari TI, Benninga MA, Barnett CP et al. Characterization of esophageal body and lower esophageal motorfunction. *J Pediatr* 1999; **135**: 517–521.
11. Fell JM, Smith VV, Milla PJ. Infantile chronic idiopathic intestinal pseudo obstruction: the role of small intestinal manometry as a diagnostic tool and prognostic indicator. *Gut* 1996; **39**: 306–311.
12. Stanghellini V, Camilleri M, Malagelada JR. Chronic idiopathic pseudo obstruction; clinical and intestinal manometric findings. *Gut* 1987; **28**: 5–12.
13. Di Lorenzo C, Floros AF, Hyman PE. Age related changes in colon manometry. *J Paediatr* 1995; **127**: 593–596.
14. Vanderwinden JM, Liu H, De Laet MH, Vanderhaeghen JJ. Study of the interstitial cells of Cajal in infantile hypertrophic pyloric stenosis. *Gastroenterology* 1996; **111**: 279–288.
15. Vanderwinden JM, Rumessen JJ, Liu H et al. Interstitial cells of Cajal in human colon and in Hirschsprung's disease. *Gastroenterology* 1996; **111**: 901–910.
16. Berdon WE, Baker DH, Blanc WA et al. Megacystitis-microcolon-intestinal hypoperistalsis syndrome: a new cause of intestinal obstruction in the new born. *Am J Roentgenol* 1976; **126**: 957–964.
17. Schuffler MD, Low CW, Bill AH. Studies of idiopathic intestinal pseudo obstruction. 1. Hereditary hollow visceral myopathy: clinical and pathological studies. *Gastroenterology* 1977; **73**: 327–338.
18. Schuffler MD, Pope CE. Studies of idiopathic intestinal pseudo obstruction. Hereditary hollow visceral myopathy: family studies. *Gastroenterology* 1977; **73**: 339–344.
19. Shaw A, Shaffer HA, Anuras S. Familial visceral myopathy: the role of surgery. *Am J Surg* 1985; **150**: 102–108.
20. Mueller LA, Camilleri M, Emslie SA. Mitochondrial neurogastrointestinal encephalo-myopathy: manometric and diagnostic features. *Gastroenterology* 1999; **116**: 959–963.
21. Anuras S, Mitros FA, Milano A et al. A familial visceral myopathy with dilatation of the entire gastrointestinal tract. *Gastroenterology* 1986; **90**: 385–390.
22. Sjogren RW. Gastrointestinal motility disorders in scleroderma. *Arthritis Rheum* 1994; **37**: 1265–1282.
23. Lenard HW, Goebel HH, Weigel W. Smooth muscle involvement in congenital myotonic dystrophy. *Neuropeadiatrie* 1976; **8**: 42–52.
24. Hoffman EP, Brown RH, Kumdel LM. Dystrophin: the protein product of the Duchenne muscular dystrophy locus. *Cell* 1987; **51**: 919–928.
25. Staiano A, Del Giudice E, Romano A et al. Upper gastrointestinal tract motility in children with progressive muscular dystrophy. *J Paediatr* 1992; **121**: 720–724.
26. Furness JB, Costa M. *The Enteric Nervous System.* Edinburgh: Churchill Livingstone,1987.
27. Wood JD. Physiology of the enteric nervous system. In Johnson LR, ed. *Physiology of the Gastrointestinal Tract*, 3rd edn. New York: Raven Press, 1994: 423–482.
28. Sanders KM. A case for interstitial cells of Cajal as pace makers and mediators of neurotransmission in the gastrointestinal tract. *Gastroenterology* 1996; **111**: 492–515.
29. Mayer EA, Schuffler MD, Rotter JI et al. Familial visceral neuropathy with autosomal dominant transmission. *Gastroenterology* 1986; **91**: 1528–1535.
30. Barnett JL, McDonnell WM, Appelman HD, Dobbins WO. Familial visceral neuropathy with neuronal intranuclear inclusions: diagnosis by rectal biopsy. *Gastroenterology* 1992; **102**: 684–691.
31. Faber J, Fich A, Steinberg A et al. Familial intestinal pseudoobstruction dominated by a progressive neurologic disease at a young age. *Gastroenterology* 1987; **92**: 786–790.
32. Schuchardt A, D'Agati V, Larsson-Blomberg L et al. Defect in the kidney and enteric nervous system of mice lacking the tyrosine kinase receptor RET. *Nature* 1994; **367**: 380–383.
33. Cote CJ, Gaged RF. Lessons learned from the management of a rare genetic career. *N Engl J Med* 2003; **399**: 1566–1568.
34. Eng C, Marsh DJ, Robinson BG et al. Germline, RET, Codon 918 mutation in apparently isolated intestinal ganglioneuromatosis. *J Endocrinol Metab* 1998; **83**: 4191–4194.
35. Smith VV, Eng C, Milla PJ. Intestinal ganglioneuromatosis and multiple neoplasia type 2B: implications for treatment. *Gut* 1999; **45**: 143–146.
36. Smith VV. Intestinal neuronal density in childhood: a baseline for the objective assessment of hypo and hyper aganglionosis. *Paediatr Pathol* 1993; **13**: 225–237.
37. Krishnamurthy S, Heng Y, Shuffler ND. Chronic intestinal pseudo obstruction in infants and children caused by diverse abnormalities of the myenteric plexus, *Gastroenterology* 1993; **104**: 1398–1408.
38. Smith VV, Milla PJ. Argyrophilia in the developing human myenteric plexus. *Br J Biomed Sci* 1996; **53**: 287–283.
39. Schoffield DE, Yunise J. Intestinal neuronal dysplasia. *J Pediatr Gastroenterol Nutr* 1991; **12**: 182–189.
40. Meier-Ruge WA, Gambazzi F, Kaufeler RE et al. The neuropathological diagnosis of neuronal intestinal dysplasia (NIDB). *Eur J Paediatr Surg* 1993; **4**: 267–273.
41. Smith VV. Isolated intestinal neuronal dysplasia: a descriptive histological pattern or a distinct clinicopathological entity. In Hadziseli Movic F, Herzog B, eds. *Inflammatory Bowel Disease & Morbus Hirschsprung.* Dordrecht: Kluwer, 1992: 203–214.
42. Cord-Udy CL, Smith VV, Ahmed S et al. An evaluation of the role of suction biopsy in the diagnosis of intestinal neuronal dysplasia. *J Pediatr Gastroenterol Nutr* 1997; **24**: 1–6.
43. Koletzko S, Jesch I, Faus-Kebetaler T et al. Rectal biopsy for diagnosis of intestinal neuronal dysplasia in children: a prospective multi-centre study on interobserver variation and clinical outcome. *Gut* 1999; **44**: 853–861.
44. Sonsino E, Mouy R, Foucaud P et al. Intestinal pseudo obstruction related to cytomegalovirus infection of the myenteric plexus. *N Engl J Med* 1984; **311**: 196–197.
45. Bruyn GA, Bots GT, Van Wijhe M et al. Chronic intestinal pseudoobstruction as a possible sequel to encephalitis. *Am J Gastroenterol* 1986; **81**: 50–54.
46. Chen JJ, Liou YM, Gershon M. Latent, lytic, reactive varicella zoster virus in the ENS of humans and guinea pigs: could intestinal singles be a hidden cause of gastrointestinal disease. *Neurogastroenterol Motil* 2004; in press.
47. Smith VV, Gregson N, Foggensteiner L et al. Acquired intestinal agangliosis and circulating auto antibodies without neoplasia or other neural involvement. *Gastroenterology* 1997; **112**: 1366–1371.

19 Gastrointestinal and nutritional problems in the neurologically handicapped child

Jan Taminiau and Marc Benninga

Introduction

The neurologically handicapped child almost invariably experiences nutritional problems.[1] They more commonly present as malnutrition, but obesity and overnutrition can also be found. Parameters to assess malnutrition and overnutrition in the handicapped child have to be adjusted. Height is a proper parameter for growth and nutritional status, but difficult in children with malformations and spasticity.[2–4] Also, disproportionate development of the head, rump and extremities makes assessment of height as a parameter of nutritional status difficult.[5–7] Therefore, crown–rump length, width, crown–heel length, distal femoral length and distal arm length (Spender growth curve) have been developed to assess growth and to relate height to developmental abnormalities or to nutrition.[8] It is clear that the Quetelet index or body mass index (BMI) have to be used with care in these children.

Different etiologies result in different growth abnormalities during development in childhood.[9]

Children with Down's syndrome, which is a genetic chromosomal disorder, have height and bone development retardation from birth. The rump or sitting height is normal in these children. The height development becomes relatively shorter each year up to the age of 15. The skull development stops at the age of 3. The growth deficit is more pronounced in height than in width and they appear microcephalic when they get older.

Children with multiple congenital anomalies, with specific histories of drug therapy, irradiation and viral infections early in gestation, and which could be considered as an environmental insult, have height curves that are normal until the age of 5 for both sexes, and then start to lag behind. By the age of 10, they slow down and seem to miss their adolescent growth spurt. Many children in this group become microcephalic, and usually there are more deficits in width than height.

In children with hypoxia, severe or prolonged deprivation of oxygen at the time of birth, in essence cerebral palsy with motor function impairment, height and trunk measurements are normal for 10 years and then slow down, perhaps reflecting a failure of the adolescent growth spurt. Head circumferences lag behind over all ages. On the other hand, children whose neurological deficit is minimal brain damage (attention deficit hyperactivity disorder, children with school and learning problems and no definite impairment of motor function), have their heights and weights within normal ranges. Therefore, body weight and BMI (kg/m^2) are more appropriate for evaluation of malnutrition in these children.

In a study on more than 2000 institutionalized children with a handicap in Tokyo, Japan,[3] height and weight were measured in four distinct groups. Groups were divided into deaf children; blind children; mentally retarded children, some of whom were completely ambulatory and 15% of whom needed crutches; and physically handicapped children, of whom 65% were non-ambulatory. Height more than 3 standard deviations below the mean was present in 2% of deaf children, 10% of blind children, 15% of children with mental retardation and 45% of physically handicapped children. Underweight more than 2 standard deviations below the mean was present in 1% of deaf children, 4% of blind children, 5% of children with mental retardation and 24% of physically handicapped children. Overweight more than 2 standard deviations above the mean was present in 8% of deaf children, 7.5% of blind children, 17% of mentally retarded children and 9% of physically handicapped children.[10] In a Finnish study of patients up to the age of 20, the BMI showed that underweight (BMI < 20 kg/m^2) was present in 30%, overweight in 10% and severe overweight in 7% (BMI > 32 kg/m^2).[11] Also, more than 20% of children being overweight was found in another survey of more than 1100 children.[12,13] Although the studies report height and weight reduction of almost 1 standard deviation in large cohorts of handicapped children, it seems more appropriate to relate the chance of malnutrition to mental retardation (5%) or physical handicap (25%). A height reduction of more than 3 standard deviations occurs in 1% of deaf children, 5% of blind children, 2% of mentally retarded children and 6% of physically handicapped children. This proportion of stagnation in height development in chromosomal, toxic and hypoxic disorders was not easily explained by nutritional depletion. Also, disproportionate development in the head, trunk and extremities were not in keeping with nutritional problems.

In the normal child, undernutrition or overnutrition is obviously undesirable. In the handicapped child, however, a proper nutritional status is of crucial importance, as it supports the ability to employ all nutrients necessary for normal body functions in biological, physiological and psychological ways. Undernourished handicapped children might not respond properly to intercurrent diseases and suffer unnecessarily. On the other hand, restoring a normal nutritional status results in a better quality of life in many.

Assessment of nutritional status requires a proper follow-up of height, body weight and assessment of the standard deviation score. By so doing, negative changes are easily discovered and appropriate nutritional intervention can be initiated. Spender et al[8] showed that upper arm length and lower leg length were as appropriate as height measurements in these children and had the same technical intra- and interobserver errors as the measurements of height, usually difficult to obtain in these children. In practice, they are easier to perform and have a better compliance for regular follow-up measurements. Triceps skin fold as indication of body fat and arm circumference as indication of muscle mass, should be measured in conjunction with height and body weight with the highly variable muscle mass in these children.[14]

Appetite

Undernutrition in children with a neurological handicap is mostly caused by a decreased appetite or intake. Increased requirements or increased losses are not reported. Eating problems or difficulties in chewing, swallowing disturbances, absent swallowing reflex, no co-ordination of oral and esophageal phases and choking of food into the nose are implicated. Also, rumination, hypersensitivity in the mouth area, food refusal or aversion contribute to eating disorders.

Nutrition is further influenced negatively by changes in taste, dry mouth, epigastric pain, nausea, sedation and hypersalivation. Specifically, anti-epileptics cause gingival hyperplasia and anorexia; antidepressants such as lithium increase thirst and appetite; mental stimulants such as Ritalin® decrease appetite; antacids might cause constipation; and aspirin and non-steroidal anti-inflammatory drugs (NSAIDs) cause pyrosis and nausea and may lead to ulcerations in the gastrointestinal tract. In the Institutional Tokyo Study it was shown that around 10% of the blind needed assistance with eating, mostly because of some chewing problems, and around 20% had poor appetite. In the mentally retarded, around 25% needed assistance during eating, 2% had swallowing disorders, around 35% had chewing disorders and 20% had poor appetite. In the physically handicapped, around 65% needed assistance with eating, 20% had swallowing disorders, 40% had chewing disorders and 30% had poor appetite. Four per cent of the mentally retarded children had a voracious appetite, which was in keeping with their overweight tendency.[15,16]

Nutrient deficiencies

Nutrient deficiencies further show a relationship between undernutrition and nutritional intake, supported by several studies.[17–20] The undernourished had a lower intake of energy, protein, fat, fiber and water. In general, the linoleic acid intake was insufficient in 39% and fiber intake overall was insufficient in 59%. The micronutrient intake showed deficiencies in vitamin B_6 (32%), vitamin C (18%), nicotinic acid (71%), sodium (61%) and iron (84%). Deficient intake of vitamins A, B_1, B_2 and B_6 was related to the undernourished group;

nicotinic acid and vitamin C were deficient in the whole group. In the undernourished, low sodium intake was more pronounced and that was also seen to a minor extent in the whole group. Sodium, potassium, calcium and phosphate intake were deficient only in the undernourished. Interestingly, iron intake was not different between the undernourished and the well-nourished group, in keeping with the laboratory assessments. Iron intake did not correlate with serum hemoglobin, serum iron and vitamin C intake. Calcium intake and milk intake showed no correlation with serum iron level. Low use of antacids was not correlated with serum iron level. Despite iron supplementation, serum iron remained deficient. Anemia occurred in 9% and, low serum iron in 24%. Anemia was more common in the undernourished (83% vs. 50%) as was the use of iron medication (67% vs. 22%) and also medication for gastroesophageal reflux (25% versus 16%). The iron resorption was not influenced by low levels of vitamin C, or high levels calcium, milk or antacid intake. The more severe the anemia, the more reflux medication was given. It is suggested that the anemia and low iron level were more related to intestinal blood loss due to reflux esophagitis than to the nutritional variations.

Nutritional intervention

In this last study a nutritional intervention was undertaken; in the well-nourished group, the nutritional intervention was compared and followed. The multiply handicapped children had spastic tetraplegia (75%), epilepsy (84%), disturbed chewing (84%), regurgitation (50%) and choking (50%). The nutritional intervention consisted more in a team approach than in taking measures specifically directed to individual needs. Milk products were maximized to 750 ml a day and were taken with meals. In between snacks, the emphasis was more on fruit and vegetable mixtures and fruit mixtures. Fiber was added to cereals in the order of 30 g a day. Those who refused bread were given porridge based on a mixture of tube feeding powder (1 kcal/ml), water and cereals. Special considerations to drinks were given: drinks were enriched with nutritional supplements. If necessary, tube feeding was added; 30% needed additional tube feeding.

This multidisciplinary approach and intervention lasted for 1 year and resulted in an increase of energy intake from 1349 kcal to 1598 kcal. The normally fed group changed from 1673 to 1683 kcal/day. Protein intake increased from 50 to 67 g and in the normally fed from 73 to 79 g/day. Carbohydrates increased in the undernourished from 170 to 212 g/day, and in the well nourished from 189 to 208 g/day. Fat increased from 52 to 54 g/day, in the well nourished it declined from 70 to 60 g/day. Linoleic acid went from 6 to 10 g/day, and in the well nourished 8 to 9 g/day. Fiber increased from 11 to 26 g/day and in the well nourished from 18 to 31 g/day. Water increased from 1077 to 1167 ml/day, and in the well nourished from 1401 to 1437 ml/day. After 1 year, the BMI improved from 18.8 to 19.3 kg/m^2, triceps skin fold did not change, 0.98 to 1.03 cm, and the upper arm muscle circumference increased from 19 to 20.1 cm. Nutritional deficiencies (in percentage less than two-thirds of the daily recommended allowance) declined in vitamin B_6 of 32 to 2%, nicotinic acid of 77 to 34%, vitamin C of 18 to 0%, sodium of 61 to 39%, and iron of 84 to 11%). The normalization of fiber intake reduced the necessity for stimulant suppositories for constipation by 56%.

Thus, nutritional intervention by a team approach seems to be beneficial in the majority, showing that appropriate feeding is helpful in overcoming nutritional problems. When tube feeding is necessary for longer periods, percutaneous endoscopic gastrostomy (PEG) has become a fashionable approach. In a 1.5-year prospective study, the change of nasogastric tube feeding to PEG tube feeding had an unsuspected side-effect in reducing nutritional problems, vomiting and respiratory infections between 30 and 40%.[21] Also, well-being was improved in 40%. Interestingly, vomiting, airway infections and also irritability diminished. The standard deviation score of weight for height improved from -3.8 to -1.8. An easier access via PEG tube feeding, as compared to the irritating tube in the nose, resulted in better daily nutrient intake than more traditional nasogastric tube feeding.

These observations are in keeping with studies in energy expenditure of children or adolescents with severe disabilities. In a study in children with cerebral palsy,[19] Stallings et al measured basic energy expenditure by indirect calorimetry and total energy expenditure by the doubly labeled water method. Physical activity including chronic spasticity of children with spastic quadriplegic cerebral palsy was estimated from the ratio of total energy expenditure to resting energy expenditure. Control children were those children with adequate weight, adequate fat-free mass and fat mass, as well as children with a lower fat-free mass and a lower body fat mass. Measurements were made by triceps skin folds and arm circumference. An interesting observation in children with severe quadriplegic cerebral palsy who were expected to have extra energy demands for involuntary muscular work showed lower total energy expenditure and lower resting energy expenditure compared to well-nourished children with this handicap and to controls. Resting energy expenditure and activity energy expenditure (estimated as total minus resting energy expenditure) were both diminished, thus not supporting the commonly held view that spastic children expend more energy because of their involuntary movements. In this study, reported dietary intake was compared to total energy expenditure measured by the doubly labeled water method. With this method, body weight before and after the test period measures exactly the number of calories expended and this can be compared with the intake. It was thus shown that the dietary intake reported was overestimated by 50% compared to the actual intake measured exactly by the total energy expenditure. This finding underlines the problems that these children face with feedings: meal duration is longer, frequently exceeding 45 min, exceeding the tolerance attention span of the patient and the available time of the caregiver. Oral motor abnormalities of varying degrees are observed in these patients. They often contribute to the symptoms and may lead to food loss. In all these children with growth failure and abnormal body composition, it was shown that the resting energy expenditure adjusted for fat-free mass was lower in the poorly nourished than in the adequately nourished group of children with severe spasticity. This suggested a basic metabolic response or adaptation to the poorly nourished condition.

Gastroesophageal reflux (GER) symptoms such as vomiting, rumination and regurgitations are found in 20–30% of the intellectually disabled population. GER-related iron deficiency anemia and hematemesis are noted in 10–20% of patients. In the Netherlands and Belgium in a large cohort of more then 1500 patients, a randomly selected intellectually disabled population was tested with pH-metry during 24 h. A pathological pH test (defined as a duration of a pH of < 4 for more than 4% of the measured time) was seen in 48% of cases.[22] These patients were subjected to endoscopy and reflux esophagitis was found in 96%: 14% had grade I esophagitis, 33% had grade II, 39% had grade III and 13% had grade IV (Savary Miller classification). Barrett's esophagus was found in 14% and peptic strictures in 4% of cases. This study was repeated for the group under the age of 14, and similar findings were seen. In fact, GER disease was found even in the absence of overt symptomatology.

A possible explanation for the high prevalence of GER disease is the increased prevalence of hiatal hernia, found in 50% of elderly patients and 76% of intellectually disabled children. In the Dutch study, 46% had hiatal hernia and no relationship with rumination. There was some association with cerebral palsy, use of anticonvulsant drugs, scoliosis and restlessness. Anticholinergics and sedatives do decrease the lower esophageal sphincter pressure, which in turn might trigger more episodes of GER. Interestingly, dental erosions were seen more frequently in individuals with a pH lower than 4 for more than 6.3% of the measured time and with an IQ of less than 35.

For the whole Dutch and Belgian group, the standardized morbidity ratio for esophageal carcinoma was 2.9; there is thus an increased risk of developing esophageal cancer, probably related to chronic GER disease and Barrett's dysplasia. For the patients who underwent anti-reflux surgery, this was found to be effective in 38%, while no symptom relief was seen in the remaining 62%. H_2-blockers were effective in 60% of patients and proton pump inhibitors were effective in 69% of patients. Surgery for the neurologically impaired children is known to have a significantly higher incidence of major complications than in intellectually normal patients with GER. It is in fact, a common notion that re-operation and relapses of GER are frequent. The mortality rate was 8.8–9.4%. The postoperative complication rate was 12–15%. In this large Dutch and Belgian cohort, omeprazole was used in a dose of 40 mg once daily and was effective in 88% independently of the severity of the esophagitis. Ten per cent of patients had symptomatic relapse after decreasing the dose to 20 mg daily as maintenance treatment; however, all these patients became symptom-free again after increasing the dose to 40 mg daily. Endoscopically, the esophagus was healed at the end of the study.[23] The occasional patient may need up to 60 mg of omeprazole: Hassal et al found that a dose of 1–4 mg/kg per day was needed in a variety of esophagitis patients with hiatal hernia, mental retardation, repaired esophageal atresia and even in apparently healthy children with esophagitis.[24] Keeping these children on a maintenance of omeprazole 20 mg daily resulted in a marked improvement of persistent vomiting, hematemesis, regurgitation, food refusal and iron deficiency anemia. The prevalence of *Helicobacter pylori* infections was also tested and found to be around 50% of children, and up to 83% in adults. No clear correlation (either direct or inverse) between *H. pylori* infection and GER symptoms was found.

Gastroesophageal reflux and percutaneus endoscopic gastrostomy

GER and aspiration in patients fed via a gastrostomy tube may be caused by relaxation of the lower esophageal sphincter (LES) secondary to gastric distension caused by rapid intragastric bolus feeding. When feeding rate was slowed, LES pressure did not diminish to incompetent levels of 2 mmHg. In general, prospective studies have shown reduction of vomiting, pneumonia, restlessness and pain in more then 60% of patients. After PEG placement, 24-h pH monitoring improved, and histological reflux esophagitis normalized in these children. Anti-reflux surgery for PEG placement considerably increased the complications and failed to improve symptomatology. Thus, there does not seem to be a place for anti-reflux surgery unless symptoms progress after PEG placement, in spite of concomitant treatment with proton pump inhibitors.

The improvement in nutritional status obtained through PEG feeding induced further improvement in reflux, as judged by 24-h pH studies, suggesting a relation between malnourishment and reflux symptoms.[25]

Constipation in mentally handicapped children

The incidence of constipation was around 61% in a large cohort of mentally handicapped children in Dutch and Belgian institutions. Constipation was defined as bowel movements less than 3 times a week. Eighty-eight per cent of the constipated, mentally handicapped, children used laxatives, in comparison to 40% of constipated controls whose constipation was easily controlled. A significant correlation was found between non-ambulancy, cerebral palsy, use of anticonvulsive medication or benzodiazepines on the one hand and use of H_2-receptor antagonists or proton pump inhibitors on the other. Also, an IQ of less than 50 correlated with food refusal, while there was no correlation with age, gender, use of cisapride, motilium, untreated GER disease or vomiting. Laxatives used were contact laxatives in 45%, and osmotic agents such as lactulose and enemas in 14%. Manual evacuation of feces was necessary in 7% of patients. In patients with cerebral palsy, anal sphincter pressures were normal. Rectal sensation was reduced and rectal size was increased, possibly contributing to the constipation so commonly seen in these children. Cisapride did not influence colonic transit time, but slightly and non-significantly increased the frequency of defecation from 2.5 to four times weekly. Thus, in summary, constipation in mentally handicapped children is frequently encountered, but seems to respond to laxative treatment without major sequelae.[26,27]

REFERENCES

1. Eyman RK, Grossman HJ, Chaney RH et al. The life expectancy of profoundly handicapped people with mental retardation. *N Engl J Med* 1990; **323**: 584–589.
2. Amundson JA, Sherbondy A, Dyke van DC, Alexander R. Early identification and treatment necessary to prevent malnutrition in children and adolescents with severe disabilities. *J Am Diet Assoc* 1994; **94**: 880–883.
3. Miller F, Koreska J. Height measurement of patients with neuromuscular disease and contractures. *Dev Med Child Neurol* 1991; **33**: 55–58.
4. Garn S, Weir HF. Assessing the nutritional status of the mentally retarded. *Am J Clin Nutr* 1971; **24**: 853–854.
5. Roche AF. Growth assessment in abnormal children. *Kidney Int* 1978; **14**: 369–377.
6. Mosier HD, Grossman HJ, Dingman HF. Physical growth in mental defectives: a study in an institutionalised population. *Pediatrics* 1995; **36**: 465–473.
7. Rimmer JH, Kelly LE, Rosentswieg J. Accuracy of anthropometric equations for estimating body composition of mentally retarded adults. *Am J Ment Def* 1987; **91**: 626–632.
8. Spender QW, Cronk CE, Charney EB, Stallings VA. Assessment of linear growth of children with cerebral palsy: use of alternative measures to height or length. *Dev Med Child Neurol* 1989; **31**: 206–214.
9. Pryor HB, Thelander HE. Growth deviations in handicapped children. *Clin Pediatr* 1967; **6**: 501–512.
10. Suzuki M, Saitoh S, Tasaki Y et al. Nutritional status and daily physical activity of handicapped students in Tokyo metropolitan schools for deaf, blind, mentally retarded, and physically handicapped individuals. *Am J Clin Nutr* 1991; **54**: 1101–1111.
11. Similä S, Niskanen P. Underweight and overweight cases among the mentally retarded. *J Ment Def Res* 1991; **35**: 160–164.
12. Fox R, Rotatori A. Prevalence of obesity in mentally retarded adults. *Am J Ment Retard* 1982; **87**: 228–230.
13. Perry M. Treating obesity in people with learning disabilities. *Nursing Times* 1996; **92**: 37–38.
14. Cole HS, Lopez R, Epel R et al. Nutritional deficiencies in institutionalised mentally retarded and physically disabled individuals. *Am J Ment Def* 1985; **89**: 552–555.
15. Ault MM, Guy B, Rues J et al. Some educational implications for students with profound disabilities at risk for inadequate nutrition and the nontherapeutic effects of medication. *Ment Retard* 1994; **32**: 200–205.
16. Karle IP, Bleiler RE, Ohlson MA. Nutritional status of cerebral-palsied children. *J Am Diet Assoc* 1960; **38**: 22–26.
17. Couriel JM, Bisset R, Miler R et al. Assessment of feeding problems in neurodevelopmental handicap: a team approach. *Arch Dis Child* 1993; **69**: 609–613.
18. Ellman G, Salfi M, Fong A et al. Vitamin B6 status measures of an institutionalised mentally retarded population. *Am J Ment Def* 1986; **91**: 30–34.
19. Stallings VA, Zemel BS, Davies JC et al. Energy expenditure of children and adolescents with severe disabilities: a cerebral palsy model. *Am J Clin Nutr* 1996; **64**: 627–634.
20. Hordijk R. De waarde van diverse parameters (antropometrische en laboratoriumgegevens, nutriënten) bij het bepalen van de voedingstoestand van ernstig meervoudig gehandicapten. 1992
21. Mathus-Vliegen EM, Koning H, Taminiau JA, Moorman Voestermans CG. Percutaneous endoscopic gastrostomy and gastrojejunostomy in psychomotor retarded subjects: a follow-up covering 106 patient years. *J Pediatr Gastroenterol Nutr* 2001; **33**: 488–494.
22. Bohmer CJ, Niezen-de Boer MC, Klinkenberg-Knol EC et al. Gastro-oesophageal reflux disease in institutionalised intellectually disabled individuals. *Neth J Med* 1997; **51**: 134–139.
23. Clarisse JM, Böhmer CJ, Riet C et al. Omeprazole. Therapy of choice in intellectually disabled children. *Arch Pediatr Adolesc Med* 1998; **152**: 1113–1118.
24. Hassal E, Israel D, Shepherd R et al. Omeprazole for treatment of chronic erosive esophagitis in children: a multicenter study of efficacy, safety, tolerability and dose requirements. International Pediatric Omeprazole Study Group. *J Pediatr* 2000; **137**: 800–807.
25. Van Winckel M, Vander Stichele R, De Bacquer D, Bogaert M. Use of laxatives in institutions for the mentally retarded. *Eur J Clin Pharmacol* 1999; **54**: 965–969.
26. Staiano A, del Giudice E, Simeone D et al. Cisapride in neurologically impaired children with chronic constipation. *Dig Dis Sci* 1996; **41**; 870–874.
27. Böhmer CJ, Taminiau JA, Klinkenberg-Knol EC, Meuwissen SG. The prevalence of constipation in institutionalized people with intellectual disability. *J Intellect Disabil Res* 2001; **45**: 212–218.

20 Cyclic vomiting syndrome

Bhanu Sunku and B UK Li

Introduction

Cyclic vomiting syndrome (CVS) is a disorder of unknown etiology and pathogenesis characterized by recurrent, stereotypical episodes of vomiting with varying intervals of baseline or normal health in between.[1] Various recent articles and proceedings of two international conferences on CVS published in the past decade have defined this disorder in detail and proposed potential mechanisms and treatment. These publications and symposia have provided critical steps in recognizing and understanding a disorder that has been poorly recognized and commonly misdiagnosed. Typical misdiagnoses include gastroenteritis, gastroesophageal reflux, food poisoning, recurrent 'flu' and eating disorders.[2] Although CVS can begin in infancy, the median age of onset in our cohort is 4.8 years of age. As a measure of misdiagnosis, the median interval from onset of symptoms to the proper recognition is 1.9 years, during which time the child has suffered through about 15 or so episodes. Although the prevalence and incidence of CVS are unknown, current estimates in a school-based survey of Caucasian children 5–15 years of age report a prevalence of 2%.[3] Although CVS is clearly misdiagnosed, in our experience this figure appears to be excessive, perhaps because the study was based on a questionnaire that did not involve exclusionary testing and because milder cases that did not require medical intervention were detected. In any case, in our reported pediatric gastroenterology experience, CVS was second only to gastroesophageal reflux disease as a cause of recurrent vomiting.[4] Similar to the gender profile in migraine headaches, there is a slight predominance of girls over boys (57:43).[5]

Although cyclic vomiting was first reported in France by Heberden in 1806,[6] Samuel Gee in England in 1882 is credited with the most accurate 'modern' description.[7] In the past decade, greater recognition and mechanistic understanding of this disorder have been achieved. Prior to this recent period, an association with migraine headaches was noted as early as 1898 by Whitney[8] and in 1904 by Rachford.[9] Recently, pathophysiological connections have been made with mitochondrial disease, autonomic dysfunction and the stress response. Current research, including our own, is focused on the identification of neuroendocrine mechanisms mediating vomiting in these patients, with a specific emphasis on the role of hypothalamic corticotropin releasing factor (CRF).

Clinical patterns

CVS is distinguished by recurrent, severe, discrete episodes of vomiting. Episodes are stereotypical in regards to time of onset, duration and symptomatology. This disorder is also distinguished by an on–off pattern with intervals of returning to completely normal or baseline health between episodes.[2] The duration of episodes is generally from hours to days, with a median duration of 27 h. The median frequency of episodes is 4 weeks. Because nearly 47% of all patients have regular intervals and the remaining have sporadic attacks at unpredictable intervals, 'cyclic' is a slight misnomer.

The most common time of onset is during nighttime or early morning hours with 42% of patients having onset from 01.00 to 07.00.[10] Of patients, 67% have a well-described prodrome that precedes the episodes of vomiting. The parents often characterize both the onset and the resolution as sudden. The warning period typically lasts a median of 0.5–1.5 h. Despite the similarities to migraines, these prodromes rarely have visual disturbances and are characterized by pre-vomiting autonomic symptoms of pallor, nausea, abdominal pain and lethargy. Many parents have noted a rapid 'shut-off' of symptoms from the end of vomiting to the point of resuming oral intake and near-normal function that generally lasts a median of 8 h with a range of 0 h to 1 week.

The vomiting itself has been described as rapid-fire in nature, peaking at an average of six times per hour or once every 10 min during the worst episode.[4] The vomiting is typically projectile, and contains bile, mucus and occasionally blood. The latter generally occurs late in the episode as a result of prolapse gastropathy from repetitive vomiting which can also produce epigastric pain.[11] Although a threshold of more than four emeses per hour at the peak originally identified 92% of those with CVS, we have detected increasing numbers who fit the consensus historical criteria with a lower intensity of vomiting of two to four times per hour.[4] These children can appear remarkably debilitated during episodes. They are often curled up into the fetal position from pain, which is often accompanied by pallor, listlessness and unresponsiveness, and therefore appear much more ill than children with gastroenteritis.[2]

Even though children return to baseline health between episodes and are well about 90% of the time, CVS can have a significant impact on the quality of life of affected children.[10] Over half (58%) of all affected patients require intravenous hydration during episodes and 19% require this with every episode. School-age children miss an average of 24 days of school per year, owing to episodes of vomiting. The high medical morbidity is reflected by the average annualized cost of management of $17 000, including doctor visits, emergency department visits, in-patient hospitalizations, biochemical, radiographic, endoscopic testing and missed work by the parents.[12]

There are many symptoms that typically accompany vomiting during CVS episodes (Table 20.1). Abdominal pain, retching, anorexia and nausea are the most common gastrointestinal symptoms. The abdominal pain can be excruciating occasionally to the point of requiring narcotics and/or laparotomy.

By the patient's report, nausea is generally the most persistent and distressing symptom: it is minimally relieved by vomiting, often receding only while sleeping or with sedation. Typical behaviors (assuming a fetal position, social withdrawal, compulsive drinking, and avoiding lights and sounds) represent attempts to alleviate the nausea.[10]

The most common autonomic symptoms are lethargy and pallor. Other autonomic symptoms include fever, flushing, drooling, diarrhea, hypothermia and hypertension. Less than half of the patients have migraine features including headache (42%), photophobia (38%) and phonophobia (30%). However, these numbers are significantly higher than in those with the chronic vomiting pattern who primarily have upper gastrointestinal tract disorders.[13] Other symptoms

Table 20.1 Clinical features

- Median age of onset: 4.8 years
- Female/male: 57/43
- Vomiting: 6 emesis/h at peak, with bile (81%), mucus (68.6%) and blood (34%)
- Average emesis per episode: 31
- Duration of episodes: 27 h
- Typical time of onset: 01.00–07.00
- Median interval between episodes: 4 weeks
- Associated symptoms: lethargy (93%), nausea (82%), abdominal pain (81%), anorexia (81%), retching (79%), headache (42%), photophobia (38%), phonophobia (30%)
- Associated signs: pallor (91%), social withdrawal (54%), fever (30%), diarrhea (30%), drooling (27%)

during episodes include sensory hypersensitivity and vertigo.

The largest fraction (32%) have a seasonal clustering of episodes with more during the winter and fewer during the summer. Although this pattern correlates with the school year, we can only speculate that less school-related stress and less exposure to infections trigger fewer episodes. Winter holidays including Thanksgiving, Christmas and New Year can serve as a positive stress for some.

Various stressors have been noted to precipitate episodes of CVS. In 76% of patients, the parents can identify a recurring trigger preceding the vomiting episodes. These triggers consist of psychological, infectious and physical stressors (Table 20.2). Stress and infections are the most common triggers (44% and 31%, respectively). Interestingly, two-thirds of the stress is positive rather than negative. Various infections can trigger episodes, especially chronic sinusitis. Other triggers include dietary (23%), physical exhaustion (24%), atopic symptoms (6%), motion sickness (12%) and menses (22% of menstruating girls).

Evaluating the family history of patients with CVS is helpful in diagnosis because of the much higher rate of positive migraines (82%) compared to that obtained in those with chronic vomiting due to gastrointestinal disorders or to the general population (15%).[5] Also, a family history of food allergies or atopy can be a clue for food triggers of attacks. In our series, we have found an unusually high percentage of patients with a family history of depression (40%) compared to the general population. How this plays a role in possible susceptibility to CVS of patients is currently unknown.

Cyclic versus chronic patterns of vomiting

An important clinical clue to the diagnosis of CVS is the pattern of vomiting. Based on a temporal pattern, children with recurrent vomiting can be delineated into cyclic and chronic groups (Figure 20.1). The cyclic group has an intense, but intermittent pattern of vomiting with peak emeses of ≥ 4/h and 2 episodes per week.[13] The chronic group has a low-grade, daily pattern of emeses with <4 emeses/h and >2 episodes per week[13] (Table 20.3). These criteria are 92% sensitive and 100% specific for identifying children with CVS.[2] Two-thirds of all children with recurrent vomiting fit into the chronic or continuous pattern of vomiting. These children rarely appear acutely ill or become dehydrated. Conversely, the cyclical pattern is associated with more intense vomiting and affected children more often require intravenous hydration (62% vs. 18%) compared with the chronic group.[4]

These two patterns are important because both of these groups differ in symptom and diagnostic profile. In those with the cyclical vomiting pattern,

Table 20.2 Common triggers for episodes of cyclic vomiting syndrome
Infections (urinary tract infection, streptococcal throat, flu, sinusitis, gastroenteritis)
Positive stress (birthdays, holidays, vacations)
Negative stress (school, family, deaths)
Dietary intake (cheese, chocolate, caffeine, monosodium glutamate)
Physical exhaustion (lack of sleep)
Motion sickness (car rides, roller-coasters, air travel)
Asthma
Allergies (seasonal, inhalants, foods)
Menses
Surgery/anesthesia
Weather (temperature or pressure changes)

non-gastrointestinal disorders including neurological (including abdominal migraine), renal, endocrine and metabolic disorders predominate over gastrointestinal disorders by a ratio of 5 : 1.[2,13] In contrast, in the chronic group, gastrointestinal disorders (mostly peptic disease) predominate over non-gastrointestinal causes of vomiting by a ratio of 7 : 1.[2,13] This implies the need to center the diagnostic work-up on extraintestinal disorders in cyclic vomiting, and on upper gastrointestinal tract disorders in chronic vomiting. Consistent with proposed migraine association with CVS, the cyclic pattern of vomiting has a higher prevalence of family members with migraine headache (72% vs. 14%), associated headache (41% vs. 19%) and photophobia (18% vs. 4%).[4]

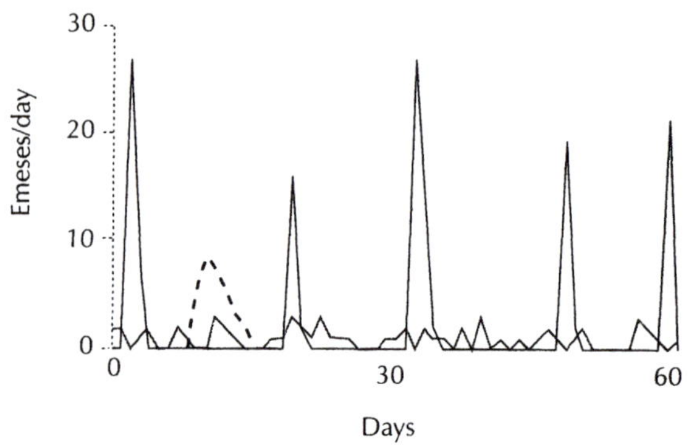

Figure 20.1 Temporal patterns of vomiting: cyclic versus chronic. The number of emeses is plotted over a 2-month period. The chronic pattern represented by a dashed line has low-grade, nearly daily episodes, whereas the cyclic pattern represented by the solid line has many emeses over a 1–2-day period that recurs every few weeks. (Adapted from reference 46).

Differential diagnosis

Differentiating a cyclic versus a chronic pattern of vomiting is the first step in narrowing the differential diagnosis (Table 20.4). Although the majority of patients (88%) with a cyclical pattern ultimately are diagnosed with CVS, the remaining 12% have specific causes for vomiting found on diagnostic testing. The majority of disorders that can mimic CVS include non-gastrointestinal as well as gastrointestinal disorders.

Of the gastrointestinal disorders, the most serious are anatomic anomalies of the gastrointestinal tract including malrotation with intermittent volvulus, which can cause ischemic necrosis. Although not typically cyclical, we have found a few children with eosinophilic esophagitis related to significant food allergies to mimic CVS. Lucarelli et al have described seven children with a positive radioallergosorbent test (RAST) to foods (milk, egg

Table 20.3 Characteristics of chronic and cyclic vomiting

	Chronic pattern	Cyclic pattern
Time of onset	daytime	night-time or early morning
Number of emeses/h	<4 emeses	≥4 emeses
Frequency of recurrence	>2 episodes/week	″2 episodes/week, typically 2–4 weeks
Family history of migraine	uncommon (14%)	common (82%)
Ill-appearing	no	yes (pale, lethargic)
Headaches	infrequent (19%)	frequent (41%)
Photophobia	infrequent (4%)	frequent (18%)
Vertigo	infrequent (7%)	frequent (24%)
Intravenous hydration required	uncommon (18%)	common (62%)
Esophagitis on EGD	common (59%)	uncommon (15%)

EGD, esophagogastroduodenoscopy

Table 20.4 Differential diagnosis of cyclic vomiting

	Chronic pattern	Cyclic pattern
Gastrointestinal	peptic injury (GERD esophagitis, gastritis, duodenitis) inflammatory bowel disease celiac disease chronic appendicitis pancreatitis eosinophilic gastroenteritis/esophagitis	anatomic (malrotation, volvulus, duplication cyst) pseudo-obstruction cholelithiasis/gallbladder dyskinesia
Infectious	chronic sinusitis giardiasis	sinusitis/other infections may be a trigger
Genitourinary	pyelonephritis, pregnancy	acute hydronephrosis due to uretopelvic junction obstruction or stones
Metabolic	rare	mitochondrial disorders (MELAS) organic acidemias aminoacidurias fatty acid oxidation defects urea cycle defects acute intermittent porphyria
Endocrine	adrenal hyperplasia	Addison's disease diabetic ketoacidosis pheochromocytoma
Neurological	Chiari malformation subtentorial neoplasm	migraine (headaches/abdominal) abdominal epilepsy familial dysautonomia
Psychiatric	Münchausen-by-proxy pscyhogenic vomiting	Münchausen-by-proxy anorexia nervosa bulimia nervosa CVS

GERD, gastroesophageal reflux disease; CVS, cyclic vomiting syndrome

white and soy) whose episodes diminished after specific food elimination.[14]

The most common extraintestinal cause is acute hydronephrosis resulting from proximal or distal ureteral obstruction. Metabolic causes include mitochondrial disorders (disorders of fatty acid oxidation, mitochondrial encephalopathy, lactic acid and stroke-like syndrome), urea cycle defects (partial ornithine transcarbamylase deficiency), organic acidurias (proprionic acidemia), aminoacidurias and porphyrin degradation disorders (acute intermittent porphyria).[15,16]

Neurosurgical causes include various lesions of the subtentorial region including cerebellar medulloblastoma, brain stem glioma and Chiari malformation.[2]

Pathophysiology

CVS is considered an idiopathic disorder because no etiopathogenesis has been documented. However, although no specific cause has been identified, several tenable hypotheses and associations have been raised to explain this unique disorder. The current concept is that CVS is a functional brain–gut disorder involving central neuroendocrine mediation and peripheral gastrointestinal manifestations.

Migraines

An association with migraines was identified over a century ago.[8,9] Previous reports demonstrated the association CVS has with migraine headaches, a positive family history of migraines,[5] and progression of clinical episodes of CVS to migraine headaches with advancing age.[5,17] In the absence of definitive diagnostic tests for migraines and CVS, a putative causal relationship is further supported by similar symptomatology (e.g. pallor, lethargy, nausea, photophobia, phonophobia) and positive responses in both groups to anti-migraine therapy.

Data from our series of over 440 patients show that the majority (87%) of patients with CVS do have a migraine association based on either a positive family history or concomitant or subsequent development of migraines in the patient. The progression of cyclic vomiting in childhood to abdominal migraines and eventually migraine headaches in adulthood has been labeled by Barlow as the periodic syndrome.[18] Many studies have confirmed this observation including reports of adults with migraines whose headache symptoms started with recurrent vomiting.[19,20] Compared with the 13% who have non-migraine CVS, these migraine-associated CVS patients generally have milder episodes with significantly fewer emeses/episode, more symptoms of abdominal pain, headache, photophobia and social withdrawal, a greater association with psychological stress and significantly higher response rates to anti-migraine therapy (79% vs. 36%).[5,17]

Among the anti-migraine drugs that achieve such a positive response is sumatriptan (52%), a selective 1B/1D serotonin agonist. This action on serotonin receptors with similar rates of response to patients with migraine headaches suggests a central role of action presumably by decreasing cerebrovascular dilatation. Since less than half of patients with a migraine association actually have headaches, a family history of migraines and the development of headaches over time are important in supporting this etiological linkage. Abdominal migraine shares many of the clinical features of CVS with midline abdominal pain being the most consistent and distressing symptom during episodes.[13] Migraine headaches, abdominal migraine and CVS differ in their primary symptoms but all have similar rates of secondary symptoms of pallor, lethargy, anorexia and nausea.

Recent studies on migraine headaches have identified the periaqueductal gray (PAG) matter as a site of dysfunction in migraine attacks. Previous work with electrode stimulation on PAG,[21] positron emission tomography (PET) scan data demonstrating increased blood flow,[22] and altered iron homeostasis[23] all suggest PAG involvement in migraine patients. Welch et al have speculated that similar mechanisms could be involved in CVS: PAG dysfunction may fail to attenuate afferent signals for vomiting and other autonomic symptoms during attacks.[23] Until we have a clearer delineation of mechanisms involved in migraine and CVS, we cannot be certain whether the CVS patients who do not fit under the migraine umbrella have distinct or similar pathophysiologic cascades.

Mitochondrial dysfunction

An association with mitochondrial DNA (mtDNA) mutations has been noted in children with CVS. Although the precise functional defects are unknown, Boles and Willians have proposed that altered mitochondrial metabolism may be involved.[16] They reported a large mtDNA rearrangement associated with CVS and subsequently demonstrated nine mutations in the hypervariable region of the D-loop (control region) of the mtDNA.[16] Some migraines and cyclic vomiting appear to result from disordered energy metabolism in mitochondrial encephalopathy lactic acidosis and stroke-like (MELAS) syndrome.[24] Since mtDNA is maternally derived, the findings of a matrilineal predominance of migraines (64% maternal side only vs. 16% paternal side) in children with CVS further suggested an association.[10] Many of the affected children with identified mutations have a clinical presentation with developmental delay, poor growth and seizures. However, based on non-specific lactate elevations and organic acid abnormalities (ethylmalonic acid), we suspect that there could be subtle underlying mitochondrial dysfunction evident during CVS episodes even in patients without identified mutations.

Neuroendocrine dysfunction

Activation of the hypothalamic–pituitary–adrenal (HPA) axis was first described in CVS by Wolfe and Adler[25] and Sato et al.[25,26] Stressors in the form of infectious disorders, psychological perturbations and physical triggers have been well documented as precipitants of CVS episodes.[2] Sato et al described elevated levels of adrenocorticotropic hormone (ACTH), antidiuretic hormone (ADH), cortisols, prostaglandin E_2, and serum and urinary catecholamines during episodes of CVS.[27] This finding may partially explain the symptoms of hypertension and profound lethargy in this subset of patients.

The role of CRF as a brain–gut mediator in foregut function has been extensively described in animals by Taché et al.[28] In animal models, these authors demonstrated convincingly that central CRF acting on CRF-R2 receptors stimulated the dorsal motor nucleus (proximal end) of the vagus and delayed gastric emptying.[28,29] Clinical CVS in humans is precipitated by parallel stimuli that augment CRF release in animals. Also, the same hormones in a subset of Sato's group reflected a stimulated HPA axis presumably initiated by CRF release, and appeared to give rise to the prominent symptoms of hypertension, anorexia and delayed gastric emptying. Our current studies examining the role of CRF in CVS may not only elucidate the pathophysiological cascade but could also open potential therapeutic avenues involving CRF antagonists.

Despite the coherent hypothesis of CRF as a main mediator of vomiting, there may be another layer of dysfunction needed to explain why CVS episodes tend to be prolonged for hours. This added dysfunction could explain why most stressed individuals simply have 'butterflies in their stomach' or a single emesis, whereas children with CVS vomit for days on end. This could represent a dysfunctional PAG area that permits afferent autonomic signals to persist unattenuated, or augmented HPA axis stimulation or CRF receptor sensitivity in CVS patients.

Autonomic dysfunction

Symptoms of fever, lethargy, pallor, flushing, drooling and diarrhea occur commonly during episodes of CVS and are mediated by the autonomic nervous system. There are several lines of evidence that support the role of autonomic dysfunction in CVS, including clinical parallels in familial dysautonomia, documented alterations in autonomic tone and evidence of dysmotility on electrogastrography. Children with familial dysautonomia (FD, also known as Riley–Day syndrome), can manifest episodes of autonomic crises which resemble a sympathetic storm including discrete episodes of vomiting associated with tachycardia, hypertension, diffuse sweating, and emotional lability. Given the similarities, there may be commonalities in autonomic dysfunction between CVS episodes and FD crises. Studies using single photon emission computed tomography (SPECT) (cerebral perfusion) have localized enhanced temporal lobe perfusion during symptoms of nausea and retching that support that region's involvement in ictal vomiting.[30]

To et al have observed heightened sympathetic cardiovascular tone and diminished parasympathetic vagal modulation via spectral analysis of R–R interval variability in CVS patients compared to controls.[31] Rashed et al demonstrated similar adrenergic autonomic abnormalities between CVS and migraine patients by showing lowered postural adjustment ratios.[32] Although the significance is still controversial, there is some electrogastrographic evidence of baseline gastric dysmotility in children with CVS that may respond to medium-dose erythromycin acting like motilin to enhance gastric motility and prevent vomiting episodes.[33–35]

Potential subtypes of cyclic vomiting syndrome and common associations

The vast majority (87%) of patients with CVS have a migraine association either based most commonly on a family history of migraine or, less frequently, on the subsequent development of migraines in the affected child. Because these associated symptoms occurred less than half the time, we did not use headache, photophobia and phonophobia as specific criteria to determine who had migraine-associated CVS. When we examined the remainder with non-migraine-associated CVS (13%), they appeared to have longer episodes, had more emeses per episode and were far less likely to respond to anti-migraine therapy (79 vs. 36%).[5] At present, we cannot determine whether the non-migraine CVS is pathophysiologically distinct or simply resides at the severe end of the same mechanistic spectrum.

Are there more subtypes of CVS? Although we have been able to differentiate other subgroups based on precipitating events, clinical pattern and associated symptomatology, there are too few subjects in each to know whether there are significant differences. In Sato's subtype, described patients have hypertension and profound lethargy to the point of inability to walk, talk or respond. We have found that these patients generally have more prolonged episodes (102 h vs. 50 h) and increased vomiting per episode (75 vs. 31 emeses).

Several children with developmental and growth delay, seizures and mild lactic acidosis are suspected of having underlying mitochondrial enzymopathy from a mtDNA mutation. Indeed, nine patients with this clinical picture have been found to have mutations in the D-loop or control region of the mtDNA.[36] Others with CVS have been found to a have either a large rearrangement or a single point mutation (MELAS).[16,24]

There are several other clinical patterns that can be identified. Again, it is unclear whether they simply represent various inciting stimuli that initiate the same pathophysiological cascade, or whether they represent distinct effector pathways. We hope that delineation of clinical patterns into subgroups may ultimately point us towards potential treatment approaches. For instance, some appear to have episodes that occur after periods of fasting, often induced by illness. They appear to respond rapidly to intravenous glucose and are suspected of being heterozygote carriers of disorders of fatty acid oxidation. Others have a stable periodicity (e.g. 60 days) to their episodes independent of stress or infectious triggers. Stable periodicity has been observed in some postmenarchal girls who have episodes at the onset of their menses and often respond to birth control pills with a low estrogen dose.[2] Some respond to prokinetic agents, but because of the lack of motility studies, it is not known whether they have documented gastric dysmotility.[37] Finally, in a group of children, dietary triggers of their episodes can be identified. Some are initiated by typical migraine precipitants including cheese, chocolate and monosodium glutamate, whereas others are triggered by food allergies identified by RAST testing.[14]

Diagnostic evaluation

At present, there are no specific laboratory changes to diagnose CVS, and the diagnosis depends on fulfilling key historical criteria (Table

Table 20.5 Diagnostic criteria (from the First International Symposium on Cyclic Vomiting Syndrome)

Essential criteria
≥3 recurrent, severe, discrete episodes of vomiting
Varying intervals of normal or baseline health between episodes
Duration of episodes from hours to days
No apparent cause for vomiting (negative laboratory, radiographic and endoscopic testing)
Supportive criteria
Stereotypical episodes are similar in regards to time of onset, intensity, duration, frequency and associated symptoms and signs
Self-limited in that episodes will resolve if left untreated
Associated symptoms and signs

20.5). In the absence of positive laboratory findings, most of the testing with recurrent vomiting is directed towards excluding other treatable causes. Potentially treatable underlying gastrointestinal, neurological, renal, metabolic and endocrine causes are not rare, and are found in 12% of those who present with a cyclic pattern of vomiting. In addition, 12% (many overlapping) have an identifiable surgical disorder.[2] The challenge is to determine what and how much testing should be done, because a 'shot-gun' approach can be costly, time-consuming and invasive. We conducted a cost-decision analysis and concluded that an upper gastrointestinal tract X-ray with a small bowel follow-through followed by 2 months of empiric anti-migraine therapy was the most cost-effective initial treatment strategy for CVS.[12] If no therapeutic response occurs, more systematic testing should be performed (Figure 20.2).

The first step is to identify a recurrent pattern versus a single acute vomiting illness typical of gastroenteritis. The next is to distinguish between a low-grade, nearly daily chronic and explosive, intermittent cyclic pattern of vomiting. Once identified, the diagnostic evaluation involves evaluation for both gastrointestinal and non-gastrointestinal causes. In our experience, the most potentially devastating causes are sought including anatomic anomalies of the gastrointestinal tract and renal hydronephrosis by upper gastrointestinal series with small bowel follow-through and renal ultrasound examination, respectively. Metabolic and endocrine testing must be performed *before* intravenous glucose and fluids are administered, because these can alter respective findings on metabolic screening and evaluation of the HPA axis metabolites. The endoscopy and the head magnetic resonance imaging (MRI) are reserved for those in whom therapy has failed or who have specific symptoms suggesting peptic or allergic gastrointestinal disease or intractable headaches, respectively. Laboratory testing and a proposed algorithm for evaluation are presented in Figure 20.2.

Natural history and complications

There are limited data on the natural history of CVS. From our data of over 440 patients, the median age of resolution of symptoms is 9.9 years and one-third (28%) of the children have thus far undergone the transition from CVS into migraine headaches as they reached early adolescence. Our projection analysis estimates that 75% of patients will develop migraine headaches by the of age 18. Other long-term studies have shown that up to half of CVS patients will continue with CVS or migraine headaches.[17] Several studies have noted the mean duration of illness to be around 6 years,[13,38] but in our cohort, the younger the age of onset, the longer the duration. Also, 5% of patients will progress through all three phases of periodic disease including CVS to abdominal migraine and finally to migraine headaches.[13]

Complications and medical morbidity include iatrogenic tests and interventions from the misdiagnoses that were often applied to recurrent vomiting. Most are mislabeled as gastroenteritis, gastroesophageal reflux and food poisoning, and are treated in urgent care settings. Some with severe pain, bilious vomiting and intractability have undergone inappropriate laparotomy, appendectomy, cholecystectomy and Nissen fundoplication. Others have been labeled with psychiatric disorders including bulimia and psychogenic vomiting, and have been hospitalized on psychiatric wards, and a few parents have been suspected of Münchausen-by-proxy.[39]

Complications can also occur from the frequent and often severe episodes of vomiting that occur with CVS. Dehydration and electrolyte disturbances are common and intravenous rehydration is required in 58% of patients, which can be compared to less than 1% in rotavirus infection. Hematemesis can occur towards the end of attacks and is usually related to prolapse gastropathy or Mallory–Weiss tears.[11] Although not common, frequent vomiting can lead to secondary peptic injury. Aspiration and growth failure fortunately seem to be uncommon occurrences.

Treatment

Current treatment for CVS can be divided into supportive (during episodes), prophylactic (to prevent episodes) (Table 20.6) and abortive therapy (to stop episodes) (Table 20.7). Other strategies for management of CVS include avoidance of identified triggers (e.g. dietary cheese),

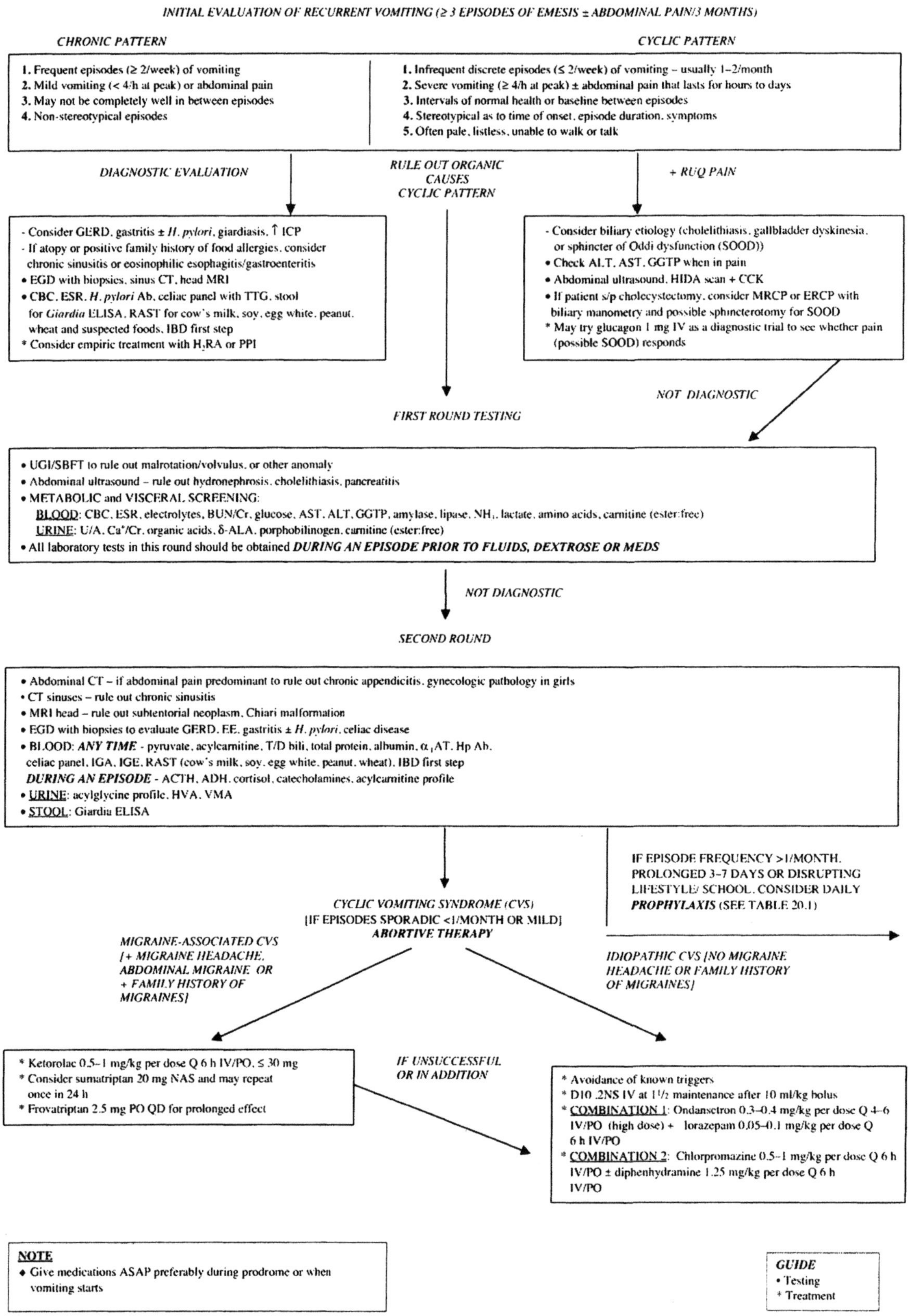

Figure 20.2 Algorithm for diagnostic evaluation and acute management of recurrent (chronic and cyclic) vomiting.

Table 20.6 Prophylactic therapy

Drug	Side-effects
Anti-migraine	
Amitryptyline (1–2 mg/kg per day) qhs	sedation, anticholinergic
Propranalol (0.5–1 mg/kg per day) bid or tid	hypotension, bradycardia, fatigue
Cyproheptadine (0.25–0.5 mg/kg per day) bid or tid	sedation, weight gain, anticholinergic
Anticonvulsants	
Phenobarbital (2–3 mg/kg per day) qd or bid	sedation
Valproate (500–1000 mg ER qhs)	somnolence, hepatotoxicity
Carbamezapine (5–10 mg/kg per day) bid	sedation, anticholinergic
Prokinetic	
Erythromycin (10–20 mg/kg per day) qid	gastric cramps in larger doses
Birth control	
Norethindrone (1.5 mg) ethinylestradiol (20–30 μg) qd	estrogen-related, nausea, abdominal pain

qhs, at bed-time: bid, twice a day; tid, three times a day; qd, every day

Table 20.7 Abortive therapy

Drug	Side-effects
Anti-migraine	
Sumatriptan 20 mg NAS and may repeat x1 or 25 mg po x1	chest and neck burning (po form), headache
Frovatriptan 2.5 mg po and may repeat x1	coronary vasospasm, dizziness
Rizatriptan 5–10 mg po x1, may repeat q 2 h	arrythmias, chest pain
Ketorolac 0.5–1 mg/kg per dose q 6 h iv/po	GI bleeding, dyspepsia
Antiemetic	
Ondansetron 0.3–0.4 mg/kg per dose q 4–6 h iv/po	headache, drowsiness, dry mouth
Granisetron 10 μg/kg iv q 4–6 h	pancytopenia, headache
Sedative	
Lorazepam 0.05–0.1 mg/kg per dose q 6 h iv/po (useful adjunct to ondansetron)	sedation, respiratory depression
Chlorpromazine 0.5–1 mg/kg per dose q 6 h iv/po	drowsiness, hypotension, seizures
Diphenhydramine 1.25 mg/kg per dose q 6 h iv/po (useful adjunct to chlorpromazine)	hypotension, sedation, dizziness

NAS, intranasally ; po, orally; q, every; iv, intravenous; GI, gastrointestinal

psychological interventions (e.g. stress management) and supportive care during attacks when all else fails.[40] Avoidance of known triggers, especially dietary, can reduce the episode frequency. In some cases, stress management strategies through the aid of a psychologist can attenuate the effects of positive or negative stressors.[41]

Daily use of prophylactic medications is based on empiric therapy that is traditionally used to treat other disorders, including migraines, epilepsy, gastrointestinal dysmotility and birth control. Although there are no evidence-based guidelines, we generally consider prophylaxis in children who have either frequent episodes, e.g. more than one episode per month, or severe episodes (prolonged for more than 3–5 days), debilitating (associated with hospitalization) or disabling (e.g. missing school days).[2] The goal of prophylaxis is to prevent attacks altogether, and if unsuccessful to at least to reduce the frequency, duration or intensity (number of emeses) of episodes.

A family history of migraines is a strong indicator (79%) of a positive response to anti-migraine therapy.[5] In addition, associated symptoms of headache, photophobia and phonophobia should make one consider starting anti-migraine prophylaxis with propranolol, cyproheptadine, or amitriptyline with respective efficacy (more than 50% reduction in frequency or severity of episodes) rates of 52%, 39% and 67%, respectively, based on our data. Propranolol is contraindicated in asthmatics, has side-effects of tiredness and can be monitored by a resting pulse decline of 15–20 beats/min. Cyproheptadine can cause tiredness and an increase in appetite and weight.[4] Pizotifen, available in Europe, Canada and Australia, acts similarly but with fewer side-effects.[42] Amitriptyline has been the most effective prophylactic agent in our experience, but it can cause arrhythmias, especially in those with a prolonged QTc interval.[43] Based on current recommendations, prior to starting amitriptyline, we evaluate all candidate patients by checking their QTc interval on electrocardiogram.

Other prophylactic agents that have been used include phenobarbital, valproate, gabapentin and carbamazepine.[44] Although they are specifically indicated when spike and waves are noted on the electroencephalogram, they are increasingly used in both migraine and CVS prophylaxis. Erythromycin has been useful as a prokinetic agent[34] and low-dose estrogen birth control can be useful in teenage girls who have catemenial CVS. We also note that the efficacy rates in the open-label trials above must be interpreted cautiously, because of the large placebo effect (70%) that has been described from consultation alone prior to instituting therapy.

Abortive therapy is medication taken at the onset of an episode or even earlier during the prodromal phase, ideally to abort the episode altogether or reduce the duration or severity of the episode. Abortive therapy should be considered for those who have sporadic episodes that occur less than once per month and who prefer not taking prophylaxis or those who have breakthrough episodes while on prophylaxis.[2,40] Because patients with intractable emesis are unable to tolerate oral medication, these medications usually have to be administered parenterally.

The primary anti-migraine therapy includes 5-$HT_{1B/1D}$ agonists commonly used for migraine headaches. In our experience, success rates are higher in those children with migraine-associated CVS, when used early in the episode, and in those with episodes less than 24 h. In our patients, sumatriptan administered via oral, subcutaneous or intranasal routes has a 51% efficacy rate, as compared with 65% in headaches. The sensation of substernal and neck burning rarely occurs with intranasal administration.

Supportive care is used whenever the child is in a break-through episode that fails to respond to abortive therapy. Supportive care includes intravenous fluids, non-stimulating environment, antiemetics, sedation and analgesia.[2,40] Intravenous fluids with high dextrose concentration (10%) and electrolytes have a 42% efficacy alone in our experience. A quiet, dark single room may be helpful. Analgesia is not routinely used in our experience but occasionally can include narcotic agents.

Ondansetron, a 5-HT_3 antagonist, is primarily used as an antiemetic with efficacy rates around 62%.[45] More effective at the higher dosing of 0.3–0.4 mg/kg per dose, the side-effect profile has been excellent with few reports of drowsiness, dry mouth and headache.[10] It generally reduces both nausea and vomiting, but only rarely aborts the episode. The addition of a γ-aminobutyric acid (GABA) inhibitor, lorazepam, provides sedation that relieves intractable nausea. When all else fails, we use a combination of chlorpromazine and diphenhydramine primarily to provide sleep for relief from symptoms. In our experience, phenothiazine antiemetics (D_2 antagonists), have poor (15%) efficacy in this disorder, even less than our placebo responses, suggesting that dopaminergic pathways are not involved.

Summary

Recurrent vomiting is one of the most common causes for referral to the pediatric gastroenterologist. Improved recognition of CVS as a definable disorder with established criteria for diagnosis has come with time, and support of two recent scientific symposia. The Cyclic Vomiting Syndrome Association has been invaluable in providing family support for CVS patients as well as supporting research efforts in CVS. As work in understanding metabolic defects and the pathophysiological cascade(s) responsible for brain–gut interactions in CVS continues to define this disorder better, greater understanding will no doubt result in improved therapeutic strategies for patients suffering from CVS.

Acknowledgments

We would like to acknowledge Abid Kagalwalla for managing our CVS database and providing us with the appropriate data for this chapter. Dr Li was supported by funding from the Cyclic Vomiting Syndrome Association, Grant Healthcare Foundation and NINS.

REFERENCES

1. Li BUK. Cyclic vomiting syndrome and abdominal migraine. *Int Semin Pediatr Gastroenterol* 2000; **9**: 1–9.
2. Li BUK, Balint J. Cyclic vomiting syndrome: evolution in our understanding of a brain–gut disorder. In *Adv Pediatr* 2000; **47**: 117–160.
3. Abu-Arafeh I, Russel G. Cyclic vomiting syndrome in children: a population based study. *J Pediatr Gastroenterol Nutr* 1995; 21:454–458.
4. Pfau BT, Li BUK, Murray RD et al. Differentiating cyclic from chronic vomiting patterns in children: quantitative criteria and diagnostic implications. *Pediatr* 1996; **97**: 364–368.
5. Li B UK, Murray RD, Heitlinger LA. Is cyclic vomiting syndrome related to migraine? J *Pediatrics* 1999; **134**: 567–572.
6. Heberden W. *Commentaries on the History and Causes of Diseases*, 3rd edn. London: Payne & Foss, 1806, cited by Hammond J. The late sequelae of recurrent vomiting of childhood. *Dev Med Child Neurol* 1974; **16**: 15–22.
7. Gee S. On fitful or recurrent vomiting. *St Bartholemew Hosp Rev* 1882; **18**: 1–6.
8. Whitney HB. Cyclic vomiting: a brief review of this affection as illustrated by a typical case. *Arch Pediatr* 1898; **15**: 839–845.
9. Rachford BK. Recurrent vomiting. *Arch Pediatr* 1904; **21**: 881–891.
10. Li BUK, Fleisher DR. Cyclic vomiting syndrome: features to be explained by a pathophysiologic model. *Dig Dis Sci* 1999; **44**: 13S–18S.
11. Shepherd HA, Harvey J, Jackson A et al. Recurrent retching and gastric mucosal prolapse: a proposed prolapse gastropathy syndrome. *Dig Dis Sci* 1984; **29**: 121–128.
12. Olson AD, Li BUK. The diagnostic evaluation of children with cyclic vomiting: a cost-effectiveness assessment. *J Pediatr* 2002; **141**: 724–728.
13. Li BUK. Cyclic vomiting: the pattern and syndrome paradigm. *J Pediatr Gastroenterol Nutr* 1995; **21**(Suppl 1): S6–S10.
14. Lucarelli S, Corrado G, Pelliccia A et al. Cyclic vomiting syndrome and food allergy/intolerance in seven children: a possible association. *Eur J Pediatr* 2000; **159**: 360–363.
15. Rinaldo P. Mitochondrial fatty acid oxidation disorders and cyclic vomiting syndrome. *Dig Dis Sci* 1999; **44**: 97S–102S.
16. Boles RG, Williams JC. Mitochondrial disease and cyclic vomiting syndrome. *Dig Dis Sci* 1999; **44**: 103S–107S.
17. Symon DNK. Is cyclical vomiting an abdominal form of migraine in children? *Dig Dis Sci* 1999; **44**: 23S–25S.
18. Barlow CF. The periodic syndrome: cyclic vomiting and abdominal migraine. *Clin Dev Med* 1984; **91**: 76–92.
19. Lance JW, Anthony M. Some clinical aspects of migraine. *Arch Neurol* 1966; **15**: 356–361.
20. Salmon MA. The evolution of adult migraine through childhood migraine equivalents. In Lanzi G, Balottin U, Cernibori A, eds. *Headache in Children and Adolescents.* Amsterdam: Elvesier Science Publishers, 1989: 27–32.
21. Raskin NH, Hosobuchi Y, Lamb S. Headache may arise from perturbation of the brain. *Headache* 1987; **27**: 416–420.
22. Weiller C, May A, Limmroth V et al. Brain stem activation in spontaneous human migraine attacks. *Nat Med* 1995; **1**: 658–660.
23. Welch KM, Nagesh V, Aurora SK. Periaqueductal gray matter dysfunction in migraine: cause or the burden of illness? *Headache* 2001; **41**: 629–637.
24. Hirano M, Pavlakis SG. Mitochondrial myopathy: encephalopathy, lactic acidosis, and strokelike episodes (MELAS): current concepts. *J Child Neurol* 1994; **9**: 4–13.
25. Wolfe SM, Adler R. A syndrome of periodic hypothalamic discharge. *Am J Med* 1964; **36**: 956–967.
26. Sato T, Uchigata Y, Uwadana N et al. A syndrome of periodic adrenocorticotropin and vasopressin discharge. *J Clin Endocrinol Metab* 1982; **54**: 517–522.
27. Sato T, Igarashi M, Minami S et al. Recurrent attacks of vomiting, hypertension, and psychotic depression: a syndrome of periodic catecholamine and prostaglandin discharge. *Acta Endocrinol* 1988; **117**: 189–197.

28. Taché Y, Martinez V, Million M et al. Stress and the gastrointestinal tract III. Stress–related alterations of gut motor function: role of brain corticotropin-releasing factor receptors. *Am J Physiol-Gastrointest Liver Physiol* 2001; **280**: G173–G177.
29. Taché Y. Cyclic vomiting syndrome: the corticotropin-releasing-factor hypothesis. *Dig Dis Sci* 1999; **44**: 79S–86S.
30. Axelrod FB, Zupanc M, Hilz MJ et al. Ictal SPECT during autonomic crisis in famial dysautonomia. *Neurology* 2000; **55**: 122–125.
31. To J, Issenman RM, Kamath MV et al. Evaluation of neurocardiac signals in pediatric patients with cyclic vomiting syndrome through power spectral analysis of heart rate variability. *J Pediatr* 1999; **135**: 363–366.
32. Rashed R, Abell TL, Familoni BO et al. Autonomic function in cyclic vomiting syndrome and classic migraine. *Dig Dis Sci* 1999; **44**: 74S–78S.
33. Chong SKF. Electrogastrography in cyclic vomiting syndrome. *Dig Dis Sci* 1999; **44**: 64S–73S.
34. Vanderhoof JA, Young R, Kaufmann SS et al. Treatment of cyclic vomiting syndrome in childhood with erythromycin. *J Pediatr Gastroenterol Nutr* 1993; **17**: 387–391.
35. Wood JD. Enteric nervous control of motility in the upper gastrointestinal tract in defensive states. *Dig Dis Sci* 1999; **44**: 44S–52S.
36. Boles RG, Adams K, Ito M, Li BUK. Maternal inheritance in cyclic vomiting syndrome with neuromuscular disease. *Am J Med Genet* 2003; **120A**: 474–482.
37. Abell TL, Chung HK, Malagelada JR. Idiopathic cyclic nausea and vomiting – a disorder of gastrointestinal motility? *Mayo Clin Proc* 1988; **63**: 1169–1175.
38. Fleisher DR, Matar M. The cyclic vomiting syndrome: a report of 71 cases and literature review. *J Pediatr Gastroenterol Nutr* 1993; **17**: 361–369.
39. Brown JB, Li BUK. Recurrent vomiting in children. *Clin Perspect Gastroenterol* 2002; 35–39.
40. Li BUK. Cyclic vomiting syndrome. *Curr Treat Options Gastroenterol* 2000; **3**: 395–402.
41. Forbes D, Withers G, Silburn S et al. Psychological and social characteristics and precipitants of vomiting in children with cyclic vomiting syndrome. *Dig Dis Sci* 1999; **44**: 19S–22S.
42. Symon DNK. Double-blind placebo-controlled trial of pizotifen syrup in the treatment of abdominal migraine. *Arch Dis Child* 1995; **72**: 48–50.
43. Prakash C, Clouse RE. Cyclic vomiting syndrome in adults: clinical features and response to tricyclic antidepressants. *Am J Gastroenterol* 1999; **94**: 2855–2859.
44. Gokhale R, Huttenlocher PR, Brady L et al. Use of barbiturates in the treatment of cyclic vomiting during childhood. *J Pediatr Gastroenterol Nutr* 1997; **25**: 64–67.
45. Li BUK, Robbins JL, Vu KT et al. Morbidity and treatment in cyclic vomiting syndrome. *Gastroenterology* 1996; **110**: 25A.
46. Li BUK. Cyclic vomiting syndrome: new understanding of an old disorder. *Contemp Pediatr* 1996; **13**: 49.

21 Acute and chronic pancreatitis

Michelle M Pietzak

Introduction

Pancreatitis commonly occurs in the pediatric population, but it mostly remains undiagnosed. The clinician treating acute cases must have a low threshold to test for the non-specific and common symptoms that occur with this inflammatory process. Often, the symptoms are dismissed as occurring from an acute gastroenteritis or viral infection.

Pancreatitis can be defined as an inflammatory process of the pancreas which occurs in the clinical setting of characteristic abdominal and back pain, accompanied by elevations of the pancreatic enzymes. The different types of pancreatitis can be characterized into five main categories according to the timing of the illness, clinical symptoms, family history and radiographic findings (acute, chronic, hereditary, hemorrhagic and necrotic).

Acute pancreatitis is usually a short, self-limited process characterized by the classic symptoms of nausea, vomiting, anorexia, epigastric pain and back pain. Levels of serum amylase and lipase are markedly elevated in the acute inflammatory response. Although a child may suffer from repeated bouts of acute pancreatitis, the symptoms and enzyme elevations should completely resolve between attacks. Pancreatic function remains intact and the pancreatic morphology is undisturbed.

If the signs and symptoms of inflammation are progressive, this may lead to chronic pancreatitis. Chronicity may be accompanied by either temporary or permanent loss of both exocrine and endocrine function. The severe pain that accompanies this condition can be debilitating and lead to dependence upon narcotics. Within the gland itself, protein plugs may calcify, indicating advanced and chronic disease (Figure 21.1).

Patients with hereditary pancreatitis, by definition, will have a family history of the disease. These diseases are autosomal dominant; affected family members will often present with recurrent bouts of acute pancreatitis starting in childhood.

Hemorrhagic and necrotic pancreatitis are uncommon in the pediatric population, but are a significant cause of morbidity and mortality from the disease. A secondary bacterial infection can occur within the gland, leading to bacteremia, shock and resultant multi-organ system failure.

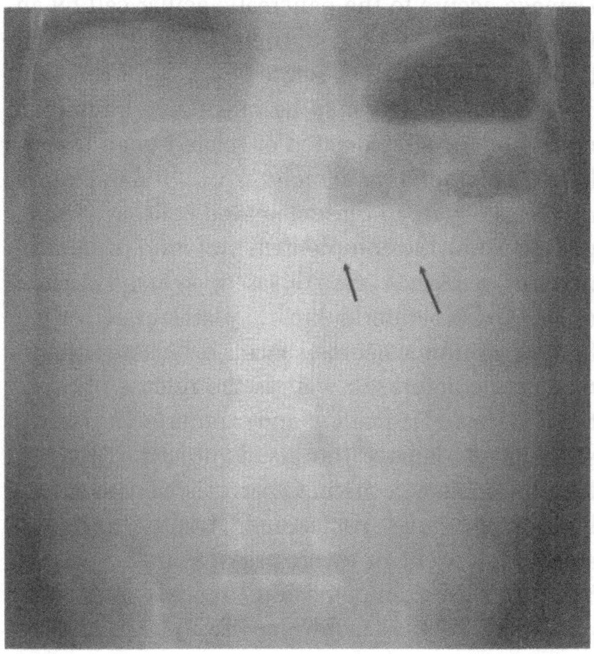

Figure 21.1 Kidney, ureters and bladder radiograph with calcified pancreas of a 6-year-old female who presented to the emergency department with a 3-month history of abdominal pain and distension due to severe pancreatitis. Plain film revealed ascites and extensive pancreatic calcifications (arrows). Ascitic fluid was markedly hemorrhagic and the endoscopic retrograde cholangiopancreatogram was normal. Patient was later discovered to have two different mutations in the *CFTR* gene.

Incidence and prevalence

Although pancreatitis is seen more often in the adult rather than the pediatric population, it is likely to be underdiagnosed. Its true identification requires a high index of suspicion on the part of the clinician with a prompt evaluation before its resolution. In the literature, most publications on this disease in childhood are restricted to reports of either an isolated patient or small clusters of patients. Because of this, the true incidence and prevalence of the disease in this population are unknown. The most common pancreatic disorder in children is thought to be acute pancreatitis, with cystic fibrosis the second most common.

Etiology and pathophysiology

The clinical characteristics of acute pancreatitis follow a similar pattern, despite its varied causes. Damage occurs to the pancreatic acinar cell by an inciting event, leading to premature activation of the digestive enzymes while still within the cell. This inciting event may be infectious, traumatic, metabolic, drug-associated or related to an underlying anatomic anomaly. An inflammatory response occurs to these damaged cells, activating platelets and the complement system. Pro-inflammatory cytokines are released, which include nitric oxide, interleukin-1, platelet activating factor and tumor necrosis factor-α.[1] These inflammatory mediators, as well as the release of additional free radicals and other vasoactive substances, damage the gland directly. This can lead to edema, ischemia, necrosis and eventual loss of glandular tissue and atrophy. Systemic shock may occur in severe cases, as demonstrated by tachycardia, hypotension, hypoxia and adult respiratory distress syndrome (ARDS).

While the majority of adult cases of pancreatitis are related to either alcohol consumption or gallstone disease, the causes of pediatric pancreatitis are more varied. In adolescent females, gallstone pancreatitis is not uncommon. However, young children with this disease have often been exposed to a recent trauma, infection, or medication as the inciting event. Recurrent pancreatitis in childhood can be attributed to hereditary pancreatitis, an anatomic variant of the pancreatic or biliary tree, or an underlying systemic or metabolic disorder. Despite exhaustive investigation, up to 25% of pediatric patients will not have an attributable cause for their acute pancreatitis. The conditions associated with acute and chronic pancreatitis in childhood are outlined in Table 21.1.[1–17]

Anatomic abnormalities

Congenital defects in the pancreas are rare, but if left uncorrected they can lead to chronic pancreatitis. Pancreatic divisum is the most common anatomic variant.[18] It occurs when the dorsal and ventral pancreatic ducts fail to fuse during fetal development, directing flow primarily to the dorsal duct.[19] Some believe this variant to be a significant cause of recurrent pancreatitis, which requires either endoscopic or surgical correction. Others think that pancreatic divisum is a variant of normal, and that most people with this anatomy will not experience pancreatitis.

Changes in anatomy which result in duodenal obstruction can also lead to pancreatitis. Reasons for this include strictures, tumors, duplications or diverticula of the duodenum or pancreas, and duodenal hematoma from either accidental or non-accidental trauma (child abuse).

Traumatic causes

Trauma is possibly the most common cause of pancreatitis in childhood, and is probably underestimated. Motor vehicle and bicycle accidents can result in blunt trauma to the pancreas from seatbelts and handlebars. Findings on physical examination consistent with trauma, in the absence of a reliable history, should raise suspicion for child abuse. There are often other associated intra-abdominal injuries in cases of significant blunt abdominal trauma. Duodenal hematoma and intestinal perforation are not uncommon.

Infectious causes

A variety of organisms account for a significant number of cases of pancreatitis worldwide, including bacteria, viruses and parasites. The *Escherichia coli* strain which produces verotoxin and is associated with hemolytic uremic syndrome can also cause pancreatitis. Viruses such as varicella and

Table 21.1 Conditions associated with pancreatitis in the pediatric population (from references 1–17)

Idiopathic
Up to 25% of cases

Anatomic
Ampullary diverticulum
Ampullary stenosis
Annular pancreas
Biliary tract malformations
Choledochal cyst
Choledochocele
Choledochopancreaticoductal junction anomaly
Cholelithiasis
Common bile duct: absence or anomalous insertion
Duodenal obstruction from diverticulum, hematoma, tumor or stricture
Duodenal ulcer – perforated
Duplication cyst of the common bile duct, duodenum, gastropancreatic area
Gastric trichobezoar
Pancreatic aplasia
Pancreatic divisum
Pancreatic duct: absence or anomalous insertion
Pancreatic dysplasia
Pancreatic heterotopy
Pancreatic hypoplasia
Pancreatic pseudocyst
Pancreatic tumors
Sclerosing cholangitis
Sphincter of Oddi dysfunction

Traumatic
Blunt injury to the abdomen
Burns
Contrast from ductal imaging (endoscopic retrograde cholangiopancreatography, percutaneous transhepatic cholangiography)
Head trauma
Non-accidental trauma (child abuse)
Radiation to the abdomen
Surgical trauma
Total body cast

Infectious
Ascaris lumbricoides (duct obstruction)
Campylobacter fetus
Clonorchis sinensis (duct obstruction)
Coxsackie B virus
Cryptosporidium
Cytomegalovirus
Echovirus
Enterovirus
Escherichia coli (verotoxin-producing)
Hepatitis A virus
Hepatitis B virus
Human immunodeficiency virus (HIV)
Influenza A virus
Influenza B virus
Legionnaire's disease
Leptospirosis
Malaria
Measles
Mumps
Mycobacteria
Mycoplasma
Rubella
Rubeola
Toxoplasma
Typhoid fever
Varicella
Yersinia

Hereditary/Metabolic/Systemic
α_1-Antitrypsin deficiency
Anorexia nervosa
Autoimmune disease
Brain tumor
Bulimia
Collagen vascular disease
Congenital partial lipodystrophy
Crohn's disease
Cystic fibrosis
Dehydration
Dermatomyositis
Diabetes mellitus (ketoacidosis)
Glycogen storage disease types Ia and Ib
Hemochromatosis
Hemolytic–uremic syndrome
Honoch–Schönlein purpura
Hereditary pancreatitis
Hyperalimentation
Hypercalcemia
Hyperlipidemia types I, IV and V
Hyperparathyroidism
Hypertriglyceridemia
Hypothermia
Hypovolemia
Inborn errors of metabolism (organic academia, cytochrome-C oxidase deficiency)
Juvenile tropical pancreatitis
Kawasaki disease
Liver disease
Malnutrition
Organic acidemias (homocystinuria, isovaleric acidemia, methylmalonic acidemia, maple syrup urine disease)
Periarteritis nodosa
Peritonitis
Refeeding syndrome
Renal failure with uremia
Reye's syndrome
Sarcoidosis
Sepsis
Shock
Systemic lupus erythematosus
Transplantation (bone marrow, heart, kidney, liver, pancreas)
Ulcerative colitis
Vascular diseases
Uremia
Wilson's disease

influenza B, associated with Reye's syndrome, have also been implicated in causing acute pancreatitis in childhood. Parasites that are more common in developing areas, such as *Ascaris* and *Clonorchis*, can migrate into the biliary tree, leading to obstructive jaundice and pancreatitis. Left untreated, this obstruction can lead to severe portal hypertension, liver failure and death.

Children with AIDS are at higher risk for developing acute pancreatitis. One Italian study in symptomatic HIV-infected children demonstrated pancreatic biochemical abnormalities in 15% of the patients.[20] However, the elevated enzymes did not correlate with clinical evidence of acute pancreatitis. Although an adult autopsy series showed pancreatic lesions in about 30% of AIDS patients, fewer than 10% had clinical symptoms.[21] In children with HIV at autopsy, pancreatic involvement, defined as edema, inflammation, fibrosis, inspissated material and enlarged Langerhan's islets, was frequent.[22] However, tumors and involvement of opportunistic infectious was rare. HIV-positive patients can develop elevated enzymes, owing to the HIV infection itself, or owing to other co-infections, such as cytomegalovirus (CMV), *Toxoplasma*, mycobacteria and *Cryptosporidium*.[17] Many of the pharmacological agents used to inhibit HIV can cause pancreatitis (see Medications). Hyperamylasemia without pancreatitis can occur from renal failure, AIDS-associated nephropathy, or salivary hyperamylasemia from parotid gland disease due to HIV.[23] Kaposi's sarcoma and lymphoma can also affect the pancreas.[24]

Hereditary, metabolic and systemic diseases

The most common inherited disease of the exocrine pancreas is thought to be cystic fibrosis (CF).[25] This autosomal recessive disease is caused by mutations in the CF transmembrane conductance regulator gene (*CFTR*). *CFTR* is located on the apical membrane of the epithelial cells that line the pancreatic ducts. The transporter promotes dilution and alkalinization of the pancreatic secretions and they flow through the ductular network. CF may be one of the most common causes of pancreatitis in childhood, but pancreatitis itself is a rare presenting feature of CF.[26] It is believed that up to 2% of individuals with CF experience pancreatitis as a result of ductal plugging due to mutant *CFTR*.[27] CF is the only known hereditary disease in which there can be both pancreatitis, and exocrine insufficiency in the absence of pancreatic inflammation.[28] However, those patients with CF and pancreatic insufficiency do not develop acute relapsing pancreatitis, presumably because of the loss of functional acinar tissue.[7] Even in the absence of lung disease, there appears to be a strong correlation between specific *CFTR* mutations and idiopathic and chronic pancreatitis.[29–31] Patients with recurrent pancreatitis without an obvious cause should be screened for CF with a sweat chloride test. *CFTR* mutational analysis is also commercially available. The role of CFTR in pancreatitis and other diseases of the pancreas is the subject of ongoing research.

The second most common cause of chronic pancreatitis in childhood is believed to be hereditary pancreatitis.[32] The gene defects were reported in 1996,[33] and help explain some of the pathophysiology of the non-hereditary forms of both acute and chronic pancreatitis.[34,35] The two known types of hereditary pancreatitis are clinically similar, and involve different mutations within the same gene. Both types are autosomal dominant with 80% penetrance.[36] The majority of affected patients report symptoms before the age of 15 years, with some symptomatic even before the age of 5 years. The gene involved is located on chromosome 7q35, and codes for cationic trypsinogen (*PRSS1*). Both mutations result in a form of trypsin that resists degradation by mesotrypsin and enzyme Y,[26] allowing trypsinogen to become activated to trypsin within the pancreas instead of within the duodenum. This leads to uncontrolled activation of other pancreatic enzymes within the acinar cell, resulting in autodigestion and inflammation. The attacks of acute pancreatitis are remarkably only intermittent. It is thought that this uncontrolled activation of other enzymes occurs only when trypsin exceeds the capacity of pancreatic secretory trypsin inhibitor, the 'secondary brake' within the pancreatic gland. Identification of those with hereditary pancreatitis is critical, as affected patients are at increased risk for pseudocysts, pancreatic adenocarcinoma, and exocrine and endocrine failure.[37]

Since the discovery that hereditary pancreatitis can be caused by mutations in *PRSS1*, researchers have been searching for other potential candidate genes that may predispose patients to chronic pancreatitis. Given that the proposed mechanism for pancreatitis with *PRSS1* mutations is decreased inactivation, one candidate gene is that encoding for pancreatic secretory trypsin inhibitor or serine protease inhibitor, Kazal type 1 (*SPINK1*).[38] *SPINK1* mutations have been reported in a wide phenotype of conditions, including familial, hereditary, tropical and idiopathic chronic pancreatitis.[39–42] Whether or not *SPINK1* mutations modify an already underlying genetic disease has yet to be elucidated.[38]

Pancreatitis has been a reported complication in children who have received heart, kidney, liver, pancreas or bone marrow transplants.[8] Following liver transplantation, it can be life-threatening, and is associated with a higher risk for infectious peritonitis and emergency retransplantation.[9] As with autoimmune and collagen–vascular diseases, it is difficult to distinguish between the contributions of medications versus the primary disease process to the development of the pancreatitis.

Medications

Numerous medications and naturally occurring toxins have been reported as a cause of pancreatitis (Table 21.2).[1–4,6,17,23,43–45] Often, however, the

Table 21.2 Drugs and toxins associated with pancreatitis (from references 1–4,6,17,23,43–45)

Acetaminophen overdose	Meprobamate
Alcohol	Mercaptopurine
Amphetamines	Mesalamine
Anticoagulants	Methotrexate
Asparaginase	Methyldopa
Azathioprine	Metronidazole
Boric acid	Non-steroidal anti-inflammatory drugs
Bumetanide	Nitrofurantoin
Calcium	Octreotide
Carbamazepine	Opiates
Chlorthalidone	Oxyphenbutazone
Cholestyramine	Organophosphates
Cimetidine	Paromomycin
Cisplatin	Penicillin
Clonidine	Pentamidine
Clozapine	Phenformin
Corticosteroids	Piroxicam
Corticotropin	Procainamide
Cyclophosphamide	Propoxyphene
Cyproheptadine	Propylthiouracil
Cytarabine	Ranitidine
Cytosine arabinoside	Rifampin
Diazoxide	Salicylates
Didanosine	Scorpion venom
Dideoxycinosine	Spider venom
Dideoxycytidine	Sulfasalazine
Diphenoxylate	Sulfonamides
Enalapril	Sulindac
Erythromycin	Tetracycline
Estrogen	Thiazides
Ethacrynic acid	Tretinoin
Furadantin	Trimethoprim–sulfamethoxazole
Furosemide	Valproic acid
Heroin	Vincristine
Histamine	Vitamin D
Indomethacin	
Isoniazid	
Lamivudine	

relationship between drugs and pancreatitis is more of association than causation. Classes of medications most likely to cause pancreatitis include antibiotics (erythromycin, metronidazole, nitrofurantoin, penicillin, rifampin), anticonvulsants (carmbamazepine, valproic acid), antihypertensives (clonidine, diazoxide, enalapril), anti-inflammatories (corticosteroids, ibuprofen, indomethacin, sulfasalazine and acetaminophen when overdosed) and antineoplastic agents (asparaginase, azathioprine, mercaptopurine, cyclophosphamide, vincristine). Most of the drugs mentioned in this chapter have a proposed but unproven pathophysiology, and very few documented an established causal relationship to pancreatitis.

Clinical signs and symptoms

In the pediatric population, the classic signs of acute pancreatitis include nausea, vomiting, anorexia and abdominal pain. The pain is classically located in the epigastrium, with radiation to the back. However, the pain could also be located in the periumbilical region, right upper quadrant or lower chest.[46,47] Eating usually exacerbates the abdominal discomfort and emesis, which may progress to biliousness. In the review of systems, the physician should inquire about rashes, diarrhea, joint pain and other signs of vasculitis. A family history of pancreatitis should raise suspicion for hereditary and metabolic diseases (see Table 21.1).

More common causes of acute abdominal pain in childhood may be differentiated from pancreatitis by a thorough physical examination. If fever is present, it is usually of low grade. However, tachycardia and hypotension may be present early in the course of the disease. Tachypnea with hypoxemia can indicate developing pulmonary edema. The child may be icteric and ill-appearing, with a distended abdomen and decreased bowel sounds, owing to an ileus, ascites or a mass from a pancreatic phlegmon or pseudocyst. While lying supine on the examination table, the patient may experience some relief of pain when the knees are drawn up to a flexed trunk. In advanced disease, where there has been pancreatic hemorrhage or necrosis, two signs may be present: Grey Turner sign, which is a blue discoloration of the flank; and Cullen's sign, where there is blue discoloration around the pancreas. The child should be examined for physical findings of child abuse, especially if there is an unclear history of trauma to the abdomen.

Evaluation

Laboratory tests

Routine blood tests can usually differentiate acute pancreatitis from the more common causes of abdominal pain in childhood. A complete blood cell count with white cell differential usually demonstrates leukocytosis with a left shift, and hemoconcentration from dehydration. Frequent findings in a routine chemistry panel include hyperglycemia and elevated levels of total bilirubin, alanine aminotransferase and aspartate aminotransferase. Anemia, azotemia, hypoalbuminemia, hypocalcemia and an elevated lactate dehydrogenase level suggest advanced disease with hemorrhage and pancreatic damage.

The most frequently used laboratory tests to screen for acute pancreatitis are serum amylase and lipase. Amylase levels begin to rise within 2–12 h, and peak at 12–72 h after the initial pancreatic insult.[48] However, an isolated serum amylase level has a relatively low sensitivity (75–92%) and specificity (20–60%).[5] This is because normal amylase levels may be seen with pancreatitis, and hyperamylasemia can result from many diseases that are not of pancreatic origin (Table 21.3).[5,23,48,49] If the amylase level is three to six times above the upper limit of normal for that laboratory, the specificity increases for pancreatitis, but at the expense of sensitivity.[5] More discriminatory are the measurements of serum isoamylase levels, which differentiate between enzymes of salivary and pancreatic origin. Isoamylase levels should be determined if parotitis from a viral infection is suspected (such as with HIV), in the presence of some cancers, and if ovarian disease is present (Table 21.3).

After serum amylase, serum lipase is the test most frequently used to confirm acute pancreatitis. Lipase levels begin to increase 4–8 h after the onset of symptoms, and also peak at about 24 h.[50] However, lipase levels remain elevated for a longer period of time than amylase levels, decreasing over

Table 21.3 Conditions other than pancreatitis associated with elevated serum amylase (from references 5,23,48,49)

Abdominal aortic aneurysm (pancreatic amylase elevation only)	Lung cancer (salivary amylase elevation only)
Alcoholism	Macroamylasemia
Anorexia nervosa (salivary amylase elevation only)	Opiates
Appendicitis (pancreatic amylase elevation only)	Ovarian cyst (salivary amylase elevation only)
Biliary duct obstruction (parasite, stone, tumor) (pancreatic amylase elevation only)	Ovarian tumor (salivary amylase elevation only)
Biliary tract disease (pancreatic amylase elevation only)	Pancreatic duct obstruction (parasite, stone, tumor) (pancreatic amylase elevation only)
Bulimia (salivary amylase elevation only)	Pancreatic tumor (pancreatic amylase elevation only)
Burns	Parotitis (salivary amylase elevation only)
Cardiopulmonary bypass	Peptic ulcer – perforated (pancreatic amylase elevation only)
Choledocholithiasis (pancreatic amylase elevation only)	Peritonitis (pancreatic amylase elevation only)
Cirrhosis	Pneumonia (salivary amylase elevation only)
Cystic fibrosis	Prostate tumors (salivary amylase elevation only)
Diabetic ketoacidosis	Renal insufficiency
Drugs	Renal transplant
Hepatitis	Ruptured ectopic pregnancy
Heroin addiction	Salivary duct obstruction (salivary amylase elevation only)
Intestinal infarction (pancreatic amylase elevation only)	Salpingitis (salivary amylase elevation only)
Intestinal obstruction (pancreatic amylase elevation only)	Trauma (to the head or abdomen)
Intestinal perforation (pancreatic amylase elevation only)	Viral infections (mumps) (salivary amylase elevation only)

8–14 days. Serum lipase levels have a reported clinical sensitivity of 86–100% and specificity of 50–99%.[51] If the serum lipase level is greater than three times the upper limit of normal for that laboratory, sensitivity and specificity can be increased to 99–100%.[5] However, a significantly elevated lipase level, in the presence of a normal amylase level, has been reported in esophagitis, hypertriglyceridemia, renal insufficiency, acute cholecystitis and non-pancreatic sources of lipolytic enzymes due to malignant tumors.[52]

Clinical sensitivity for the diagnosis of acute pancreatitis increases to 94% by using serum amylase and lipase level determinations in parallel.[5,52] It is important to note, however, that the degrees of elevation of the amylase and lipase levels in the plasma in no way reflect the severity of the pancreatic disease process itself. There are serum enzymes more sensitive than amylase which do correlate with disease severity, such as plasma immunoreactive cationic trypsin, pancreatic elastase I and phospholipase A_2.[5] However, these tests are not readily available outside research centers.

The diagnosis of chronic pancreatitis relies not only on clinical and radiographic findings (see next section), but also on tests of pancreatic function.[53] The 'gold standard' for the assessment of pancreatic function involves direct testing for pancreatic insufficiency. This is accomplished via the administration of intravenous secretin or cholecystokinin, and measuring the levels of bicarbonate and pancreatic enzymes from the pancreatic ductal secretions. To perform this in a pediatric patient requires endoscopic intubation of the duodenum, with accurate placement of a catheter to collect the secretions, under appropriate anesthesia. If performed correctly, the sensitivity and specificity of this procedure for the diagnosis of chronic pancreatitis ranges from 90 to 100%.[54]

Because of the challenges in performing and interpreting these examinations, they are usually available only in tertiary centers.

Although not as accurate, non-invasive tests of pancreatic function are more readily available. Chronic pancreatitis can be demonstrated by decreased enzymes in the blood (amylase, lipase, isoamylase, immunoreactive trypsinogen) or stool (trypsin, pancreatic elastase I), or increased amounts of malabsorbed food products (primarily fat). A recent pediatric study showed that testing for fecal pancreatic elastase I compared favorably to the secretin–pancreozymin test, reporting 100% sensitivity and 96% specificity for pancreatic insufficiency due to CF. However, because of the generally poor negative predictive value of these tests, chronic pancreatitis cannot be excluded with certainty. False-positive results can be seen with bacterial overgrowth and other mucosal diseases of the small bowel.

Radiographic studies

Although the study of choice to delineate pancreatic changes is abdominal ultrasonography,[55] a plain abdominal radiograph (kidney, ureters and bladder; KUB) may demonstrate anomalies. Acute pancreatitis may result in an ileus, with either colonic distension or a 'sentinel' loop of dilated small bowel. Obscured psoas margins or a radiolucent 'halo' around the left kidney are also suggestive of pancreatitis. Calcifications can be seen in the area of the pancreatic parenchyma and ductal system with chronic pancreatitis (Figure 21.1).

Changes in pancreatic size, contour and texture are best appreciated with ultrasound. This modality is also excellent at identifying ascites, abscesses, pseudocysts, dilated ducts and gallstone disease (Figures 21.2–21.5).

Computed tomography (CT), with oral and intravenous contrast, is useful in managing the complications of long-standing pancreatitis.[55] CT can provide more accurate guidance in the aspiration and drainage of an abscess, phlegmon or pseudocyst. Prior to any type of surgical intervention, such as necrostomy (surgical debridement for necrosis), CT may be utilized for further definition of the peripancreatic anatomy, and to rule out other complications, such as a portal vein thrombosis (Figures 21.6–21.15).

KUB, ultrasound and CT are not adequate in clinical circumstances under which a detailed anatomy of the pancreatic and biliary tree is necessary, such as in chronic pancreatitis and recurrent attacks of acute pancreatitis. Cholangiopancreatography may be accomplished by endoscopic retrograde cholangiopancreatography (ERCP), magnetic resonance cholangiopancreatography (MRCP), or via a direct cholangiogram performed either percutaneously or

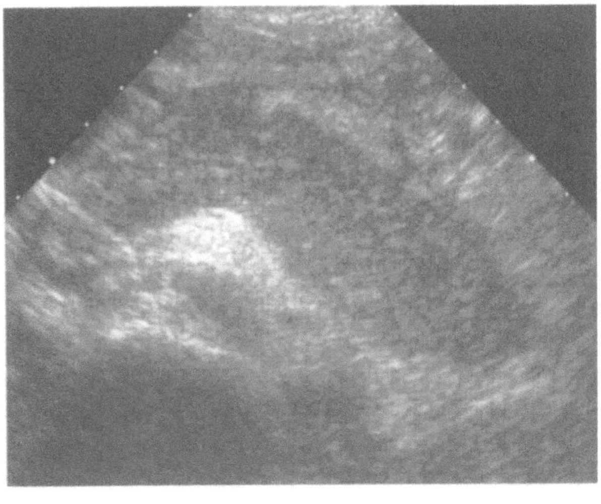

Figure 21.2 Ultrasound demonstrating acute pancreatitis in a 9-year-old HIV-positive girl. The head and the body of the pancreas are decreased in echogenicity and diffusely enlarged.

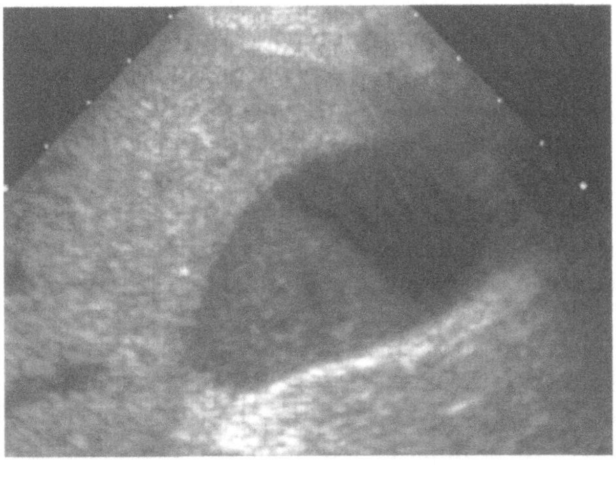

Figure 21.3 Ultrasound demonstrating sludge in the gallbladder of the same patient as in Figure 21.2. There is no gallbladder wall thickening or pericholecystic fluid. No calculi were identified, but they could be obscured by the sludge.

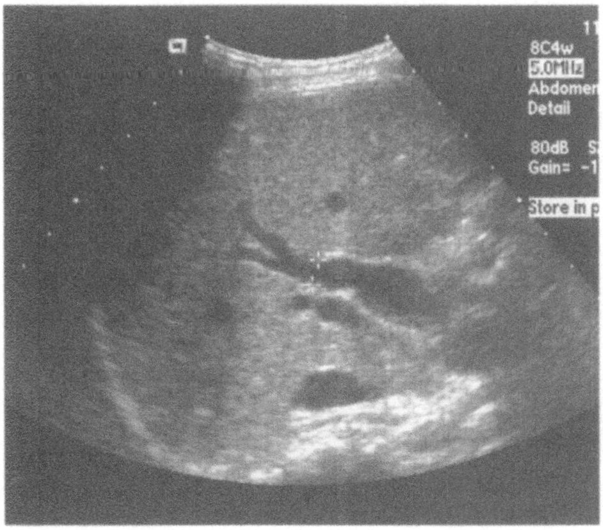

Figure 21.4 Ultrasound demonstrating biliary ductal dilatation in a 7-year-old girl with chronic pancreatitis. The common bile duct is abnormally dilated, measuring 1.2 cm in diameter. This fusiform enlargement of the common bile duct, proximal to its bifurcation just at the hilus of the liver, is suggestive of a choledochal cyst.

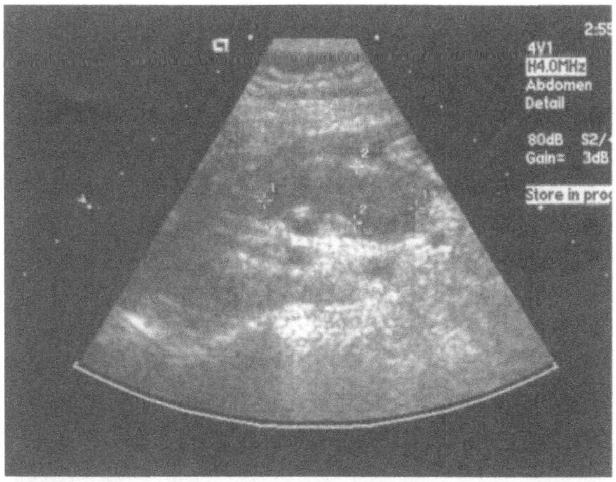

Figure 21.5 Ultrasound of a pseudocyst in an 18-year-old female with chronic pancreatitis after a severe upper gastrointestinal bleed, respiratory failure and septic shock. The pancreas was normal in echogenicity, but a pseudocyst was seen in the body measuring 2.8 x 1.9 x 1 cm.

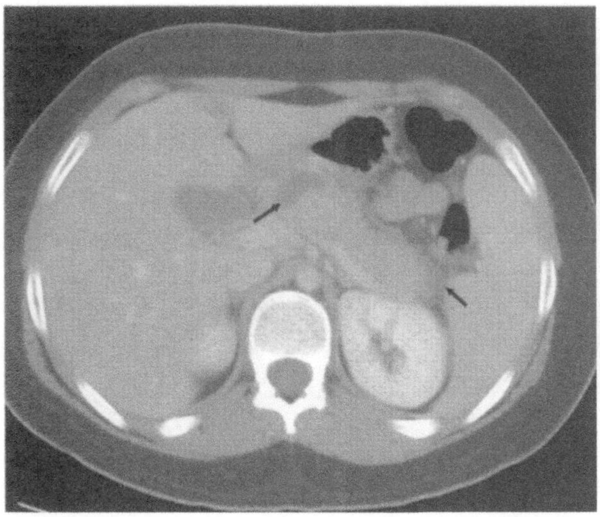

Figure 21.6 Computed tomography scan of acute pancreatitis in the abdomen of a 4-year-old boy. Fluid collections are seen near the pancreatic head and tail (arrows), consistent with inflammatory changes. There are areas of hypodensity within the pancreas, representative of acute pancreatitis.

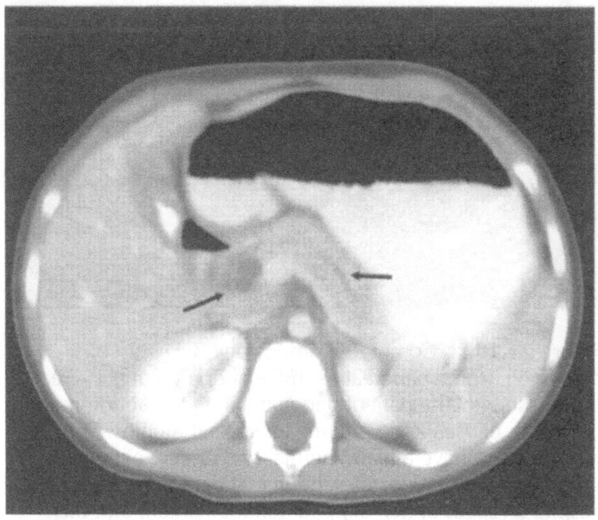

Figure 21.7 Computed tomography scan demonstrating biliary ductal dilatation in the abdomen of the patient in Figure 21.4. There is extrahepatic bile duct and pancreatic duct dilatation (arrows). The pancreas has a normal density. Intrahepatic ductal dilatation was seen on other sections. The differential diagnosis in this patient includes choledochal cyst, Caroli's disease and sclerosing cholangitis.

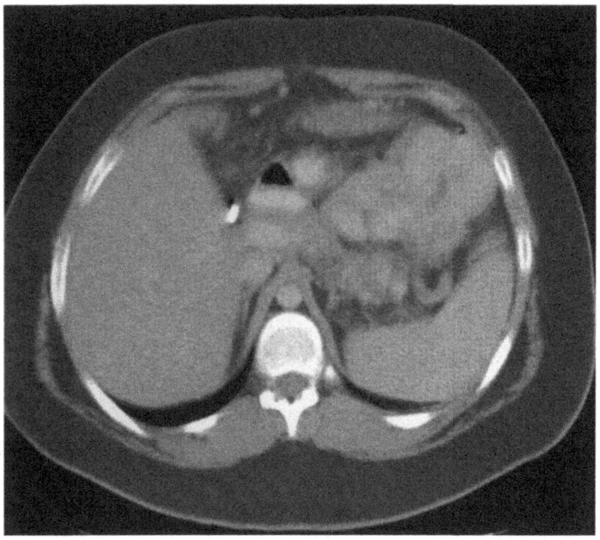

Figure 21.8 Computed tomography scan of the abdomen of a 16-year-old morbidly obese male with chronic pancreatitis. The pancreas demonstrates enhancements with focal lesions. The head was poorly visualized. The body and tail are enlarged, consistent with chronic pancreatitis. Endoscopic retrograde cholangiopancreatography demonstrated pancreatic divisum.

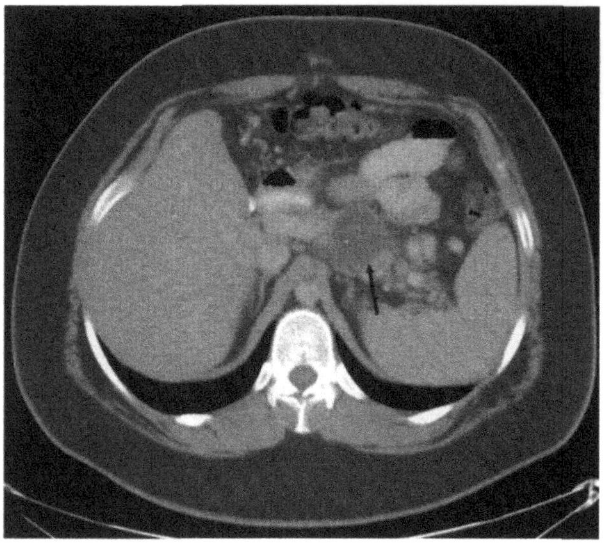

Figure 21.9 Computed tomography scan of an atrophic pancreas in the same patient as in Figure 21.8, 1 year later. The pancreas is essentially absent, with only minimal tissue identified in the tail. A 4x3.6x3.8cm cystic mass is present in the region of the former body of the pancreas, consistent with a pseudocyst (arrow). This patient went on to develop cirrhosis with portal hypertension due to portal vein thrombosis. Esophageal, gastric, splenic and retroperitoneal varices were seen on other sections. Recanalization of the portal and umbilical veins was also visualized. Pancreatic atrophy rendered this patient dependent upon insulin and pancreatic enzyme replacements.

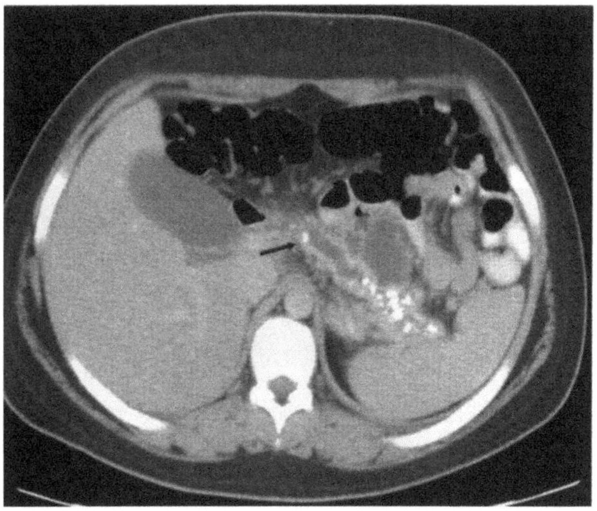

Figure 21.10 Computed tomography (CT) scan of calcified chronic pancreatitis in the abdomen of a 14-year-old obese girl. The patient had complained of abdominal pain with nausea and vomiting for several months. She was found to have a hiatal hernia, and underwent laparoscopic fundoplication. The abdominal pain persisted, despite a repeat of her 'slipped' fundoplication, and this CT scan was ordered. There is fatty atrophy of the pancreas with multiple punctuate and small calcifications consistent with chronic pancreatitis. The pancreatic duct is dilated, measuring 1.2 cm at the uncinate process. There is a calcification in the duct near the ampulla of Vater (arrow), which appears to be lodged in the common bile duct, causing proximal dilatation. There are several small pseudocysts in the upper abdomen. The largest is in the lesser sac just inferior to the stomach, measuring 3x4x 3 cm, with inflammation present. This patient remains dependent upon parenteral nutrition.

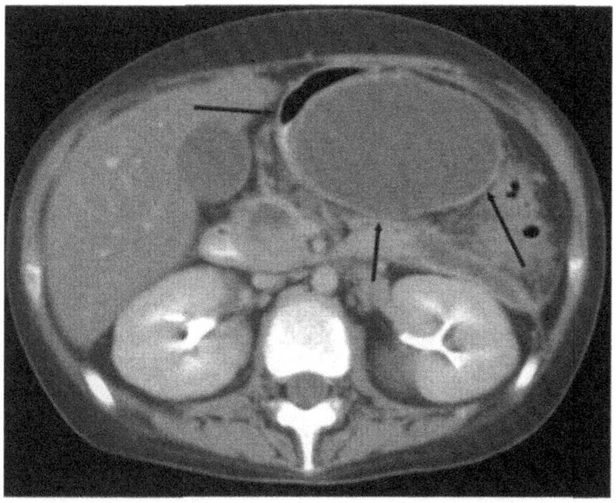

Figure 21.11 Computed tomography scan of the abdomen in an 11-year-old girl with chronic pancreatitis undergoing treatment for acute lymphoblastic leukemia. A massive 19x5.5x8.5cm pseudocyst is seen in the left upper quadrant (arrows). There is edema and necrosis within the pancreatic tissue, and a smaller pseudocyst within the pancreatic head. There is free fluid within the abdomen and stranding within the mesentery of the left upper quadrant consistent with chronic inflammation. The liver shows fatty infiltration with a normal gallbladder. This pseudocyst resolved without surgical intervention.

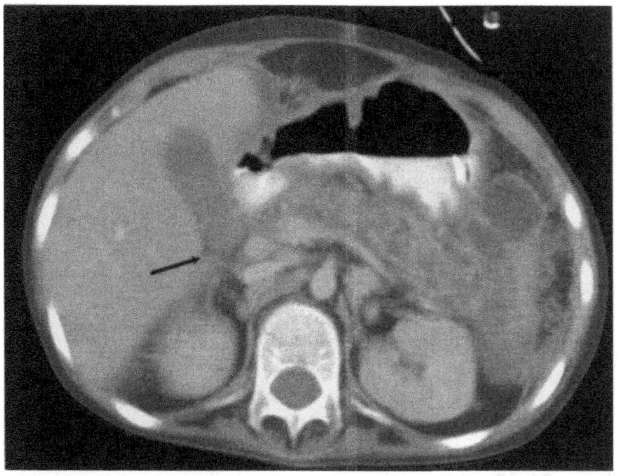

Figure 21.12 Computed tomography scan of the abdomen in a 10-year-old girl with end-stage renal disease, found to have bloody drainage from her peritoneal dialysis catheter. There are diffuse inflammatory changes around the pancreas which extend up and around the lateral aspect of the stomach. The pancreas is low in attenuation and heterogeneous, suggestive of necrosis. There are multiple fluid collections in the region of the tail of the pancreas. There is a small amount of pericholecystic fluid surrounding the anterior wall of the gallbladder (arrow). Other sections delineated superior mesenteric and portal vein thrombosis. The kidneys did not concentrate or excrete contrast, consistent with the patient's renal failure.

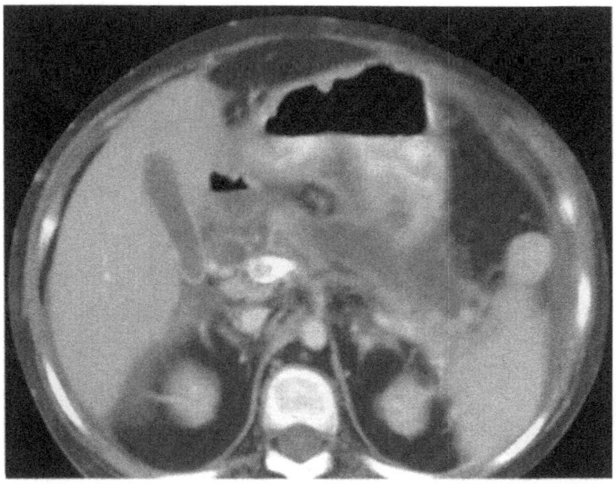

Figure 21.13 Computed tomography scan of chronic pancreatitis with cystic changes in the same patient as in Figure 21.12, taken 5 months later, demonstrating pseudocyst formation with extensive cystic changes within the body and tail of the pancreas. Owing to an intracranial bleed, the patient's nutritional status was maintained on an elemental liquid diet (appropriate for a patient with renal failure) via a gastrostomy tube.

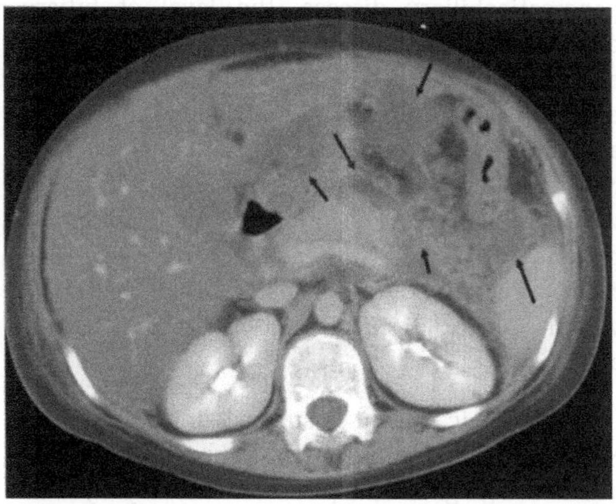

Figure 21.14 Computed tomography scan of the abdomen of a teenage boy with recurrent pancreatitis. He had received high-dose steroids for treatment of non-Hodgkin's lymphoma. The pancreas is edematous and there are multiple, small pseudocysts (arrows) which have enhancing rims. These findings are consistent with severe hemorrhagic pancreatitis. The liver is enlarged with low attenuation consistent with fatty infiltration.

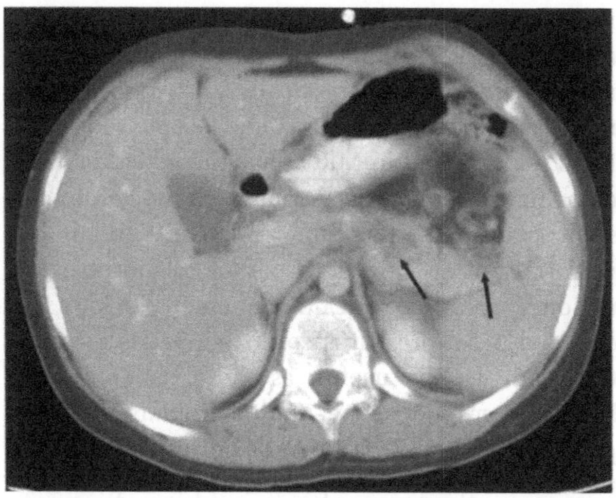

Figure 21.15 Repeat computed tomography scan of the abdomen of the patient in Figure 21.14, performed 8 months later. There are areas of necrosis within the pancreatic body and tail (arrows). A pseudocyst is present at the pancreatic tail near the splenic hilum. Bones demonstrate osteopenia, also consistent with high-dose steroids.

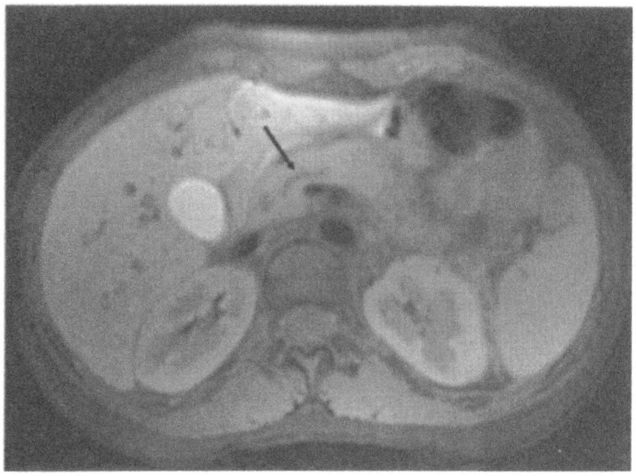

Figure 21.16 Magnetic resonance imaging (MRI) demonstrating pancreatitis with ductal dilatation in a previously healthy 16-year-old female with a 1-month history of nausea and epigastric pain after meals. Initial ultrasound examination revealed pancreatic edema and ductal dilatation. The patient's amylase and lipase levels continued to rise, despite the pancreatic rest. MRI revealed a dilated pancreatic duct (arrow) with increased signal intensity at the junction of the body and the tail, consistent with edema.

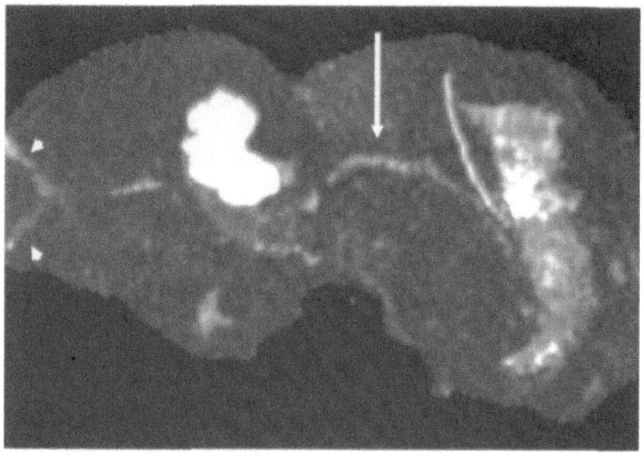

Figure 21.17 Magnetic resonance cholangiopancreatography demonstrating pancreatitis with ductal dilatation in the same patient as in Figure 21.16. Dilatation of the pancreatic duct (arrow), common bile duct, and the right and left main hepatic ducts (arrowheads) are seen, consistent with an impacted stone at the ampulla of Vater.

intraoperatively. These studies may reveal cholelithiasis, anatomic malformations or biliary strictures.

ERCP is the study of choice to visualize anatomic malformations, such as pancreas divisum or anomalous pancreaticobiliary duct junction.[15,18] ERCP may be difficult in very small children, owing to the large diameter of the endoscope required. ERCP, as opposed to MRCP, has the added benefit of being a therapeutic modality. Sphincterotomy, stent placement and stone removal can all be performed at the time of the initial diagnostic evaluation.[56] Sphincter of Oddi manometry to look for elevated basal pressures consistent with dysfunction can also be useful, as these patients may benefit from endoscopic sphincterotomy.[15] These procedures should be undertaken only at centers that have significant experience both in performing the studies and in managing severe cases of childhood pancreatitis. A pediatric surgeon should be available at the center, as complications of ERCP can include duct perforation or a worsening of the pancreatitis from the contrast, leading to abscess, phlegmon or pseudocyst formation requiring surgical drainage. However, when performed by experienced endoscopists, therapeutic ERCP in selected pediatric patients has been reported to have a lower rate of complications than in the adult population.[57]

MRCP should be reserved for patients who are too small or too clinically unstable to receive general anesthesia to undergo ERCP. This modality has proved useful in determining the presence of pancreaticobiliary disease, the level of biliary obstruction, and the presence of malignancy or bile duct calculi (Figures 21.16 and 21.17).[58,59] The quality of the MRCP images depend upon the ability of the patient to remain still (which may require light sedation in small children), and whether the MRCP equipment and computer programs are regularly updated. Interpretation also requires a skilled radiologist familiar with the various potential pancreaticobiliary tree anomalies.

If an anatomic variant is suspected, and ERCP or MRCP are not possible, the next appropriate step is direct imaging of the pancreaticobiliary system with contrast, performed either percutaneously or intraoperatively. A percutaneous cholangiogram may be performed in the presence of dilated ducts, or through a biliary drain. Biliary drains may have been placed postoperatively from pancreatic surgical debridement or orthotopic liver transplant. This type of study requires a skilled interventional radiologist. In the absence of dilated ducts or a biliary drain, transduodenal exploration with intraoperative pancreatography should be performed. Like ERCP, intraoperative imaging can likewise be a therapeutic modality at the time of initial diagnostic evaluation. If minor or major stenosis of papillae is found, surgical sphincteroplasty can be performed concurrently.[60]

Treatment

The management of acute, uncomplicated pancreatitis in childhood is mainly supportive. The patient should be provided adequate hydration, pain relief and pancreatic rest.[55] The child should be made nil per os in severe cases, which will decrease the cephalic, gastric and intestinal phases of pancreatic secretion. Continuous or intermittent nasogastric suction may be required in cases with ileus or persistent emesis. If the child is expected to be without enteral feedings for more than 3 days, parenteral nutrition should be initiated to prevent protein catabolism. Recent studies have suggested that nasojejunal feedings with an elemental diet, which bypass the duodenum completely and therefore do not potently stimulate pancreatic secretion, are just as safe as parenteral nutrition in adults with severe, acute pancreatitis. Nasojejunal feeds are also less costly, have fewer metabolic complications, and may shorten the length of stay.[61] Antibiotics are not normally indicated, unless there are signs of sepsis, necrotic pancreatitis, or multiorgan system failure. Histamine (H_2) receptor antagonists may help to prevent stress ulceration by reducing duodenal acidification. Current research targeting the inflammatory cascade as described in the Pathophysiology section of this chapter may also lead to therapies that are beneficial for acute pancreatitis, regardless of the etiology.

Adequate treatment of pain in acute, severe pancreatitis in childhood can be challenging. It may be difficult to relieve a child's pain completely. Opiates have been reported to worsen symptoms by increasing spasms of the sphincter of Oddi. Meperidine (Demerol®) is the analgesic of choice of all the pure opiate agonists for acute pancreatitis, because it produces the least increase in enterobiliary pressure. We have also used hydromorphone hydrochloride (Dilaudid®) as a continuous infusion in many children with severe, acute pancreatitis, as well as in chronic and complicated pancreatitis, with excellent pain control.

Complications of chronic pancreatitis include pancreatic atrophy with resultant exocrine and/or endocrine insufficiency. Severe, prolonged cases may require insulin, pancreatic enzyme replacement and an elemental or low-fat diet to optimize absorption once enteral feedings are reinitiated.

The major cause of mortality in pediatric patients with acute pancreatitis is septic complications. These are believed to arise from bacteria that have translocated across the intestinal epithelium and disseminated systemically via the mesenteric lymph nodes and lymphatics. This can result in pancreatic abscess, infected pseudocyst, or even necrosis of the gland. Evidence of infection within a defined area can be obtained with fine-needle aspiration under ultrasound or CT guidance. Gram stain and culture of the aspirate are clinically useful. Often, enteric organisms are recovered, such as *Escherichia coli*, *Klebsiella* species and other Gram-negative rods.[62] In the patient with necrotizing pancreatitis and organ failure, it is reasonable to initiate treatment with an antibiotic that has broad-spectrum activity against both aerobic and anaerobic bacteria.[55]

These infections necessitate surgical intervention. However, whether a sterile abscess, pseudocyst or necrosis requires operative management is still controversial.[55] Antibiotics and intensive care usually provide adequate support for the patient who has sterile necrosis. The presence of persistent ileus, bowel perforation, portal vein thrombosis and multisystem organ failure are 'red flags' that indicate urgent surgical intervention. Infected pancreatic necrosis is an absolute surgical indication, requiring necrosectomy (surgical debridement). Necrosectomy is thought to stop the progression of the necrotizing process and resultant multi-organ failure. Debridement, rather than total or partial pancreatic resection, is preferred, as it preserves exocrine and endocrine function. It may be necessary for the patient to undergo multiple reoperations, or continuous lavage with catheters left in the retroperitoneum. Necrosectomy itself may cause further complications, such as sepsis, hemorrhage, wound infection and fistulas of the pancreas, intestine and biliary system.

Short- and long-term prognosis

Most cases of acute pancreatitis in childhood are isolated and uncomplicated, persisting for usually less than a week, and rarely progress to chronic pancreatitis. The chances of surviving a severe or complicated course of pancreatitis are directly related to the other organ systems involved. Associated complications can affect virtually all organ systems (Table 21.4).[2–4,6,15,17–19,21,23,26,34,36,37,45,53,60–63] The primary morbidity and mortality arise from septic shock, renal failure, respiratory failure and inflammatory masses of the pancreas.

The APACHE-II and Ranson criteria, which have been developed to predict the outcome from acute pancreatitis in adults, are not as reliable in young children. Pediatric studies have shown a mortality rate of 5–17.5% from an initially mild presentation of acute pancreatitis to upwards of 80–100% from hemorrhagic pancreatitis or severe multisystem disorders. After a bout of necrotizing pancreatitis, exocrine and endocrine insufficiency are common. The degree of dysfunction correlates directly with the extent of parenchymal damage.

For patients with traumatic pancreatitis, in the absence of complete duct transection, non-operative management is believed to be safe, and there are usually no long-term complications.[63] Identification of those with hereditary pancreatitis is critical, as affected family members are at increased risk for pseudocysts, pancreatic adenocarcinomas, and exocrine and endocrine failure.

Table 21.4 Complications associated with pancreatitis (from references 2–4,6,15,17–19,21,23,26,34, 36,37,45,53,60–63)

Pancreatic	*Systemic/metabolic*
Abscess	Acidosis
Ascites	Atelectasis
Calculi	Adult respiratory distress syndrome
Carcinoma	Disseminated intravascular coagulation
Diabetes mellitus	Electrocardiographic changes
Duct strictures	Encephalopathy
Exocrine insufficiency	Fat emboli
Fibrosis	Fat necrosis
Fistula	Hyperglycemia
Necrosis	Hyperkalemia
Phlegmon	Hypertriglyceridemia
Pseudocyst	Hypoalbuminemia
	Hypocalcemia
Gastrointestinal/hepatic	Hypotension
Biliary obstruction	Mediastinal abscess
Bowel infarction	Pericardial effusion
Gastritis	Pleural effusion
Gastrointestinal fistula	Pneumonitis
Hemorrhage	Psychosis
Hepatic vein thrombosis	Renal failure
Hepatorenal syndrome	Renal vessel thrombosis
Ileus	Respiratory failure
Jaundice	Sepsis
Peptic ulcer	Sudden death
Portal vein thrombosis	Thrombosis
Splenic vein varices	

Conclusion

The clinician needs to have a high index of suspicion for pancreatitis in the child who presents with the non-specific but common symptoms of nausea, vomiting and abdominal pain. A thorough history that emphasizes recent infections, medications, trauma and any underlying medical condition may make the diagnosis clearer. The traditional use of enzyme testing alone (serum amylase and lipase) for the diagnosis of both acute and chronic pancreatitis may not be adequate, since the clinical specificity remains suboptimal.

Unlike pancreatitis in adults, in which the majority of cases are due to either gallstone disease or alcoholism, this disease in childhood can be from a variety of disparate causes. No identifying factor is present in up to 25% of cases. Common known etiologies include infection, trauma, medications, abnormal anatomy and hereditary or systemic diseases. A family history of pancreatitis, especially occurring at a young age, should prompt the physician to look for evidence of anatomic abnormalities or inherited biochemical defects.

Ultrasound remains the initial radiographic study of choice in acute pancreatitis in childhood, to screen for infection, cholelithiasis, congenital abnormalities and biliary ductal dilatation. If the course of the pancreatitis is complicated or recurrent, further detailed imaging of the biliary system should be performed with ERCP, MRCP or percutaneous or intraoperative cholangiogram.

Treatment of acute, uncomplicated pancreatitis in the pediatric population is basically supportive, and most children will recover without sequelae. Complications, when they occur, can involve every major organ system and be life-threatening. Children with severe or complicated pancreatitis should be managed at a center with expertise in pediatric biliary surgery and non-operative radiological and endoscopic interventions.

REFERENCES

1. Karne S, Gorelick FS. Etiopathogenesis of acute pancreatitis. *Surg Clin North Am* 1999; **79**: 699-710.
2. Lerner A. Acute pancreatitis in children and adolescents. In Lebenthal E, ed. *Gastroenterology and Nutrition in Infancy*, 2nd edn. New York: Raven Press, 1989: 897–906.
3. Robertson MA, Durie PR. Pancreatitis. In Walker WA, Durie PR, Hamilton JS, Walker-Smith JA, Watkins JB, eds. *Pediatric Gastrointestinal Disease*, 2nd edn. St Louis: Mosby, 1996: 1436–1465.
4. Roy CC, Silverman A, Alagille D. Pancreatitis and pancreatic tumors. In Roy CC, Silverman A, Alagille D, eds. *Pediatric Clinical Gastroenterology*, 4th edn. St. Louis: Mosby, 1995: 986–1004.
5. Tietz NW. Support of the diagnosis of pancreatitis by enzyme tests – old problems, new techniques. *Clin Chim Acta* 1997; **257**: 85–98.
6. Weizman Z. Acute pancreatitis. In Wyllie R, Hyams JS, eds. *Pediatric Gastrointestinal Disease*. Philadelphia: WB Saunders, 1993: 873–879.
7. Durie PR. Pancreatitis and mutations of the cystic fibrosis gene. *N Engl J Med* 1998; **339**: 687–688.
8. Werlin SL, Casper J, Antonson D et al. Pancreatitis associated with bone marrow transplantation in children. *Bone Marrow Transplant* 1992; **10**: 65–69.
9. Tissieres P, Simon L, Debray D et al. Acute pancreatitis after orthotopic liver transplantation in children: incidence, contributing factors and outcome. *J Pediatr Gastroenterol Nutr* 1998; **26**: 315–320.
10. Collins JE, Brenton DP. Pancreatitis and homocystinuria. *J Inherit Metab Dis* 1990; **13**: 232–233.
11. Kahler SG, Sherwood G, Woolf D et al. Pancreatitis in patients with organic acidemias. *J Pediatr* 1994; **124**: 239–243.
12. Lévy P, Menzelxhiu A, Paillot B et al. Abdominal radiotherapy is a cause for chronic pancreatitis. *Gastroenterology* 1993; **105**: 905–909.
13. Keljo DJ, Sugerman KS. Pancreatitis in patients with inflammatory bowel disease. *J Pediatr Gastroenterol Nutr* 1997; **25**: 108–112.
14. See Y, Martin K, Rooney M et al. Severe juvenile dermatomyositis complicated by pancreatitis. *Br J Rheumatol* 1997; **36**: 912–916.
15. Guelrud M, Morera C, Rodriguez M et al. Sphincter of Oddi dysfunction in children with recurrent pancreatitis and anomalous pancreaticobiliary union: an etiologic concept. *Gastrointest Endosc* 1999; **50**: 194–199.
16. Mattioli G, Buffa P, Pesce F et al. Pancreatitis caused by duodenal duplication. *J Pediatr Surg* 1999; **34**: 645–648.
17. Dassopoulos T, Ehrenpreis ED. Acute pancreatitis in human immunodeficiency virus-infected patients: a review. *Am J Med* 1999; **107**: 78–84.
18. Kamelmaz I, Elitsur Y. Pancreas divisum – the role of ERCP in children. *W V Med J* 1999; **95**: 14–16.
19. Lerner A, Branski D, Lebenthal E. Pancreatic diseases in children. *Pediatr Clin North Am* 1996; **43**: 125–156.
20. Carroccio A, Fontana M, Spagnuolo MI et al. Serum pancreatic enzymes in human immunodeficiency virus-

infected children. A collaborative study of the Italian Society of Pediatric Gastroenterology and Hepatology. *Scand J Gastroenterol* 1998; **33**: 998–1001.
21. Brivet FG, Naneau SH, Lemaigre GF et al. Pancreatic lesions in HIV-infected patients. *Ballières Clin Endocrinol Metab* 1994; **8**: 859–877.
22. Kahn E, Anderson VM, Greco A et al. Pancreatic disorders in pediatric acquired immune deficiency syndrome. *Hum Pathol* 1995; **26**: 765–770.
23. Aboulafia DM. Acute pancreatitis: a fatal complication of AIDS therapy. *J Clin Gastroenterol* 1997; **25**: 640–645.
24. Friedman SL. Kaposi's sarcoma and lymphoma of the gut in AIDS. *Ballières Clin Gastroenterol* 1990; **4**: 455–475.
25. Welsh MJ, Tsui LC, Boat TF et al. Cystic fibrosis. In Scriver CR, Beaudet AL, Sly WS, Valle D, eds. *The Metabolic and Molecular Basis of Inherited Disease*. New York: McGraw-Hill, 1995: 3799–3876.
26. Dodge JA. Paediatric and hereditary aspects of chronic pancreatitis. *Digestion* 1998; **59 (Suppl 4)**: 49–59.
27. Uomo G, Manes G, Rabitti PR. Role of hereditary pancreatitis and CFTR gene mutations in the aetiology of acute relapsing pancreatitis of unknown origin. How are they important? *J Pancreas* (Online) 2001; **2**: 368–372.
28. Rosenstein MG, Cutting GR. The diagnosis of cystic fibrosis: a consensus statement. *J Pediatr* 1998; **132**: 589–595.
29. Cohn JA, Friedman KJ, Noone PG et al. Relation between mutations of the cystic fibrosis gene and idiopathic pancreatitis. *N Engl J Med* 1998; **339**: 653–658.
30. Cohn JA, Jowell PS. Are mutations in the cystic fibrosis gene important in chronic pancreatitis? *Surg Clin North Am* 1999; **79**: 723–731.
31. Sharer N, Schwarz M, Malone G et al. Mutations of the cystic fibrosis gene in patients with chronic pancreatitis. *N Engl J Med* 1998; **339**: 645–652.
32. Elitsur Y, Chertow BC, Jewell RD et al. Identification of a hereditary pancreatitis mutation in four West Virginia families. *Pediatr Res* 1998; **44**: 927–930.
33. Whitcomb DC, Gorry MC, Preston RA et al. A gene for hereditary pancreatitis maps to chromosome 7q35. *Gastroenterology* 1996; **110**: 1975–1980.
34. Gates LK, Ulrich CD II, Whitcomb DC. Hereditary pancreatitis. *Surg Clin North Am* 1999; **79**: 711–722.
35. Whitcomb DC. Hereditary pancreatitis: a model for understanding the genetic basis of acute and chronic pancreatitis. *Pancreatology* 2001; **1**: 565–570.
36. Perrault J. Hereditary pancreatitis. *Gastroenterol Clin North Am* 1994; **23**: 743–752.
37. Uretsky G, Goldschmiedt M, James K, Childhood pancreatitis. *Am Fam Physician* 1999; **59**: 2507–2512.
38. Pfützer RH, Whitcomb DC. SPINK1 mutations are associated with multiple phenotypes. *Pancreatology* 2001; **1**: 457–460.
39. Pfützer RH, Barmada MM, Brunskill APJ et al. SPINK1/PSTI polymorphisms act as disease modifiers in familial and idiopathic chronic pancreatitis. *Gastroenterology* 2000; **119**: 615–623.
40. Chen JM, Mercier B, Audrezet MP et al. Mutational analysis of the human pancreatic secretory trypsin inhibitor (PSTI) gene in hereditary and sporadic chronic pancreatitis (letter). *J Med Genet* 2000; **37**: 67–69.
41. Rossi L, Pfützer RH, Parvin S et al. SPINK1/PSTI mutations are associated with tropical pancreatitis in Bangladesh: a preliminary report. *Pancreatology* 2001; **1**: 242–245.
42. Teich N, Ockenga J, Hoffmeister A et al. Chronic pancreatitis associated with an activation peptide mutation that facilitates trypsin activation. *Gastroenterology* 2000; **119**: 461–465.
43. Sahu S, Saika S, Pai SK et al. L-Asparaginase (Leunase) induced pancreatitis in childhood acute lymphoblastic leukemia. *Pediatr Hematol Oncol* 1998; **15**: 533–538.
44. Sammett D, Greben C, Sayeed-Shah U. Acute pancreatitis caused by penicillin. *Dig Dis Sci* 1998; **43**: 1778–1783.
45. Tobias JD, Capers C, Sims P et al. Necrotizing pancreatitis after 10 years of therapy with valproic acid. *Clin Pediatr* 1995; **34**: 446–448.
46. Oberlander TF, Rappaport LA. Recurrent abdominal pain during childhood. *Pediatr Rev* 1993; **14**: 313-319.
47. Stevenson RJ, Ziegler MM. Abdominal pain unrelated to trauma. *Pediatr Rev* 1993; **14**: 302–311.
48. Pieper-Bigelow C, Strocchi A, Levitt MD. Where does serum amylase come from and where does it go? *Gastroenterol Clin North Am* 1990; **19**: 793–810.
49. Murthy UK, DeGregorio F, Oates RP et al. Hyperamylasemia in patients with the acquired immunodeficiency syndrome. *Am J Gastroenterol* 1992; **87**: 332–336.
50. Gwodz GP, Steinberg WM, Werner M et al. Comparative evaluation of the diagnosis of acute pancreatitis based on serum and urine enzyme assays. *Clin Chim Acta* 1990; **187**: 243–248.
51. Agarwal N, Pitchumoni CS, Sivaprasad AV. Evaluating tests for acute pancreatitis. *Am J Gastroenterol* 1990; **85**: 356–360.
52. Frank B, Gottlieb K. Amylase normal, lipase elevated: is it pancreatitis? A case series and review of the literature. *Am J Gastroenterol* 1999; **94**: 463–469.
53. Clain JE, Pearson RK. Diagnosis of chronic pancreatitis. *Surg Clin North Am* 1999; **79**: 829–845.
54. Heiji HA, Obertop H, Schmitz PIM et al. Evaluation of the secretin–cholecystokinin test for chronic pancreatitis by discriminant analysis. *Scand J Gastroenterol* 1986; **21**: 35–42.
55. Banks PA. Practice guidelines in acute pancreatitis. *Am J Gastroenterol* 1997; **92**: 377–386.
56. Samavedy R, Sherman S, Lehman GA. Endoscopic therapy in anomalous pancreatobiliary duct junction. *Gastrointest Endoscop* 1999; **50**: 623–627.
57. Guelrud M, Endoscopic therapy of pancreatic disease in children. *Gastrointest Endoscop Clin North Am* 1998; **8**: 195–219.
58. Fulcher AS, Turner MA, Capps GW et al. Half-Fourier RARE MR cholangiopancreatography: experience in 300 subjects. *Radiology* 1998; **207**: 21–32.
59. Hirohashi S, Hirohashi R, Uchida H et al. Pancreatitis: evaluation with MR cholangiopancreatography in children. *Radiology* 1997; **203**: 411–415.
60. O'Rourke RW, Harrison MR. Pancreas divisum and stenosis of the major and minor papillae in an 8 year old girl: treatment by dual sphincteroplasty. *J Pediatr Surg* 1998; **33**: 789–791.
61. Abou-Assi S, Craig K, O'Keefe SJ. Hypocaloric jejunal feeding is better than total parenteral nutrition in acute pancreatitis: Results of a randomized, comparative study. *Am J Gastroenterol* 2002; **97**: 2255–2262.
62. Luiten EJ, Hop WC, Lange JF et al. Differential prognosis of gram-negative versus gram-positive infected and sterile pancreatic necrosis: results of a randomized trial in patients with severe, acute pancreatitis treated with adjuvant selective decontamination. *Clin Infect Dis* 1997; **25**: 811–818.
63. Holland AJ, Davey RB, Sparnon AL et al. Traumatic pancreatitis: long-term review of initial non-operative management in children. *Paediatr Child Health* 1999; **35**: 78–81.

22 Food allergies

Simon Murch

Introduction

During the past half century, allergies of all kinds have become much more common within the developed world. Dietary allergies are no exception, and up to 5% of children develop allergy to cow's milk and other proteins (reviewed by Walker-Smith and Murch[1] and Wood[2]). There has also been a change in patterns of presentation. As dietary exposures in infancy and early childhood have altered, previously unusual reactions to antigens such as peanut and sesame have become much more common.[3–5] There are important geographical differences, with different incidence of specific allergies varying from country to country.[5] This may relate to genetic differences in immune responses amongst different ethnic groups, or to local dietary customs – exemplified most strikingly by reports of anaphylaxis to birds' nest soup in Singaporean infants.[6] However, a broader context is provided by recent evidence from the direction of basic science, which highlights the importance of infectious exposures of the innate immune system in early life in inducing tolerance to dietary antigens (oral tolerance). This chapter attempts to encompass both the clinical aspects of food allergy and some of the relevant scientific background.

Early life exposures, possibly even prenatal exposures, have changed substantially within countries of the developed world, in the past two generations. Birth in disadvantaged conditions within the developing world is protective against most forms of allergy, and predisposition to allergy may manifest only once a certain threshold of improved material conditions is passed.[7,8] Allergies occur because of breakdown of immunological tolerance. The immune system must differentiate between all foreign molecules, reacting only to potentially harmful pathogens while remaining unresponsive (tolerant) to the commensal bacterial flora and to foods. The role of the bacterial flora in establishing immune tolerance has only recently become apparent, and will be discussed in more detail later, together with evidence that manipulation of the bacterial flora may provide a novel approach to the management of dietary and other allergies.[8–11]

First, however, it is important to clarify the difference between food intolerance and food allergy (Table 22.1). As there may however be an overlap in the symptomatology, an accurate history and

Table 22.1 Food intolerance reactions which may be confused with true allergy

Direct toxic effects Bacterial contamination; heavy metals or toxins; some food additives
Intolerance due to enzyme deficiency Inborn metabolic abnormalities (e.g. phenylketonuria, tyrosinemia, galactosemia) inducing adverse responses to specific dietary components. Enterocyte gene deficiencies (lactase deficiency, sucrase–isomaltase deficiency or glucose–galactose malabsorption) inducing diarrhea after ingestion of relevant sugars. Enteropathy causing down-regulated expression of lactase and sucrase
Symptoms due to pharmacological properties of foods For example tyramine contained in cheese or red wine; histamine in strawberries

supportive investigations are needed for secure diagnosis of true food allergy.

Food allergies – classification

There are two major classes of food allergic reactions: IgE-mediated and non-IgE-mediated. IgE-mediated allergies usually present soon after ingestion, and thus the causative antigen is often readily identifiable. In addition, there are usually supportive diagnostic tests such as skin prick tests. These reactions are those of type I hypersensitivity (Table 22.2).[12,13] They can be very severe, and may cause death through anaphylaxis in severe cases. Non-IgE-mediated allergies usually present later after ingestion, and the causative antigen may be more difficult to detect, particularly as tests for immediate allergies are often negative. These may include type IV hypersensitivity (Table 22.2), or may be caused by local eosinophil recruitment. They can be an important cause of morbidity, which may go unrecognized. The immunological basis of such reactions is discussed later.

Food allergic reactions may also be divided clinically into quick-onset reactions, occurring within an hour of food ingestion, and slow-onset reactions, taking hours or days. In general, quick onset symptoms are IgE-mediated and slow-onset symptoms are non-IgE-mediated. However, this is by no means invariable, and many children with clear quick-onset responses to foods have a low or even undetectable serum total IgE level and absent food-specific IgE level.[14] It is also notable that mice totally deficient in IgE owing to gene knockout may still suffer anaphylaxis, as IgG1 bound to FCγRIII on mast cells may induce antigen-specific degranulation.[15,16] Such a phenomenon may explain why investigations such as skin prick tests may be positive in children despite undetectable specific IgE for that antigen.

Differentiation between IgE-mediated and non-IgE-mediated reactions may therefore be difficult. The Melbourne Milk Allergy Study, conducted by Hill and colleagues,[17] identified three types of reaction in sensitized children – immediate reactions (rapid skin reactions with perioral erythema, facial angioedema and urticaria, some developing anaphylaxis), intermediate reactions (gastrointestinal symptoms such as vomiting or diarrhea occurring 1–24 h after ingestion) and delayed reactions (eczema flares or respiratory symptoms such as cough and wheeze, occurring between 1 and 5 days after challenge). The volume of milk required

Table 22.2 The classical forms of hypersensitivity (after reference 12)

Type I: anaphylactic or immediate hypersensitivity

This occurs within minutes of exposure, as seen in quick-onset food allergy. The allergen binds to, and cross-links IgE (occasionally IgG1) on the mast cell surface, inducing its degranulation and release of vasoactive agents (histamine, tryptase, etc.) and cytokines (tumor necrosis factor-α). Responses to some antigens (classically peanut) are usually of this kind.

Type II: cytotoxic hypersensitivity

This reaction occurs when antibody binds to an epitope on the cell surface, then fixes complement, causing complement-mediated cell death. This is not a reaction usually described for food allergy, but complement activation can be detected in celiac disease.

Type III: immune complex hypersensitivity

In this type of reaction, antigen complexes with antibody (IgG or IgM) in the presence of antigen excess, to induce complement fixation and a consequent local inflammatory response, several hours after exposure to the antigen. The expression of Fc receptors for immunoglobulin appears to determine tissue damage.[13]

Type IV: delayed hypersensitivity or cell-mediated immunity

This reaction is essentially mediated by T lymphocytes, with tissue damage also caused by macrophages responding to T-cell cytokines. The pattern of T-cell responses (Th1 or Th2) may determine overall immunopathology. The classic type IV reaction is a Th1 response, as in Crohn's disease, while both Th1 and Th2 reactions occur in food allergy.

to elicit these symptoms increased between groups, and classic allergy tests such as skin prick tests were helpful only for the first group of early reactors. Knowledge of the time course and likely immunopathogenesis indicates that the early reactions are due to IgE responses and mast cell degranulation, the intermediate reactions follow eosinophil recruitment and the delayed responses are likely to relate to T-cell responses.[18] These concepts will be discussed later, in the sections on immunopathogenesis. The Melbourne group have also played an important role in the recognition of the increasing incidence of multiple food allergies, and of the role of food allergy in inducing a spectrum of symptoms not previously associated with allergy.[5] The role of food allergy in inducing visceral dysmotility syndromes such as infant colic, gastroesophageal reflux and recurrent abdominal pain will be discussed later.

In a recent study of 121 children with allergy to two or more foods, including both those with IgE-mediated and those with non-IgE-mediated allergies,[14] children with early-onset symptoms had a significant overall increase in serum IgE compared to those with late-onset symptoms. However, 30% of those with early-onset symptoms had no elevation of IgE concentration above the normal range, while 10% of those with only delayed symptoms did have an elevated IgE concentration. Over 90% of those with early-onset symptoms additionally demonstrated late-onset symptoms. Although the groups differed in IgE responses, they shared, regardless of speed of reaction, a pattern of immune deviation, with increased serum IgG1 and circulating B cells, but reduced IgG2 and IgG4, CD8 cells and natural killer cells. IgA concentrations were at the low end of the normal range or below. This raises the question of whether the propensity to sensitize to food antigens is associated with minor immunodeficiency, a concept first suggested by Soothill,[19] who postulated that demonstrated maturational delay in IgA responses predisposed to food allergic sensitization. Further data in support of a link with a developmental delay in IgA maturation was provided by a population survey from Iceland, in which an IgA level at the lower end of the normal range was more predictive of allergic sensitization than was elevated IgE concentration,[20] and from other studies of food allergic infants, in which increased B cells and decreased CD8 cells and decreased IgA, IgG2 and IgG4 were associated with milk allergies and food-sensitive colitis.[21,22] These data suggest that there may be a consistent pattern of minor immunodeficiency associated with the process of sensitization in early life, and that the manifestation of that sensitization (quick- or slow-onset) may depend on whether the child has inherited a tendency to high IgE production. Thus, a high IgE level may not cause food allergy *per se*, but may determine how that allergy is expressed. Most of the early literature on food allergy, however, understandably focuses on IgE and quick-onset responses.

Later in the chapter, the role of infectious exposures in maturation of mucosal immune responses and immune tolerance will be explored. Whether food allergy can be fully explained by the Clean Child Hypothesis[7] remains uncertain, but there is substantial circumstantial evidence that these infectious exposures are probably an important contributory factor in the pathogenesis of allergies. Recent recognition of the role of infectious exposures in the generation of cells producing the regulatory cytokine transforming growth factor (TGF)-β, and of the central requirement for TGF-β in both IgA responses and oral tolerance, may provide some explanation for the consistent links with slow IgA maturation.[8,19,23]

Patterns of food allergic responses

Quick-onset symptoms

These often follow the ingestion of a single food, such as egg, peanut or sesame. Within minutes the sufferer may notice tingling of the tongue, and there may be the rapid development of skin rash, urticaria or wheezing. One localized variant, the oral allergy syndrome, is often seen in older pollen-sensitized individuals and is characterized by lip tingling and mouth swelling after ingestion of certain fruits and vegetables.[24] More serious reactions, however, can occur at any age, and antigens such as peanut, tree nuts, fish and shellfish can cause exquisite sensitization from early childhood. Swelling of the mucous membranes of the mouth and upper airway (angioneurotic edema) can develop extremely quickly, and the airway may become compromised. In cases where appropriate therapy is not available, life-saving tracheostomy has even been performed in the presence of gross laryngeal edema. Anaphylactic shock may also occur, with dramatic systemic hypotension accompanying the airway obstruction. A grading system for anaphylaxis has been suggested by Sampson,[25] with a severity score based on the worst symptom present (Table 22.3).

Specific therapy for mild cases of immediate hypersensitivity would include antihistamines such as chlorpheniramine, together with inhaled bronchodilators as appropriate. It is notable that some patients can have a biphasic response, with a relatively modest initial reaction followed several hours later by a more profound and potentially life-threatening response, and therefore care should be taken in the assessment to ensure that adequate instructions and therapy are administered before allowing the patient home. There have indeed been several cases of anaphylactic death in patients discharged home after initial resuscitation, up to 6 h after food ingestion, and it is therefore prudent to maintain observation for several hours if there are any clear risk factors, such as active asthma or a history of a severe reaction.[25,26] The presence of wheezing on examination should suggest caution; a bronchodilator should certainly be prescribed, and in many cases a few days' course of oral prednisolone.

More severe reactions should be assessed very rapidly, and any evidence of airway obstruction or systemic hypotension warrants the immediate use of intramuscular epinephrine (adrenaline) (Table 22.3). Use of a preloaded syringe pen, such as a pediatric or adult EpiPen®, prior to transfer to hospital, may be life-saving, and avoids potential

Table 22.3 A grading for anaphylactic reactions, proposed by Sampson.[25] The severity score should be based on the most severe symptom in any domain. Symptoms in bold are absolute indications for the use of epinephrine (adrenaline)

Grade	Skin	Gastrointestinal tract	Respiratory	Cardiovascular	Neurological
1	Localized itching, flushing, urticaria, angioedema	oral itching or tingling, mild lip swelling			
2	Generalized itching, flushing, urticaria, angioedema	any of the above, nausea and/or single vomiting episode	nasal congestion and/or sneezing		change in activity level
3	Any of the above	any of the above plus repetitive vomiting	rhinorrhea, marked congestion, **sensation of throat itching or tightness**	tachycardia (increase >15 beats/min)	change in activity level plus anxiety
4	Any of the above	any of the above plus diarrhea	any of the above, **hoarseness, 'barky' cough, difficulty swallowing, dyspnea, wheezing, cyanosis**	any of the above, **dysrhythmia and/or mild hypotension**	'light headedness,' feeling of 'impending doom'
5	Any of the above	any of the above, loss of bowel control	any of the above, **respiratory arrest**	**severe bradycardia and/or hypotension or cardiac arrest**	**loss of consciousness**

dosage errors at such a time of extreme stress. Any child thought to be at risk of an anaphylactic reaction to food should be prescribed such injection devices (at least two or three should be prescribed, so that all those caring for the child are equipped), and parents and carers should be trained in their use. Any severe immediate reaction to foods necessitates urgent transfer to an appropriate medical setting, such as an Accident and Emergency Department. Other treatments that may be needed include oxygen, intravenous hydrocortisone, chlorpheniramine and inhaled β-adrenergic bronchodilator therapy.[25] Supportive treatment for hypotension or cardiac dysrrhythmia may be required, and in the most severe cases the patient may need to be transferred to an intensive therapy unit.

The true incidence of anaphylactic death due to food allergy is unknown. A recent UK report suggested a low incidence of 0.006 deaths per 100000 children per year,[27] but this is thought to be a significant underestimate, as many cases were unlikely to be identified from the study of death certificates and clinical reporting alone.[25]

In the follow-up of a patient who has had an immediate hypersensitive response to food antigens, a decision needs to be taken about the level of prophylaxis required, and whether or not to prescribe an epinephrine pen. Clearly the severity of the first response will inform this decision, and it is probably better to err on the side of caution if foods such as peanuts are implicated, because of their propensity for triggering particularly severe episodes. If there is doubt about the food involved, both skin prick tests and specific IgE radioallergosorbent test (RAST) may be very helpful. However, these should be postponed for several weeks after an episode of anaphylaxis, as they may be artifactually negative in the immediate aftermath of a severe reaction.

Late-onset symptoms

Slow-onset symptoms may be more insidious and their true allergic nature may not be recognized (Table 22.4). These may include failure to thrive or chronic diarrhea due to enteropathy or colitis, eczema, rhinitis, or rectal bleeding.[1,24] As these are likely to be mediated by T cells in a delayed hypersensitive reaction, they may not be so clearly linked to food ingestion. Children may, however, manifest both delayed and immediate-onset symptoms. Analysis of IgG subclasses and peripheral lymphocyte subsets may identify the child at increased risk of delayed food allergic reactions.[14] Certain specific presentations can be recognized, as discussed below.

Food protein-induced enterocolitis

This disorder is most common in young infants below the age of 3 months, and usually presents with blood streaking of stools in the absence of marked weight loss or systemic upset. Anemia is

Table 22.4 Clinical manifestations in food allergic responses

1. Quick onset	wheezing, urticaria, angioedema, rashes, vomiting, gastroesophageal reflux, anaphylaxis
2. Late onset	diarrhea, abdominal pain, allergic rhinitis, atopic eczema, food-sensitive enteropathy or colitis, rectal bleeding, constipation, protein-losing enteropathy
3. Less clear responses	irritable bowel syndrome, chronic fatigue, attention-deficit with hyperactivity, autistic symptoms
4. Secondary general effects	eosinophilia, iron deficiency anemia, hypoproteinemia

For group 3 conditions, there are anecdotal reports of clinical improvement with dietary exclusions. However, there are as yet few properly validated studies, and it is likely that only a proportion of such patients will benefit. While many maintain an open-minded approach, it is important to ensure that any such diet is nutritionally adequate (joint management with dietitians is ideal), and that clinical responses to exclusion and challenge are sufficiently striking to justify continuing exclusion diets.

unusual, but an elevated platelet count ($>450\times10^9$/l) is characteristic. Cow's milk or soy proteins are the most common causative antigens, and it is common for such symptoms to occur in exclusively breast-fed infants, triggered by milk protein in the mother's diet.[28] It is important to recognize that negative skin prick tests do not exclude this diagnosis, and indeed most cases are negative.[24] If colonoscopy is performed, the colitic changes are usually milder than with classic inflammatory bowel disease, and the macroscopic findings are dominated by loss of vascular pattern, prominent lymphoid follicles with a rim of perifollicular erythema (red halo sign) and an easily traumatized mucosa. Histological changes include mononuclear cell infiltration, mucosal eosinophilia with evidence of degranulation and the presence of lymphoid follicles in the majority of colonic biopsies. If the ileum is visualized, lymphoid hyperplasia is usually seen. Recent data suggest a concordance between the endoscopic finding of ileocolonic lymphoid hyperplasia and food allergies (Figure 22.1), not restricted to those infants with allergic enterocolitis alone,[29] which may be associated with an increase in mucosal $\gamma\delta$ T-cell infiltration.[30] See also Chapter 30.

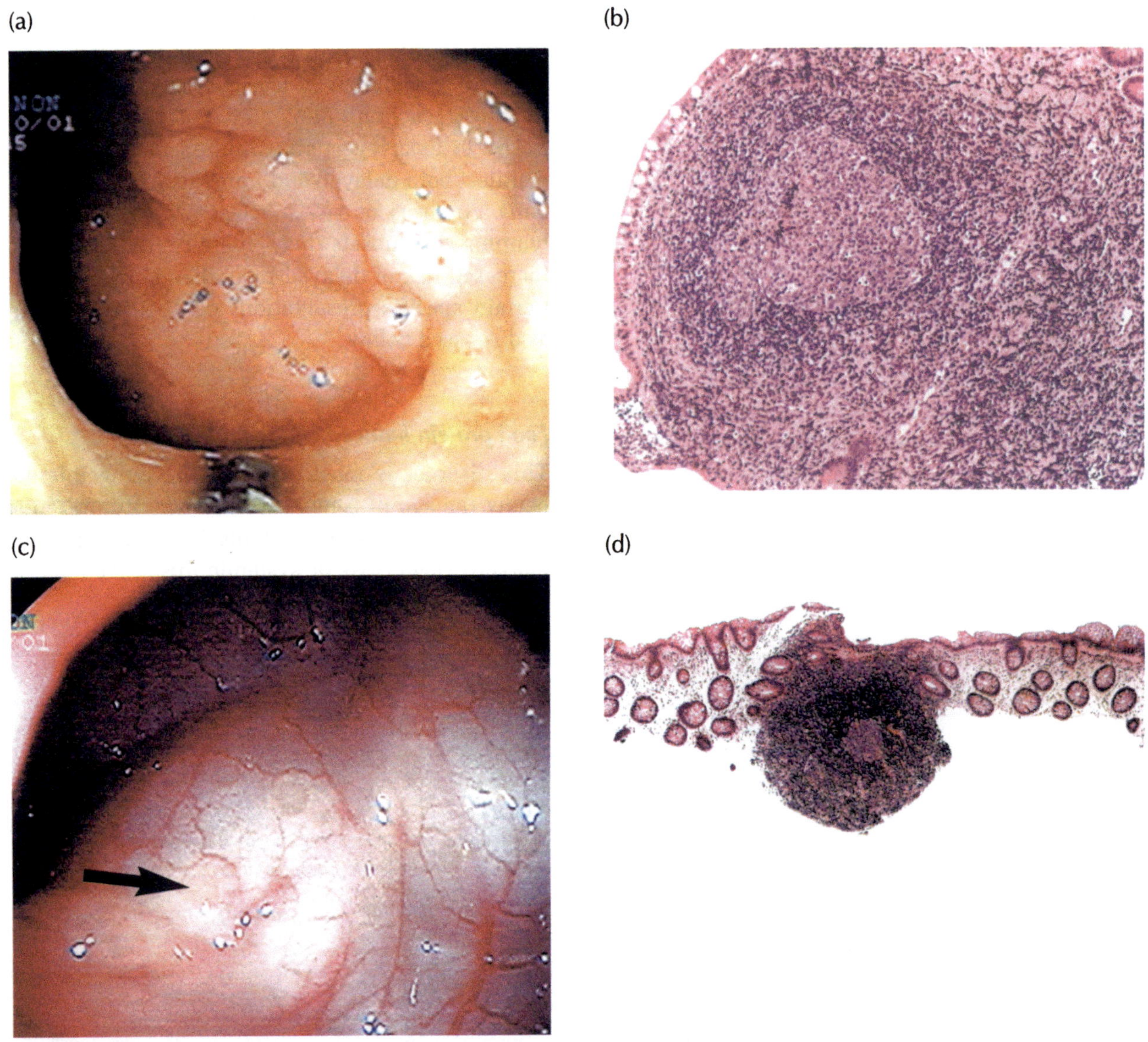

Figure 22.1 Lymphoid hyperplasia is an important endoscopic feature in food allergies.[29] This ileocolonoscopy was performed in a 2-year-old girl with multiple food allergies, and demonstrated ileal lymphonodular hyperplasia (a), with prominent reactive germinal centers on histology (b), together with multiple colonic lymphoid follicles (c – a typical follicle is arrowed). Histology of each biopsy in her colonic series demonstrated a lymphoid follicle (d).

Some infants manifest a form of food protein-induced enterocolitis that is more severe than the classic variant, and is less often induced by cow's milk.[24] The histological response is more severe, with evidence of frank colitis including crypt abscesses, and the response to food challenge may include shock.

Food protein enteropathy

The most common and best described mucosal manifestation of food allergy is food-sensitive enteropathy, in which there is an immunologically mediated abnormality of the small intestinal mucosa, which may include excess lymphocyte infiltration, epithelial abnormality or architectural disturbance. This may often impair absorption and less commonly causes a frank malabsorption syndrome. This continues while the food remains in the diet and remits on an exclusion diet. This is best described for cow's milk, and cow's milk-sensitive enteropathy (CMSE) has been recognized for over two decades.[32] Enteropathy can also occur in response to other antigens, notably soy. The lesion is less severe than celiac disease, but is characterized by similar findings of crypt elongation and villus shortening, giving a reduction of overall crypt/villus ratio. There is usually an increase of mononuclear cell density within the mucosal lamina propria, often including prominent eosinophils, and the intraepithelial lymphocyte density is often increased (Figures 22.2 and 22.3). The lesion is not associated directly with systemic IgE responses, and skin prick tests are often negative. Analysis of mucosal lymphocytes confirms excess T-cell activation, with either a Th1 dominated or mixed Th1/Th2 response.[31,33,34] The consequences of this mucosal T-cell activation include reduction in brush-border disaccharidase expression, leading to impaired carbohydrate absorption, and a secondary reduction in pancreatic enzyme release,[35] both contributing to malabsorption. There is evidence that some children do not grow out of CMSE in early childhood, and an abnormal mucosa may be seen in later childhood.[36]

In cases of diagnostic uncertainty, it may be necessary to confirm the return of mucosal abnormality by food challenge. This was a more common practice in the past, when the very existence of food-sensitive enteropathies other than celiac disease was uncertain. Improvements in infant formulas have led to a change in the mucosal appearances of CMSE, so that celiac-like villous atrophy is now very rare in the developed world. Morphometry of recent cases of CMSE confirms a less severe lesion than archival biopsies from the 1980s.[14] This causes some histopathological difficulty, as there is no international consensus in the reporting of subtle lesions such as villous blunting or mild mucosal eosinophilia.

Eczema/atopic dermatitis

There seems little doubt that food-allergic responses may contribute to the clinical presentation of eczema in infancy, but considerable uncertainty about whether adults have anything to gain from exclusion diets.[37] There is evidence that children with eczema have elevated food-specific IgE in serum, and that food challenges of eczematous children induce increases in circulating eosinophil and mast cell products.[38] There is evidence of enhanced intestinal permeability in infants with eczema, potentially contributing to sensitization through bypass of enterocyte antigen-handling mechanisms.[39] The response within the skin is dominated by Th2 cytokines, and characterized by influx of both T lymphocytes, which express skin-homing markers such as the cutaneous lymphocyte antigen (CLA), and eosinophils.[37,40] The mechanisms by which skin-homing markers become expressed on gut sensitized cells remains uncertain, as expression of the gut-homing marker β7 integrin is likely to have been required for initial homing to the intestine.[1] There remains the intriguing possibility that bacterial products, particularly superantigens from staphylococci and streptococci, may specifically up-regulate CLA expression in an interleukin (IL)-12-dependent fashion, and thus promote skin homing of lymphocytes sensitized to dietary antigens.[41] *Staphylococcus aureus* may be an important specific complicating factor, as 24 and 28 kD proteins within the toxins may directly induce an IgE-mediated response and thus contribute to allergic immunopathology.[42,43] Deficiency in innate immune responses, in particular production of β-defensins, may contribute to the propensity for superinfection with toxin-producing staphylococci in children with allergic eczema.[44] Therefore, an important consideration in the infant or young child with eczema is whether both the diet and the

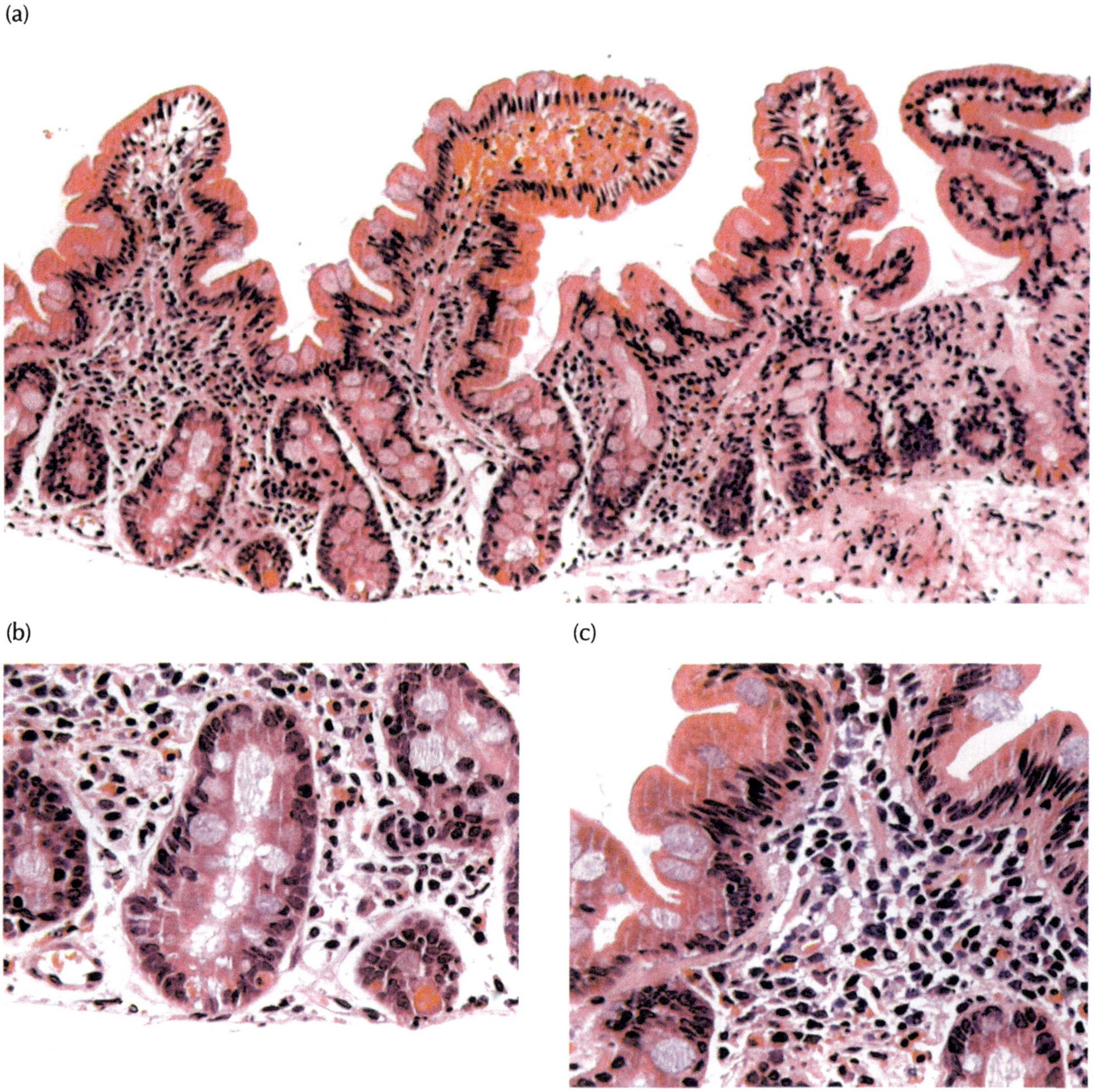

Figure 22.2 The relatively subtle appearances of food-sensitive enteropathy. Duodenal biopsy of the same patient as shown in Figure 22.1, showing minimal evidence of duodenal blunting, but with a patchy increase in mononuclear cell infiltration within the lamina propria (a). High-power views (b, c) show infiltration of eosinophils within the lamina propria and epithelium, together with a moderate increase in mononuclear cells.

bacteriological status of the child have been optimized.

A recent large study of skin prick reactivity to dietary antigen in infants with eczema identified positive skin prick tests for cow's milk, egg or peanut in 22% of 6-month-old infants with eczema, compared to only 5% without eczema.[45] At 1 year the incidences were 36% and 11%, respectively, giving a calculated attributable risk of 65%. This supports data by Kjellman and Hattevig[46] that the development of infantile, but not later-onset eczema, is associated with IgE antibodies to food antigens. Whether the IgE antibodies are directly causative, or alternatively a marker of dietary sensitization in infants

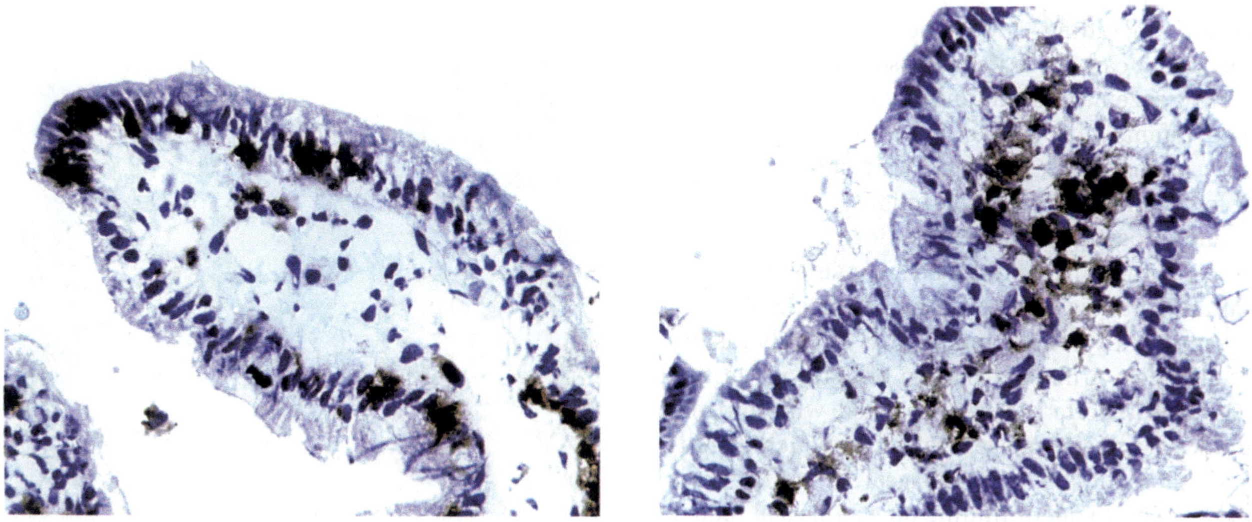
(a) (b)

Figure 22.3 There may be an increase of intraepithelial lymphocytes in food-allergic children. This child with cow's milk-sensitive enteropathy showed normal villous architecture, but increase in CD8 intraepithelial lymphocytes (a). The CD4 cell population lies essentially within the lamina propria (b). Photomicrographs courtesy of Dr Franco Torrente.

predisposed to high IgE levels, remains uncertain. However, there is clear evidence that manipulation of the diet of the eczematous child may be beneficial. A double-blind study by Atherton et al in 1978[47] found that two-thirds of 2–8-year-old children with atopic eczema were improved by exclusion diets. Subsequent studies have broadly confirmed this finding, although in most cases the response was not so striking, except in younger infants.[37] The dominant inducing antigens of food allergy-induced childhood eczema are eggs, milk, soy, and peanut in young infants, with the addition of wheat, tree nuts and fish in older infants. Most children tend to outgrow allergies to eggs, milk, wheat and soy, but tend to have persistent reactions to peanuts, tree nuts, shellfish and fish. The use of skin patch testing has suggested that multiple sensitizations are common in affected infants below 2 years, and thus exclusion of single antigens may not give satisfactory clinical responses.[48]

In addition to antigen exclusion, the use of probiotic treatment has been reported to improve the symptoms of chronic eczema in food-allergic infants.[49] Whether this is because of a direct effect on epithelial integrity, or competitive reduction of toxin-producing staphylococci is as yet unknown. Probiotics are considered in further depth later in this chapter, as well as in Chapter 32. For the affected infant who is exclusively breast fed, maternal dietary exclusions can improve the eczema, but potentially at the cost of maternal nutritional inadequacy if multiple exclusions are required.[50] In addition, some infants may not respond completely to extensively hydrolyzed formulas, due to response to the residual milk antigens, and these may show improvement only with an amino acid formula.[51,52]

Allergic dysmotility

The concept that food allergies might trigger intestinal dysmotility in pediatric patients is relatively new, but there is mounting evidence that dietary antigens (most commonly cow's milk, soy or wheat) can induce gastroesophageal reflux or constipation.[8,53–55] Gastrointestinal investigation of children with delayed food allergic responses frequently uncovers a history of infant colic, gastroesophageal reflux and chronic abdominal pain.[5,14,24,51,52] Conversely, amongst infants presenting with colic, there is a significant incidence of underlying cow's milk allergy.[56,57] There may additionally be evidence of small-intestinal enteropathy or allergic colitis. However, it is not uncommon for food allergy to be overlooked because 'the investigations are negative'.

In infancy, food allergy-induced gastroesophageal reflux is often accompanied by a complex presentation, including low-grade enteropathy with secondary carbohydrate malabsorption, colic, irritability, eczema and prolonged viral infections.[5,8,14] The infants may fail to thrive, and show food-aversive behavior, or weight gain may be acceptable.[5,14] In many cases, reactions to hydrolysate formulas occur, and a therapeutic trial of an amino acid formula should be considered.[5,52,58,59] Dermatographia may be a useful clinical pointer in an apparently colicky infant, as is a family history of allergies. A distinct pattern on 24-h pH testing has been reported to be associated with antigen-induced gastroesophageal reflux, in which there is gradual reduction in esophageal pH following a feed.[53] The frequent finding on esophageal biopsy is mucosal eosinophilia, which may be related to expression of the chemokine eotaxin in milk-induced gastroesophageal reflux.[55]

Even in the older child, milk responses may be a cause of continuing symptoms, including chronic abdominal pain, with endoscopic findings of lymphonodular hyperplasia.[60] There is some evidence that delayed allergic responses to milk in infancy are not always outgrown, and thus the diagnosis should be considered in the older child with an atopic history who presents with chronic abdominal pain.[36] There is also evidence that constipation can be triggered by delayed allergic responses to cow's milk protein in older children.[54] Once again, mucosal eosinophil infiltration was characteristic. Studies using anorectal manometry suggested that this pattern of constipation was caused by antigen-induced spasm of the anal spincter muscles, rather than a more widespread colonic dysmotility.[61] The use of radio-opaque markers may confirm the pattern of normal colonic transit with impaction within the rectum. Clinically the children often demonstrate avoidance posturing, leaning forward during defecation in an attempt to stop the large rectal hard mass from bearing down, while passing the softer stool from above. Clinical examination may be difficult, and even a sizeable acquired megarectum may be difficult to palpate. In cases of clinical doubt, a plain abdominal X-ray may be helpful (Figure 22.4). One characteristic pattern is of fecal impaction within the rectum, together with abundant gas within the small intestine, related to malabsorption of carbohydrates plus constipation-associated small-bowel bacterial overgrowth.

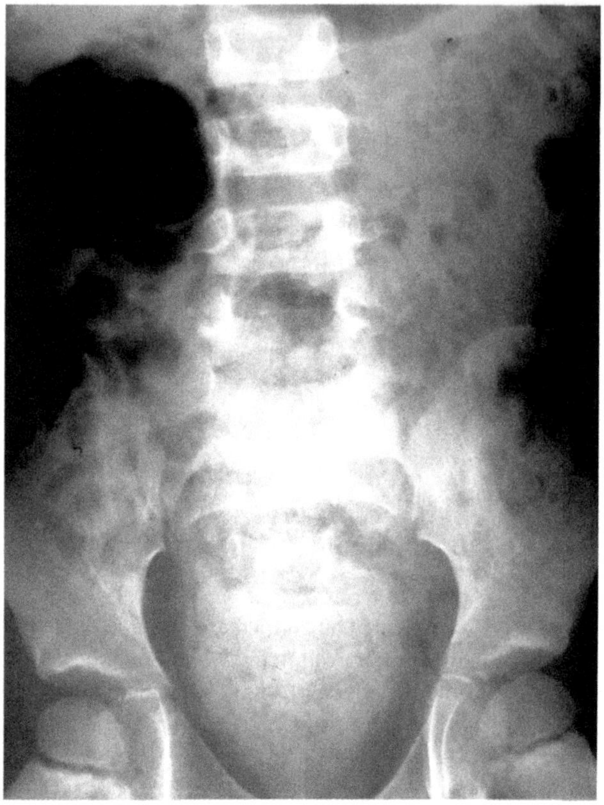

Figure 22.4 Plain abdominal X-ray of a child with non-IgE-mediated food allergies, demonstrating acquired megarectum with fecal impaction. Conventional constipation therapy was ineffective, and a cow's milk- and wheat-free diet were required.

Eosinophilic esophagitis and eosinophilic enteropathy

Eosinophilic esophagitis and eosinophilic enterocolitis are emerging clinical entities, which overlap with non-IgE-mediated food allergy, but which may also occur without recognizable food responses.[62] While an apparently increasing cause of infant gastroesophageal reflux disease, eosinophilic esophagitis is also increasingly seen in older children, who often present with abdominal pain, dysphagia or vomiting, sometimes with associated loose stools.[63,64] In some cases, eosinophil recruitment is confined to the serosa, and may be missed on mucosal biopsies. In many cases, symptoms of esophagitis are severe and prolonged.

At endoscopy, the esophagus shows a distinctive finding of linear furrows or transverse rings, and the mucosa appears granular.[64] The mucosa is traumatized unusually easily.[65] Histological diagnosis is based on the detection of five or more eosinophils per high-powered field. Recent reports of endoscopic ultrasound examination show increased thickness of the esophageal wall.[66] The results of 24-h pH testing are variable, and novel techniques such as luminal impedance testing suggest that much non-acid reflux may occur.[67] Skin prick testing is often negative, but a combination of skin prick and skin patch testing may be helpful in identifying cases of food-induced eosinophilic esophagitis.[68]

Later in the chapter, the potential mechanisms of eosinophil recruitment within the mucosa will be addressed. The eosinophil chemokine eotaxin is clearly important in this process, and indeed this chemokine was up-regulated within the basal esophageal epithelium in infants with milk-induced reflux, in comparison to those with simple mechanical gastroesophageal reflux.[55]

Management of eosinophilic esophagitis

Particularly in younger infants, it is important to perform adequate dietary exclusions. In a significant minority of affected infants, symptoms are not adequately relieved using hydrolysate formulas, and an amino acid-based formula may be required.[58] Effective acid reduction therapy with ranitidine or omeprazole, together with a prokinetic such as domperidone, are frequently used in conjunction.[67] An important clinical finding is the rapid symptomatic worsening during viral illnesses, which is unresponsive to dietary exclusion. This often requires a temporary increase in antacid therapy.

For the older child, dietary exclusions are often less helpful, but a therapeutic trial of a 'few foods' diet may determine whether this is an avenue worth exploring. Topical corticosteroids such as inhaled fluticasone have proved effective in cases where diet has proved ineffective.[69] More recent evidence suggests that leukotriene antagonists such as montelukast may be helpful in corticosteroid-resistant eosinophilic esophagitis.[70]

Respiratory symptoms

Respiratory allergies, particularly asthma, are increasingly common in young children. It is also well recognized that the immediate hypersensitive response to a food allergen includes respiratory symptoms such as wheeze (Table 22.4). What has been less clear is whether delayed responses to food antigens may include worsening of respiratory status in asthma, or can be implicated in upper airway disorders such as rhinitis.[71] Food-induced wheezing appears most common in young infants.[5,17] The estimated prevalence of food-induced wheezing is under 6% of the total population of children with asthma, but it occurs much more frequently in children with cow's milk allergy (29%) or atopic dermatitis (17–27%[71]). Whether antigen-induced gastroesophageal reflux can contribute to respiratory symptoms is an important consideration, and there is potentially important recent evidence suggesting that effective treatment of gastroesophageal reflux may significantly diminish the requirements for bronchodilator therapy in an unselected population of childhood asthmatics.[72] However, it is not clear how many children had straightforward mechanical gastroesophageal reflux and how many may have had an underlying allergic dysmotility.

Testing for food allergies

Food challenge testing

The essential criterion for diagnosis of food allergy is a response to an elimination diet, and other diagnostic tests are secondary to this. If there is allergy to a single food, exclusion should induce relief of all symptoms, and restore normal growth. For secure diagnosis, a positive response to challenge with the food antigen is strongly supportive of the diagnosis of food allergy. This is not always practicable in routine practice, if diagnostic tests were positive at diagnosis, and many parents may refuse challenge if their child has improved dramatically. Insurance companies, however, may require evidence of positive food challenge for reimbursement.

In addition to initial challenge for first diagnosis, subsequent challenge may be performed when it is reasonably likely that tolerance has been regained.

This is usually after 2 years, but often later, especially in multiply allergic children. The European Society for Paediatric Gastroenterology, Hepatology and Nutrition[73] made recommendations for challenge criteria for children with predominant gastrointestinal symptoms, suggesting that blinded challenge is not always necessary in younger children, but that small-bowel biopsy should be performed in cases with failure to thrive or diarrhea. Skin prick testing (see later) may provide more specific guidance for children with immediate reactions.

In children with multiple food allergies, the response to elimination of single antigens is incomplete, and lengthy assessment with a very restricted diet is often required. Such situations may become complicated, particularly since the advent of Internet sites that implicate food allergies in an unfeasibly broad spectrum of disorders, and it may be difficult to persuade some parents to broaden their child's diet. For the child who manifests the symptoms of only non-IgE-mediated allergy, it may become extraordinarily difficult to obtain a clear picture of the true state of current true allergy. This situation is complicated by the minor immunodeficiency often associated with multiple food allergies, and the exacerbating effects of intercurrent viral illnesses.[14,19,20] It is important not to perform food challenges while a child is systemically unwell. For cases of multiple sensitization, with delayed responses, it becomes logistically difficult to perform lengthy blinded challenges. Close teamwork with an experienced dietitian is essential in management of any such complicated cases.

The open food challenge is the most common form of diagnostic challenge, and is performed either in the out-patient clinic or in a day ward, depending on the severity and type of reaction expected.[74] Many centers will use a graded challenge in those children who manifest immediate reactions, initially placing a single drop of milk or other antigen on the skin, then on the lips, and then giving increasing amounts by mouth, leaving a period of several minutes between each stage. For the child with a history of severe reaction, it is mandatory that there be adequate medical supervision with the presence of appropriate resuscitation and drugs. For those with a history of anaphylaxis, an intravenous line is usually inserted prior to the procedure.

For the child who makes delayed reactions only, the test may have to be completed at home for logistic reasons. False-negative results have been reported if late reactions are not taken into account. In a study of 370 challenges in 242 children, five exhibited mild immediate reactions that manifested only on the second day at home.[75] These reactions were subsequently confirmed by skin prick test and double-blind placebo-controlled food challenge, and the authors suggested supervised feeding of antigen on the second day to identify late reactors. Hill et al[17] identified very late reactions (up to 3 days) which required up to 120 ml to elicit. Recent data suggest that even later reactions may occur during cow's milk challenges, with the onset of gastrointestinal, respiratory or cutaneous responses beyond 1 week after reintroduction.[76] Therefore, caution and judgement are needed to interpret food challenge tests, to prevent the missing of true late phenomena, but also to exclude over-reporting of symptoms by parents convinced that food allergy is responsible for all their child's various symptoms.

The 'gold-standard' challenge test, the double-blind placebo-controlled food challenge is a cumbersome and time-consuming intervention, but is clearly necessary for assessment of cases with genuine uncertainty about sensitization.[24,73,77] In cases of true uncertainty, the test can firmly establish tolerance or persistent reactivity in a way that no other test can. Its value is much lower when there are large numbers of foods to be tested, and the child makes delayed responses only. Normal day-to-day variation may then be overinterpreted, the situation can become stressed if performed on an in-patient basis, or intercurrent viral illness induces symptoms interpreted as due to the food allergy. This test requires extremely good teamwork between pediatrician, dietitian, pediatric nursing staff and the child's family. No universally accepted protocol exists,[78] but in general the suspected allergen or placebo is given in disguised form, either by capsule or hidden in a liquid over a period of around 2 h. The child should not be receiving antihistamines and should not have received the antigen for at least 2 weeks, and should be well. A total dose of around 10 g is normally taken as sufficient, although this would not pick up some of the delayed reactors identified by Hill et al,[17] Carroccio et al[76] or Caffarelli and Petroccione.[75] Nevertheless, for immediate allergies, the test is highly specific and of very high prognostic value, with a suggested false-positive rate below 1% and false-negative rate below 5%.[78]

Skin prick testing

The skin prick test remains a cornerstone of the diagnosis of immediate allergic reactions, but is usually negative in those who manifest delayed reactions only.[14,74] This is performed by placing a drop of the potential antigen on the skin (usually a commercially obtained solution, although some units use freshly prepared foods) and introducing it into the skin through a puncture device such as a lancet. A positive control (histamine) and negative control (saline) are used at the same time, and the results read at 15–20 min. The test is based on the induced degranulation of cutaneous mast cells by antigen binding and cross-linking of their surface IgE molecules. The size of wheal elicited determines whether the test is regarded as positive. Usually a wheal of 3 mm or more is taken as a positive reading, although in young infants the test can be falsely negative, as the histamine-induced positive control is much smaller in infancy than later childhood, owing to the smaller numbers of cutaneous mast cells.[79] Recent data suggest that the size of wheal obtained may be an important predictor of reaction, and large wheals (> 8 mm) may be so highly predictive of sensitization that unnecessary food challenges can be avoided.[80,81] The study by Sporik et al,[80] of 467 children aged from 1 month to 16 years, correlated the size of the wheal elicited to cow's milk, egg or peanut with clinical outcome. Using the traditional cut-off value of 3 mm was not found to be helpful in predicting a response to challenge, and many false-positive and false-negative results were obtained. However, using a cut-off value of 8 mm for cow's milk and peanut and 7 mm for egg, they found no children with a negative response on challenge. Their calculations suggest that they could avoid clinical testing of 33% of milk-allergic, 56% of egg-allergic and 68% of peanut-allergic patients. These are potentially very important results, but clearly do require local replication, as testing solutions and technique will vary from center to center, and a negative test will not rule out a delayed non-IgE-mediated response to an antigen.

Roberts and Lack[79] have extrapolated from the data from Sporik et al to suggest that a more precise risk value can be obtained using the Fagan likelihood nomogram,[82] in which the risk of true reaction based on history is used together with the result of the skin prick to determine the overall likelihood of true sensitization. They provide an example where a child with low pre-test likelihood of peanut sensitization (headache and vomiting 4 h after a peanut butter sandwich) would have a 0.2% likelihood of true peanut allergy with a 3 mm wheal, rising to 5% with a 6 mm wheal and > 99% only at 10 mm, in contrast to a child with a high pre-test likelihood (urticaria and wheeze on two occasions within minutes of accidental peanut exposure), who would have a 15% likelihood of true peanut allergy with a negative skin prick test, rising to 70% with a 3 mm reaction and 96% with a 6 mm reaction.

Skin patch testing

The use of the skin patch (atopy patch) test, in which the relevant antigen is maintained against the skin under a sealed patch for 48 h, has been suggested to identify cases of non-IgE-mediated delayed allergy. A positive test is signaled by the finding of erythema and induration at 72 h. Combination of patch testing with either skin prick testing or specific IgE testing has identified significant numbers of food-sensitized children who may have been negative on classic testing.[83,84] Of children with delayed reactions to antigen, 89% were identified by patch test in one study.[83] This test has not become widely used and remains under evaluation. Recent reports do, however suggest that patch testing may be clinically useful, particularly in the presence of eczema.[85,86] There are some logistic difficulties, in that the test should be read only after 3 days, requiring a second clinic visit, and some children will not tolerate an occlusive dressing for so long. It is also potentially open to artifact due to lack of supervision, and our unit has had at least one case of factitious illness, in which irritants were introduced beneath the occlusive dressing by the mother. However, it appears that the test induces a specific T-cell response to dietary antigen,[87] and thus a properly performed patch test may be helpful in confirming delayed food allergic responses in cases of diagnostic difficulty.

Specific IgE testing

Testing of specific IgE production to individual foods can be helpful. Formerly known as RAST testing, the technique is now usually based on enzyme-linked immunosorbent assay (ELISA) or the Pharmacia Cap system. It provides results that are complementary to skin prick testing, but at greater cost and with more delay. However, there is evidence that the information provided can be clinically predictive. Using the Pharmacia Cap system, positive predictive values of 95% were found for egg at 6 kUA/l, milk at 32 kUA/l, peanut at 15 kUA/l and fish at 20 kUA/l.[88] These tests are frequently reported on a semiquantitative scale of 0 (no specific IgE) to 6 (high titers), with increasing likelihood of clinical relevance above level 3. However, there is wide variance between centers, and it is important to perform local audit to determine the clinical relevance of reported specific IgE. There is an increased likelihood of long-lasting allergy in children with higher titers of specific IgE for milk, casein or β-lactoglobulin.[89]

Potentially important prognostic information may be allowed in future by study of the specific sequence of epitopes bound by food-specific IgE. Cooke and Sampson[90] identified two forms of IgE binding to ovomucoid (the dominant egg allergen). Binding to linear peptide sequences within the ovomucoid molecule was associated with long-lasting allergy, whereas binding to discontinuous sequences, which are brought into apposition only by protein folding, was seen in those who outgrew their allergies. This may explain the phenomenon whereby some children will be tolerant of cooked egg, where the tertiary sequence has been disrupted in the cooking process, but still react to raw egg white. For cow's milk, too, IgE reaction to linear sequences in casein, rather than the whey proteins α-lactalbumin and β-lactoglobulin, appears to be predictive of long-lasting milk allergy. IgE binding sites in specific sequences of α_{S1}-casein, α_{S2}-casein and κ-casein were identified in those whose allergy was not outgrown.[91,92] It is possible that this may provide the basis for future testing of milk-allergic infants, to identify those for whom immunotherapy may be necessary to prevent lifelong sensitization.

In vitro testing

In vitro tests for lymphocyte response remains so far a research tool, and simple proliferation assays have given quite unreliable results. However, analysis of cytokine production patterns, using single-cell techniques such as ELISPOT or flow cytometry, represents a promising approach for the future. Lymphocytes from food-allergic children produce a pattern of cytokines associated with Th2 responses (IL-4, IL-5, IL-13) on antigen challenge, whereas those from healthy controls may make a more Th1-dominated response, with higher interferon-γ production.[93] However, studies have reported quite contradictory results when based on derived T-cell lines or clones, which may not represent true *in vivo* responses.

A promising novel technique has recently been reported, in which peripheral blood mononuclear cells were tagged with a fluorescent molecule called carboxyfluorescein succinimidyl ester, before stimulation with peanut antigen.[94] This allowed simple identification of peanut-responding T cells by flow cytometry, and confirmed that T-cell responses to peanut in children with active allergies are indeed skewed towards Th2 (producing IL-4, IL-5 and IL-13, but not interferon-γ or TNF-α), in contrast to findings of a Th1-dominated response with high interferon-γ and tumor necrosis factor (TNF)-α in healthy controls or those who had outgrown their allergies.[94] The authors reported similar skewing in milk- and egg-allergic children compared to controls, suggesting that this is likely to be a common mechanism in IgE-mediated food allergies. These findings imply that it is the host immune response, rather than a fundamental property of individual food antigens, that determines whether a Th2-skewed response occurs and allergy is induced.

It should be noted that mucosal responses appear quite different from systemic responses, and there are as yet no validated tests that might help in the diagnosis of non-IgE-mediated food allergies (Figure 22.5). TNF-α production is stimulated within the mucosa by milk challenge of allergic patients,[38,95] which would not be expected from study of circulating T cells,[94] but may reflect its release from mucosal mast cells. Studies of mucosal T-cell responses agree in showing that Th1 responses are maintained in intraepithelial,

(a) (b)

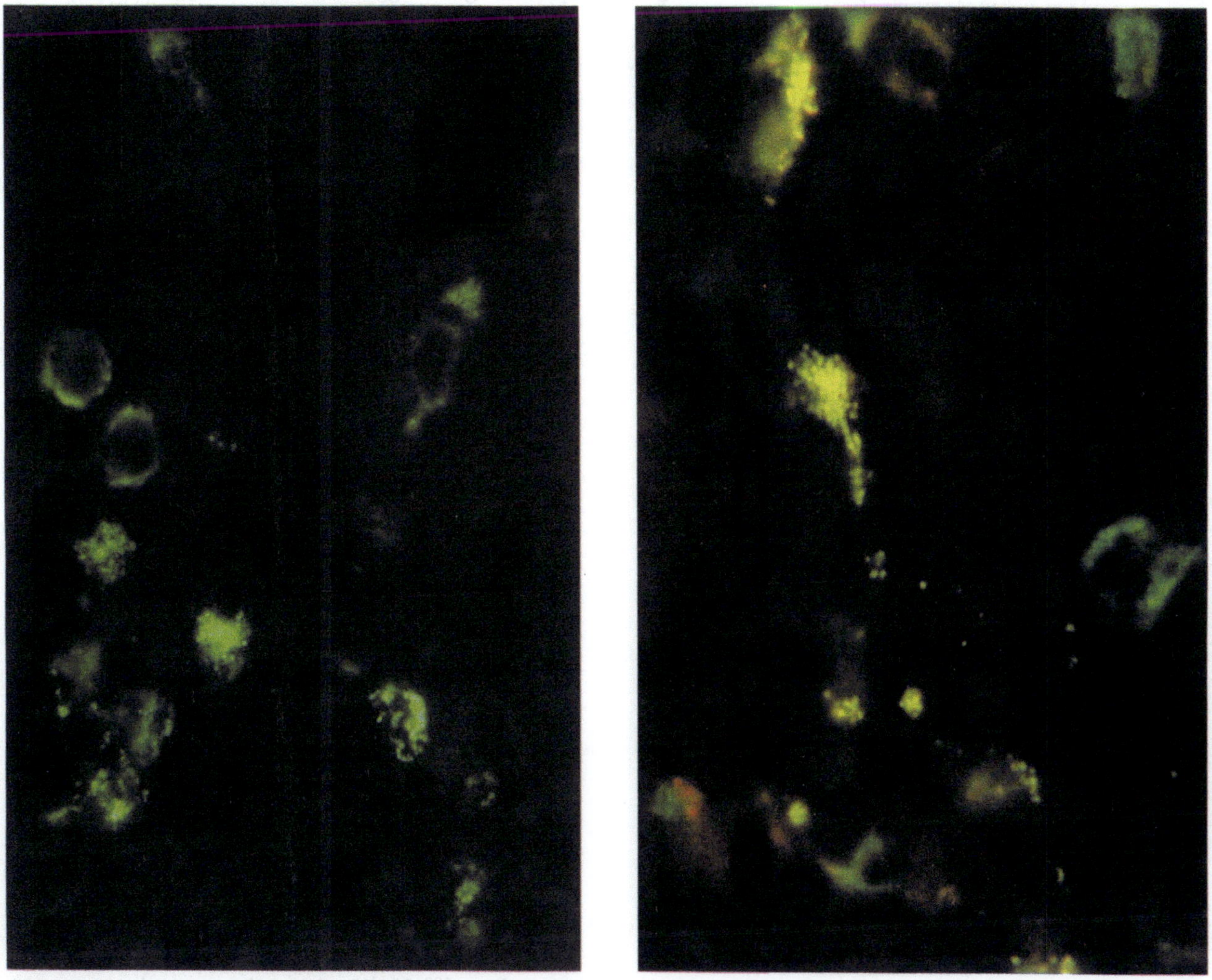

Figure 22.5 Mucosal IgE responses may be distinct from those in other sites. (a) IgE immunohistochemistry of the duodenal mucosa of a child with milk-induced dysmotility, but negative skin prick testing, a serum IgE below 5 kIU/l and no circulating specific IgE. Two types of IgE-positive cell are seen: round cells with a large nucleus and strong surface staining (IgE plasma cells) and irregularly shaped cells with intense granular staining (mast cells). (b) Confirmation that these granular cells are mast cells, as double staining for mast cell tryptase (red) and IgE (green) gives a resultant yellow color. Photomicrographs courtesy of Dr Franco Torrente.

lamina propria and Peyer's patch lymphocytes of food-allergic children.[23,31,96]

Specific food allergies

Allergic responses to many food proteins have been described. The most common in childhood are to cows' milk, soy, eggs and fish, with peanut allergy rapidly becoming more common.[1,3,4,24] However, intolerance to fruits, vegetable, meats, chocolate, nuts, shellfish and cereals has been described. In adult life there is a different spectrum, with allergy to nuts, fruits and fish relatively more common than in childhood. However, as the dietary exposures of UK children broaden, the range of reported allergens also increases: thus sesame, kiwi fruit, mango, avocado and other allergies have increased in frequency. Such sensitization may depend as much on a combination of genetics, infectious challenges and timing and dose of exposure as on innate antigenicity of individual foodstuffs.

There are no consistent associations between any particular food and specific syndromes, although some foods are more likely than others to induce enteropathy, such as cow's milk and soy, and others usually induce immediate hypersensitivity, such as peanut. The incidence of gastrointestinal food allergy is greatest in early life and appears to decrease with age. However, analogy with celiac disease, in which late-onset enteropathy is more likely to be clinically subtle, suggests that the increase in colonic salvage that occurs with age may mask true food-sensitive enteropathy. Although enteropathy can cause significant failure to thrive, complex multiple allergies may also occur in the presence of normal growth.[5]

Cow's milk

Cow's milk allergy may commonly present either as an immediate response, including anaphylaxis, or with delayed responses within the gut or skin. CMSE was frequently diagnosed in the past because of failure to thrive following an episode of gastroenteritis,[97] and the consequent lactose intolerance often inappropriately managed with reduced-lactose formulas without cow's milk antigen exclusion (still common practice in some developing world countries). Modern adapted formulas are now much less sensitizing, and the mucosal lesions less severe. While positive skin prick tests and milk-specific IgE may be seen in some children with enteropathy, they are much more frequent in children who have immediate reactions to milk. Cow's milk colitis is most common in breast-fed babies, whose mothers are consuming milk in their diet, and usually presents with low-grade rectal bleeding. For reasons unknown, it is unusual for one infant to develop both cow's milk enteropathy and colitis. Milk-induced dysmotility is discussed above.

Egg

By contrast to cow's milk, egg allergy usually presents either as an acute hypersensitive response or with delayed respiratory or cutaneous reactions, with worsening of asthma or eczema. While vomiting may occur soon after ingestion, or diarrhea ensue after a few hours, there is little evidence that egg can induce small-intestinal enteropathy.[1] Skin prick tests, patch tests and specific IgE to egg are more often positive than for other antigens,[86] and may be predictive of time taken to outgrow egg allergy. About half of under-2-year-old children who develop egg allergy will tolerate it during 3 years of follow-up, with the size of skin prick reaction and specific IgE potentially predictive of those children who are unlikely to outgrow allergy.[79,98]

Soy

Soy-based formulas have for some years been used in infants with cow's milk allergy, although more commonly by general pediatricians than pediatric gastroenterologists. However, recommendation of soy milk use by the American Academy of Pediatrics Committee on Nutrition[99] may increase the use of soy in comparison to hydrolysates. Soy-based formulas are as antigenic as cow's milk formulas,[100] and the reported reactions span the range from anaphylaxis to enteropathy, eczema and respiratory symptoms.[1] A 30 kD protein in soy may induce cross-reactivity to cow's milk caseins,[101] potentially explaining the high incidence of soy intolerance in cow's milk-allergic children. An important consideration is that antigenicity of soy-derived products is strongly influenced by methods of preparation, and thus children may react to some soy-based products and not others.[102] Unlike in antigens such as peanut and egg, skin prick testing is frequently not a good predictor of subsequent clinical reactions to soy.[79] Patch testing may provide more clinically relevant information, particularly in a child with eczema.[85]

Wheat

Acute allergic reactions to wheat are very uncommon, although wheat anaphylaxis has been described,[103] and an ω-gliadin has been characterized as the likely sensitizing antigen in children with immediate reactions.[104] By contrast to the relative rarity of immediate reactions, delayed hypersensitive reactions are common and clinically important. Celiac disease is particularly important, and affects at least 1% of European and North American populations.[105] Celiac disease is discussed in Chapter 27 in depth. However, it is important to recognize that a low IgA predisposes to both celiac disease and food allergies. It is thus advisable that serological testing for celiac disease should be performed in all food-allergic patients at some stage during their diagnostic evaluation.

There is increasing recognition that wheat products may play a disproportionate role in inducing intestinal dysmotility, such as gastroesophageal reflux and constipation. There are also reports that wheat and cow's milk may induce behavioral effects, possibly because of their natural content of morphine-like exorphins such as β-casomorphine and gliadomorphine.[106,107] While this may also contribute to constipation, such a response would technically be an intolerance rather than a true allergy. However, further work is clearly needed in what is a poorly understood but potentially important area.

Peanut

Peanut allergy is concerning, because of its rising incidence and its propensity to induce severe anaphylaxis.[3,4,24,25] It is particularly important in childhood allergy as a cause of fatal anaphylactic reaction.[108] Even trace amounts of peanut can cause death in those severely sensitized. The surge in peanut hypersensitivity may relate to novel patterns of exposure, and there is recent evidence to suggest that percutaneous sensitization may be more important than simple ingestion.[108] Analysis of the Avon Longitudinal Study of Parents and Children identified that prenatal sensitization was extremely uncommon, but that peanut allergy was associated with intake of soy milk, rash over joints or a crusted oozing rash, and in particular use of skin creams for eczema that contained peanut oil.[109] In this study, cases were initially identified on the basis of a questionnaire, and then subsequently the diagnosis was confirmed by double-blind placebo-controlled food challenge. From a studied cohort of just under 14000 children, 49 were identified with a history of peanut allergy and the diagnosis confirmed in 23 of 36 children tested.

T-cell responses appear important in determining sensitization to peanut, and indeed there has been one report of peanut anaphylaxis transferred to the recipient of a liver transplant.[110] Intriguingly, chimerism was noted in the skin, but not the blood, of the recipient, which implies that lymphocyte homing had occurred. The T-cell response of peanut-allergic, but not tolerant, children is skewed towards Th2 cytokines,[94] suggesting that there is no innate property of peanuts that is responsible for allergic sensitization. However, the severity of peanut reactions does argue for some additional factor beyond simple Th2 skewing, and it is thus notable that the peanut-derived lectin peanut agglutinin is used by pathologists to identify germinal centers in lymphoid follicles. In a rodent model of food allergic sensitization, peanut agglutinin was notable amongst dietary antigens for its ability to induce high IgE responses.[111] Whether the presence of peanut agglutinin affects the level of response to the recognized sensitizing epitopes for humans is currently unknown. Similar evidence from this model that a wheat lectin, wheat germ agglutinin, has a modulating effect on ovalbumin responses,[112] suggests that the presence of lectins within foods may contribute to immune sensitization events.

In the UK, it is recommended that children from an atopic background should not be given peanut products until after the age of 6.[3,4] However, as most children may be sensitized early in life by non-classical routes,[109] this may not be as effective as was initially hoped. There is evidence that many children may outgrow peanut allergy, and that skin prick testing may identify those with a good chance of a successful peanut challenge (see above). For those with established allergy and a history of anaphylaxis, monoclonal anti-IgE therapy is a promising option.[113] This is discussed in more depth in the section on basic mechanisms later in the chapter.

Multiple food allergy

Many infants develop gastrointestinal and other symptoms related to a wide variety of foods. The condition of multiple food allergy[5] provides great challenges for the family, the child and the allergist. Reactions may be immediate or delayed, and do not differ significantly from those described above for individual foods. Affected children often have a family history of atopy, may have increased eosinophils in the peripheral blood, with elevated serum IgE and positive specific IgE, and skin tests to specific foods.[8,14,24,51] Many cases appear to sensitize through maternally ingested antigens during exclusive breast feeding, with the small amounts of dietary proteins either sufficient to sensitize or insufficient to tolerize. A specific defect in oral tolerance for low-dose antigen has been postulated as a cause of this phenomenon,[114] supported by recent data of a defective generation of Th3 cells within the mucosa of affected children.[34] Affected children may show residual intolerance of hydrolysates.[5,14,52]

Recommendations for food allergen avoidance

There remains controversy about the stringency of allergen avoidance required in food allergies, recently reviewed by Zeiger.[115] Two position statements have been published, by the American Academy of Pediatrics (AAP)[99] and a joint statement by the European Society for Pediatric Allergology and Clinical Immunology (ESPACI) and the European Society for Pediatric Gastroenterology, Hepatology, and Nutrition (ESPGHAN).[116] These statements deal with two areas of importance: the primary prevention of development of food allergies, and the treatment of the affected child.

With respect to primary prevention, there are areas of clear concordance, and both statements support the limitation of primary prevention to high-risk infants only, and the use of hypoallergenic formulas (ideally extensively hydrolyzed) but not soy milk for bottle-fed high-risk infants. High risk is defined on family history grounds rather than any perinatal testing, although the AAP defines a positive family history as two first-degree relatives with atopic disease and the ESPACI/ESPGHAN definition requires only one. Neither recommend maternal exclusion diets during pregnancy and both recommend exclusive breast feeding (AAP 6 months, ESPACI/ESPGHAN 4–6 months). While the European bodies do not recommend a maternal exclusion diet during lactation, the American body recommends exclusion of peanuts and nuts, and consideration of further exclusions. The European regulations are also less restrictive about the introduction of solid foods, suggesting introduction at 5 months, rather than the much later introduction of cow's milk and eggs suggested in the AAP report.

For treatment of established food allergies, both statements recommend complete exclusion of the causative antigen, and show broad consensus in the management of a formula-fed cow's milk-sensitized infant, with recommendation of an extensively hydrolyzed but not partially hydrolyzed formula. However, the AAP guidelines also suggest that soy is an alternative in this circumstance, which is not supported by the European guidelines. Both recommend an amino acid formula for the infant who is intolerant of hydrolysates. Neither support the use of unmodified goat's or sheep's milk. For the infant who becomes sensitized while breast fed, both statements concord in support of maternal exclusion of the relevant antigen, while the AAP further recommends weaning to an extensively hydrolyzed formula or soy milk. For the infant with concomitant malabsorption due to enteropathy, both recommend extensively hydrolyzed or amino acid formulas.

An important recent report from the German Infant Nutrition Intervention (GINI) study group[117] assessed 2252 at-risk infants, who were randomly assigned at birth to receive one of four blinded formulas, either cow's milk-based, partially hydrolyzed whey, extensively hydrolyzed whey, or extensively hydrolyzed casein. The primary endpoint at 1 year of age was the presence of one or more of atopic dermatitis, gastrointestinal food allergy or urticaria. The drop-out rate was high, as 865 remained exclusively breast fed for 4 months, 304 left the study and 138 did not comply. Study of the 945 remaining treated infants showed a significant protective effect of extensively hydrolyzed casein compared to unmodified cow's milk (9% vs. 16% had allergies) and atopic dermatitis was significantly reduced with extensively hydrolyzed casein or partially hydrolyzed whey formulas. The protective effect of hydrolysates was attenuated in those with a strong family history of atopy.

The basic mechanisms of immune response to dietary antigen

The intestine is an organ that shows the traces of evolutionary longevity, and indeed Cambrian period fossils from over 600 million years ago show a recognizable gastrointestinal tract.[118] There is much current interest on the links between innate and adaptive immune responses, in particular pattern receptor molecules such as toll-like receptors and nod proteins that induce an immune response within innate cells, such as dendritic cells, that polarize subsequent T-cell responses.[119,120] Evidence that oral tolerance cannot be established normally in germ-free mice suggests that the normal flora plays an important role in the generation of tolorogenic lymphocytes and the prevention of food allergies.[121,122] The potential role for probiotics in prevention of food allergies in susceptible infants is thus likely to be based on the role of luminal bacteria in inducing a tolerant lymphocyte response.[8,9] Transgenic mice whose only T cells responded to ovalbumin were in fact entirely tolerant of ovalbumin feeds, unless innate immune responses to the flora were blocked using cyclo-oxygenase-2 antagonists, when food-sensitive enteropathy was induced.[123] Further study of dendritic cell populations within the intestine is likely to shed light on basic mechanisms of tolerance and sensitization. Genetic variation in receptors for bacterial products, such as toll-like receptors and nod proteins, is known to occur, and is likely to be related to allergic sensitizations,[124] particularly as toll receptors are also expressed on mast cells.[125]

In addition to innate immune cells, the intestine also contains large numbers of primitive T and B cells, such as peritoneal B1 lymphocytes, $\gamma\delta$ T cells, natural killer T cells and atypical CD8 cells with two α and no β chains.[9] Little is known about the role of these primitive lymphocyte types in food allergies, although it is intriguing that $\gamma\delta$-deficient mice have low mucosal IgA levels,[126] while their numbers are increased within the mucosa in food allergies.[30] There is also evidence that these types of T cell can react to lipid and glycolipid antigens, presented by non-classical MHC molecules such as CD1d, which are expressed by the enterocyte.[127–129] It is thus notable that IgE responses to β-lactoglobulin in a rodent model of sensitization were substantially enhanced when the animals were sensitized to whole milk than to β-lactoglobulin alone.[130]

The role of extrathymically derived T cells, which mature within the gut epithelium, is also unknown but likely to be significant, particularly in infants born preterm. Given the numbers and situation of these cells, it is likely that further studies will unmask a relevant role in the induction of tolerance to dietary antigen. It is probably not coincidence that infants with a variety of immunodeficiencies have a high incidence of dietary sensitizations, chronic enteropathy and failure to thrive.[131] It is likely that T-cell responses play a large role in determining tolerance or sensitization to dietary antigen. There are differences in racial susceptibility to sensitization to individual antigens, which do not relate to simple early life exposure.[5]

Antigen presentation by the epithelium

One cell type that is likely to play a more significant role in food allergies than was previously recognized is the small-intestinal enterocyte, which separates the immune system from both dietary antigens and bacteria. Their role in antigen presentation and production of an array of cytokines has recently been recognized.[32,128,129,132] An important role in induction of tolerance has thus been suggested. Recent data suggest that intestinal epithelium may directly induce a regulatory phenotype in CD8 cells.[133] Increased paracellular permeability, allowing transfer of antigen to the immune system without epithelial processing and presentation, may underlie the phenomenon of sensitization to food antigens during conditions such as rotavirus gastroenteritis.[32,97] Formal confirmation of the sensitizing role of excess paracellular permeability was provided in a transgenic mouse model where an intercellular adhesion molecule called cadherin was mutated, inducing severe enteropathy.[134]

Skewing of B cells towards IgE

While non-IgE-mediated responses to dietary antigen may cause chronic symptomatology, IgE-mediated mechanisms account for the majority of immediate hypersensitive reactions to foods. Transient IgE responses to foods are seen in normal children, so this is unlikely to be clinically relevant.[135] By contrast, high-level IgE responses are usually pathological and may be important in severe food allergies and anaphylaxis.

Production of IgE is favored by dominance of Th2 responses, particularly due to IL-4 and IL-13 secretion.[136] The receptors for IL-4 and IL-13 share a common α chain (IL-4Rα), mutations in which increased signaling is associated with increased atopy.[137,138] Intracellular signaling downstream of this receptor is mediated through Stat-6 (signal transducer and activator of transcription-6), and blockade of either IL-4Rα or Stat-6 appears promising as a therapeutic target for IgE-mediated allergic reactions.[139,140]

Lineage commitment of B cells towards IgE is favored by the presence of IL-4 and IL-13, and inhibited by Th1-associated cytokines.[136] This may potentially occur within the Peyer's patches in circumstances of Th2-skewed local responses, and lead to generation of mucosal IgE-producing plasma cells without necessarily affecting the commitment of circulating B-cell populations. Mucosally produced IgE may also be transported into the lumen of the gut or airway by a mechanism distinct from secretory component-mediated IgA transport.[141,142] It is thus possible that a compartmentalized response may occur within the intestine, in which mucosal IgE responses may be elicited by dietary antigen, even if cutaneous IgE responses do not occur, leading to negative skin prick tests, and in the absence of circulating specific IgE.

Mast cells and eosinophils in food allergies

There are undoubted links between intestinal food allergic responses and the infiltration of both eosinophils and mast cells, which produce a variety of vasoactive and neuroactive mediators. Both cell types have been particularly implicated in dysmotility responses, and it is likely that these products may directly affect the function of enteric nerves.[143] During the food allergic response, both mast cell tryptase and cationic protein (ECP) are released into the lumen and may be detected in stools.[144–146] However, although mast cells and eosinophils produce a similar spectrum of mediators, their responses show a different time-course. Mast cells induce rapid responses through immediate degranulation of mediators stored in intracellular granules, whereas eosinophil responses are often delayed for several hours, as they are recruited from the peripheral circulation into tissues.

Two molecules are very clearly implicated in mucosal eosinophilia – the chemokine eotaxin and the cytokine IL-5. Important studies by Rothenberg et al, using targeted gene deletion in mice, have clarified the relative contributions of both mediators. Mice were sensitized to ovalbumin, and then challenged with oral administration of ovalbumin-coated beads.[147] Wild-type mice mounted an allergen-specific Th2 response, showing mucosal eosinophilia with increased circulating IgE and IgG1, while eotaxin-deficient mice had preserved systemic IgE and IgG1 responses but did not recruit eosinophils to the mucosa. By contrast, IL5-deficient mice had reduced circulating eosinophils.[147] In additional studies of gastric eosinophil recruitment, it was possible to confirm that antigen-coated beads induced delayed gastric emptying, and again eotaxin-deficient mice were protected.[148] Further studies from this group have identified the esophagus as an apparent target for eosinophil recruitment, either as a consequence of inhalation of aeroallergens such as aspergillus[149] or in circumstances of excess systemic IL-5 expression.[150] This targeting may presumably have some as yet unclear evolutionary basis, but these findings have potentially important clinical implications. First, there may be more than one factor inducing esophageal eosinophilia, and there may be only a partial response to antigen exclusion if the child is also responding to inhaled aspergillus. Second, an intercurrent systemic viral illness in an allergic child with a Th2-deviated immune response may promote esophageal eosinophilia in an antigen non-specific manner. The increased frequency of viral infections in food-allergic children, probably due to low immunoglobulins, CD8 and natural killer cells,[14] may make this a clinically difficult scenario, as appropriate food exclusions may give an apparently poor clinical response.

In adults, IL-5 mRNA is increased within the small-bowel mucosa of food-allergic patients, but not in atopic or non-allergic controls.[151] T cells from food antigen sensitized children produce IL-5 on food challenge, whereas those from tolerant children do not.[93,94] Thus, there is evidence for a final common pathway in the mucosal allergic response to dietary antigen, which is dependent on up-regulation of IL-5 production and expression of the chemokine eotaxin.

T-cell responses in oral tolerance

The phenomenon of oral tolerance lies at the heart of food allergy, which by its nature implies a breakdown or failure of establishment of oral tolerance mechanisms. There has been much recent progress in the understanding of oral tolerance mechanisms. The dose of ingested antigen appears to be particularly important in determining how tolerance is established.[152] The bulk of dietary antigen is absorbed by enterocytes for nutritional purposes, and this antigen is presented by the epithelium in such a way that lymphocyte reactivity is suppressed and the lymphocytes become anergic.[128,129] The absent expression of co-stimulatory molecules by enterocytes and production of suppressor cytokines may both play a role, although little is known about these processes in human infancy and childhood. Food antigens have also been shown to induce apoptosis of antigen-specific lymphocytes in the Peyer's patches of mice, but this has not yet been shown in humans.[153] More recent data suggest that a more complex state is induced in tolerogenic lymphocytes by food administration, in which pro-apoptotic and anti-apoptotic factors are simultaneously up-regulated while T-cell receptor signaling molecules are down-regulated.[154]

In contrast, tolerance to low doses of antigen requires uptake by the antigen-sampling M cells that overlie Peyer's patches. This form of tolerance requires an active generation of suppressor lymphocytes within the Peyer's patches, and in particular Th3 cells that produce the anti-inflammatory cytokine TGF-β.[8,155,156] Other regulatory T-cell populations that are likely to be very important in preventing food allergies include T regulator-1 (Tr1) cells, which produce IL-10, and CD4+CD25+ cells.[9,129,156] The transcription factor *Foxp3* appears to be central in the commitment of naive T cells towards the regulatory pathway in mice.[157] Similar relevance in humans is suggested by the development of a multifocal inflammatory condition (IPEX syndrome) in infants with mutations in *Foxp3*.[158] Thus, *Foxp3* may be a molecule that is of critical importance in maintaining oral and systemic tolerance. There are currently no clear data to determine which regulatory cell type is most relevant in prevention of childhood food allergy. There is certainly evidence that a multiply exposed population of elderly circulating CD4+CD25+ cells inhibits milk responses in adult humans.[159] However, which would be unlikely to be the case in early life, when most T cells are initially of the naive phenotype? Analysis of circulating CD4+CD25+ in adults shows that the majority express the skin-homing marker CLA, but not the gut-homing β7 integrin, while cord blood CD25+CD4+ cells express neither CLA nor β7 integrin.[160] Evidence of functional immaturity of the neonatal CD4+CD25+ cell population, at least in mice, is provided by data showing that adult CD4+CD25+ cells prevent an autoimmune response to the autoantigen myelin oligodendrocyte protein, whereas cord blood cells do not.[161] This is likely to be functionally important in responses to ingested antigen, as neonatal animals show impaired low-dose oral tolerance and may even paradoxically sensitize.[162]

There are now extensive data to suggest that oral tolerance is not innate, and that the mechanisms are not present at birth but develop postnatally. The expression of a specific array of toll receptors on CD4+CD25+ regulatory T cells, and increase of their suppressor functions by bacterial lipopolysaccharide,[163] suggest that the early infectious exposures of the young infant are indeed likely to be important in the generation of oral tolerance and the prevention of allergy. The current data on human infants point to a particular role for TGF-β rather than IL-10 in the prevention of infant allergy. Study of spontaneous and cow's milk-stimulated cytokine production of cord blood mononuclear cells identified a reduced TGF-β but not IL-10 response in children of allergic mothers.[164] The dominant cytokine abnormality in the mucosa of food-allergic children does not appear to be diminished Th1 or excess Th2 responses, but reduced numbers of TGF-β secreting Th3 cells.[34] Other studies have confirmed that Th1 responses are normal or even increased within the mucosa in childhood food allergy,[31,33,34] but that TGF-β responses are impaired: expression of TGF-β1 and its receptor are diminished within the mucosa in food-allergic enterocolitis,[165] while milk-reactive T-cell clones from milk-allergic children show a Th2-deviated response but with minimal TGF-β production.[166] The factors involved in early life generation of TGF-β1-producing Th3 cells are thus likely to be of great importance in determining whether food-allergic sensitization occurs. Infectious exposures are certainly one such factor, and it is notable that the density of TGF-β-producing cells within the duodenal mucosa of infants in rural Gambia was an order of magnitude higher than in healthy UK infants.[167] It is likely that early-life immunomodulation of regulatory responses, rather than alteration of dietary exposures, will prove the way ahead in childhood food allergies.

Future challenges and opportunities in food allergy

There have been substantial recent advances in the basic science of food allergies. There has been a broadening of the concepts of food allergy, away from simple focus on IgE and towards a consideration of overall mucosal tolerance. Could a genetic tendency to high IgE responses simply make adverse immunological reactions to foods more noticeable? As many practitioners are uncomfortable without supporting diagnostic tests, non-IgE-mediated allergy may remain a difficult and controversial clinical area. Absence of specific tests can also lead to overdiagnosis of allergies, or inappropriate blaming of non-specific symptoms on food allergy – as can be seen on large numbers of Internet sites.

The advances in basic research, which encompass both gut inflammation and allergy because of shared tolerance mechanisms, may explain some of the recent demographic shifts in allergy. Inappropriate infectious priming of the nascent mucosal immune system may affect the development of normal gut tolerance. Handling of the newborn infant has been shown in one study to affect allergy in young adulthood.[168] There is also clear evidence that the early gut colonization of allergic infants differs from those without allergies.[169] One study which thus demonstrated great promise was the recent placebo-controlled trial by Isolauri's group in which neonatal administration of a probiotic organism (*Lactobacillus GG*) led to a 50% reduction in the later development of eczema, although without alteration of systemic IgE responses at either 1 year or 4 years.[10,11] The use of probiotics at birth may be more effective than later, as it may allow stable long-term colonization, which does not occur if probiotics are administered even at the age of 10 months.[170] As interaction between bacterial exposures in early infancy and genetically determined responses in innate immune cells may determine whether an adequate tolerogenic response occurs, probiotics may represent an important new class of immunomodulators, particularly if used in early infancy. However, much work remains to be done to determine the dosage, timing and nature of the probiotics to be used.[9] An alternative approach to programming a Th1 or tolerant response is to use bacterial products, such as mycobacterial peptides. A suspension made from killed *Mycobacterium vaccae* inhibited airway eosinophilia in a murine model of allergy, through the induction of an allergen-specific regulatory T-cell response, dependent on TGF-β and IL-10.[171] Such therapy may offer a refined alternative to probiotic therapy, in which regulatory T-cell generation is the therapeutic goal. However, much safety information needs to be accumulated, and placebo-controlled trials completed, before such therapies can become more widely used.

There are other exciting potential therapies for food allergies, some of which have been subject to clinical trials in humans.[172] The area of immunotherapy is well established for systemic allergies such as bee-sting allergy, and has depended on increasing the dose of antigen gradually until an allergy-suppressing Th1 response is made. For food allergies, the use of small peptides, foods with altered protein sequences, DNA immunizations and IgE-blocking agents represent future targets for immunotherapy. For small peptide vaccines, an antigenic peptide is sequenced and synthetic 10–20 amino acid portions are then produced, covering the entire protein sequence. While able to block IgE binding sites, they are not long enough to cross-link IgE on mast cells. Food proteins can also be engineered, which are able to bind to T cells but not mast cells. In recent studies, the major peanut proteins Ara h1, ara h2 and ara h3 have been purified, their T-cell and IgE-binding domains elicited, and mutations made in the IgE-binding domain.[173]

While much of the data outlined above suggests that IL-5 responses may be critical in food allergies, the therapeutic credentials of a highly promising anti-IL-5 monoclonal antibody were dented by a study in asthmatic patients, in which peripheral eosinophilia was reduced, but without any significant modulation of the late bronchoconstrictor response in asthma.[174] The results of clinical trials in severe food allergy will be extremely interesting, provided that such agents remain in clinical development after such a setback. Similarly, a monoclonal antibody that blocks eotaxin chemoattraction may prevent the migration of eosinophils into the mucosa in response to food allergens.

Relevant therapeutic antibodies that have reached clinical trials include two anti-IgE monoclonals. The humanized monoclonal anti-IgE rhu Mab E-25, which binds to the constant region of IgE, and thus prevents IgE binding to its high- or low-affinity receptors, has shown promising effects in allergic asthma.[175] In a potentially very important study, the humanized IgG1 anti-IgE monoclonal TNX-901 showed clear promise in the treatment of established peanut allergy.[113] Using a dose of 450 mg, given subcutaneously at 4-weekly intervals for 16 weeks, treated patients showed an increase in reaction threshold to peanut from 178 to 2805 g, essentially the difference between half a peanut and nine peanuts. A dose-dependent increase in reaction threshold was seen from 150–450 mg doses. This represents a clinically worthwhile increase in reaction threshold, and would substantially reduce the chances of inadvertent consumption of sufficient peanut to trigger anaphylaxis.

In addition to such radical advances in therapy, one future challenge in the field of food allergy will be provided by the advent of genetically modified foods, which have so far an unknown propensity for causing allergic reactions. Genes may be introduced into plants either through use of a bacterial vector or by direct physical methods, while alternatively naturally occurring genes may be silenced.[176] Important lessons have already been learned. In an attempt to increase the nutritional component of cattle feed, the brazil nut 2S albumen protein was introduced transgenically into soy. Unfortunately, this protein turned out to be a major brazil nut allergen, and indeed the transgenic soy was able to induce hypersensitivity in brazil nut-allergic patients.[177] Therefore, avoidance of similar adverse events for the future must be minimized by appropriate predictions. Recognition of potentially allergic molecules can be attempted, on the basis that many are large and heavily glycosylated molecules that are resistant to breakdown by proteolysis or digestion.[178] However, some antigens, particularly fruit allergens, do not follow these rules. One suggestion has thus been to test proteins from genes considered for transgenic insertion by immunoassay against sera from a variety of allergic patients.[179]

Even if genetically modified foods do not reach the market place in large amounts, there still remains the major challenge of ensuring that modern food manufacturing processes do not leave food-allergic patients at risk of anaphylaxis. Taylor et al[180] have published an important call for the determination of the minimal doses of antigen required to trigger reactions, and for international legislation to ensure that food manufacturers do not exceed these doses. The dietary exposure of infants and young children have changed out of all recognition within developing countries in the past decades, at a time when their infectious exposures have also been altered in a way that evolution has not prepared them for. The challenge of preventing food-allergic deaths is one in which food manufacturers may have to work together with basic scientists, and in which microbiologists may have as much to offer as immunologists. These are interesting times.

REFERENCES

1. Walker-Smith JA, Murch SH. Gastrointestinal food allergy. In *Diseases of the Small Intestine in Childhood*, 4th edn. Oxford: Isis Medical Media, 1999: 205–234.
2. Wood RA. The natural history of food allergy. *Pediatrics* 2003; **111**: 1631–1637.
3. Ewan P. Clinical study of peanut and nut allergy in 62 consecutive patients: new features and associations. *BMJ* 1996; **312**: 1074–1078.
4. Hourihane JO. Peanut allergy – current status and future challenges. *Clin Exp Allergy* 1997; **27**: 1240–1246.
5. Hill DJ, Hosking CS, Heine RG. Clinical spectrum of food allergy in children in Australia and South-East Asia: identification and targets for treatment. *Ann Med* 1999; **31**: 272–281.
6. Goh DL, Chew FT, Chua KY et al. Edible 'bird's nest'-induced anaphylaxis: an under-recognized entity? *J Pediatr* 2000; **137**: 277–279.
7. Rook GAW, Stanford JL. Give us this day our daily germs. *Immunol Today* 1998; **19**: 113–116.
8. Murch SH. The immunologic basis for intestinal food allergy. *Curr Opin Gastroenterol* 2000; **16**: 552–557.
9. Murch SH. Toll of allergy reduced by probiotics. *Lancet* 2001; **357**: 1057–1059.
10. Kalliomaki M, Salminen S, Arvillomi H et al. Probiotics in primary prevention of atopic disease: a randomised placebo-controlled trial. *Lancet* 2001; **357**: 1076–1079.
11. Kalliomaki M, Salminen S, Poussa T et al. Probiotics and prevention of atopic disease: 4-year follow-up of a randomised placebo-controlled trial. *Lancet* 2003; **361**: 1869–1871.
12. Gell PGH, Coombs RRA. Classification of allergic reactions responsible for hypersensitivity and disease. In Gell PGH, Coombs RRA, eds. *Clinical Aspects of Immunol.* Oxford: Blackwell, 1968: 575.
13. Clynes R, Dumitru C, Ravetch JC. Uncoupling of immune complex formation and kidney damage in autoimmune glomerulonephritis. *Science* 1998; **279**: 1052–1054.
14. Latcham F, Merino F, Lang A et al. A consistent pattern of minor immunodeficiency and subtle enteropathy in children with multiple food allergy. *J Pediatr* 2003; **43**: 39–47.
15. Oettgen HC, Martin TR, Wynshaw-Boris A et al. Active anaphylaxis in IgE-deficient mice. *Nature* 1994; **370**: 367–370.
16. Miyajima I, Dombrowicz D, Martin TR et al. Systemic anaphylaxis in the mouse can be mediated largely through IgG1 and FcgRIII. Assessment of the cardiopulmonary changes, mast cell degranulation and death associated with active or IgE- or IgG1-dependent passive anaphylaxis. *J Clin Invest* 1997; **99**: 901–914.
17. Hill DJ, Firer MA, Shelton MJ, Hosking CS. Manifestations of milk allergy in infancy: clinical and immunologic findings. *J Pediatr* 1986; **109**: 270–276.
18. Hill DJ, Ball G, Hosking CS, Wood PR. Gamma-interferon production in cow milk allergy. *Allergy* 1993; **48**: 75–80.
19. Soothill JF, Stokes CR, Turner MW et al. Predisposing factors and the development of reaginic allergy in infancy. *Clin Allergy* 1976; **6**: 305–319.
20. Ludviksson BR, Elriksson TH, Ardal B et al. Correlation between serum immunoglobulin A concentrations and allergic manifestations in infants. *J Pediatr* 1992; **121**: 23–27.
21. Järvinen KM, Aro A, Juntunen-Backman K, Suomalainen H. Large number of $CD19^+/CD23^+$ B cells and small number of $CD8^+$ T cells as early markers for cow's milk allergy (CMA). *Pediatr Allergy Immunol* 1998; **9**: 139–142.
22. Ojuawo A, St Louis D, Lindley KJ, Milla PJ. Non-infective colitis in infancy: evidence in favour of minor immunodeficiency in its pathogenesis. *Arch Dis Child* 1997; **76**: 345–348.
23. Pérez-Machado MA, Ashwood P, Thomson MA et al. Reduced transforming growth factor-β1 producing T cells in the duodenal mucosa of children with food allergy. *Eur J Immunol* 2003; **33**: 2307–2315.
24. Sicherer SH. Clinical aspects of gastrointestinal food allergy in childhood. *Pediatrics* 2003; **111**: 1609 –1616.
25. Sampson HA. Anaphylaxis and emergency treatment. *Pediatrics* 2003; **111**: 1601–1608.
26. Pumphrey RS. Lessons for management of anaphylaxis from a study of fatal reactions. *Clin Exp Allergy* 2000; **30**: 1144–1150.
27. Macdougall CF, Cant AJ, Colver AF. How dangerous is food allergy in childhood? The incidence of severe and fatal allergic reactions across the UK and Ireland. *Arch Dis Child.* 2002; **86**: 236–239.
28. Anveden HL, Finkel Y, Sandstedt B, Karpe B. Proctocolitis in exclusively breast-fed infants. *Eur J Pediatr* 1996; **155**: 464–467.
29. Kokkonen J, Karttunen TJ. Lymphonodular hyperplasia on the mucosa of the lower gastrointestinal tract in children: an indication of enhanced immune response? *J Pediatr Gastroenterol Nutr* 2002; **34**: 42–46.
30. Kokkonen J, Ruuska T, Karttunen TJ, Maki M. Lymphonodular hyperplasia of the terminal ileum associated with colitis shows an increase γδ+ T cell density in children. *Am J Gastroenterol* 2002; **97**: 667–672.
31. Hauer AC, Breese E, Walker-Smith JA, MacDonald TT. The frequency of cells secreting interferon-γ, interleukin-4, interleukin-5 and interleukin-10 in the blood and duodenal mucosa of children with cow's milk hypersensitivity. *Pediatr Res* 1997; **42**: 629–638.
32. Walker-Smith JA, Murch SH. Enterocyte proliferation and functions. In *Diseases of the Small Intestine in Childhood*, 4th edn. Oxford: Isis Medical Media, 1999: 29–43.
33. Veres G, Westerholm-Ormio M, Kokkonen J et al. Cytokines and adhesion molecules in duodenal mucosa of children with delayed-type food allergy. *J Pediatr Gastroenterol Nutr* 2003; **37**: 27–34.
34. Pérez-Machado MA, Ashwood P, Torrente F et al. Spontaneous Th1 cytokine production by intraepithelial, but not circulating T cells, in infants with or without food allergies. *Allergy* 2004; **59**: 346–353.
35. Schappi MG, Smith VV, Cubitt D et al. Faecal elastase 1 concentration is a marker of duodenal enteropathy. *Arch Dis Child* 2002; **86**: 50–53.
36. Kokkonen J, Haapalahti M, Laurila K et al. Cow's milk protein-sensitive enteropathy at school age. *J Pediatr* 2001; **139**: 797–803.
37. Burks W. Skin manifestations of food allergy. *Pediatrics* 2003; **111**: 1617–1624.
38. Sampson HA, Broadbent KR, Bernhisel-Broadbent J. Spontaneous release of histamine from basophils and histamine-releasing factor in patients with atopic dermatitis and food hypersensitivity. *N Engl J Med* 1989; **321**: 228–232.
39. Majamaa H, Isolauri E. Evaluation of the gut mucosal barrier: evidence for increased antigen transfer in children with atopic eczema. *J Allergy Clin Immunol* 1996; **97**: 985–990.

40. Abernathy-Carver KJ, Sampson HA, Picker LJ, Leung DY. Milk-induced eczema is associated with the expansion of T cells expressing cutaneous lymphocyte antigen. *J Clin Invest* 1995; **95**: 913–918.
41. Leung DY, Gately M, Trumble A et al. Bacterial superantigens induce T cell expression of the skin-selective homing receptor, the cutaneous lymphocyte-associated antigen, via stimulation of interleukin 12 production. *J Exp Med* 1995; **181**: 747–753.
42. Nissen D, Pedersen LJ, Skov PS et al. IgE-binding components of staphylococcal enterotoxins in patients with atopic dermatitis. *Ann Allergy Asthma Immunol* 1997; **79**: 403–408.
43. Sohn MH, Kim CH, Kim WK et al. Effect of staphylococcal enterotoxin B on specific antibody production in children with atopic dermatitis. *Allergy Asthma Proc* 2003; **24**: 67–71.
44. Ong PY, Ohtake T, Brandt C et al. Endogenous antimicrobial peptides and skin infections in atopic dermatitis. *N Engl J Med* 2002; **347**: 1151–1160.
45. Hill DJ, Sporik R, Thorburn J, Hosking CS. The association of atopic dermatitis in infancy with immunoglobulin E food sensitization. *J Pediatr* 2000; **137**: 475–479.
46. Kjellman B, Hattevig G. Allergy in early and late onset atopic dermatitis. *Acta Pediatr* 1994; **83**: 229–231.
47. Atherton DJ, Sewell M, Soothill JF et al. A double-blind controlled crossover trial of an antigen-avoidance diet in atopic eczema. *Lancet* 1978; **1**: 401–403.
48. Kekki OM, Turjanmaa K, Isolauri E. Differences in skin-prick and patch-test reactivity are related to the heterogeneity of atopic eczema in infants. *Allergy* 1997; **52**: 755–759.
49. Isolauri E, Arvola T, Sutas Y et al. Probiotics in the management of atopic eczema. *Clin Exp Allergy* 2000; **30**: 1604–1610.
50. Isolauri E, Tabvanainen A, Peltola T, Arvola T. Breast-feeding of allergic infants. *J Pediatr* 1999; **134**: 27–32.
51. Hill DJ, Cameron DJ, Francis DE et al. Challenge confirmation of late-onset reactions to extensively hydrolyzed formulas in infants with multiple food protein intolerance. *J Allergy Clin Immunol* 1995; **96**: 386–394.
52. de Boissieu D, Dupont C. Time course of allergy to extensively hydrolyzed cow's milk proteins in infants. *J Pediatr* 2000; **136**: 119–120.
53. Cavataio F, Iacono G, Montalto G et al. Clinical and pH-metric characteristics of gastroesophageal reflux secondary to cows' milk protein allergy. *Arch Dis Child* 1996; **75**: 51–56.
54. Iacono G, Cavataio F, Montalto G et al. Intolerance of cow's milk and chronic constipation in children. *N Engl J Med* 1998; **339**: 1100–1104.
55. Butt AM, Murch SH, Ng C et al. Upregulated eotaxin expression and T cell infiltration in the basal oesophageal epithelium in cow's milk-associated reflux esophagitis. *Arch Dis Child* 2002; **87**: 124–130.
56. Iacono G, Carroccio A, Montalto G et al. Severe infantile colic and food intolerance: a long-term prospective study. *J Pediatr Gastroenterol Nutr* 1991; **12**: 332–335.
57. Heine RG, Elsayed S, Hosking CS, Hill DJ. Cow's milk allergy in infancy. *Curr Opin Allergy Clin Immunol* 2002; **2**: 217–225.
58. Kelly KJ, Lazenby AJ, Rowe PC et al. Eosinophilic esophagitis attributed to gastroesophageal reflux: improvement with an amino acid-based formula. *Gastroenterology* 1995; **109**: 1503–1512.
59. Vanderhoof JA, Murray ND, Kaufman SS et al. Intolerance to protein hydrolysate infant formulas: an underrecognized cause of gastrointestinal symptoms in infants. *J Pediatr* 1997; **131**: 741–744.
60. Kokkonen J, Tikkanen S, Karttunen TJ, Savilahti E. A similar high level of immunoglobulin A and immunoglobulin G class milk antibodies and increment of local lymphoid tissue on the duodenal mucosa in subjects with cow's milk allergy and recurrent abdominal pains. *Pediatr Allergy Immunol* 2002; **13**: 129–136.
61. Shah N, Lindley K, Milla P. Cow's milk and chronic constipation in children. *N Engl J Med* 1999; **340**: 891–892.
62. Furuta GT. Eosinophilic esophagitis: an emerging clinicopathologic entity. *Curr Allergy Asthma Rep* 2002; **2**: 67–72.
63. Khan S, Orenstein SR. Eosinophilic gastroenteritis: epidemiology, diagnosis and management. *Paediatr Drugs* 2002; **4**: 563–570.
64. Orenstein SR, Shalaby TM, Di Lorenzo C et al. The spectrum of pediatric eosinophilic esophagitis beyond infancy: a clinical series of 30 children. *Am J Gastroenterol* 2000; **95**: 1422–1430.
65. Vasilopoulos S, Murphy P, Auerbach A et al. The small-caliber esophagus: an unappreciated cause of dysphagia for solids in patients with eosinophilic esophagitis. *Gastrointest Endosc* 2002; **55**: 99–106.
66. Fox VL, Nurko S, Teitelbaum JE et al. High-resolution EUS in children with eosinophilic 'allergic' esophagitis. *Gastrointest Endosc* 2003; **57**: 30–36.
67. Thomson MA. The pediatric esophagus comes of age. *J Pediatr Gastroenterol Nutr* 2002; **34**: S40–45.
68. Spergel JM, Beausoleil JL, Mascarenhas M, Liacouras CA. The use of skin prick tests and patch tests to identify causative foods in eosinophilic esophagitis. *J Allergy Clin Immunol* 2002; **109**: 363–368.
69. Teitelbaum JE, Fox VL, Twarog FJ et al. Eosinophilic esophagitis in children: immunopathological analysis and response to fluticasone propionate. *Gastroenterology* 2002; **122**: 1216–1225.
70. Attwood SE, Lewis CJ, Bronder CS et al. Eosinophilic esophagitis: a novel treatment using Montelukast. *Gut* 2003; **52**: 181–185.
71. James JM. Respiratory manifestations of food allergy. *Pediatrics* 2003; **111**: 1625–1630.
72. Khoshoo V, Le T, Haydel RM Jr et al. Role of gastroesophageal reflux in older children with persistent asthma. *Chest* 2003; **123**: 1008–1013.
73. The European Society for Paediatric Gastroenterology and Nutrition Group for the diagnostic criteria for food allergy. Diagnostic criteria for food allergy with predominantly intestinal symptoms. *J Pediatr Gastroenterol Nutr* 1992; **14**: 108–112.
74. Bock SA. Diagnostic evaluation. *Pediatrics* 2003; **111**: 1638–1644.
75. Caffarelli C, Petroccione T. False-negative food challenges in children with suspected food allergy. *Lancet* 2001; **358**: 1871–1872.
76. Carroccio A, Montalto G, Custro N et al. Evidence of very delayed clinical reactions to cow's milk in cow's milk-intolerant patients. *Allergy* 2000; **55**: 574–579.
77. Sampson HA, Sicherer SH, Bimbaum AH. AGA technical review on the evaluation of food allergy in gastrointestinal disorders. American Gastroenterological Association. *Gastroenterology* 2001; **120**: 1026–40.
78. Sampson HA. Use of food challenge tests in children. *Lancet* 2001; **358**: 1832–1833.
79. Roberts G, Lack G. Getting more out of your skin prick tests. *Clin Exp Allergy* 2000; **30**: 1495–1498.
80. Sporik R, Hill DJ, Hosking CS. Specificity of allergen skin testing in predicting positive open food challenges to milk, egg and peanut in children. *Clin Exp Allergy* 2000; **30**: 1540–1546.

81. Hill DJ, Hosking CS, Reyes-Benito MLV. Reducing the need for food allergen challenges in young children: comparison of *in vitro* with *in vivo* tests. *Clin Exp Allergy* 2001; **31**: 1031–1035.
82. Fagan TJ. Nomogram for Bayes's theorem. *N Engl J Med* 1975; **293**: 257.
83. Isolauri E, Turjanmaa K. Combined skin prick and patch testing enhances identification of food allergy in infants with atopic dermatitis. *J Allergy Clin Immunol* 1996; **97**: 9–15.
84. Roehr CC, Reibel S, Ziegert M et al. Atopy patch tests, together with determination of specific IgE levels, reduce the need for oral food challenges in children with atopic dermatitis. *J Allergy Clin Immunol* 2001; **107**: 548–553.
85. Niggemann B, Reibel S, Wahn U. The atopy patch test (APT) – a useful tool for the diagnosis of food allergy in children with atopic dermatitis. *Allergy* 2000; **55**: 281–285.
86. Stromberg L. Diagnostic accuracy of the atopy patch test and the skin-prick test for the diagnosis of food allergy in young children with atopic eczema/dermatitis syndrome. *Acta Paediatr* 2002; **91**: 1044–1049.
87. Wistokat-Wulfing A, Schmidt P, Darsow U et al. Atopy patch test reactions are associated with T lymphocyte-mediated allergen-specific immune responses in atopic dermatitis. *Clin Exp Allergy* 1999; **29**: 513–521.
88. Sampson HA, Ho DG. Relationship between food-specific IgE concentrations and the risk of positive food challenges in children and adolescents. *J Allergy Clin Immunol* 1997; **100**: 444–451.
89. Sicherer SH, Sampson HA. Cow's milk protein-specific IgE concentrations in two age groups of milk-allergic children and in children achieving clinical tolerance. *Clin Exp Allergy* 1999; **29**: 507–512.
90. Cooke SK, Sampson HA. Allergenic properties of ovomucoid in man. *J Immunol* 1997;159: 2026–2032.
91. Vila L, Beyer K, Jarvinen KM et al. Role of conformational and linear epitopes in the achievement of tolerance in cow's milk allergy. *Clin Exp Allergy* 2001; **31**: 1599–1606.
92. Järvinen KM, Beyer K, Vila L et al. B-cell epitopes as a screening instrument for persistent cow's milk allergy. *J Allergy Clin Immunol* 2002; **110**: 293–297.
93. Schade RP, Van Leperen-Van Dijk AG, Van Reijsen FC. Differences in antigen-specific T-cell responses between infants with atopic dermatitis with and without cow's milk allergy: relevance of Th2 cytokines. *J Allergy Clin Immunol* 2000; **106**: 1155–1162.
94. Turcanu V, Maleki SJ, Lack G. Characterization of lymphocyte responses to peanuts in normal children, peanut-allergic children, and allergic children who acquired tolerance to peanuts. *J Clin Invest* 2003; **111**: 1065–1072.
95. Heyman M, Darmon N, Dupont C et al. Mononuclear cells from infants allergic to cow's milk secrete tumor necrosis factor α, altering intestinal function. *Gastroenterology* 1994; **106**: 1514–1523.
96. Nagata S, McKenzie C, Pender SL et al. Human Peyer's patch T cells are sensitized to dietary antigen and display a Th cell type 1 cytokine profile. *J Immunol* 2000; **165**: 5315–5321.
97. Kilby A, Walker-Smith JA, Wood CBS. Small intestinal mucosa in cow's milk allergy. *Lancet* 1975; **1**: 53.
98. Boyano-Martinez T, Garcia-Ara C, Diaz-Pena JM, Martin-Esteban M. Prediction of tolerance on the basis of quantification of egg white-specific IgE antibodies in children with egg allergy. *J Allergy Clin Immunol* 2002; **110**: 304–309.
99. American Academy of Pediatrics, Committee on Nutrition. Hypoallergenic infant formulas. *Pediatrics* 2000; **106**: 346–349.
100. Eastham EJ, Lichanco T, Pang K, Walker WA. Antigenicity of infant formulas and the induction of systemic immunological tolerance by oral feeding: cow's milk versus soy milk. *J Pediatr Gastroenterol Nutr* 1982; **1**: 23–28.
101. Rozenfeld P, Docena GH, Anon MC, Fossati CA. Detection and identification of a soy protein component that cross-reacts with caseins from cow's milk. *Clin Exp Immunol* 2002; **130**: 49–58.
102. Franck P, Moneret Vautrin DA, Dousset B et al. The allergenicity of soybean-based products is modified by food technologies. *Int Arch Allergy Immunol* 2002; **128**: 212–219.
103. Rudd P, Manuel PD, Walker-Smith JA. Anaphylactic shock in an infant after feeding with a wheat rusk. A transient phenomenon. *Postgrad Med J* 1981; **57**: 794–795.
104. Palosuo K, Varjonen E, Kekki OM et al. Wheat omega-5 gliadin is a major allergen in children with immediate allergy to ingested wheat. *J Allergy Clin Immunol* 2001; **108**: 634–638.
105. Catassi C, Ratsch IM, Fabiani E et al. Coeliac disease in the year 2000: exploring the iceberg. *Lancet* 1994; **343**: 200–203.
106. Knivsberg AM, Reichelt KL, Hoien T, Nodland M. A randomised, controlled study of dietary intervention in autistic syndromes. *Nutr Neurosci* 2002; **5**: 251–261.
107. Wakefield AJ, Puleston JM, Montgomery SM et al. Entero-colonic encephalopathy, autism and opioid receptor ligands. *Aliment Pharmacol Therapeut* 2002; **16**: 663–674.
108. Sampson HA, Mendelson L, Rosen JP. Fatal and near-fatal anaphylactic reactions to food in children and adolescents. *N Engl J Med* 1992; **327**: 380–384.
109. Lack G, Fox D, Northstone K, Golding J, for the Avon Longitudinal Study of Parents and Children Study Team. Factors associated with the development of peanut allergy in childhood. *N Engl J Med* 2003; **348**: 977–985.
110. Legendre C, Caillat-Zucman S, Samuel D et al. Transfer of symptomatic peanut allergy to the recipient of a combined liver-and-kidney transplant. *N Engl J Med* 1997; **337**: 822–824.
111. Dearman RJ, Caddick H, Stone S et al. Characterization of antibody responses induced in rodents by exposure to food proteins: influence of route of exposure. *Toxicology* 2001; **167**: 217–231.
112. Watzl B, Neudecker C, Hansch GM et al. Dietary wheat germ agglutinin modulates ovalbumin-induced immune responses in Brown Norway rats. *Br J Nutr* 2001; **85**: 483–490.
113. Leung DYM, Sampson HA, Yunginger JW et al, for the TNX-901 Peanut Allergy Study Group. Effect of anti-IgE therapy in patients with peanut allergy. *N Engl J Med* 2003; **348**: 986–993.
114. Murch S. Diabetes and cows' milk. *Lancet* 1996; **348**: 1656.
115. Zeiger RS. Food allergen avoidance in the prevention of food allergy in infants and children. *Pediatrics* 2003; **111**: 1662–1671.
116. Host A, Koletzko B, Dreborg S et al. Joint Statement of the European Society for Paediatric Allergology and Clinical Immunology (ESPACI) Committee on Hypoallergenic Formulas and the European Society for Paediatric Gastroenterology, Hepatology and Nutrition (ESPGHAN) Committee on Nutrition. *Arch Dis Child* 1999; **81**: 80–84.

117. von Berg A, Koletzko S, Grubl A, Filipiak-Pittroff B, Wichmann HE, Bauer CP, Reinhardt D, Berdel D; German Infant Nutritional Intervention Study Group. The effect of hydrolyzed cow's milk formula for allergy prevention in the first year of life: the German Infant Nutritional Intervention Study, a randomized double-blind trial. *J Allergy Clin Immunol* 2003; **111**: 533–540.
118. Zhu D, Zhang X, Chen L. Reinterpretation of Yunnanozoon as the earliest known hemichordate. *Nature* 1996; **380**: 428–430.
119. Medzhitov R, Janeway CA Jr. Innate immunity: impact on the adaptive immune response. *Curr Opin Immunol* 1997; **9**: 4–9.
120. Aderem A, Ulevitch RJ. Toll-like receptors in the induction of the innate immune response. *Nature* 2000; **406**: 782–787.
121. Sudo N, Sawamura S, Tanaka K et al. The requirement of intestinal bacterial flora for the development of an IgE production system susceptible to oral tolerance induction. *J Immunol* 1997; **159**: 1739–1745.
122. Cebra JJ. Influences of microbiota on intestinal immune system development. *Am J Clin Nutr* 1999; **69** (Suppl): 1046S–1051S.
123. Newberry RD, Stenson WF, Lorenz RG. Cycloxygenase-2-dependent arachidonic acid metabolites are essential modulators of the immune response to dietary antigen. *Nature Med* 1999; **5**: 900–906.
124. Tlaskalova-Hogenova H, Tuckova L, Lodinova-Zadnikova R et al. Mucosal immunity: its role in defense and allergy. *Int Arch Allergy Immunol* 2002; **128**: 77–89.
125. Supajatura V, Ushio H, Nakao A et al. Differential responses of mast cell Toll-like receptors 2 and 4 in allergy and innate immunity. *J Clin Invest* 2002; **109**: 1351–1359.
126. Fujihashi K, McGhee JR, Kweon MN et al. γδ T cell-deficient mice have impaired mucosal immunoglobulin A responses. *J Exp Med* 1996; **183**: 1929–1935.
127. Ulrichs T, Porcelli SA. CD1 proteins: targets of T cell recognition in innate and adaptive immunity. *Rev Immunogenet* 2000; **2**: 416–432.
128. Mayer L. Mucosal immunity and gastrointestinal antigen processing. *J Pediatr Gastroenterol Nutr* 2000; **30**: S4–S12.
129. Mayer L. Mucosal immunity. *Pediatrics* 2003; **111**: 1595–1600.
130. Miller K, Meredith C, Selo I, Wal JM. Allergy to bovine beta-lactoglobulin: specificity of immunoglobulin E generated in the Brown Norway rat to tryptic and synthetic peptides. *Clin Exp Allergy*1999; **29**: 1696–1704.
131. Fischer A. Primary immunodeficiency diseases: an experimental model for molecular medicine. *Lancet* 2001; **357**: 1863–1869.
132. Eckmann L, Kagnoff MF, Fierer J. Epithelial cells secrete the chemokine interleukin-8 in response to bacterial entry. *Infection Immun* 1993; 61: 4569–4574.
133. Allez M, Brimnes J, Dotan I, Mayer L. Expansion of CD8+ T cells with regulatory function after interaction with intestinal epithelial cells. *Gastroenterology* 2002; **123**: 1516–1526.
134. Hermiston ML, Gordon JI. Inflammatory bowel disease and adenomas in mice expressing a dominant negative N-cadherin. *Science* 1995; **270**: 1203–1207.
135. Sigurs N, Hattevig G, Kjellman B et al. Appearance of atopic disease in relation to serum IgE antibodies in children followed from birth for 4 to 15 years. *J Allergy Clin Immunol* 1994; **94**: 757–763.
136. Corry DB, Kheradmand F. Induction and regulation of the IgE response. *Nature* 1999; **402** (Suppl): B18–B23.
137. Hershey GK, Friedrich MF, Esswein LA et al. The association of atopy with a gain-of-function mutation in the α subunit of the interleukin-4 receptos. *N Engl J Med* 1997; **337**: 1720–1725.
138. Mitsuyasu H, Izuhara K, Mao XQ et al. Ile50val variant of IL4Rα upregulates IgE synthesis and associates with atopic asthma. *Nature Genet* 1998; **19**: 119–120.
139. Grunewald SM, Werthmann A, Schnarr B et al. An antagonistic IL-4 mutant prevents type I allergy in the mouse: inhibition of the IL-4/IL-13 receptor system completely abrogates humoral immune response to allergen and development of allergic symptoms *in vivo*. *J Immunol* 1998; **160**: 4004–4009.
140. Shimoda K, van Deursen J, Sangster MY et al. Lack of IL-4-induced T cell response and IgE class switching in mice with disrupted Stat6 gene. *Nature* 1996; **380**: 630–633.
141. Ramaswamy K, Hakimi J, Bell RG. Evidence for an interleukin-4 inducible immunoglobulin E uptake and transport mechanism in the intestine. *J Exp Med* 1994; **180**: 1793–1803.
142. Negrao-Correa D, Adams LS, Bell RG. Intestinal transport and catabolism of IgE: a major blood-independent pathway of IgE dissemination during a *Trichinella spiralis* infection of rats. *J Immunol* 1996; **157**: 4037–4044.
143. Collins SM. The immunomodulation of enteric neuromuscular function: implications for motility and inflammatory disorders. *Gastroenterology* 1996; **111**: 1683–1699.
144. Majamaa H, Miettinen A, Laine S, Isolauri E. Intestinal inflammation in children with atopic eczema: fecal eosinophil cationic protein and tumor necrosis factor-α as non-invasive indicators of food allergy. *Clin Exp Allergy* 1996; **26**: 181–187.
145. Kapel N, Matarazzo P, Haouchine D et al. Fecal tumor necrosis factor α, eosinophil cationic protein and IgE levels in infants with cows milk allergy and gastrointestinal manifestations. *Clin Chem Lab Med* 1998; **37**: 29–32.
146. Santos J, Bayarri C, Saperas E et al. Characterisation of immune mediator release during the immediate response to segmental mucosal challenge in the jejunum of patients with food allergy. *Gut* 1999; **45**: 553–558.
147. Hogan SP, Mishra A, Brandt EB et al. A critical role for eotaxin in experimental oral antigen-induced eosinophilic gastrointestinal allergy. *Proc Natl Acad Sci USA* 2000; **97**: 6681–6686.
148. Hogan SP, Mishra A, Brandt EB, et al. A pathological function for eotaxin and eosinophils in eosinophilic gastrointestinal inflammation. *Nature Immunol* 2001; **2**: 353–360.
149. Mishra M, Hogan SP, Brandt EB, Rothenberg ME. An etiological role for aeroallergens and eosinophils in experimental esophagitis. *J Clin Invest* 2001; **107**: 83–90.
150. Mishra A, Hogan SP, Brandt EB, Rothenberg ME. IL-5 promotes eosinophil trafficking to the esophagus. *J Immunol* 2002; **168**: 2464–2469.
151. Vandenzande LM, Wallaert B, Desreumaux P et al. Interleukin-5 immunoreactivity and mRNA expression in gut mucosa from patients with food allergy. *Clin Exp Allergy* 1999; **29**: 652–659.
152. Weiner HL. Oral tolerance: immune mechanisms and treatment of autoimmune diseases. *Immunol Today* 1997; **18**: 335–343.

153. Chen Y, Inobe J, Marks R et al. Peripheral deletion of antigen-reactive T cells in oral tolerance. *Nature* 1995; **376**: 177–180.
154. Kaji T, Hachimura S, Ise W, Kaminogawa S. Proteome analysis reveals caspase activation in hyporesponsive CD4 T lymphocytes induced *in vivo* by the oral administration of antigen. *J Biol Chem* 2003; **278**: 27836–27843.
155. Groux H, Powrie F. Regulatory T cells and inflammatory bowel disease. *Immunol Today* 1999; **20**: 442–446.
156. Strobel S. Oral tolerance, systemic immunoregulation, and autoimmunity. *Ann NY Acad Sci* 2002; **958**: 47–58.
157. Hori S, Nomura T, Sakaguchi S. Control of regulatory T cell development by the transcription factor *Foxp3*. *Science* 2003; **299**: 1057–1061.
158. Wildin RS, Smyk-Pearson S, Filipovich AH. Clinical and molecular features of the immunodysregulation, polyendocrinopathy, enteropathy, X linked (IPEX) syndrome. *J Med Genet* 2002; **39**: 537–545.
159. Taams LS, Vukmanovic-Stejic M, Smith J et al. Antigen-specific T cell suppression by human CD4+CD25+ regulatory T cells. *Eur J Immunol* 2002; **32**: 1621–1630.
160. Iellem A, Colantonio L, D'Ambrosio D. Skin- versus gut-skewed homing receptor expression and intrinsic CCR4 expression on human peripheral blood CD4+CD25+ suppressor T cells. *Eur J Immunol* 2003; **33**: 1488–1496.
161. Wing K, Lindgren S, Kollberg G et al. CD4 T cell activation by myelin oligodendrocyte glycoprotein is suppressed by adult but not cord blood CD25+ T cells. *Eur J Immunol* 2003; **33**: 579–587.
162. Miller A, Lider O, Abramsky O, Weiner HL. Orally administered myelin basic protein in neonates primes for immune responses and enhances experimental autoimmune encephalomyelitis in adult animals. *Eur J Immunol* 1994; **24**: 1026–1032.
163. Caramalho I, Lopes-Carvalho T, Ostler D et al. Regulatory T cells selectively express toll-like recptors and are activated by lipopolysaccharide. *J Exp Med* 2003; **197**: 403-411.
164. Hauer AC, Rieder M, Griessl A et al. Cytokine production by cord blood mononuclear cells stimulated by cows milk protein *in vitro*: interleukin-4 and transforming growth factor β-secreting cells detected in the CD45RO T cell population in children of atopic mothers. *Clin Exp Allergy* 2003; **33**: 615–623.
165. Chung HL, Hwang JB, Park JJ, Kim SG. Expression of transforming growth factor β1, transforming growth factor type I and II receptors, and TNF-α in the mucosa of the small intestine in infants with food-protein induced enterocolitis syndrome. *J Allergy Clin Immunol* 2002; **109**: 150–154.
166. Beyer K, Castro R, Birnbaum A et al. Human milk-specific mucosal lymphocytes of the gastrointestinal tract display a Th2 cytokine profile. *J Allergy Clin Immunol* 2002; **109**: 707–713.
167. Campbell DI, Murch SH, Lunn PG et al. Chronic T cell-mediated enteropathy in rural West African children: Relationship with nutritional status and small bowel function. *Pediatr Res* 2003; **54**: 306–311.
168. Montgomery SM, Wakefield AJ, Morris DL et al. The initial care of newborn infants and subsequent hayfever. *Allergy* 2000; **55**: 916–922.
169. Björksten B, Sepp E, Julge K et al. Allergy development and the intestinal microflora during the first year of life. *J Allergy Clin Immunol* 2001; **108**: 516–520.
170. Heilig HG, Zoetendal EG, Vaughan EE et al. Molecular diversity of *Lactobacillus* spp. and other lactic acid bacteria in the human intestine as determined by specific amplification of 16S ribosomal DNA. *Appl Environ Microbiol* 2002; **68**: 114–123.
171. Zuany-Amorim C, Sawicka E, Manlius C et al. Suppression of airway eosinophilia by killed *Mycobacterium vaccae*-induced allergen-specific regulatory T-cells. *Nature Med* 2002; **8**: 625–629.
172. Nowak-Wegrzyn A. Future approaches to food allergy. *Pediatrics* 2003; **111**: 1672–1680.
173. Rabjohn P, Helm EM, Stanley JS et al. Molecular cloning and epitope analysis of the peanut allergen Ara h 3. *J Clin Invest* 1999; **103**: 535–542.
174. Leckie MJ, ten Brinke A, Khan J et al. Effects of an interleukin-5 blocking monoclonal antibody on eosinophils, airway hyper-responsiveness, and the late asthmatic response. *Lancet* 2000; **356**: 2144–2148.
175. Milgrom H, Fick RBJ, Su JQ et al. Treatment of allergic asthma with monoclonal anti-IgE antibody. rhuMAb-E25 Study Group. *N Engl J Med* 1999; **341**: 1966–1973.
176. BSACI Working Party: Lack G, Chapman M, Kalsheker N, King V, Robinson C, Venables K. Report on the potential allergenicity of genetically modified organisms and their products. *Clin Exp Allergy* 2002; **32**: 1131–1143.
177. Nordlee JA, Taylor SL, Townsend JA et al. Identification of a Brazil-nut allergen in transgenic soybeans. *N Engl J Med* 1996; **334**: 688–692.
178. Taylor SL, Lehrer SB. Principles and characteristics of food allergens. *Crit Rev Food Sci Nutr* 1996; **36(S)**: 91–118.
179. Lack G. Clinical risk assessment of GM foods. *Toxicol Lett* 2002; **127**: 337–340.
180. Taylor SL, Hefle SL, Bindslev-Jensen C et al. Factors affecting the determination of threshold doses for allergenic foods: how much is too much? *J Allergy Clin Immunol* 2002; **109**: 24–30.

23 Crohn's disease

Qian Yuan and Harland S Winter

Introduction

New knowledge continues to impact on the pathogenesis and treatment of the chronic inflammatory intestinal disorder described by Dr Burrill Bernard Crohn in the early 1930s.[1] However, for over a century prior to this report physicians knew of the existence of a non-tuberculous ileitis. Characterized by transmural, chronic mucosal inflammation involving any portion of the gastrointestinal tract from the lips to the perineum, Crohn's disease frequently involves the small intestine, especially the terminal ileum. Diarrhea, abdominal pain, malnutrition and growth delay are common features of disease that involves the small intestine. Rectal bleeding and extraintestinal manifestations are more commonly associated with colonic involvement. Although the clinical features of the disease are similar in adults and children, complications of chronic inflammation are most frequently seen in adults who by nature of their age, have had inflammation for a longer period of time. Growth retardation and delays in sexual maturation are issues faced primarily by children with Crohn's disease.

The diagnosis of Crohn's disease remains a clinical–pathological diagnosis. Despite the availability of new serological tests, radiological and pathological features are needed to establish a diagnosis. Granulomata or chronic inflammation involving the small and large intestine will enable an experienced pathologist to establish the diagnosis with some certainty. However, if only colonic involvement is present, one may have difficulty distinguishing Crohn's colitis from ulcerative colitis. The distribution of the inflammation, such as rectal sparing or predominantly right-sided disease, may favor Crohn's over ulcerative colitis.

Inflammatory bowel disease (IBD) is thought to result from inappropriate and ongoing activation of the mucosal immune system driven by the presence of normal luminal flora.[2] Despite many advances, the relationship between the environment and the immunogenetics of the host remains unclear. Crohn's disease and ulcerative colitis are collectively referred to as inflammatory bowel diseases, and they are thought to be distinct entities with significant overlap in pathogenesis, clinical presentation and therapeutic management. Understanding the potential mechanism of mucosal immune dysregulation and developing effective therapies in children will not only improve our management of Crohn's disease, but may also prevent the complications of chronic inflammation seen in adults with Crohn's disease. This new knowledge will ultimately improve the life quality of all patients with Crohn's disease.

Epidemiology

General incidence and prevalence

A recent systematic review by Loftus et al[3] analyzed the epidemiology and natural history of Crohn's disease in population-based cohorts from North America. The prevalence rates of Crohn's disease ranged from 26.0 to 198.5 cases per 100 000 persons. The incidence rates ranged from 3.1 to 14.6 cases per 100 000 person-years. Based on an estimate of 300 million people in North America, there are approximately 400 000 to 600 000 patients living with Crohn's disease and approximately 9000 to 44 000 people are newly diagnosed in North America with Crohn's disease each year.[3] There appears to be a slight female predominance, with the percentage of females with Crohn's disease ranging from 48% to 66%.[3]

The prevalence and incidence of IBD is higher in North America and Northern Europe than in Asia,

Africa and southern Europe.[4–9] This geographic difference is also observed within individual countries including the USA.[10] Despite the low incidence and prevalence of IBD in Africa,[11] similar rates for Crohn's disease have been observed between African-American and Caucasian people.[12] Both Crohn's disease and ulcerative colitis appear to have a higher incidence among the Jewish people.[13,14]

Incidence and prevalence in children with inflammatory bowel disease

There is significantly less information about prevalence and incidence rates in children with Crohn's disease. From a study in Sweden,[15] the incidence of Crohn's disease in children appears to be increasing, from 2.4 per 100 000 persons between 1990 and 1992 to 5.4 per 100 000 persons between 1996 and 1998. Similar findings have also been observed by other investigators.[15–17] The peak incidence occurs between the ages of 15 and 25 years, and about 25–30% of patients with Crohn's disease develop the illness before the age of 20 years.[5] In a recent study performed in Wisconsin,[18] the incidence of Crohn's disease was 4.56 per 100 000 children, more than twice the rate of ulcerative colitis (2.14 per 100 000 children). An equal incidence occurred among all ethnic groups, and children from sparsely and densely populated counties were equally affected.[18] A report from the British Pediatric Surveillance Unit revealed an estimated incidence of IBD in the UK of 5.3 per 100 000 children under the age of 16, with Crohn's disease being at least twice as common as ulcerative colitis.[19] The mean age at diagnosis was 11.8 years (median 12.6 years) and 13% of cases occurred in children aged less than 10 years of age.[19] There was a median delay of 5 months from the onset of symptoms to a diagnosis; furthermore, 25% of children experienced symptoms for more than 1 year prior to diagnosis.[19]

Etiology

Genetic factors

Recent studies in identifying susceptibility genes for human IBD have supported the hypothesis that genetic factors play an important role in the development of IBD. Several clinical observations with variations in incidence and prevalence among different populations, co-segregation of IBD in rare kindreds with various genetic disorders and familial aggregation of IBD have suggested that genetic factors contribute to an individual's susceptibility to IBD.[2] First-degree relatives of an affected patient with IBD are 4–20 times more likely to develop the disease than are the background population.[20–23] The absolute risk of IBD is approximately 7% among first-degree family members.[24] In addition, a family history of Crohn's disease is associated with an earlier age of diagnosis in affected patient.[25–27] Observations in twin studies have strongly supported the role of genetic factors in the development of Crohn's disease.[24,28] However, the absence of simple Mendelian inheritance suggests that multiple gene products contribute to a person's risk of IBD.[2]

DNA linkage analyses have identified an area on chromosome 16, designated *IBD1*, with apparent linkage to Crohn's disease but not ulcerative colitis.[29] Several other genomic loci have also been identified in patients with both Crohn's disease and ulcerative colitis.[30–32] Detailed mapping analysis revealed that the *NOD2* gene on chromosome 16 was linked to Crohn's disease.[33,34] The *NOD2* gene encodes a cytoplasmic protein expressed in macrophages known as CARD 15 (caspase activation and recruitment domain). CARD 15 is thought to function as a pattern-recognition receptor for bacterial lipopolysaccharide and to regulate nuclear factor-κB (NFκB) activation and macrophage apoptosis.[2] European and North American patients with Crohn's disease, including those without a family history of IBD are more likely to have a variant of *NOD2* than are persons without Crohn's disease;[2] however, the number of individuals with Crohn's disease who also have a variant of *NOD2* remains very small. A more than 20-fold increase in susceptibility to Crohn's disease (ileal disease in particular) is observed in individuals homozygous for variant *NOD2*.[35–37] In children with Crohn's disease, not only are *NOD2/CARD15* variants associated with ileal disease, but they are also associated with lower weight percentiles at the time of diagnosis.[37] Another putative locus on chromosome 5 has been identified in strong association with early-onset Crohn's disease.[38,39] A list of putative genes identified for IBD is given in Table 23.1.

Table 23.1 Putative genes for inflammatory bowel disease (IBD)

IBD	Locus	Chromosome	Putative genes	Reference
CD				
	IBD1	16q12	NOD2	29
	IBD4	14q11	TCR α/δ complex	32, 164
	IBD5	5q31-33	IL-3, 4, 5, 13, and CSF-2	38
CD, UC				
	IBD6	19p13	ICAM-1, C3, TBXA2R, LTB4H	38
	other	1p36	TNF-R family, CASP9	165
	other	7q	MUC-3	30
	other	3p	HGFR, EGFR, GNAI2	30
UC				
	IBD2	12q13	VDR, INF-γ	30

CD, Crohn's disease; UC, ulcerative colitis

Environmental factors

Despite the genetic association of Crohn's disease, lack of total concordance among monozygotic twins indicates that additional factors may contribute to the pathogenesis of Crohn's disease. Multiple environmental factors have been studied, but when critically evaluated, many do not provide consistent results. The evolving role of epigenetics may be significant in explaining some of these observations.

Dietary component

To date, no specific dietary component has been consistently identified as a cause for IBD. Diets high in refined sugar appear to be associated with the development of Crohn's disease,[40] but not ulcerative colitis.[41] Decreased dietary consumption of fruits and vegetables may be associated with an increased risk of developing Crohn's disease.[40] Increased dietary n-6 polyunsaturated fatty acids relative to n-3 polyunsaturated fatty acids also may be associated with Crohn's disease.[42] Dietary components may alter intestinal flora, which then may modify the mucosal immune response in the susceptible host. Modified carbohydrate diets are used by many patients with Crohn's disease and one should not disregard patients' observations about the impact of specific foods on disease activity. As long as dietary restriction does not impact on nutritional well-being, patient observation will guide these therapies in the absence of randomized controlled studies.

Breast feeding and perinatal exposures

The data supporting the positive or negative association of breast feeding with IBD is not strong. Although studies on children with Crohn's disease and their unaffected siblings suggest that children with Crohn's disease are three to four times less likely to have been breast fed,[43] no apparent association existed between breast feeding and the development of ulcerative colitis.[44] Other data do not indicate an association between breast feeding and Crohn's disease.[45] The negative association between breast feeding and Crohn's disease may be related to early exposure to pathogens. Children with Crohn's disease are three times more likely to have had a diarrheal illness in infancy.[43] Furthermore, in a Swedish study, a four-fold increased risk of IBD was observed in patients who had a history of illness in early infancy.[46]

Cigarette smoking

Cigarette smoking appears to have different effects on the development of Crohn's disease and ulcerative colitis. Smoking doubles the risk for developing Crohn's disease,[47,48] and cessation of smoking may decrease the risk of exacerbation in patients with established Crohn's disease.[49] In contrast, smoking decreases the risk of developing ulcerative colitis.[48,50,51] Although current smokers have about a 40% lower risk of developing ulcerative colitis than non-smokers, former smokers are about 1.5 times more likely to develop ulcerative colitis than those individuals who have never smoked.[51]

Non-steroidal anti-inflammatory drugs

Taking non-steroidal anti-inflammatory drugs (NSAIDs) has been associated with an increased risk for the development and exacerbation of IBD.[52–55] A retrospective study by Bonner et al failed to demonstrate an association between NSAID use and an increased risk for active IBD;[56] however, there may be subsets of IBD patients who can tolerate NSAIDs with less likelihood of an exacerbation of disease.[57] Although the mechanisms of NSAID-associated gastric toxicity have been extensively studied, the mechanisms leading to intestinal damage are poorly understood, but may be related to damage of enterocyte mitochondria causing enhanced intestinal permeability,[58] inhibition of cyclo-oxygenase (COX),[59] enterohepatic recirculation,[60] and formation of drug enterocyte adducts.[61,62]

Both COX-1 and COX-2 serve as constitutive and inducible enzymes in inflammation and cytoprotection.[63] Although selective inhibition of COX-1 or COX-2 is not ulcerogenic, the combined inhibition of COX-1 and COX-2 induced severe lesions in the stomach and small intestine in rats, suggesting an important role for COX-2 in the maintenance of gastrointestinal mucosal integrity.[64,65] While COX-2 selective inhibitors have been shown to cause less gastrointestinal injury than standard NSAIDs in healthy animals and humans,[66,67] their effect on pre-existing gastrointestinal inflammation is not completely clear. COX-1 expression is detected in both non-inflamed and inflamed gastrointestinal mucosa. In contrast, COX-2 is expressed in epithelial cells in the upper portions of the crypts as well as on the surface of colonic enterocytes in Crohn's colitis and ulcerative colitis and in villous epithelial cells in Crohn's ileitis. COX-2 is not detectable in the epithelium of the normal ileum or colon,[68,69] but is up-regulated in the colonic mucosa in both experimental and human colitis[68] and appears to have a beneficial effect in healing experimental colitis. On the other hand, COX products are an important part of the inflammatory process and COX inhibition by agents such as mesalamine might be beneficial.[70]

Oral contraceptive drugs

Data relating oral contraceptive drugs to the development of inflammatory bowel disease have been inconsistent. In two prospective studies,[47,71] oral contraceptive use has been associated with increased risk for developing both Crohn's disease and ulcerative colitis. Women who currently use oral contraceptives are 2.5 times more likely to develop ulcerative colitis and 1.7 times more likely to develop Crohn's disease.[47] Other case–control studies have not found a strong association between the use of oral contraceptives and the development of either Crohn's disease[72] or ulcerative colitis.[73]

Infectious agents

Although available data do not convincingly incriminate a single, persistent pathogen as a universal cause of IBD, the role of infectious agents is still considered a strong possibility as a trigger for the development of IBD. Many infectious agents including *Mycobacterium*, *Chlamydia*, *Listeria monocytogenes*, cell-wall-deficient *Pseudomonas* species and reovirus have been proposed as the causative organism of Crohn's disease. Paramyxovirus (measles virus) has been implicated etiologically in Crohn's disease as a cause of granulomatous vasculitis and microinfarcts of the intestine.[74] However, the tissue evidence for persistent measles infection in patients with Crohn's disease remains controversial.[75,76] One Swedish study demonstrated an increased incidence of Crohn's disease but not ulcerative colitis among individuals born during measles epidemics;[77] however, two other studies from the UK failed to establish an association between the development of Crohn's disease and birth during measles epidemics.[78,79] The relationship between measles vaccination and the development of Crohn's disease has evoked even more acrimonious discussion. Although one initial study reported that the relative risk for developing Crohn's disease and ulcerative colitis was 3.0 and 2.5, respectively, in children who received the measles vaccine,[80] subsequent studies failed to confirm these findings.[81,82] *Mycobacterium paratuberculosis* has been cultured from the bowel of patients with IBD, but definitive evidence to link a mycobacterium to Crohn's disease is lacking.[83–85]

Commensal bacterial flora is an important etiological factor in IBD. Bacteria within the enteric lumen have a complex ecosystem that is in contact with the external environment. There are 10^{12} bacteria/g feces in the colon, of 400 different species, with anaerobes predominating.[86] The numbers of anaerobic bacteria and *Lactobacillus* are significantly decreased in patients with active, but not inactive, IBD.[87] Genetically altered animals that are susceptible to acquiring IBD do not express the phenotype when raised in a germ-free environment.[88,89] Furthermore, experimental colitis is attenuated when animals are treated with broad-spectrum antibiotics.[90] Further studies by Duchmann et al demonstrated that mucosal, but not peripheral blood mononuclear cells from patients with IBD proliferate when exposed to autologous intestinal bacteria. These data support the hypothesis that normal flora function as a modulator of 'physiological inflammation'.[91,92] Patients with IBD have increased numbers of surface-adherent and intracellular bacteria in the colonic epithelium,[93,94] and these commensal organisms may be playing a role in the development and maintenance of mucosal inflammation.

Others factors

Several studies have suggested that appendectomy may protect against the occurrence and severity of ulcerative colitis.[95–99] However, appendectomy does not affect the disease course of ulcerative colitis.[100] The relationship between appendectomy and the risk of developing Crohn's disease is controversial.[99,100] In a large, retrospective cohort study, Andersson et al demonstrated that an increased risk of Crohn's disease was found for more than 20 years after appendectomy. This increased risk was dependent on the patient's gender, age and the diagnosis at operation (non-perforated vs. perforated appendicitis).[101] In T cell receptor (TCR)-α-deficient mice, appendectomy is protective against the development of colitis.[102]

Pathophysiology

Growing evidence suggests that inflammatory bowel disease is the result of a dysregulated immune response to common luminal flora. The intestinal inflammation of IBD may be viewed as an exaggeration of the 'physiological' inflammatory response always present in the normal lamina propria of the intestine and colon.[103] An intact mucosal barrier and regulatory mechanisms normally prevent the immune and inflammatory responses from causing tissue injury.[103] A defect in either mucosal barrier function, antigen processing or immunoregulation could result in a chronic inflammation, lymphocyte proliferation, cytokine release, neutrophil recruitment and tissue damage.[103] The factors that trigger activation of the immune system are unclear, but could be related to an intrinsic defect (either constitutive activation or the failure of down-regulatory mechanisms) or ongoing stimulation resulting from a change in the epithelial mucosal barrier.[2]

Data from studies on tissue samples from patients with IBD and experimental animal models of colitis have demonstrated unbalanced Th1 vs. Th2 responses in the intestinal mucosa.[84,104,105] The mucosa of patients with established Crohn's disease is dominated by $CD4^+$ lymphocytes with a Th1 phenotype, characterized by the production of interferon-γ and interleukin (IL)-2;[2] whereas the mucosa in patients with ulcerative colitis may be dominated by $CD4^+$ lymphocytes with an atypical Th2 phenotype, characterized by the production of transforming growth factor (TGF)-β and IL-5, but not IL-4.[2] $CD4^+$ lymphocytes clearly play an important role in the pathogenesis of tissue damage in inflammatory bowel disease, particularly in Crohn's disease.[84,106] Patients with disorders such as glycogen storage disease 1b, which are associated with abnormalities in neutrophil function may exhibit clinical manifestations of IBD. These observations suggest that the mechanisms leading to mucosal injury are not always lymphocyte dependent.

Loss of tolerance towards the luminal commensal bacterial flora appears to be an important factor in the pathophysiology of IBD. Concomitant decrease of production of TGF-β and IL-10 by regulatory T lymphocytes may be partially responsible for the loss of tolerance to luminal flora and activation of

Th1 cells.[107–109] Results from murine studies have shown that Th1 cytokines activate macrophages, which in turn, produce IL-12, IL-18 and macrophage migration inhibitor factor, thereby stimulating a Th1 response in a self-sustaining cycle.[110,111] Activated macrophages produce a variety of potent proinflammatory cytokines including tumor necrosis factor (TNF)-α, IL-1 and IL-6. TNF-α has a variety of biological effects, including: macrophage activation and induction of protease, both of which can play a role in tissue destruction;[112] up-regulation of adhesion molecule expression, facilitating recruitment of monocytes, lymphocytes and granulocytes;[113] enhancement of chloride secretion from intestinal epithelial cells;[114] increase of epithelial cell permeability;[115] and enhancement of production of acute-phase reactants.[112] The inflammatory process and tissue destruction of the intestine are further promoted by generation of various proinflammatory mediators including other cytokines, chemokines, growth factors, arachidonic acid metabolites (prostaglandins and leukotrienes) and reactive oxygen metabolites such as nitric oxide.[2] Activation of this destructive process results in the mucosal injury and clinical manifestations of IBD.

Clinical signs and symptoms

The initial clinical presentation of Crohn's disease may be subtle, variable, non-specific and easily overlooked. Common symptoms include abdominal pain, diarrhea and/or weight loss.[103] A plateau in linear growth, delayed pubertal development, perianal lesions, fever, pallor, hematochezia and digital clubbing may also be present.[103] Crohn's disease may affect any area of the gastrointestinal tract from the lips to the perianal area. In a study on Scottish children and adolescents with Crohn's disease,[116] approximately 30% of patients had disease limited to the terminal ileum, 20% of patients had exclusive colonic involvement and 50% of patients had both ileal and colonic involvement. In a more recent population-based study in Wisconsin, at the time of diagnosis isolated ileal disease was identified in 25% and ileocolonic involvement was found in 29%. About one-third of children had colonic involvement and 14% had disease in the upper gastrointestinal tract.[18] The inflammation associated with ulcerative colitis is limited to the colon, with the exception of mild inflammation in the ileum, termed 'backwash ileitis'.

The constellation of abdominal pain, diarrhea, poor appetite and weight loss represents the classic presentation of Crohn's disease in children of any age group.[103] Frequently, the onset of pain is insidious and intermittent. Families and care providers often dismiss the symptoms as an acute illness, or a condition related to anxiety. In some individuals, anorexia may be the primary manifestation prompting an evaluation for anorexia nervosa or an eating disorder. Laboratory studies may suggest chronic inflammation, but up to 20% of children with IBD have a normal erythrocyte sedimentation rate. A summary of the prevalence of various clinical presentations from two separate studies is shown in Table 23.2. Abdominal pain is the most common single symptom at presentation, and may be periumbilical or localized to the right lower quadrant or to the lower abdomen. Grossly bloody diarrhea or extraintestinal manifestations signify colonic involvement. When diarrhea is predominant without visible blood or the patient has clubbing, one should suspect small-bowel involvement. Uncontrolled gastrointestinal hemorrhage is rare in Crohn's disease, but may occur with an ileal ulcer.

Clinical case 1

A 6-year-old boy developed swollen lips (Figure 23.1) and painful ulcers in his mouth. He denied any history of abdominal pain, but his weight was decreased. An upper gastrointestinal series with small-bowel follow-through was normal. He had a history of anal fissures in the past and because of hard stools, he had been treated with stool softeners. An upper endoscopy and colonoscopy did not reveal evidence of inflammation, but a biopsy of the buccal mucosa demonstrated granulomatous cheilitis. He was treated with oral prednisone and metronidazole, with an initial improvement. He developed hepatitis while taking 6-mercaptopurine. Three infusions of infliximab were not effective. His perianal disease improved with a course of 20 hyperbaric oxygen sessions. Nutritional therapy with nightly nasogastric tube feedings for 2

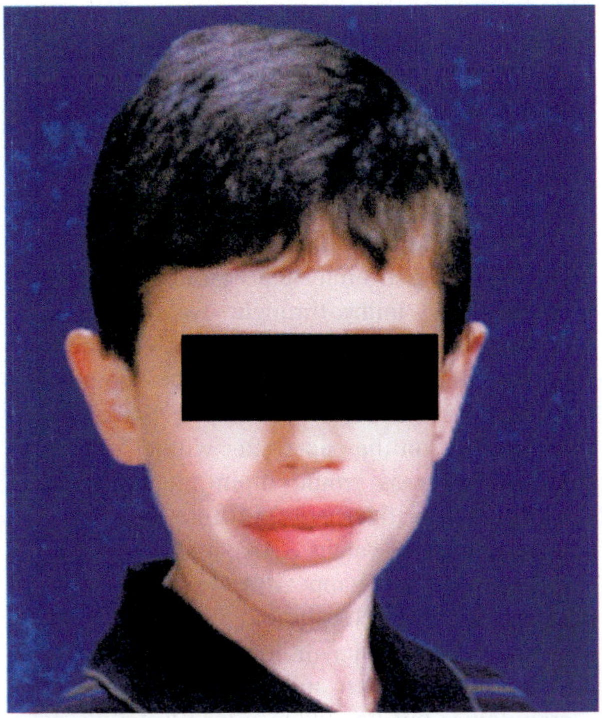

Figure 23.1 Swollen lips in a child with Crohn's disease involving the oral mucosa.

years has contributed to his maintaining his weight and growth, but he has been unable to tolerate sufficient caloric intake to have catch-up growth. Five years after his initial presentation, he has developed chronic inflammatory changes in the colon.

Points of interest

(1) Crohn's disease may present in any region of the gastrointestinal tract;

(2) One-third of patients with Crohn's disease do not respond to infliximab;

(3) Nutritional therapy is important adjunctive therapy.

Impaired linear growth and concomitant delay in sexual maturation are important clinical manifestations in children with Crohn's disease, that may precede the onset of intestinal symptoms by 12–18 months.[103] In a prospective study of children with IBD,[117] 30% of children with Crohn's disease had growth delay, which was defined as a fall in the height centile of more than 0.3 standard deviation per year, a growth velocity of less than 5 cm per year, or a decrease in the growth velocity of ≥ 2 cm compared with the preceeding year. About 50% of children had evidence of decreased height velocity prior to the diagnosis of Crohn's disease.[118] Delayed linear growth velocity and sexual maturation may be related to a chronically insufficient dietary intake and/or an increased energy requirements related to chronic inflammation or fever.[118,119] Anorexia occurs in 30% of children with Crohn's disease and may be related to upper gastrointestinal tract involvement.[120] Studies in a rat colitis model demonstrated that TNF-α inhibited maturation of growth plate chondrocytes,[121] suggesting that some proinflammatory cytokines

Table 23.2 Prevalence of clinical presentations in Crohn's disease from two studies (references 103 and 166)

Clinical symptoms	Percentage (n=386)[103]	Percentage (n=40)[166]
Abdominal pain	86	95
Weight loss	80	80
Diarrhea	78	77
Blood in the stool	49	60
Perianal lesions	44	*
Fevers	38	*
Growth failure	*	30
Mouth ulcers	28	*
Arthralgia/arthritis	17	*
Skin lesions	8	*

*Prevalence was not specified

may be a factor in the growth delay observed in children with Crohn's disease.

Anemia is present in 25–85% of patients with Crohn's disease,[122] many of whom have anemia of chronic disease. Iron deficiency anemia is microcytic and may result from gastrointestinal blood loss, malabsorption of iron in the duodenum and jejunum because of inflammation and/or a lack of adequate oral intake. Folate deficiency causes a megaloblastic anemia, but frequently folate deficiency is associated with iron deficiency as well, and the indices may not be macrocytic. Folate deficiency is most commonly due to nutritional causes, but patients who take sulfasalazine are at increased risk for developing folate deficiency. For that reason, sulfasalazine is always prescribed with folate supplementation. Vitamin B_{12} is absorbed in the ileum; deficiencies are usually related to lack of absorption, related to inflammatory changes, fibrosis or resection. Because many years may be required to deplete vitamin B_{12} stores in an individual who has a normal reserve, the development of deficiency is often insidious. Children with ileal disease should be monitored for vitamin B_{12} deficiency by measuring serum levels. Clinical manifestations of the disease – anemia, dermatitis, cheilitis, decreased serum transaminases, peripheral neuritis, irritability and posterior column signs – do not develop for many months.

Clinical case 2

A 13-year-old girl was referred for evaluation of lower abdominal pain, diarrhea and a perirectal abscess. She had had intermittent abdominal pain from infancy but about 1 year prior to evaluation noted an increase in frequency and intensity. Her pediatrician recommended a lactose-restricted diet and the pain completely resolved. Two months prior to her referral to a pediatric gastroenterologist, she developed a perirectal abscess that was drained by a surgeon. The abscess healed slowly. She reported having 4–5 loose stools daily, but never noticed any blood. Her appetite was good and her rate of growth was not changed. There was no family history of IBD but her mother has Sjögren's syndrome, a maternal second cousin has juvenile dermatomyositis and her maternal grandfather has rheumatoid arthritis. Her physical examination was normal with the exception of a well-healed surgical incision about 4cm from the anus. Her weight was 25% for age; her height was 50% for age. A complete blood count (CBC), erythrocyte sedimentation rate (ESR) and liver function tests were normal. An upper gastro-intestinal radiograph with small-bowel follow-through was read as normal. Over the next 10 weeks she continued to experience intermittent crampy abdominal pain and occasional loose stools. She noted some blood on the paper after wiping and the perianal abscess would drain intermittently. However, over this period of time she continued to gain weight. An ileocolonoscopy revealed a normal-appearing ileum and right colon with multiple aphthoid lesions in the left colon and erythema in the rectum. Biopsies identified an active and chronic ileitis with granulomas but no evidence for ulceration, as well as microscopic changes of chronic and active inflammatory changes in the left colon with erosions.

She was started on mesalamine and metronidazole. She began to feel better after 1 week of therapy, but then had recurrence of crampy abdominal pain with nausea and increased frequency of stooling up to seven loose bowel movements daily. Two weeks after starting therapy, prednisone 20mg twice a day was prescribed. Metronidazole was discontinued because of dysesthesia in her hands. After 3 weeks of taking prednisone, she was quite Cushingoid, but she was passing three formed bowel movements daily and the perianal abscess was not draining. She began to taper the dose of prednisone by 5mg/day every week. When she reached 30mg of prednisone daily, she began to have increased frequency of stooling and crampy abdominal pain. Because of concerns for steroid dependence, she was started on 50mg daily of 6-mercaptopurine after it was checked that her thiopurine methyltransferase (TPMT) activity was in the normal range. A CBC and differential, liver function tests and amylase were checked weekly for 3 weeks and then monthly. She tolerated the 6-mercaptopurine well and was able to discontinue prednisone after 5 months. She was maintained on mesalamine and 6-mercaptopurine.

After 18 months of therapy, she began to develop intermittent abdominal pain and diarrhea. Her symptoms increased despite therapy with metronidazole and ciprofloxacin. She began to lose weight. Infliximab was started and 1 week after the initial infusion, she began to improve. She completed a second infusion 2 weeks after the first and a third infusion 6 weeks after the second infusion. She is now maintained on 6-mercaptopurine and an infliximab infusion every 8 weeks and remains without gastrointestinal symptoms.

Points of interest

(1) The onset of Crohn's disease is often insidious;

(2) Radiographic studies in the early stages of Crohn's disease may appear normal;

(3) Mucosal biopsy of normal-appearing endoscopic areas may provide evidence for inflammatory bowel disease;

(4) Mesalamine with or without antibiotics may be effective therapy in some children with new-onset mild-to-moderate Crohn's disease, but therapy should be changed if there is not a response within 2–4 weeks;

(5) The inability to tolerate a taper of corticosteroids is an indication to begin 6-mercaptopurine;

(6) Therapy with 6-mercaptopurine may take at least 3 months to become effective;

(7) When 6-mercaptopurine fails to control symptoms of Crohn's disease, infliximab should be considered. About two-thirds of adults will have an initial response to infliximab.

Perianal lesions may be the first presenting feature of Crohn's disease. Perianal disease associated with Crohn's disease is frequently mild with small perianal skin tags or anal fissures, but more severe problems such as perianal fistulae and abscesses may develop. Fortunately, less than 5% of children with Crohn's disease will develop a highly destructive form of perianal disease with recurrent abscesses and fistulae (Figure 23.2) involving the genitalia, and often resulting in rectal strictures.[123,124] As illustrated in Case 2, the patient was thought to have a perirectal abscess, but after surgical intervention, the area did not heal. With the exception of the first 2 years of life, children with persistent perianal abscess, fissure or fistula that does not respond to topical treatment and antibiotics should be evaluated for Crohn's disease prior to the initiation of surgical therapy. Approximately one-third of children with Crohn's disease can have significant perianal abnormalities during the course of their disease.[123] The most common perianal problem is skin tags which may become quite large. Some may become inflamed and painful, but for many adolescents they become a source of embarrassment. Perianal inflammatory disease may respond to antibiotics that have good anaerobic coverage, such as metronidazole, but intravenous administration is frequently required to achieve maximal healing. Non-inflamed skin

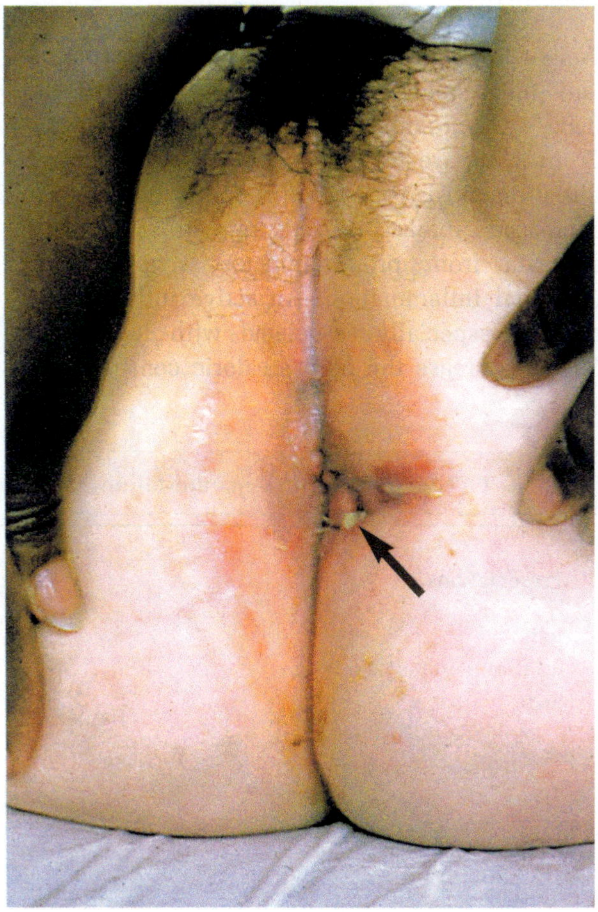

Figure 23.2 Perianal fistula in a child with Crohn's disease. Arrow marks the opening of the fistula. The erythema is commonly seen because of the excoriation to the skin caused by the drainage onto the perineum.

tags usually do not resolve with medical treatment, and the use of topical tacrolimus or corticosteroids has not proved to be beneficial in reducing the size of the skin tags. Immunomodulators or corticosteroids may be necessary to control mucosal inflammation which may be a contributing factor to the growth of perianal skin tags.

Extraintestinal manifestations are usually associated with colonic involvement of Crohn's disease, and may precede intestinal symptoms by many months. The commonly involved organs are joints, skin, liver, eye and bone; the manifestations are listed in Table 23.3.[125,126] At least one extraintestinal manifestation is present in about 25–35% of adults with IBD.[125]

Complications

Malnutrition

Weight loss and malnutrition are the most prevalent nutritional disturbances in patients with IDB.[103] Approximately 85% of children with Crohn's disease have a history of weight loss at initial diagnosis.[127] Malnutrition is mainly due to decreased intake caused by either primary anorexia from proinflammatory cytokines, or intestinal inflammation. An active inflammatory process, especially associated with fever, may further increase the body's caloric consumption. Estimates suggest that an increase in 1°C increases the metabolic rate by 7%. For this reason, children with Crohn's disease who experience recurrent febrile episodes often need to receive additional calories.

As the result of the location of chronic intestinal inflammation in Crohn's disease, a variety of micronutrient deficiencies may occur. These deficiencies include water-soluble vitamins (mainly folic acid and vitamin B_{12}), fat-soluble vitamin D, and minerals (iron, copper and zinc).[103] Deficiency of these micronutrients may be subclinical or associated with specific clinical signs and symptoms (Table 23.4). The following factors may create or potentiate specific nutrient deficiencies: inadequate intake, the inflammatory/immunological response, poor absorption, increased nutrient demand for tissue repair or concurrent usage of specific medications. The severity of nutrient deficiency is often associated with the duration of disease and the degree of Crohn's disease activity.

Hepatobiliary and pancreatic complications

Bile salts are absorbed in the distal ileum via an enterohepatic circulation. Malabsorption of bile salts caused by ileal inflammation or resection results in increased colonic bile salts and diarrhea. Bile salt malabsorption also may predispose towards gallstone formation. Agents that bind bile acids may be beneficial in these clinical situations.

Table 23.3 Extraintestinal manifestations of Crohn's disease

Presentations	Percentage	Reference
Joint		
arthritis/arthralgia	2*, 15 (adult data)	126
Skin		
erythema nodosum	1*, 8–15 (adult data)	18, 125
pyoderma gangrenosum	0.5*, 1.3 (adult data)	
Eye		
episcleritis		125, 126
uveitis		
orbital myositis		
Hepatobiliary involvement	3*	18
PSC	<1*	
Pancreatitis	1*	18

* At time of diagnosis. PSC, primary sclerosing cholangitis

Table 23.4 Micronutrient deficiencies

Micronutrient	Prevalence	Clinical presentations	Laboratory test	RDA	Reference
Water-soluble vitamins					
Vitamin B_{12}	20–60%	macrocytic anemia, neuropathy	plasma vitamin B_{12} level	1.5–3 µg for children; 3 µg for adults	168 169 170
Vitamin C	*	scurvy (ecchymoses, gingival bleeding, petechiae, hyperkeratosis, arthralgia, poor wound healing	plasma vitamin C level	40–45 mg for children 60–125 mg for adults	171 172 173 174
Folate	34–54%	macrocytic anemia	plasma folate level	200–400 µg for children; 400 µg for adults	127 168 175
Thiamine (vitamin B_1)	*	beriberi-like symptoms (neuropathy, cardiomyopathy, encephalopathy, gastrointestinal symptoms)	erythrocyte thiamine transketolase (ETKA), or blood thiamine concentration, or transketolase urinary thiamine excretion	0.9–1.5 mg for children; 1–1.4 mg for adults	122 169
Nicotinic acid	*	pellagra (dermatitis, diarrhea and dementia)	? plasma nicotinic acid level	12–20 mg for children and adults	122 169 176 177
Riboflavin (B_2)	*	photophobia, angular stomatitis, dermatitis	plasma riboflavin level	0.4 mg for infants; 1.1–1.8 mg for children and adults	122 169 177 178
Pyridoxine (vitamin B_6)	*	neuropathy, glossitis, dermatitis	plasma pyrodoxal-5-phophate (PLP) level, or erythrocyte transaminase activity, or urinary 4-pyridoxic acid excretion, or urinary excretion of xanthurenic acid	0.9–2 mg for children; 2 mg for adults	122 169 178
Fat-soluble vitamins					
Vitamin A	11%	xerophthalmia (dry eyes and skin, blindness)	plasma retinol level	2500–4000 IU for children; 4000–5000 IU for adults	171 172 179 180 181
Vitamin D	75%	osteomalacia, rickets	plasma vitamin D level	400 IU for children and adults	122 182
Vitamin E	*	neuromuscular disorders, hemolysis and anemia	plasma vitamin E level	9–15 IU for children and 30 IU for adults	171 172 173
Vitamin K	*	bleeding diathesis		20–80 µg for children; 65–80 µg for adults	168

continued

Table 23.4 continued Micronutrient deficiencies

Micronutrient	Prevalence	Clinical presentations	Laboratory test	RDA	Reference
Minerals					
Calcium	13%	osteopenia, rickets	plasma calcium level	800–1200 mg for children and adults	168 173
Copper	*	skin and hair abnormalities	plasma copper level	0.4–0.6 mg for infants; 1.5–3 mg for children and adults	183
Iron	39–81%	microcytic anemia	plasma iron level	10–18 mg for children and adults	168 184
Magnesium	14–33%	myopathy	plasma magnesium level	200–400 mg for children; 300–350 mg for adults	122 168 169 185 186 187
Selenium	*	cardiomyopathy, encephalopathy, immune dysfunction	plasma selenium level	20-50 µg for children; 55–70 µg for adults	173 188 189 190 191
Zinc	40–50%	growth retardation, alopecia, dysgeusia, acrodermatitis, impaired wound healing	plasma zinc level	10–15 µg for children; 15 mg for adults	122 168 192 193

* Not specified
RDA, recommended daily allowance

Pancreatitis can occur as a result of inflammation in the duodenum or by medications such as azathioprine, 6-mercaptopurine or 5-aminosalicylic acid.[103] In some patients, the cause of pancreatitis is unknown and may be recurrent. Pancreatic insufficiency and carbohydrate intolerance are rare in Crohn's disease, but a trial of pancreatic enzyme supplementation may be beneficial in treating inflammation.

Nephrolithiasis

Patients with Crohn's disease have an increased risk of developing calcium oxalate and uric acid renal stones as a result of chronic steatorrhea and diarrhea. Under normal circumstances, free dietary calcium binds to oxalate in the intestinal lumen and is eliminated in the stool. In patients with steatorrhea, increased luminal fatty acids competitively bind free dietary calcium and leave oxalate free to be absorbed. The increased oxalate absorption results in hyperoxaluria. Dehydration and metabolic acidosis potentiate the formation of uric acid stones.

Thromboembolic events

Venous and arterial thromboembolism can result from hypercoaguability caused by thrombocytosis, hyperfibrinogenemia, elevated factor V and factor VII, and depression of antithrombin III.[128,129] A retrospective study by Talbot et al in 7199 adult patients with either chronic ulcerative colitis or Crohn's disease demonstrated that thromboembolic complications developed in 92 (1.3%) of these patients.[130] An additional four patients had cutaneous vasculitis, and 17 had an arteritis-associated diagnosis. Of the thromboembolic complications, 61 were deep vein thromboses or pulmonary emboli.[130] Peripheral arterial thrombosis, coronary thrombosis, and mesenteric and portal vein thrombosis were predominantly post-surgical complications, but 77% of peripheral venous thromboses occurred spontaneously.[130,131] In isolated case reports, cerebrovascular accidents have occurred in children with Crohn's disease with seizures being the primary presenting symptom.[132–134] Retinal vascular disease can also occur in patients with Crohn's disease.[129,135,136] Children with clinical evidence of a hypercoagulable state should be evaluated for underlying causes. Dehydration and indwelling catheters are the main risk factors that should be avoided.

Metabolic bone disease

Decreased bone density is an important and probably underdiagnosed complication in children with Crohn's disease. Multiple factors, including inflammatory cytokines that inhibit osteoclast activity, vitamin D deficiency and chronic systemic steroid therapy, may contribute to osteopenia or osteoporosis. Therefore, in children with Crohn's disease, it is crucial to assess bone density and decrease the risk factors for osteoporosis such as lack of physical exercise, chronic steroid use, lack of hormonal therapy of chronic secondary amenorrhea in adolescent girls, and deficient calcium and vitamin D supplementation.[103] Bisphosphonates are synthetic analogs of inorganic pyrophosphate that inhibit bone resorption (Table 23.5). In a recent randomized study of 84 adult patients with Crohn's disease and osteopenia/osteoporosis, the efficacy of ibandronate and sodium fluoride as adjuncts to calcium and vitamin D treatment was evaluated.[137] The results showed that both ibandronate and sodium fluoride were effective, safe and well tolerated in inducing an increase in lumbar bone density.[137] Experience is very limited with bisphosphonate therapy in children who have metabolic bone disease associated with Crohn's disease. Results from ongoing multicenter trials of bisphosphonate in children with Crohn's disease will provide valuable information.

Local intestinal complications

Intestinal obstruction, severe hemorrhage, perforation, fistulae, intra-abdominal abscesses and toxic megacolon can occur as a result of chronic intestinal inflammation. Mucosal ulceration may result in bleeding and perforation depending on the site and size of the ulcer. Fibrosis, a complication of inflammation, may result in stricture formation that

Table 23.5 Bisphosphonate preparations

Preparations	Potency within generation	Potency across generation
First generation		low
Etidronate		↓
Second generation	high	
Pamidronate	↓	
Clodronate		
Tiludronate	low	
Third generation	high	
Zolendronate	↓	
Ibandronate		
Risedronate		
Olpadronate		
Alendronate		
Neridronate		
Incadronate	low	high

predisposes the patient to fistula, abscess, obstruction and perforation. In contrast to fibrosis, which usually accompanies Crohn's disease, perforation and toxic megacolon are unusual and most commonly associated with ulcerative colitis. These conditions may require surgical intervention.

Diagnosis

The list of conditions that should be considered in the differential diagnosis for Crohn's disease is extensive, and is related to the various clinical presentations of Crohn's disease (Table 23.6). A high index of clinical suspicion is crucial if the clinician is to make a diagnosis in the early phases of the illness. Delay in growth is often a clue that the presenting symptoms are not caused by an acute illness.

Clinical suspicion for Crohn's disease

It is important to rule out Crohn's disease in any child with recurrent abdominal pain, chronic diarrhea, weight loss, blood in stools, growth delay, pubertal delay, unexplained anemia and perianal disease. Growth failure can be an important initial clue in suspecting Crohn's disease, since approximately half the children with Crohn's disease have a delay in height velocity prior to obvious intestinal manifestation.[118] For patients with abdominal pain or growth delay, accompanying anorexia, change in diet, diarrhea or extraintestinal manifestations should raise the possibility of Crohn's disease. If fecal leukocytes are found in a patient with hematochezia, inflammatory/infectious causes should be considered. Although 20% of patients with Crohn's disease may have a normal ESR, if it is abnormal, this non-specific marker of inflammation may have relevance.

Table 23.6 Differential diagnosis of Crohn's disease

Symptoms	Differential diagnosis
Constitutional	
recurrent fever, malaise, pallor	collagen vascular disease, infection, malignancy, especially lymphoma
Intestinal	
abdominal pain	lactose intolerance, constipation, peptic ulcer disease, *Helicobacter pylori*, irritable bowel syndrome or psychosocial stress
diarrhea	infectious colitis/enteritis (*Salmonella, Shigella, Campylobacter, Yersinia*); immunodeficiency (HIV, primary immune deficiency)
heme-positive stool/hematochezia	ulcerative colitis, infectious colitis including *Shigella, Salmonella, Campylobacter, Escherichia coli* O157:H7 and amebiasis, *Clostridium difficile* colitis, CMV colitis, vasculitis, Henoch–Schönlein purpura; juvenile polyp, Meckel's diverticulum, fissure, hemorrhoid
fever, acute severe abdominal pain	appendicitis, diverticulitis, intestinal perforation
perianal disease	histiocytosis, immunodeficiency
Abnormal liver profile	viral hepatitis, toxin, cholelithiasis
Abnormal pancreatic enzymes	idopathic pancreatitis, familial pancreatitis, cystic fibrosis
Growth failure	celiac disease, cystic fibrosis, endocrinopathy (thyroid, adrenal, pituitary, especially growth hormone), anorexia nervosa,
Pubertal delay	anorexia nervosa; bulimia; chromosomal abnormality
Arthritis	juvenile rheumatoid arthritis, acute rheumatic fever

CMV, cytomegalovirus

Findings on physical examination such as pallor and abdominal tenderness are most often not specific for Crohn's disease, but abdominal mass, aphthoid oral ulcers, erythema nodosum, pyoderma gangrenosum, digital clubbing, arthritis, or perianal skin tags are highly suggestive of Crohn's disease.

Laboratory studies

A number of laboratory tests can offer useful and supportive information in facilitating diagnosis, although they are generally non-specific. An initial screening evaluation with CBC with differential, platelet count, ESR, serum albumin, stool hemoccult test, and stool culture are often obtained. Serum iron studies and serum levels of vitamins A, E, B_{12} and folate can be helpful in assessing specific nutritional deficiencies.

Serological markers

Several serological markers have been reported to facilitate the diagnosis of IBD and in distinguishing between Crohn's disease and ulcerative colitis. Although these tests may have benefit in some clinical situations, the diagnosis remains to be determined by clinical–pathological criteria. Atypical perinuclear antineutrophil cytoplasmic antibodies (atypical P-ANCA, i.e. not directed against myeloperoxidase) can be detected in 60–80% of adult patients with ulcerative colitis and 10–20% of adult patients with Crohn's disease.[138–140] In children with IBD, a positive test for P-ANCA and a negative test for anti-*Saccharomyces cerevisiae* antibody (ASCA) are indicative of increased likelihood of ulcerative colitis rather than Crohn's disease (sensitivity 57%, specificity 97%).[139] Conversely, a negative P-ANCA test and a positive ASCA test in children with IBD are suggestive of Crohn's disease (sensitivity 49%, specificity 97%). The relatively low sensitivities of these serological markers for establishing a diagnosis of Crohn's disease and ulcerative colitis limit their widespread clinical utility.[103] Antibody against *Escherichia coli* outer membrane porin (anti-OmpC antibody) has been reported as a potential serological marker for Crohn's disease. It is a curious finding that the markers that are associated with Crohn's disease are related to a host response to luminal organisms (i.e. yeast and bacteria). As experience increases in the pediatric population with the relationship between phenotype and serological markers, they may become more clinically relevant.

Radiographic studies

Barium upper gastrointestinal series with small-bowel follow-through is a useful tool in diagnosing gastroduodenal and ileal involvement of Crohn's disease (Figure 23.3). Radiographic features in patients with Crohn's disease include narrowing of the lumen of the small intestine or colon with nodularity and ulceration, a 'string' sign when luminal narrowing becomes more advanced or with severe spasm, a cobblestone appearance, fistulae and abscess formation, and separation of bowel loops, a manifestation reflecting the transmural inflammation and bowel wall thickening. Antral narrowing and segmental structuring of the duodenum can be seen with gastroduodenal Crohn's disease.

Air-contrast barium enema may be helpful in detecting colonic lesions such as ulcers, strictures and fistulae, but these colonic radiographs have been largely replaced by colonoscopy. In specific clinical situations, such as a distal stricture that does not permit visual inspection of the more proximal colon, virtual colonoscopy may be of benefit. Inflammation limited to the colon may make it difficult to distinguish ulcerative colitis from Crohn's colitis; however, radiographic disease in the small intestine, stomach or esophagus strongly supports a diagnosis of Crohn's disease.

Computerized tomography (CT) scans have become extremely valuable in the assessment of the child with established Crohn's disease who presents with abdominal pain or fever. The use of oral, rectal and or intravenous contrast increases the likelihood of finding a fistula, stricture or abscess. For the child with perianal disease, a careful CT scan with narrow cuts may identify a small perirectal abscess.

Scintigraphy

Scintigraphy with the 99mTc hexamethyl, propylene amino oxime (HMPAO)-labeled leukocyte scan (99mTc white blood cell (WBC) scan) has been

(a) (b)

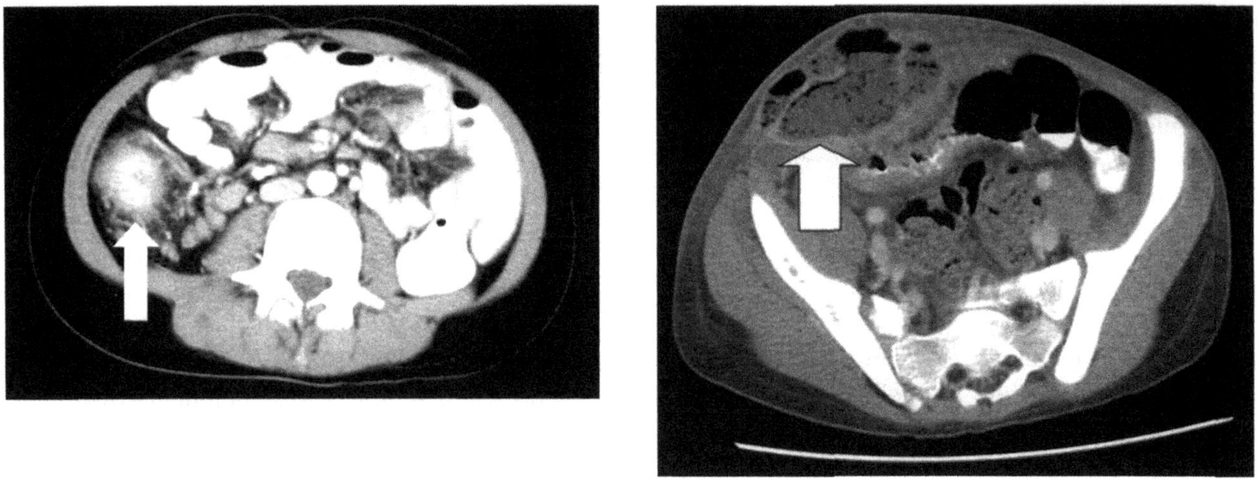

(c)

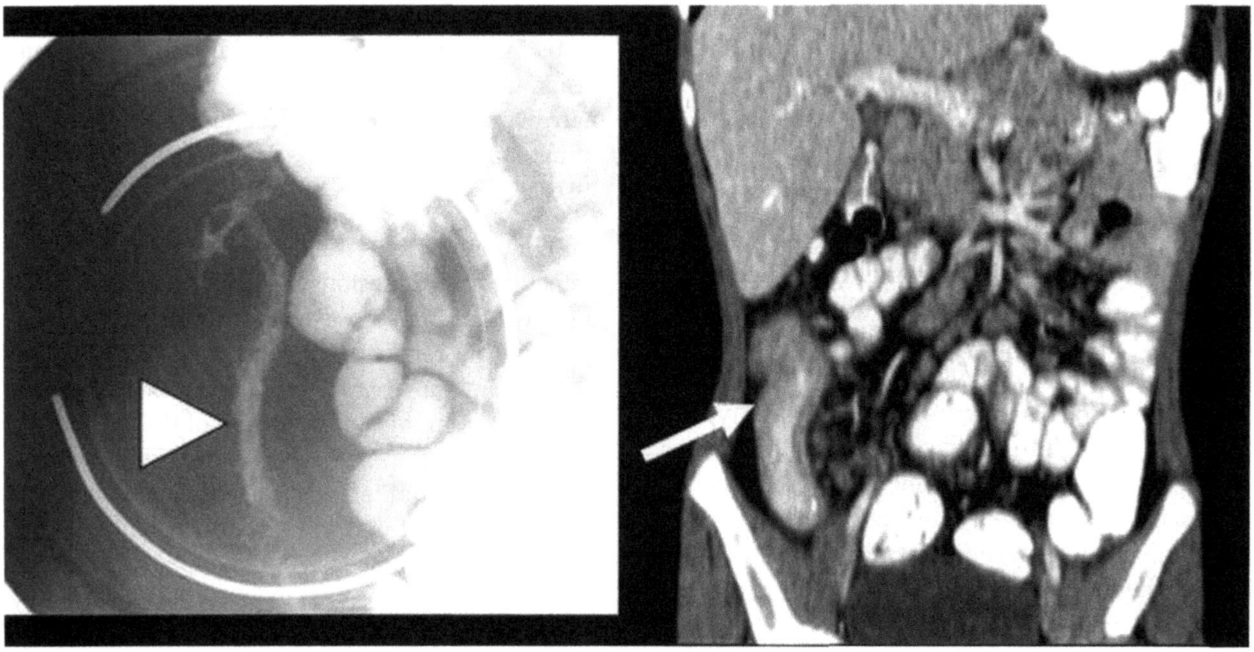

(d)

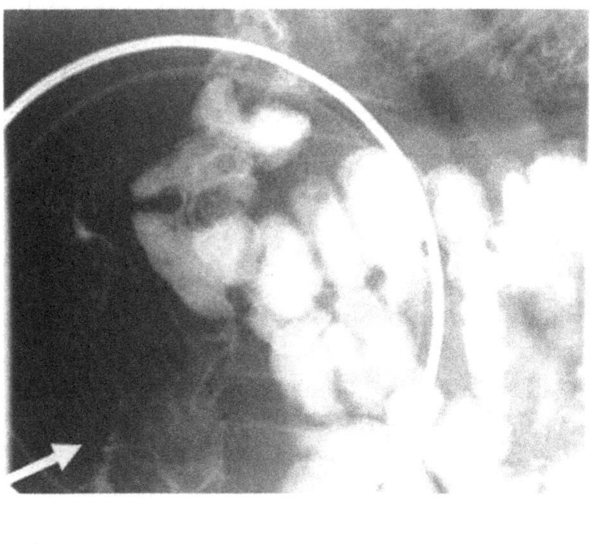

Figure 23.3 (a) Axial computerized tomography (CT) images with intravenous and oral contrast revealing abnormal mucosal thickening of the cecum with abnormal enhancement. Numerous enlarged mesenteric lymph nodes are present (arrow). (b) This 15-year-old child with Crohn's disease developed a large abscess in the anterior abdominal wall (arrow).(c) Markedly narrowed terminal ileum with ulcerations seen on a barium study (arrowhead). The same small bowel loop is seen on a coronal reformatted CT image (white arrow). (d) Small fistula tracks are seen extending from a thickened, inflamed terminal ileum to the ascending colon (arrow). (Courtesy of Dr Sudha Anupindi).

used as an alternative, non-invasive diagnostic test to determine the extent and distribution of inflammation in children with IBD.[142–144] In one study,[141] the result of the 99mTc WBC scan correlated with histological findings on endoscopic and colonoscopic biopsies in 128 of 137 children. The sensitivity and specificity were 90% and 97%, respectively.[141] Nevertheless, the value of this study for diagnosis is limited.

Endoscopic studies and histologic features

Compared with the continuous distribution of ulcerative colitis, Crohn's disease is characteristically segmental, with areas of sparing throughout the intestinal tract; the terminal ileum is the most commonly affected site.[103] Data from a study in 389 children and adolescents with Crohn's disease[103] revealed that 29% of patients had involvement of the terminal ileum with or without cecal disease, 9% had more isolated proximal (ileal or jejunal) disease, 42% had ileocolonic inflammation and 20% had only colonic involvement.

Endoscopic examination is an important diagnostic tool for Crohn's disease and colonoscopy is the most effective test to determine whether the colon is affected. Crohn's disease often spares the rectosigmoid region, but this pattern of involvement may also be seen in early ulcerative colitis, especially in young patients. The colonoscopic features of Crohn's disease range from subtle focal aphthoid ulcerations adjacent to areas of normal appearing mucosa (Figure 23.4) to diffuse areas of edema and ulceration that create a polypoid mucosa and give a cobblestone appearance (Figure 23.5). Discontinuous colonic involvement with intervening normal appearing mucosa, often referred to as skip areas, is a key feature of Crohn's disease. Deep linear ulcerations may evolve into mucosal bridges with relatively normal-appearing mucosa traversing ulcers (Figure 23.6). Non-specific gastritis and duodenitis may be seen in patients with Crohn's disease on esophagogastroduodenoscopy, but histological findings are often most helpful in establishing a diagnosis.

Mucosa that appears grossly normal may reveal abnormalities on histological examination. Edema and an increase in mononuclear cell density in the lamina propria are relatively non-specific findings.[103]

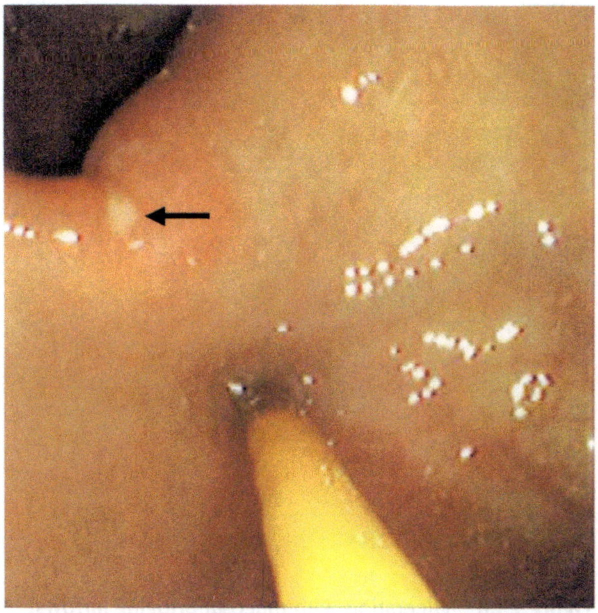

Figure 23.4 Focal aphthous lesion in Crohn's disease with surrounding area of erythema (arrow).

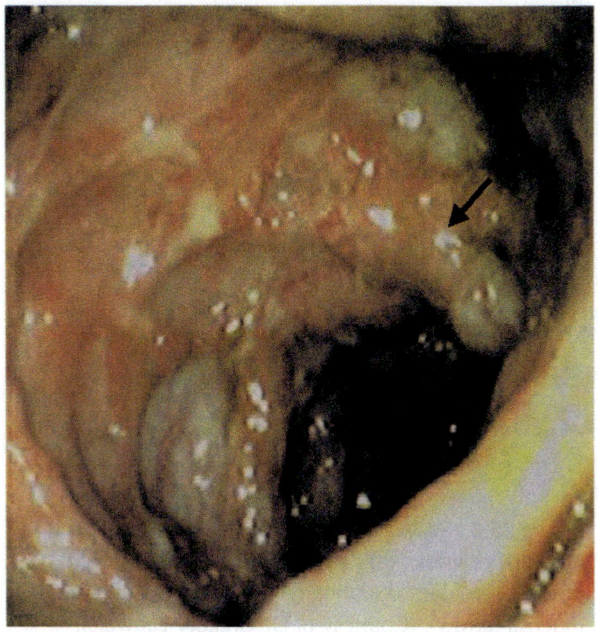

Figure 23.5 Cobblestone appearance (arrow) and mucosal ulcerations with mucopurulent exudate of the colon in Crohn's disease. (Courtesy of Dr Esther J. Israel).

In the early phases of Crohn's disease, microscopic changes may resemble an infectious colitis with infiltration of the crypts by polymorphonuclear leukocytes (cryptitis or crypt abscesses), and distortion of crypt architecture[103] (Figure 23.7). Focal

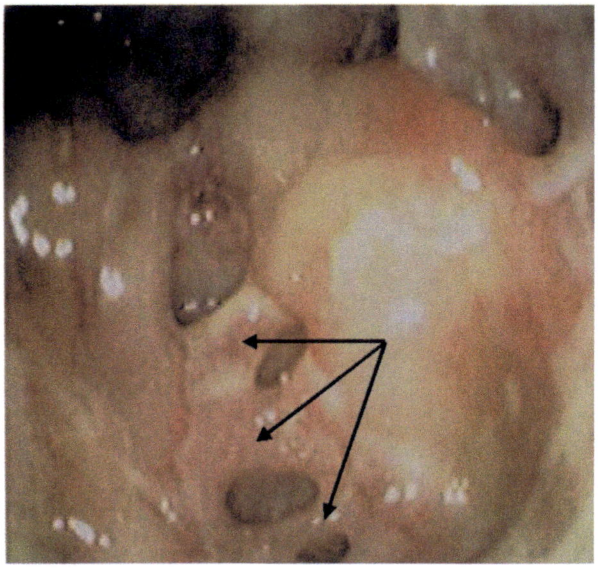

Figure 23.6 Ulceration with mucosal bridging (arrows) caused by undermining ulcerations of the colon in Crohn's disease. (Courtesy of Dr Esther J. Israel).

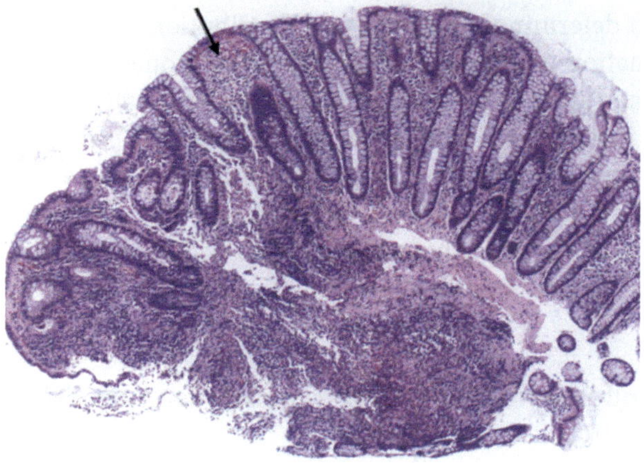

Figure 23.7 Active colitis in Crohn's disease (arrow) with area of relatively preserved mucosa without mucin depletion. (Courtesy of Dr Gregory Lauwers).

(a)

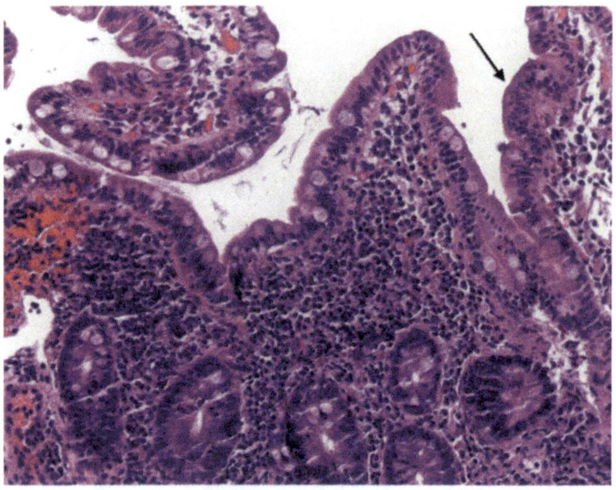

(b)

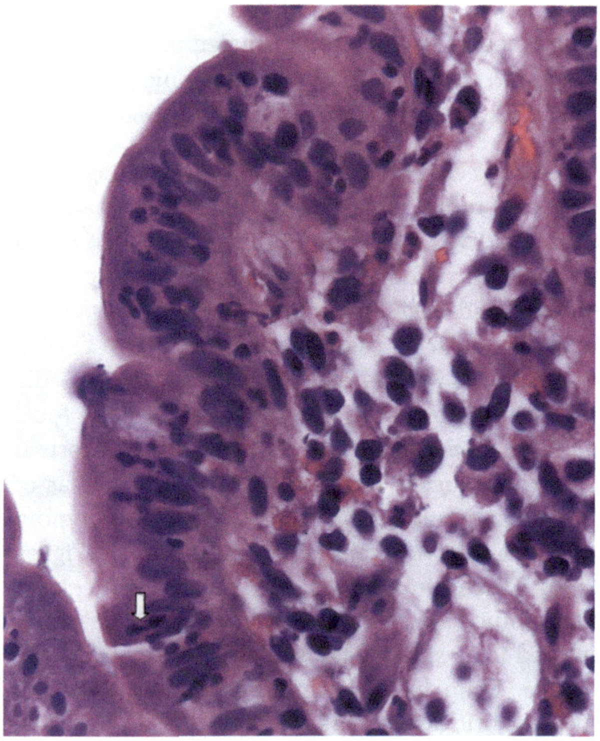

Figure 23.8 (a) Focal ileitis in Crohn's disease (arrow) (low-power view). (b) Ileitis in Crohn's disease (high-power view) demonstrating neutrophilic infiltrate into the mucosa (arrow). (Courtesy of Dr Gregory Lauwers).

ileitis is characteristic of Crohn's disease (Figure 23.8). The presence of fibrosis and histiocytic proliferation in the submucosa suggests Crohn's disease. The pathological hallmark of Crohn's inflammation is focal inflammation or transmural extension involving all layers of the bowel wall. Non-necrotizing granulomas are seen in 60% of surgical specimens and 20–40% of mucosal biopsies[145,146] (Figure 23.9). Microscopic focal enhancing lesions in the stomach (Figure 23.10) were thought to be indicative of Crohn's disease, but they can be seen in ulcerative colitis as well. However, they are supportive of a chronic inflammatory process.

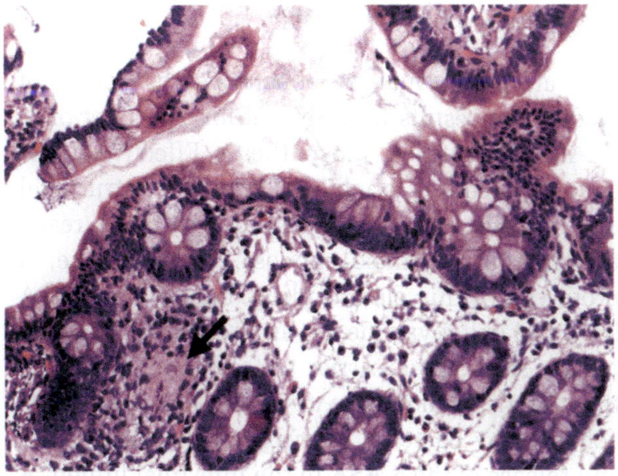

Figure 23.9 Focal granuloma (arrow) in the colon of a child with Crohn's disease. (Courtesy of Dr Gregory Lauwers).

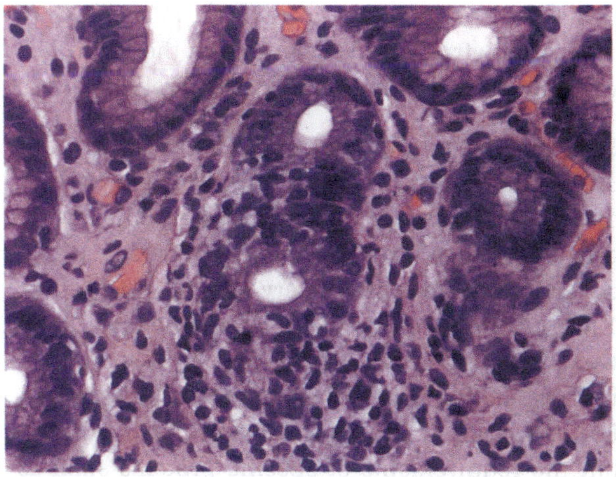

Figure 23.10 Focal enhancing lesions of the stomach in a patient with Crohn's disease. (Courtesy of Dr Gregory Lauwers).

Treatment

Management of children with Crohn's disease includes medical therapy, potential surgical intervention as well as nutritional and psychiatric support. Education of the patient and the family is a critical aspect of care that should not be overlooked. The *IBD Notebook* that is available through the North American Society for Pediatric Gastroenterology, Hepatology and Nutrition is a valuable resource empowering patients to understand and control their disease. The general guiding principles for treatment are to control inflammation and achieve normal growth while maintaining a high quality of life. For patients with mild-to-moderate disease, initial therapy with 5-aminosalicylic acid (5-ASA) and antibiotics may induce remission. For patients with more active disease, corticosteroids may provide a more rapid response. Initial treatment with 6-mercaptopurine seems to decrease steroid dependency, but most clinicians reserve immunomodulator therapy for patients who fail to maintain a remission.

Nutrition support

Nutritional therapy is a necessary and essential aspect of therapy for all children with Crohn's disease; achieving normal growth potential is one of the major therapeutic challenges. Nutrition has been used as a primary therapy for children with Crohn's disease, but when compared to corticosteroids, children treated with nutritional therapy relapsed sooner. Although the impact on linear growth was less in the nutrition group, compliance with nutritional regimens is more difficult. Suboptimal intake related to anorexia or fear of symptoms with eating, stool losses of nutrients caused by inflammation, ulceration or resection, increased nutritional requirements secondary to fever or increased metabolic requirements, treatment with corticosteroids that inhibit insulin-like growth factor-1, or circulating cytokines that delay linear growth are all relevant factors that impair growth. Medical or surgical therapy may correct or in some situations exacerbate some of the causes of undernutrition, but finding a tolerable nutritional supplement is the key to successful nutritional therapy.

Careful plotting of weight, height and rate of growth, and calculation of the body mass index (BMI) (weight in kg/(height in m)^2) is a critical part of the evaluation that enables one to assess when growth delay began. Anthropometric measurements such as triceps skin-fold thickness and mid-arm circumference provide an estimation of body fat and muscle mass. CT scans and magnetic resonance imaging (MRI) may also be beneficial in assessing body composition. Bioelectric impedance analysis (BIA) and total body electrical conductance (TOBEC) assess total body water and fat mass, but have not been validated in the pediatric IBD population. Dual energy X-ray absorptiometry (DEXA) scanning of the spine is a valuable tool to assess bone mineralization.

Daily energy requirements are increased in children with Crohn's disease, and during a flare of disease energy requirements increase while energy generation decreases. Catch-up growth is possible, but may require daily dietary energy intakes over 130% of the recommended values for ideal body weight. In practical terms, this corresponds to intakes ranging between 60 and 75 kcal/kg per day. Daily protein intake should approximate 3 g/kg, but the requirements of specific proteins such as glutamine is not substantiated. Amino acid-based, hydrolyzed or intact protein diets appear to be equally beneficial although there is a theoretical immunological benefit to giving protein that is less antigenic. In practice this does not seem to be beneficial for most patients. Total amount of protein rather than composition appears most relevant.

Growing children with Crohn's disease who are treated with corticosteroids stimulate osteoclastic bone resorption, inhibit osteoblast proliferation, decrease calcitriol synthesis and do not absorb calcium efficiently. These processes result in decreased bone mineralization. Patients who are at greatest risk for decreased bone mineralization seem to be those who take more than 7.5 mg/day, have a greater than 5 g lifetime cumulative dose or more than 1 year lifetime exposure. For a growing adolescent 1300 mg/day of calcium is recommended along with 400 IU/day of vitamin D.

Other minerals and vitamins should be replaced if deficient. Zinc is decreased with inflammation and serum zinc may not reflect intracellular stores. Many patients with Crohn's disease take zinc along with selenium and vitamin E as an antioxidant cocktail without strong supportive evidence for efficacy. Folate requirements may increase in active Crohn's disease, but the folic acid requirement for children with Crohn's disease is not known. Many clinicians recommend a dose of 1 mg daily, but the dose is not based on sound evidence. Vitamin B_{12} deficiency may need to be treated with subcutaneous injections as ileal absorption is often impaired. Release in 2003 of a nasal form of vitamin B_{12} may permit children who require vitamin B_{12} to avoid painful injections.

5-Aminosalicylic acid drugs

The anti-inflammatory effects of this class of medication results from the inhibitory effect of 5-ASA on leukotriene biosynthesis. Effective delivery of these drugs is achieved by various structural modifications that permit the medication to reach the area of inflamed mucosa. Sulfasalazine, a prototype of this class of drug, consists of 5-ASA linked to sulfapyridine via an azo bond. The sulfa moiety serves as a carrier to facilitate delivery of therapeutically active 5-ASA to the colon, which is achieved by bacterial cleavage of the diazo bond and release of the 5-ASA in the intestinal lumen. A number of different 5-ASA preparations have been developed based on a similar strategy. A summary of the different chemical modifications of 5-ASA preparations, and their release mechanisms are listed in Table 23.7. The dosage and site of effect as well as side-effects are listed in Tables 23.8 and 23.9, respectively. A profile of release within the gastrointestinal tract of the different 5-ASA preparations is shown in Figure 23.11. The medication should be selected that targets the areas of inflammation. The dose ranges between 30–60 mg/kg per day, but some clinicians use higher doses. Pediatric dosing should not exceed the adult recommended dose. Topical 5-ASA preparations (enema or suppository) are used more commonly in ulcerative colitis or in those patients with Crohn's disease who do not have rectal sparing.

Corticosteroids

Systemic corticosteroid treatment remains an important and effective therapy for children with Crohn's disease, but side-effects often limit their use. The anti-inflammatory effect of corticosteroids is related to inhibition of cell-mediated immunity, decreased cytokine production, decreased capillary permeability, impaired neutrophil and monocyte chemotaxis and stabilization of lysosomal membranes.[147,148] Prednisone or prednisolone is commonly used in children with Crohn's disease who have active mucosal inflammation that does not respond to initial therapy with 5-ASA and antibiotics. Prednisone is a synthetic glucocorticoid of intermediate potency, and is converted to its active form, prednisolone, in the liver.[103] Prednisone or prednisolone is administrated orally or intravenously at 1–2 mg/kg

Table 23.7 Chemical modification and release mechanisms of 5-aminosalicylic acid (5-ASA) preparations

Preparation	Trade name	Chemical modification	Release mechanism
Sulfasalazine	Azulfidine	azo bond to sulfapyridine	bacterial cleavage
Olsalazine	Dipentum	5-ASA attaches to 5-ASA	bacterial cleavage
Ipsalazide		azo bond to inert carrier	bacterial cleavage
Balsalazide	Colazal	azo bond to inert carrier	bacterial cleavage
Mesalamine/mesalazine	Asacol	attach to acrylic-based resins	pH-dependent release (pH >7)
Mesalamine/mesalazine	Salofalk, Claversal	attach to acrylic-based resins	pH-dependent release (pH >5.6)
Mesalamine/mesalazine	Pentasa	coated with ethyl cellulose	time and moisture-dependent release
Mesalamine/mesalazine enema/suppository	Rowasa, Canasa	uncoated	direct local effect (rectum to left colon)

Table 23.8 Dosage and site of effect of 5-aminosalicylic acid preparations

Preparation	Trade name	Dosage	Site of effect
Sulfasalazine	Azulfidine	C: 40–60 mg/kg per day ÷ BID. For maintenance 30 mg/kg per day ÷ QID (max 2 g/day) A: 3-4 g/day ÷ QID For maintenance 2 g/day ÷ QID	colon
Olsalazine	Dipentum	C: not available A: 1.5–3 g/day ÷ BID – QID	colon
Balsalazide	Colazal	C: not available A: 6.75 g/day ÷ TID. For maintenance 3–4 g/day ÷ BID	colon
Mesalamine	Asacol	C: 25–50 mg/kg per day ÷ BID – TID A: 2.4–4.8 g/day ÷ TID – QID	distal ileum or right colon
Mesalamine	Salofalk, Claversal	C: not available A: 2.4–4 g/day ÷ TID – QID	mid- to small bowel
Mesalamine	Pentasa	C: 25–50 mg/kg per day ÷ BID – TID A: 4 g/day ÷ TID – QID	small bowel and colon
Mesalamine enema/suppository	Rowasa enema, Canasa suppository	C: not available A: 4 g enema nightly; 500 mg suppository BID	rectum and left colon

C, children; A, adults; BID, twice a day; QID, four times a day; TID, three times a day

Table 23.9 Side-effects of 5-aminosalicylic acid preparations

Preparation	Side-effect
Sulfasalazine (mainly related to sulfa moiety)	dose-dependent (nausea, vomiting, headaches, hemolysis)
	hypersensitivity (fever, rashes, Stevens–Johnson syndrome, agranulocytosis, pulmonary fibrosis, hepatotoxicity)
	male fertility impairment
	folate deficiency
Mesalamine/mesalazine	acute pancreatitis
Olsalazine	diarrhea

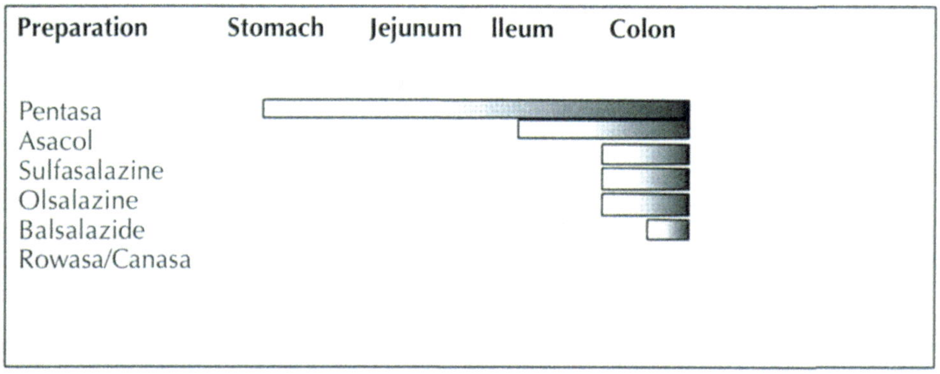

Figure 23.11 Gastrointestinal release profile of 5-aminosalicylic acid preparations. The diagram of gradient indicates increased release.

per day to a maximum of 40–60 mg/day, and gradually tapered after establishment of remission. A typical adolescent patient who required corticosteroids might start on 40 mg of prednisone once daily (or 2 mg/kg per day, whichever was less). If the clinical response is suboptimal, the dose may be divided twice a day. Splitting the dose further has little proven efficacy and increases adrenal suppression. Although some clinicians may increase the dose to a maximum of 60 mg/day for those patients who do not respond, there is no evidence that higher doses are beneficial and they are associated with increased untoward events. Systemic corticosteroid therapy is generally not used as a maintenance regimen. The adverse effects of systemic corticosteroid therapy are summarized in Table 23.10. Topical intrarectal corticosteroids (hydrocortisone enemas or foam) are also available for those patients with rectal disease.

Oral budesonide is designed for release in the ileum, cecum and right colon and is usually prescribed at 9 mg/day initially for an adult for 8 weeks and then tapered by 3-mg increments. Budesonide is not approved by the Food and Drug Administration (FDA) for use in children. Because of its high first-pass hepatic metabolism, budesonide has significant local effect with much less systemic effect.[149] The incidence of overall adverse effects is less than with prednisolone as noted in clinical trials with adult patients with Crohn's disease.[150] However, long-term use of oral budesonide may still cause significant systemic glucocorticoid effects, since budesonide has an affinity for the glucocorticoid receptor 50–100 times more than that of prednisone.[2] Experience with pediatric patients with Crohn's disease has demonstrated that growth failure remains an active issue in long-term treatment with budesonide, because

Table 23.10 Adverse effect of systemic corticosteroid therapy

Common	Rare	Long term
Acne	seizure	growth failure
Moon facies	pseudotumor cerebri	nephrolithiasis (hypercalciuria)
Hirsutism	psychosis	osteopenia
Cutaneous striae	myopathy	osteoporosis
	aseptic necrosis of femoral head	diabetes
	cataracts	secondary hyperparathyroidism
	increased intraocular pressure	

of either direct suppression of linear growth or an inability to control disease activity fully.[151]

Immunoregulatory agents

Azathioprine and 6-mercaptopurine

Growing evidence supports the use of the immunoregulatory agents azathioprine and 6-mercaptopurine in treating Crohn's disease as effective therapy to maintain control of intestinal inflammation. These agents are particularly useful in patients who are steroid-dependent. 6-Mercaptopurine is a purine analog capable of interfering with DNA and RNA synthesis by competing with endogenous purines. Azathio-purine is a prodrug that exerts its immunosuppressive effect through its metabolite 6-mercaptopurine. 6-Mercaptopurine undergoes extensive transformations to form cytotoxic intracellular metabolites responsible for the immunosuppressive effect. Studies suggest that the intracellular levels of the metabolite 6-thioguanine (6-TG) correlate with efficacy, and the intracellular levels of the metabolite 6-methyl mercaptopurine (6-MMP) with hepatotoxicity.[152] Genetic polymorphisms of thiopurine methyltransferase (TPMT), an enzyme that catabolizes 6-mercaptopurine to 6-MMP, controls the baseline enzymatic activity of TPMT. One in 300 subjects has very low enzyme activity or none at all, and 11% of the population has intermediate enzyme activity. Inherited low TPMT activity appears to be a risk factor for acute bone marrow failure by leaving more 6-mercaptopurine available for conversion to cytotoxic 6-TG.

In a prospective, double-blind, placebo-controlled pediatric trial, 55 children (mean age of 13 years) with newly diagnosed Crohn's disease were randomly assigned to receive prednisone plus either 6-mercaptopurine (1.5 mg/kg per day) or placebo.[153] Markowitz et al found that the duration of steroid use and the cumulative steroid dose was significantly decreased in the group that received steroids plus 6-mercaptopurine. Although the rate of remission achieved in both groups was similar (89%), relapse was less frequent in the group that received 6-mercaptopurine.[153] Base on these findings, 6-mercaptopurine should be considered as part of the initial treatment prescribed for children with newly diagnosed moderate-to-severe Crohn's disease activity who are started on corticosteroids.[153] The dosages, adverse effects, and monitoring parameters for azathioprine and 6-mercaptopurine are listed in Table 23.11. The monitoring of 6-TG and 6-MMP remains controversial, as discussed by Dubinsky and Griffiths.[154]

Methotrexate

Methotrexate exerts its cytotoxic effect by interfering with thymidine synthesis, by inhibiting the conversion of the folic acid to its active form tetrahydrofolate. Intramuscular administration of methotrexate weekly has proved effective in inducing and maintaining remission in adult patients with Crohn's disease who are either steroid-refractory or -dependent,[155] or in pediatric patients with Crohn's disease intolerant or refractory to azathioprine/6-mercaptopurine treatment.[156] Common adverse effects of methotrexate include nausea and abnormal liver serum transaminase levels. Concerns about possible hepatic fibrosis may limit the long-term use of methotrexate.

Table 23.11 6-Mercaptopurine and azathioprine therapy

Dosage			
Azathioprine	**6-Mercaptopurine**	**Potential adverse effects**	**Monitoring program**
1.5–2.5 mg/kg per day	1–2 mg/kg per day	fever pancreatitis rash	TPMT level before therapy
		arthralgia nausea vomiting diarrhea, leukopenia thrombocytopenia opportunistic infection	weekly for 4 weeks, then every 3 months: CBC with differential, liver function tests, amylase, lipase
		hepatitis malignancy	consider: monitoring 6-TG and 6-MMP

TPMT, thiopurine methyltransferase; CBC, complete blood count; 6-TG, 6-thioguanine; 6-MMP, 6-methyl mercaptopurine

Anti-tumor necrosis factor-α agents

TNF-α is a pro-inflammatory cytokine produced by activated macrophages, and is thought to play an important role in the pathogenesis and clinical manifestations of IBD. Several reagents have been developed as antagonists of TNF-α in the treatment of Crohn's disease. Infliximab (Remicade®) is a chimeric monoclonal antibody composed of a complement-fixing 'human' IgG1 constant region and a mouse-derived antigen-binding variable region, and binds directly to soluble TNF-α.[2] Infliximab is efficacious as therapy in about two-thirds of adult patients with moderately to severely active Crohn's disease resistant to corticosteroid and azathioprine/6-mercaptopurine therapy. However, about half of those who respond initially will have a sustained response over the first year. Infliximab is also effective in patients with fistulae that are refractory to antibiotic and/or azathioprine/6-mercaptopurine treatment.[157–159] Infliximab is administered intravenously with a recommended regimen for treatment of fistulae of three initial doses at 0, 2 and 6 weeks, followed by repeat infusions at 2-month intervals, for patients who demonstrate response to the initial doses.[160] Although this regimen is not FDA approved, most patients with Crohn's disease including those without fistulae are treated thus. Common side-effects associated with infliximab therapy include fever, rash, vomiting and chest pain.[160] Rarely, a serious hypersensitivity reaction may also occur with repeat infusion. Reactivation of tuberculosis associated with infliximab therapy has been reported as a potential lethal complication.[160] Therefore, all patients must receive tuberculosis screening prior to initiation of therapy. Lymphoma has developed in a small number of patients receiving infliximab, although a causal relationship has not been established.[2,160]

In a retrospective open-labeled pediatric study, 19 children with Crohn's disease (mean age 14.4 years) received 1–3 infusions of infliximab (5 mg/kg per dose) over a 12-week period for corticosteroid-resistant ($n = 7$) or corticosteroid-dependent disease ($n = 12$).[161] Significant initial improvement (first 4 weeks after infusion) was noted in all subjects, with pediatric Crohn's disease activity index (PCDAI) values decreasing significantly (42.1 ± 13.7 to 10.0 ± 5.6, $p < 0.0001$), but over the subsequent 8 weeks, eight of 19 treated children had worsening of symptoms, although none deteriorated to a level of severe disease activity.[161] The requirement of prednisone was also significantly reduced with infliximab treatment. Adverse effects were noted in three children during infusion (dyspnea, rash) and were self-limited.[161] In a recent prospective multicenter, open-label, dose-blinded clinical trial, 21 children with Crohn's disease (aged 8–17 years) were randomized to receive a single infusion of infliximab 1 mg/kg ($n = 6$), 5 mg/kg ($n = 7$), or 10 mg/kg ($n = 8$).[162] Improvement in the PCDAI, ESR and C-reactive protein (CRP) was observed with all infliximab doses, beginning at week 1. All treated patients experienced approximately 50% improvement in the PCDAI by week 2, and by week 12, the PCDAI remained approximately 30% improved from baseline.[162] During the study, all 21 patients (100%) achieved a clinical response, and ten patients (48%) achieved clinical remission; there were no infusion reactions in any of the treated patients.[162] Appropriately powered pediatric studies of infliximab are needed to establish safety and efficacy.[163]

Antibiotics

Antibiotics are often used to treat newly diagnosed or relapsed patients with Crohn's disease or patients with perianal fistulae/abscesses. There are no randomized clinical trials to support efficacy in the pediatric population. Commonly used antibiotics and their dosage and side-effects are listed in Table 23.12.

Surgery

The most common reasons for surgery are intractable symptoms despite medical therapy, obstruction, intra-abdominal abscess, fistula refractory to medical therapy, or intractable hemorrhage. In patients with a well-defined region of disease that has not been progressive over time, surgical resection can be a highly effective therapy. The potential benefits of surgery include rapid resolution of symptoms, enhanced growth and pubertal development, and improved quality of life. Postoperative recurrence of disease is a significant risk. Data from adults have indicated that the incidence of clinical recurrence following resection is about 10% per year.

Supportive measures

Psychological support and psychiatric counseling are important adjunctive therapies to cope with chronic disease. Children with Crohn's disease may have to face delayed sexual maturation and short stature. Missing school impacts on social maturation and relationships. Psychiatric and psychological support is a critical aspect of a pediatric IBD program; anti-anxiety or antidepressant medications may be beneficial. Long-term therapy should be considered for any child having difficulty in school or with interpersonal relationships.

Follow-up management

The PCDAI is a useful monitoring tool for disease activity, but it is time-consuming to use in a routine clinical setting.[194–198] A numerical score (0–100) based on general well-being, clinical symptoms and objective measurements of weight, height and clinical examination, as well as laboratory tests provides an objective means to follow disease activity and response to therapy (Table

Table 23.12 Commonly used antibiotics for Crohn's disease

Antibiotic	Dosage	Side-effects
Metronidazole	30–50 mg/kg per day, TID	metallic taste, disulfiram reaction with alcohol, peripheral neuropathy, potential birth defect
Ciprofloxacin	20–30 mg/kg per day, BID	skin rash, headache, nausea, vomiting, renal failure, seizures, arthropathy
Augmentin	20–40 mg/kg per day, TID	skin rash, nausea, vomiting, diarrhea, hypersensitivity reactions, seizures, interstitial nephritis

TID, three times a day; BID, twice a day

23.13). A score of 0–10 indicates inactive disease, 11–30 mild-to-moderate disease, and over 30 moderate-to-severe disease. Signs of pubertal development and nutritional assessment should be an important part of ongoing care. Annual ophthalmological examination is important for all patients who have been exposed to corticosteroids. In addition to dietary supplement of vitamin D and calcium to prevent development of osteopenia and osteoporosis, regular bone density study using DEXA is recommended for patients on prolonged corticosteroid therapy. There are no proven therapeutic interventions in children with Crohn's disease that have been shown to prevent recurrence of disease or maintain remission. Nevertheless, immunomodulator therapy and 5-ASA are often used in this role.

Table 23.13 Pediatric Crohn's Disease Activity Index (PCDAI) (adapted from reference 194)

History (recall, 1 week)	**Score**
Abdominal pain	
None	0
Mild (brief, does not interfere with activities	5
Moderate (daily, prolonged, nocturnal, interfering with activities)	10
Stools (per day)	
0–1 (liquid, no blood)	0
1–2 (semi-formed with small amount of blood)	5
or 2–5 (liquid)	
≥6 (liquid or gross bleeding or nocturnal diarrhea)	10
Patient functioning, general well-being (recall, 1 week)	
No limitation of activities, well	0
Occasional difficulty in maintaining age-appropriate activities	5
Frequent limitation of activity	10
Laboratory tests	
Hematocrit (%)	
<10 years	
value >33	0
28–32	2.5
<28	5
11–19-year-old girl	
value >34	0
29–33	2.5
<29	5
11–14-year-old boy	
value ≥35	0
30–34	2.5
<30	5
15–19-year-old boy	
value ≥37	0
32–36	2.5
<32	5
ESR (mm/h)	
< 20	0
20–50	2.5
>50	5
Albumin (g/dl)	
≥3.5	0
3.1–3.4	2.5
″3.0	5

ESR, erythrocyte sedimentation rate

Prognosis

Crohn's disease is a chronic inflammatory process that cannot be cured by current medical therapy or by resection. Nevertheless, children with Crohn's disease can manage their disease and achieve their goals. General Eisenhower had Crohn's disease and he was elected President of the United States. Athletes with Crohn's disease perform effectively and children should be encouraged to pursue their dreams. Education, recognition of early manifestations of disease and compliance will enable children to reach their potential and maximize benefit from medical therapy.

Acknowledgments

We would like to thank Dr Gary J. Russell for critical reading of the manuscript, Dr Gregory Lauwers for contributing the histology photographs, Dr Esther Israel for endosopic photographs and Dr Sudha Anupindi for providing the radiographic figures.

REFERENCES

1. Haubich WS. Crohn of Crohn's disease. *Gastroenterology* 1999; **116**: 1034.
2. Podolsky DK. Inflammatory bowel disease. *N Engl J Med* 2002; **347**: 417–429.
3. Loftus EV, Jr, Schoenfeld P, Sandborn WJ. The epidemiology and natural history of Crohn's disease in population-based patient cohorts from North America: a systematic review. *Aliment Pharmacol Ther* 2002; **16**: 51–60.
4. Moum B, Vatn MH, Ekbom A et al. Incidence of Crohn's disease in four counties in southeastern Norway, 1990-93. A prospective population-based study. The Inflammatory Bowel South-Eastern Norway (IBSEN) Study Group of Gastroenterologists. *Scand J Gastroenterol* 1996; **31**: 355–361.
5. Shivananda S, Lennard-Jones J, Logan R et al. Incidence of inflammatory bowel disease across Europe: is there a difference between north and south? Results of the European Collaborative Study on Inflammatory Bowel Disease (EC-IBD). *Gut* 1996; **39**: 690–697.
6. Ranzi T, Bodini P, Zambelli A et al. Epidemiological aspects of inflammatory bowel disease in a north Italian population: a 4-year prospective study. *Eur J Gastroenterol Hepatol* 1996; **8**: 657–661.
7. Tragnone A, Corrao G, Miglio F et al. Incidence of inflammatory bowel disease in Italy: a nationwide population-based study. Gruppo Italiano per lo Studio del Colon e del Retto (GISC). *Int J Epidemiol* 1996; **25**: 1044–1052.
8. Tragnone A, Hanau C, Bazzocchi G, Lanfranchi GA. Epidemiological characteristics of inflammatory bowel disease in Bologna, Italy – incidence and risk factors. *Digestion* 1993; **54**: 183–188.
9. Manousos ON, Koutroubakis I, Potamianos S et al. A prospective epidemiologic study of Crohn's disease in Heraklion, Crete. Incidence over a 5-year period. *Scand J Gastroenterol* 1996; **31**: 599–603.
10. Sonnenberg A, McCarty DJ, JacobsenSJ. Geographic variation of inflammatory bowel disease within the United States. *Gastroenterology* 1991; **100**: 143–149.
11. Mayberry J, Mann R. Inflammatory bowel disease in rural sub-Saharan Africa: rarity of diagnosis in patients attending mission hospitals. *Digestion* 1989; **44**: 172–176.
12. Kurata JH, Kantor-Fish S, Frankl H et al. Crohn's disease among ethnic groups in a large health maintenance organization. *Gastroenterology* 1992; **102**: 1940–1948.
13. Calkins BM, Lilienfeld AM, Garland CF, Mendeloff AI. Trends in incidence rates of ulcerative colitis and Crohn's disease. *Dig Dis Sci* 1984; **29**: 913–920.
14. Roth MP, Petersen GM, McElree C et al. Geographic origins of Jewish patients with inflammatory bowel disease. *Gastroenterology* 1989; **97**: 900–904.
15. Askling J, Grahnquist L, Ekbom A, Finkel Y. Incidence of paediatric Crohn's disease in Stockholm, Sweden. *Lancet* 1999; **354**: 1179.
16. Barton JR, Gillon S, Ferguson A. Incidence of inflammatory bowel disease in Scottish children between 1968 and 1983; marginal fall in ulcerative colitis, three-fold rise in Crohn's disease. *Gut* 1989; **30**: 618–622.
17. Armitage E, Drummond H, Ghosh S, Ferguson A. Incidence of juvenile-onset Crohn's disease in Scotland. *Lancet* 1999; **353**: 1496–1497.
18. Kugathasan S, Judd RH, Hoffman RG et al. Epidemiologic and clinical characteristics of children with newly diagnosed inflammatory bowel disease in Wisconsin: a statewide population-based study. *J Pediatrics* 2003; **143**: 525–531.
19. Jenkins, H. R. Inflammatory bowel disease. *Arch Dis Child* 2001; **85**: 435–437.

20. Roth MP, Petersen GM, McElreeC et al. Familial empiric risk estimates of inflammatory bowel disease in Ashkenazi Jews. *Gastroenterology* 1989; **96**: 1016–1020.
21. Monsen U, Brostrom O, Nordenvall B et al. Prevalence of inflammatory bowel disease among relatives of patients with ulcerative colitis. *Scand J Gastroenterol* 1987; **22**: 214–218.
22. Fielding JF. The relative risk of inflammatory bowel disease among parents and siblings of Crohn's disease patients. *J Clin Gastroenterol* 1986; **8**: 655–657.
23. Yang H, McElree C, Roth MP et al. Familial empirical risks for inflammatory bowel disease: differences between Jews and non-Jews. *Gut* 1993; **34**: 517–524.
24. Orholm M, Munkholm P, Langholz E et al. Familial occurrence of inflammatory bowel disease. *N Engl J Med* 1991; **324**: 84–88.
25. Lee JC, Lennard-Jones JE. Inflammatory bowel disease in 67 families each with three or more affected first-degree relatives. *Gastroenterology* 1996; **111**: 587–596.
26. Polito JM 2nd, Childs B, Mellits ED et al. Crohn's disease: influence of age at diagnosis on site and clinical type of disease. *Gastroenterology* 1996; **111**: 580–586.
27. Colombel JF, Grandbastien B, Gower-Rousseau C et al. Clinical characteristics of Crohn's disease in 72 families. *Gastroenterology* 1996; **111**: 604–607.
28. Tysk C, Lindberg E, Jarnerot G, Floderus-Myrhed B. Ulcerative colitis and Crohn's disease in an unselected population of monozygotic and dizygotic twins. A study of heritability and the influence of smoking. *Gut* 1988; **29**: 990–996.
29. Hugot JP, Laurent-Puig P, Gower-Rousseau C et al. Mapping of a susceptibility locus for Crohn's disease on chromosome 16. *Nature* 1996; **379**: 821–823.
30. Satsangi J, Parkes M, Louis E et al. Two stage genome-wide search in inflammatory bowel disease provides evidence for susceptibility loci on chromosomes 3, 7 and 12. *Nat Genet* 1996; **14**: 199–202.
31. Brant SR, Fu Y, Fields CT et al. American families with Crohn's disease have strong evidence for linkage to chromosome 16 but not chromosome 12. *Gastroenterology* 1998; **115**: 1056–1061.
32. Ma Y, Ohmen JD, Li Z et al. A genome-wide search identifies potential new susceptibility loci for Crohn's disease. *Inflamm Bowel Dis* 1999; **5**: 271–278.
33. Hugot J, Chamaillard PM, Zouali H et al.Association of NOD2 leucine-rich repeat variants with susceptibility to Crohn's disease. *Nature* 2001; **411**: 599–603.
34. Ogura Y, Bonen DK, Inohara N et al. A frameshift mutation in NOD2 associated with susceptibility to Crohn's disease. *Nature* 2001; **411**: 603–606.
35. Cuthbert AP, Fisher SA, Mirza MM et al. The contribution of NOD2 gene mutations to the risk and site of disease in inflammatory bowel disease. *Gastroenterology* 2002; **122**: 867–874.
36. Lesage S, Zouali H, Cezard JP et al. CARD15/NOD2 mutational analysis and genotype–phenotype correlation in 612 patients with inflammatory bowel disease. *Am J Hum Genet* 2002; **70**: 845–857.
37. Tomer G, Ceballos C, Concepcion E, Benkov KJ. NOD2/CARD15 variants are associated with lower weight at diagnosis in children with Crohn's disease. *Am J Gastroenterology* 2003; **98**: 2479–2484.
38. Rioux JD, Silverberg MS, Daly MJ et al. Genomewide search in Canadian families with inflammatory bowel disease reveals two novel susceptibility loci. *Am J Hum Genet* 2000; **66**: 1863–1870.
39. Rioux JD, Daly MJ, Silverberg MS et al. Genetic variation in the 5q31 cytokine gene cluster confers susceptibility to Crohn disease. *Nat Genet* 2001; **29**: 223–228.
40. Thornton JR, Emmett PM, Heaton KW. Diet and Crohn's disease: characteristics of the pre-illness diet. *Br Med J* 1979; **2**: 762–764.
41. Jarnerot G, Jarnmark I, Nilsson K. Consumption of refined sugar by patients with Crohn's disease, ulcerative colitis, or irritable bowel syndrome. *Scand J Gastroenterol* 1983; **18**: 999–1002.
42. Shoda R, Matsueda K, Yamato S, Umeda N. Epidemiologic analysis of Crohn disease in Japan: increased dietary intake of n-6 polyunsaturated fatty acids and animal protein relates to the increased incidence of Crohn disease in Japan. *Am J Clin Nutr* 1996; **63**: 741–745.
43. Koletzko S, Sherman P, Corey M et al. Role of infant feeding practices in development of Crohn's disease in childhood. *Br Med J* 1989; **298**: 1617–1628.
44. Koletzko S, Griffiths A, Corey M et al. Infant feeding practices and ulcerative colitis in childhood. *Br Med J* 1991; **302**: 1580–1581.
45. Gilat T, Hacohen D, Lilos P, Langman MJ. Childhood factors in ulcerative colitis and Crohn's disease. An international cooperative study. *Scand J Gastroenterol* 1987; **22**: 1009–1024.
46. Ekbom A, Adami HO, Helmick GC et al. Perinatal risk factors for inflammatory bowel disease: a case–control study. *Am J Epidemiol* 1990; **132**: 1111–1119.
47. Vessey M, Jewell D, Smith A et al. Chronic inflammatory bowel disease, cigarette smoking, and use of oral contraceptives: findings in a large cohort study of women of childbearing age. *Br Med J (Clin Res Ed)* 1986; **292**: 1101–1103.
48. Calkins BM. A meta-analysis of the role of smoking in inflammatory bowel disease. *Dig Dis Sci* 1989; **34**: 1841–1845.
49. Cosnes J, Beaugerie L, Carbonnel F, Gendre JP. Smoking cessation and the course of Crohn's disease: an intervention study. *Gastroenterology* 2001; **120**: 1093–1099.
50. Harries AD, Jones L, Heatley RV, Rhodes J. Smoking habits and inflammatory bowel disease: effect on nutrition. *Br Med J (Clin Res Ed)* 1982; **284**: 1161.
51. Boyko EJ, Koepsell TD, Perera DR, Inui TS. Risk of ulcerative colitis among former and current cigarette smokers. *N Engl J Med* 1987; **316**: 707–710.
52. Tanner AR, Raghunath AS. Colonic inflammation and nonsteroidal anti-inflammatory drug administration. An assessment of the frequency of the problem. *Digestion* 1988; **41**: 116–120.
53. Kaufmann HJ, Taubin HL. Nonsteroidal anti-inflammatory drugs activate quiescent inflammatory bowel disease. *Ann Intern Med* 1987; **107**: 513–516.
54. Evans JM, McMahon AD, Murray FE et al. Non-steroidal anti-inflammatory drugs are associated with emergency admission to hospital for colitis due to inflammatory bowel disease. *Gut* 1997; **40**: 619–622.
55. Felder JB, Korelitz BI, Rajapakse R et al. Effects of non-steroidal anti-inflammatory drugs on inflammatory bowel disease: a case–control study. *Am J Gastroenterol* 2000; **95**: 1949–1954.
56. Bonner GF, Walczak PA, Kitchen L, Bayona M. Tolerance of nonsteroidal antiinflammatory drugs in patients with inflammatory bowel disease. *Am J Gastroenterol* 2000; **95**: 1946–1948.
57. O'Brien J. Nonsteroidal anti-inflammatory drugs in patients with inflammatory bowel disease. *Am J Gastroenterol* 2000; **95**: 1859–1861.
58. Bjarnason I, Hayllar J, MacPherson AJ, Russell AS. Side effects of nonsteroidal anti-inflammatory drugs on the small and large intestine in humans. *Gastroenterology* 1993; **104**: 1832–1847.

59. Wallace JL. Nonsteroidal anti-inflammatory drugs and gastroenteropathy: the second hundred years. *Gastroenterology* 1997; **112**: 1000–1016.
60. Reuter BK, Davies NM, Wallace JL. Nonsteroidal anti-inflammatory drug enteropathy in rats: role of permeability, bacteria, and enterohepatic circulation. *Gastroenterology* 1997; **112**: 109–117.
61. Pumford NR, Myers TG, Davila JC et al. Immunochemical detection of liver protein adducts of the nonsteroidal antiinflammatory drug diclofenac. *Chem Res Toxicol* 1993; **6**: 147–150.
62. Atchison CR, West AB, Balakumaran A et al. Drug enterocyte adducts: possible causal factor for diclofenac enteropathy in rats. *Gastroenterology* 1996; **119**: 1537–1547.
63. Halter F, Tarnawski AS, Schmassmann A, Peskar BM. Cyclooxygenase 2–implications on maintenance of gastric mucosal integrity and ulcer healing: controversial issues and perspectives. *Gut* 2001; **49**: 443–453.
64. Wallace JL, McKnight W, Reuter BK, Vergnolle N. NSAID-induced gastric damage in rats: requirement for inhibition of both cyclooxygenase 1 and 2. *Gastroenterology* 2000; **119**: 706–714.
65. Tanaka A, Hase S, Miyazawa T, Takeuchi K. Up-regulation of cyclooxygenase-2 by inhibition of cyclooxygenase-1: a key to nonsteroidal anti-inflammatory drug-induced intestinal damage. *J Pharmacol Exp Ther* 2002; **300**: 754–761.
66. Silverstein FE, Faich G, Goldstein JL et al. Gastrointestinal toxicity with celecoxib vs nonsteroidal anti-inflammatory drugs for osteroarthritis and rheumatoid arthritis: the CLASS study: a randomized controlled trial. Celecoxib long-term arthritis safety study. *J Am Med Assoc* 2000; **284**: 1247–1255.
67. Watson DJ, Harper SE, ZhaoPL et al. Gastrointestinal tolerability of the selective cyclooxygenase-2 (COX-2) inhibitor rofecoxib compared with nonselective COX-1 and COX-2 inhibitors in osteoarthritis. *Arch Intern Med* 2000; **160**: 2998–3003.
68. Singer II, Kawka DW, Schloemann S et al. Cyclooxygenase 2 is induced in colonic epithelial cells in inflammatory bowel disease. *Gastroenterology* 1998; **115**: 297–306.
69. Handel J, Nielsen OH. Expression of cyclooxygenase-2 mRNA in active inflammatory bowel disease. *Am J Gastroenterol* 1997; **92**: 1170–1173.
70. Bantel H, Berg C, Vieth M et al. Mesalazine inhibits activation of transcription factor NF-kappaB in inflamed mucosa of patients with ulcerative colitis. *Am J Gastroenterol* 2000; **95**: 3452–3457.
71. Logan RF. Inflammatory bowel disease incidence: up, down or unchanged? *Gut* 1998; **42**: 309–311.
72. Lashner BA, Kane SV Hanauer SB. Lack of association between oral contraceptive use and Crohn's disease: a community-based matched case-control study. *Gastroenterology* 1989; **97**: 1442–1447.
73. Lashner BA, Kane SV, Hanauer SB. Lack of association between oral contraceptive use and ulcerative colitis. *Gastroenterology* 1990; **99**: 1032–1036.
74. Wakefield AJ, Ekbom A, Dhillon AP et al. Crohn's disease: pathogenesis and persistent measles virus infection. *Gastroenterology* 1995; **108**: 911–916.
75. Wakefield AJ, Pittilo RM, Sim R et al. Evidence of persistent measles virus infection in Crohn's disease. *J Med Virol* 1993; **39**: 345–353.
76. Haga Y, Funakoshi O, Kuroe K et al. Absence of measles viral genomic sequence in intestinal tissues from Crohn's disease by nested polymerase chain reaction. *Gut* 1996; **38**: 211–215.
77. Ekbom A, Wakefield AJ, Zack M, Adami HO. Perinatal measles infection and subsequent Crohn's disease. *Lancet* 1994; **344**: 508–510.
78. Thompson NP, Pounder RE, Wakefield AJ. Perinatal and childhood risk factors for inflammatory bowel disease: a case–control study. *Eur J Gastroenterol Hepatol* 1995; **7**: 385–390.
79. Haslam N, Mayberry JF, Hawthorne AB et al. Measles, month of birth, and Crohn's disease. *Gut* 2000; **47**: 801–803.
80. Thompson NP, Montgomery SM, Pounder RE, Wakefield AJ. Is measles vaccination a risk factor for inflammatory bowel disease? *Lancet* 1995; **345**: 1071–1074.
81. Feeney M, Ciegg A, Winwood P, Snook J. A case–control study of measles vaccination and inflammatory bowel disease. The East Dorset Gastroenterology Group. *Lancet* 1997; **350**: 764–766.
82. Davis RL, Kramarz P, Bohlke K et al. Measles–mumps–rubella and other measles-containing vaccines do not increase the risk for inflammatory bowel disease: a case–control study from the Vaccine Safety Datalink project. *Arch Pediatr Adolesc Med* 2001; **155**: 354–359.
83. Lisby G, Andersen J, Engbaek K, Binder V. *Mycobacterium paratuberculosis* in intestinal tissue from patients with Crohn's disease demonstrated by a nested primer polymerase chain reaction. *Scand J Gastroenterol* 1994; **29**: 923–929.
84. Fiocchi C. Inflammatory bowel disease: etiology and pathogenesis. *Gastroenterology* 1998; **115**: 182–205.
85. Shanahan F. Crohn's disease. *Lancet* 2002; **359**: 62–69.
86. Ardizzone S, Bianchi Porro G. Inflammatory bowel disease: new insights into pathogenesis and treatment. *J Intern Med* 2002; **252**: 475–496.
87. Fabia R, Ar'Rajab A, Andersson ML et al. Impairment of bacterial flora in human ulcerative colonic and experimental colitis in the rat. *Digestion* 1993; **54**: 248–255.
88. Contractor NV, Bassiri H, Reya T et al. Lymphoid hyperplasia, autoimmunity, and compromised intestinal intraepithelial lymphocyte developement in colitis-free gnotobiotic IL-12-deficient mice. *J Immunol* 1998; **160**: 385–394.
89. Taurog JD, Richardson JA, Croft JT et al. The germfree state prevents development of gut and joint inflammatory disease in HLA-B27 transgenic rats. *J Exp Med* 1994; **180**: 2359–2364.
90. Sartor R. Microbial factors in the pathogenesis of Crohn's disease, ulcerative colitis, and experimental intestinal inflammation. In Kirsner JB, ed. *Inflammatory Bowel Disease*. Philadelphia: WB Saunders, 2000: 153.
91. Duchmann R, Kaiser I, Hermann E et al. Tolerance exists towards resident intestinal flora but is broken in active inflammatory bowel disease. *Clin Exp Immunol* 1995; **102**: 448–455.
92. Duchmann R, May E, Heike M et al. T cells specificity and cross reactivity towards enterobacteria, bacteroides, bifidobacterium, and antigens from resident intestinal flora in humans. *Gut* 1999; **44**: 812–818.
93. Darfeuille-Michaud A, Neut C, Barnich N et al. Presence of adherent *Escherichia coli* strains in ileal mucosa of patients with Crohn's disease. *Gastroenterology* 1998; **115**: 1405–1413.
94. Swidsinski A, Ladhoff A, Pernthaler A et al. Mucosal flora in inflammatory bowel disease. *Gastroenterology* 2002; **122**: 44–54.
95. Rutgeerts P, D'Haens G, Hiele M, et al. Appendectomy protects against ulcerative colitis. *Gastroenterology* 1994; **106**: 1251–1253.
96. Sandler RS. Appendicectomy and ulcerative colitis. *Lancet* 1998; **352**: 1797–1798.

97. Andersson RE, Olaison G, Tysk C, Ekbom A. Appendectomy and protection against ulcerative colitis. *N Engl J Med* 2001; **344**: 808–814.
98. Cosnes J, Carbonnel F, Beaugerie L et al. Effects of appendicectomy on the course of ulcerative colitis. *Gut* 2002; **51**: 803–807.
99. Radford-Smith GL, Edwards JE, Purdie DM et al. Protective role of appendicectomy on onset and severity of ulcerative colitis and Crohn's disease. *Gut* 2002; **51**: 808–813.
100. Selby WS, Griffin S, Abraham N, Solomon MJ. Appendectomy protects against the development of ulcerative colitis but does not affect its course. *Am J Gastroenterol* 2002; **97**: 2834–2838.
101. Andersson RE, Olaison G, Tysk C, Ekbom A. Appendectomy is followed by increased risk of Crohn's disease. *Gastroenterology* 2003; **124**: 40–46.
102. Mizoguchi A, Mizoguchi E, Chiba C, Bhan AK. Role of appendix in the development of inflammatory bowel disease in TCR-a mutant mice. *J Exp Med* 1996; **184**: 707–715.
103. Griffiths AM, Buller HB. Inflammatory bowel disease. In Walker WA, Durie PR, Hamilton JR et al., eds. *Pediatric Gastrointestinal Disease*. Ontario, BC: Decker, 2000: 613.
104. Monteleone I, Vavassori P, Biancone L et al. Immunoregulation in the gut: success and failures in human disease. *Gut* 2002; **50**(Suppl 3): III60–III64.
105. De Winter H, Cheroutre H, Kronenberg M. Mucosal immunity and inflammation. II. The yin and yang of T cells in intestinal inflammation: pathogenic and protective roles in a mouse colitis model. *Am J Physiol* 1999; **276**: G1317–G1321.
106. MacDonald TT, Monteleone G, Pender SL. Recent developments in the immunology of inflammatory bowel disease. *Scand J Immunol* 2000; **51**: 2–9.
107. Singh B, Read S, Asseman C et al. Control of intestinal inflammation by regulatory T cells. *Immunol Rev* 2001; **182**: 190–200.
108. Toms C, Powrie F. Control of intestinal inflammation by regulatory T cells. *Microbes Infect* 2001; **3**: 929–935.
109. Read S, Powrie F. CD4(+) regulatory T cells. *Curr Opin Immunol* 2001; **13**: 644–649.
110. Micallef MJ, Ohtsuki T, Kohno K et al. Interferon-gamma-inducing factor enhances T helper 1 cytokine production by stimulated human T cells: synergism with interleukin-12 for interferon-gamma production. *Eur J Immunol* 1996; **26**: 1647–1651.
111. Matsui K, Yoshimoto T, Tsutsui H et al. Propionibacterium acnes treatment diminishes CD4+ NK1.1+ T cells but induces type I T cells in the liver by induction of IL-12 and IL-18 production from Kupffer cells. *J Immunol* 1997; **159**: 97–106.
112. Dinarello CA. Interleukin-1 and tumor necrosis factor: effector cytokines in autoimmune diseases. *Semin Immunol* 1992; **4**: 133–145.
113. Mackay F, Loetscher H, Stueber D et al. Tumor necrosis factor alpha (TNF-alpha)-induced cell adhesion to human endothelial cells is under dominant control of one TNF receptor type, TNF-R55. *J Exp Med* 1993; **177**: 1277–1286.
114. Schmitz H, Fromm M, Bode H et al. Tumor necrosis factor-alpha induces Cl- and K+ secretion in human distal colon driven by prostaglandin E2. *Am J Physiol* 1996; **271**: G669–G674.
115. Mullin JM, Snock KV. Effect of tumor necrosis factor on epithelial tight junctions and transepithelial permeability. *Cancer Res* 1990; **50**: 2172–2176.
116. Barton JR, Ferguson A. Clinical features, morbidity and mortality of Scottish children with inflammatory bowel disease. *Q J Med* 1990; **75**: 423–439.
117. Motil KJ, Grand RJ, Davis-Kraft L et al. Growth failure in children with inflammatory bowel disease: a prospective study. *Gastroenterology* 1993; **105**: 681–691.
118. Kanof ME, Lake AM, Bayless TM. Decreased height velocity in children and adolescents before the diagnosis of Crohn's disease. *Gastroenterology* 1988; **95**: 1523–1527.
119. Cezard JP, Touati G, Alberti C et al. Growth in paediatric Crohn's disease. *Horm Res* 2002; **58** (Suppl 1): 11–15.
120. Lenaerts C, Roy CC, Vaillancourt M et al. High incidence of upper gastrointestinal tract involvement in children with Crohn disease. *Pediatrics* 1989; **83**: 777–781.
121. Ballinger A. Fundamental mechanisms of growth failure in inflammatory bowel disease. *Horm Res* 2002; **58** (Suppl 1): 7–10.
122. Zurita VF, Rawls DE, Dyck WP. Nutritional support in inflammatory bowel disease. *Dig Dis Sci* 1995; **13**: 92–107.
123. Markowitz J, Grancher K, Rosa J et al. Highly destructive perianal disease in children with Crohn's disease. *J Pediatr Gastroenterol Nutr* 1995; **21**: 149–153.
124. Tolia V. Perianal Crohn's disease in children and adolescents. *Am J Gastroenterol* 1996; **91**: 922–926.
125. Greenstein AJ, Janowitz HD, Sachar DB. The extra-intestinal complications of Crohn's disease and ulcerative colitis: a study of 700 patients. *Medicine (Baltimore)* 1976; **55**: 401–412.
126. Hyams JS. Extraintestinal manifestations of inflammatory bowel disease in children. *J Pediatr Gastroenterol Nutr* 1994; **19**: 7–21.
127. Seidman E, LeLeiko N, Ament M et al. Nutritional issues in pediatric inflammatory bowel disease. *J Pediatr Gastroenterol Nutr* 1991; **12**: 424–438.
128. Bernstein CN, Blanchard JF, Houston DS, Wajda A. The incidence of deep venous thrombosis and pulmonary embolism among patients with inflammatory bowel disease: a population-based cohort study. *Thromb Haemost* 2001; **85**: 430–434.
129. Markowitz RL, Ment LR, Gryboski JD. Cerebral thromboembolic disease in pediatric and adult inflammatory bowel disease: case report and review of the literature. *J Pediatr Gastroenterol Nutr* 1989; **8**: 413–420.
130. Talbot RW, Heppell J, Dozois RR, Beart RWJ. Vascular complications of inflammatory bowel disease. *Mayo Clin Proc* 1986; **61**: 140–145.
131. Sanghavi P, Paramesh A, Dwivedi A, et al. Mesenteric arterial thrombosis as complication of Crohn's disease. *Dig Dis Sci* 1999; **46**: 2344–2346.
132. Gormally SM, Bourke W, Kierse B et al. Isolated cerebral thrombo-embolism and Crohn's disease. *Eur J Pediatr* 1995; **154**: 815–818.
133. Akobeng A, Miller V, Thomas AG. Epilepsy and Crohn's disease in children. *J Pediatr Gastroenterol Nutr* 1998; **26**: 458–460.
134. Ertem D, Ozguven E, Acar Y et al. Thromboembolic complications in children with Crohn's disease. *J Pediatr Gastroenterol Nutr* 1999; **28**: 540–541.
135. Garcia-Diaz M, Mira M, Nevado L et al. Retinal vasculitis associated with Crohn's disease. *Postgrad Med J* 1995; **71**: 170–172.
136. Greenfield SM, Teare JP, Whitehead MW, Thompson RP. Amaurosis fugax, Crohn's disease and the cardiolipin antibody. *Lupus* 1993; **2**: 271–273.
137. van Tirpitz C, Klaus J, Steinkamp M et al. Therapy of osteoporosis in patients with Crohn's disease: a randomized study comparing sodium fluoride and ibandronate. *Aliment Pharmacol Ther* 2003; **17**: 807–816.
138. Winter HS, Landers CJ, Winkelstein A et al. Anti-neutrophil cytoplasmic antibodies in children with ulcerative colitis. *J Pediatr* 1994; **125**: 707–711.

139. Ruemmele FM, Targan SR, Levy G et al. Diagnostic accuracy of serological assays in pediatric inflammatory bowel disease. *Gastroenterology* 1998; **115**: 822–829.
140. Terjung B, Spengler U, Sauerbruch T, Worman HJ. "Atypical p-ANCA" in IBD and hepatobiliary disorders react with a 50-kilodalton nuclear envelope protein of neutrophils and myeloid cell lines. *Gastroenterology* 2000; **119**: 310–322.
141. Charron M, del Rosario FJ, Kocoshis SA. Pediatric inflammatory bowel disease: assessment with scintigraphy with 99mTc white blood cells. *Radiology* 1999; **212**: 507–513.
142. Alberini JL, Badran A, Freneaux E et al. Technetium-99m HMPAO-labeled leukocyte imaging compared with endoscopy, ultrasonography, and contrast radiology in children with inflammatory bowel disease. *J Pediatr Gastroenterol Nutr* 2001; **32**: 278–286.
143. Charron M, Di Lorenzo C, Kocoshis S. Are 99mTc leukocyte scintigraphy and SBFT studies useful in children suspected of having inflammatory bowel disease? *Am J Gastroenterol* 2000; **95**: 1208–1212.
144. Charron M, del Rosario JF, Kocoshis S. Use of technetium-tagged white blood cells in patients with Crohn's disease and ulcerative colitis: is differential diagnosis possible? *Pediatr Radiol* 1998; **28**: 871–877.
145. Surawicz CM, Meisel JL, Ylvisaker T et al. Rectal biopsy in the diagnosis of Crohn's disease: value of multiple biopsies and serial sectioning. *Gastroenterology* 1981; **80**: 66–71.
146. Chong SK, Blackshaw AJ, Boyle S et al. Histological diagnosis of chronic inflammatory bowel disease in childhood. *Gut* 1985; **26**: 55–59.
147. Brattsand R, Linden M. Cytokine modulation by glucocorticoids: mechanisms and actions in cellular studies. *Aliment Pharmacol Ther* 1996; **10**: 81–90.
148. Zimmerman MJ, Jewell DP. Cytokines and mechanisms of action of glucocorticoids and aminosalicylates in the treatment of ulcerative colitis and Crohn's disease. *Aliment Pharmacol Ther* 1996; **10**: 93–98.
149. Brattsand R. Overview of newer glucocorticoid preparations for inflammatory bowel disease. *Can J Gastroenterol* 1990; **4**: 407–414.
150. Rutgeerts P, Lofberg R, Malchow H et al. A comparison of budesonide with prednisolone for active Crohn's disease. *N Engl J Med* 1994; **331**: 842–845.
151. Kundhal P, Zachos M, Holmes JL, Griffiths AM. Controlled ileal release budesonide in pediatric Crohn's disease: efficacy and effect on growth. *J Pediatr Gastroenterol Nutr* 2001; **33**: 75–80.
152. Cuffari C, Theoret Y, Latour S, Seidman G. 6-Mercaptopurine metabolism in Crohn's disease. Correlation with efficacy and toxicity. *Gut* 1996; **39**: 401–406.
153. Markowitz J, Grancher K, Kohn N et al. A multicenter trial of 6-mercaptopurine and prednisone in children with newly diagnosed Crohn's disease. *Gastroenterology* 2000; **119**: 895–902.
154. Dubinsky MC, Griffiths AM. Contorversies in IBD: monitoring of AZA/6-MP treatment in children with IBD. *Inflamm Bowel Dis* 2003; **9**: 386–388.
155. Feagan BG, Fedorak RN, Irvine EJ et al. A comparison of methotrexate with placebo for the maintenance of remission in Crohn's disease. *N Engl J Med* 2000; **342**: 1627–1632.
156. Mack DR, Young R, Kaufman SS et al. Methotrexate in patients with Crohn's disease after 6-mercaptopurine. *J Pediatr* 1998; **132**: 830–835.
157. Targan SR, Hanauer SB, van Deventer SJ et al. A short-term study of chimeric monoclonal antibody cA2 to tumor necrosis factor alpha for Crohn's disease. *N Engl J Med* 1997; **337**: 1029–1035.
158. Present DH, Rutgeerts P, Targan S et al. Infliximab for the treatment of fistulas in patients with Crohn's disease. *N Engl J Med* 1999; **340**: 1398–1405.
159. Cohen RD, Tsang JF, Hanauer SB. Infiximab in Crohn's disease: first anniversary clinical experience. *Am J Gastroenterol* 2000; **95**: 3469–3477.
160. Hanauer SB, Feagan BG, Lichtenstein GR et al. Maintenance infliximab for Crohn's disease: the ACCENT I randomised trial. *Lancet* 2002; **359**: 1541–1549.
161. Hyams JS, Markowitz J, Wyllie R. Use of infliximab in the treatment of Crohn's disease in children and adolescents. *J Pediatr* 2000; **137**: 192–196.
162. Baldassano R, Braegger CP, Escher JC et al. Infliximab (REMICADE) therapy in the treatment of pediatric Crohn's disease. *Am J Gastroenterol* 2003; **98**: 833–838.
163. Cezard JP, Nouaili N, Talbotec C et al. A prospective study of the efficacy and tolerance of a chimeric antibody to tumor necrosis factors (Remicade) in severe pediatric Crohn's disease. *J Pediatr Gastroenterol Nutr* 2003; **36**: 632–636.
164. Duerr RH, Barmada MM, Zhang L et al. High-density genome scan in Crohn disease shows confirmed linkage to chromosome 14q11-12. *Am J Hum Genet* 2000; **66**: 1857–1862.
165. Cho JH, Nicolae DL, Gold LH et al. Identification of novel susceptibility loci for inflammatory bowel disease on chromosomes 1p, 3q, and 4q: evidence for epistasis between 1p and IBD1. *Proc Natl Acad Sci USA* 1998; **95**: 7502–7507.
166. Gryboski JD. Crohn's disease in children 10 years old and younger: comparison with ulcerative colitis. *J Pediatr Gastroenterol Nutr* 1994; **18**: 174–182.
167. Keljo DJ, Sugerman KS. Pancreatitis in patients with inflammatory bowel disease. *J Pediatr Gastroenterol Nutr* 1997; **25**: 108–112.
168. Perkal MF, Seashore JH. Nutrition and inflammatory bowel disease. *Gastroenterol Clin North Am* 1989; **18**: 567–578.
169. Harries AD, Jones LA, Heatley RV, Rhodes J. Malnutrition in inflammatory bowel disease: an anthropometric study. *Hum Nutr Clin Nutr* 1982; **36**: 307–313.
170. Behrend C, Jeppesen PB, Mortensen PB. Vitamin B12 absorption after ileorectal anastomosis for Crohn's disease: effect of ileal resection and time span after surgery. *Eur J Gastroenterol Hepatol* 1995; **7**: 397–400.
171. Fernandez-Banares F, Abad-Lacruz A, Xiol X et al. Vitamin status in patients with inflammatory bowel disease. *Am J Gastroenterol* 1989; **84**: 744–748.
172. Kuroki F, Iida M, Tominaga M et al. Multiple vitamin status in Crohn's disease. Correlation with disease activity. *Dig Dis Sci* 1993; **38**: 1614–1618.
173. Geerling BJ, Badart-Smook A, Stockbrugger RW, Brummer RJ. Comprehensive nutritional status in patients with long-standing Crohn disease currently in remission. *Am J Clin Nutr* 1998; **67**: 919–926.
174. Jacob RM. Vitamin C. In Shils Olson J, Shike M et al. eds. *Modern Nutrition in Health and Disease*. Philadelphia: Lippincott, 2000: 467.
175. Steger GG, Mader RM, Vogelsang H et al. Folate absorption in Crohn's disease. *Digestion* 1994; **55**: 234–238.
176. Abu-Qurshin R, Naschitz JE, Zuckermann E et al. Crohn's disease associated with pellagra and increased excretion of 5-hydroxyindolacetic acid. *Am J Med Sci* 1997; **313**: 111–113.
177. Food and Nutrition Board, Institute of Medicine. *Dietary Reference Intakes. Thiamine, Riboflavin, Niacin, Vitamin B6, Folate, Vitamin B12, Pantothenic Acid, Biotin, and Choline*. Washington, DC: National Academy Press, 1989.

178. Food and Nutrition Board, National Research Council. In *Recommended Dietary Allowances*. Washington, DC: National Academy Press, 1989.
179. Main AN, Mills PR, Russell RI et al. Vitamin A deficiency in Crohn's disease. *Gut* 1983; **24**: 1169–1175.
180. Schoelmerich J, Becher MS, Hoppe-Seyler P et al. Zinc and vitamin A deficiency in patients with Crohn's disease is correlated with activity but not with localization or extent of the disease. *Hepatogastroenterology* 1985; **32**: 34–38.
181. Janczewska I, Bartnik W, Butruk E et al. Metabolism of vitamin A in inflammatory bowel disease. *Hepatogastroenterology* 1991; **38**: 391–395.
182. Leichtmann GA, Bengoa JM, Bolt MJ, Sitrin MD. Intestinal absorption of cholecalciferol and 25-hydroxycholecalciferol in patients with both Crohn's disease and intestinal resection. *Am J Clin Nutr* 1991; **54**: 548–552.
183. Goldschmid S, Graham M. Trace element deficiencies in inflammatory bowel disease. *Gastroenterol Clin North Am* 1989; **18**: 579–587.
184. Heatley RV. Assessing nutritional state in inflammatory bowel disease. *Gut* 1986; **27** (Suppl 1): 61–66.
185. Sjogren A, Floren CH, Nilsson A. Evaluation of magnesium status in Crohn's disease as assessed by intracellular analysis and intravenous magnesium infusion. *Scand J Gastroenterol* 1988; **23**: 555–561.
186. Hessov I, Hasselblad C, Fasth S, Hulten L. Magnesium deficiency after ileal resections for Crohn's disease. *Scand J Gastroenterol* 1983; **18**: 643–649.
187. Galland L. Magnesium and inflammatory bowel disease. *Magnesium* 1988; **7**: 78–83.
188. Loeschke K, Konig A, Trebert Haeberlin S, Lux F. Low blood selenium concentration in Crohn disease. *Ann Intern Med* 1987; **106**: 908.
189. Hinks LJ, Inwards KD, Lloyd B, Clayton B. Reduced concentrations of selenium in mild Crohn's disease. *J Clin Pathol* 1988; **41**: 198–201.
190. Ringstad J, Kildebo S, Thomassen Y. Serum selenium, copper, and zinc concentrations in Crohn's disease and ulcerative colitis. *Scand J Gastroenterol* 1993; **28**: 605–608.
191. Rannem T, Ladefoged K, Hylander E et al. Selenium status in patients with Crohn's disease. *Am J Clin Nutr* 1992; **56**: 933–937.
192. Kelly DG, Fleming CR. Nutritional considerations in inflammatory bowel diseases. *Gastroenterol Clin North Am* 1995; **24**: 597–598.
193. Hendricks KM, Walker WA. Zinc deficiency in inflammatory bowel disease. *Nutr Rev* 1988; **46**: 401–408.
194. Hyams JS, Ferry GD, Mandel FS et al. Development and validation of a pediatric Crohn's disease activity index. *J Pediatr Gastroenterol Nutr* 1991; **12**: 439–447.
195. Hyams JS, Mandel F, Ferry GD et al. Relationship of common laboratory parameters to the activity of Crohn's disease in children. *J Pediatr Gastroenterol Nutr* 1992; **14**: 216–222.
196. Otley A, Loonen H, Parekh N et al. Assessing activity of pediatric Crohn's disease: which index to use? *Gastroenterology* 1999; **116**: 527–531.
197. Loonen HJ, Griffiths AM, Merkus MP, Derkx HH. A critical assessment of items on the Pediatric Crohn's Disease Activity Index. *J Pediatr Gastroenterol Nutr* 2003; **36**: 90–95.
198. Kundhal PS, Critch JN, Zachos M et al. Pediatric Crohn Disease Activity Index: responsive to short-term change. *J Pediatr Gastroenterol Nutr* 2003; **36**: 83–89.

24 Indeterminate colitis

Barbara S Kirschner

Introduction

The majority of patients with chronic inflammatory bowel disease (IBD) are diagnosed with either ulcerative colitis or Crohn's disease on the basis of established clinical, endoscopic, histological and radiological criteria.[1] However, in 5–23% of patients with chronic colitis, a definitive diagnosis of ulcerative colitis or Crohn's disease cannot be established because the initial colonoscopic and histological features overlap between ulcerative colitis and Crohn's disease.[2–6] While the condition of most of these patients eventually evolves into patterns consistent with ulcerative colitis or Crohn's disease, approximately 20–60% retain the diagnosis of indeterminate colitis over periods as long as 5–10 years after the diagnosis.[3,5,7–11] This latter observation suggests that indeterminate colitis may constitute a separate category within the spectrum of IBD. This chapter reviews the clinical features of indeterminate colitis, focusing primarily on the pediatric population.

Epidemiological aspects of indeterminate colitis

Most children with indeterminate colitis are evaluated because of recurrent abdominal pain and diarrhea, with a smaller number noting hematochezia.[12] In young children (less than 5 years of age), failure to thrive is more prominent than seen in ulcerative colitis.[13] Hassan et al noted no difference in gender, age at diagnosis or types of symptom at presentation among the 38 newly diagnosed children with ulcerative colitis, indeterminate colitis and Crohn's disease.[14]

The prevalence of indeterminate colitis in reported series of patients with IBD varies among centers from 5 to 23%[2–6] (Table 24.1). In our pediatric population of 428 children actively followed with IBD, 49 (11.4%) were diagnosed with indeterminate colitis[4] (Table 24.2). In 42.9% of those with indeterminate colitis, the histology 'favored ulcerative colitis' but these patients also had features of

Table 24.1 Prevalence of indeterminate colitis (IC)

	Total no. of IBD patients	Age group	Indeterminate colitis patients	Peak age (years) IC	Peak age (years) UC
Gupta et al[4]	420	pediatric	51 (11.9%)	10	—
Heikenen et al[5]	91	pediatric	9 (10%)	7.8	9.7
Hildebrand et al[3]	132	pediatric	36 (27%)	—	—
Stewenius et al[15]	—	—	—	10–19	20–29
Meucci et al[10]	1113	adult	50 (4.6%)	—	—
Shivananda et al[2]	2201	adult	116 (5.3%)	—	—

IBD, inflammatory bowel disease; UC, ulcerative colitis

Table 24.2 Indeterminate colitis: histological features in 49 pediatric patients at the University of Chicago (from reference 4)

'Favor ulcerative colitis': 43% – except for the presence of:

Focal colitis
Colonic granulomas adjacent to ruptured crypts
Gastroduodenal inflammation (*Helicobacter pylori* negative)
Anal fissure

'Favor Crohn's disease': 18% – except for findings of:

Absence of granulomas
No small-bowel X-ray features of Crohn's disease

No distinguishing features: 39%

Crohn's disease including areas of focal colitis, focal gastric or duodenal inflammation, anal fissures or isolated granulomas adjacent to ruptured crypts. Features 'favoring Crohn's disease' were present in 20.4% of children with indeterminate colitis, none of whom had granulomas, radiological evidence of small-bowel Crohn's disease or perianal findings. Endoscopic and histological findings of IBD without distinguishing features of ulcerative colitis or Crohn's disease were present in 36.7% of our patients with indeterminate colitis.

Heikenen et al noted a similar prevalence of indeterminate colitis (10%) in a pediatric population of IBD.[5] These authors noted that children with indeterminate colitis were diagnosed at a younger age (7.8 years) than those with either ulcerative colitis (9.7 years) or Crohn's disease (11.4 years). Similarly, in Sweden, the peak age range at diagnosis was younger (10–19 years) for patients with indeterminate colitis in comparison with ulcerative colitis (20–29 years).[15] A particularly high prevalence of indeterminate colitis (23%) has been reported from one pediatric center in Sweden.[3]

Criteria for histological diagnosis

In establishing the diagnosis of indeterminate colitis, it is essential to exclude other causes of colitis such as infections (*Clostridium difficile, Yersinia, Mycobacterium tuberculosis, Entamoeba histolytica, Escherichia coli* 0157:H7 or other verocytotoxin-producing strains), drugs (non-steroidal anti-inflammatory drugs (NSAIDs)), Behçet's disease, malignancy, vasculitis and other identifiable causes of colitis.

Riddell stated that to differentiate indeterminate colitis lesions from Crohn's disease lesions such as submucosal and subserosal lymphoid aggregates away from areas of ulceration, non-necrotizing granulomas and skip areas should be absent.[16] This is particularly true where there is nonspecific ileal involvement or gastritis and special stains for *Helibacter pylori* are negative. The most frequently used diagnostic study for distinguishing indeterminate colitis from Crohn's disease (in addition to ileocolonoscopy with biopsy) is the small-bowel X-ray.

The endoscopic and histological findings differ from classic ulcerative colitis in that there may be relative rectal sparing, focal inflammation or deep fissuring ulceration. The latter is most common in patients with fulminant colitis. It is also important to recognize that some medications, such as corticosteroids or aminosalicylic acid preparations, may change the diffuse histological appearance in ulcerative colitis to a more focal appearance.[6,16] Thus, slides from the original or pretreatment colonoscopy should be reviewed when considering a diagnosis of indeterminate colitis.

Although the above criteria would appear to allow differentiation between Crohn's disease and ulcerative colitis on the basis of pathology, Farmer et al documented disparity among pathologists reviewing cases of colonic IBD.[17] The diagnoses of gastrointestinal pathologists differed from that of the referring institution in 45% of surgical specimens and 54% of biopsy specimens. Of 70 cases initially diagnosed with ulcerative colitis, 30 (43%) were changed to Crohn's disease or indeterminate colitis; in contrast, 17% of cases initially diagnosed with Crohn's disease were changed to ulcerative colitis or indeterminate colitis.

The performance of upper gastrointestinal endoscopy and biopsy (EGD) identifies some patients with Crohn's disease whose colonoscopy biopsies were indeterminate.[12,18] Kundhal et al reported that, while diffuse non-specific gastritis occurred with similar frequency in children with either Crohn's disease or ulcerative colitis (92% vs. 75%), focal antral gastritis was significantly more common in Crohn's disease than ulcerative colitis (52% vs. 8%).[12] The authors defined focal inflammation as 'localized inflammation of the gastric pits, glands, or foveolae by mononuclear and polymorphonuclear leukocytes bordering directly on uninflamed mucosa'. This is similar to the statements previously published by Riddell.[16] Granulomas in the stomach or duodenum provided evidence confirming the diagnosis of Crohn's disease even in endoscopically normal-appearing mucosa.[12] Hence, performing an EGD should be strongly considered during the initial evaluation of patients for IBD. In order to further categorize our patients with indeterminate colitis further, an X-ray study of the upper gastrointestinal tract with small-bowel follow-through was performed in all patients to exclude the possibility of Crohn's disease. EGD with biopsy may be particularly useful in those children whose symptoms (such as nausea, vomiting, early satiety) suggest gastroduodenal Crohn's disease.[18]

Serologic markers and defining inflammatory bowel disease categories

We are currently evaluating the role of perinuclear anti-neutrophil cytoplasmic antibodies (P-ANCA) and anti-*Saccharomyces cerevisiae* antibodies (ASCA) in identifying patients with ulcerative colitis and Crohn's disease previously diagnosed with indeterminate colitis.[4] While P-ANCA was positive in 68% of those favoring ulcerative colitis, and ASCA was positive in 37% of those favoring Crohn's disease, 86% of our patients with indeterminate colitis were both p-ANCA and ASCA negative.

Recently, Joossens et al correlated serological markers with prospective follow-up evaluation in 97 adult patients with indeterminate colitis.[8] After a mean follow-up of 6 years, 32% of the adult patients with indeterminate colitis were reclassified as having ulcerative colitis or Crohn's disease, half of whom were positive for p-ANCA or ASCA. However, almost half of the patients with indeterminate colitis (48.5%) remained p-ANCA/ASCA negative and continued to have characteristics of indeterminate colitis even 10 years after the initial diagnosis.

Radiological imaging

In a further attempt to distinguish between the various forms of pediatric IBD, ^{99}m-technetium white cell scans and magnetic resonance imaging have been evaluated in children with indeterminate colitis, ulcerative colitis and Crohn's disease.[18–20] The technetium scan had a sensitivity of only 76% compared with colonoscopy and biopsy.[19] Others found that conventional magnetic resonance imaging had a low sensitivity (40%) for detecting Crohn's disease and did not correlate with the severity of inflammation.[20] However, gadolinium-enhanced magnetic resonance imaging in combination with oral polyethylene glycol (PEG) solution (used to distend the small bowel) may be more discriminating.[21] With the latter technique, increased wall thickness was noted in 26/26 children with Crohn's disease while those with indeterminate colitis and ulcerative colitis showed mild parietal contrast enhancement but not bowel wall thickening. Further confirmation of these observations is needed.

Natural history

With time, 50–72% of adult patients and 64% of pediatric patients with indeterminate colitis can be reclassified as having definite ulcerative colitis or Crohn's disease during subsequent observation[3–4,9–11,22] (Table 24.3). After a mean follow-up period of 14 months, one group reported that 33% of 36 patients with indeterminate colitis were reclassified as ulcerative colitis and 17% as Crohn's disease.[9] Meucci et al reported that 37 of 50 patients (74%) changed from indeterminate colitis to a definite diagnosis of ulcerative colitis or Crohn's disease during follow-up with a cumulative probability of 80% within 8 years of diagnosis.[10] In contrast, Wells et al followed 16 patients with indeterminate colitis for a mean of 10 years and observed that three were reclassified with ulcerative colitis, one with Crohn's disease and the rest remained indeterminate.[11] The course of indeterminate colitis in 36 Swedish children after a mean follow-up of 4.6 years was analyzed by Hildebrand et al.[3] The findings were similar to

Table 24.3 Indeterminate colitis (IC): changes in diagnosis with time

	Initial IC	Diagnosis Final IC (%)	Final UC (%)	Final CD (%)
Hildebrand et al[3]	36 (pediatric)	36	58	6
Moum et al[9]	36 (adult)	50	33	17
Meucci et al[10]	50 (adult)	20	34	40
Kangas et al[22]	6 (surgery)	50	—	50
Wells et al[11]	16 (surgery)	75	19	6
Gupta et al[4]	12 (surgery/pediatric)	33	50	17

UC, ulcerative colitis; CD, Crohn's disease

those as described above in adults: 21/36 (58%) were subsequently categorized as ulcerative colitis, 2/36 (6%) as Crohn's disease and 13/36 (36%) remaining as indeterminate colitis. In our report describing 49 children with indeterminate colitis, nine had undergone colectomy at a mean of 24 months after diagnosis. During a mean follow-up period of 42 months, 6/9 (66%) had a subsequent course, including repeat endoscopic examination consistent with ulcerative colitis, 3/9 (33%) as indeterminate colitis and 1/9 (11%) as Crohn's disease.

Medical therapy

The observation that the majority of patients with indeterminate colitis over time are reclassified as ulcerative colitis or Crohn's disease makes it difficult to know whether indeterminate colitis represents a separate form of IBD. Perhaps because of the small number of patients with indeterminate colitis, the response to various drug regimens in this population has not been specifically addressed.[7] In our program the choice of therapeutic intervention is selected depending on the severity of symptoms, extent and severity of endoscopic and histological findings and laboratory parameters[23] (Table 24.4). For most patients, drug therapy is similar to that indicated for patients with ulcerative colitis of comparable extent and severity. These include 5-aminosalicylic acid (5-ASA) preparations for mild disease and corticosteroids and immunomodulatory therapy for moderate and severe disease. However, we are more likely to use metronidazole in this population, especially where there is extensive focal colitis or those 'favoring' Crohn's disease. Immunomodulatory agents, such as azathioprine or 6-mercaptopurine, are used in approximately 60% of our pediatric population with IBD, owing to the presence of steroid dependency, resistance or toxicity.[24]

Many large series involving clinical trials of adult patients with IBD have included small numbers of patients with indeterminate colitis, although they have not specifically addressed the treatment of indeterminate colitis.[7] The response of adult patients with refractory ulcerative colitis and indeterminate colitis appears to show similar improvement to azathioprine/6-mercaptopurine and cyclo-sporin as well as newer immunomodulatory agents such tacrolimus and thalidomide.[25–27] The role of infliximab in indeterminate colitis is as yet to be determined. However, favorable outcomes in pediatric patients with ulcerative colitis suggest that it could be considered in patients with indeterminate colitis who are not responding to conventional medications.[28]

Table 24.4 Medical approach to the pediatric patient with indeterminate colitis

5-Aminosalicylic acid preparations for mild disease
Corticosteroids (moderate-to-severe disease severity)
Metronidazole if histology favors Crohn's disease
Azathioprine (AZA) or 6-mercaptopurine (6-MP)
Consider measuring red blood cell 6-thioguanine levels to reduce the risk of toxicity if increasing the dose in refractory patients
Change to AZA from 6-MP (or vice versa) for non-hypersensitivity side-effects (e.g. rash, arthralgia, headache)
Methotrexate (parenterally) if intolerant or refractory to AZA/6-MP
Cyclosporin intravenously or micro-emulsified oral formulation
Tacrolimus (0.1–0.15 mg/kg twice a day); monitor blood level
Thalidomide (50–100 mg/day in older children and adolescents)
Remicade (at conventional dosing)

Surgical treatment

Considerable conflicting data have been published regarding complication rates following medical and surgical intervention in patients with indeterminate colitis versus ulcerative colitis. Some centers reported that indeterminate colitis was more refractory to medical interventions than ulcerative colitis, resulting in a greater relapse rate[29] and subsequent need for colectomy.[30] Colectomy rates averaged 36.1/1000 person-years in patients with indeterminate colitis versus only 7.5 for those with definite ulcerative colitis.[30] In contrast, Witte et al described similar response rates to medical intervention in indeterminate colitis and ulcerative colitis.[31] The European Collaborative Study on Inflammatory Bowel Disease (EC-IBD) reported 'complete relief of complaints' in 48% of ulcerative colitis patients versus 50% of those with indeterminate colitis; in addition, 37% of patients with ulcerative colitis 'improved' versus 33% with indeterminate colitis.[31] Similarly, higher rates of pouch failure after ileal pouch–anal anastomosis (IPPA)[32,33] and colorectal cancer[34] have been reported by some groups, while others have reported lower rates of pouchitis for indeterminate colitis (29%) than ulcerative colitis (58%) and Crohn's disease (72%). However, this latter group observed a greater frequency of fistulae after IPAA in patients with indeterminate colitis (26%) versus for ulcerative colitis (10%).[35] Post-IPAA complications resulting in pouch removal were higher for indeterminate colitis (19–28%) versus ulcerative colitis (0.4–8%) in some studies[32,33] but not in others.[35–37]

It is our practice to repeat colonoscopy, usually with concurrent EGD, during selected periods of relapse to assess whether histological changes consistent with ulcerative colitis or Crohn's disease have developed. This is especially the case if colectomy and IPAA are being considered because of refractory disease. At this time, repeat small-bowel X-ray is usually obtained so that patients with ileal Crohn's disease would be excluded and patients with persistent indeterminate colitis would be counseled regarding the potentially greater risk of pouch complications. Often, patients with indeterminate colitis undergo a multi-staged operative procedure consisting of a subtotal colectomy with temporary ileostomy and Hartmann pouch. In this way, the entire resected colon can be assessed to exclude Crohn's disease prior to creating the IPAA.[36]

REFERENCES

1. Marion JF, Rubin TH, Present DH. Differential diagnosis of chronic ulcerative colitis and Crohn disease. In Kirsner JB, ed. *Inflammatory Bowel Disease*, 5th edn. Philadelphia: WB Saunders, 2000: 315–325.
2. Shivananda S, Lennard-Jones J, Logan R et al. Incidence of inflammatory bowel disease across Europe: is there a difference between north and south? Results of the European Collaborative Study on Inflammatory Bowel Disease (EC-IBD). *Gut* 1996; **39**: 690–697.
3. Hildebrand H, Brydolf M, Holmquist L et al. Incidence and prevalence of inflammatory bowel disease in children in southwestern Sweden. *Acta Paediatr* 1994; **83**: 640–645.
4. Gupta P, Hart J, Kirschner BS. Perinuclear antineutrophilic cytoplasmic antibodies (pANCA) and anti-*Saccharomyces cerevisiae* (ASCA) antibodies in children with indeterminate colitis (abstract). *Gastroenterology* 2000; **118**: 103, A687.
5. Heikenen JB, Werlin SL, Brown CW et al. Presenting symptoms and diagnostic lag in children with inflammatory bowel disease. *Inflamm Bowel Dis* 1999; **5**: 158–160.
6. Kirschner BS, Heyman MB, Clemons T et al. The Pediatric IBD Consortium Database – initial demographic data. *Gastroenterology* 2002; **122**: A-611.
7. Geboes K, DeHertogh G. Indeterminate colitis. *Inflamm Bowel Dis* 2003; **9**: 324–331.
8. Joossens S, Reinisch W, Vermeire S et al. The value of serologic markers in indeterminate colitis: a prospective follow-up. *Gastroenterology* 2002; **122**: 1242–1247.
9. Moum B, Ekbom A, Vatn MH et al. Inflammatory bowel disease: re-evaluation of the diagnosis in a prospective population based study in south eastern Norway. *Gut* 1997; **40**: 328–332.
10. Meucci G, Bortoli A, Riccioli FA et al. Frequency and clinical evolution of indeterminate colitis: a retrospective multi-centre study in northern Italy. GSMII (Gruppo di Studio per le Malattie Infiammatorie Intestinali). *Eur J Gastroenterol Hepatol* 1999; **11**: 909–913.
11. Wells AD, McMillan I, Price AB et al. Natural history of indeterminate colitis. *Br J Surg* 1991; **78**: 179–181.
12. Kundhal PS, Stormon MO, Zachos M et al. Gastric antral biopsy in the differentiation of pediatric colitides. *Am J Gastroenterol* 2003; **98**: 557–561.
13. Mamula P, Telega GW, Markowitz JE et al. Inflammatory bowel disease in children 5 years of age and younger. *Am J Gastroenterol* 2002; **97**: 2005–2010.
14. Hassan K, Cowan FJ, Jenkins HR. The incidence of childhood inflammatory bowel disease in Wales. *Eur J Pediatr* 2000; **159**: 261–263.
15. Stewenius J, Adnerhill I, Ekelund GR et al. Ulcerative colitis and indeterminate colitis in the city of Malmo, Sweden. A 25-year incidence study. *Scand J Gastroenterol* 1995; **30**: 38–43.
16. Riddell RH. Pathology of idiopathic inflammatory bowel disease. In Kirsner JB, ed. *Inflammatory Bowel Disease*, 5th edn. Philadelphia: WB Saunders, 2000: 439–441.
17. Farmer M, Petras RE, Hunt LE et al. The importance of diagnostic accuracy in colonic inflammatory bowel disease. *Am J Gastroenterol* 2000; **95**: 3184–3188.
18. Lenaerts C, Roy CC, Vaillancourt M et al. High incidence of upper gastrointestinal tract involvement in children with Crohn disease. *Pediatrics* 1989; **83**: 777–781.
19. Cucchiara S, Celentano L, deMagistris TM et al. Colonoscopy and technetium99m white cell scan in children with suspected inflammatory bowel disease. *J Pediatr* 1999; **135**: 727–732.
20. Durno CA, Sherman P, Williams T et al. Magnetic resonance imaging to distinguish the type and severity of pediatric inflammatory bowel diseases. *J Pediatr Gastroenterol Nutr* 2000; **30**: 170–174.
21. Laghi A, Borrelli O, Paolantonio P et al. Contrast enhanced magnetic resonance imaging of the terminal ileum in children with Crohn disease. *Gut* 2000; **52**: 393–397.
22. Kangas E, Matikainen M, Mattila J. Is 'indeterminate colitis' Crohn disease in the long-term follow-up? *Int Surg* 1994; **79**: 120–123.
23. Kirschner BS. Indeterminate colitis. Implications for management: medical approach. *Inflamm Bowel Dis* 2000; **6**: 516–517.
24. Kirschner BS. The safety of azathioprine and 6-mercaptopurine in children and adolescents with inflammatory bowel disease. *Gastroenterology* 1998; **115**: 813–821.
25. Fraser AG, Orchard TR, Jewell DP. The efficacy of azathioprine for the treatment of inflammatory bowel disease: a 30-year review. *Gut* 2002; **50**: 485–489.
26. Fellerman K, Tanko Z, Herrlinger KR et al. Response of refractory colitis to intravenous or oral tacrolimus (FK506). *Inflamm Bowel Dis* 2002; **8**: 317–324.
27. Bariol C, Meagher AP, Vickers CR et al. Early studies on the safety and efficacy of thalidomide for symptomatic inflammatory bowel disease. *J Gastroenterol Hepatol* 2002; **17**: 135–139.
28. Mamula P, Markowitz JE, Brown KA et al. Infliximab as a novel therapy for pediatric ulcerative colitis. *J Pediatr Gastroenterol Nutr* 2002; **34**: 307–311.
29. Stewenius J, Adnerhill I, Ekelund GR et al. Risk of relapse in new cases of ulcerative colitis and indeterminate colitis. *Dis Colon Rectum* 1996; **39**: 1019–1025.
30. Stewenius J, Adnerhill I, Ekelund GR et al. Operations in unselected patients with ulcerative colitis and indeterminate colitis. A long-term follow-up study. *Eur J Surg* 1996; **162**: 131–137.
31. Witte J, Shivananda S, Lennard-Jones et al. Disease outcome in inflammatory bowel disease: mortality, morbidity and therapeutic management of 796-person inception cohort in the European Collaborative Study on Inflammatory Bowel Disease (EC-IBD). *Scand J Gastroenterol* 2000; **35**: 1272–1277.
32. Koltun WA, Schoetz DJJ Jr, Roberts PL et al. Indeterminate colitis predisposes to perineal complications after ileal pouch–anal anastomosis. *Dis Colon Rectum* 1991; **34**: 857–860.
33. McIntyre PB, Pemberton JH, Wolff BG et al. Indeterminate colitis. Long-term outcome in patients after ileal pouch–anal anastomosis. *Dis Colon Rectum* 1995; **38**: 51–54.
34. Stewenius J, Adnerhill I, Ekelund GR et al. Incidence of colorectal cancer and all cause mortality in non-selected patients with ulcerative colitis and indeterminate colitis in Malmo, Sweden. *Int J Colorectal Dis* 1995; **10**: 117–122.
35. Rudolph WG, Uthoff SM, McAuliffe TL et al. Indeterminate colitis: the real story. *Dis Colon Rectum* 2002; **45**: 1528–1534.
36. Marcello PW, Schoetz DJ, Rogers PL et al. Evolutionary changes in the pathologic diagnosis after the ileoanal pouch procedure. *Dis Colon Rectum* 1997; **40**: 263–269.
37. Gramlich T, Delaney CP, Lynch AC et al. Pathological subgroups may predict complications but not late failure after ileal pouch–anal anastomosis for indeterminate colitis. *Colorectal Dis* 2003; **5**: 315–319.

25 Ulcerative colitis

Leslie M Higuchi and Athos Bousvaros

Introduction

Ulcerative colitis and Crohn's disease are the two most common forms of idiopathic inflammatory bowel disease (IBD). Ulcerative colitis differs from Crohn's disease in that the inflammation in ulcerative colitis is confined to the mucosal layer of the colon. In contrast, Crohn's disease is characterized by transmural inflammation in either a limited region or extensively in the bowel, and may involve any portion of the gastrointestinal tract from the mouth to the anus. The peak incidence of IBD occurs between the ages of 15 and 25 years, but ulcerative colitis may begin at any age.[1] Approximately 20% of patients with ulcerative colitis present before the age of 20 years.[2] While children and adults develop similar symptoms, children often present with more extensive disease.[3] Clinicians caring for children and adolescents with ulcerative colitis must treat both the gastrointestinal and extraintestinal complications, optimize nutrition and linear growth, and address the psychosocial ramifications of the illness. Since the majority of the published studies investigating the natural history and treatment of ulcerative colitis are in adults, we refer primarily to these studies, with reference to pediatric studies where available.

Epidemiology

Most children with ulcerative colitis present between the ages of 10 and 18 years. However, ulcerative colitis in children under the age of 5 years is well described.[1,4,5] Epidemiological studies primarily conducted in the US, GB, and Scandinavian countries, suggest that the incidence of ulcerative colitis in children ranges from 1.4 to 4.3 cases/100 000 population per year.[3,6–10] The incidence of ulcerative colitis in children has remained relatively stable[11] (Table 25.1). The majority of incidence data for Crohn's disease and ulcerative colitis in the pediatric population originates from geographic regions with higher rates of IBD.

Adult studies demonstrate that ulcerative colitis is more prevalent in North America, the UK, and Scandinavia and less common in southern Europe, Asia and Africa.[2] The data suggest a north–south gradient with higher incidence rates of both Crohn's disease and ulcerative colitis in northern locations, even within individual countries.[12,13] Ulcerative colitis is more common among Jewish than non-Jewish peoples,[14] but disease rates in people of Jewish origin vary by geographic region and parallel those of the general population.[15] The higher rates of IBD in individuals of Jewish origin across different countries support a common genetic predisposition; however, the geographic variation of IBD rates in Jews emphasizes that environmental factors (see below) influence the inherited risk.

Etiology and pathogenesis

The pathogenesis of ulcerative colitis is unknown. A widely accepted hypothesis suggests that, in the genetically susceptible individual, a combination of host and environmental factors leads to the initiation and perpetuation of an abnormal intestinal immune response, resulting in ulcerative colitis.[16] In support of this theory, colitis in animals occurs in a wide variety of genetically altered rodents, including: knockout mice for interleukin (IL)-2, IL-10 and T-cell receptor; and HLA-B27 transgenic rats.[17] Interestingly, most of these animal models do not develop colitis in germ-free environments. These findings suggest that multiple genes may contribute to the pathogenesis of IBD, and that interaction with the environment is essential.

In humans, ulcerative colitis appears to have a non-Mendelian pattern of inheritance. Current evidence suggests that genes comntribute less to the risk in individuals with ulcerative colitis than in those with Crohn's disease. In a Danish twin cohort study and a recently updated Swedish twin cohort study, the calculated pair concordance rates among monozygotic twins were 14–19% for ulcerative colitis and 50% for Crohn's disease; and among dizygotic twins, 0–5% for ulcerative colitis and 0–4% for Crohn's disease.[18,19] Although the concordance rates of disease are higher in monozygotic twins, the incomplete concordance suggests that non-genetic factors also contribute to the development of ulcerative colitis. First-degree relatives of patients with ulcerative colitis have a 9.5-fold increase in risk of developing ulcerative colitis, compared to the general population.[20] The risk of developing Crohn's disease or ulcerative colitis is increased in children of affected parents with IBD. In one study, the life-time risks for IBD in offspring ranged from 5–8% when one parent had Crohn's disease, and from 2–5% when one parent had ulcerative colitis.[21] In another study of families with two or more affected family members with IBD, there was a high concordance for the diagnosis of ulcerative colitis or Crohn's disease.[22] Of 83 families in which the proband had ulcerative colitis, 72 relatives had ulcerative colitis (81%, 72/89) and 17 had Crohn's disease (19%, 17/89).[22] Family linkage studies suggest that candidate genes may be present on chromosomes 3, 7 and 12, with the strongest association identified on chromosome 12.[23] Associations with certain HLA alleles (especially DR2) have been described.[16,24,25] However, no specific gene or protein has been identified.[17]

Environmental factors may contribute to the development of ulcerative colitis. However, most studies examining environmental risk factors have the limitations of retrospective, case–control methodology. One of the most consistent findings in multiple studies is the lower risk of ulcerative colitis among current smokers. Current smokers have approximately one-half the risk of developing ulcerative colitis compared to non-smokers.[26,27]

Table 25.1 Incidence of ulcerative colitis (UC) in children and adolescents (no. of new cases/100 000 persons per year)

First author	Location	Age range (years)	Time period studied	Incidence
Barton, 1989[6]	Scotland	>5 and ″ 16 for UC	1968–83	
			1968	1.9
			1983	1.6
Calkins, 1984[7]	Baltimore, MD, USA	<10	1977–79	M 0.34
				F 0.36
		≥10 and ″ 19	1977–79	M 2.25
				F 1.32
Langholz, 1997[3]	Copenhagen county, Denmark	<15	1962-1987	2.0
Lindberg, 2000[8]	Stockholm, Sweden	″ 15	1984–86	1.4
			1993–95	3.2
Olafsdottir, 1989[9]	Western Norway	″ 15	1984–85	4.3
Bentsen, 2002[10]	Southeastern, Norway	<16	1990–93	2.1

Several authors have suggested that exposure to infections in the perinatal period or early life may contribute to the development of ulcerative colitis. Individuals with Crohn's disease or ulcerative colitis were more likely to have experienced a diarrheal illness during infancy, when compared to their unaffected siblings.[28] Appendectomy at a young age is associated with a lower risk of ulcerative colitis.[29–31] In a population-based study, the inverse relation between appendectomy and ulcerative colitis was observed only in those individuals who underwent surgery before the age of 20 years.[29] Interestingly, the risk of ulcerative colitis was reduced only in patients who had an appendectomy performed for inflammatory conditions, such as appendicitis or mesenteric lymphadenitis, but not in patients who underwent appendectomy for non-specific abdominal pain.[29] These findings may suggest that the inflammatory condition that preceded the appendectomy, rather than the appendectomy itself, may be inversely related to the development of ulcerative colitis later in life.[29]

Some published reports suggest that non-steroidal anti-inflammatory drugs (NSAIDs) may precede the onset of IBD, lead to a reactivation of quiescent IBD, or exacerbate already active IBD in humans.[32–35] In an adult case–control study, Felder et al compared the use of NSAIDs in 60 patients hospitalized for exacerbations of IBD, either ulcerative colitis or Crohn's disease, to that of 62 out-patients with irritable bowel syndrome.[36] At least 31% of the IBD patients (35% of the ulcerative colitis patients) who used NSAIDs within 1 month of symptoms developed the onset or an exacerbation of IBD, whereas only 2% of the irritable bowel patients experienced aggravation of their symptoms after similar NSAID use. In a retrospective review of initial office visit records of adult out-patients with either Crohn's disease (112 initial visits) or ulcerative colitis (80 initial visits), Bonner et al did not find any association between NSAID use and active IBD.[37] Also, another short report suggested the possible exacerbation of IBD activity associated with the use of celecoxib, a selective cyclooxygenase (COX)-2 inhibitor, in two patients, one with ulcerative colitis and one with Crohn's disease.[35] Studies suggest that both standard NSAIDs and selective COX-2 inhibitors can exacerbate colitis in animal models of colonic inflammation.[38,39] It has been postulated that NSAIDs may worsen colitis by inhibiting the synthesis of colonic prostaglandins that may exert anti-inflammatory effects in the setting of colonic inflammation.[40] Further study is needed to clarify any true association of NSAID therapy with the onset of ulcerative colitis, to identify those individuals at most risk, and to determine the safety profile of COX-2 inhibitors in comparison to standard NSAIDs in reference to potential colonic mucosal injury. In general, given the current data, it is advisable for children with ulcerative colitis to avoid NSAID therapy if there are other reasonable alternatives for pain control (e.g. acetaminophen). In patients with arthritis, alternative anti-inflammatory medications (e.g. sulfasalazine) should be considered.

Given the constant intestinal exposure to numerous luminal dietary antigens, it seems reasonable to postulate a relationship between diet and ulcerative colitis. The data on the association of breast feeding and ulcerative colitis are inconclusive, with one published study suggesting a protective effect,[41] and two other studies showing no effect.[28,42] Ecological and case–control studies have examined the association between certain foods and ulcerative colitis,[43,44] but at present, there is no definitive evidence linking diet to the development of ulcerative colitis. Methodological issues of these retrospectively designed dietary studies, such as the collection of pre-illness dietary information, remain a problem in the interpretation of findings. As an example, the recalled dietary intake may reflect changes in the diet secondary to the effects of the disease itself, rather than the individual's dietary habits preceding the onset of disease. The association between oral contraceptive use and ulcerative colitis remains controversial.[26,45]

Current evidence suggests that colitis results when the intestinal mucosal immune system in patients with inflammatory bowel disease reacts inappropriately to intestinal bacteria. Evidence supporting this hypothesis includes the fact that most animal models of colitis do not develop disease in germ-free environments, the reports of efficacy of antibiotics in the treatment of colitis and pouchitis, and the seasonal variations in the onset of ulcerative colitis. However, no specific infectious agent has consistently been associated with exacerbations of ulcerative colitis.[17,46]

Activated cells of the mucosal immune system are present in the bowel of both Crohn's disease and ulcerative colitis patients. There is some evidence that Crohn's disease and ulcerative colitis are characterized by different mucosal immune responses, suggesting that different subsets of T cells may be involved. Crohn's disease is characterized by increased secretion of the cytokines IL-2, interferon-γ, tumor necrosis factor (TNF)-α, and IL-12, suggesting a Th1 pattern of cytokine response.[47,48] In contrast, in ulcerative colitis, the lamina propria T cells secrete increased amounts of IL-5 and possibly IL-13 and there is increased production by B cells of IgG1, suggesting a Th2 pattern of cytokine response.[46,29] Such differences may explain why anti-TNF therapies, such as infliximab, have thus far failed to show the same degree of efficacy in ulcerative colitis as in Crohn's disease. Patients with active ulcerative colitis also have increased levels of the chemokine IL-8 in biopsy specimens as well as in rectal dialysates.[50–52] IL-8 and other chemokines facilitate the recruitment and transmigration of neutrophils across mucosal surfaces.[53,54] These neutrophils in turn produce prostaglandins and leukotrienes, which cause pain, diarrhea and further intestinal inflammation.[55] Thus, alterations in function of immune system cells, particularly regulatory CD4 lymphocytes, probably result in aberrant responses to bacterial antigens, antibody production and cytotoxicity against gut epithelium, and recruitment of inflammatory cells into the colonic crypts.

Clinical signs and symptoms

The typical symptoms of ulcerative colitis include rectal bleeding, diarrhea and abdominal pain. The presentation can vary depending upon the extent of colonic involvement and the severity of inflammation. The colon in ulcerative colitis is inflamed in a diffuse, continuous distribution, extending from the rectum proximally. By convention, ulcerative colitis is classified according to the extent of disease into the following three subgroups: proctitis (disease limited to the rectum), left-sided colitis (disease extending to the sigmoid or descending colon, but not past the splenic flexure) and pancolitis (disease extending past the splenic flexure). Proctitis may present with tenesmus, urgency and the passage of formed or semi-formed stool with blood and mucus.[56] In contrast, pancolitis or left-sided disease may present with bloody diarrhea and significant abdominal pain. The majority of patients will present with a history of symptoms for several weeks; however, some will present with a more acute clinical picture.

Although adults and children with ulcerative colitis can present with similar symptoms, there are differences in the clinical presentation of these two populations. Studies suggest that children with ulcerative colitis present with more extensive colonic involvement than adults with ulcerative colitis.[3,4,10] In a Danish study of 80 patients aged less than 15 years and 1081 patients aged 15 years or more with ulcerative colitis, the younger group had more extensive disease at diagnosis compared to the older group diagnosed with ulcerative colitis.[3] Of the ulcerative colitis patients younger than 15 years, 29% had pancolitis and 25% had proctitis; in contrast, of the ulcerative colitis patients 15 years or older, 16% had pancolitis and 46% had proctitis.[3] Gryboski examined 38 children diagnosed with ulcerative colitis at ″ 10 years old and reported 71% with pancolitis, 13% with left-sided colitis and 6% with proctitis.[4] Approximately 5% of children with ulcerative colitis have evidence of delayed linear growth and/or weight loss at diagnosis, although growth failure is much less frequent than in children with Crohn's disease[4,57] (Table 25.2).

Table 25.2 Symptoms at initial presentation of ulcerative colitis in children and adolescents (from references 3, 4, 9, 57, 300)

Clinical symptoms	Range (%)
Rectal bleeding	75–98
Diarrhea	71–91
Abdominal pain	44–92
Weight loss	13–74
Arthralgia/arthritis	5–9
Fever	3–34
Growth restriction	4–5

Children with ulcerative colitis may present with varying degrees of disease severity. Approximately 50% of children with ulcerative colitis will present with a mild form of disease, characterized by an insidious onset of diarrhea and rectal bleeding, without abdominal pain or systemic symptoms such as fever. In these patients, disease may be confined to the distal colon.[58,59] Disease of moderate severity is seen in 30% of children with ulcerative colitis and is characterized by a more acute presentation with bloody diarrhea, tenesmus and urgency; systemic symptoms including low-grade fever, abdominal tenderness, weight loss and mild anemia may be present.[58,59] Approximately 10% of children will present with a severe form of ulcerative colitis.[58,59] Characteristic findings in severe disease include six or more bloody stools per day, fever, weight loss, anemia, hypoalbuminemia and diffuse abdominal tenderness on physical examination.[58–60] A very small percentage of children will present initially with extraintestinal symptoms or manifestations, without obvious intestinal symptoms.[59] These extraintestinal manifestations of IBD may include axial or peripheral arthritis, erythema nodosum, pyoderma gangrenosum, or primary sclerosing cholangitis (see Extraintestinal manifestations, p.394).

Table 25.3 Differential diagnosis of colitis

Infectious etiologies
Campylobacter
Salmonella
Shigella
Escherichia coli 0157: H7 and other enterohemorrhagic *E. coli*
Clostridium difficile
Aeromonas
Plesiomonas
Entamoeba histolytica
Cytomegalovirus
Herpes simplex virus
Yersinia
Tuberculosis
HIV and HIV-related opportunistic infections
Other
Ulcerative colitis
Crohn's disease
Henoch–Schönlein purpura
Hemolytic uremic syndrome
Intestinal ischemia
Intussusception
Allergic colitis (primarily in infancy)
Hirschsprung's enterocolitis (primarily in infancy)

Diagnosis and differential

Differential diagnosis

The diagnosis of ulcerative colitis is established by the information gathered from a detailed symptom and family history, physical examination, and a combination of laboratory, radiological, endoscopic and histological findings. It is important to exclude other etiologies, such as an infectious process, and to distinguish ulcerative colitis from Crohn's disease. Colonic inflammation is typically characterized by bloody diarrhea with abdominal cramping. The differential diagnosis of colitis depends upon the age of the child at the time of evaluation. In infancy, necrotizing enterocolitis, Hirschsprung's enterocolitis and allergic colitis are common. In contrast, in the older child and adolescent, enteric infection and IBD are the most common diagnoses. Causes of colitis are listed in Table 25.3. In patients with painless rectal bleeding, other conditions (Meckel's diverticulum, polyp) should be considered. In addition to details of the clinical presentation, the history should include family history, recent antibiotic therapy, infectious exposures, growth and sexual development and the presence of extraintestinal manifestations of ulcerative colitis. Physical examination should include assessment of height, weight and body mass index; abdominal distension, tenderness, or mass; extraintestinal manifestations (e.g. aphthous stomatitis, pyoderma gangrenosum, uveitis or arthritis); and fecal blood on rectal examination, perianal abnormalities (e.g. fistulae, fissures or tags). Findings on physical examination may help to distinguish ulcerative colitis from Crohn's disease; for example, pronounced growth failure or a perianal abscess strongly suggests the diagnosis of Crohn's disease. A severely ill child with ulcerative colitis may have tachycardia, orthostatic hypotension, fever, or dehydration.

Such findings in the presence of abdominal distension and a concerning abdominal examination, may herald a fulminant presentation of ulcerative colitis with increased risk of developing toxic megacolon.

Laboratory assessment

Initial laboratory evaluation should include appropriate blood tests, stool for occult blood, *Clostridium difficile* toxin assay and stool cultures. A complete blood cell count with differential may reveal a leukocytosis with or without left shift, anemia, or thrombocytosis. Thrombocytosis, hypoalbuminemia and elevated erythrocyte sedimentation rate (ESR) or C-reactive protein (CRP) may indicate increased disease activity.[61–63] The presence of anemia with low mean corpuscular volume (MCV), wide red cell distribution width (RDW) and low iron levels may indicate an iron-deficient anemia secondary to ongoing fecal blood losses or the anemia of chronic disease. Children with significant mucosal inflammation may have normal laboratory test results. In a study of children with ulcerative colitis or Crohn's colitis, 13 of 36 patients with ulcerative colitis (36%) had normal blood test results, including seven of 28 ulcerative colitis patients with macroscopic findings (obvious abnormalities) on colonoscopy, and 12 of 31 ulcerative colitis patients with histological moderate or severe chronic inflammation.[63] Stool examination should rule out possible enteric infections (see Table 25.3). In sexually active patients, rectal cultures for gonorrhea should be considered. In ulcerative colitis, Gram stain or methylene blue stain of stools may identify leukocytes.

It has been proposed that certain serum antibodies may be helpful for screening for IBD and discriminating ulcerative colitis from Crohn's disease.[64,65] Perinuclear antineutrophil cytoplasmic antibodies (P-ANCA) are seen in 60–80% of adults with ulcerative colitis compared to 10–27% of adults with Crohn's disease.[64,66,67] Similarly, anti-*Saccharomyces cerevisiae* antibodies (ASCA) are commonly found in individuals with Crohn's disease but are rarely seen in ulcerative colitis. In a study of 173 children, ASCA yielded a sensitivity of 55% and specificity of 95% for Crohn's disease, and ANCA had a sensitivity of 57% and specificity of 92% for ulcerative colitis.[64] In a study of 128 pediatric patients undergoing evaluation for IBD, Dubinsky et al utilized modified cut-off values to optimize the sensitivity of the ASCA and ANCA assays. For the combination of ASCA and P-ANCA, the sensitivity of detecting IBD increased to 81% with the modified values compared to the 69% with standard cut-off values; however, this was accompanied by an increase in false-positive rates among the children without IBD.[65] An overlap of ASCA and P-ANCA positive serology between patients with Crohn's disease or ulcerative colitis remains. In particular, P-ANCA tends to test positive in the serum of patients with Crohn's disease who exhibit ulcerative colitis features.[64,68] The value of these tests to supplement the routine diagnostic tests in IBD is a subject under study.

Endoscopic and radiographic evaluation

Evaluation with colonoscopy and ileoscopy with biopsies and a barium upper gastrointestinal series with small-bowel follow-through should be performed to diagnose ulcerative colitis, determine the extent and severity of ulcerative colitis presentation and distinguish ulcerative colitis from Crohn's disease or a non-IBD diagnosis. In patients with severe colitis, a limited flexible sigmoidoscopy examination with minimal air insufflation may be prudent to avoid increased risk of a full colonoscopy (perforation, hemorrhage, toxic dilatation). In order to establish the extent of disease involvement by colonoscopy, we recommend biopsies from the terminal ileum and each segment of the colon, even if there are no visible findings at a particular level of the colon. In ulcerative colitis, typical findings seen by the endoscopist include a diffuse, continuous process starting at the rectum and extending more proximally into the colon. However, in children with ulcerative colitis, rectal sparing has been reported.[69,70] The colonic mucosa often appears edematous, erythematous and friable, with minute surface erosions and ulcerations (Figure 25.1). Larger, deeper ulcerations with associated exudate may develop in more severe disease. With more chronic (longstanding) ulcerative colitis, pseudopolyps may be present. (Figure 25.2). In contrast, in Crohn's disease, colonoscopy may reveal focal ulcerations (aphthous lesions) with intervening areas of normal-appearing mucosa (skip lesions).

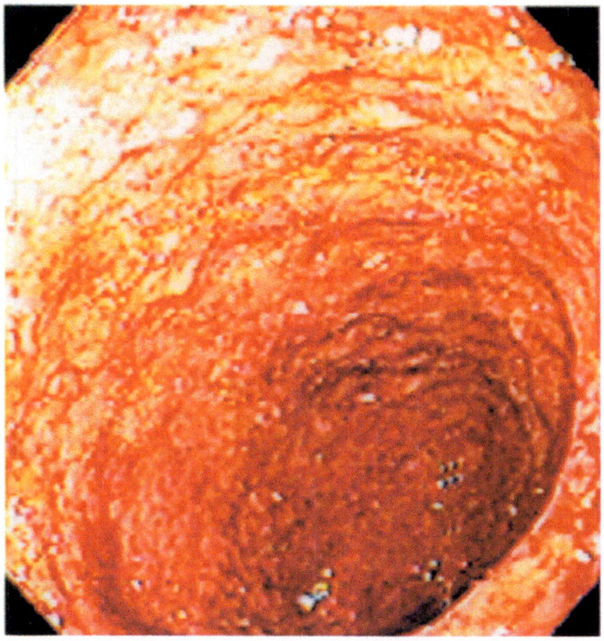

Figure 25.1 Severe colitis at initial presentation of ulcerative colitis. The colonoscopy demonstrates a featureless colon with loss of vascular pattern and hemorrhage.

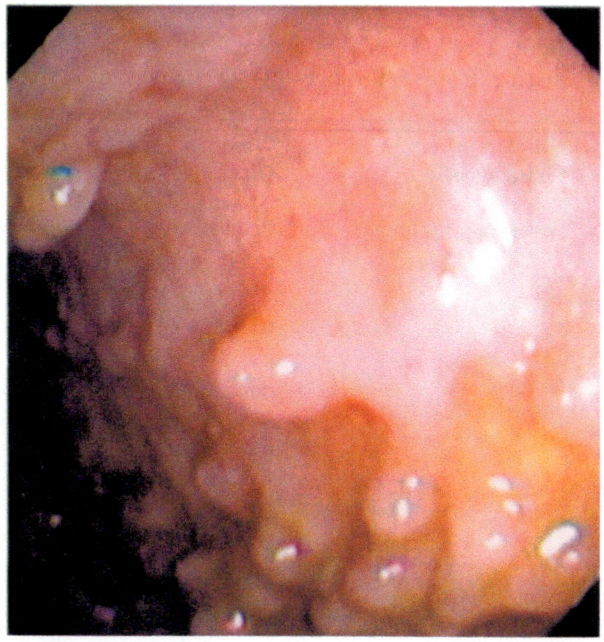

Figure 25.2 Colonic pseudopolyps present in a 16-year-old girl with an 8-year history of ulcerative colitis. The patient had persistent symptoms of diarrhea and rectal bleeding despite chronic corticosteroid and 6-mercaptopurine therapy, and subsequently underwent colectomy.

In severe or chronic Crohn's disease, linear ulcerations, nodularity (cobblestoning) and strictures or stenoses may be present. In general, the ulcerations in Crohn's disease are deeper and focal versus the diffuse, superficial ulcerations typical of ulcerative colitis (Table 25.4).[64–74]

An upper gastrointestinal series with small-bowel follow-through should be performed to look for any evidence of abnormality of the terminal ileum or more proximal gastrointestinal tract, and the presence of fistulae, which would suggest Crohn's disease. The only exception is the finding of ulcerative colitis-associated 'backwash ileitis', which should be distinguished from terminal ileal disease of Crohn's disease. With 'backwash ileitis', the ileum appears patulous and inflamed, involves only the distal ileal segment and is associated with pancolitis; there should be no evidence of extensive ulcerations or stricturing, as seen with Crohn's disease.[75]

Although by definition, the disease of ulcerative colitis is confined to the colon, children with Crohn's disease or ulcerative colitis can have inflammation of the upper gastrointestinal tract.[76–79] In a controlled, blinded study of children with ulcerative colitis or Crohn's disease, biopsies from the esophagus, gastric antrum and duodenum revealed histological evidence of esophagitis, gastritis and duodenitis in patients with either ulcerative colitis or Crohn's disease. Esophagitis occurred in 50%, gastritis in 69% and duodenitis in 23% of patients with ulcerative colitis. In contrast to ulcerative colitis patients, those with Crohn's disease had a higher prevalence of esophagitis, gastritis and duodenitis (72%, 92% and 33%, respectively).[76] Granulomas of the upper gastrointestinal tract were seen in 40% of the patients with Crohn's disease and duodenal cryptitis was noted in 26% of patients with Crohn's disease; none of these lesions was seen in the biopsies of patients with ulcerative colitis.[76] In another study, the presence of focally enhanced gastritis in children did not reliably differentiate between Crohn's disease and ulcerative colitis.[79] Except for the presence of granulomas of Crohn's disease, it may be difficult to distinguish between ulcerative

Table 25.4 Typical endoscopy and histopathology findings – ulcerative colitis (UC) vs. Crohn's disease (from references 69–74, 84)

Characteristic	Ulcerative colitis	Crohn's disease
Endoscopy findings	diffuse continuous involvement extending from the rectum	focal lesions/disease interspersed with normal-appearing mucosa (skip lesions)
	rectum usually involved*	rectal sparing possible
	diffuse, superficial, minute ulcerations; deeper ulcerations in severe disease	aphthous lesions often surrounded by normal-appearing mucosa; deep 'collar button' ulcers; linear or serpiginous ulcerations
	strictures very rare	strictures, often occurring in terminal ileum
	pseudopolyps	
Histopathology findings	no granulomas†	granulomas (36%)
	diffuse chronic inflammation limited to the mucosa††; crypt abscesses	focal chronic inflammation, transmural inflammation
	with or without architectural distortion**	

* In children, 'rectal sparing' has been seen in UC[69,70]

† Giant cell reactions can occur around damaged crypts and spilled mucin. This must be distinguished from 'true' granulomas, which by definition, are not seen in UC

†† Deeper layers of the colon may be involved in fulminant UC disease

** In children with UC, initial colonic biopsies at time of diagnosis are less likely to show architectural distortion than biopsies from adults[74]

colitis and Crohn's disease by the appearance of upper gastrointestinal lesions. Some pediatric centers routinely perform upper endoscopy in addition to colonoscopy under general anesthesia in their initial evaluation of children with suspected IBD, in order to determine the extent and severity of upper gastrointestinal inflammation.

Evaluation of plain abdominal radiographs and abdominal/pelvic computerized tomography (CT) scans may aid in the assessment for complications of ulcerative colitis, including toxic megacolon, perforation or stricture. A plain abdominal radiograph may demonstrate thumbprinting, loss of haustral patterns, colonic dilatation (i.e. toxic megacolon), obstruction, or pneumoperitoneum (i.e. perforation of the bowel).[80–82] CT is not typically performed in the initial assessment for ulcerative colitis, but may demonstrate diffuse bowel wall thickening, marked rectal wall thickening and perirectal fibrofatty proliferation.[75] A barium enema should not be performed during active ulcerative colitis as this predisposes to toxic megacolon.[83] Prior to the routine use of colonoscopy for the diagnosis of ulcerative colitis, published barium enema findings of ulcerative colitis included mucosal granularity, superficial ulcerations, thickened and nodular haustral folds (secondary to inflammation and edema) and colonic shortening.[81] With longstanding ulcerative colitis, the colon becomes featureless and markedly shortened[81] and strictures may form, which may require colonoscopy for further evaluation for possible cancer.[75]

(a) (b)

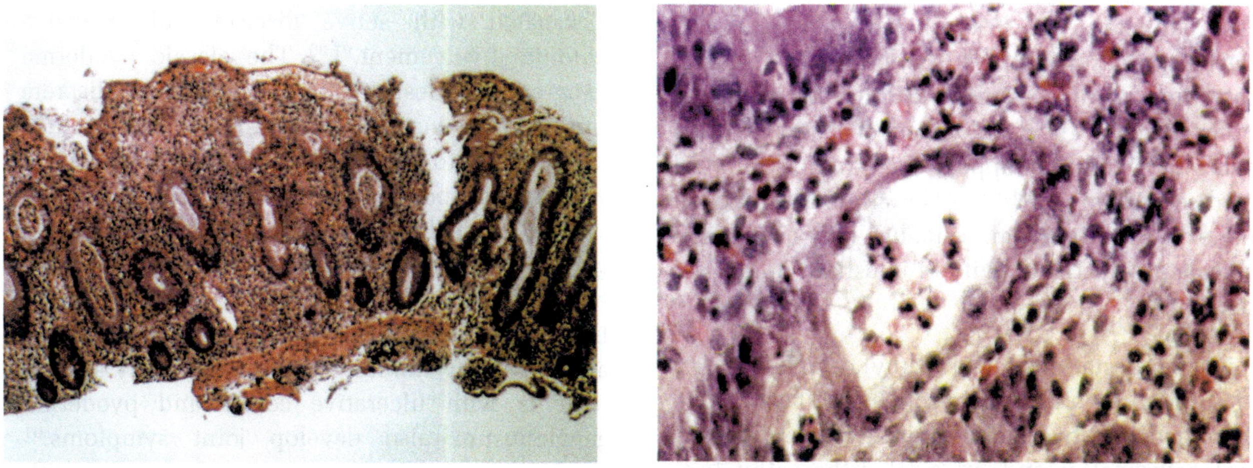

Figure 25.3 (a) Low-power view of a colonic biopsy from a patient with active ulcerative colitis. Note the increased lamina propria inflammatory infiltrate, crypt abscesses and crypt architectural distortion. The crypts are irregular in shape and placement and do not descend to the level of the muscularis mucosae. (b) High-power view of colonic crypts in a patient with active ulcerative colitis, demonstrating neutrophilic infiltration in the crypt and a crypt abscess. (Courtesy of Jonathan Glickman, MD, Department of Pathology, Children's Hospital, Boston).

Pathology of ulcerative colitis

In active ulcerative colitis, typical findings on histopathology include a diffuse inflammatory cell infiltrate of the lamina propria mostly with plasma cells, lymphocytes and neutrophils, but mast cells and eosinophils are also seen[73] (Figure 25.3a). Neutrophils invade the epithelium of the crypts, leading to cryptitis, crypt abscess formation and goblet cell mucin depletion (Figure 25.3b). The inflammatory infiltrate is typically confined to the mucosa, but in severe ulcerative colitis, ulceration may extend into the submucosa and deeper layers.[73] In quiescent (inactive) ulcerative colitis, the inflammatory infiltrate may diminish, but signs of chronic colitis (architectural distortion, crypt branching and shortening, reduction in the number of crypts and separation of crypts) can persist.[73] In children with ulcerative colitis, signs of chronic colitis (e.g. architectural distortion) are not always seen.[74]

Histological differentiation of ulcerative colitis from Crohn's disease can be difficult. The histological hallmark of Crohn's disease is the non-caseating granuloma, which may be found in up to 36% of children with Crohn's disease.[84] However, a giant cell reaction mimicking a granuloma can occur around damaged crypts and spilled mucin. These 'mucin granulomas' must be distinguished from true granulomas, which, by definition, are not seen in ulcerative colitis.[73] Histological skip areas, rectal sparing, focal inflammation and transmural inflammation also suggest the diagnosis of Crohn's disease. How-ever, in children, histological skip areas may occur both at initial presentation of ulcerative colitis and as a result of therapy.[69,85] In addition, patients with ulcerative colitis can have histological evidence of upper gastrointestinal inflammation similar to that in Crohn's disease.[76,77,79] Given the overlap of histopathology findings in ulcerative colitis and Crohn's disease, it may be difficult to distinguish between these two diagnoses if granulomas are not present.

If a clinician cannot reliably distinguish between Crohn's disease and ulcerative colitis based on the available clinical, radiographic and endoscopic data, an interim diagnosis of 'indeterminate colitis' may be given until the patient can be more clearly classified in the future. The prevalence of indeterminate colitis in adults and children with IBD is estimated to be 10–20%.[10,86] Approximately one-third of these patients will later be classified as ulcerative colitis or Crohn's disease.[87]

Extraintestinal manifestations

Approximately 25–35% of patients with IBD develop extraintestinal symptoms.[88,89] Extraintestinal manifestations of IBD may occur before, during, or after the development of gastrointestinal symptoms and may appear after surgical removal of diseased bowel.[88,90–93] The clinical activity of the extraintestinal manifestations may or may not correlate with the activity of intestinal inflammation.

Joint manifestations (arthropathy) occur in 5–20% of children with ulcerative colitis.[4,90] These can be classified into two main clinical forms: a peripheral arthropathy and an axial arthropathy (e.g. ankylosing spondylitis).[88,90] Patients with IBD develop peripheral arthropathies in approximately 5–20% of cases.[88–90,94] The peripheral arthropathy is generally asymmetrical, non-deforming and migratory, affecting mostly the large joints of the lower extremities including the knees, ankles and hips. Less commonly, the upper limb joints or hands are affected.[88,90,94] Small joints of the hands and feet are generally spared.[90]

Exacerbations of peripheral joint disease seem to parallel increased activity of bowel disease in ulcerative colitis or Crohn's disease.[95] Orchard et al, in a study of 976 adults with ulcerative colitis, suggested that there may be two subtypes of peripheral arthropathy: a pauciarticular form with fewer than five swollen joints, and a polyarticular form with more than five joints. Of these two subtypes, the pauciarticular arthropathy is more likely to be correlated with exacerbations of bowel disease.[93]

Axial arthropathies associated with HLA B27 occur in 1–4% of patients.[88–90,94] Ankylosing spondylitis associated with IBD runs a course independent of the activity of bowel disease, and may progress to permanent deformity.[88,90,94] In addition to the two main forms of joint manifestations, individuals with ulcerative colitis can develop isolated arthritis involving large joints, including the sacroiliac joints, hips and shoulders.[94]

Pyoderma gangrenosum and erythema nodosum are the two main skin manifestations associated with ulcerative colitis and Crohn's disease. Pyoderma gangrenosum occurs in <1–5% of patients with ulcerative colitis[89,91] and is often associated with active disease and extensive colonic involvement.[91,96] The classic pyoderma gangrenosum lesion often begins as a discrete pustule with surrounding erythema, then extends peripherally to develop into an ulceration with a well-defined border and a deep erythematous to violaceous color.[97] The lesions of pyoderma gangrenosum tend to be multiple and localize below the knees, and can develop at sites of trauma and previous surgical sites including scars and ileostomy stomas.[96–98] Approximately 40% of patients with ulcerative colitis and pyoderma gangrenosum also develop joint symptoms.[91] Erythema nodosum occurs more frequently with Crohn's disease (27%) in comparison to ulcerative colitis (4%)[89] and usually coincides with increased bowel disease activity.[89,91,94] Erythema nodosum lesions appear as tender, warm, red nodules or raised plaques and usually localize to the extensor surfaces of the lower extremities.[99] Both pyoderma gangrenosum and erythema nodosum can precede the development of bowel symptoms, and pyoderma gangrenosum can occur after bowel resection.[91] Other skin manifestations include Sweet's syndrome (acute febrile neutrophilic dermatosis) and oral lesions include aphthous lesions and pyostomatitis (pyoderma) vegetans.[100]

Ophthalmological abnormalities are described in approximately 1–3% of children with IBD.[88] Uveitis and episcleritis are the more common ocular disorders reported.[88,101] Uveitis associated with IBD in children may be asymptomatic, and thus the incidence of associated eye findings may be underreported in the literature.[102] Ocular inflammation appears to develop more commonly in patients with other extraintestinal manifestations,[102] including arthritis, and may be associated with genes in the HLA region.[103] In addition, corticosteroid use increases the risk of increased intraocular pressure (IOP) and the development of posterior subcapsular cataracts.[104,105] Given the potential eye complications, children with IBD should be monitored carefully at regular intervals.

Hepatic abnormalities in children with ulcerative colitis have been well described. While these are typically identified after the ulcerative colitis diagnosis, they may also precede the gastrointestinal symptoms.[92,106] Transient elevations of alanine aminotransferase (ALT) occur in 12% of children with ulcerative colitis and appear to be related to medications or disease activity.[106] Persistent ALT elevations suggest the presence of primary sclerosing cholangitis (PSC) or autoimmune chronic hepatitis.[106] Among children with ulcerative colitis, 3.5% develop sclerosing cholangitis and < 1% develop chronic hepatitis.[106] The diagnosis of PSC may be suspected based on symptoms of chronic fatigue, anorexia, pruritus or jaundice, although many children may be asymptomatic.[107] γ-Glutamyl-transpeptidase and alkaline phosphatase levels are typically elevated.[92] The diagnosis of PSC may be established through a combination of cholangiography and liver biopsy.[107] There is a paucity of literature addressing the long-term outcome of children with PSC specifically associated with ulcerative colitis.[106] In children with PSC (with or without IBD), later age at presentation, splenomegaly and prolonged prothrombin time (PT) at presentation were associated with poor outcome, defined as death or listing for transplantation.[92] Fatty changes of the liver observed on liver biopsies of patients with ulcerative colitis or Crohn's disease may be secondary to malnutrition, protein losses, anemia and corticosteroid use.[108] An increased risk of cholelithiasis has been reported in individuals with ulcerative colitis, but is more commonly observed in Crohn's disease.[109]

Thromboembolic disease, including cerebrovascular involvement, deep vein thrombosis and pulmonary emboli, can lead to significant morbidity for individuals with IBD.[110–112] Multiple coagulation abnormalities are observed in IBD including thrombocytosis; elevated levels of fibrinogen, factor V and factor VII; and depressed levels of antithrombin III and factor V Leiden.[100,110] Controversy still remains as to whether the thromboembolic complications are directly related to the altered hemostatic states observed in ulcerative colitis and Crohn's disease and whether they may involve a more complex multifactorial cascade involving gene–gene and gene–environment interactions.[113] Rarely, other hematological abnormalities associated with ulcerative colitis occur, including immune thrombocytopenic purpura[114] and autoimmune hemolytic anemia.[115]

Osteopenia (low bone mineral density; BMD) occurs in children with ulcerative colitis, but less often than in children with Crohn's disease.[116] Corticosteroid use increases the risk of osteopenia in children with IBD.[116] Other extraintestinal manifestations include nephrolithiasis,[89,117] pancreatitis (related or unrelated to medications),[118,119] and pulmonary and cardiac involvement.[88]

Complications

Complications of ulcerative colitis include massive hemorrhage, toxic megacolon, perforation of the bowel, strictures and colon cancer. Massive hemorrhage can occur with severe ulcerative colitis and is managed with blood transfusions and treatment of the underlying ulcerative colitis; urgent colectomy may be required. One consensus group suggested that an individual with ulcerative colitis who requires more than 6–8 units of blood in the first 48 h and is still actively bleeding should undergo a colectomy.[120] Colonic perforation is the most dangerous complication of ulcerative colitis. It can occur in the setting of severe ulcerative colitis with or without toxic colonic dilatation,[121–123] and requires urgent colectomy.

Toxic megacolon is a potentially life-threatening complication of ulcerative colitis and is characterized by total or segmental non-obstructive colonic dilatation of at least 6 cm in adults associated with systemic toxicity.[122,124,125] Previous reports suggest a lifetime risk of toxic megacolon complicating IBD of 1–5%, but this has decreased more recently, probably secondary to earlier recognition and improved management of severe colitis.[122,126] The pathogenesis of toxic megacolon is most likely to be multifactorial.[122] In contrast to typical ulcerative colitis, in which the inflammatory changes are limited to the mucosa, in toxic megacolon, the severe inflammation extends into the deeper layers of the colonic wall.[121] It is thought that the spread of the inflammatory process to the smooth-muscle layer may lead to the paralysis of the colonic smooth muscle and subsequent dilatation of the colon.[122] Nitric oxide, an inhibitor of smooth muscle tone, may be involved in the pathogenesis of this condition.[127]

Several triggering factors have been reported to precede the development of toxic megacolon.[121,122] Medications that can impair colonic motility should be avoided. They have been implicated as precipitating factors, including narcotic agents for pain or antidiarrheal effects, anticholinergic agents, drugs that decrease motility, or antidepressants with significant anticholinergic effects.[121,128,129] A barium enema or colonoscopy may cause distension that can further impair the colonic wall blood supply and may increase the mucosal uptake of bacterial products.[122] Barium enema examinations have been reported in proximity to the development of toxic megacolon.[83,129] The early discontinuation or rapid tapering of steroids or 5-aminosalicylic acid (5-ASA) may contribute to the development of toxic megacolon.[121,122] Electrolyte abnormalities, such as hypokalemia, have been observed in the setting of toxic megacolon, although it is not clear whether this finding is a causative factor or secondary to the illness itself.[121] Along with colonic dilatation, patients with toxic megacolon present with systemic findings, including fever, tachycardia, leukocytosis and anemia.[124] A decrease in the number of stools may herald the onset of toxic megacolon. With progressive disease, these individuals can develop dehydration, mental status changes, electrolyte disturbances, hypotension and increasing abdominal distension and tenderness, with or without signs of peritonitis.[122,124]

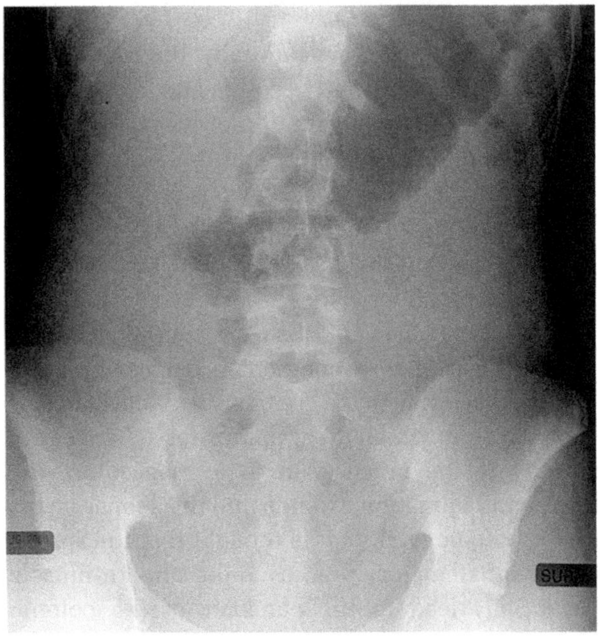

Figure 25.4 Toxic megacolon in a teenager with fulminant ulcerative colitis. There is a massively dilated loop of transverse colon in the upper quadrants, with a paucity of bowel gas in the remainder of the abdomen. This patient developed the megacolon despite corticosteroid therapy, and subsequently underwent emergent surgery for a colonic perforation. (Courtesy of Carlo Buonomo, MD, Department of Radiology, Children's Hospital, Boston).

Abdominal X-ray reveals colonic dilatation, most frequently involving the transverse colon, sometimes accompanied by inflammatory changes including an absent or markedly edematous haustral pattern[130] (Figure 25.4). In two series of adults with toxic megacolon, the diameter of the colon varied, with a range of 5.8–16 cm.[125,129] Because the transverse colon is the most anterior portion of the colon, air will tend to accumulate in this segment of the colon when the patient is in the supine position; however, with repositioning of the patient, the colonic air will redistribute, filling other segments of the bowel.[131]

The management of toxic megacolon is detailed in multiple reviews elsewhere.[121,122] If toxic megacolon is present, surgical consultation is essential, and the patient will probably require a colectomy. Some authors have utilized medical management of this condition; however, this requires very close monitoring to avoid complications.[132] Early surgical intervention is indicated in the setting of failed medical therapy with progressive colonic dilatation, worsening systemic toxicity, perforation or uncontrolled hemorrhage.[122]

Both benign and malignant colonic strictures can develop in longstanding ulcerative colitis.[75,133,134] Benign strictures present most commonly in the rectum and the sigmoid, are due to smooth-muscle hypertrophy and are thought to be potentially reversible.[133] Colonic strictures should be evaluated for possible malignancy, but the majority of strictures in ulcerative colitis are benign.[75,133,134] There is an increased risk of dysplasia and colon cancer in patients with longstanding ulcerative colitis, which is addressed later in this chapter (see Prognosis and follow-up, p.407).

Treatment options

The treatment goals for children with ulcerative colitis are the control of active disease and induction of remission, the long-term maintenance of remission, and provision of education and psychosocial support for the patient and family. The initial treatment of ulcerative colitis is medical, with surgery reserved for patients with severe disease, patients with medically refractory disease, or patients who develop adverse effects of medical therapy.

Knowledge of the extent and severity of disease involvement will enable the clinician to choose the appropriate therapy for each individual patient. Distal ulcerative colitis (left-sided ulcerative colitis or proctitis) is characterized by involvement limited to the area distal to the splenic flexure, and potentially may be treated with topical agents (e.g. aminosalicylate or hydrocortisone enemas or suppositories). Extensive ulcerative colitis is defined by involvement extending proximally to the splenic flexure and requires systemic therapies with or without additional topical agents. Severity of disease is usually simple to ascertain, and can be determined by assessing stool frequency and consistency, abdominal pain, nocturnal diarrhea, hematocrit, albumin level and feeding intolerance. Separate published disease severity criteria for adults and children have been developed by Truelove and Witts,[135] and Werlin and Grand,[60] respectively (Tables 25.5 and 25.6). Other clinical scoring systems have been utilized in clinical trials to quantify disease severity of ulcerative colitis, but are less useful for day-to-day clinical management.[136–139] Typically, severe colitis requires hospitalization and administration of either intravenous corticosteroids or other immunosuppressive agents (e.g. cyclosporin). Many patients with severe colitis will require colectomy.

Induction therapy

Mild-to-moderate colitis

In the child with mild-to-moderate ulcerative colitis, with no or only minimal systemic signs

Table 25.6 Characteristics of severe colitis in children* (from reference 60)

Grossly bloody diarrhea, ≥ 5 stools per a day
Oral temperature >37.8°C during the first hospital day
Tachycardia (pulse ≥ 90)
Anemia (hematocrit ″ 30%)
Hypoalbuminemia (serum albumin ″ 3.0 g/100 ml)
Toxic megacolon

* Patients need to fulfill four of the first five criteria or the 6th criterion alone

Table 25.5 Severity of ulcerative colitis in adults* (from reference 135)

Characteristic	Mild	Severe
Grossly bloody diarrhea	″ 4 stools per day (″ small amounts of blood)	≥ 6 stools per day
Fever	none	mean evening temperature >37.5°C, or temperature ≥37.8°C, at least 2 out of 4 days
Tachycardia	none	>90 beats/min
Anemia	not severe; hemoglobin essentially normal	present; hemoglobin ″ 75% of normal value
Erythrocyte sedimentation rate	″ 30 mm/h	>30 mm/h

* Moderate severe – intermediate between severe and mild

Table 25.7 Aminosalicylate agents* (from references 325, 326)

Oral preparations	Dosage form	Mechanism of release	Site of delivery
Azo-bond			
sulfasalazine (Azulfidine)	500-mg tablet	bacterial cleavage of azo bond	colon
olsalazine (Dipentum)	250-mg capsule	bacterial cleavage of azo bond	colon
balsalazide (Colazal/Colazide)	750-mg capsule	bacterial cleavage of azo bond	colon
Delayed-release			
mesalamine (Asacol)	400 mg/800 mg tablets	pH-dependent breakdown (pH >7)	distal ileum to colon
mesalamine (Salofalk/ Mesasal/Claversal)	250 mg/500 mg tablets	pH-dependent breakdown (pH >6)	ileum to colon
Sustained-release			
mesalamine (Pentasa)	250 mg/500 mg/ 1000 mg tablets	ethylcellulose-controlled time-release	small intestine to colon
Rectal preparations			
mesalamine suppository (Canasa – 500 mg)	400 mg/500 mg/ 1000 mg		rectum
mesalamine enema (Rowasa – 4 g/60 ml)	1 g/4 g; 60-ml/ 100-ml suspension		rectum to splenic flexure

* Availability of different preparations and dosage forms varies between different markets/countries

(such as elevated ESR or mild anemia), aminosalicylates (ASAs) (e.g. sulfasalazine, olsalazine, mesalamine, balsalazide) are usually the first line of therapy (Tables 25.7 and 25.8). ASAs have multiple immunological effects. Potential mechanisms of action include the inhibition of the synthesis of leukotriene B_4, a potent chemotactic and chemokinetic agent, and the inhibition of the activation of nuclear transcription factor κB (NF-κB), an important mediator of the immune response in inflammatory processes.[140–142] Controlled studies suggest that currently available ASAs are superior to placebo for induction of remission and prevention of relapse.[143–146] However, there do not appear to be any differences in efficacy between the older agent, sulfasalazine, and newer ASA drugs.[146,147] There are very few trials of ASA therapy in children with ulcerative colitis. One pediatric multicenter, randomized, double-blind study compared the efficacy and safety of olsalazine (30 mg/kg per day; maximum 2 g/day) to sulfasalazine (60 mg/kg per day; maximum 6 g/day) in the treatment of mild-to-moderate ulcerative colitis. The findings demonstrated clinical remission after 3 months in 79% of the sulfasalazine-treated children, in comparison to 39% of the olsalazine-treated children.[148] The authors suggested the low dosage of olsalazine as a possible explanation for the difference in efficacy between sulfasalazine and osalazine.[148]

Potential advantages of the non-sulfa ASA agents include better tolerance compared to sulfasalazine[147,149] and the availability of a non-sulfa

Table 25.8 Medical therapies for ulcerative colitis

Medication	Dosage	Major side-effects
Sulfasalazine	50–75 mg/kg per day PO divided qid, bid or tid (maximum 6 g/day) adult dose: 3–4 g/day divided bid or tid	nausea, headaches, diarrhea, photosensitivity, hypersensitivity reaction, pancreatitis, azoospermia, hemolytic anemia, neutropenia
Mesalamine		
oral formulation	50–75 mg/kg per day PO divided qid, tid, or bid (may vary according to preparation) (maximum 6 g/day); adult dose: 3–4 g/day divided qid, tid, or bid	nausea, headaches, diarrhea, pancreatitis, nephritis, pericarditis, pleuritis
enema formulation	2–4 g PR q 12–24 h	
suppository formulation	500 mg PR q 12–24 h	
Corticosteroids		
intravenous or oral formulation	1–2 mg/kg per day of prednisone or equivalent, IV or PO, divided q 12 to 24 h (maximum 60 mg/day)	numerous; including Cushing's syndrome, growth suppression, immunosuppression, hypertension, hyperglycemia, increased
enema formulation	50–100 mg of hydrocortisone PR qhs	appetite, osteoporosis, aseptic
suppository formulation	25 mg of hydrocortisone acetate PR qhs	necrosis (hip), cataracts
Azathioprine*	1.5–2.5 mg/kg per day PO qd	nausea, emesis, immunosuppression, hepatotoxicity, pancreatitis, myelosuppression
6-Mercaptopurine*	1.0–2.0 mg/kg per day PO qd	nausea, emesis, immunosuppression, hepatotoxicity, pancreatitis, myelosuppression
Cyclosporin	induction regimen for fulminant colitis: initial dose, 4 mg/kg per day IV continuous or bid; maintenance oral dose varies according to oral preparation	nephrotoxicity, hypertension, headache, hirsutism, nausea, emesis, diarrhea, tremor, hypomagnesemia, hyperkalemia, hepatotoxicity, seizures, gingival hyperplasia, possibly lymphoproliferative disorder

PO, orally; bid, twice a day; tid, three times a day; qid, four times a day; PR, per rectum; q, every; qd, every day; IV, intravenously; qhs, at bedtime

* Thiopurine methyltransferase (TPMT) genotype determines metabolism and blood levels of metabolites; may help to determine risk of myelosuppression and optimal dosage of azathioprine or 6-mercaptopurine

ASA agent for sulfa-sensitive individuals. In adult-onset ulceratimve colitis, balsalazide at higher doses (6.75 g/day) may provide a faster improvement in active, mild-to-moderate ulcerative colitis than lower doses of balsalazide (2.25 g/day) or mesalamine (2.4 g/day).[150,151] Although some studies suggest an advantage of azo-bond ASA agents (e.g. balsalazide) in comparison to delayed-release ASA agents (e.g. mesalamine), the overall data suggest equivalence between the different oral ASAs, when comparable amounts of the ASA are released at the site of disease activity.[152]

Common side-effects of sulfasalazine include headache, nausea and fatigue, which improve with reduction of the dose[152] (Table 25.8). The sulfa moiety can cause hypersensitivity reactions resulting in rash, fever, hepatitis, hemolytic anemia, bone marrow suppression and pneumonitis.[152,153] Other side-effects include neutropenia, oligospermia, pancreatitis and the exacerbation of colitis.[60,154] Folic acid supplementation is recommended, given that sulfasalazine impairs the absorption of folic acid and may lead to anemia.[152] To decrease side-effects, sulfasalazine is started at a dose of 10–20 mg/kg per day and gradually increased to the full dose (50–75 mg/kg per day) over 5–7 days. Mesalamine and the other non-sulfa ASA agents have also been associated with adverse reactions, including pancreatitis, hepatitis, nephritis, exacerbation of colitis, and pneumonitis.[152,155,156]

In addition to medical therapy, a low-residue diet (no popcorn, nuts, seeds, raw fruits and vegetables) and avoidance of spicy foods during acute symptoms has been anecdotally reported to reduce symptoms during a flare-up of disease.[157]

Moderate-to-severe colitis

Children with moderate disease are usually managed with oral corticosteroids (usually 1 mg/kg per day, up to 60 mg/day of prednisone) as out-patients. In an uncontrolled study of 20 children with active ulcerative colitis (three with mild, 13 with moderate, four with severe activity), 85% of the children achieved clinical remission with combination therapy of corticosteroids (oral prednisolone for pancolitis or topical prednisolone for distal colitis) and mesalamine (20–40 mg/kg per day).[158] Reassessment with colonoscopy at 8 weeks demonstrated complete endoscopic remission in 40% and full histological remission in only 15%, suggesting that clinical remission may not correlate with endoscopic or histological remission.[158] Potential short-term complications of steroid therapy in patients with ulcerative colitis include increased appetite, weight gain, fluid retention, mood swings, hyperglycemia, hypertension, insomnia, acne and facial swelling.

Complications of long-term steroid therapy (usually of more than 3 months) include growth restriction, osteopenia with compression fractures, aseptic necrosis of the hip, and cataracts.[152,159] Given these reasons and the suppression of the hypothalamic–pituitary–adrenal axis, corticosteroids should be tapered shortly after remission is achieved. A standard taper utilized by the authors is reduction by 5 mg/week of prednisone down to 20 mg/day, and then a more gradual taper on alternate days, aiming for 10 mg every other day with further taper and cessation if remission is maintained.[159] Budesonide, a steroid with a high first-pass metabolism and fewer systemic side-effects, is available in capsule form for treatment of ileocecal Crohn's disease.[160] In Europe and Canada, there is an enema form of budesonide for treatment of distal colitis.[161] Unfortunately, there is no available oral budesonide preparation shown to treat patients with pancolitis effectively.[162]

Children with severe disease (e.g. more than five bowel movements/day, liquid bloody stools, or severe pain with defecation, anemia and hypoalbuminemia) require intravenous corticosteroids (methylprednisolone at 40–60 mg/day, divided into two doses/day, approximately 1–2 mg/kg per day) and hospitalization for further evaluation, observation and management.[157,163] Rectal corticosteroids or 5-ASA agents may be used as an adjunctive therapy with parenteral corticosteroids for patients with severe tenesmus.[152] Intravenous fluid for rehydration and correction of electrolyte imbalances should be provided. Blood transfusions and albumin infusions may be required. If bowel rest is indicated, the child may require central venous access for parenteral nutrition support. In addition to high-dose steroids, empiric antibiotics are sometimes used in severe colitis, although the efficacy of antibiotics has not been proven.[164–167] Assessment for response to intensive medical therapy includes resolution of fever, tachycardia, abdominal tenderness and macroscopic blood per rectum. Stools should be decreasing in frequency, but may still be unformed. Once the child shows significant improvement, diet is advanced to a low-residue diet, intravenous methylprednisolone is switched to oral prednisone, and similar parameters for steroid wean are followed as outlined above. The optimal duration of intravenous corticosteroid therapy is unclear, but most children will respond within 7–10 days.

If the child has not responded to steroid therapy after 7–10 days, the options of surgery or more intensive immunosuppression (intravenous cyclosporin or oral tacrolimus) should be considered and discussed with the family. Intensive immunosuppression should not be started if surgery is believed imminent, such as in a septic patient, a patient with toxic megacolon, or a patient with a suspected perforation. Intravenous or oral cyclosporin therapy has successfully induced remission in children with steroid-refractory ulcerative colitis.[168–170] The exact dosage of cyclosporin varies in different protocols, depending upon whether intravenous or oral medication is utilized.[136,169–171] In a study of 14 children treated with oral cyclosporin therapy for severe active colitis, unresponsive to high-dose intravenous steroids, 80% achieved clinical remission within 2–9 days; however, the majority of children who initially responded to cyclosporin eventually required colectomy within a year.[170] In these studies, most of the children who improved with cyclosporin induction relapsed or underwent colectomy within a year.[169,170] Cyclosporin may be most useful in delaying emergency colectomy at a time when the child's health status is most compromised (high-dose steroids, anemia, hypoalbuminemia, poor nutrition) and may allow time to improve the child's health and mental status in preparation for future 'elective' colectomy.[170] A recent review outlines specific recommendations on the initiation and monitoring of cyclosporin therapy in children with IBD.[171]

Oral tacrolimus can also induce remission of disease activity in children with severe active colitis.[172] If either cycloporin or tacrolimus is utilized as induction therapy, the aim should be the transition of patients off these potentially toxic agents and onto a maintenance medication (e.g. 6-mercaptopurine, azathioprine) over a 3–6-month period. Azathioprine or 6-mercaptopurine may be effective in preventing relapse after cyclosporin-induced remission in children with ulcerative colitis.[173] Children on cyclosporin or tacrolimus should receive prophylaxis for *Candida* and *Pneumocystis carinii*, and have careful monitoring of electrolytes, blood glucose, renal function, blood pressure and neurological status.

The timing of colectomy in a child who is not responding to intravenous corticosteroids or other immunosuppression can be difficult. It should be emphasized that, even if a child responds to immunosuppression, such as cyclosporin, there is a high likelihood that he/she will require a colectomy within a year.[170,172] If immunosuppression with cyclosporin is used and the child does not respond to these medications within 10–14 days, surgery should be strongly recommended.

Close monitoring of patients with severe colitis for the development of fulminant colitis and associated complications including hemorrhage, toxic megacolon and perforation is essential, using serial abdominal examinations, complemented by serial abdominal films or other imaging as necessary. Physical examination should look for evidence of worsening abdominal tenderness, distension and hypoactive bowel sounds; these may herald the development of toxic megacolon. The appearance of persistent abdominal pain and distension, diffuse abdominal tenderness and rebound, fever and tachycardia are worrisome signs of an acute abdomen and may signal the need for emergency surgical intervention. Opiates and loperamide should be avoided, given the increased risk of developing toxic megacolon.[128] Steroid therapy may mask the typical symptoms and signs of perforation, but these may be detected by serial upright abdominal films (see Complications, p.395).

Left-sided colitis/proctitis

Topical ASA or topical corticosteroids are effective in the treatment of proctitis, proctosigmoiditis, or left-sided ulcerative colitis[174–176] (see Tables 25.7 and 25.8). To be effective, topical therapy must reach the most proximal extent of the disease activity. Mesalamine enemas or suppositories are effective as first-line therapy/maintenance therapy for mild or moderately active left-sided ulcerative colitis or proctitis, respectively.[152] Rectal mesalamine may be superior to oral mesalamine in the treatment of active ulcerative proctitis.[177] Mesalamine enemas may be superior to rectal corticosteroids[178] and are also effective in treating distal colitis that is unresponsive to oral ASAs or corticosteroids.[179,180] Combination therapy with oral and topical mesalamine is more effective than one agent alone in the treatment of mild-to-moderate distal colitis.[181] Mesalamine suppositories spread to the upper rectum, and enemas and foams can reach the splenic flexure or into the distal transverse colon.[179,180]

Corticosteroid suppositories or enemas also can be used as first-line induction therapy in patients with mild or moderately active ulcerative proctitis or left-sided ulcerative colitis.[152] Rectal administration of hydrocortisone or prednisolone permits more direct delivery of steriods to distal ulcerative colitis sites; however, as with oral steroid therapy, prolonged treatment with topical steroids may induce systemic steroid side-effects, including adrenal suppression.[176,180] Topical agents such as budesonide enemas, may induce remission in distal colitis with fewer systemic steroid side-effects.[161,182] In a randomized, double-blind, placebo-controlled trial, budesonide enema therapy (2.0 mg or 8.0 mg/enema, once per evening) effectively induced remission, with significant improvement in sigmoidoscopy and histopathology scores, compared to placebo in adults with active distal ulcerative colitis/proctitis.[161] However, in another controlled trial, less frequent dosing of twice weekly budesonide enemas (2.0 mg/enema) was not superior to placebo in the maintenance of remission.[183] Some evidence suggests that ASA enemas may be superior to hydrocortisone enemas.[175,178,180] Cyclosporin-A enemas have been used in the treatment of severe refractory distal ulcerative colitis,[184] but were not found to be effective in a placebo-controlled trial for mildly to moderately active left-sided ulcerative colitis.[185]

Maintenance therapy

5-Aminosalicylic acid agents

Medication for the prevention of relapse after induction of remission is often started before the induction therapy is discontinued. The clinician usually aims towards a transition of the patient from corticosteroids onto sulfasalazine or another ASA agent. Multiple studies of adults with ulcerative colitis demonstrate the effectiveness of sulfasalazine and other ASA agents in preventing relapse.[147] Mesalamine is well tolerated in the long-term treatment of children with IBD, with the principal adverse event being exacerbation of diarrhea.[186] Sulfasalazine and newer ASAs are all effective in maintaining remission in ulcerative colitis.[149] Balsalazide, at a higher dose (6 g/day), may be more effective in preventing relapses of ulcerative colitis in adults, compared to lower-dose balsalazide (3 g/day) and mesalamine (1.5 g/day).[187] Topical mesalamine can effectively prevent relapse of active distal ulcerative colitis,[188] but because of the rectal route of administration, patients may prefer oral mesalamine for maintenance therapy. The combination of oral and topical 5-ASA therapy may be more effective in preventing relapse than oral 5-ASA therapy alone, especially for distal disease.[189] Some authors suggest that 5-ASA agents may reduce the risk of colorectal cancer.[190–192] Children with ulcerative colitis require years of maintenance therapy. The exact duration that an ulcerative colitis patient in remission should remain on maintenance therapy is unclear, and there are no formal guidelines on when or whether maintenance therapy should be discontinued. The risk of discontinuing maintenance medication is the possibility of relapse. In addition, maintenance with 5-ASA or other agents may reduce the risk of colorectal neoplasia.[193]

6-Mercaptopurine and azathioprine

The immunomodulatory drugs azathioprine and its metabolite 6-mercaptopurine can reduce disease activity and allow the withdrawal of steroid therapy in children with steroid-dependent ulcerative colitis.[194,195] In a small, open-label trial of children with Crohn's disease or ulcerative colitis, six of nine patients with ulcerative colitis reduced their steroid use by at least 75% with azathioprine therapy.[194] In another series of 16 children with severe, steroid-dependent or steroid-refractory ulcerative colitis, 6-mercaptopurine or azathioprine therapy allowed the discontinuation of steroid use in 75%, and 67% remained without steroid therapy for 3–65 months.[195] Given their steroid-sparing effects[194,195] and reasonable tolerance by children with IBD,[196] azathioprine and 6-mercaptopurine offer an alternative maintenance treatment of IBD in children. In a study of 95 children with either Crohn's disease or ulcerative colitis, only 18% required discontinuation of the medication; the majority of side-effects responded to dose reduction, or improved spontaneously.[196] Side-effects reported include aminotransferase elevations or hepatitis, pancreatitis, bone marrow depression, hypersensitivity reactions and recurrent infections;[196,197] children should be monitored for the development of these complications. Some clinicians have utilized 6-mercaptopurine metabolite levels to monitor responsiveness, compliance and potential toxicity.[198,199] Evaluation for thiopurine methyltransferase genetic polymorphism should be obtained prior to the institution of 6-mercaptopurine or azathioprine therapy as it can identify those children at higher risk for drug toxicity[200] and guide the clinician to prescribe lower doses of azathioprine and 6-mercaptopurine, if appropriate.

Given the high relapse rate with withdrawal of 6-mercaptopurine in adults with ulcerative colitis,[201] the majority of children requiring azathioprine or 6-mercaptopurine to suppress disease activity will probably require long-term maintenance therapy with these agents. There are no good data in ulcerative colitis addressing the question of when (or whether) immunomodulators should be discontinued after a patient has entered remission. Most patients are continued on the medication for several years if they respond to 6-mercaptopurine or azathioprine. At the present time, evidence does not suggest any definitive increased risk of malignancy secondary to long-term use of azathioprine in adults.[202–204] However, one paper has identified a slightly increased risk of Epstein–Barr virus-associated lymphoma in a large cohort of patients treated with long-term 6-mercaptopurine or azathioprine.[205]

Methotrexate

Methotrexate appears to be less effective for the treatment of ulcerative colitis than for Crohn's disease.[206,207] Although open-label trials in adults with ulcerative colitis suggested a benefit of methotrexate in the induction of remission,[137,208] a double-blind, randomized trial failed to show any advantage of methotrexate in the induction or maintenance of remission in adults with chronic active ulcerative colitis in comparison to placebo.[209] Another study of two different dosages of parenteral methotrexate in adults with IBD showed a remission rate of approximately 20%.[210] While methotrexate can be useful in treating children with Crohn's disease intolerant to 6-mercaptopurine, there are currently no published studies describing its efficacy in children with ulcerative colitis.[211]

Other therapies

Despite the potential role of infectious agents in the pathogenesis of ulcerative colitis,[17] the use of antibiotic therapy in the treatment of ulcerative colitis remains controversial. There is a lack of consistent evidence of the effectiveness of antibiotics in the induction and maintenance of remission in ulcerative colitis.[165,212–215] In one study, oral tobramycin therapy improved short-term clinical and histological outcomes,[212] but there was no advantage in the prevention of relapse compared to placebo.[213] In two studies of active ulcerative colitis, the addition of 10–14 days of oral or intravenous ciprofloxacin to corticosteroid therapy did not improve rates of remission.[167,216] In another placebo-controlled study, the administration of 6 months of treatment with ciprofloxacin, in addition to standard therapy with prednisone and mesalamine, resulted in a greater clinical response compared to placebo; however, this advantage was not sustained after the cessation of ciprofloxacin.[217] Empiric broad-spectrum antibiotics are often administered in the setting of severe active ulcerative colitis,[60,164] especially if there is concern for potential fulminant colitis or toxic megacolon.[122]

In open, uncontrolled trials, infliximab (chimeric monoclonal antibody to TNF-α) therapy resulted in clinical improvement in adults and children with ulcerative colitis.[218–222] However, the clinical response of infliximab therapy may not be sustained.[223] In an open-label study of nine children and adolescents with moderate-to-severe ulcerative colitis, seven children (77%) showed a decrease in disease activity measured by the Physician Global Assessment, and corticosteroid therapy was discontinued in six children (66%).[222] A small, double-blind, placebo-controlled clinical trial of infliximab in 11 adults with severe, active steroid-refractory ulcerative colitis suggested a clinical benefit for patients treated with one dose of infliximab (5 mg, 10 mg or 20 mg/kg per dose), compared to those who received placebo.[224] In this study, four of eight ulcerative colitis patients receiving infliximab improved, compared to none of three receiving placebo. Because of poor recruitment, the trial was terminated prematurely and no statistical analysis was performed. In a larger, randomized, double-blind, placebo-controlled study of 43 adults with moderately active glucocorticoid-resistant ulcerative colitis, there was no significant difference in remission rate or sigmoidoscopic score between the infliximab-treated group (5 mg/kg per dose, at weeks 0 and 2) and the placebo group.[225] Thus, the therapeutic benefit of infliximab in ulcerative colitis remains unclear at this time, and the treatment does carry a risk of infusion reactions, antinuclear antibody formation and opportunistic infections.[226–230]

Studies evaluating the effectiveness of mycophenolate mofetil therapy for ulcerative colitis show mixed results and may suggest increased side-effects compared to other immunomodulatory agents such as azathioprine.[231–233]

Probiotics have been studied in the maintenance of remission in adults with ulcerative colitis.[234–236] In an open-label trial of the probiotic VSL no. 3, performed in adults with inactive ulcerative colitis, 75% of patients remained in remission during the 12-month study,[234] but no controlled trials with VSL no. 3 for maintenance therapy for ulcerative colitis have been performed. In two randomized controlled comparison trials, non-pathogenic *E. coli* strains and mesalamine maintained similar rates of remission in adults with quiescent ulcerative colitis.[235,236] There are no formal studies on the effectiveness of probiotics in children with ulcerative colitis.

In adults with ulcerative colitis, transdermal nicotine therapy, combined with mesalamine or corticosteroids, may result in clinical improvement, but is associated with unwanted side-effects.[237,238] Transdermal nicotine therapy does not appear to be effective in the maintenance of remission of ulcerative colitis.[239] An open-label trial of nicotine enema therapy in adults with ulcerative colitis showed improvement in symptoms of urgency and stool frequency, and sigmoidoscopic and histological scores,[240] but controlled studies are needed to determine true efficacy.

Several placebo-controlled studies suggested a benefit of adjunctive therapy with fish oil supplementation containing eicosapentaenoic acid, a potent inhibitor of leukotriene B_4 synthesis, in the treatment of active ulcerative colitis.[241–243] However, fish oil supplementation did not appear to show any benefit in maintenance therapy.[243,244] Unfortunately, given the large number of capsules required for daily therapy and the intolerance to unwanted fishy odor, patients' compliance has been suboptimal.

Randomized, controlled trials in adults with active distal ulcerative colitis suggest that therapy with topical short-chain fatty acid (SCFA) preparations result in clinical symptomatic improvement, but there is no statistically significant advantage in comparison to placebo.[245–247] In one double-blind, placebo-controlled, 6-week trial of rectal SCFA, 103 patients with distal ulcerative colitis were entered and those on SCFA had larger, but statistically non-significant, reductions in every component of their clinical and histological activity scores.[246]

In several open-label trials, adults with steroid-resistant ulcerative colitis showed a clinical response to heparin therapy;[248–250] however, a controlled trial did not show any advantage of heparin treatment for moderate-to-severe ulcerative colitis, compared to corticosteroid therapy.[251] In an open-label pilot study, daclizumab (humanized anti-IL-2R antibody; CD25) resulted in clinical and endoscopic improvement in adults with refractory ulcerative colitis;[252] further study is needed to determine the effectiveness of this novel therapy.

Nutritional therapy

The importance of nutrition in the management of ulcerative colitis is extensively reviewed elsewhere.[253,254] Children with ulcerative colitis can develop nutritional deficits with poor oral intake secondary to symptoms; and thus, promotion of continued good nutritional intake is essential for appropriate healing and nutritional repletion.[255] Enteral nutrition is preferred to total parenteral nutrition when possible. In contrast to Crohn's disease, enteral nutrition is not an effective primary therapy for active ulcerative colitis.[152,171] Studies suggest no advantage of total nutritional support and bowel rest in addition to conventional medical therapy alone in the treatment of ulcerative colitis.[256,257] In a randomized, controlled trial of corticosteroid therapy combined with either polymeric enteral nutrition or total parenteral nutrition, adults with moderate or severe ulcerative colitis showed no differences in remission rate, need for colectomy, or changes in anthropometric parameters.[258] Total parenteral nutrition is often utilized for nutritional repletion in severe ulcerative colitis, especially if the patient develops severe cramps and diarrhea when challenged with enteral nutrition.

Surgical therapy

In the majority of cases, medical therapy remains the first-line treatment for ulcerative colitis. However, colectomy may be required for patients with severe or medically refractory disease, or to prevent colon cancer. Since the inflammation in ulcerative colitis is limited to the colon, colonic resection will most often result in resolution of symptoms. However, colectomy is not without potential complications, such as the development of pouchitis in patients who undergo ileoanal anastomosis.[259,260] It is important to consider timely surgical intervention in the appropriate setting to avoid complications of ulcerative colitis. Indications for colectomy in a patient with ulcerative colitis include fulminant colitis or a complication of colitis, such as massive hemorrhage, perforation, or toxic megacolon; medical therapy failure; steroid dependency, which may lead to undesired side-effects; and the presence of colonic dysplasia.[261] Prepubertal children may experience catch-up growth after colectomy for ulcerative colitis. In one series, 11 of 18 children increased their median height velocity from 3.85 cm/year preoperatively to 7.35 cm/year postoperatively.[262] As medical treatment for ulcerative colitis was developed, the frequency of colectomy decreased. At one center, a retrospective review of children and adolescents with ulcerative colitis revealed a decrease in the frequency of colectomy from 48.9% (between 1955 and 1964) to 26.2% (between 1965 and 1974).[263]

There are no early predictors to help determine who will proceed to colectomy. Hyams et al, in a retrospective review, reported that the 5-year colectomy rate in patients with mild disease at presentation was 8%, compared to 26% in patients with moderate-to-severe disease at presentation.[264] In another retrospective review of 73 children with ulcerative colitis between the ages of 1 and 18 years, the combination of steroid dependency and pancolitis was associated with an increased need for colectomy.[265] Seventy-three per cent of the children with steroid-dependent pancolitis required colectomy within 3 years of diagnosis.[265]

Except in the setting of emergency colectomy, a complete evaluation should be performed to ensure that there is no evidence of Crohn's disease prior to colectomy. If there is evidence suggesting the possibility of Crohn's disease, the patient and family need to be informed of the potential for postoperative recurrence, and the relative contraindications of ileoanal pull-through procedures in patients with known Crohn's disease. The authors recommend an upper gastrointestinal series with small-bowel follow-through and upper gastrointestinal endoscopy, in addition to a full colonoscopy with ileoscopy, if there is no clinical contraindication. Prior endoscopies and pathology reports should be carefully reviewed to establish that there is no evidence of Crohn's disease.

The surgical options available for ulcerative colitis are reviewed in detail elsewhere.[261] The ileal pouch–anal canal anastomosis (IPAA) is the operation most commonly performed in the majority of patients with ulcerative colitis. The IPAA removes the entire colon and the rectal mucosa, avoids permanent ileostomy, and preserves anorectal function. Several types of ileal pouches can be constructed, including the J-shaped, S-shaped, W-shaped and the lateral–lateral pouch.[261] The J-pouch design is now most commonly used for the IPAA operation.[266,267] If the rectal mucosa is in good condition, many centers use the two-stage operative approach. During the first stage, a subtotal colectomy of the cecum to proximal rectum, the removal of the distal rectal and proximal anal mucosa, and the formation of the ileal pouch are performed. In this initial stage, a diverting loop ileostomy is performed in order to allow the pouch to heal. The second stage involves closure of the loop ileostomy with restoration of fecal flow to the pouch. Surgeons at some surgical centers also complete the IPAA in one stage, without the loop ileostomy;[268] however, this would not be the procedure of choice in patients receiving high-dose corticosteroids.[267] Some authors[261] believe that the omission of the diverting ileostomy may increase the risk of anastomotic leaks and prolong recovery;[269] thus, candidate patients for the one-stage IAPP should be selected carefully.[270]

If the patient presents for emergency surgical intervention, such as with fulminant colitis, a three-stage operative approach is often utilized. At the time of acute presentation, a subtotal colectomy is performed with formation of a rectal stump (the so-called Hartman pouch) and Brooke ileostomy. After the first operation, the rectal mucosa is treated with topical therapies (e.g. hydrocortisone, aminosalicylates) to induce mucosal healing. At the second operation, the distal rectal and proximal anal mucosa is removed and the ileal pouch is created. The ileostomy is reversed at the third operation.

The potential complications of IPAA include small-bowel obstruction, pelvic sepsis, anastomotic leak, fecal incontinence, pouchitis, strictures or fistulae.[261,270,271] The development of fistulae raises the suspicion of Crohn's disease.[261] In one series of children aged 9–16 who underwent proctocolectomy with IPAA, 12/29 (41%) of patients with ulcerative colitis developed early complications (wound infection, early bowel obstruction, prolonged fever).[272] Late complications (bowel obstruction, pouch fistula) occurred in 11/29 (38%) and pouchitis developed in 9/29 (31%) of the children with ulcerative colitis. Median follow-up was 4 years (range 6 months to 9 years). In this same study, daytime continence was noted in 100% and night-time continence in 93%. The median frequency of bowel movements was four in 24 h, and 7% of patients had night-time bowel movements.

Pouchitis, or inflammation of the newly created reservoir, is the most significant chronic complication in ulcerative colitis patients undergoing IPAA; as many as 44–53% of children and young adults with ulcerative colitis and ileoanal anastomosis will develop pouchitis on long-term follow-up.[259,260] The etiology of pouchitis is unknown, but theories involve the role of genetic susceptibility, fecal stasis, bacterial overgrowth, disruption of the balance of luminal bacteria, nutritional deficiencies, ischemia and IBD recurrence.[273] Symptoms of pouchitis include diarrhea, rectal bleeding, abdominal cramping, urgency and incontinence of stool, malaise and fever.[261,273,274] Patients with ulcerative colitis who undergo IPAA develop pouchitis more commonly than patients with familial polyposis who undergo the same procedure.[275] Pouchitis may occur more frequently in children and adults with primary sclerosing cholangitis (PSC)-associated ulcerative colitis[276,277] and in individuals with extraintestinal manifestations of ulcerative colitis.[273] Laboratory studies may demonstrate anemia and an elevated ESR. The definitive diagnosis is established by flexible endoscopy of the pouch with biopsies (Figure 25.5). In some patients, a contrast enema may be useful in identifying fistulae.

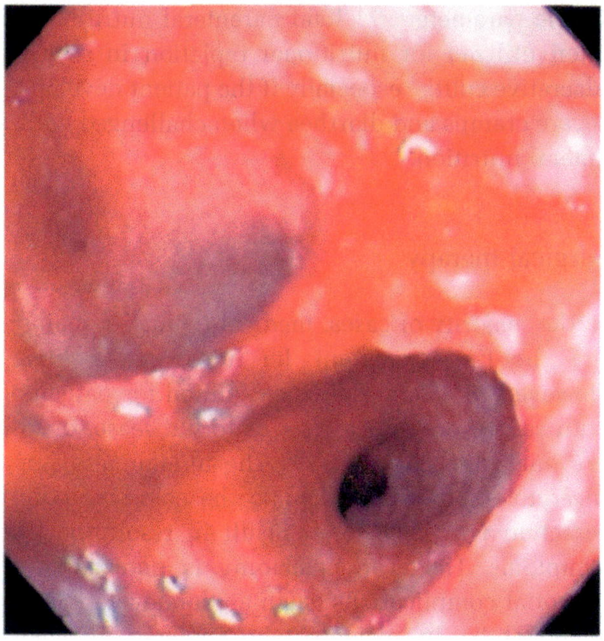

Figure 25.5 Chronic active inflammation of an ileal J-pouch (pouchitis) in a patient with a history of ulcerative colitis. Note that both limbs of the ileal reservoir are erythematous with exudate.

Broad-spectrum antibiotics are usually the first-line treatment for pouchitis.[273,278] Metronidazole is the most commonly used antibiotic, but alternative therapies include ciprofloxacin, amoxicillin–clavulanic acid, erythromycin and tetracycline.[274,279] If there is no improvement with antibiotics, other options include mesalamine enemas and steroid enemas or oral therapy with mesalamine, sulfasalazine or steroids.[274,280,281] Other therapies examined include cyclosporin enemas, SCFA enemas, butyrate suppositories and glutamine suppositories.[184,274,282,283]

Probiotic therapy may prevent the onset of acute pouchitis after ileostomy closure[284] and effectively maintain remission after chronic pouchitis.[285] A double-blind, placebo-controlled study evaluated the efficacy of a probiotic preparation VSL no. 3, (containing 5 x 10^{11} per gram of viable lyophilized bacteria of four strains of lactobacilli, three strains of bifidobacteria, and one strain of *Streptococcus salivarius* subsp. *thermophilus*), compared with placebo in maintenance of remission of chronic pouchitis in 40 patients in clinical and endoscopic remission. Three patients (15%) in the VSL no. 3 group had relapses within the 9-month follow-up period, compared with 20 (100%) in the placebo group.[285] In another double-blind, placebo-controlled study performed by the same authors in 40 patients, VSL no. 3, administered immediately after ileostomy closure for 1 year, effectively reduced the onset of acute pouchitis in the VSL no. 3 group (10%) in comparison to the placebo group (40%).[284]

Several studies have suggested that the risk of dysplasia in the ileal pouch appears to be low[286,287] and may be associated with chronic pouchitis.[288] The development of adenocarcinoma has been reported in the ileal pouch.[289] In a follow-up study (mean of 5 years) of 76 children and adolescents with ulcerative colitis who had an IPAA, no dysplasia was identified in screening pouch biopsy specimens.[286] The authors cautioned that the long-term risk of development of dysplasia is not yet known and recommended screening of the pouch for dysplasia. In the rare patient who has undergone an ileorectal anastomosis without rectal mucosectomy, surveillance of the rectum should be performed to screen for rectal cancer.

Psychosocial support

The social impact of ulcerative colitis on the lives of children with the disease needs to be considered. Ulcerative colitis often has its onset in adolescence, a time when body image issues are paramount. Children and teenagers with IBD may often experience anxiety over the diagnosis of a chronic disease, the need for invasive procedures and the uncertainty of the future. In addition, there may be struggles with parents about proper diet, and 'medication fatigue' from having to take more than ten pills per day. Social, school-related and extracurricular activities may be affected and may need appropriate modification. For example, a self-limited reduction of physical education activities and permission for special bathroom privileges may be needed.

Previous studies report an increased risk of psychiatric and behavioral issues in children with IBD including depression, anxiety and low self-esteem.[290–294] Burke and colleagues reported that children are at increased risk for depression as early as the time of diagnosis.[290] The physician caring for these patients needs to discuss the above issues openly with the patient and family, and be alert to the possibility that a patient may develop anxiety or depressive symptoms. More recently, two patient-generated, disease-specific, health-related quality of life (HRQoL) questionnaires for children with IBD have been validated: the IMPACT and Impact-II questionnaires.[295,296] Impact-II is a modified version of the IMPACT questionnaire. The use of these instruments may provide important information to improve the care of children with IBD. Referral to an educational support group, such as those sponsored by the Crohn's and Colitis Foundation of America (www.ccfa.org), may be helpful for patients and their famililies.

Prognosis and follow-up

Whether children with ulcerative colitis are treated medically or surgically, they have an excellent long-term prognosis and good quality of life. The majority of children with ulcerative colitis respond to medical therapy. In one American retrospective study of 171 children ranging in age from 1.5 to 17.7 years, diagnosed with ulcerative colitis between 1967 and 1994, 43% had mild disease at presentation and 57% had moderate or severe ulcerative colitis. With treatment, 70% of all the children were in remission within 3 months of diagnosis and, by 6 months, 90% of the children with mild disease and 81% of the children with moderate-to-severe ulcerative colitis experienced resolution of their symptoms. In each yearly follow-up period, approximately 55% of the children were symptom free, 38% experienced chronic intermittent symptoms and 7% had continuous symptoms.[264] In this same study, children with mild ulcerative colitis at presentation had a lower frequency of colectomy than children with moderate-to-severe ulcerative colitis (9% vs. 26% at 5 years, respectively). Patients with left-sided disease had comparable rates of colectomy at 5 years to patients with pancolitis.[264] However, the authors cautioned that the number of patients in each subgroup of disease extent was small, and a true difference in colectomy rates may have been missed secondary to insufficient power of the study.[264] Another study of 80 children diagnosed with ulcerative colitis before the age of 15 years reported a slightly higher rate of remission of 60–70% in each of the first 10 years, after the year of diagnosis.[3] In the same study, the cumulative probability of colectomy was 6% after 1 year and 29% after 20 years.[3]

Limited distal ulcerative colitis (proctitis or proctosigmoiditis) diagnosed in adults and children can extend further to involve more proximal colon with time.[297–300] In a retrospective study of 38 children (mean age 11.6 years; range 4.2–17.7 years) diagnosed with ulcerative colitis proctitis between 1975 and 1994, 29% of the children developed extension of disease involvement beyond the rectosigmoid.[299] Another retrospective evaluation of 85 patients under 21 years of age, diagnosed with ulcerative colitis proctosigmoiditis between 1958 and 1983, demonstrated the extension of disease to the descending colon in 20% and to the hepatic flexure or beyond in another 38% of the patients.[300] The extension of disease may warrant a change in medical therapy to control disease activity and may have implications for an increased risk of potential colorectal cancer in the future.[301]

Women with ulcerative colitis generally experience similar rates of fertility to those of the general population; however, an increased risk of preterm births has been reported in some studies.[302–304] In contrast, women with ulcerative colitis who undergo proctocolectomy with IPAA may experience reduced fertility.[305]

Individuals with longstanding ulcerative colitis are at increased risk of developing colorectal cancer.[301,306,307] Risk of colorectal cancer increases with more extensive colonic involvement and longer duration of disease since diagnosis.[301,306–309] Therefore, children with ulcerative colitis will potentially be at risk for colorectal cancer over a longer period of time, compared to individuals with adult-onset ulcerative colitis. In a population-based cohort study in Sweden, Ekbom et al reported standardized incidence ratios for colorectal cancer of 1.7 for ulcerative colitis proctitis, 2.8 for left-sided ulcerative colitis and 14.8 for ulcerative colitis pancolitis.[307] The absolute risk (cumulative risk) of colorectal cancer 35 years after diagnosis was 30% for patients with pancolitis at diagnosis for the entire cohort (adults and children), but 40% for individuals diagnosed with pancolitis at less than 15 years of age.[307]

Individuals with PSC and ulcerative colitis have a higher risk of developing colorectal neoplasia compared to those with ulcerative colitis alone, and of developing cholangiocarcinoma.[310–314] Ursodeoxycholic acid (UDCA) may decrease the risk for developing colorectal dysplasia or cancer in patients with ulcerative colitis and PSC.[315] Other risk factors reported for colorectal cancer in patients with ulcerative colitis include a family history of colorectal cancer[316] and the occurrence of backwash ileitis.[317] In contrast, some retrospective studies suggest that 5-ASA agents may provide a protective effect in the development of colorectal cancer in patients with ulcerative colitis, but not all studies support these findings.[190,191,193,318] A retrospective, case–control study suggested a risk reduction of colorectal cancer in ulcerative colitis with folate supplementation, but the findings were not statistically significant.[319] The role of pharmacological therapy and vitamin supplements in the development of colorectal cancer in patients with ulcerative colitis remains controversial.[320] Further prospective studies are needed to evaluate the potential risk reduction (preventive) effects of folate and 5-ASA agents.[192,321,322]

There are no randomized controlled trials examining the effectiveness of surveillance colonoscopy for dysplasia and colorectal cancer in patients with ulcerative colitis.[323,324] The reported general current practice includes surveillance colonoscopy every 1–2 years beginning at 8 years after the diagnosis of disease for pancolitis and 15 years in those with left-sided colitis.[324] However, it may be prudent to perform the initial surveillance colonoscopy beginning at 8–10 years after diagnosis in all patients with ulcerative colitis, in order to reassess the true extent of disease.[324] The consensus recommendations suggest that biopsy specimens should be taken every 10 cm in all four quadrants and additional biopsies should be performed for strictures and mass lesions.[324] It is not clear whether surveillance practice should differ for patients with younger-onset ulcerative colitis. There are no published formal recommendations to guide surveillance colonoscopy in children.[323]

Conclusions

Ulcerative colitis in children presents in a similar manner to that in adults, although children often have more extensive disease at diagnosis. Once the diagnosis is established by colonoscopy, the first line of induction treatment in mild disease is usually an aminosalicylate, with corticosteroids reserved for moderate-to-severe disease. If a patient responds to induction therapy, the maintenance agent most commonly used is aminosalicylates or 6-mercaptopurine. In severe steroid-unresponsive colitis, the clinician is faced with the challenge of recommending either colectomy or more aggressive immunosuppression (e.g. cyclosporin). Even if a patient responds to cyclosporin, there is a high likelihood of proceeding to colectomy within a year. Surgery will eradicate the disease, but patients may develop chronic pouchitis requiring additional medical treatment. In addition to medical care of these patients, nutritional counseling, monitoring of growth, and psychosocial support are essential. If the medical team can give proper care and support, the patient's long-term prognosis is usually excellent.

REFERENCES

1. Chong SK, Blackshaw AJ, Morson BC et al. Prospective study of colitis in infancy and early childhood. *J Pediatr Gastroenterol Nutr* 1986; **5**: 352–358.
2. Mendeloff AI, Calkins BM. The epidemiology of idiopathic inflammatory bowel disease. In Kirsner JB, Shorter RG, eds. *Inflammatory Bowel Disease*. Philadelphia: Lea & Febiger, 1988: 3–34.
3. Langholz E, Munkholm P, Krasilnikoff PA et al. Inflammatory bowel diseases with onset in childhood. Clinical features, morbidity, and mortality in a regional cohort. *Scand J Gastroenterol* 1997; **32**: 139–147.
4. Gryboski JD. Ulcerative colitis in children 10 years old or younger. *J Pediatr Gastroenterol Nutr* 1993; **17**: 24–31.
5. Mamula P, Telega GW, Markowitz JE et al. Inflammatory bowel disease in children 5 years of age and younger. *Am J Gastroenterol* 2002; **97**: 2005–2010.
6. Barton JR, Gillon S, Ferguson A. Incidence of inflammatory bowel disease in Scottish children between 1968 and 1983; marginal fall in ulcerative colitis, three-fold rise in Crohn's disease. *Gut* 1989; **30**: 618–622.
7. Calkins BM, Lilienfeld AM, Garland CF et al. Trends in incidence rates of ulcerative colitis and Crohn's disease. *Dig Dis Sci* 1984; **29**: 913–920.
8. Lindberg E, Lindquist B, Holmquist L et al. Inflammatory bowel disease in children and adolescents in Sweden, 1984–1995. *J Pediatr Gastroenterol Nutr* 2000; **30**: 259–264.
9. Olafsdottir EJ, Fluge G, Haug K. Chronic inflammatory bowel disease in children in western Norway. *J Pediatr Gastroenterol Nutr* 1989; **8**: 454–458.
10. Bentsen BS, Moum B, Ekbom A. Incidence of inflammatory bowel disease in children in southeastern Norway: a prospective population-based study 1990–94. *Scand J Gastroenterol* 2002; **37**: 540–545.
11. Askling J, Grahnquist L, Ekbom A et al. Incidence of paediatric Crohn's disease in Stockholm, Sweden. *Lancet* 1999; **354**: 1179.
12. Sonnenberg A, McCarty DJ, Jacobsen SJ. Geographic variation of inflammatory bowel disease within the United States. *Gastroenterology* 1991; **100**: 143–149.
13. Shivananda S, Lennard-Jones J, Logan R et al. Incidence of inflammatory bowel disease across Europe: is there a difference between north and south? Results of the European Collaborative Study on Inflammatory Bowel Disease (EC-IBD). *Gut* 1996; **39**: 690–697.
14. Acheson ED. The distribution of ulcerative colitis and regional enteritis in United States veterans with particular reference to the Jewish religion. *Gut* 1960; **1**: 291–293.
15. Gilat T, Grossman A, Fireman Z et al. Inflammatory bowel disease in Jews. *Front Gastrointest Res* 1986; **11**: 141–145.
16. Fiocchi C. Inflammatory bowel disease: etiology and pathogenesis. *Gastroenterology* 1998; **115**: 182–205.

17. Hendrickson BA, Gokhale R, Cho JH. Clinical aspects and pathophysiology of inflammatory bowel disease. *Clin Microbiol Rev* 2002; **15**: 79–94.
18. Orholm M, Binder V, Sorensen TI et al. Concordance of inflammatory bowel disease among Danish twins. Results of a nationwide study. *Scand J Gastroenterol* 2000; **35**: 1075–1081.
19. Halfvarson J, Bodin L, Tysk C et al. Inflammatory bowel disease in a Swedish twin cohort: a long-term follow-up of concordance and clinical characteristics. *Gastroenterology* 2003; **124**: 1767–1773.
20. Orholm M, Munkholm P, Langholz E et al. Familial occurrence of inflammatory bowel disease. *N Engl J Med* 1991; **324**: 84–88.
21. Yang H, McElree C, Roth MP et al. Familial empirical risks for inflammatory bowel disease: differences between Jews and non-Jews. *Gut* 1993; **34**: 517–524.
22. Annese V, Andreoli A, Astegiano M et al. Clinical features in familial cases of Crohn's disease and ulcerative colitis in Italy: a GISC study. Italian Study Group for the Disease of Colon and Rectum. *Am J Gastroenterol* 2001; **96**: 2939–2945.
23. Satsangi J, Parkes M, Louis E et al. Two stage genome-wide search in inflammatory bowel disease provides evidence for susceptibility loci on chromosomes 3, 7 and 12. *Nature Genet* 1996; **14**: 199–202.
24. Farrell RJ, Peppercorn MA. Ulcerative colitis. *Lancet* 2002; **359**: 331–340.
25. Papadakis KA, Targan SR. Current theories on the causes of inflammatory bowel disease. *Gastroenterol Clin North Am* 1999; **28**: 283–296.
26. Vessey M, Jewell D, Smith A et al. Chronic inflammatory bowel disease, cigarette smoking, and use of oral contraceptives: findings in a large cohort study of women of childbearing age. *Br Med J (Clin Res Ed)* 1986; **292**: 1101–1103.
27. Calkins BM. A meta-analysis of the role of smoking in inflammatory bowel disease. *Dig Dis Sci* 1989; **34**: 1841–1854.
28. Koletzko S, Griffiths A, Corey M et al. Infant feeding practices and ulcerative colitis in childhood. *BMJ* 1991; **302**: 1580–1581.
29. Andersson RE, Olaison G, Tysk C et al. Appendectomy and protection against ulcerative colitis. *N Engl J Med* 2001; **344**: 808–814.
30. Duggan AE, Usmani I, Neal KR et al. Appendicectomy, childhood hygiene, *Helicobacter pylori* status, and risk of inflammatory bowel disease: a case control study. *Gut* 1998; **43**: 494–498.
31. Feeney MA, Murphy F, Clegg AJ et al. A case–control study of childhood environmental risk factors for the development of inflammatory bowel disease. *Eur J Gastroenterol Hepatol* 2002; **14**: 529–534.
32. Evans JM, McMahon AD, Murray FE et al. Non-steroidal anti-inflammatory drugs are associated with emergency admission to hospital for colitis due to inflammatory bowel disease. *Gut* 1997; **40**: 619–622.
33. Kaufmann HJ, Taubin HL. Nonsteroidal anti-inflammatory drugs activate quiescent inflammatory bowel disease. *Ann Intern Med* 1987; **107**: 513–516.
34. Rampton DS, Sladen GE. Relapse of ulcerative proctocolitis during treatment with non-steroidal anti-inflammatory drugs. *Postgrad Med J* 1981; **57**: 297–299.
35. Bonner GF. Exacerbation of inflammatory bowel disease associated with use of celecoxib. *Am J Gastroenterol* 2001; **96**: 1306–1308.
36. Felder JB, Korelitz BI, Rajapakse R et al. Effects of nonsteroidal antiinflammatory drugs on inflammatory bowel disease: a case–control study. *Am J Gastroenterol* 2000; **95**: 1949–1954.
37. Bonner GF, Walczak M, Kitchen L et al. Tolerance of nonsteroidal antiinflammatory drugs in patients with inflammatory bowel disease. *Am J Gastroenterol* 2000; **95**: 1946–1948.
38. Reuter BK, Asfaha S, Buret A et al. Exacerbation of inflammation-associated colonic injury in rat through inhibition of cyclooxygenase-2. *J Clin Invest* 1996; **98**: 2076–2085.
39. Wallace JL, Keenan CM, Gale D et al. Exacerbation of experimental colitis by nonsteroidal anti-inflammatory drugs is not related to elevated leukotriene B4 synthesis. *Gastroenterology* 1992; **102**: 18–27.
40. Wallace JL. Nonsteroidal anti-inflammatory drugs and gastroenteropathy: the second hundred years. *Gastroenterology* 1997; **112**: 1000–1016.
41. Corrao G, Tragnone A, Caprilli R et al. Risk of inflammatory bowel disease attributable to smoking, oral contraception and breastfeeding in Italy: a nationwide case–control study. Cooperative Investigators of the Italian Group for the Study of the Colon and the Rectum (GISC). *Int J Epidemiol* 1998; **27**: 397–404.
42. Gilat T, Hacohen D, Lilos P et al. Childhood factors in ulcerative colitis and Crohn's disease. An international cooperative study. *Scand J Gastroenterol* 1987; **22**: 1009–1024.
43. The Epidemiology Group of the Research Committee of Inflammatory Bowel Disease in Japan. A case–control study of ulcerative colitis in relation to dietary and other factors in Japan. The Epidemiology Group of the Research Committee of Inflammatory Bowel Disease in Japan. *J Gastroenterol* 1995; **30**: 9–12.
44. Jarnerot G, Jarnmark I, Nilsson K. Consumption of refined sugar by patients with Crohn's disease, ulcerative colitis, or irritable bowel syndrome. *Scand J Gastroenterol* 1983; **18**: 999–1002.
45. Lashner BA, Kane SV, Hanauer SB. Lack of association between oral contraceptive use and ulcerative colitis. *Gastroenterology* 1990; **99**: 1032–1036.
46. Bouma G, Strober W. The immunological and genetic basis of inflammatory bowel disease. *Nat Rev Immunol* 2003; **3**: 521–533.
47. Plevy S. The immunology of inflammatory bowel disease. *Gastroenterol Clin North Am* 2002; **31**: 77–92.
48. Sartor RB. Current concepts of the etiology and pathogenesis of ulcerative colitis and Crohn's disease. *Gastroenterol Clin North Am* 1995; **24**: 475–507.
49. Fuss IJ, Neurath M, Boirivant M et al. Disparate CD4+ lamina propria (LP) lymphokine secretion profiles in inflammatory bowel disease. Crohn's disease LP cells manifest increased secretion of IFN-gamma, whereas ulcerative colitis LP cells manifest increased secretion of IL-5. *J Immunol* 1996; **157**: 1261–1270.
50. Izzo RS, Witkon K, Chen AI et al. Interleukin-8 and neutrophil markers in colonic mucosa from patients with ulcerative colitis. *Am J Gastroenterol* 1992; **87**: 1447–1452.
51. Daig R, Andus T, Aschenbrenner E et al. Increased interleukin 8 expression in the colon mucosa of patients with inflammatory bowel disease. *Gut* 1996; **38**: 216–222.
52. Keshavarzian A, Fusunyan RD, Jacyno M et al. Increased interleukin-8 (IL-8) in rectal dialysate from patients with ulcerative colitis: evidence for a biological role for IL-8 in inflammation of the colon. *Am J Gastroenterol* 1999; **94**: 704-712.
53. MacDermott RP. Chemokines in the inflammatory bowel diseases. *J Clin Immunol* 1999; **19**: 266–272.
54. Luster AD. Chemokines – chemotactic cytokines that mediate inflammation. *N Engl J Med* 1998; **338**: 436–445.

55. Wallace JL. Prostaglandin biology in inflammatory bowel disease. *Gastroenterol Clin North Am* 2001; **30**: 971–980.
56. Rao SS, Holdsworth CD, Read NW. Symptoms and stool patterns in patients with ulcerative colitis. *Gut* 1988; **29**: 342–345.
57. Heikenen JB, Werlin SL, Brown CW et al. Presenting symptoms and diagnostic lag in children with inflammatory bowel disease. *Inflamm Bowel Dis* 1999; **5**: 158–160.
58. Motil KJ, Grand RJ. Ulcerative colitis and Crohn disease in children. *Pediatr Rev* 1987; **9**: 109–120.
59. Grand RJ, Homer DR. Approaches to inflammatory bowel disease in childhood and adolescence. *Pediatr Clin North Am* 1975; **22**: 835–850.
60. Werlin SL, Grand RJ. Severe colitis in children and adolescents: diagnosis. Course, and treatment. *Gastroenterology* 1977; **73**: 828–832.
61. Sachar DB, Smith H, Chan S et al. Erythrocytic sedimentation rate as a measure of clinical activity in inflammatory bowel disease. *J Clin Gastroenterol* 1986; **8**: 647–650.
62. Macfarlane PI, Miller V, Wells F et al. Laboratory assessment of disease activity in childhood Crohn's disease and ulcerative colitis. *J Pediatr Gastroenterol Nutr* 1986; **5**: 93–96.
63. Holmquist L, Ahren C, Fallstrom SP. Relationship between results of laboratory tests and inflammatory activity assessed by colonoscopy in children and adolescents with ulcerative colitis and Crohn's colitis. *J Pediatr Gastroenterol Nutr* 1989; **9**: 187–193.
64. Ruemmele FM, Targan SR, Levy G et al. Diagnostic accuracy of serological assays in pediatric inflammatory bowel disease. *Gastroenterology* 1998; **115**: 822–829.
65. Dubinsky MC, Ofman JJ, Urman M et al. Clinical utility of serodiagnostic testing in suspected pediatric inflammatory bowel disease. *Am J Gastroenterol* 2001; **96**: 758–765.
66. Duerr RH, Targan SR, Landers CJ et al. Anti-neutrophil cytoplasmic antibodies in ulcerative colitis. Comparison with other colitides/diarrheal illnesses. *Gastroenterology* 1991; **100**: 1590–1596.
67. Winter HS, Landers CJ, Winkelstein A et al. Anti-neutrophil cytoplasmic antibodies in children with ulcerative colitis. *J Pediatr* 1994; **125**: 707–711.
68. Rutgeerts P, Vermeire S. Serological diagnosis of inflammatory bowel disease. *Lancet* 2000; **356**: 2117–2118.
69. Markowitz J, Kahn E, Grancher K et al. Atypical rectosigmoid histology in children with newly diagnosed ulcerative colitis. *Am J Gastroenterol* 1993; **88**: 2034–2037.
70. Bousvaros A, Glickman JN, Farraye FA et al. Pediatric patients with untreated ulcerative colitis may present initially with unusual morphologic findings. *Gastroenterology* 2002; **122**: A-11.
71. Seidman EG. Role of endoscopy in inflammatory bowel disease. *Gastrointest Endosc Clin North Am* 2001; **11**: 641–657, vi.
72. Chutkan RK, Scherl E, Waye JD. Colonoscopy in inflammatory bowel disease. *Gastrointest Endosc Clin North Am* 2002; **12**: 463–483, viii.
73. Domizio P. Pathology of chronic inflammatory bowel disease in children. *Baillières Clin Gastroenterol* 1994; **8**: 35–63.
74. Washington K, Greenson JK, Montgomery E et al. Histopathology of ulcerative colitis in initial rectal biopsy in children. *Am J Surg Pathol* 2002; **26**: 1441–1449.
75. Horton KM, Jones B, Fishman EK. Imaging of the inflammatory bowel diseases. In Kirsner JB, ed. *Inflammatory Bowel Diseases*, 5th edn. Philadelphia: WB Saunders, 2000: 479–500.
76. Tobin JM, Sinha B, Ramani P et al. Upper gastrointestinal mucosal disease in pediatric Crohn disease and ulcerative colitis: a blinded, controlled study. *J Pediatr Gastroenterol Nutr* 2001; **32**: 443–448.
77. Kaufman SS, Vanderhoof JA, Young R et al. Gastroenteric inflammation in children with ulcerative colitis. *Am J Gastroenterol* 1997; **92**: 1209–1212.
78. Ruuska T, Vaajalahti P, Arajarvi P et al. Prospective evaluation of upper gastrointestinal mucosal lesions in children with ulcerative colitis and Crohn's disease. *J Pediatr Gastroenterol Nutr* 1994; **19**: 181–186.
79. Sharif F, McDermott M, Dillon M et al. Focally enhanced gastritis in children with Crohn's disease and ulcerative colitis. *Am J Gastroenterol* 2002; **97**: 1415–1420.
80. Scotiniotis I, Rubesin SE, Ginsberg GG. Imaging modalities in inflammatory bowel disease. *Gastroenterol Clin North Am* 1999; **28**: 391–421, ix.
81. Aideyan UO, Smith WL. Inflammatory bowel disease in children. *Radiol Clin North Am* 1996; **34**: 885–902.
82. Langmead L, Rampton DS. Plain abdominal radiographic features are not reliable markers of disease extent in active ulcerative colitis. *Am J Gastroenterol* 2002; **97**: 354–359.
83. Koudahl G, Kristensen M. Toxic megacolon in ulcerative colitis. *Scand J Gastroenterol* 1975; **10**: 417–421.
84. Chong SK, Blackshaw AJ, Boyle S et al. Histological diagnosis of chronic inflammatory bowel disease in childhood. *Gut* 1985; **26**: 55–59.
85. Odze R. Diagnostic problems and advances in inflammatory bowel disease. *Mod Pathol* 2003; **16**: 347–358.
86. Hildebrand H, Fredrikzon B, Holmquist L et al. Chronic inflammatory bowel disease in children and adolescents in Sweden. *J Pediatr Gastroenterol Nutr* 1991; **13**: 293–297.
87. Joossens S, Reinisch W, Vermeire S et al. The value of serologic markers in indeterminate colitis: a prospective follow-up study. *Gastroenterology* 2002; **122**: 1242–1247.
88. Hyams JS. Extraintestinal manifestations of inflammatory bowel disease in children. *J Pediatr Gastroenterol Nutr* 1994; **19**: 7–21.
89. Greenstein AJ, Janowitz HD, Sachar DB. The extra-intestinal complications of Crohn's disease and ulcerative colitis: a study of 700 patients. *Medicine (Baltimore)* 1976; **55**: 401–412.
90. Lindsley CB, Schaller JG. Arthritis associated with inflammatory bowel disease in children. *J Pediatr* 1974; **84**: 16–20.
91. Mir-Madjlessi SH, Taylor JS, Farmer RG. Clinical course and evolution of erythema nodosum and pyoderma gangrenosum in chronic ulcerative colitis: a study of 42 patients. *Am J Gastroenterol* 1985; **80**: 615–620.
92. Wilschanski M, Chait P, Wade JA et al. Primary sclerosing cholangitis in 32 children: clinical, laboratory, and radiographic features, with survival analysis. *Hepatology* 1995; **22**: 1415–1422.
93. Orchard TR, Wordsworth BP, Jewell DP. Peripheral arthropathies in inflammatory bowel disease: their articular distribution and natural history. *Gut* 1998; **42**: 387–391.
94. Das KM. Relationship of extraintestinal involvements in inflammatory bowel disease: new insights into autoimmune pathogenesis. *Dig Dis Sci* 1999; **44**: 1–13.
95. Passo MH, Fitzgerald JF, Brandt KD. Arthritis associated with inflammatory bowel disease in children. Relationship of joint disease to activity and severity of bowel lesion. *Dig Dis Sci* 1986; **31**: 492–497.
96. Levitt MD, Ritchie JK, Lennard-Jones JE et al. Pyoderma gangrenosum in inflammatory bowel disease. *Br J Surg* 1991; **78**: 676–678.

97. Callen JP. Pyoderma gangrenosum. *Lancet* 1998; **351**: 581–585.
98. Finkel SI, Janowitz HD. Trauma and the pyoderma gangrenosum of inflammatory bowel disease. *Gut* 1981; **22**: 410-412.
99. Requena L, Requena C. Erythema nodosum. *Dermatol Online J* 2002; **8**: 4.
100. Su CG, Judge TA, Lichtenstein GR. Extraintestinal manifestations of inflammatory bowel disease. *Gastroenterol Clin North Am* 2002; **31**: 307–327.
101. Rychwalski PJ, Cruz OA, Alanis-Lambreton G et al. Asymptomatic uveitis in young people with inflammatory bowel disease. *J AAPOS* 1997; **1**: 111–114.
102. Hofley P, Roarty J, McGinnity G et al. Asymptomatic uveitis in children with chronic inflammatory bowel diseases. *J Pediatr Gastroenterol Nutr* 1993; **17**: 397–400.
103. Orchard TR, Chua CN, Ahmad T et al. Uveitis and erythema nodosum in inflammatory bowel disease: clinical features and the role of HLA genes. *Gastroenterology* 2002; **123**: 714–718.
104. Tripathi RC, Kipp MA, Tripathi BJ et al. Ocular toxicity of prednisone in pediatric patients with inflammatory bowel disease. *Lens Eye Toxic Res* 1992; **9**: 469–482.
105. Tripathi RC, Kirschner BS, Kipp M et al. Corticosteroid treatment for inflammatory bowel disease in pediatric patients increases intraocular pressure. *Gastroenterology* 1992; **102**: 1957–1961.
106. Hyams J, Markowitz J, Treem W. Characterization of hepatic abnormalities in children with inflammatory bowel disease. *Inflamm Bowel Dis* 1995; **1**: 27.
107. Roberts EA. Primary sclerosing cholangitis in children. *J Gastroenterol Hepatol* 1999; **14**: 588–593.
108. Raj V, Lichtenstein DR. Hepatobiliary manifestations of inflammatory bowel disease. *Gastroenterol Clin North Am* 1999; **28**: 491–513.
109. Lorusso D, Leo S, Mossa A et al. Cholelithiasis in inflammatory bowel disease. A case–control study. *Dis Colon Rectum* 1990; **33**: 791–794.
110. Markowitz RL, Ment LR, Gryboski JD. Cerebral thromboembolic disease in pediatric and adult inflammatory bowel disease: case report and review of the literature. *J Pediatr Gastroenterol Nutr* 1989; **8**: 413–420.
111. Talbot RW, Heppell J, Dozois RR et al. Vascular complications of inflammatory bowel disease. *Mayo Clin Proc* 1986; **61**: 140–145.
112. Schapira M, Henrion J, Ravoet C et al. Thromboembolism in inflammatory bowel disease. *Acta Gastroenterol Belg* 1999; **62**: 182–186.
113. Koutroubakis IE. Unraveling the mechanisms of thrombosis in inflammatory bowel disease. *Am J Gastroenterol* 2001; **96**: 1325–1327.
114. Higuchi LM, Joffe S, Neufeld EJ et al. Inflammatory bowel disease associated with immune thrombocytopenic purpura in children. *J Pediatr Gastroenterol* Nutr 2001; **33**: 582–587.
115. Giannadaki E, Potamianos S, Roussomoustakaki M et al. Autoimmune hemolytic anemia and positive Coombs test associated with ulcerative colitis. *Am J Gastroenterol* 1997; **92**: 1872–1874.
116. Gokhale R, Favus MJ, Karrison T et al. Bone mineral density assessment in children with inflammatory bowel disease. *Gastroenterology* 1998; **114**: 902–911.
117. Clark JH, Fitzgerald JF, Bergstein JM. Nephrolithiasis in childhood inflammatory bowel disease. *J Pediatr Gastroenterol Nutr* 1985; **4**: 829–834.
118. Keljo DJ, Sugerman KS. Pancreatitis in patients with inflammatory bowel disease. *J Pediatr Gastroenterol Nutr* 1997; **25**: 108–112.
119. Huang C, Lichtenstein DR. Pancreatic and biliary tract disorders in inflammatory bowel disease. *Gastrointest Endosc Clin North Am* 2002; **12**: 535–559.
120. Jewell DP, Caprilli R, Mortensen N et al. Indications and timing of surgery for severe ulcerative colitis. *Gastroenterol Int* 1991; **4**: 161–164.
121. Present DH. Toxic megacolon. *Med Clin North Am* 1993; **77**: 1129–1148.
122. Sheth SG, LaMont JT. Toxic megacolon. *Lancet* 1998; **351**: 509–513.
123. Greenstein AJ, Barth JA, Sachar DB et al. Free colonic perforation without dilatation in ulcerative colitis. *Am J Surg* 1986; **152**: 272–275.
124. Jalan KN, Sircus W, Card WI et al. An experience of ulcerative colitis. I. Toxic dilation in 55 cases. *Gastroenterology* 1969; **57**: 68–82.
125. Fazio VW. Toxic megacolon in ulcerative colitis and Crohn's colitis. *Clin Gastroenterol* 1980; **9**: 389–407.
126. Grieco MB, Bordan DL, Geiss AC et al. Toxic megacolon complicating Crohn's colitis. *Ann Surg* 1980; **191**: 75–80.
127. Mourelle M, Casellas F, Guarner F et al. Induction of nitric oxide synthase in colonic smooth muscle from patients with toxic megacolon. *Gastroenterology* 1995; **109**: 1497–1502.
128. Brown JW. Toxic megacolon associated with loperamide therapy. *JAMA* 1979; **241**: 501–502.
129. Norland CC, Kirsner JB. Toxic dilatation of colon (toxic megacolon): etiology, treatment and prognosis in 42 patients. *Medicine (Baltimore)* 1969; **48**: 229–250.
130. Halpert RD. Toxic dilatation of the colon. *Radiol Clin North Am* 1987; **25**: 147–155.
131. Kramer P, Wittenberg J. Colonic gas distribution in toxic megacolon. *Gastroenterology* 1981; **80**: 433–437.
132. Present DH, Wolfson D, Gelernt IM et al. Medical decompression of toxic megacolon by 'rolling'. A new technique of decompression with favorable long-term follow-up. *J Clin Gastroenterol* 1988; **10**: 485–490.
133. Caroline DF, Evers K. Colitis: radiographic features and differentiation of idiopathic inflammatory bowel disease. *Radiol Clin North Am* 1987; **25**: 47–66.
134. Gumaste V, Sachar DB, Greenstein AJ. Benign and malignant colorectal strictures in ulcerative colitis. *Gut* 1992; **33**: 938–41.
135. Truelove SC, Witts LJ. Cortisone in ulcerative colitis. Final report on a therapeutic trial. *BMJ* 1955; **2**: 1041.
136. Lichtiger S, Present DH, Kornbluth A et al. Cyclosporine in severe ulcerative colitis refractory to steroid therapy. *N Engl J Med* 1994; **330**: 1841–1845.
137. Kozarek RA, Patterson DJ, Gelfand MD et al. Methotrexate induces clinical and histologic remission in patients with refractory inflammatory bowel disease. *Ann Intern Med* 1989; **110**: 353–356.
138. Harvey RF, Bradshaw JM. A simple index of Crohn's-disease activity. *Lancet* 1980; **1**: 514.
139. Kane SV, Sandborn WJ, Rufo PA et al. Fecal lactoferrin is a sensitive and specific marker in identifying intestinal inflammation. *Am J Gastroenterol* 2003; **98**: 1309–1314.
140. Leichtner AM. Aminosalicylates for the treatment of inflammatory bowel disease. *J Pediatr Gastroenterol Nutr* 1995; **21**: 245–252.
141. Wahl C, Liptay S, Adler G et al. Sulfasalazine: a potent and specific inhibitor of nuclear factor kappa B. *J Clin Invest* 1998; **101**: 1163–1174.
142. Bantel H, Berg C, Vieth M et al. Mesalazine inhibits activation of transcription factor NF-kappaB in inflamed mucosa of patients with ulcerative colitis. *Am J Gastroenterol* 2000; **95**: 3452–3457.

143. Dick AP, Grayson MJ, Carpenter RG et al. Controlled trial of sulfasalazine in the treatment of ulcerative colitis. *Gut* 1964; **5**: 437–442.
144. Sninsky CA, Cort DH, Shanahan F et al. Oral mesalamine (Asacol) for mildly to moderately active ulcerative colitis. A multicenter study. *Ann Intern Med* 1991; **115**: 350–355.
145. Sutherland LR, May GR, Shaffer EA. Sulfasalazine revisited: a meta-analysis of 5-aminosalicylic acid in the treatment of ulcerative colitis. *Ann Intern Med* 1993; **118**: 540–549.
146. Gisbert JP, Gomollon F, Mate J et al. Role of 5-aminosalicylic acid (5-ASA) in treatment of inflammatory bowel disease: a systematic review. *Dig Dis Sci* 2002; **47**: 471–488.
147. Sutherland LR, Roth DE, Beck PL, Alternatives to sulfasalazine: a meta-analysis of 5-ASA in the treatment of ulcerative colitis. *Inflamm Bowel Dis* 1997; **3**: 65–78.
148. Ferry GD, Kirschner BS, Grand RJ et al. Olsalazine versus sulfasalazine in mild to moderate childhood ulcerative colitis: results of the Pediatric Gastroenterology Collaborative Research Group Clinical Trial. *J Pediatr Gastroenterol Nutr* 1993; **17**: 32–38.
149. Barden L, Lipson A, Pert P. Mesalazine in childhood inflammatory bowel disease. *Aliment Pharmacol Ther* 1989; **3**: 597.
150. Levine DS, Riff DS, Pruitt R et al. A randomized, double blind, dose–response comparison of balsalazide (6.75 g), balsalazide (2.25 g), and mesalamine (2.4 g) in the treatment of active, mild-to-moderate ulcerative colitis. *Am J Gastroenterol* 2002; **97**: 1398–1407.
151. Green JR, Lobo AJ, Holdsworth CD et al. Balsalazide is more effective and better tolerated than mesalamine in the treatment of acute ulcerative colitis. The Abacus Investigator Group. *Gastroenterology* 1998; **114**: 15–22.
152. Hanauer SB. Inflammatory bowel disease. *N Engl J Med* 1996; **334**: 841–848.
153. Boyer DL, Li BU, Fyda JN et al. Sulfasalazine-induced hepatotoxicity in children with inflammatory bowel disease. *J Pediatr Gastroenterol Nutr* 1989; **8**: 528–532.
154. Garau P, Orenstein SR, Neigut DA et al. Pancreatitis associated with olsalazine and sulfasalazine in children with ulcerative colitis. *J Pediatr Gastroenterol Nutr* 1994; **18**: 481–485.
155. Paerregaard A, Krasilnikoff PA. Pancreatitis in a child after rectal administration of 5-aminosalicylic acid. *Inflamm Bowel Dis* 1997; **3**: 20.
156. Sturgeon JB, Bhatia P, Hermens D et al. Exacerbation of chronic ulcerative colitis with mesalamine. *Gastroenterology* 1995; **108**: 1889–1893.
157. Kirschner BS. The medical management of inflammatory bowel disease in children. In Kirsner JB, ed. *Inflammatory Bowel Disease*. Philadelphia: Saunders, 2000: 578–597.
158. Beattie RM, Nicholls SW, Domizio P et al. Endoscopic assessment of the colonic response to corticosteroids in children with ulcerative colitis. *J Pediatr Gastroenterol Nutr* 1996; **22**: 373–379.
159. Truhan AP, Ahmed AR. Corticosteroids: a review with emphasis on complications of prolonged systemic therapy. *Ann Allergy* 1989; **62**: 375–391.
160. Greenberg GR, Feagan BG, Martin F et al. Oral budesonide for active Crohn's disease. Canadian Inflammatory Bowel Disease Study Group. *N Engl J Med* 1994; **331**: 836–841.
161. Hanauer SB, Robinson M, Pruitt R et al. Budesonide enema for the treatment of active, distal ulcerative colitis and proctitis: a dose-ranging study. US Budesonide enema study group. *Gastroenterology* 1998; **115**: 525–532.
162. Hanauer SB, New steroids for IBD: progress report. *Gut* 2002; **51**: 182–183.
163. Bousvaros A. Immunosuppression. In Walker WA, Durie PR, Hamilton JR, Walker-Smith JA, Watkins JB, eds. *Pediatric Gastrointestinal Disease*. Hamilton, Ontario, Canada: BC Decker, 2000: 1769–1794.
164. Peppercorn MA. Are antibiotics useful in the management of nontoxic severe ulcerative colitis? *J Clin Gastroenterol* 1993; **17**: 14–17.
165. Chapman RW, Selby WS, Jewell DP. Controlled trial of intravenous metronidazole as an adjunct to corticosteroids in severe ulcerative colitis. *Gut* 1986; **27**: 1210–1212.
166. Mantzaris GJ, Hatzis A, Kontogiannis P et al. Intravenous tobramycin and metronidazole as an adjunct to corticosteroids in acute, severe ulcerative colitis. *Am J Gastroenterol* 1994; **89**: 43–46.
167. Mantzaris GJ, Petraki K, Archavlis E et al. A prospective randomized controlled trial of intravenous ciprofloxacin as an adjunct to corticosteroids in acute, severe ulcerative colitis. *Scand J Gastroenterol* 2001; **36**: 971–974.
168. Treem WR, Davis PM, Hyams JS. Cyclosporine treatment of severe ulcerative colitis in children. *J Pediatr* 1991; **119**: 994–997.
169. Benkov KJ, Rosh JR, Schwersenz AH et al. Cyclosporine as an alternative to surgery in children with inflammatory bowel disease. *J Pediatr Gastroenterol Nutr* 1994; **19**: 290–294.
170. Treem WR, Cohen J, Davis PM et al. Cyclosporine for the treatment of fulminant ulcerative colitis in children. Immediate response, long-term results, and impact on surgery. *Dis Colon Rectum* 1995; **38**: 474–479.
171. Escher JC, Taminiau JA, Nieuwenhuis EE et al. Treatment of inflammatory bowel disease in childhood: best available evidence. *Inflamm Bowel Dis* 2003; **9**: 34–58.
172. Bousvaros A, Kirschner BS, Werlin SL et al. Oral tacrolimus treatment of severe colitis in children. *J Pediatr* 2000; **137**: 794–799.
173. Ramakrishna J, Langhans N, Calenda K et al. Combined use of cyclosporine and azathioprine or 6-mercaptopurine in pediatric inflammatory bowel disease. *J Pediatr Gastroenterol Nutr* 1996; **22**: 296–302.
174. Marshall JK, Irvine EJ. Rectal aminosalicylate therapy for distal ulcerative colitis: a meta-analysis. *Aliment Pharmacol Ther* 1995; **9**: 293–300.
175. Marshall JK, Irvine EJ. Rectal corticosteroids versus alternative treatments in ulcerative colitis: a meta-analysis. *Gut* 1997; **40**: 775–781.
176. Mulder CJ, Tytgat GN. Review article: topical corticosteroids in inflammatory bowel disease. *Aliment Pharmacol Ther* 1993; **7**: 125–130.
177. Gionchetti P, Rizzello F, Venturi A et al. Comparison of oral with rectal mesalazine in the treatment of ulcerative proctitis. *Dis Colon Rectum* 1998; **41**: 93–97.
178. Cohen RD, Woseth DM, Thisted RA et al. A meta-analysis and overview of the literature on treatment options for left-sided ulcerative colitis and ulcerative proctitis. *Am J Gastroenterol* 2000; **95**: 1263–1276.
179. Allgayer H. Sulfasalazine and 5-ASA compounds. *Gastroenterol Clin North Am* 1992; **21**: 643–658.
180. Sutherland LR. Topical treatment of ulcerative colitis. *Med Clin North Am* 1990; **74**: 119–131.
181. Safdi M, DeMicco M, Sninsky C et al. A double-blind comparison of oral versus rectal mesalamine versus combination therapy in the treatment of distal ulcerative colitis. *Am J Gastroenterol* 1997; **92**: 1867–1871.

182. Danielsson A, Lofberg R, Persson T et al. A steroid enema, budesonide, lacking systemic effects for the treatment of distal ulcerative colitis or proctitis. *Scand J Gastroenterol* 1992; **27**: 9–12.
183. Lindgren S, Lofberg R, Bergholm L et al. Effect of budesonide enema on remission and relapse rate in distal ulcerative colitis and proctitis. *Scand J Gastroenterol* 2002; **37**: 705–710.
184. Winter TA, Dalton HR, Merrett MN et al. Cyclosporin A retention enemas in refractory distal ulcerative colitis and 'pouchitis'. *Scand J Gastroenterol* 1993; **28**: 701–704.
185. Sandborn WJ, Tremaine WJ, Schroeder KW et al. A placebo-controlled trial of cyclosporine enemas for mildly to moderately active left-sided ulcerative colitis. *Gastroenterology* 1994; **106**: 1429–1435.
186. D'Agata ID, Vanounou T, Seidman E. Mesalamine in pediatric inflammatory bowel disease: A 10-year experience. *Inflamm Bowel Dis* 1996; **2**: 229–235.
187. Kruis W, Schreiber S, Theuer D et al. Low dose balsalazide (1.5g twice daily) and mesalazine (0.5g three times daily) maintained remission of ulcerative colitis but high dose balsalazide (3.0g twice daily) was superior in preventing relapses. *Gut* 2001; **49**: 783–789.
188. d'Albasio G, Paoluzi P, Campieri M et al. Maintenance treatment of ulcerative proctitis with mesalazine suppositories: a double-blind placebo-controlled trial. The Italian IBD Study Group. *Am J Gastroenterol* 1998; **93**: 799–803.
189. d'Albasio G, Pacini F, Camarri E et al. Combined therapy with 5-aminosalicylic acid tablets and enemas for maintaining remission in ulcerative colitis: a randomized double-blind study. *Am J Gastroenterol* 1997; **92**: 1143–1147.
190. Eaden J, Abrams K, Ekbom A et al. Colorectal cancer prevention in ulcerative colitis: a case-control study. *Aliment Pharmacol Ther* 2000; **14**: 145–153.
191. Pinczowski D, Ekbom A, Baron J et al. Risk factors for colorectal cancer in patients with ulcerative colitis: a case–control study. *Gastroenterology* 1994; **107**: 117–120.
192. Ekbom A, Kornfield D. Sulfasalazine use as a preventative factor in colorectal cancer in ulcerative colitis patients: a review. *Inflamm Bowel Dis* 1996; **2**: 276.
193. Ryan BM, Russel MG, Langholz E et al. Aminosalicylates and colorectal cancer in IBD: a not-so bitter pill to swallow. *Am J Gastroenterol* 2003; **98**: 1682–1687.
194. Verhave M, Winter HS, Grand RJ. Azathioprine in the treatment of children with inflammatory bowel disease. *J Pediatr* 1990; **117**: 809–814.
195. Kader HA, Mascarenhas MR, Piccoli DA et al. Experiences with 6-mercaptopurine and azathioprine therapy in pediatric patients with severe ulcerative colitis. *J Pediatr Gastroenterol Nutr* 1999; **28**: 54–58.
196. Kirschner BS. Safety of azathioprine and 6-mercaptopurine in pediatric patients with inflammatory bowel disease. *Gastroenterology* 1998; **115**: 813–821.
197. Present DH, Meltzer SJ, Krumholz MP et al. 6-Mercaptopurine in the management of inflammatory bowel disease: short- and long-term toxicity. *Ann Intern Med* 1989; **111**: 641–649.
198. Cuffari C, Theoret Y, Latour S et al. 6-Mercaptopurine metabolism in Crohn's disease: correlation with efficacy and toxicity. *Gut* 1996; **39**: 401–406.
199. Dubinsky MC, Lamothe S, Yang HY et al. Pharmacogenomics and metabolite measurement for 6-mercaptopurine therapy in inflammatory bowel disease. *Gastroenterology* 2000; **118**: 705–713.
200. Lennard L, Van Loon JA, Weinshilboum RM. Pharmacogenetics of acute azathioprine toxicity: relationship to thiopurine methyltransferase genetic polymorphism. *Clin Pharmacol Ther* 1989; **46**: 149–154.
201. George J, Present DH, Pou R et al. The long-term outcome of ulcerative colitis treated with 6-mercaptopurine. *Am J Gastroenterol* 1996; **91**: 1711–1714.
202. Fraser AG, Orchard TR, Robinson EM et al. Long-term risk of malignancy after treatment of inflammatory bowel disease with azathioprine. *Aliment Pharmacol Ther* 2002; **16**: 1225–1232.
203. Korelitz BI, Mirsky FJ, Fleisher MR et al. Malignant neoplasms subsequent to treatment of inflammatory bowel disease with 6-mercaptopurine. *Am J Gastroenterol* 1999; **94**: 3248–3253.
204. Connell WR, Kamm MA, Dickson M et al. Long-term neoplasia risk after azathioprine treatment in inflammatory bowel disease. *Lancet* 1994; **343**: 1249–1252.
205. Dayharsh GA, Loftus EV Jr, Sandborn WJ et al. Epstein–Barr virus-positive lymphoma in patients with inflammatory bowel disease treated with azathioprine or 6-mercaptopurine. *Gastroenterology* 2002; **122**: 72–77.
206. Feagan BG, Rochon J, Fedorak RN et al. Methotrexate for the treatment of Crohn's disease. The North American Crohn's Study Group Investigators. *N Engl J Med* 1995; **332**: 292–297.
207. Schroder O, Stein J, Low dose methotrexate in inflammatory bowel disease: current status and future directions. *Am J Gastroenterol* 2003; **98**: 530–537.
208. Paoluzi OA, Pica R, Marcheggiano A et al. Azathioprine or methotrexate in the treatment of patients with steroid-dependent or steroid-resistant ulcerative colitis: results of an open-label study on efficacy and tolerability in inducing and maintaining remission. *Aliment Pharmacol Ther* 2002; **16**: 1751–1759.
209. Oren R, Arber N, Odes S et al. Methotrexate in chronic active ulcerative colitis: a double-blind, randomized, Israeli multicenter trial. *Gastroenterology* 1996; **110**: 1416–1421.
210. Egan LJ, Sandborn WJ, Tremaine WJ et al. A randomized dose–response and pharmacokinetic study of methotrexate for refractory inflammatory Crohn's disease and ulcerative colitis. *Aliment Pharmacol Ther* 1999; **13**: 1597–1604.
211. Mack DR, Young R, Kaufman SS et al. Methotrexate in patients with Crohn's disease after 6-mercaptopurine. *J Pediatr* 1998; **132**: 830–835.
212. Burke DA, Axon AT, Clayden SA et al. The efficacy of tobramycin in the treatment of ulcerative colitis. *Aliment Pharmacol Ther* 1990; **4**: 123–129.
213. Lobo AJ, Burke DA, Sobala GM et al. Oral tobramycin in ulcerative colitis: effect on maintenance of remission. *Aliment Pharmacol Ther* 1993; **7**: 155–158.
214. Gilat T, Suissa A, Leichtman G et al. A comparative study of metronidazole and sulfasalazine in active, not severe, ulcerative colitis. An Israeli multicenter trial. *J Clin Gastroenterol* 1987; **9**: 415–417.
215. Dickinson RJ, O'Connor HJ, Pinder I et al. Double blind controlled trial of oral vancomycin as adjunctive treatment in acute exacerbations of idiopathic colitis. *Gut* 1985; **26**: 1380–1384.
216. Mantzaris GJ, Archavlis E, Christoforidis P et al. A prospective randomized controlled trial of oral ciprofloxacin in acute ulcerative colitis. *Am J Gastroenterol* 1997; **92**: 454–456.
217. Turunen UM, Farkkila MA, Hakala K et al. Long-term treatment of ulcerative colitis with ciprofloxacin: a prospective, double-blind, placebo-controlled study. *Gastroenterology* 1998; **115**: 1072–1078.

218. Chey WY, Hussain A, Ryan C et al. Infliximab for refractory ulcerative colitis. *Am J Gastroenterol* 2001; **96**: 2373–2381.
219. Su C, Salzberg BA, Lewis JD et al. Efficacy of anti-tumor necrosis factor therapy in patients with ulcerative colitis. *Am J Gastroenterol* 2002; **97**: 2577–2584.
220. Kohn A, Prantera C, Pera A et al. Anti-tumour necrosis factor alpha (infliximab) in the treatment of severe ulcerative colitis: result of an open study on 13 patients. *Dig Liver Dis* 2002; **34**: 626–630.
221. Serrano MS, Schmidt-Sommerfeld E, Kilbaugh TJ et al. Use of infliximab in pediatric patients with inflammatory bowel disease. *Ann Pharmacother* 2001; **35**: 823–828.
222. Mamula P, Markowitz JE, Brown KA et al. Infliximab as a novel therapy for pediatric ulcerative colitis. *J Pediatr Gastroenterol Nutr* 2002; **34**: 307–311.
223. Actis GC, Bruno M, Pinna-Pintor M et al. Infliximab for treatment of steroid-refractory ulcerative colitis. *Dig Liver Dis* 2002; **34**: 631–634.
224. Sands BE, Tremaine WJ, Sandborn WJ et al. Infliximab in the treatment of severe, steroid-refractory ulcerative colitis: a pilot study. *Inflamm Bowel Dis* 2001; **7**: 83–88.
225. Probert CS, Hearing SD, Schreiber S et al. Infliximab in moderately severe glucocorticoid resistant ulcerative colitis: a randomised controlled trial. *Gut* 2003; **52**: 998–1002.
226. Keane J, Gershon S, Wise RP et al. Tuberculosis associated with infliximab, a tumor necrosis factor alpha-neutralizing agent. *N Engl J Med* 2001; **345**: 1098–1104.
227. Farrell RJ, Alsahli M, Jeen YT et al. Intravenous hydrocortisone premedication reduces antibodies to infliximab in Crohn's disease: a randomized controlled trial. *Gastroenterology* 2003; **124**: 917–924.
228. Baert F, Noman M, Vermeire S et al. Influence of immunogenicity on the long-term efficacy of infliximab in Crohn's disease. *N Engl J Med* 2003; **348**: 601–608.
229. Crandall WV, Mackner LM. Infusion reactions to infliximab in children and adolescents: frequency, outcome and a predictive model. *Aliment Pharmacol Ther* 2003; **17**: 75–84.
230. Sandborn WJ, Hanauer SB. Infliximab in the treatment of Crohn's disease: a user's guide for clinicians. *Am J Gastroenterol* 2002; **97**: 2962–2972.
231. Orth T, Peters M, Schlaak JF et al. Mycophenolate mofetil versus azathioprine in patients with chronic active ulcerative colitis: a 12-month pilot study. *Am J Gastroenterol* 2000; **95**: 1201–1207.
232. Fellermann K, Steffen M, Stein J et al. Mycophenolate mofetil: lack of efficacy in chronic active inflammatory bowel disease. *Aliment Pharmacol Ther* 2000; **14**: 171–176.
233. Skelly MM, Logan RF, Jenkins D et al. Toxicity of mycophenolate mofetil in patients with inflammatory bowel disease. *Inflamm Bowel Dis* 2002; **8**: 93–97.
234. Venturi A, Gionchetti P, Rizzello F et al. Impact on the composition of the faecal flora by a new probiotic preparation: preliminary data on maintenance treatment of patients with ulcerative colitis. *Aliment Pharmacol Ther* 1999; **13**: 1103–1108.
235. Kruis W, Schutz E, Fric P et al. Double-blind comparison of an oral *Escherichia coli* preparation and mesalazine in maintaining remission of ulcerative colitis. *Aliment Pharmacol Ther* 1997; **11**: 853–858.
236. Rembacken BJ, Snelling AM, Hawkey PM et al. Non-pathogenic *Escherichia coli* versus mesalazine for the treatment of ulcerative colitis: a randomised trial. *Lancet* 1999; **354**: 635–639.
237. Pullan RD, Rhodes J, Ganesh S et al. Transdermal nicotine for active ulcerative colitis. *N Engl J Med* 1994; **330**: 811–815.
238. Sandborn WJ, Tremaine WJ, Offord KP et al. Transdermal nicotine for mildly to moderately active ulcerative colitis. A randomized, double-blind, placebo-controlled trial. *Ann Intern Med* 1997; **126**: 364–371.
239. Thomas GA, Rhodes J, Mani V et al. Transdermal nicotine as maintenance therapy for ulcerative colitis. *N Engl J Med* 1995; **332**: 988–992.
240. Green JT, Thomas GA, Rhodes J et al. Nicotine enemas for active ulcerative colitis – a pilot study. *Aliment Pharmacol Ther* 1997; **11**: 859–863.
241. Stenson WF, Cort D, Rodgers J et al. Dietary supplementation with fish oil in ulcerative colitis. *Ann Intern Med* 1992; **116**: 609–614.
242. Aslan A, Triadafilopoulos G. Fish oil fatty acid supplementation in active ulcerative colitis: a double-blind, placebo-controlled, crossover study. *Am J Gastroenterol* 1992; **87**: 432–437.
243. Hawthorne AB, Daneshmend TK, Hawkey CJ et al. Treatment of ulcerative colitis with fish oil supplementation: a prospective 12 month randomised controlled trial. *Gut* 1992; **33**: 922–928.
244. Greenfield SM, Green AT, Teare JP et al. A randomized controlled study of evening primrose oil and fish oil in ulcerative colitis. *Aliment Pharmacol Ther* 1993; **7**: 159–166.
245. Scheppach W. Treatment of distal ulcerative colitis with short-chain fatty acid enemas. A placebo-controlled trial. German–Austrian SCFA Study Group. *Dig Dis Sci* 1996; **41**: 2254–2259.
246. Breuer RI, Soergel KH, Lashner BA et al. Short chain fatty acid rectal irrigation for left-sided ulcerative colitis: a randomised, placebo controlled trial. *Gut* 1997; **40**: 485–491.
247. Vernia P, Marcheggiano A, Caprilli R et al. Short-chain fatty acid topical treatment in distal ulcerative colitis. *Aliment Pharmacol Ther* 1995; **9**: 309–313.
248. Evans RC, Wong VS, Morris AI et al. Treatment of corticosteroid-resistant ulcerative colitis with heparin – a report of 16 cases. *Aliment Pharmacol Ther* 1997; **11**: 1037–1040.
249. Torkvist L, Thorlacius H, Sjoqvist U et al. Low molecular weight heparin as adjuvant therapy in active ulcerative colitis. *Aliment Pharmacol Ther* 1999; **13**: 1323–1328.
250. Folwaczny C, Wiebecke B, Loeschke K. Unfractioned heparin in the therapy of patients with highly active inflammatory bowel disease. *Am J Gastroenterol* 1999; **94**: 1551–1555.
251. Panes J, Esteve M, Cabre E et al. Comparison of heparin and steroids in the treatment of moderate and severe ulcerative colitis. *Gastroenterology* 2000; **119**: 903–908.
252. Van Assche G, Dalle I, Noman M et al. A pilot study on the use of the humanized anti-interleukin-2 receptor antibody daclizumab in active ulcerative colitis. *Am J Gastroenterol* 2003; **98**: 369–376.
253. Motil KJ, Grand RJ. Nutritional management of inflammatory bowel disease. *Pediatr Clin North Am* 1985; **32**: 447–469.
254. Burke A, Lichtenstein GR, Rombeau JL. Nutrition and ulcerative colitis. *Baillières Clin Gastroenterol* 1997; **11**: 153–174.
255. Kleinman RE, Balistreri WF, Heyman MB et al. Nutritional support for pediatric patients with inflammatory bowel disease. *J Pediatr Gastroenterol Nutr* 1989; **8**: 8–12.
256. Dickinson RJ, Ashton MG, Axon AT et al. Controlled trial of intravenous hyperalimentation and total bowel rest as an adjunct to the routine therapy of acute colitis. *Gastroenterology* 1980; **79**: 1199–1204.

257. McIntyre PB, Powell-Tuck J, Wood SR et al. Controlled trial of bowel rest in the treatment of severe acute colitis. *Gut* 1986; **27**: 481–485.
258. Gonzalez-Huix F, Fernandez-Banares F, Esteve-Comas M et al. Enteral versus parenteral nutrition as adjunct therapy in acute ulcerative colitis. *Am J Gastroenterol* 1993; **88**: 227–232.
259. Durno C, Sherman P, Harris K et al. Outcome after ileoanal anastomosis in pediatric patients with ulcerative colitis. *J Pediatr Gastroenterol Nutr* 1998; **27**: 501–507.
260. Perrault J, Berry R, Greseth J et al. Pouchitis in young patients after the ileal-pouch anal anastomosis. *Inflamm Bowel Dis* 1997; **3**: 181–185.
261. Dozois RR, Kelly KA, The surgical management of ulcerative colitis. In Kirsner JB, ed. *Inflammatory Bowel Disease*. Philadelphia: WB Saunders, 2000: 626–657.
262. Nicholls S, Vieira MC, Majrowski WH et al. Linear growth after colectomy for ulcerative colitis in childhood. *J Pediatr Gastroenterol Nutr* 1995; **21**: 82–86.
263. Michener WM, Farmer RG, Mortimer EA. Long-term prognosis of ulcerative colitis with onset in childhood or adolescence. *J Clin Gastroenterol* 1979; **1**: 301–305.
264. Hyams JS, Davis P, Grancher K et al. Clinical outcome of ulcerative colitis in children. *J Pediatr* 1996; **129**: 81–88.
265. Falcone RA Jr, Lewis LG, Warner BW. Predicting the need for colectomy in pediatric patients with ulcerative colitis. *J Gastrointest Surg* 2000; **4**: 201–206.
266. Kettlewell MGW. Recent advances in surgical therapy. In Tytgat GNJ, Bartelsman JFWM, van Deventer SJH, eds. *Inflammatory Bowel Diseases*. Boston: Kluwer Academic Publishers, 1995: 508–516.
267. Farouk R, Pemberton JH. Surgical options in ulcerative colitis. *Surg Clin North Am* 1997; **77**: 85–94.
268. Mowschenson PM, Critchlow JF. Outcome of early surgical complications following ileoanal pouch operation without diverting ileostomy. *Am J Surg* 1995; **169**: 143–145; discussion 145–146.
269. Cohen Z, McLeod RS, Stephen W et al. Continuing evolution of the pelvic pouch procedure. *Ann Surg* 1992; **216**: 506–511; discussion 511–512.
270. Fonkalsrud EW, Thakur A, Beanes S. Ileoanal pouch procedures in children. *J Pediatr Surg* 2001; **36**: 1689–1692.
271. Telander RL, Spencer M, Perrault J et al. Long-term follow-up of the ileoanal anastomosis in children and young adults. *Surgery* 1990; **108**: 717–723; discussion 723–725.
272. Rintala RJ, Lindahl HG. Proctocolectomy and J-pouch ileo-anal anastomosis in children. *J Pediatr Surg* 2002; **37**: 66–70.
273. Mahadevan U, Sandborn WJ. Diagnosis and management of pouchitis. *Gastroenterology* 2003; **124**: 1636–1650.
274. Sandborn WJ. Pouchitis following ileal pouch–anal anastomosis: definition, pathogenesis, and treatment. *Gastroenterology* 1994; **107**: 1856–1860.
275. Kartheuser AH, Parc R, Penna CP et al. Ileal pouch–anal anastomosis as the first choice operation in patients with familial adenomatous polyposis: a ten-year experience. *Surgery* 1996; **119**: 615–623.
276. Faubion WA Jr, Loftus EV, Sandborn WJ et al. Pediatric 'PSC-IBD': a descriptive report of associated inflammatory bowel disease among pediatric patients with PSC. *J Pediatr Gastroenterol Nutr* 2001; **33**: 296–300.
277. Penna C, Dozois R, Tremaine W et al. Pouchitis after ileal pouch-anal anastomosis for ulcerative colitis occurs with increased frequency in patients with associated primary sclerosing cholangitis. *Gut* 1996; **38**: 234–239.
278. Gionchetti P, Amadini C, Rizzello F et al. Treatment of mild to moderate ulcerative colitis and pouchitis. *Aliment Pharmacol Ther* 2002; **16** (Suppl 4): 13–19.
279. Shen B, Achkar JP, Lashner BA et al. A randomized clinical trial of ciprofloxacin and metronidazole to treat acute pouchitis. *Inflamm Bowel Dis* 2001; **7**: 301–305.
280. Miglioli M, Barbara L, Di Febo G et al. Topical administration of 5-aminosalicylic acid: a therapeutic proposal for the treatment of pouchitis. *N Engl J Med* 1989; **320**: 257.
281. Sambuelli A, Boerr L, Negreira S et al. Budesonide enema in pouchitis – a double-blind, double-dummy, controlled trial. *Aliment Pharmacol Ther* 2002; **16**: 27–34.
282. de Silva HJ, Ireland A, Kettlewell M et al. Short-chain fatty acid irrigation in severe pouchitis. *N Engl J Med* 1989; **321**: 1416–1417.
283. Wischmeyer P, Pemberton JH, Phillips SF. Chronic pouchitis after ileal pouch–anal anastomosis: responses to butyrate and glutamine suppositories in a pilot study. *Mayo Clin Proc* 1993; **68**: 978–981.
284. Gionchetti P, Rizzello F, Helwig U et al. Prophylaxis of pouchitis onset with probiotic therapy: a double-blind, placebo-controlled trial. *Gastroenterology* 2003; **124**: 1202–1209.
285. Gionchetti P, Rizzello F, Venturi A et al. Oral bacteriotherapy as maintenance treatment in patients with chronic pouchitis: a double-blind, placebo-controlled trial. *Gastroenterology* 2000; **119**: 305–309.
286. Sarigol S, Wyllie R, Gramlich T et al. Incidence of dysplasia in pelvic pouches in pediatric patients after ileal pouch–anal anastomosis for ulcerative colitis. J Pediatr Gastroenterol Nutr 1999; **28**: 429–434.
287. Thompson-Fawcett MW, Marcus V, Redston M et al. Risk of dysplasia in long-term ileal pouches and pouches with chronic pouchitis. *Gastroenterology* 2001; **121**: 275–281.
288. Veress B, Reinholt FP, Lindquist K et al. Long-term histomorphological surveillance of the pelvic ileal pouch: dysplasia develops in a subgroup of patients. *Gastroenterology* 1995; **109**: 1090–1097.
289. Heuschen UA, Heuschen G, Autschbach F et al. Adenocarcinoma in the ileal pouch: late risk of cancer after restorative proctocolectomy. *Int J Colorectal Dis* 2001; **16**: 126–130.
290. Burke PM, Neigut D, Kocoshis S et al. Correlates of depression in new onset pediatric inflammatory bowel disease. *Child Psychiatry Hum Dev* 1994; **24**: 275–283.
291. Szajnberg N, Krall V, Davis P et al. Psychopathology and relationship measures in children with inflammatory bowel disease and their parents. *Child Psychiatry Hum Dev* 1993; **23**: 215–232.
292. Engstrom I. Mental health and psychological functioning in children and adolescents with inflammatory bowel disease: a comparison with children having other chronic illnesses and with healthy children. *J Child Psychol Psychiatry* 1992; **33**: 563–582.
293. Engstrom I, Lindquist BL. Inflammatory bowel disease in children and adolescents: a somatic and psychiatric investigation. *Acta Paediatr Scand* 1991; **80**: 640–647.
294. Loonen HJ, Grootenhuis MA, Last BF et al. Quality of life in paediatric inflammatory bowel disease measured by a generic and a disease-specific questionnaire. *Acta Paediatr* 2002; **91**: 348–354.
295. Otley A, Smith C, Nicholas D et al. The IMPACT questionnaire: a valid measure of health-related quality of

life in pediatric inflammatory bowel disease. *J Pediatr Gastroenterol Nutr* 2002; **35**: 557–563.
296. Loonen HJ, Grootenhuis MA, Last BF et al. Measuring quality of life in children with inflammatory bowel disease: the impact-II (NL). *Qual Life Res* 2002; **11**: 47–56.
297. Langholz E, Munkholm P, Davidsen M et al. Changes in extent of ulcerative colitis: a study on the course and prognostic factors. *Scand J Gastroenterol* 1996; **31**: 260–266.
298. Meucci G, Vecchi M, Astegiano M et al. The natural history of ulcerative proctitis: a multicenter, retrospective study. Gruppo di Studio per le Malattie Infiammatorie Intestinali (GSMII). *Am J Gastroenterol* 2000; **95**: 469–473.
299. Hyams J, Davis P, Lerer T et al. Clinical outcome of ulcerative proctitis in children. *J Pediatr Gastroenterol* Nutr 1997; **25**: 149–152.
300. Mir-Madjlessi SH, Michener WM, Farmer RG. Course and prognosis of idiopathic ulcerative proctosigmoiditis in young patients. *J Pediatr Gastroenterol Nutr* 1986; **5**: 571–575.
301. Ekbom A. Risk factors and distinguishing features of cancer in IBD. *Inflamm Bowel Dis* 1998; **4**: 235–243.
302. Kane S. Inflammatory bowel disease in pregnancy. *Gastroenterol Clin North Am* 2003; **32**: 323–340.
303. Baird DD, Narendranathan M, Sandler RS. Increased risk of preterm birth for women with inflammatory bowel disease. *Gastroenterology* 1990; **99**: 987–994.
304. Norgard B, Fonager K, Sorensen HT et al. Birth outcomes of women with ulcerative colitis: a nationwide Danish cohort study. *Am J Gastroenterol* 2000; **95**: 3165–3170.
305. Ording Olsen K, Juul S, Berndtsson I et al. Ulcerative colitis: female fecundity before diagnosis, during disease, and after surgery compared with a population sample. *Gastroenterology* 2002; **122**: 15–19.
306. Devroede GJ, Taylor WF, Sauer WG et al. Cancer risk and life expectancy of children with ulcerative colitis. *N Engl J Med* 1971; **285**: 17–21.
307. Ekbom A, Helmick C, Zack M et al. Ulcerative colitis and colorectal cancer. A population-based study. *N Engl J Med* 1990; **323**: 1228–1233.
308. Brostrom O, Lofberg R, Nordenvall B et al. The risk of colorectal cancer in ulcerative colitis. An epidemiologic study. *Scand J Gastroenterol* 1987; **22**: 1193–1199.
309. Gilat T, Fireman Z, Grossman A et al. Colorectal cancer in patients with ulcerative colitis. A population study in central Israel. *Gastroenterology* 1988; **94**: 870–877.
310. Broome U, Lofberg R, Veress B et al. Primary sclerosing cholangitis and ulcerative colitis: evidence for increased neoplastic potential. *Hepatology* 1995; **22**: 1404–1408.
311. Brentnall TA, Haggitt RC, Rabinovitch PS et al. Risk and natural history of colonic neoplasia in patients with primary sclerosing cholangitis and ulcerative colitis. *Gastroenterology* 1996; **110**: 331–338.
312. Shetty K, Rybicki L, Brzezinski A et al. The risk for cancer or dysplasia in ulcerative colitis patients with primary sclerosing cholangitis. *Am J Gastroenterol* 1999; **94**: 1643–1649.
313. Jayaram H, Satsangi J, Chapman RW. Increased colorectal neoplasia in chronic ulcerative colitis complicated by primary sclerosing cholangitis: fact or fiction? *Gut* 2001; **48**: 430–434.
314. Soetikno RM, Lin OS, Heidenreich PA et al. Increased risk of colorectal neoplasia in patients with primary sclerosing cholangitis and ulcerative colitis: a meta-analysis. *Gastrointest Endosc* 2002; **56**: 48–54.
315. Pardi DS, Loftus EV Jr, Kremers WK et al. Ursodeoxycholic acid as a chemopreventive agent in patients with ulcerative colitis and primary sclerosing cholangitis. *Gastroenterology* 2003; **124**: 889–893.
316. Askling J, Dickman PW, Karlen P et al. Family history as a risk factor for colorectal cancer in inflammatory bowel disease. *Gastroenterology* 2001; **120**: 1356–1362.
317. Heuschen UA, Hinz U, Allemeyer EH et al. Backwash ileitis is strongly associated with colorectal carcinoma in ulcerative colitis. *Gastroenterology* 2001; **120**: 841–847.
318. Lindberg BU, Broome U, Persson B. Proximal colorectal dysplasia or cancer in ulcerative colitis. The impact of primary sclerosing cholangitis and sulfasalazine: results from a 20-year surveillance study. *Dis Colon Rectum* 2001; **44**: 77–85.
319. Lashner BA, Heidenreich PA, Su GL et al. Effect of folate supplementation on the incidence of dysplasia and cancer in chronic ulcerative colitis. A case–control study. *Gastroenterology* 1989; **97**: 255–259.
320. Judge TA, Lewis JD, Lichtenstein GR. Colonic dysplasia and cancer in inflammatory bowel disease. *Gastrointest Endosc Clin North Am* 2002; **12**: 495–523.
321. Bernstein CN, Eaden J, Steinhart AH et al. Cancer prevention in inflammatory bowel disease and the chemoprophylactic potential of 5-aminosalicylic acid. *Inflamm Bowel Dis* 2002; **8**: 356–361.
322. van Hogezand RA, Eichhorn RF, Choudry A et al. Malignancies in inflammatory bowel disease: fact or fiction? *Scand J Gastroenterol Suppl* 2002: 48–53.
323. Griffiths AM, Sherman PM. Colonoscopic surveillance for cancer in ulcerative colitis: a critical review. *J Pediatr Gastroenterol Nutr* 1997; **24**: 202–210.
324. Winawer S, Fletcher R, Rex D et al. Colorectal cancer screening and surveillance: clinical guidelines and rationale. Update based on new evidence. *Gastroenterology* 2003; **124**: 544–560.
325. Hanauer SB, Kane S. The pharmacology of anti-inflammatory drugs in inflammatory bowel disease. In Kirsner JB, ed. *Inflammatory Bowel Diseases*. Philadelphia: WB Saunders, 2000: 510–518.
326. Makins RJ, Cowan RE. 5-amino-salicylate in the management of inflammatory bowel disease. *Colorectal Dis* 2001; **3**: 218–222.

26 Vasculitides

Salvatore Cucchiara and Osvaldo Borrelli

Introduction

Vasculitides is a general term for a group of diseases characterized by inflammation within or around the wall of blood vessels, with alteration of the vascular blood flow and deranged integrity of the vessels, leading to ischemia and necrosis of the dependent organs. Blood vessels of all sizes may be affected, from the largest vessel in the body (the aorta) to the smallest vessels in the skin (capillaries). The size of the affected blood vessels varies according to the specific type of vasculitis.[1–3] The symptoms of vasculitides depend on the blood vessels involved in the inflammatory process. However, vasculitides are a systemic illness, and patients have fever, weight loss, fatigue, a rapid pulse, and diffuse aches and pains. In some cases, identifying the source and underlying cause of the pain is extremely challenging. In addition to these diffuse, poorly localized systemic symptoms, vasculitides may involve virtually every organ system in the body.

It should be stressed that, although several specific entities are identified, different vasculitides may also have overlapping features. Table 26.1 reports a classification that takes into account the heterogeneity of vasculitides, and also the fact that some syndromes are mainly systemic, leading to progressive organ system dysfunction, whereas

Table 26.1 Classification of the vasculitic syndromes

Systemic necrotizing vasculitis
polyarteritis nodosa (PAN) (classic PAN, microscopic polyangiitis)
allergic angiitis and granulomatosis of Churg–Strauss
polyangiitis overlap syndrome
Wegener's granulomatosis
Temporal arteritis
Takayasu's arteritis
Henoch–Schönlein purpura
Predominantly cutaneous vasculitis (hypersensitivity vasculitis)
exogenous stimuli proven or suspected (drug-induced, serum sickness and serum sickness-like reactions, associated with infectious diseases)
endogenous antigens likely to be involved (associated with neoplasms, with connective tissue diseases, with other underlying diseases, or with congenital deficiencies of the complement system)
Other vasculitic syndromes
Kawasaki disease
isolated central nervous system vasculitis
thromboangiitis obliterans (Buerger's disease)
Behçet's syndrome
miscellaneous vasculitis

others are predominantly localized to the skin and rarely cause dysfunction of vital organs. Organ systems that can be affected by the vasculitic process are: skin, joints, lungs, kidneys, gastrointestinal tract, blood, sinuses, nose and ears, eyes, brain and nerves. In general, however, any type of systemic vasculitis can affect the gastrointestinal tract. For practical clinical work, vasculitides can also be differentiated into 'primary' and 'secondary'. Primary vasculitides are not associated with systemic entities and the type of the disease depends on the caliber of the involved vessels. Secondary vasculitides are associated with underlying diseases, mainly rheumatic or connective tissue diseases, malignancy, infections, drugs and toxic agents. Rheumatic and autoimmune diseases, a cause of intestinal vasculitides, are systemic lupus erythematosus (SLE), rheumatoid arthritis, systemic sclerosis, dermatomyositis, primary biliary cirrhosis and autoimmune hepatitis. However, the most common infectious diseases underlying vasculitides are bacterial (streptococci, borrelia, mycobacteria, mycoplasms), viral (hepatitis, cytomegalovirus, herpes, HIV) and fungal.

Vasculitides involving the gastrointestinal tract are part of a systemic process, although signs and symptoms may initially be limited. The onset of clinical manifestations may be acute and severe (mesenteric infarction) or chronic, due to mesenteric ischemia.[4] Acute intestinal vasculitides present as a rapidly evolving disorder, with a clinical picture mimicking embolic or thrombotic ischemia: intensive abdominal pain, signs of peritonitis and ileus. Chronic intestinal vasculitides can mimic each type of gastrointestinal disorder and require a detailed diagnostic procedure. The main symptoms of chronic vasculitides involving the intestine include abdominal pain, weight loss, nausea, vomiting, diarrhea, hematochezia and tenesmus. Endoscopy of both the upper and lower gastrointestinal tract often shows signs of inflammation such as petechiae, erosions and small ulcerations. Affected patients may also present acute episodes of small-bowel obstruction secondary to strictures, resembling Crohn's disease or intussusceptions, or with massive gastrointestinal bleeding, secondary to aneurysm formation.[4] In addition to mesenteric ischemia, systemic vasculitides can also cause ischemic damage to the liver, pancreas, gallbladder and, less commonly, esophagus or stomach.

Epidemiology

Certain forms of vasculitis occur more commonly in specific age groups. Vasculitides in childhood are dominated by Kawasaki disease and Henoch–Schönlein purpura, whereas primary systemic vasculitides, as well as conditions that can be complicated by a vasculitic process (e.g. SLE and juvenile dermatomyositis) are rarely reported in children. Furthermore, certain ethnic groups are at higher risk than others. The incidence of Kawasaki disease in children younger than 5 years doubled from 4.0 per 100000 in 1991–92 to 8.1 per 100000 in 1999–2000, whereas for Henoch–Schönlein purpura the annual incidence is about 20 per 100000.[5] Recent data from the West Midlands of the UK indicated an incidence of 0.24 per 100000 for primary systemic vasculitides including cases of polyarteritis nodosa (PAN), microscopic polyangiitis, Wegener's granulomatosis and Behçet's disease.[6]

Pathogenesis

Most of the vasculitides are thought to be mediated by immunopathogenetic mechanisms, although the evidence for this is mainly indirect. Three potential mechanisms of vessel damage in vasculitides have been suggested.[7]

Pathogenetic immune-complex formation

The mechanism of tissue damage in immune complex diseases is derived from the occurrence of antigen–antibody complexes formed in antigen excess and deposited in vessel walls, whose permeability is increased by several vasoactive amines. The deposition of complexes determines the activation of complement components, mainly C5a, that recruit neutrophils. Neutrophils infiltrate the vessel wall, phagocytose the immune complexes and release enzymes that damage the vessel wall. When the process becomes subacute or chronic, an infiltrate of mononuclear cells predominates. The causal role of deposition of immune complexes in the wall of vessels has not been clearly defined in most vasculitides. Indeed, many patients with vasculitides do not show circulating or deposited immune complexes.

Antineutrophil cytoplasmic antibodies

These are antibodies directed against certain proteins of the neutrophil cytoplasm, and are detected in a high percentage of patients with systemic vasculitides (particularly Wegener's granulomatosis), microscopic polyangiitis and in those with necrotizing and crescentic glomerulonephritis. Two main categories of antineutrophil cytoplasmic antibodies (ANCA) are recognized, based on different targets: cytoplasmic ANCA (c-ANCA) have a diffuse cytoplasmic staining pattern at immunofluorescence microscopy, when proteinase-3 (located in neutrophil azurophilic granules) is the c-ANCA antigen; and perinuclear ANCA (p-ANCA) which have a perinuclear or nuclear staining pattern when the targets are myeloperoxidase, elastase, cathepsin G, lactoferrin, lysozyme or bactericidal/permeability-increasing protein. It is not clear why patients with certain vasculitides develop ANCA, but, once ANCA are present, they can contribute to the pathogenesis of the vasculitides. It is conceivable that when neutrophils are primed by tumor necrosis factor (TNF)-α or interleukin (IL)-1, intracytoplasmatic proteinase-3 translocates to the cell membrane, where it interacts with extracellular ANCA. The neutrophils degranulate and reactive oxygen species are delivered, causing tissue damage. Tanslocation of proteinase-3 close to the cell membrane also occurs in the endothelial cells upon priming with TNF-α, IL-1, or interferon (IFN)γ, thus making them susceptible to interaction with ANCA and consequent tissue damage due to complement-mediated cytotoxicity or antibody-dependent cellular toxicity. Although these in vitro data are attractive as explanations, there are no conclusive data that ANCA play a direct role in the pathogenesis of vasculitides, as they may represent epiphenomena.

Pathogenic T-lymphocyte responses and granuloma formation

Vascular endothelial cells can express HLA class II molecules following activation by cytokines such as IFNγ. They can take part in immunological reactions, such as interaction with CD4+ lymphocytes, similarly to antigen-presenting macrophages. They can also secrete IL-1, which is a powerful inducer of adhesion molecules such as endothelial leukocyte adhesion molecule 1 (ELAM-1) and vascular cell adhesion molecule 1 (VCAM-1) with consequent adhesion of leukocytes to the endothelial cells in the blood vessel wall. There is no strong evidence that other mechanisms, such as direct cellular cytotoxicity or antibodies directed against vessel components or antibody-dependent cellular cytotoxicity, have a causal contribution to the pathogenesis of vasculitides.

Many aspects of the pathogenesis of vasculitides remain unclear. Other variables certainly implicated in the development of vasculitides are: genetic predisposition; defects of the regulatory factors of the immune responses to certain antigens; the ability of the reticuloendothelial system in clearing circulating complexes; the size and physicochemical properties of immune complexes; the degree of turbulence of blood flow; and the intravascular hydrostatic pressure in different vessels.

Clinical manifestations

It is clinically useful to distinguish between acute and chronic intestinal vasculitides, although both may have a severe course with deleterious effects. Acute intestinal vasculitis is a rapidly evolving disease, which presents with intense abdominal pain, followed by signs of peritonitis and ileus, and progressive cardiovascular shock syndrome with high lethality. It is often difficult to distinguish mesenteric ischemia due to vasculitides clinically from embolic or thrombotic ischemia in patients complaining of severe abdominal pain. It is therefore necessary to collect the patient's history carefully, as well as clinical and laboratory parameters, in order to reach the diagnosis and begin treatment. Standard emergency laboratory values, serum concentration of lactate and coagulation parameters as well as disease-specific values must be measured. Table 26.2 gives a number of tests that are useful in establishing a link between 'vasculitis' and an underlying disease. Every patient suspected of having ischemia should receive an abdominal ultrasonography including Doppler examination of the mesenteric arteries and an X-ray of the abdomen for assessing ileus, intestinal edema and perforation. If findings of mesenteric ischemia are evident or suspected,

Table 26.2 Clinical features that raise suspicion of vasculitides

General clinical feature	Signs or presenting disorders	Type of vasculitis
Constitutional symptoms	fever, fatigue, malaise, anorexia, weight loss	any type of vasculitis
Polymyalgia rheumatica	proximal muscle pain with morning stiffness	giant cell arteritis; less commonly other vasculitides
Non-destructive oligoarthritis	joint swelling, warmth, painful range of motion	polyarteritis, Wegener's granulomatosis, Churg–Strauss vasculitis
Skin lesions	livedo reticularis, necrotic lesions, ulcers, nodules, digital tip infarcts	polyarteritis, Wegener's granulomatosis, Churg–Strauss vasculitis, hypersensitivity vasculitis
	palpable purpura	any type of vasculitis except giant cell arteritis and Takayasu's arteritis
Multiple mononeuropathy (mononeuritis multiplex)	injury to two or more separate peripheral nerves (e.g. patient presents with both right foot drop and left wrist drop)	polyarteritis, Takayasu's arteritis; less commonly, Churg–Strauss vasculitis and Wegener's granulomatosis
	glomerulonephritis	microscopic polyangiitis, Wegener's granulomatosis, cryoglobulinemia, Churg–Strauss vasculitis, Henoch–Schönlein purpura

angiography and subsequent surgery should be planned.

The diagnosis of chronic vasculitis should be considered in young children and adolescents with systemic symptoms and evidence of single and/or multiorgan specific dysfunction. In these cases, common complaints are fatigue, weakness, fever, arthralgia and abdominal pain. Common signs include fever, hypertension, neurological dysfunction and renal abnormalities with an active urine sediment (containing red cells, other cellular and granular casts). The above findings are neither sensitive nor specific for vasculitides, and the diagnosis is often delayed because the clinical manifestations of the vasculitides mimic those of other more common disorders. In addition, although each type of vasculitis usually has a characteristic pattern of organ involvement, a single approach to the diagnosis is difficult, owing to the variability of the manifestations of the vasculitides. All children suspected of having vasculitides should undergo a complete history and physical examination and certain basic laboratory tests (Figure 26.1). Both upper and lower intestinal endoscopy frequently reveal signs of mucosal inflammation, such as multiple petechiae, friability, erosions and small ulcers. A number of serological markers, such as antinuclear antibodies (ANA) and ANCA are associated with specific types of vasculitis, but tissue biopsy is often required to establish the diagnosis.

History

Diagnostic work-up starts with a detailed patient history. Postprandial abdominal pain that usually begins 30–60 min after meals is a predominant symptom. Other aspects of the history include

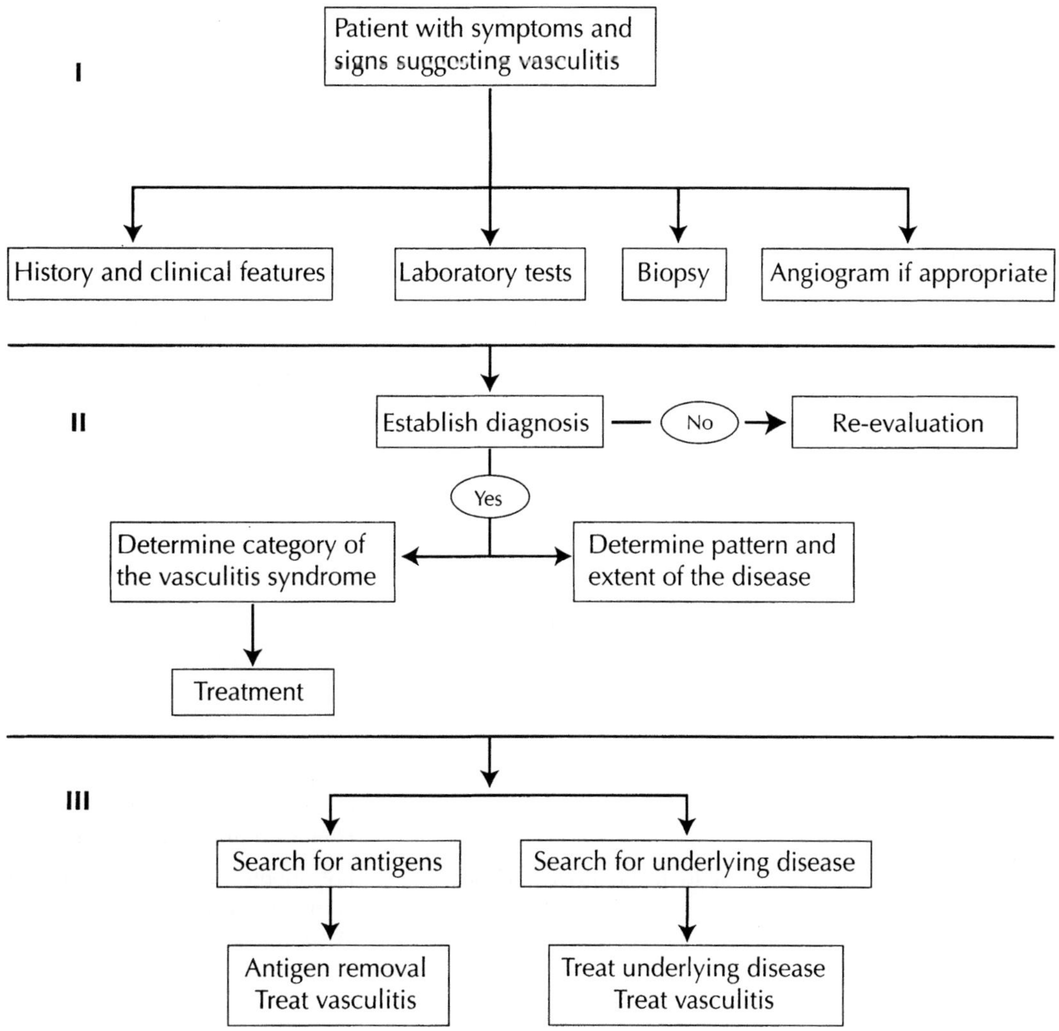

Figure 26.1 Suggested algorithm for the approach to patients with suspected vasculitis.

whether the patient has recently been ill or taken medications or drugs, has a history of hepatitis (virus C), or has been diagnosed with any disorder known to be associated with vasculitis. Knowing the propensity of certain disorders to occur in specific ages, gender, or ethnic groups can be useful in making the diagnosis. Table 26.2 outlines clinical features that raise the suspicion of vasculitis.

Physical examination

A careful physical examination helps in determining the extent of vascular lesions, the distribution of affected organs and the presence of additional disease processes. The type and extent of organ involvement in vasculitis can be helpful in determining the specific type of vasculitides and the degree of urgency in initiating treatment. The clinical features in a given patient can be used to discern the size of vessels affected by vasculitis (Table 26.3). Table 26.4 reports the frequency of intestinal involvement in different vasculitides. Incomplete stenosis of one of the major vessels (e.g. mesenteric artery) may cause changes in the Doppler ultrasound flow pattern, as well as typical bruits at abdominal auscultation. In three series with a total of 351 patients, approximately one-third had gastrointestinal manifestations.[8] In a large series of patients with PAN or Churg–Strauss syndrome, for example, the following frequency of

Table 26.3 Clues for identifying the type of vessel involvement in vasculitides

Clinical feature	Vessels most likely to be affected	Most commonly associated systemic vasculitis
Cutaneous		
Palpable purpura	post-capillary venules	any type of vasculitis except giant cell arteritis and Takayasu's arteritis
Skin ulcers	arterioles to small arteries	polyarteritis, Churg–Strauss vasculitis Wegener's granulomatosis, hypersensitivity vasculitis
Gangrene in an extremity	small to medium-sized arteries	polyarteritis, Churg–Strauss vasculitis, Wegener's granulomatosis
Gastrointestinal tract		
Abdominal pain or mesenteric ischemia	small to medium-sized arteries	Henoch–Schönlein purpura, polyarteritis, Churg–Strauss vasculitis
Gastrointestinal bleeding	capillaries to medium-sized arteries	Henoch–Schönlein purpura, polyarteritis, Churg–Strauss vasculitis
Renal		
Glomerulonephritis	capillaries	microscopic polyangiitis, Wegener's granulomatosis, cryoglobulinemia, Churg–Strauss vasculitis, Henoch–Schönlein purpura
Ischemic renal failure	small to medium-sized arteries	polyarteritis, Takayasu's arteritis; less commonly, Churg–Strauss vasculitis, Wegener's granulomatosis
Pulmonary		
Pulmonary hemorrhage	capillaries; less commonly small to medium-sized arteries	microscopic polyangiitis, Wegener's granulomatosis
Pulmonary infiltrate	small to medium-sized arteries or cavities	Churg–Strauss vasculitis, microscopic polyangiitis
Neurological		
Peripheral neuropathy	small arteries	polyarteritis, Churg–Strauss vasculitis, Wegener's granulomatosis, cryoglobulinemia
Stroke	small, medium-sized or large arteries	giant cell arteritis, SLE-associated vasculitis

SLE, systemic lupus erythematosus

gastrointestinal symptoms and findings was noted: abdominal pain (25%), gastrointestinal bleeding (7%), peritonitis (4%), intestinal infarction (2%), pancreatitis (2%), duodenal ulcer (2%) and cholecystitis (1%), while ischemic hepatitis, gastritis and esophagitis occurred more rarely (<1%).[4]

Laboratory evaluation

Laboratory tests are helpful in determining the type of vasculitis as well as the type and extent of the organs affected. Standard laboratory analyses include a complete blood count, urinalysis, blood

Table 26.4 Frequency of intestinal involvement in different vasculitides (from references 24, 38–47)

Type of vasculitis	Frequency of intestinal involvement (%)
Primary vasculitis	
Polyarteritis nodosa (PAN) (classic PAN, microscopic polyangiitis)	30–50
Churg–Strauss syndrome	25–50
Behçet's disease	up to 30
Takayasu's arteritis	up to 15
Wegener's granulomatosis	5–10
Giant cell arteritis	1
Secondary vasculitis	
Henoch–Schönlein purpura	50–90
Systemic lupus erythematosus	50
Rheumatoid arthritis vasculitis	10

urea nitrogen, creatinine, liver enzymes, erythrocyte sedimentation rate (ESR), hepatitis serological markers and chest radiograph. Additional tests that may be required are cerebrospinal fluid analysis, central nervous system imaging, pulmonary function testing, and blood and tissue culture. These tests assess the extent of organ involvement and may suggest, confirm, or exclude additional diagnostic considerations. More specific laboratory tests may be indicated, depending upon the diagnosis being considered (Table 26.5).

Imaging studies

Imaging studies, such as computed tomography (CT) scanning or barium studies, are frequently normal in patients with symptomatic intestinal vasculitides and, when abnormal, reveal nonspecific abnormalities such as a thickened edematous bowel wall, unless a mesenteric infarction has occurred. Angiography may be useful in diagnosing small and medium vessel vasculitides, such as PAN. Nuclear medicine scanning using white blood cell markers such as indium-111 may localize bowel inflammation in vasculitis, but its clinical utility is uncertain.

Endoscopy

Endoscopy should be performed with great caution in patients with vasculitides because of an elevated risk of perforation of an edematous and ischemic bowel. In these cases, magnetic resonance imaging (MRI) of the intestinal tract can be used. As demonstrated recently, the two techniques show a good correlation in detecting inflammation of the intestinal mucosa.[9]

Tissue biopsy

Biopsy examination of the involved tissue is almost always necessary for diagnosis. Obviously, specimens are more likely to yield a diagnosis when they are of adequate size and obtained from an involved area of an organ. The histological findings evolve as lesions progress and may vary from acute inflammation to healing and repair. The biopsy findings in the various vasculitides are discussed below (see Specific disorders). The decision to obtain a tissue biopsy is based upon the overall clinical assessment of the patient and complications associated with the procedure. As an example, the skin, which characteristically is involved in children with leukocytoclastic vasculitis, is easily accessible for biopsy, and skin biopsy in this setting has low morbidity. However, in this scenario, the biopsy adds little, if any, new information. The biopsy findings of leukocytoclastic vasculitis (inflammation of the small blood vessels most prominent in the post-capillary venules) are relatively non-specific, unless accompanied by vascular IgA deposition, which establishes a diag-

Table 26.5 Laboratory parameters useful in the diagnostic approach to vasculitis

Laboratory parameters	Purpose of interpretation
Routine tests (including complete blood cell count, liver enzymes, creatinine, urinalysis)	evaluate for hematologic, renal and other organ involvement
Blood cultures	rule out infection
ESR, C-reactive protein	high values suggest active inflammatory disease
Eosinophilia	Churg–Strauss syndrome
Anti-nuclear antibodies	screen for SLE and Sjögren's syndrome
Anti-double-stranded DNA antibodies	suggest SLE
Rheumatoid factor	very high titers in rheumatoid arthritis, Sjögren's syndrome and cryoglobulinemia-associated vasculitis
Complement (C3, C4, CH50)	low complement levels suggest consumption by immune complexes, which are commonly found in SLE and cryoglobulinemia
Cytoplasmic anti-neutrophil cytoplasmic (anti-proteinase-3) antibodies	Wegener's granulomatosis
Perinuclear anti-neutrophil cytoplasmic antibodies (anti-myeloperoxidase)	panarteritis nodosa, microscopic polyangiitis
Creatine phosphokinase	elevation suggests myositis, which can occur in many vasculitis syndromes
Anti-glomerular basement membrane	rule out Goodpasture's syndrome, which can mimic vasculitis and cause pulmonary hemorrhage and glomerulonephritis
Circulating immune complexes	immune complex vasculitides
HLA B51	suggests Behçet's syndrome
HLA B8	suggests SLE

ESR, erythrocyte sedimentation rate; SLE, systemic lupus erythematosus

nostic of Henoch–Schönlein purpura.[10] However, the diagnosis of Henoch–Schönlein purpura in children is usually made on clinical grounds, and biopsy may not be necessary.

Arteriography

Arteriograms can identify and characterize vasculitides of large and medium-sized arteries and giant cell arteritis with an aortic arch syndrome, whereas they are not helpful in the evaluation of vasculitides involving small vessels, because these are not visible with routine angiograms. Angiographic abnormalities may not be pathognomonic, but usually support a diagnosis when combined with other clinical data. The decision to perform angiography in a patient with suspected vasculitis depends on the overall clinical judgement and assessment of the risk for complications associated with the procedure. Arteriography alone is usually performed to confirm the diagnosis of Takayasu's arteritis: the arteriography changes tend to be most pronounced in the region of the aortic arch and its primary branches, which are relatively inaccessible for biopsy. In the patient with suspected PAN without an obvious area for biopsy, a mesenteric angiogram should be planned, particularly in the presence of abdominal pain: angiograms of mesenteric or renal arteries may show aneurysms, occlusions and vascular wall irregularities. Magnetic resonance arteriography of the aorta and great vessels including some major branches such as the coronaries and renal arteries may be an alternative to contrast arteriography in children. When the two techniques were compared in ten children with various vascular lesions (age range: 1 month to 16 years), excellent correlation was found between them.[11]

Specific disorders

Primary vasculitides

Polyarteritis nodosa

PAN affects medium and small-sized arteries and can cause a wide spectrum of gastrointestinal symptoms and signs, which are mainly due to visceral ischemia and are detected in about two-thirds of patients. Common intestinal features are: epigastric pain, nausea, anorexia, mucosal ulcerations (Figure 26.2), bleeding and diarrhea. The most severe intestinal findings are infarction, perforation, pneumatosis intestinalis and pseudomembranous colitis.[4] Survival after bowel infarction requiring surgery is poor. Typical aneurysmal dilatation of small and medium-sized arteries on arteriogram will provide a definite diagnosis. In a series of 16 patients with severe PAN, five developed an abdominal crisis related to the disease: at laparotomy, all had evidence of mesenteric arteritis with infarcted bowel and intestinal perforation.[12] In another series of 165 patients with PAN or Churg–Strauss syndrome, 31% of deaths occurring at the follow-up were attributable to gastrointestinal disease (bleeding, peritonitis and pancreatitis).[12] Vasculitis of the hepatic arteries may cause elevated levels of transaminases, bilirubin and alkaline phosphatase.

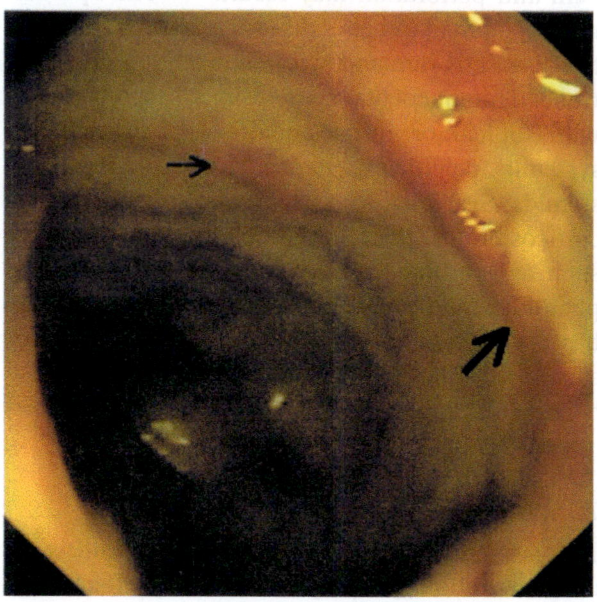

Figure 26.2 A large (thick arrow) and a small (thin arrow) ulceration in a 14-year-old boy with polyarteritis nodosa at the level of the descending colon. The large ulceration is surrounded by hyperemic and friable mucosa.

Treatment with corticosteroids and cyclophosphamide has relieved symptoms and improved the overall survival of these patients.[13] Adequate therapy for patients with PAN related to hepatitis B virus infection or hairy cell leukemia may require treatment of these underlying disorders.[12] The tendency of PAN to involve large vessels has an important long-term implication. Some patients with PAN have gastrointestinal symptoms and other manifestations at a time when the disease is clinically inactive, owing to effective immunosuppressive therapy. In this setting, healing of inflamed vessels has led to progressive narrowing of the vascular bed.

Churg–Strauss syndrome

The Churg–Strauss syndrome (also called 'allergic angiitis and granulomatosis') is a multisystemic disease characterized by hypereosinophilia, pulmonary infiltration, extravascular granulomas and necrotizing vasculitis affecting small and medium-sized arteries and veins.[12] Involvement of the intestinal vasculature ranges from 25 to 50% and any intestinal organ can be affected with features such as ulcerations, bleeding, ileus, perforation and cholecystitis. Interestingly, microscopic polyangiitis resembles Churg–Strauss syndrome for the spectrum of gastrointestinal features as well as for its similar response to corticosteroids and cyclophosphamide.[14] Intestinal histology can reveal both eosinophilic infiltrates around the vessels and eosinophilic gastroenteritis. The syndrome commonly occurs in middle-aged adults and is rare in children. A 15-year-old girl with multiple colonic ulcers has recently been described. This patient also had vasculitic involvement of the major organs including migratory pulmonary infiltrates, myocarditis and central nervous system disease with hemiparesis.[15]

Wegener's granulomatosis

Wegener's granulomatosis is characterized by a granulomatous (peri)vascular inflammation of the upper and lower airways combined with glomerulonephritis. It appears to be a disorder restricted to Caucasians, since only 3% of patients with Wegener's granulomatosis are of other ethnic groups. Interestingly, although c-ANCA is considered a specific marker, it is not yet an accepted criterion for the diagnosis of Wegener's granulomatosis. Gastrointestinal involvement seems to be rare, mostly producing granulomatous colitis and gastritis.[4] An unusual presentation of Wegener's granulomatosis has been reported in a 16-year-old girl with symptoms and signs suggesting an inflammatory bowel disease (diarrhea, fever, weight loss, abdominal pain, arthralgias and mouth ulcers). However, biopsy specimens of rectal mucosa, oro- and nasopharynx, and skin conclusively demonstrated the vasculitic lesion of Wegener's granulomatosis.[16]

Behçet's disease

Behçet's disease is a necrotizing vasculitis of unknown etiology primarily affecting young adult males. The predominant features are recurrent oral and genital ulcerations (more than three times per year) in combination with other signs, such as uveitis, iritis, retinal vasculitis, skin lesions (erythema nodosum, acneiform or papulopustulous lesions, pseudofolliculitis) and pathergy (papulopustulous lesions 24–48 h after cutaneous injection of 0.9% sodium chloride). A strong genetic component is thought to be part of the disorder, owing to the association with HLA B51.[17] The disease has the highest incidence in Turkey (up to 3000 per million), and in southern Mediterranean and Asiatic regions. Gastrointestinal involvement is found frequently and includes major intestinal arteries as well as upper and lower parts of the gut. Oral lesions resemble aphthous ulcers commonly observed in Crohn's disease and may be single or multiple; esophageal ulcerations and erosions are found frequently at endoscopy (Figure 26.3), although they do not

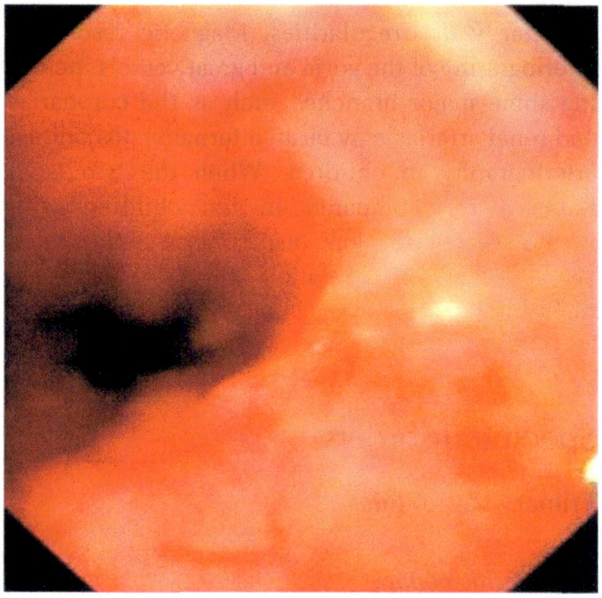

Figure 26.3 Mucosa of the distal esophagus in an 8-year-old girl with Behçet's disease. Diffuse hyperemia, erosions and ulcerations are evident, together with an open cardia.

cause bleeding or perforation. Intestinal involvement at the level of both small and large bowel can resemble Crohn's disease; bleeding, abdominal pain and perforation may result.[18,19] The optimal management of Behçet's disease is uncertain, since the disease is rare and symptoms tend to wax and wane. The mucocutaneous lesions can be treated with topical or intralesional corticosteroids, or systemic colchicine, dapsone, thalidomide, or steroids. Systemic disease is typically treated with corticosteroids and immunosuppressive drugs such as azathioprine, cyclosporin, or cyclophosphamide. Interestingly, systemic Behçet's disease has been successfully treated with anti-TNF-α agents such as thalidomide and monoclonal antibodies (infliximab).[20]

Takayasu's arteritis

Takayasu's arteritis is a rare chronic vasculitis of unknown etiology that predominantly affects the aorta and its primary branches.[21,22] It characteristically affects young women, with an age of onset usually between 10 and 40 years (this is one of the major criteria for diagnosis). The prevalence is greatest in Asians. Gastrointestinal features result from involvement of the large branches of the abdominal aorta such as the celiac trunk and the upper mesenteric artery. Although not a major feature, mesenteric ischemia can occur, leading to abdominal pain, diarrhea and gastrointestinal hemorrhage. An association of Takayasu's arteritis with ulcerative colitis has also been reported.[23] Severe cerebral, intestinal and coronary circulatory disturbances as well as an insufficient blood supply in both arms have been described in a 9-month-old infant with extensive inflammatory lesions in the large arterial trunks originating at the aorta.[24]

Giant cell arteritis and polymyalgia rheumatica

These two closely related vasculitides mainly affect the vessels of the shoulder girdle and the intra- and extra-cranial arteries; however, involvement of mesenteric vessels can also occur.[25] Disseminated fibrinoid necrosis of small vessels can result in visceral ischemia, abdominal pain, nausea, anorexia, weight loss, bleeding and perforation. Hepatic artery involvement can determine disturbances of liver function and hepatitis with fibrin-ring granulomas.[26]

Kawasaki's disease

Also called mucocutaneous lymph node syndrome, Kawasaki's disease is a multisystem vasculitis affecting children under the age of 5 years. The principal symptoms are high fever for more than 5 days and resistance to antibiotics; polymorphonuclear cell exanthema, skin lesions in peripheral extremities (reddening, indurative edema, membranous desquamation), oral lesions (pharyngitis, enanthema, 'strawberry tongue'), bilateral conjunctive congestion and acute cervical lymphadenopathy. In addition to these symptoms, gastrointestinal complications can determine deterioration of the overall condition of the patient. Intestinal features during the acute phase are abdominal pain, vomiting and diarrhea; whereas small-bowel obstruction has been reported as a consequence of acquired ischemic stricture.[27,28] The vasculitic process underlying intestinal involvement in Kawasaki's disease includes four stages: intensive perivasculitis, focal panvasculitis, ongoing inflammation and granulation and stenosis with aneurysms. The spectrum of gastroenterological complications also includes hepatitis, cholangitis, gallbladdor hydrops and pancreatic ductitis.

Secondary vasculitides

Henoch–Schönlein purpura and leukocytoclastic vasculitis

Henoch–Schönlein purpura is a generalized vasculitis of small to medium-sized vessels which characteristically occurs in children of all ages. It is secondary to an immune process that generates circulating immune complexes containing large amounts of IgA. Patients classically present lower extremity purpura, arthritis and acute glomerulonephritis. The gastrointestinal tract is frequently involved and intramural hemorrhages, bloody diarrhea or colic may result; erythema, friability and ulcerations of the gastrointestinal mucosa can be observed at endoscopy (Figure 26.4). Intestinal obstruction and intussusception have also been described. Gastrointestinal signs may have a recurrent course and may precede the onset of the characteristic purpuric rash,[29,30] which rarely may even be lacking. The clinical spectrum of gastro-

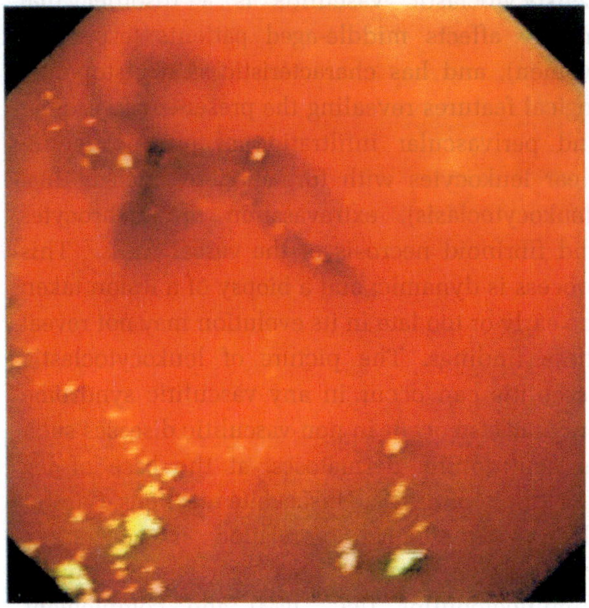

Figure 26.4 Diffuse hyperemia and congestion with small erosions in a 6-year-old girl with Henoch–Schönlein purpura at the level of the gastric antrum.

intestinal involvement in Henoch–Schönlein purpura ranges from a dull periumbilical pain to severe courses with intestinal perforation and necrosis of the bile ducts. Ultrasonography and CT provide useful information to support the diagnosis, which is commonly strongly suspected on clinical grounds. Confirmation of the diagnosis requires evidence by immunofluorescence microscopy of tissue deposition in the skin or kidney of IgA. Biopsy of the skin lesions reveals inflammation of the small blood vessels, called leukocytoclastic vasculitis (see below) that is most prominent in the post-capillary venules. The prognosis of this disease is good, except for cases with severe renal involvement. The efficacy of corticosteroids and immunosuppressants (azathioprine, cyclophosphamide) in the treatment of Henoch–Schönlein purpura is debated, especially when the kidneys are involved.[31] Some cases of Henoch–Schönlein purpura have been successfully treated by plasmapheresis.[32] Little experience concerning treatment of Henoch–Schönlein purpura during pregnancy exists, although corticosteroids and plasmapheresis have been used in these cases.[31]

Leukocytoclastic vasculitis

Leukocytoclastic vasculitis is a disorder that mainly affects middle-aged patients (especially women), and has characteristic skin histopathological features revealing the presence of vascular and perivascular infiltration of polymorphonuclear leukocytes with formation of nuclear dust (leukocytoclasis), extravasation of erythrocytes and fibrinoid necrosis of the vessel walls.[7] This process is dynamic; and a biopsy of a lesion taken too early or too late in its evolution may not reveal these findings. The picture of leukocytoclastic vasculitis can occur in any vasculitic syndrome but may also occur in non-vasculitic diseases such as neutrophilic dermatoses, at the base of leg ulceration, or in some insect bite reactions. Careful clinical–pathological correlation is necessary.[7] Immuno-fluorescent staining may reveal immunoglobulins (IgG, IgM) and complement components (C3, C4) deposited on the skin basement membrane, which are suggestive of immune complex deposition.[12]

Vasculitides in connective tissue diseases

The term connective tissue disease includes numerous entities such as SLE, systemic sclerosis, polymyositis, dermatomyositis or Sjögren's syndrome. Most clinical signs of these disorders are attributed to a small-vessel vasculitis, and gastrointestinal clinical problems most frequently occur in SLE.

Systemic lupus erythematosus

The vasculitis associated with SLE involves small and medium-sized vessels, and affects the gastrointestinal tract in up to 50% of patients. Lower abdominal pain secondary to mesenteric vasculitis is generally an insidious symptom that may be intermittent for months prior to the development of an acute abdomen with nausea, vomiting, diarrhea, bleeding and fever. Risk factors for the development of mesenteric vasculitis are peripheral vasculitis and central nervous system involvement. Patients with an acute presentation may also have mesenteric thrombosis and infarction, often in association with antiphospholipid antibodies. Mesenteric vasculitis is a potentially life-threatening disorder. In addition to the possible development of necrotic segments of bowel, patients may have septic complications and bowel perforation. In a series published in 1982, 15 of 140 patients with SLE who required hospitalization developed a disease-related abdominal event and 11 underwent laparotomy.[33] The majority of the patients in this study had prodromic signs, such as insidious onset of intermittent, lower quadrant cramping and abdominal pain, which were present for an average of 34 days prior to the hospitalization. The presence of these symptoms in patients with SLE should raise suspicion of possible mesenteric vasculitis, thereby permitting early diagnosis and treatment. Interestingly, abdominal features such as pain, rectal bleeding by mucosal ulcers and protein-losing enteropathy due to increased mucosal permeability have been described as sole and initial manifestations in patients with SLE.[34,35] Chronic intestinal pseudo-obstruction of the myogenic type has also been described to complicate the course of SLE.[36] Simple laboratory tests may be helpful in making the diagnosis or in evaluating a flare-up. However, the diagnosis is mostly dependent on the historical and physical findings. Antinuclear antibody, an antibody to nucleosomal DNA–histone complexes, is highly sensitive but not specific; anti-double-stranded DNA is more specific for SLE. This test may correlate with the degree of disease activity. Antiphospholipid antibodies are present in 30% of SLE patients.

Antiphospholipid antibody syndrome

The antiphospholipid antibody syndrome (APS), also known as Hughes syndrome, is a disorder characterized by multiple different antibodies that are associated with both arterial and venous thrombosis. There are three primary classes of antibodies associated with the APS: anticardiolipin antibodies; the lupus anticoagulant; and antibodies directed against specific molecules including a molecule known as β_2-glycoprotein-1. The APS can occur in patients with SLE or as an isolated disorder. There are two main classifications of the APS: if there is an underlying autoimmune disorder, such as SLE, the patient is said to have secondary APS; if the patient has no known underlying autoimmune disorder, it is termed primary APS. Of the APS patients, over half of them have the primary form. In persons with SLE, around 30% will develop the APS. In general, anticardiolipin antibodies occur approximately five times more often than the lupus anticoagulant in patients with the APS. Approximately 10% of patients with an initial presentation of primary APS will eventually be diagnosed with an autoimmune disorder such as SLE or a mixed connective tissue disorder. The APS represents a hypercoagulable state, which can be associated with a variety of clinical features including arterial and venous thrombosis, livedo reticularis and spontaneous abortions. The exact mechanism by which the antiphospholipid antibodies and anticardiolipin antibodies induce the thrombophilic state is not known. Gastrointestinal manifestations of APS are due to ischemia involving any part of the intestinal tube, and resulting in bleeding, abdominal pain, acute abdomen, esophageal necrosis with perforation, or giant gastric ulceration.[37,38]

Juvenile dermatomyositis and juvenile polymyositis

These are uncommon disorders. Juvenile dermatomyositis has an incidence of 2–3 per 100 000 per year. The clinical manifestations resemble those of adult dermatomyositis and polymyositis and include symmetric proximal muscle weakness, myalgias, muscle tenderness, fever and rash (the latter commonly detected in juvenile dermatomyositis). In addition, calcinosis is seen in one-third of patients. Functional outcomes have become good with modern treatments, but the diseases remain chronic in a large number of children and sequelae are often seen. Affected children typically present prodromic non-specific signs such as malaise, muscle aching, fever and irritability that are often interpreted as a viral illness. A change in gait may be a clue to muscle disease at this stage.[39] Gastrointestinal tract involvement can also occur, and includes mucosal ulcerations due to vascular occlusion. Affected patients may present with abdominal pain, gastrointestinal bleeding, or perforation.[39] In a recently revised series of 25 patients aged between 1.5 and 15 years, dysphagia and abdominal pain were present in 32% and 40% of cases, respectively.[40] A case of atonic esophagus and gastroparesis has been described in a child with juvenile dermatomyositis.[41] Juvenile dermatomyositis can usually be diagnosed on a clinical basis in the child with a characteristic rash and proximal muscle weakness. The diagnosis of juvenile dermatomyositis can be more difficult with the lack of cutaneous manifestations. Certain laboratory features such as elevated muscle enzyme levels, increase in von Willebrand's factor 8 antigen (vWF) and autoantibodies are frequently present in both disorders: they provide confirmatory evidence of the disease and a means of following patients. Electromyography can assist in making the diagnosis in equivocal cases (e.g. those without a typical rash or with normal muscle enzyme levels). Muscle biopsy may also be necessary in these instances, and is often the definitive test. The mainstays of therapy are corticosteroids; some children require additional immunosuppressive agents because of corticosteroid resistance or intolerance.

Rheumatoid vasculitis

A small-vessel vasculitis can complicate the course of rheumatoid arthritis. Small arteries in the peripheral organs are usually affected, resulting in gastrointestinal vasculitis in up to 10% of the patients with rheumatoid arthritis.[42] In contrast to PAN, vasculitis in rheumatoid arthritis shows few signs of inflammation, but intensive intimal proliferation and vascular occlusion.[43] The gastrointestinal symptoms of rheumatoid vasculitis range from slight recurrent abdominal pain to severe bleeding, intestinal ischemia and necrosis.[4] It should be observed that, in rheumatoid arthritis, abdominal pain is not necessarily due to vasculitis, but can arise from mucosal lesions such as ulcers or bleeding, as a consequence of the administration of anti-inflammatory drugs.

Thromboangiitis obliterans (Winiwarter–Buerger's disease)

A non-atherosclerotic, segmental, inflammatory disorder, Winiwarter–Buerger's disease most commonly affects the small and medium-sized arteries, veins and nerves of the extremities.[4] This condition is distinguished from other forms of vasculitis by the highly cellular and inflammatory thrombus with relative sparing of the blood vessel wall. ESR and serum C-reactive protein are usually normal; commonly measured autoantibodies (e.g. antinuclear antibody and rheumatoid factor) are normal, as are other serological tests such as circulating immune complexes, complement levels and cryoglobulins, despite an immune reaction in the arterial intima. Winiwarter–Buerger's disease usually begins with ischemia of the distal small arteries and veins, followed by more proximal arterial involvement as the disease advances. Patients usually note ischemia of the digits, which may manifest as claudication of the feet, legs, hands or arms.[44] The disease can progress to include ischemic ulcerations of the fingers or toes, with accompanying ischemic pain at rest. Buerger's disease should be suspected in passive or active smokers who present with distal ischemia of the hands and/or feet. Obliteration of the intestinal vasculature can occur with abdominal angina, resulting in bowel infarction that requires immediate surgery.[45,46] A definitive diagnosis is made when the histopathology identifies the acute phase lesion in a patient with a clinical history of smoking. Typical arteriographic findings help to exclude proximal atherosclerotic disease and to meet the criteria for thromboangiitis obliterans.

Treatment and follow-up

Childhood vasculitides, particularly Kawasaki disease and PAN, require prompt recognition, because they can be life-threatening in the absence of appropriate therapy. The diagnosis can be laborious and cumbersome, since the clinical features of the various disorders overlap. Furthermore, although the disorders usually have a characteristic pattern of organ involvement, each organ system can be affected. Available treatments are helpful, particularly in the acute phase. When chronic therapy is required, the adverse effects of drugs and secondary infections are clinically relevant. Mortality data suggest that early deaths in vasculitides are due to active disease, whereas late deaths mainly result from the complications of therapy. The treatment of vasculitides depends upon the nature and severity of the disorder, and may include antihistamines, corticosteroids, non-steroidal anti-inflammatory drugs, or cytotoxic agents. Patients with systemic vasculitis usually need at least corticosteroid therapy. As an example, glucocorticoid therapy is used for the treatment of vasculitis accompanying connective tissue disease. In most patients, the dose can be reduced and gradually discontinued, but some patients require chronic long-term administration of low-dose corticosteroids. Patients with rapidly progressive vasculitic diseases, such as PAN, are likely to require therapy consisting of a combination of a cytotoxic drug (usually cyclophosphamide) and corticosteroids. Both oral and pulse cyclophosphamide are used, depending upon the physician's experience and the disease severity. After 1–2 months of combined therapy, the corticosteroid dose may be reduced if symptoms improve; therapy is usually continued for 6–12 months to decrease the risk of relapse. Azathioprine and methotrexate have been used in less severe forms of vasculitides and as maintenance therapy, after remission has been induced by cyclophosphamide. Corticosteroid therapy, even in low doses, can produce substantial toxicity. The risk is greater as the dose increases, with complications ranging from minor skin bruising to life-threatening infections and fractures. Some of these complications can be prevented with appropriate patient monitoring. Some manifestations of vasculitis such as neuropathy can take months to recede, even if the underlying vasculitis has abated, whereas others may be permanent. Patients in whom a chronic course is expected may become discouraged about their lack of rapid improvement and possible poor outcome. These patients may benefit from extra support and encouragement. Once the treatment has been initiated, patient monitoring is based on most of the procedures used during the diagnostic approach. There are two main long-term concerns: most forms of vasculitis (except for drug-induced hypersensitivity vasculitis) can relapse; and vascular injury during the acute phase can heal with scarring and narrowing of the affected vessels, leading to signs of ischemia that do not reflect recurrent active disease.[47] Therefore, prolonged monitoring is indicated, even though it may be difficult to determine whether a change in findings results from the disease, the medications, or scarring.

REFERENCES

1. Langford CA. Vasculitis. *J Allergy Clin Immunol* 2003; **111** (2 Suppl): S602–S612.
2. Jennette JC, Falk RJ. Do vasculitis categorization systems really matter? *Curr Rheumatol Rep* 2000; **2**: 430–438.
3. Yalcindag A, Sundel R. Vasculitis in childhood *Curr Opin Rheumatol* 2001; **13**: 422–427.
4. Müller-Ladner U. Vasculitides of the gastrointestinal tract. *Best Pract Res Clin Gastroenterol* 2001; **15**: 59–82.
5. Gardner-Medwin JM, Dolezalova P, Cummins C et al. Incidence of Henoch–Schönlein purpura, Kawasaki disease, and rare vasculitides in children of different ethnic origins. *Lancet* 2002; **360**: 1197–1202.
6. Watts RA, Scott DGI. Epidemiology of the vasculitides. *Curr Opin Rheumatol* 2003; **15**: 11–16.
7. Weyand CM, Goronzy JJ. Multisystem interactions in the pathogenesis of vasculitis. *Curr Opin Rheumatol* 1997; **9**: 3–11.
8. Guillevin L, Du LT, Godeau P et al. Clinical findings and prognosis of polyarteritis nodosa and Churg–Strauss angiitis: a study of 165 patients. *Br J Rheumatol* 1988; **27**: 258–264.
9. Laghi A, Borrelli O, Paolantonio P et al. Contrast enhanced magnetic resonance imaging of the terminal ileum in children with Crohn's disease. *Gut* 2003; **52**: 393–397.
10. Koutkia P, Mylonakis E, Rounds S et al. Leucocytoclastic vasculitis: an update for the clinician. *Scand J Rheumatol* 2001; **30**: 315–322.
11. Katayama H, Shimizu T, Tanaka Y et al. Three-dimensional magnetic resonance angiography of vascular lesions in children. *Heart Vessels* 2000; **15**: 1–6.
12. Ozen S. The spectrum of vasculitis in children. *Best Pract Res Clin Rheumatol* 2002; **16**: 411–425.
13. Guillevin L, Pagnoux C. When should immunosuppressants be prescribed to treat systemic vasculitides. *Intern Med* 2003; **42**: 313–317.
14. Noth I, Strek ME, Leff AR. Churg–Strauss syndrome. *Lancet* 2003; **361**: 587–594.
15. Lin TL, Wang CR, Liu MF et al. Multiple colonic ulcers caused by Churg–Strauss syndrome in a 15-year-old girl. *Clin Rheumatol* 2001; **20**: 362–364.
16. Sokol RJ, Farrell MK, McAdams AJ. An unusual presentation of Wegener's granulomatosis mimicking inflammatory bowel disease. *Gastroenterology* 1984; **87**: 426–432.
17. Bang D. Clinical spectrum of Behçet's disease. *J Dermatol* 2001; **28**: 610–613.
18. Terrin G, Borrelli O, Di Nardo G et al. A child with aphthae and diarrhoea. *Lancet* 2002; **359**: 316.
19. Geboes K. Crohn's disease, ulcerative colitis or indeterminate colitis – how important is it to differentiate? *Acta Gastroenterol Belg* 2001; **64**: 197–200.
20. Rozenbaum M, Rosner I, Portnoy E. Current therapy for Behçet's disease. *Am J Ther* 2002; **9**: 465–470.
21. Lupi-Herrera E, Sanchez-Torres G, Marcushamer J et al. Takayasu's arteritis. Clinical study of 107 cases. *Am Heart J* 1997; **93**: 94–103.
22. Johnston SL, Lock RJ, Gompels MM, Takayasu arteritis: a review. *J Clin Pathol* 2002; **55**: 481–486.
23. Sakhuja V, Gupta KL, Bhasin DK et al. Takayasu's arteritis associated with idiopathic ulcerative colitis. *Gut* 1990; **31**: 831–833.
24. Westphal J, Lobbecke F, Mietens C. Arteritis of the large vessels originating at the aorta (Takayasu's arteritis) in childhood. *Klin Padiatr* 1976; **188**: 570–577.
25. Salvarani C, Cantini F, Boiardi L et al. Polymyalgia rheumatica and giant-cell arteritis. *N Engl J Med* 2002; **347**: 261–271.
26. De Bayser L, Roblot P, Ramassamy A et al. Hepatic fibrin-ring granulomas in giant cell arteritis. *Gastroenterology* 1993; **105**: 272–273.
27. Mele T, Evans M. Intestinal obstruction as a complication of Kawasaki disease. *J Pediatr Surg* 1996; **31**: 985–986.
28. Beiler HA, Schmidt KG, von Herbay A et al. Ischemic small bowel strictures in a case of incomplete Kawasaki disease. *J Pediatr Surg* 2001; **36**: 648–650.
29. Saulsbury FT. Epidemiology of Henoch–Schönlein purpura. *Cleve Clin J Med* 2002; **69** (Suppl 2): SII87–89.
30. Esaki M, Matsumoto T, Nakamura S et al. GI involvement in Henoch–Schönlein purpura. *Gastrointest Endosc* 2002; **56**: 920–923.
31. Dillon MJ. Henoch–Schönlein purpura (treatment and outcome). *Cleve Clin J Med* 2002; **69** (Suppl 2): SII121–123.
32. Hattori M, Ito K, Konomoto T et al. Plasmapheresis as the sole therapy for rapidly progressive Henoch–Schönlein purpura nephritis in children. *Am J Kidney Dis* 1999; **33**: 427–433.

33. Zizic TM, Classen JN, Stevens MB. Acute abdominal complications of systemic lupus erythematosus and polyarteritis nodosa. *Am J Med* 1982; **73**: 525–31.
34. Yuasa S, Suwa A, Hirakata M et al. A case of lupus erythematosus presenting with rectal ulcers as the clinical manifestation of disease. *Clin Exp Rheumatol* 2002; **20**: 407–410.
35. Northcott KA, Yoshida EM, Streinbrecher UP. Primary protein-losing enteropathy in anti-double-stranded DNA disease: the initial and sole clinical manifestation of occult systemic lupus erythematosus? *Clin Gastroenterol* 2001; **33**: 340–341.
36. Perlemuter G, Chaussade S, Wechsler B et al. Chronic intestinal pseudo-obstruction in systemic lupus erythematosus. *Gut* 1998; **43**: 117–122.
37. Love PE, Santoro SA. Antiphospholipid antibodies: anticardiolipin and the lupus anticoagulant in systemic lupus erythematosus (SLE) and non-SLE disorders. *Ann Intern Med* 1990; **112**: 682–698.
38. Mihas AA. Gastrointestinal bleeding and intestinal ischemia associated with anticardiolipin antibodies. *Dig Dis Sci* 1995; **40**: 1039–1040.
39. Ramanan AV, Feldman BM. Clinical outcomes in juvenile dermatomyositis. *Curr Opin Rheumatol* 2002; **14**: 658–662.
40. Shehata R, Al-Mayouf S, Al-Dalaan A et al. Juvenile dermatomyositis: clinical profile and disease course in 25 patients. *Clin Exp Rheumatol* 1999; **17**: 115–118.
41. Laskin BL, Choyke P, Keenan et al. Novel gastrointestinal tract manifestations in juvenile dermatomyositis. *J Pediatr* 1999; **135**: 371–374.
42. Babian M, Nesef Sand Soloway G. Gastrointestinal infarction as a manifestation of rheumatoid vasculitis. *Am J Gastroenterol* 1998; **93**: 119–120.
43. Achkar AA, Stanson AW, Johnson CM et al. Rheumatoid vasculitis manifesting as intra-abdominal hemorrhage. *Mayo Clin Proc* 1995; **70**: 565–569.
44. Olin, JW, Thromboangiitis obliterans (Buerger's disease). *N Engl J Med* 2000; **343**: 864–869.
45. Adem C, Benamouzig R, Royer I et al. Buerger's disease or thromboangiitis obliterans revealed by an enteric ischemia. Case report and literature review. *Gastroenterol Clin Biol* 2002; **26**: 409–411.
46. Schellong SM, Bernhards J, Ensslen F et al. Intestinal type of thrombangitis obliterans (Buerger's disease). *J Intern Med* 1994; **235**: 69–73.
47. Gonzales-Gay MA, Garcia Porrua C. Systemic vasculitides. *Best Pract Res Clin Rheumatol* 2002; **16**: 833–845.

27 Celiac disease

Stefano Guandalini

Introduction

Important advances have occurred in the past few years in our understanding of celiac disease, its pathogenesis, its manifestations, its complications and its treatment. This fascinating condition is now regarded as a true autoimmune disorder, triggered by a well-known autoantigen, and affecting primarily the small intestine, where it progressively leads to severe villous blunting. However, it has clinical implications that reach far beyond the gut.

Celiac disease occurs only in genetically susceptible individuals, and is triggered by the ingestion of gliadins contained in wheat, rye and barley. Wheat gluten and similar alcohol-soluble proteins in other grains (called prolamines) cause – when ingested – the intestinal damage in individuals who are genetically predisposed. Indeed, almost 100% of celiacs are positive for either HLA DR3 (or DR5/DR7), or HLA DR4.[1] Although gluten is clearly the major environmental factor inducing celiac disease, other less known agents may be at play in modulating its onset, including the amount and type of gluten, and the utilization and duration of breast feeding.[2,3] An intriguing relationship between birth time and prevalence of celiac disease also suggests the influence of other environmental factors, such as infections.[4]

Epidemiology

The estimated prevalence of celiac disease varies according to the method of defining the condition. Earlier investigations that included only florid cases of celiac disease with overt gastrointestinal manifestations found an overall low but highly variable incidence throughout several European countries. With the availability of tests for malabsorption and of the pediatric peroral biopsy techniques, an increased incidence of celiac disease, to about 1:500, was reported in studies in Europe. Subsequently, sensitive serological tests have made it possible also to detect minimally symptomatic or even asymptomatic cases with the typical mucosal changes (thus fulfilling the definition of celiac disease). When these types of tool, and in particular the anti-endomysium antibodies, are utilized for screening studies, the prevalence of celiac disease soars to the current estimates of approximately 1:130 to 1:300 of the general European population.[5–8]

Until recently it was believed that celiac disease was a rare disorder in the USA, and rates of prevalence of lower than 1:10000 were often quoted. However, a recent multicenter investigation throughout the USA that screened more than 13000 individuals with anti-endomysium antibodies and/or human tissue transglutaminase antibodies, found a prevalence of 1:133,[9] i.e. identical to that found in Europe. It is clear, however, that the current rates of diagnosis of celiac disease in the USA are well below those in Europe, perhaps owing to an overall later onset of the disease and more frequent extraintestinal manifestations. This, in turn, may be linked to various factors, with the more prolonged and more widespread use of breast feeding being a likely cause of postponing the onset of celiac disease.[2] The prevalence of celiac disease in other areas of the world has been less studied. Data are, however, available from Latin America, North Africa, the Near and Middle East and Northwest India: in all these areas celiac disease has been reported, and where prevalence data were sought, they do not differ significantly from those indicated above. In some ethnicities, such as in the Saharawi population, celiac disease has been found in as many as 5% of the general population.[10] Thus, it is fair to assume that celiac disease constitutes one of the most common genetically induced chronic diseases. However, celiac disease is considered extremely rare or non-existing in people with African, Chinese or Japanese descent.

Pathophysiology

Celiac disease is an autoimmune disorder. The initial event in the pathogenesis of the celiac lesion is thought to be abnormal permeability, allowing the entry of gliadin peptides not entirely degraded by the intraluminal and brush-border bound-peptidases. Interestingly, the initial 'theory' on celiac disease pathogenesis was the enzymatic one: for many years, research focused on 'the missing enzyme', unable properly to digest gluten and thus creating an indigestible, toxic fragment. However, there is no missing peptidase in celiac disease; simply, the most toxic amongst the fractions of gliadin that have been shown to be harmful to the celiac mucosa are remarkably resistant to digestion by gastric, pancreatic and mucosa-associated enzymes.[11] Under normal circumstances, the intestinal epithelium would act as a barrier to the passage of such macromolecules, but in celiac disease, a well-documented loosening of the intestinal tight junctions,[12] possibly even triggered by gliadin itself,[13] leads to increased permeability to macromolecules. The role of altered expression of zonulin, a novel human protein that induces tight junction disassembly and a subsequent increase in intestinal permeability, has been suggested. Zonulin expression was found to be elevated in intestinal tissues from patients with florid celiac disease.[14]

There are two pathways involved in the pathogenesis of celiac disease: an early one, involving mainly the innate immune system; and a subsequent one, involving T cells. Soon after reaching the serosal side of the intestinal epithelium, the toxic gliadin peptides elicit an early response that causes crucial modifications of the mucosal microenvironment that precede and prime the subsequent involvement of the pathogenic T cells. A recent elegant study by Maiuri et al[15] brings important new information on this early response, by showing that a non-immunodominant gliadin fragment can activate the innate immune system, affecting the *in situ* T-cell recognition of dominant gliadin epitopes. Although more than 50 epitopes have been identified, the dominant α-gliadin T-cell epitope appears to be a single tissue transglutaminase-modified peptide.[16]

During the first phase, there is a marked increase of HLA-DR expression on both the epithelium and the adjacent lamina propria macrophages; this is followed by overexpression of intercellular adhesion molecule 1 (ICAM-1). Finally, $CD8^+$ T cells invaded epithelial cells (intraepithelial lymphocytes).

About 95% of all celiac patients belong to the DR3 (or DR5/DR7 heterozygous) genotype and express the DQ2 α,β-heterodimer, encoded by DQA1*0501/DQB1*0201, while almost all of the remaining 5% are DR4 and show the DQ8 α,β-heterodimer, encoded by DQA1*0301/DQB1*0302. This strong association implies that the adaptive branch of the immune system, and in particular $CD4^+$ T lymphocytes, must play a crucial role in the pathogenesis. In fact, DQ2 and DQ8 molecules are located on the surface of antigen-presenting cells and bind peptides to be presented to $CD4^+$ T lymphocytes. The DQ2 or DQ8 molecules expressed by the antigen-presenting cells (mostly macrophages) possess unique peptide-binding properties. They typically bind peptides of 12–20 amino acid residues, with a core region of nine amino acids being bound to the peptide-binding groove on the HLA class-II molecule via interactions between side chains of amino acids and pockets of the binding groove. The autoantigen in celiac disease, a major target of all autoantibodies such as anti-endomysium and anti-reticulin, has been found to be the ubiquitous enzyme tissue transglutaminase. This enzyme, among other functions, selectively converts glutamine residues within gluten to glutamic acid. Such deamidation increases the negative charges on the gliadin peptides,[17] thus resulting in a strong enhancement of DQ binding and T-cell recognition.

From a morphological point of view, small-bowel mucosal damage occurs as a result of gradual changes from normal mucosa to overt mucosal atrophy with crypt hyperplasia. It is crucial to understand that these changes occur in a progressive manner, so that the 'flat' mucosa, for a long time thought to be the necessary key finding in celiac disease, is only the last stage in a continuum of morphological changes. At lest three degrees of change are recognized, as classically described by Marsh.[18] The infiltrative (type 1) lesion, seen in the latent phase, is characterized by morphologically normal mucosa and is not usually associated with gastrointestinal symptoms. Initial changes seen include an increase in the number of intraepithelial lymphocytes, followed by infiltration of the lamina propria with plasma cells and lymphocytes. The hyperplastic (type 2) lesion is similar to type 1, but with elongation of crypts, owing to a marked increase in undifferentiated crypt cells. The destructive (type 3) lesion is synonymous with villous atrophy, the original lesion described in celiac disease.

The mechanisms leading to such changes have been the matter of extensive research in past years, and are currently still largely obscure. Several hypotheses coexist, each supported by experimental evidence. The ultimate agent responsible for villous flattening appears to be the enterocyte expression of FAS (the prototype of the 'death receptor') and apoptosis. Indeed, the element that differentiates patchy lesions from areas with normal histology is the specific lack of expression of FAS in morphologically normal mucosa.[19] It is also thought[20] that interleukin (IL)-15 may be involved in both the proliferating and the atrophic epithelial phases of celiac disease. In an organ culture model, IL-15 was in fact able to induce proliferation in crypts and FAS expression in enterocytes. In the active phase of celiac disease, a specific increase of intraepithelial lymphocytes expressing CD94 has been demonstrated,[21] possibly induced by IL-15. In essence, it would appear that intraepithelial lymphocytes migrate into the epithelium to induce apoptosis of the enterocytes. A scheme of the main events currently thought to occur in the mucosa of celiac patients is shown in Figure 27.1.

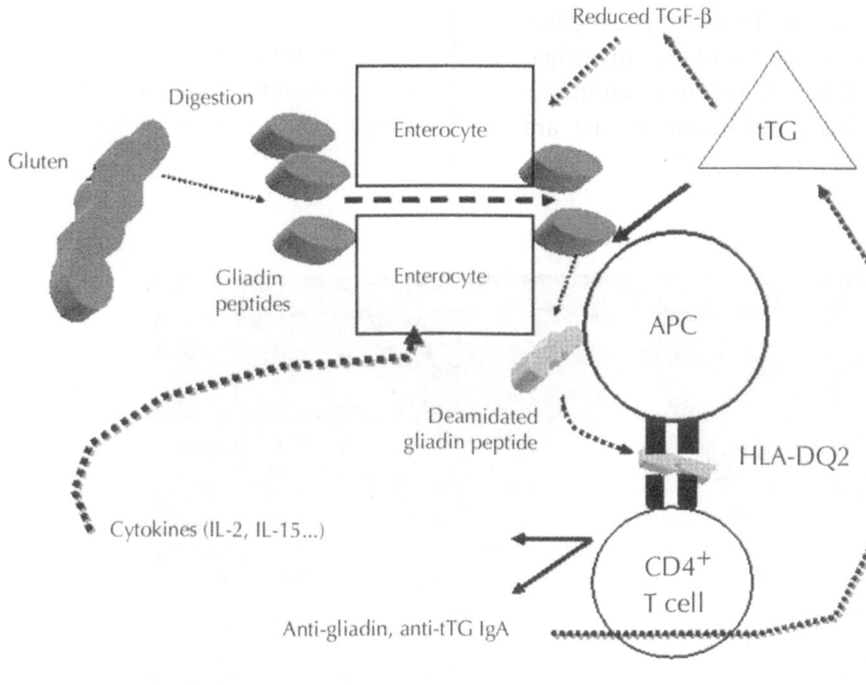

Figure 27.1 Scheme of the epithelial damage in celiac disease. After gluten is digested into gliadin peptides, they enter through an abnormally increased intestinal permeability and reach the serosal side, where they interact with tissue transglutaminase (tTG). Among several effects of this interaction is the deamidation of such peptides, a process that strongly enhances their affinity for the HLA-DQ2 or DQ8 heterodimer expressed at the surface of the antigen-presenting cell (APC). The peptide is thus presented to the T lymphocyte. This initiates a chain of events, including release of toxic lymphokines such as interleukin (IL)-2 and IL-15 that have a direct damaging effect on the epithelium. Interaction with B lymphocytes also leads (by unclear mechanisms) to the production of antibodies against the enzyme tTG (utilized in the diagnostic process). The reduced activation of the epithelium-protective peptide transforming growth factor (TGF)-β further contributes to the damage of the epithelium.

Clinical presentations

One of the most important advances in the past decade has been the understanding that, although characterized by intestinal damage, celiac disease may present with signs and symptoms not necessarily related to the gastrointestinal tract. Moreover, it may well remain asymptomatic, or oligosymptomatic, for many years or indeed for life.

Thus, we have come to distinguish four forms of celiac disease:

(1) Typical;

(2) Atypical (or more exactly 'extraintestinal');

(3) Silent;

(4) Latent.

Table 27.1 reports the corresponding definitions, and Figure 27.2 illustrates the so-called 'celiac iceberg' that depicts the relation between HLA status, duodenal morphology and clinical expression in these different forms. Interestingly, there is evidence from many epidemiological investigations that the less clinically evident conditions (silent, latent and oligosymptomatic forms) are much more common that the clinically overt ones.

Table 27.1 Definitions of the various forms of celiac disease

Typical
Gastrointestinal signs/symptoms predominate:
- diarrhea
- vomiting
- failure to thrive
- anorexia
- constipation
- recurrent abdominal pain

Atypical or extraintestinal
Gastrointestinal signs/symptoms are minimal or absent. Most common signs/symptoms are:
- fatigue
- malaise
- anemia

Silent
No signs/symptoms. Gluten-dependent duodenal mucosal changes consistent with celiac disease

Latent
No signs/symptoms. Duodenal mucosa normal. Gluten-dependent changes with or without symptoms to appear later in time

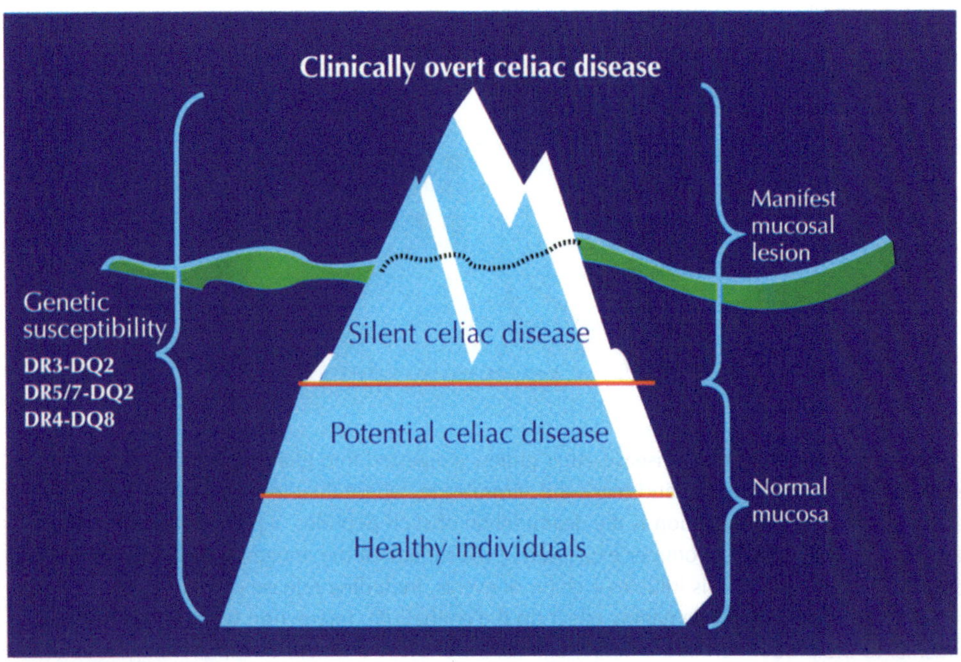

Figure 27.2 The 'celiac iceberg'. See text for details.

It should be noted that the factors ultimately responsible in any single individual for the expressivity of the disease (i.e. developing typical vs. extraintestinal vs. silent, etc.) are not known. It is, however, known that age influences the prevalence of the various forms, as schematically indicated in Figure 27.3.

The typical form of celiac disease presents with gastrointestinal symptoms typically between 6 and 24 months of age. Symptoms begin at various time intervals after the introduction of gluten in the diet, also depending on its amount and on other environmental factors such as the concomitant presence of breast feeding, occurrence of viral enteritis, etc. Affected infants have poor appetite, chronic diarrhea, abdominal distension, muscle wasting and failure to thrive. Vomiting is also common. As spontaneous avoidance of gluten-containing foods does not occur, symptoms may progress to serious malnutrition, even cachexia, if diagnosis is delayed. Behavioral changes are also often found: celiac infants and young children become less talkative, more irritable, avoid company and are sad. In the most severely affected infants, the clinical picture of the so-called 'celiac crisis' may develop. This acute syndrome, now rarely seen, is characterized by explosive watery diarrhea often followed by no passage of stools, impressive abdominal distension, dehydration, hypotension and lethargy. This severe picture is accompanied by profound electrolyte abnormalities including dangerously low potassium levels.

Atypical or extraintestinal celiac disease

In recent years an increasing number of patients have been diagnosed without typical gastrointestinal manifestations at an older age.[22,23] It is currently believed that almost 50% of patients with newly diagnosed celiac disease, and up to two-thirds of the adults, do not present with gastrointestinal symptoms and have either atypical or silent celiac disease. Table 27.2 reports the main presentations of 'atypical' or 'extraintestinal' celiac disease.

Dermatitis herpetiformis

This variant of celiac disease presents with a blistering skin rash involving elbows, knees and buttocks associated with dermal granular

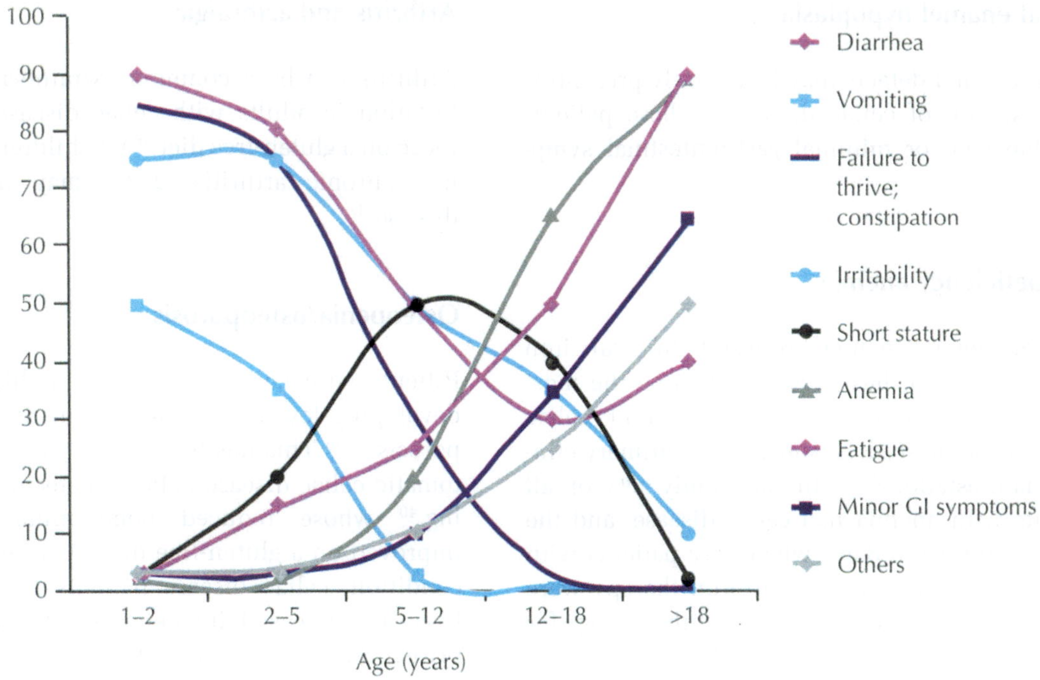

Figure 27.3 Celiac disease presentations vary with age. Most gastrointestinal (GI) signs and symptoms are more common in early years, while anemia, fatigue and minor GI symptoms predominate later in life.

Table 27.2 Main presentations of so-called 'atypical' (or 'extraintestinal') celiac disease

Dermatitis herpetiformis
Permanent enamel hypoplasia
Iron-deficient anemia resistant to oral iron intake
Short stature, delayed puberty
Chronic hepatitis with hypertransaminasemia
Primary biliary cirrhosis
Arthritis
Osteopenia/osteoporosis
Epilepsy with occipital calcifications
Primary ataxia, white-matter focal lesions
Psychiatric disorders
Infertility of women

immunoglobulin (Ig) A deposits. Rash as well as mucosal morphology improve on a gluten-free diet.[24] Previously considered a skin disease occurring often concomitantly with celiac disease, but overall a rare occurrence, it is now thought to be a common although often unrecognized problem in celiac patients.[25]

Dental enamel hypoplasia

Dental enamel defects may be the only presenting manifestation of celiac disease.[26] These patients may have no or minimal gastrointestinal symptoms.

Iron-deficiency anemia

Iron-deficiency anemia, resistant to oral iron supplementation, has been found to be the most common extraintestinal manifestation of celiac disease in some studies, and often its primary clinical manifestation.[23,27] In one study 5% of all patients with anemia had celiac disease, and the prevalence rose to 8.5% when only patients with microcytic anemia resistant to iron therapy were considered.[28] Recently, screening with serology for celiac disease a large number of adult patients who were found to have either folate or iron deficiency (in the absence of gastrointestinal manifestations) detected 11% positive.[29] In spite of these well-known data, general screening of this type of patient is still rarely conducted.

Short stature and delayed puberty

Short stature may be the only manifestation of celiac disease.[30] As many as 8–10% of children with 'idiopathic' short stature may have celiac disease that can be detected on serologic testing.[31] Adolescents with untreated celiac disease may have delayed onset of menarche.[32]

Chronic hepatitis and hypertransaminasemia

Elevated transaminase levels are a frequent finding in untreated patients with celiac disease. In the majority of cases liver enzymes normalize on a gluten-free diet.[33] As many as 9% of patients with elevated transaminase levels of unclear etiology may have silent celiac disease.[34] Liver biopsies in these patients showed non-specific reactive hepatitis. Transaminases returned to normal on a gluten-free diet. Very recently, celiac disease has been described as causing severe liver disease, indeed hepatic failure, that was further shown to be responsive to a gluten-free diet.[35]

Arthritis and arthralgia

Arthritis can be a common extraintestinal manifestation in adults with celiac disease including those on a gluten-free diet.[36] Of children with juvenile chronic arthritis, 2–3% may have celiac disease.[37]

Osteopenia/osteoporosis

Patients with celiac disease are at high risk for developing low bone mineral density and osteoporosis.[38,39] This has been found even for asymptomatic celiac disease patients detected at screening,[40] whose reduced bone mineral density improved on a gluten-free diet. As a result of this condition, celiac disease patients are known to have an increased incidence of fractures.[41] The British Society of Gastroenterology recommended measuring bone mineral density in all patients with celiac disease.[42] Recently however, a survey conducted in the UK in 244 adult patients and 169 controls showed no statistically increased prevalence of fractures, and concluded that screening for bone mineral density in all celiac patients may not be warranted.[43] Thus, this issue is still open. Bone mineral density improves in the majority of patients on a gluten-free diet.[44–46] The pathogenesis of osteoporosis is complex, and only partially understood. It seems clear that poor absorption of calcium and/or vitamin D is not the most important factor. Recently, some evidence has been provided that an autoimmune aggression of the bone matrix may take place in celiac disease.[47]

Neurological problems

Celiac disease can be the underlying cause of idiopathic cerebellar ataxia.[48] Celiac disease may also be associated with occipital calcifications and intractable epilepsy. These patients can be resistant to anti-seizure medicines but can benefit from a gluten-free diet if started soon after the onset of seizures.[49] Interestingly, a new neurological presentation of celiac disease has recently been described: focal brain white-matter lesions leading to multiple neurological manifestations such as seizures, muscle hypotonia and mild ataxia.[50]

Psychiatric disorders

Although in recent years a large number of behavioral problems and disorders, such as autism, attention deficit hyperactivity disorder, etc., have been thought to be caused by celiac disease, there is no evidence to date that this is the case.[51] Celiac disease nevertheless can certainly present with some psychiatric disorders, such as depression[52] and anxiety.[53,54] These conditions can be severe, but will usually respond to a gluten-free diet.

Infertility

Celiac disease may be responsible for unexplained infertility in women.[55] Ciacci et al[56] reported that the relative risk of abortion in women affected by celiac disease was 8.9 times higher than in healthy subjects, and that a gluten-free diet reduced the relative risk of abortion. Of interest, a recent study showed that not only fetuses from celiac mothers, but also those from celiac fathers suffered adverse effects in pregnancy, resulting in lower birth weight and perhaps shorter duration of pregnancy.[57]

Associated diseases

In addition to being responsible for various presentations, as described above, celiac disease is also known to be more commonly associated with a number of other diseases. Although the mechanisms of such links are still largely obscure, it is important to be aware of such associations in order to detect celiac disease as early as possible.

Table 27.3 lists the main medical disorders that are associated with celiac disease. It is evident that many disorders are also of the autoimmune type. The association of celiac disease with autoimmune conditions is well established.[58] Recently, even autoimmune myocarditis was added to the list of such disorders.[59] An important multicenter study

Table 27.3 Conditions associated with an increased prevalence of celiac disease

Condition	Approximate prevalence of celiac disease (%)
Insulin-dependent diabetes mellitus	6%
Thyroiditis	4%
Sjögren's syndrome and other connective tissue diseases	5%
Primary biliary cirrhosis	3%
Down's syndrome	12%
Williams' syndrome	6%
Turner's syndrome	6%
First-degree relatives of celiac patients	8–10%

established a strong positive correlation between age at diagnosis of celiac disease and prevalence of autoimmune disorders such as type 1 diabetes, thyroiditis and alopecia,[60] thus suggesting that it is indeed the presence of celiac disease that acts as a trigger for the development of other autoimmune conditions.[61]

Type 1 (insulin-dependent) diabetes

Up to 8% of patients with type-1 or insulin-dependent diabetes mellitus have been found to have typical features of celiac disease on duodenal biopsy. However, it is thought that the 'real' percentage is higher, as studies of such patients in serial screening over a period of years have documented that many individuals who initially had negative serological tests eventually developed positive tests and characteristic intestinal changes.[62] Typically (90% of cases), diagnosis of diabetes precedes by years that of celiac disease, most commonly presenting with mild to only moderate gastrointestinal symptoms.[63] As some of these symptoms are also seen in patients with diabetes (e.g. bloating or diarrhea), the diagnosis of celiac disease may be missed, unless screening is performed. Laboratory abnormalities such as anemia, and iron and folate deficiency are also common.

It is still debated whether or not diabetic individuals found to be celiacs at screening (i.e. essentially asymptomatic) need to be put on a gluten-free diet. So far there is no convincing evidence that the diet has any obvious effect on diabetes. Indeed, the same considerations apply to all of the other associated autoimmune conditions. However, the following two considerations seem to suggest that adherence to a gluten-free diet should be recommended. First, a gluten-free diet has been shown in some cases to help improve glycemic control and improve gastrointestinal symptoms in patients with both conditions. Second, it can be argued that complications of untreated celiac disease known to be prevented by adherence to gluten-free diet (including osteopenia, infertility and malignancy – all documented occurrences in diabetic individuals) may be prevented by the diet in asymptomatic celiacs. As a consequence, the case for screening a type 1 diabetic for celiac disease seems well founded.

Down's syndrome

Perhaps the best documented and most widely reported association of celiac disease with a non-autoimmune disorder is that with Down's syndrome. The prevalence of Down's syndrome in celiac disease, as assessed by screening methods, has been found to be between 5 and 12% in studies from both Europe[64–66] and more recently also North America.[9,67,68] Unlike patients with type-1 diabetes, the majority with Down's syndrome and celiac disease have other gastrointestinal symptoms, such as abdominal bloating, intermittent diarrhea, anorexia and failure to thrive. However, in a large multicenter study, it was found that about one-third of all Down's syndrome patients with celiac disease had no gastrointestinal symptoms;[66] the patients with celiac disease as a group, more commonly than their counterparts, had anemia, low serum iron and calcium, and a tendency to be mildly stunted in height and weight.[66] It seems highly desirable that patients with Down's syndrome be screened for celiac disease and, whenever found positive, they should begin the gluten-free diet. As celiac disease may start at any age, patients with Down's syndrome who test negative for serological markers (see below) would have to be re-tested again and again. To avoid this, since celiac disease occurs only in specific HLA haplotypes (see Epidemiology, p.435), an algorithm based on first determining the HLA haplotypes (thus leaving out of the re-screening process all those with the HLA haplotypes inconsistent with celiac disease) has been proposed.[69] An analogous strategy might be applied to screen for celiac disease patients with the rarer Williams' syndrome, where an increased incidence of celiac disease has been reported.[70]

Complications

Untreated, celiac disease can lead to a number of complications. Some, such as chronic liver disease, osteopenia/osteoporosis, infertility or psychiatric disorders, have been discussed under clinical presentations. Other important complications include hyposplenism, non-responsive celiac disease (including refractory sprue) and malignancy.

Hyposplenism

Often seen in older patients, less commonly in children, this condition is detected by the presence of Howell–Jolly bodies and thrombocytosis[71] and confirmed by imaging techniques.

Non-responsive celiac disease

Uncommonly, patients who have been diagnosed with celiac disease either fail to respond to the diet, continuing to present the same symptoms and signs, or they soon relapse, after a brief apparent improvement. This condition can be defined as 'non-responsive celiac disease' with initial or subsequent failure of what appears to be a strict gluten-free diet to improve symptoms and/or to restore normal intestinal architecture and function in patients who have celiac-like enteropathy. This syndrome, which includes true refractory sprue, can be due to a number of causes, which are reported in Table 27.4.

It should be stressed that, in any population of celiacs reported to fail to respond to a gluten-free diet, whether pediatric or adult, by far the most common cause remains the continued ingestion of gluten, often inadvertent. Thus, a meticulous search for hidden sources of gluten is the recommended first-line investigative approach.

Table 27.4 Main causes of apparently non-responsive celiac disease ('refractory sprue')

Continued ingestion of gluten
Incorrect diagnosis, e.g.
Crohn's disease
autoimmune enteropathy
eosinophilic gastroenteritis
giardiasis
cow's milk protein allergic enteropathy
Presence of a concomitant food allergy
Lactose intolerance
secondary to reduced absorptive surface (transient)
adult-type lactase deficiency (permanent)
Irritable bowel syndrome
Pancreatic insufficiency

Second, an erroneous diagnosis of celiac disease is to be suspected. Particular care should be used in all cases to rule out other conditions that also present with morphological changes in the duodenal mucosa (see Table 27.4 for some examples). Among them, Crohn's disease is a growing concern.

Third, particularly in pediatric cases of celiac disease apparently unresponsive to a gluten-free diet, a concomitant food allergy, such as to milk or egg protein, must be sought. Indeed, the high prevalence of cow's milk protein allergy makes the coincidental overlapping of the two conditions a not uncommon occurrence.

Also, in cases with overt gastrointestinal symptoms, lactase deficiency is commonly present at diagnosis, as a result of the reduction of the absorptive area and hence of enough available enzymatic activity. Under these circumstances, it is not surprising that for some time a secondary lactose intolerance causes symptoms such as abdominal bloating, gassiness and diarrhea. Unless lactase deficiency is the result of the permanent loss of this enzymatic activity ('adult-type' or 'late-onset' lactase deficiency), the problem is self-limited and within a few weeks in the majority of patients lactose can be reintroduced in the diet.

Irritable bowel syndrome, whose recently proposed association with celiac disease in a proportion of cases[72] has spurred much debate, is not uncommonly found in celiac disease patients, mostly teenagers or young adults. Clearly, this remains a diagnosis of exclusion, and needs to be supported by evidence of lack of any problem with adequate weight gain or maintenance. Once irritable bowel syndrome is diagnosed in a celiac patient, obviously the gluten-free diet must be maintained, and any of the currently available modalities of management can be utilized.

Pancreatic insufficiency, found also in patients who do not have an underlying important condition of malabsorption and malnutrition,[73] has been shown in newly diagnosed celiac patients to cause failure of an adequate response to the diet, particularly in terms of growth,[74] and can of course be treated with adequate pancreatic enzyme supplementation.[75]

Refractory sprue

A condition of persistence of severe symptoms (typically malabsorption), high serum autoantibodies and enteropathy in spite of a strict gluten-free diet and in the documented absence of any of the disorders mentioned above, is rare, and has never been described in pediatric age. It is termed refractory sprue. In a multicenter study conducted in France, it has been shown in the majority of cases to be characterized by abnormal monoclonal intraepithelial T lymphocytes expressing a cytoplasmic CD3 chain (CD3c), lacking CD3 and CD8 surface expression, and showing T cell receptor-γ gene rearrangements.[76] These authors suggested that refractory sprue associated with an aberrant clonal population of intraepithelial lymphocytes may be classified as cryptic enteropathy-associated T-cell lymphoma. The same group subsequently developed an immunohistochemical technique that would allow rapid identification of this condition.[77] Refractory sprue is a difficult condition to treat, and multiple aggressive immunosuppressive regimens have been suggested, ranging from cyclosporine to infliximab.[78–83]

Malignancy

The development of malignancy, particularly lymphoma of the small bowel, but also carcinoma of any segment of the esophagus and stomach, is the most serious complication to affect patients with celiac disease.[84] The association has been known for about 40 years, yet many questions are still unanswered. In particular, it is unclear why only some celiac patients develop malignancy. Development of malignancy is the main explanation for the well-documented shorter life expectancy of celiac patients who are either untreated, or diagnosed very late in the course of their disease, especially when presenting severe malabsorption.[85]

Diagnosis

The European Society of Paediatric Gastroenterology, Hepatology and Nutrition (ESPGHAN) established the criteria for diagnosis of celiac disease more than 30 years ago.[86] These original criteria, which have been widely followed by both adult and pediatric gastroenterologists for more than two decades, stated that diagnosis of celiac disease would require:

(1) The presence of compatible symptoms and demonstration of a structurally abnormal small-intestinal mucosa when taking a diet containing gluten;

(2) A clear clinical response to a gluten-free diet;

(3) Documentation of unequivocal improvement of the villous structure after having taken a gluten-free diet for 1 year;

(4) Deterioration of the mucosa and reappearance of symptoms during challenge with gluten.

With increasing availability of serological tests for diagnosis, and following a report of an Italian multicenter investigation in more than 3000 celiac children,[87] ESPGHAN in 1990 proposed new diagnostic criteria. According to them, the diagnosis of celiac disease can be established on a definitive basis when the characteristic changes of the duodenal mucosa are found in a child with signs and/or symptoms consistent with celiac disease, provided that a full and unequivocal clinical remission after withdrawal of gluten is seen, associated with the disappearance of circulating antibodies. These criteria are currently universally utilized, and it can be seen that, although the emerging role of serology testing was recognized and taken into crucial consideration, diagnosis still clearly relies on intestinal biopsy findings.[88] The role of the serological markers of celiac disease will be discussed later, but it should be clear that they must be considered an important means of screening and of monitoring compliance, offering only supportive evidence for the diagnosis.[89]

Duodenal biopsy

Currently, most of the bioptic samples are obtained from the duodenal mucosa during endoscopy. Endoscopic changes described in untreated celiac patients include scalloping, a mosaic pattern and flattening or paucity of the folds.[90] However, these findings are not specific[91] and occur only infrequently in the pediatric age. Adequate biopsy specimens can be obtained at endoscopy or with a suction biopsy tube. Specimens should be obtained from the distal duodenum. Obtaining multiple biopsies is crucial for a correct diagnosis. In fact, the old teaching that celiac disease results in a continuum of lesions has recently been proved incorrect. The typical flattening of villi can be patchy, with blunted villi juxtaposed to normal mucosa.[92] The diagnosis therefore can be easily missed if at least four or five bioptic samples are not obtained. Histological examination of involved areas confirms the loss of normal villous structure with severe shortening up to complete absence (flat mucosa) of the villi. The intestinal crypts are markedly elongated and hyperplastic. Unlike the well-differentiated, mature absorptive cells, the undifferentiated crypt cells are markedly increased in number in untreated celiac disease, and this accounts for the obvious lengthening of crypts. The cellularity of the lamina propria is increased and the thickness of the mucosa is overall also increased. The cellular infiltrate consists largely of plasma cells and lymphocytes. Another typical (but not pathognomonic) change that occurs in the small intestinal mucosa of untreated celiac patients is the increase in the number of intraepithelial lymphocytes, particularly T cells expressing the $\gamma\delta$ receptors.[93] This change (Figure 27.4) is considered an early and subtle sign of celiac disease and, if supported by concordant serology and clinical findings, can be considered sufficient to finalize the diagnosis. Indeed, it was shown that these patients would benefit from a gluten-free diet.[94] Some patients may also have only minor morphometric changes on jejunal biopsies with changes in mean surface/volume ratio without gross histological abnormalities.[95,96] As it can be seen therefore, it is imperative that an experienced pathologist carefully review intestinal biopsies for intraepithelial lymphocytes and morphometric changes in a patient with positive celiac antibodies before labeling serology results as false positive.

Furthermore, to complicate matters, some studies have demonstrated that patients with totally normal histology but positive celiac serology who are labeled as false positive may develop typical celiac morphological changes on follow-up.[97,98] Thus, development of serum antibodies seems to precede, at least in some well-documented cases, that of the morphological lesions. For this reason, it appears wise to continue to follow up patients who have high levels of anti-endomysium or tissue transglutaminase antibodies, even with a normal mucosa, and to repeat the endoscopy if clinical signs or symptoms consistent with celiac disease appear.

Serology

Serologic testing for celiac disease has included testing for food protein-directed antibodies (antigliadin (AGA)) and for an autoantibody (anti-endomysium).[99] It should be recognized that, in spite of high potential in clinical settings, particularly for screening purposes, the sensitivity and specificity of serology have varied widely, in part because of the lack of standardized protocols and of reference sera. Inter-laboratory variations have been wide, particularly for AGA, as pointed out by

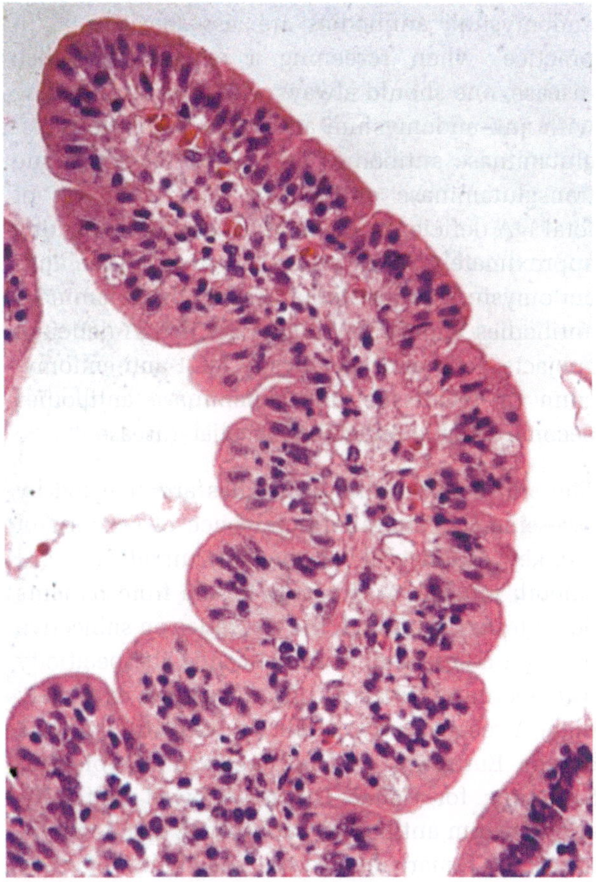

Figure 27.4 Morphologically normal villus with increased intraepithelial lymphocytes. In the early stage of the changes induced by celiac disease, an otherwise normal villus can be seen to have an increased intraepithelial infiltration of lymphocytes.

multicenter studies performed both in Europe[100] and in the USA.[101] AGA have been widely utilized since the early 1980s, having soon become widely available and inexpensive. Two classes are currently measured: IgG and IgA. The former, even though considered of high sensitivity (85–98% in most large series from Europe), has been repeatedly shown to be extremely non-specific. Indeed, AGA-IgG can be found in about 30% of a control population, and thus their positive value is of little use. AGA-IgA, on the other hand, are known to be generally much more specific (95–100%), but are unfortunately also less sensitive (sensitivities reported range between 70 and 92%). The value of measuring AGA for screening purposes is therefore at best doubtful. However, this class of antibodies maintains its usefulness in monitoring the compliance to the gluten-free diet in an already established celiac patient, as it is known that AGA are more prone to reappear in the presence of even minimal dietary transgressions, where anti-endomysium antibodies are less sensitive.[102] In practice, when screening a patient for celiac disease, one should always obtain total IgA, along with anti-endomysium antibodies or tissue transglutaminase antibodies (see below for anti-tissue transglutaminase antibodies). If a condition of total IgA deficiency is found (a condition affecting approximately 3% of celiac patients[103]), then anti-endomysium antibodies or tissue transglutaminase antibodies should be sought, as, in IgA-deficient subjects, IgG- and specifically IgG1-anti-endomysium or IgG-tissue transglutaminase antibodies become reliable indicators of celiac disease.[104]

The anti-endomysium antibodies are detected by assessing the immunofluorescence of sections of monkey esophageal or human umbilical cord smooth muscle on exposure to sera from patients being tested. Although the test relies on subjective operator assessment of fluorescence, its specificity in detecting untreated celiac disease is extremely high. A recent study conducted with strict criteria by the European working group on Serological Screening for Celiac Disease showed that anti-endomysium antibodies had, among seven laboratories, a remarkable mean specificity of 99% (93.9–99.9%), while the mean sensitivity proved to be 90% (82.7–92.5%).[105] Also, the inter-laboratory reliability proved to be quite good for this test, unlike the poor reproducibility of AGA. This assay is relatively costly, and its utilization of monkey esophagus further limits its use for the screening of large populations.

Tissue transglutaminase antibodies

In 1997 Dieterich et al identified tissue transglutaminase as the autoantigen of celiac disease.[106] In a subsequent study by the same group, an enzyme-linked immunosorbent assay (ELISA) for guinea-pig IgA tissue transglutaminase antibodies was found to be 98.1% sensitive and 94.7% specific in patients with biopsy-proved celiac disease.[107] Since then, many studies have confirmed the high sensitivity and specificity of these antibodies in the diagnosis of celiac disease. Sensitivity and specificity have been subsequently further improved by utilizing the human antigen instead of the guinea pig antigen.[108–110] A simple non-invasive immunological dot blot assay based on recognition of recombinant human transglutaminase has also recently been proposed as a practical, reliable alternative to both the immunofluorescence-based anti-endomysium test and tissue transglutaminase ELISA for the diagnosis of celiac disease.[111]

In summary, even though currently anti-endomysium antibody tests can still be considered more specific, it is likely that serological (or whole blood) tests based on human tissue transglutaminase antibodies will become the gold standard for celiac disease screening in the very near future, eventually replacing the semiquantitative, observer-dependent, costly and time-consuming anti-endomysium antibody test.

Currently, however, it seems that anti-tissue transglutaminase antibodies are less specific than anti-endomysium antibodies for celiac disease.[112]

Treatment

Total lifelong avoidance of gluten ingestion is the cornerstone treatment for celiac disease. Wheat, rye and barley are the grains containing toxic peptides. For a long time, oats were also considered toxic, and their elimination from the diet was recommended. However, during the past few years a growing body of scientific evidence obtained from *in vitro* studies as well as from clinical investigations, particularly in adults[113–115] but also recently in children,[116] allows us to conclude that oats are indeed totally safe. This makes sense based on the genetics of the grains, showing that oats are genetically entirely unrelated to the group of wheat, rye and barley.[117] Indeed, a recent *in vitro* study looking at the specificity of tissue transglutaminase further supported the lack of toxicity of oats.[118] However, because of uncontrolled harvesting and milling procedures, cross-contamination of oats with gluten is still a concern, which will have to be addressed in the context of a more general policy concerning labeling of food certified to be gluten-free.

Often in the initial phases of dietary treatment, lactose is also eliminated. This has its basis in the lactase deficiency that is thought to accompany the flat mucosa.[119] However, it should be pointed out that, as we have seen, today most new celiacs are diagnosed in the absence of overt malabsorptive symptoms, and in these circumstances clinically significant lactose malabsorption or intolerance is rarely seen. Furthermore, even in cases with obvious malabsorption, the recovery of lactase activity is typically fast, so that the use of a lactose-free diet even in these cases must be on a short-term basis only. The possibility of an association between celiac disease and milk protein allergy has been repeatedly raised in the past, but it is now clear that the two conditions may simply coexist as a result of a statistical association, so that again there is no need to recommend avoidance of 'dairy products'.

A commonly asked question is 'how strict must the diet be'? This implies that there could be a threshold, below which 'some gluten' might be tolerated. We know that the morphological damage is dose-related,[120] and that amounts of gluten as low as 100 mg/kg per day may induce damage at the clinical, histological or laboratory level.[121] Thus, there is no scientific answer to the question of how low a dose is safe. In addition, tolerance is highly variable between celiac individuals, making predictions in single cases impossible. This is the basis of the only reasonable dietetic recommendation for celiac patients: 'zero tolerance'. Currently, there is wide availability of resources to assist celiac patients and their families: recipe books, newsletters from support groups that continuously update lists of 'safe' products and hospital-affiliated specific programs. Clearly, however, a close interaction between families on the one hand and the dietitian–doctor team on the other is necessary to achieve optimal compliance. This need is especially important during adolescence, a time when dietetic compliance can be difficult,[122–124] and requires attention to possible dietetic deficiencies,[124] but also in adults, who commonly end up by only partially adhering to the diet.[125] It is indeed important to realize that a close adherence to the gluten-free diet is associated with improved quality of life, both for patients with symptom-detected celiac disease and for those – mostly asymptomatic – in whom the diagnosis was reached as a result of a screening program.[126]

REFERENCES

1. Sollid LM. Molecular basis of celiac disease. *Annu Rev Immunol* 2000; **18**: 53–81.
2. Hernell O, Ivarsson A, Persson LA. Coeliac disease: effect of early feeding on the incidence of the disease. *Early Hum Dev* 2001; **65 Suppl**: S153–S160.
3. Ivarsson A, Hernell O, Stenlund H, Persson LA. Breast-feeding protects against celiac disease. *Am J Clin Nutr* 2002; **75**: 914–921.
4. Ivarsson A, Hernell O, Nystrom L, Persson LA. Children born in the summer have increased risk for coeliac disease. *J Epidemiol Community Health* 2003; **57**: 36–39.
5. Ascher H, Krantz I, Kristiansson B. Increasing incidence of coeliac disease in Sweden. *Arch Dis Child* 1991; **66**: 608–611.
6. Catassi C, Ratsch IM, Fabiani E et al. Coeliac disease in the year 2000: exploring the iceberg. *Lancet* 1994; **343**: 200–203.
7. Maki M, Kallonen K, Lahdeaho ML, Visakorpi JK. Changing pattern of childhood coeliac disease in Finland. *Acta Paediatr Scand* 1988; **77**: 408–412.
8. Kolho KL, Farkkila MA, Savilahti E. Undiagnosed coeliac disease is common in Finnish adults. *Scand J Gastroenterol* 1998; **33**: 1280–1283.

9. Fasano A, Berti I, Gerarduzzi T et al. Prevalence of celiac disease in at-risk and not at-risk groups in the United States. *Arch Intern Med* 2003; **163**: 286–292.
10. Catassi C, Tarsch IM, Gandolfi L et al. Why is coeliac disease endemic in the people of the Sahara? *Lancet* 1999; **354**: 647–648.
11. Shan L, Molberg O, Parrot I et al. Structural basis for gluten intolerance in celiac sprue. *Science* 2002; **297**: 2275–2279.
12. Schulzke JD, Bentzel CJ, Schulzke I et al. Epithelial tight junction structure in the jejunum of children with acute and treated celiac sprue. *Pediatr Res* 1998; **43**: 435–441.
13. Clemente M, De Virgiliis S, Kang JS et al. Early effects of gliadin on enterocyte intracellular signalling involved in intestinal barrier function. *Gut* 2003; **52**: 218–223.
14. Fasano A, Not T, Wang W et al. Zonulin, a newly discovered modulator of intestinal permeability, and its expression in coeliac disease. *Lancet* 2001; **355**: 1518–1519.
15. Maiuri L, Ciacci C, Ricciardelli I et al. Association between innate response to gliadin and activation of pathogenic T cells in coeliac disease. *Lancet* 2003; **362**: 30–37.
16. Anderson RP, Degano P, Godkin AJ et al. *In vivo* antigen challenge in celiac disease identifies a single transglutaminase-modified peptide as the dominant A-gliadin T-cell epitope. *Nature Med* 2000; **6**: 337–342.
17. Wucherpfennig K. Insights into autoimmunity gained from structural analysis of MHC–peptide complexes. *Curr Opin Immunol* 2001; **13**: 650–656.
18. Marsh MN. Gluten, major histocompatibility complex, and the small intestine. A molecular and immunobiologic approach to the spectrum of gluten sensitivity ('celiac sprue'). *Gastroenterology* 1992; **102**: 330–354.
19. Maiuri L, Ciacci C, Raia V et al. FAS engagement drives apoptosis of enterocytes of coeliac patients. *Gut* 2001; **48**: 418–424.
20. Maiuri L, Ciacci C, Auricchio S et al. Interleukin 15 mediates epithelial changes in celiac disease. *Gastroenterology* 2000; **119**: 996–1006.
21. Jabri B, de Serre NP, Cellier C et al. Selective expansion of intraepithelial lymphocytes expressing the HLA-E-specific natural killer receptor CD94 in celiac disease. *Gastroenterology* 2000; **118**: 867–879.
22. Visakorpi JK, Maki M. Changing clinical features of coeliac disease. *Acta Paediatr Suppl* 1994; **83**: 10–13.
23. Bottaro G, Cataldo F, Rotaolo N et al. The clinical pattern of subclinical/silent celiac disease: an analysis on 1026 consecutive cases. *Am J Gastroenterol* 1999; **94**: 691–696.
24. Andersson H, Mobacken H. Dietary treatment of dermatitis herpetiformis. *Eur J Clin Nutr* 1992; **46**: 309–315.
25. Collin P, Reunala T. Recognition and management of the cutaneous manifestations of celiac disease: a guide for dermatologists. *Am J Clin Dermatol* 2003; **4**: 13–20.
26. Aine L. Coeliac-type permanent-tooth enamel defects. *Ann Med* 1996; **28**: 9–12.
27. Mody RJ, Brown PI, Wechsler DS. Refractory iron deficiency anemia as the primary clinical manifestation of celiac disease. *J Pediatr Hematol Oncol* 2003; **25**: 169–172.
28. Corazza GR, Valentini RA, Andreani ML et al. Subclinical coeliac disease is a frequent cause of iron-deficiency anaemia. *Scand J Gastroenterol* 1995; **30**: 153–156.
29. Howard MR, Turnbull AJ, Morley P et al. A prospective study of the prevalence of undiagnosed coeliac disease in laboratory defined iron and folate deficiency. *J Clin Pathol* 2002; **55**: 754–757.
30. Stenhammar L, Fallstrom SP, Jansson G et al. Coeliac disease in children of short stature without gastrointestinal symptoms. *Eur J Pediatr* 1986; **145**: 185–186.
31. Tumer L, Hasanoglu A, Aybay C. Endomysium antibodies in the diagnosis of celiac disease in short-statured children with no gastrointestinal symptoms. *Pediatr Int* 2001; **43**: 71–73.
32. Smecuol E, Maurino E, Vazquez H et al. Gynaecological and obstetric disorders in coeliac disease: frequent clinical onset during pregnancy or the puerperium. *Eur J Gastroenterol Hepatol* 1996; **8**: 63–89.
33. Bardella MT, Fraquelli M, Quatrini et al. Prevalence of hypertransaminasemia in adult celiac patients and effect of gluten-free diet. *Hepatology* 1995; **22**: 833–836.
34. Volta U, De Franceschi L, Lari F et al. Coeliac disease hidden by cryptogenic hypertransaminasaemia. *Lancet* 1998; **352**: 26–29.
35. Kaukinen K, Halme L, Collin P et al. Celiac disease in patients with severe liver disease: gluten-free diet may reverse hepatic failure. *Gastroenterology* 2002; **122**: 881–888.
36. Lubrano E, Ciacci C, Ames PR et al. The arthritis of coeliac disease: prevalence and pattern in 200 adult patients. *Br J Rheumatol* 1996; **35**: 1314–1318.
37. Lepore L, Martelossi S, Pennesi M et al. Prevalence of celiac disease in patients with juvenile chronic arthritis. *J Pediatr* 1996; **129**: 311–313.
38. Kemppainen T, Kroger H, Janatuinen E et al. Osteoporosis in adult patients with celiac disease. *Bone* 1999; **24**: 249–255.
39. Meyer D, Stavropolous S, Diamond B et al. Osteoporosis in a north american adult population with celiac disease. *Am J Gastroenterol* 2001; **96**: 112–119.
40. Mustalahti K, Collin P, Sievanen H et al. Osteopenia in patients with clinically silent coeliac disease warrants screening. *Lancet* 1999; **354**: 744–745.
41. Vasquez H, Mazure R, Gonzalez D et al. Risk of fractures in celiac disease patients: a cross-sectional, case-control study. *Am J Gastroenterol* 2000; **95**: 183–189.
42. Scott E, Gaywood I, Scott B. Guidelines for osteoporosis in coeliac disease and inflammatory bowel disease. *Gut* 2000; **46(Suppl 1)**: 1–8.
43. Thomason K, West J, Logan RF et al. Fracture experience of patients with coeliac disease: a population based survey. *Gut* 2003; **52**: 518–522.
44. Kalayci A, Kansu A, Girgin N et al. Bone mineral density and importance of a gluten-free diet in patients with celiac disease in childhood. *Pediatrics* 2001; **108**: E89.
45. Kemppainen T, Kroger H, Janatuinen E et al. Bone recovery after a gluten-free diet: a 5-year follow-up study. *Bone* 1999; **25**: 355–360.
46. Sategna-Guidetti C, Grosso SB, Grosso S et al. The effects of 1-year gluten withdrawal on bone mass, bone metabolism and nutritional status in newly-diagnosed adult coeliac disease patients. *Aliment Pharmacol Ther* 2000; **14**: 35–43.
47. Sugai E, Chernavsky A, Pedreira S et al. Bone-specific antibodies in sera from patients with celiac disease: characterization and implications in osteoporosis. *J Clin Immunol* 2002; **22**: 353–362.
48. Hadjivassiliou M, Grunewald R, Sharrack B et al. Gluten ataxia in perspective: epidemiology, genetic susceptibility and clinical characteristics. *Brain* 2003; **126**: 685–691.
49. Gobbi G, Bouquet F, Greco L et al. Coeliac disease, epilepsy, and cerebral calcifications. The Italian

Working Group on Coeliac Disease and Epilepsy [see comments]. *Lancet* 1992; **340**: 439–443.

50. Kieslich M, Errazuriz G, Posselt HG et al. Brain white matter lesions in celiac disease: a prospective study of 75 diet-treated patients. *Pediatrics* 2001; **108**: E21.
51. Black C, Kaye J, Jick H. Relation of childhood gastrointestinal disorders to autism: nested case-control study using data from the UK General Practice Research Database. *BMJ* 2002; **325**: 419–421.
52. Ciacci C, Iavarone A, Mazzacca G, De Rosa A. Depressive symptoms in adult coeliac disease. *Scand J Gastroenterol* 1998; **33**: 247–250.
53. Addolorato G, Capristo E, Ghittoni G et al. Anxiety but not depression decreases in coeliac patients after one-year gluten-free diet: a longitudinal study. *Scand J Gastroenterol* 2001; **36**: 502–506.
54. Carta MG, Hardoy MC, Boi MF et al. Association between panic disorder, major depressive disorder and celiac disease: a possible role of thyroid autoimmunity. *J Psychosom Res* 2002; **53**: 789–793.
55. Collin P, Vilska S, Heinonen PK et al. Infertility and coeliac disease. *Gut* 1996; **39**: 382–384.
56. Ciacci C, Cirillo M, Auriemma G et al. Celiac disease and pregnancy outcome. *Am J Gastroenterol* 1996; **91**: 718–722.
57. Ludvigsson JF, Ludvigsson J. Coeliac disease in the father affects the newborn. *Gut* 2001; **49**: 169–175.
58. Petaros P, Martelossi S, Tommasini A et al. Prevalence of autoimmune disorders in relatives of patients with celiac disease. *Dig Dis Sci* 2002; **47**: 1427–1431.
59. Frustaci A, Cuoco L, Chimenti C et al. Celiac disease associated with autoimmune myocarditis. *Circulation* 2002; **105**: 2611–2618.
60. Ventura A, Magazzu G, Greco L. Duration of exposure to gluten and risk for autoimmune disorders in patients with celiac disease. SIGEP Study Group for Autoimmune Disorders in Celiac Disease. *Gastroenterology* 1999; **117**: 297–303.
61. James M, Scott B. Coeliac disease: the cause of the various associated disorders? *Eur J Gastroenterol Hepatol* 2001; **13**: 1119–1121.
62. Barera G, Bonfanti R, Viscardi M et al. Occurrence of celiac disease after onset of type 1 diabetes: a 6-year prospective longitudinal study. *Pediatrics* 2002; **109**: 833–838.
63. Holmes G. Coeliac disease and type 1 diabetes mellitus: the case for screening. *Diabet Med* 2001; **18**: 169–177.
64. Carlsson A, Axelsson I, Borulf S et al. Prevalence of IgA-antigliadin antibodies and IgA-antiendomysium antibodies related to celiac disease in children with Down syndrome. *Pediatrics* 1998; **101**: 272–275.
65. Gale L, Wimalaratna H, Brotodiharjo A, Duggan JM. Down's syndrome is strongly associated with coeliac disease. *Gut* 1997; **40**: 492–496.
66. Bonamico M, Mariani P, Danesi HM et al. Prevalence and clinical picture of celiac disease in italian down syndrome patients: a multicenter study. *J Pediatr Gastroenterol Nutr* 2001; **33**: 139–143.
67. Book L, Hart A, Black J et al. Prevalence and clinical characteristics of celiac disease in Downs syndrome in a US study. *Am J Med Genet* 2001; **98**: 70–74.
68. Zachor DA, Mroczek-Musulman E, Brown P. Prevalence of celiac disease in Down syndrome in the United States. *J Pediatr Gastroenterol Nutr* 2000; **31**: 275–279.
69. Csizmadia C, Mearin ML, Oren A et al. Accuracy and cost-effectiveness of a new strategy to screen for celiac disease in children with Down syndrome. *J Pediatr* 2000; **137**: 756–761.
70. Giannotti A, Tiberio G, Castro M et al. Coeliac disease in Williams syndrome. *J Med Genet* 2001; **38**: 767–768.
71. O'Grady JG, Steens FM, Harding B et al. Hyposplenism and gluten-sensitive enteropathy: natural history, incidence, and relationship to diet and small bowel morphology. *Gastroenterology* 1984; **87**: 1326–1331.
72. Wahnschaffe U, Ullrich R, Riecken EO, Schulzke JD. Celiac disease-like abnormalities in a subgroup of patients with irritable bowel syndrome. *Gastroenterology* 2001; **121**: 1329–1338.
73. Carroccio A, Iacono G, Montalto G et al. Pancreatic insufficiency in celiac disease is not dependent on nutritional status. *Dig Dis Sci* 1994; **39**: 2235–2242.
74. Carroccio A., Iacono G, Lerro P et al. Role of pancreatic impairment in growth recovery during gluten-free diet in childhood celiac disease. *Gastroenterology* 1997; **112** 1839–1844.
75. Carroccio A, Iacono G, Montalto G et al. Pancreatic enzyme therapy in childhood celiac disease. A double-blind prospective randomized study. *Dig Dis Sci* 1995; **40**: 2555–2560.
76. Cellier C, Delabesse E, Helmer C et al. Refractory sprue, coeliac disease, and enteropathy-associated T-cell lymphoma. French Coeliac Disease Study Group. *Lancet* 2000; **356**: 203–208.
77. Patey-Mariaud De Serre N, Cellier C, Jabri B et al. Distinction between coeliac disease and refractory sprue: a simple immunohistochemical method. *Histopathology* 2000; **37**: 70–77.
78. Longstreth GF. Successful treatment of refractory sprue with cyclosporine. *Ann Intern Med* 1993; **119**: 1014–1016.
79. Mandal A, Mayberry J. Elemental diet in the treatment of refractory coeliac disease. *Eur J Gastroenterol Hepatol* 2001; **13**: 79–80.
80. Maurino E, Niveloni S, Chernavsky A et al. Azathioprine in refractory sprue: results from a prospective, open-label study. *Am J Gastroenterol* 2002; **97**: 2595–2602.
81. Gillett HR, Amott ID, McIntyre M et al. Successful infliximab treatment for steroid-refractory celiac disease: a case report. *Gastroenterology* 2002; **122**: 800–805.
82. Mulder CJ, Wahab PJ Meijer JW et al. A pilot study of recombinant human interleukin-10 in adults with refractory coeliac disease. *Eur J Gastroenterol Hepatol* 2001; **13**: 1183–1188.
83. Wahab PJ, Crusius JB, Meijer JW et al. Cyclosporin in the treatment of adults with refractory coeliac disease – an open pilot study. *Aliment Pharmacol Ther* 2000; **14**: 767–774.
84. Holmes GK. Coeliac disease and malignancy. *Dig Liver Dis* 2002; **34**: 229–237.
85. Corrao G, Corazza GR, Bagnardi V et al. Mortality in patients with coeliac disease and their relatives: a cohort study. *Lancet* 2001; **358**: 356–361.
86. Meeuwisse G. Round table discussion. Diagnostic criteria in coeliac disease. *Acta Paediatr Scand* 1970; **59**: 461–463.
87. Guandalini S, Ventura A, Ansaldi N et al. Diagnosis of coeliac disease: time for a change? *Arch Dis Child* 1989; **64**: 1320–4; discussion 1324–5.
88. Working Group of European Society of Paediatric Gastroenterology and Nutrition. Revised criteria for diagnosis of coeliac disease. *Arch Dis Child* 1990; **65**: 909–911.
89. Guandalini S, Gupta P. Do you still need a biopsy to diagnose celiac disease? *Curr Gastroenterol Opin* 2001; **3**: 385–391

90. Jabbari M, Wild G, Goresky CA et al. Scalloped valvulae conniventes: an endoscopic marker of celiac sprue. *Gastroenterology* 1988; **95**: 1518–1522.
91. Shah VH, Rotterdam H, Kotler DP et al. All that scallops is not celiac disease. *Gastrointest Endosc* 2000; **51**: 717–720.
92. Maiuri L, Ciacci C, Raia V et al. FAS engagement drives apoptosis of enterocytes of coeliac patients. *Gut* 2001; **48**: 418–424.
93. Iltanen S, Hol, K, Ashom M et al. Changing jejunal gamma delta T cell receptor (TCR)-bearing intraepithelial lymphocyte density in coeliac disease. *Clin Exp Immunol* 1999; **117**: 51–55.
94. Arranz E, Ferguson A. Intestinal antibody pattern of celiac disease: occurrence in patients with normal jejunal biopsy histology. *Gastroenterology* 1993; **104**: 1263–1272.
95. Corazza G, Valentini RA, Frisoni et al. Gliadin immune reactivity is associated with overt and latent enteropathy in relatives of celiac patients. *Gastroenterology* 1992; **103**: 1517–1522.
96. Vazquez H, Cabanne A, Sugai E et al. Serological markers identify histologically latent coeliac disease among first-degree relatives. *Eur J Gastroenterol Hepatol* 1996; **8**: 15–21.
97. Collin P, Helin H, Maki M et al. Follow-up of patients positive in reticulin and gliadin antibody tests with normal small-bowel biopsy findings. *Scand J Gastroenterol* 1993; **28**: 595–598.
98. Niveloni S, Pedreira S, Sugai E et al. The natural history of gluten sensitivity: report of two new celiac disease patients resulting from a long-term follow-up of nonatrophic, first-degree relatives. *Am J Gastroenterol* 2000; **95**: 463–468.
99. Lerner A, Kumar V, Iancu TC. Immunological diagnosis of childhood coeliac disease: comparison between antigliadin, antireticulin and antiendomysial antibodies. *Clin Exp Immunol* 1994; **95**: 78–82.
100. Volta U, Lazzari R, Guidetti CS et al. Multicenter study on the reproducibility of antigliadin (AGA) and antiendomysial antibodies (EmA) in celiac sprue screening. The Tenue Club Group. *J Clin Gastroenterol* 1994; **19**: 81–82.
101. Murray JA, Herlein J, Mitros F et al. Serologic testing for celiac disease in the United States: results of a multilaboratory comparison study. *Clin Diagn Lab Immunol* 2000; **7**: 584–587.
102. Troncone R, Mayer M, Spagnuolo F et al. Endomysial antibodies as unreliable markers for slight dietary transgressions in adolescents with celiac disease. *J Pediatr Gastroenterol Nutr* 1995; **21**: 69–72.
103. Cataldo F, Marino V, Ventura A et al. Prevalence and clinical features of selective immunoglobulin A deficiency in coeliac disease: an Italian multicentre study. *Gut* 1998; **42**: 362–365.
104. Cataldo F, Lio D, Marino V et al. IgG(1) antiendomysium and IgG antitissue transglutaminase (anti-tTG) antibodies in coeliac patients with selective IgA deficiency. Working Groups on Celiac Disease of SIGEP and Club del Tenue. *Gut* 2000; **47**: 366–369.
105. Stern M. Comparative evaluation of serologic tests for celiac disease: a European initiative toward standardization. Working Group on Serologic Screening for Celiac Disease. *J Pediatr Gastroenterol Nutr* 2000; **31**: 513–519.
106. Dieterich W, Ehnis T, Bauer M et al. Identification of tissue transglutaminase as the autoantigen of celiac disease. *Nature Med* 1997; **3**: 797–801.
107. Dieterich W, Laag E, Schopper H et al. Autoantibodies to tissue transglutaminase as predictors of celiac disease. *Gastroenterology* 1998; **115**: 1317–1321.
108. Seissler J, Boms S, Wohlrab U et al. Antibodies to human recombinant tissue transglutaminase measured by radioligand assay: evidence for high diagnostic sensitivity for celiac disease. *Horm Metab Res* 1999; **31**: 375–379.
109. Sblattero D, Berti I, Trevisiol C et al. Human recombinant tissue transglutaminase ELISA: an innovative diagnostic assay for celiac disease. *Am J Gastroenterol* 2000; **95**: 1253-1257.
110. Hansson T, Dahlbom I, Hall J et al. Antibody reactivity against human and guinea pig tissue transglutaminase in children with celiac disease. *J Pediatr Gastroenterol Nutr* 2000; **30**: 379–384.
111. Baldas V, Tommasini A, Trevisiol C et al. Development of a novel rapid non-invasive screening test for coeliac disease. *Gut* 2000; **47**: 628–631.
112. Carroccio A, Vitale G, Di Prima L et al. Comparison of anti-transglutaminase ELISAs and an anti-endomysial antibody assay in the diagnosis of celiac disease: a prospective study. *Clin Chem* 2002; **48**: 1546–1550.
113. Janatuinen EK, Kemppainen TA, Julkunen RJ et al. No harm from five year ingestion of oats in coeliac disease. *Gut* 2002; **50**: 332–335.
114. Storsrud S, Olsson M, Arvidsson Lenner R et al. Adult coeliac patients do tolerate large amounts of oats. *Eur J Clin Nutr* 2003; **57**: 163–169.
115. Hardman CM, Garioch JJ, Leonard JN et al. Absence of toxicity of oats in patients with dermatitis herpetiformis. *N Engl J Med* 1997; **337**: 1884–1887.
116. Hoffenberg EJ, Haas J, Drescher A et al. A trial of oats in children with newly diagnosed celiac disease. *J Pediatr* 2000; **137**: 361–366.
117. Devos KM, Gale MD. Comparative genetics in the grasses. *Plant Mol Biol* 1997; **35**: 3–15.
118. Vader LW, de Ru A, van der Wal Y et al. Specificity of tissue transglutaminase explains cereal toxicity in celiac disease. *J Exp Med* 2002; **195**: 643–649.
119. Srinivasan U, Jones E, Weir DG et al. Lactase enzyme, detected immunohistochemically, is lost in active celiac disease, but unaffected by oats challenge. *Am J Gastroenterol* 1999; **94**: 2936–2941.
120. Catassi C, Rossini M, Ratsch IM et al. Dose dependent effects of protracted ingestion of small amounts of gliadin in coeliac disease children: a clinical and jejunal morphometric study. *Gut* 1993; **34**: 1515–1519.
121. Laurin P, Wolving M, Falth-Magnusson K. Even small amounts of gluten cause relapse in children with celiac disease. *J Pediatr Gastroenterol Nutr* 2002; **34**: 26–30.
122. Fabiani E, Catassi C, Villari A et al. Dietary compliance in screening-detected coeliac disease adolescents. *Acta Paediatr Suppl* 1996; **412**: 65–67.
123. Mayer M, Greco L, Troncome R et al. Compliance of adolescents with coeliac disease with a gluten free diet. *Gut* 1991; **32**: 881–885.
124. Mariani P, Viti MG, Monturori M et al. The gluten-free diet: a nutritional risk factor for adolescents with celiac disease? *J Pediatr Gastroenterol Nutr* 1998; **27**: 519–523.
125. Ciacci C, Cirillo M, Cavallaro R, Mazzacca G. Long-term follow-up of celiac adults on gluten-free diet: prevalence and correlates of intestinal damage. *Digestion* 2002; **66**: 178–185.
126. Mustalahti K, Lohiniemi S, Collin P et al. Gluten-free diet and quality of life in patients with screen-detected celiac disease. *Eff Clin Pract* 2002; **5**: 105–113.

28 Protein-losing enteropathy

Jorge Amil Dias and Eunice Trindade

Introduction

A number of pathological conditions cause excessive leakage of protein into the gastrointestinal tract. This common mechanism has been called protein-losing enteropathy (PLE) although the site of protein leakage may also be located in the stomach.

The major clinical features of these diseases are edema and hypoalbuminemia, as the intestinal loss outweighs protein synthesis, therefore causing reduced oncotic pressure in the vascular space. This mechanism is different from maldigestion or malabsorption where nutrients escape intestinal absorption, owing to enzyme deficiencies, or mucosal lesions.

Historically, the pioneer work of Albright et al[1] in 1949 showed that hypoalbuminemia in PLE was caused by excess catabolism of intravenous albumin rather than abnormal synthesis. Later, Citrin et al[2] demonstrated that the gastrointestinal tract was the site of the protein loss. Usually, the digestive tract (stomach or intestine) is the sole source of protein loss in PLE, although nephrotic syndrome may coexist in some cases.[3]

Albumin is a water-soluble molecule with molecular weight of 60 000 Da. This protein acts as the major component of plasma oncotic pressure and is also a transporter for various substances, such as bilirubin, ions, metals or hormones.

Synthesis of albumin occurs in the liver at a rate of approximately 150 mg/kg per day (higher in the first year of life: 180–300 mg/kg per day). In the absence of liver disease, synthesis depends mostly on protein intake, although hormones such as cortisol, thyroid hormone and insulin, also affect the rate of synthesis. Approximately one-third of the body albumin pool circulates in the intravascular space. In health, less than 10% of daily albumin degradation occurs through the gastrointestinal tract. However, in conditions causing PLE there is a marked leakage of protein into the bowel lumen, without an equivalent increase in hepatic synthesis. Reasons for increased loss of protein include lymphatic obstruction, mucosal inflammation and ulceration. When the loss of protein exceeds the limited hepatic adaptation there is a decrease in the vascular pool that leads to hypoalbuminemia and edema.

The loss of protein in the gastrointestinal tract is independent of molecular weight and includes albumin, immunoglobulins and ceruloplasmin; this is different from abnormal losses from the kidneys, where molecular weight determines which proteins are lost. In fact, in PLE there are also losses of minerals, such as iron, copper and calcium, of lipids and even of cells, such as lymphocytes. However, most of these proteins are readily digested in the gut and the resulting amino acids are reabsorbed by the intact segments of bowel and reused for protein synthesis. The plasma levels of different proteins in PLE depend on the adaptative capacity to increase synthesis. As mentioned before, there is little response from the liver in albumin production and the same occurs with IgG, IgM or IgA. On the other hand, the plasma levels of proteins with increased turnover, such as IgE or insulin, may be sustained despite intestinal loss.

In conditions affecting the lymphatic system, such as intestinal lymphangiectasia, there may also be lymphocyte losses leading to lymphopenia.[4–6]

Signs and symptoms of conditions associated with PLE may reflect the cause for hypoproteinemia. However, the common link among these diseases is the loss of proteins causing hypoalbuminemia and edema. As mentioned before, albumin is the major element for oncotic pressure but there may be loss of other proteins. Although decrease in immunoglobulins, transferrin or ceruloplasmin may be documented by biochemical assay, rarely are there clinical manifestations from these abnormalities. If lymphatic obstruction is the major cause of PLE then malabsorption of fat may occur.

Investigations

Assessing protein loss from the gastrointestinal tract is not easy, because proteins secreted into the gut are readily degraded and reabsorbed. Therefore, alternative methods have been designed. One approach makes use of proteins tagged with radioactive labels injected intravenously. Several markers were used in the past (iodine,[7,8] chromium,[9,10] iron[11] and niobium[12]) bound to several proteins, usually albumin, but also dextran or ceruloplasmin. Assessment of protein loss can be made by plasma clearance or stool content of the marker. However, these studies apart from demanding several days' collections of stool or blood, had other drawbacks. It was required that the marker should not alter the metabolic pathway of the protein, that it should not be reabsorbed from the intestine and that it should not be excreted by the glands into the digestive fluids. The radiolabels used fulfill most of these aims, but calculations of catabolic rate are complex and stools free of urine must be collected for several days. These requirements, and the questionable use of radioactive elements, made these methods unpopular in pediatrics.

The other approach to diagnosis made use of a protein resistant to digestive proteolysis. Crossley and Elliott[13] suggested α_1-antitrypsin for this purpose. This protein has a molecular weight of 50 000 Da, similar to albumin, and is resistant to proteolysis, therefore fulfilling the required needs. Several studies compared this method with the radiolabel tests and confirmed that it gave reliable results.[14–16] However, α_1-antitrypsin may be degraded in the stomach by acid, and therefore has limited value in the assessment of gastric losses.

The method has been widely accepted for clinical purposes. The contamination of collected stools with urine is not a problem, as the protein is not eliminated in urine. For exact assessment of α_1-antitrypsin enteric loss, 24–72 h of stool collection may be required. Clearance is calculated by the formula:

$$Clearance = \frac{(\text{fecal } \alpha_1\text{-antitryspin concentration}) \times (\text{24-h stool volume})}{(\text{serum } \alpha_1\text{-antitryspin concentration})}$$

However, it has been proposed that random sample determination also gives reliable results for clinical use.[17,18] Magazzu et al also showed that stools may be heat-dried rather than lyophilized, with comparable results, thus adding further simplicity to the method. The normal value of α_1-antitrypsin is below 3–4 mg/g dry stools.[14,17] In some conditions there may be overestimation of protein loss from the assessment of α_1-antitrypsin: in normal newborns, α_1-antitrypsin may be increased in stools probably owing to meconium clearance of the gut[19]; gross bleeding into the gastrointestinal tract may lead to a measurable amount of the protein in the stools.[16]

If the protein exudation comes from abnormal lymphatics, as in intestinal lymphangiectasia, imaging techniques may help locate the lesion. Several methods, such as lymphangiography, contrast radiology and computed tomography (CT) have been used. This will be discussed below under specific conditions.

Diseases causing protein-losing enteropathy

The main causes are shown in Table 28.1.

Diseases related to lymphatics

Intestinal lymphangiectasia

This disease affects males and females equally and may present from birth, although the mean age is 11 years. Even prenatal diagnosis has been reported.[20] Most cases are sporadic.

Several rare diseases and syndromes have associated dyplasia of lymphatics leading to PLE. These include nephrotic syndrome[3] and other rare conditions (Table 28.2).[21–23] Familial clustering suggests genetic etiology at least in some cases with early onset of manifestations.[8]

Patients have abnormally dilated lymphatics in the mucosa, submucosa or subserosa that cause

Table 28.1 Main causes of protein-losing enteropathy

Related to lymphatics
Primary
intestinal lymphangiectasia
Secondary
cardiac disease
constrictive pericarditis
congestive heart failure
cardiomyopathy
post-Fontan procedure
obstruction of lymphatics
vena cava obstruction
tuberculosis
sarcoidosis
radiation therapy
retroperitoneal fibrosis or tumor
Related to mucosa
Gastroenteritis
Crohn's disease
Celiac disease
Parasitosis (e.g. *Giardia*)
Ménétrier's disease
Eosinophilic gastritis
Graft-versus-host disease
Langerhan's histiocytosis
Vasculitides
Systemic lupus erythematosus
Connective diseases
Henoch–Schönlein purpura
Vena cava obstruction
Related to defective cellular synthesis
Deficiency of enterocyte heparan sulfate
Congenital disorders of glycosylation

leakage of lymphatic fluid and cells into the gut, thus causing PLE with hypoproteinemia, hypogammaglobulinemia and lymphopenia, especially depletion of CD4 T cells.[5] This may lead to abnormal delayed hypersensitivity skin tests or reduced allograft rejection tests,[4,24] but these patients do not appear to be more sensitive to infections. Hyposplenism, thymic hypoplasia and neutrophil dysfunction have also been reported.[25–27]

Signs and symptoms include edema that may be asymmetric, variable diarrhea and steatorrhea related to impaired fat absorption by abnormal lymphatics. Leakage of fluid into other body cavities may also cause chylous effusions such as ascites that may lead to intestinal adhesions and obstruction. Reversible blindness has been reported, due to macular edema. Tetany secondary to hypocalcemia can occur and is usually associated with severe steatorrhea. Growth restriction reflects the increased loss of protein and other elements. The presence of a lymphatic–venous anastomosis may also cause gastrointestinal bleeding.[28]

Table 28.2 Uncommon causes of protein-losing enteropathy

Noonan's syndrome[21]
Congenital glaucoma
Peliosis hepatis
Charcot–Marie–Tooth syndrome
Klippel–Trénaunay–Weber syndrome
Hennekam syndrome[22]
Hypobetalipoproteinemia[23]

Examination of patients may be unremarkable except for edema and malnutrition. The coexistence of hypoalbuminemia, edema, lymphopenia and steatorrhea may suggest the diagnosis. Tetany may also be present, related to hypocalcemia. Fat-soluble vitamins may be deficient.

Demonstration of intestinal protein loss can be made from increased α_1-antitrypsin in stools. A number of imaging techniques have been used to demonstrate the effects of abnormal intestinal lymphatics or to show localization of segmental disease. Lymphangiography may show abnormal lymphatics, absence of the thoracic duct or drainage of contrast into the bowel, but this procedure is difficult to perform in children. Contrast radiology with barium may reveal thickening of intestinal folds, or flocculation of barium due to intestinal hypersecretion. The use of radiolabeled Tc-99m incorporated in to a microcolloid may show localized accumulation of the marker on scintigraphy. CT may also show signs suggestive of intestinal lesions causing PLE.[29–31] The use of CT may even allow identification of segmental lymphangiectasia, as recently reported.[32]

When the proximal intestine is involved, endoscopy may show an abnormal mucosal pattern with scattered white plaques (Figure 28.1a). Diagnosis may then be confirmed from biopsy specimens showing subepithelial dilated lacteals (Figure 28.1b). Although a small intestinal biopsy would reveal these typical features, there are some limitations: the use of a biopsy capsule may miss the lesion, owing to its focal distribution, making endoscopic guidance preferable when the diagnosis is suspected; and normal histology does not preclude the diagnosis in patients on a low-fat diet or with deeper lesions not available to superficial mucosal biopsy.

Treatment When disease is confined to a segment of intestine, surgery may be curative by resecting the affected part or allowing anastomosis of abnormal lymphatics to the circulatory system. Unfortunately, surgical treatment is not available for the majority of patients and reducing the lymphatic flow may decrease the leak into the gut. This may be achieved by reducing the intake of long-chain fatty acids. Medium-chain triglycerides (6–10 atoms of carbon) are absorbed and passed directly into the portal vein and bypass the lymphatic system. Therefore, part of the dietary lipid may be given using medium-chain triglycerides as oil or in formulas. It must be kept in mind that medium-chain triglycerides do not contain essential fatty acids and some long-chain fatty acids must be ingested regularly. The diet should contain high protein to circumvent ongoing minor losses.

Dietary treatment must be permanent and guided by clinical symptoms. As mentioned above, other losses must be born in mind, and supplementation with calcium and vitamins, both water-soluble and fat-soluble must be provided. Octreotide has

(a) (b)

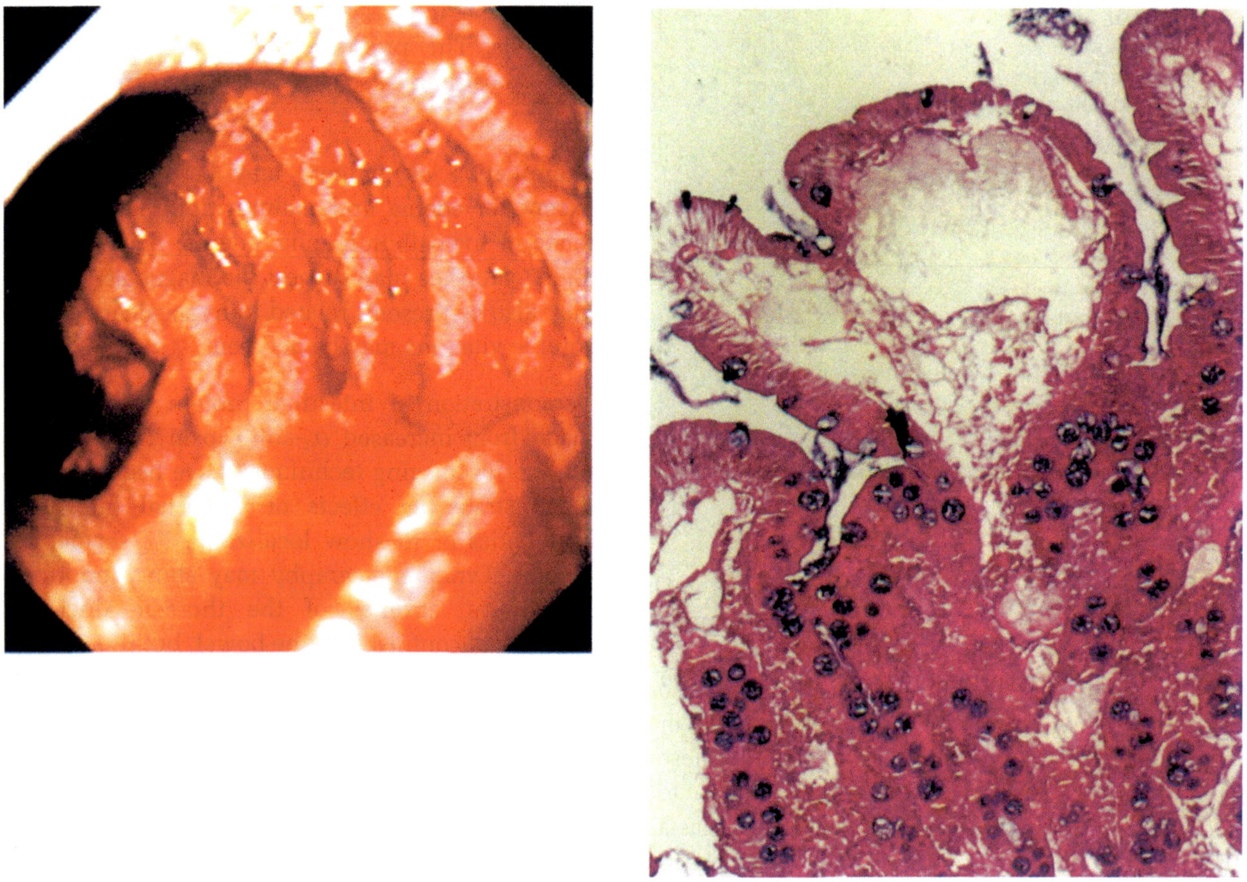

Figure 28.1 Intestinal lymphangiectasia. (a) Endoscopic view of duodenum showing numerous dilated lymphatics within the mucosa. (b) Histology of the small intestine of the same patient with a dilated lymphatic along the villus axis and normal surface epithelium. (Courtesy of F. Pereira).

shown effects in reducing the thoracic duct lymph flow and fluid loss in the enteric vasculature.[33] This effect has been used to treat patients with considerable success.[34]

In the rare occurrence of gastrointestinal bleeding, the beneficial effect of the low-fat diet may be enough to reduce the vascular pressure causing hemorrhage.[28] In adults antiplasmin therapy was reported in patients with persisting bleeding[35] but this has not been used in children.

Protein-losing enteropathy secondary to increased lymphatic pressure

PLE may arise from increased lymphatic pressure that causes leakage of fluid and protein into the bowel. This has been widely known after the Fontan operation for complex congenital cardiac disease. In this procedure the systemic venous circulation is directly connected to the pulmonary veins, bypassing the abnormal heart; the left ventricle is the only pumping mechanism for circulation. Therefore, there is an overall increase in venous pressure and lymphatic pressure causing congestion and leakage of fluid. PLE has been reported in 2.5–10% of patients.[36] The pathophysiology of PLE in this situation is not fully known, although mechanisms have been proposed, such as raised central venous pressure and increase in mesenteric vascular resistance.[37] A longer cardiopulmonary bypass time and single right ventricle anatomy may be risk factors.[38]

The first symptoms may occur weeks to years after the operation and severity is variable determining morbidity and mortality.[39] Common signs and symptoms are similar to other forms of PLE. Edema is the most frequent; half of affected patients have diarrhea and one-third also have steatorrhea. Investigations reveal hypoproteinemia, hypoalbuminemia, hypogammaglobulinemia, increased α_1-antitrypsin and fat in stools. There may also be dilatation of intestinal lymphatics similar to intestinal lymphangiectasia.[8] Immunological alterations have also been described, although these may be quantitative rather than qualitative.[40]

The therapeutic strategy in affected patients depends on the severity of each case. Diuretics, albumin infusions and nutritional supplementation with protein and medium-chain triglycerides may provide symptomatic relief. Conversion enzyme inhibitors, e.g. captopril, reduce afterload pressure and facilitate hemodynamic improvement. Stabilization of intestinal membranes with high doses of steroids[41,42] or high molecular heparin[43–45] showed improvement in protein loss. Various vascular surgical options including cardiac transplantation have also been used.[46,47]

Other cardiac and vascular diseases causing elevation of systemic pressure may lead to PLE: constrictive pericarditis, restrictive cardiomyopathy, congenital pulmonary stenosis, ventricular septal defect, tricuspid regurgitation in rheumatic disease[48] and vena cava obstruction.[49]

Protein-losing enteropathy related to the mucosa

Diseases causing extensive lesions of the gastric or intestinal mucosa may damage the mucosal barrier and allow leakage of protein. Common intestinal infections such as rotavirus gastroenteritis, giardiasis or shigellosis usually cause mild protein loss that can be documented[50–52] but the magnitude of the loss is proportional to the severity of the mucosal lesion. Crohn's disease also causes PLE although the level of stool α_1-antitrypsin does not correlate with disease activity.[53,54]

Patients with untreated celiac disease also may have PLE.[55] Langerhans histiocytosis usually does not involve the intestine but in rare instances may cause severe lesions in the mucosa with considerable loss of albumin (Figure 28.2).[56,57]

In food allergy there may be involvement of the stomach, causing PLE.[58] In these patients there are the common features of increased protein loss – edema, microcytic anemia due to iron loss, hypoalbuminemia, hypogammaglobulinemia – plus eosinophilia. Digestive symptoms may be mild and particularly related to the ingestion of the offending foods. Other signs and symptoms of allergy, such as eczema, asthma and rhinitis, as well as a positive family history may help in directing the diagnosis. Gastric and intestinal biopsy may show an eosinophilic infiltrate of the lamina propria. Patients usually recover on a restricted diet, usually cow's milk-free.

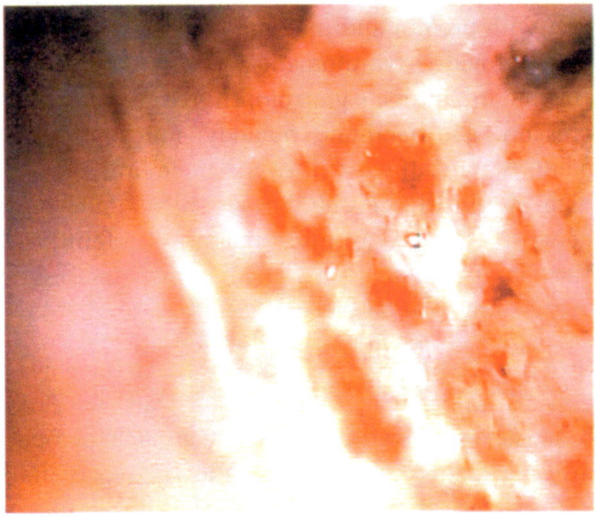

Figure 28.2 Langerhan's histiocytosis. Endoscopy of the duodenum revealing multiple mucosal erosions.

Ménétrier's disease

Ménétrier's disease is a particular form of gastropathy causing PLE. It is usually caused by cytomegalovirus infection, although there may be an underlying abnormality of regulation of gastric epithelial growth, as suggested by animal models and clinical evidence.[59,60] Most cases occur before 10 years of age. Clinical manifestations include digestive symptoms – vomiting, abdominal pain and edema. Laboratory investigations show mild anemia and hypoalbuminemia without proteinuria. As mentioned above, the use of stool α_1-antitrypsin to demonstrate digestive protein loss may not be used in this case because of the rapid inactivation in the acidic gastric environment. In this case it may be necessary to use radiolabeled proteins. Ultrasonographic and radiological patterns have been described to reveal the thickened gastric folds but endoscopy is the method of choice as it reveals abnormal inflamed folds covered with thick mucus and allows diagnostic biopsy (Figure 28.3).

Vasculitides

Among uncommon causes of PLE, syndromes due to vasculitic processes (vasculitides; see also Chapter 26) have been described. Systemic lupus erythematosus (SLE) involves various organs, but the digestive system is seldom involved. However, various cases have been reported starting in childhood. PLE may occur before the diagnosis of SLE or present years later.[61,62] The likely pathophysiology of PLE is probably immunological involving cytokines rather than mechanical disruption of lymphatics.[63,64] Clinical manifestations are similar to other forms of PLE, namely abdominal pain, diarrhea, edema and hypoalbuminemia. Diagnosis rests on demonstration of increased protein loss. Intestinal biopsy may show lymphangiectasia. Interestingly, these patients

(a) (b)

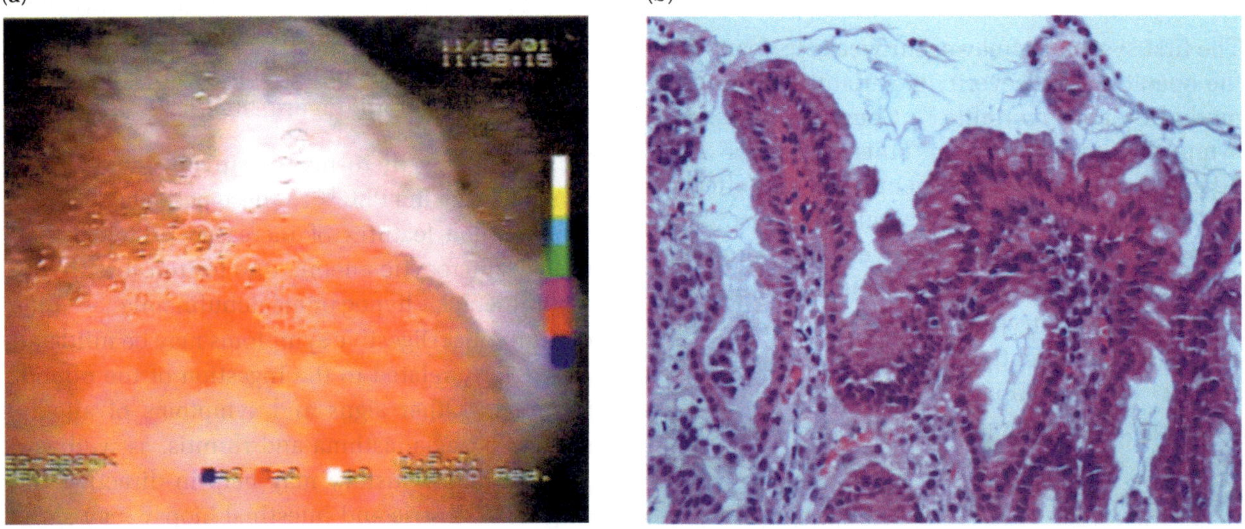

Figure 28.3 Ménétrier's disease. (a) Endoscopic view of the stomach showing inflamed mucosa of thickened folds covered by a thick layer of viscous mucus. (b) Histology of the stomach of the same patient. There is marked elongation and tortuosity of the gastric pits with cystic dilatation of some glands. (Courtesy of F. Carneiro).

may respond to steroids without relapse after stopping treatment. In severe cases pulses of cyclophosphamide,[65] plasmapheresis[66] and octreotide[67] have been used.

PLE has also been associated with Henoch–Schönlein purpura in as many as 1.3% of cases.[68,69] It may be underdiagnosed, especially in severe multivisceral cases.

Protein-losing enteropathy related to defective cellular synthesis

Recent advances in molecular biology have uncovered the etiology of many previously unclarified conditions and allowed reclassification of some diseases.[70]

The epithelial expression of sulfated glycosaminoglycans (GAGs) seems to be essential in the maintenance of albumin homeostasis. This expression may be compromised in inflammatory states. Congenital defects may cause absence of synthesis,[71] and congenital glycosylation defects may lead to mislocation of sulfated GAGs.[72] This group of diseases must also be considered in otherwise unexplained PLE, as the histology may be unspecific.

Deficiency of enterocyte heparan sulfate

Deficiency of enterocyte heparan sulfate is a rare cause of congenital severe PLE described by Murch et al[71] in three patients with malabsorption, secretory diarrhea and normal intestinal histology. There was almost complete absence of sulfated GAGs in the basolateral membrane of enterocytes despite normal distribution in vascular cells and in the lamina propria. The pathophysiology is probably similar to that of congenital nephrotic syndrome, where protein loss is due to decreased negative charges of heparan sulfate.[73] The reduced expression of sulfated GAGs allows abundant loss of albumin and water due to the reduced electrostatic interaction between anion sites of GAG and arginine residues within the albumin molecules.[74,75]

Congenital disorders of glycosylation

Congenital disorders of glycosylation are multisystemic diseases with variable clinical expression and several subtypes. The common feature is the alteration of *N*-glycosylation which may be defective in several points. This is a fundamental mechanism that regulates protein folding and allows intracellular quality control.[76,77] Most secretory and membrane proteins require glycosylation for proper folding and subsequent transport via the secretory pathway. In congenital disorders of glycosylation there is underglycosylation of several proteins including antithrombin III, factor IX or protein C, leading to cytoplasmic retention of the abnormal protein. The common screening test is identification of carbohydrate transferrin deficiency by isoelectric focusing analysis of serum transferrin. It is likely that the high turnover rate of epithelial cells may render them particularly vulnerable to this type of disease.[72] PLE is common in congenital disorders of glycosylation type 1b (mutation of phosphomannose isomerase) and type 1c (mutation of α-1,3-glucosyltransferase).[72,78] Patients with type 1b have severe diarrhea, vomiting and PLE. Intestinal biopsy shows partial villous atrophy, and the enterocyte endoplasmic reticulum is distended and engorged with precipitated abnormal protein. Mannose is effective in the treatment of these patients, correcting both symptoms and biochemical abnormalities.[79,80]

Patients with congenital disorders of glycosylation type 1c have variable clinical expression and may present features of types 1a and 1b. Westphal et al described one patient with recurrent PLE after acute gastroenteritis starting at the age of 3 months. Intestinal biopsies showed marked reduction of epithelial heparan sulfate in the basolateral membrane during exacerbations and normalization in remission.[72] It is probable that increased cellular turnover during exacerbations cause intracellular retention rather than defective synthesis. The authors speculated that the already inefficient glycosylation was overwhelmed by the increased epithelial turnover in gastroenteritis, effectively leading to complete loss of heparan sulfate in the small-intestinal epithelium. Heparin may have a role in the stabilization of the cellular membrane.

REFERENCES

1. Albright F, Bartter FC, Forbes AP. The fate of human serum albumin administered intravenously to a patient with idiopathic hypoalbuminemia and hypoglobulinemia. *Trans Assoc Am Phys* 1949; **62**: 204
2. Citrin Y, Sterling K, Halsted J. Mechanisms of hypoproteinemia associated with giant hypertrophy of gastric mucosa. *N Engl J Med* 1957; **257**: 906–912
3. de Sousa JS, Guerreiro O, Cunha A et al. Association of nephrotic syndrome with intestinal lymphangiectasia. *Arch Dis Child* 1968; **43**: 245–248.
4. Weiden PL, Blaese RM, Strober W et al. Impaired lymphocyte transformation in intestinal lymphangiectasia: evidence for at least two functionally distinct lymphocyte populations in man. *J Clin Invest* 1972; **51**: 1319–1325.
5. Fuss IJ, Strober W, Cuccherini BA et al. Intestinal lymphangiectasia, a disease characterized by selective loss of naive CD45RA+ lymphocytes into the gastrointestinal tract. *Eur J Immunol* 1998; **28**: 4275–4285.
6. Arato A, Savilahti E, Balogh L. The distribution of lymphocyte subpopulations in an infant with primary intestinal lymphangiectasia. *Acta Paediatr Hung* 1992; **32**: 309–317.
7. Gordon RSJ. Exudative enteropathy: abnormal permeability of the gastrointestinal tract demonstrable with labelled polyvinylpyrrolidone. *Lancet* 1959; **1**: 325–326.
8. Waldmann TA. Protein-losing gastroenteropathies. In Haubrich WS, Kalser MA, Roth, JL et al., eds. *Bockus Gastroenterology*, vol 4. Philadelphia: WB Saunders, 1985: 1814–1837.
9. van Tongeren JH, Reichert WJ. Demonstration of protein-losing gastroenteropathy. The quantitative estimation of gastrointestinal protein loss, using ^{51}Cr-labelled plasma proteins. *Clin Chim Acta* 1966; **14**: 42–48.
10. Waldmann TA, Wochner RD, Strober W. The role of the gastrointestinal tract in plasma protein metabolism. Studies with ^{51}Cr-albumin. *Am J Med* 1969; **46**: 275–285.
11. Jarnum S, Westergaard H, Yssing M et al. Quantitation of gastrointestinal protein loss by means of FE59-labeled iron dextran. *Gastroenterology* 1968; **55**: 229–241.
12. Jeejeebhoy KN, Jarnum S, Singh B et al. ^{95}Nb-labelled albumin for the study of gastrointestinal albumin loss. *Scand J Gastroenterol* 1968; **3**: 449–457.
13. Crossley JR, Elliott RB. Simple method for diagnosing protein-losing enteropathies. *Br Med J* 1977; **1**: 428–429.
14. Bernier JJ, Florent C, Desmazures C et al. Diagnosis of protein-losing enteropathy by gastrointestinal clearance of alpha1-antitrypsin. *Lancet* 1978; **2**: 763–764.
15. Hill RE, Hercz A, Corey ML et al. Fecal clearance of alpha 1-antitrypsin: a reliable measure of enteric protein loss in children. *J Pediatr* 1981; **99**: 416–418.
16. Thomas DW, Sinatra FR, Merritt RJ. Random fecal alpha-1-antitrypsin concentration in children with gastrointestinal disease. *Gastroenterology* 1981; **80**: 776–782.
17. Magazzu G, Jacono G, Di Pasquale G et al. Reliability and usefulness of random fecal alpha 1-antitrypsin concentration: further simplification of the method. *J Pediatr Gastroenterol Nutr* 1985; **4**: 402–407.
18. Catassi C, Cardinali E, D'Angelo G et al. Reliability of random fecal alpha 1-antitrypsin determination on nondried stools. *J Pediatr* 1986; **109**: 500–502.
19. Keller KM, Knobel R, Ewe K. Fecal alpha 1-antitrypsin in newborn infants. *J Pediatr Gastroenterol Nutr* 1997; **24**: 271–275.
20. Schmider A, Henrich W, Reles A et al. Isolated fetal ascites caused by primary lymphangiectasia: a case report. *Am J Obstet Gynecol* 2001; **184**: 227–228.
21. Vallet HL, Holtzapple PG, Eberlein WR et al. Noonan syndrome with intestinal lymphangiectasis. A metabolic and anatomic study. *J Pediatr* 1972; **80**: 269–274.
22. Van Balkom ID, Alders M, Allanson J et al. Lymphedema-lymphangiectasia-mental retardation (Hennekam) syndrome: a review. *Am J Med Genet* 2002; **112**: 412–421.
23. Dobbins WO 3rd. Hypo-beta-lipoproteinemia and intestinal lymphangiectasia. A new syndrome of malabsorption and protein-losing enteropathy. *Arch Intern Med* 1968; **122**: 31–38.
24. Strober W, Wochner RD, Carbone PP et al. Intestinal lymphangiectasia: a protein-losing enteropathy with hypogammaglobulinemia, lymphocytopenia and impaired homograft rejection. *J Clin Invest* 1967; **46**: 1643–1656.
25. Foster PN, Bullen AW, Robertson DA et al. Development of impaired splenic function in intestinal lymphangiectasia. *Gut* 1985; **26**: 861–864.
26. Sorensen RU, Halpin TC, Abramowsky CR et al. Intestinal lymphangiectasia and thymic hypoplasia. *Clin Exp Immunol* 1985 **59**: 217–226.
27. Bolton RP, Cotter KL, Losowsky MS. Impaired neutrophil function in intestinal lymphangiectasia. *J Clin Pathol* 1986; **39**: 876–880.
28. Perisic VN, Kokai G. Bleeding from duodenal lymphangiectasia. *Arch Dis Child* 1991; **66**: 153–154.
29. Fakhri A, Fishman EK, Jones B et al. Primary intestinal lymphangiectasia: clinical and CT findings. *J Comput Assist Tomogr* 1985; **9**: 767–770.
30. Puri AS, Aggarwal R, Gupta RK et al. Intestinal lymphangiectasia: evaluation by CT and scintigraphy. *Gastrointest Radiol* 1992; **17**: 119–121.
31. Stevens RL, Jones B, Fishman EK. The CT halo sign: a new finding in intestinal lymphangiectasia. *J Comput Assist Tomogr* 1997; **21**: 1005–1007.
32. Yang DM, Jung DH. Localized intestinal lymphangiectasia: CT findings. *Am J Roentgenol* 2003; **180**: 213–214.
33. Nakabayashi H, Sagara H, Usukura N et al. Effect of somatostatin on the flow rate and triglyceride levels of thoracic duct lymph in normal and vagotomized dogs. *Diabetes* 1981; **30**: 440–445.
34. Ballinger AB, Farthing MJ. Octreotide in the treatment of intestinal lymphangiectasia. *Eur J Gastroenterol Hepatol* 1998; **10**: 699–702.
35. MacLean JE, Cohen E, Weinstein M. Primary intestinal and thoracic lymphangiectasia: a response to antiplasmin therapy. *Pediatrics* 2002; **109**: 1177–1180.
36. Mertens L, Hagler DJ, Sauer U et al. Protein-losing enteropathy after the Fontan operation: an international multicenter study. PLE Study Group. *J Thorac Cardiovasc Surg* 1998; **115**: 1063–1073.
37. Rychik J, Spray TL. Strategies to treat protein-losing enteropathy. *Semin Thorac Cardiovasc Surg Pediatr Card Surg Annu* 2002; **5**: 3–11.
38. Powell AJ, Gauvreau K, Jenkins KJ et al. Perioperative risk factors for development of protein-losing enteropathy following a Fontan procedure. *Am J Cardiol* 2001; **88**: 1206–1209.

39. Marino BS. Outcomes after the Fontan procedure. *Curr Opin Pediatr* 2002; **14**: 620–626.
40. Cheung YF, Tsang HY, Kwok JS. Immunologic profile of patients with protein-losing enteropathy complicating congenital heart disease. *Pediatr Cardiol* 2002 **23**: 587–593.
41. Rychik J, Piccoli DA, Barber G. Usefulness of corticosteroid therapy for protein-losing enteropathy after the Fontan procedure. *Am J Cardiol* 1991; **68**: 819–821.
42. Zellers TM, Brown K. Protein-losing enteropathy after the modified fontan operation: oral prednisone treatment with biopsy and laboratory proved improvement. *Pediatr Cardiol* 1996; **17**: 115–117.
43. Donnelly JP, Rosenthal A, Castle VP et al. Reversal of protein-losing enteropathy with heparin therapy in three patients with univentricular hearts and Fontan palliation. *J Pediatr* 1997; **130**: 474–478.
44. Kelly AM, Feldt RH, Driscoll DJ et al. Use of heparin in the treatment of protein-losing enteropathy after fontan operation for complex congenital heart disease. *Mayo Clin Proc* 1998; **73**: 777–779.
45. Facchini M, Guldenschuh I, Turina J et al. Resolution of protein-losing enteropathy with standard high molecular heparin and urokinase after Fontan repair in a patient with tricuspid atresia. *J Cardiovasc Surg (Torino)* 2000; **41**: 567–570.
46. Rychik J. Management of protein-losing enteropathy after the Fontan procedure. *Semin Thorac Cardiovasc Surg Pediatr Card Surg Annu* 1998; **1**: 15–22.
47. Holmgren D, Berggren H, Wahlander H et al. Reversal of protein-losing enteropathy in a child with Fontan circulation is correlated with central venous pressure after heart transplantation. *Pediatr Transplant* 2001; **5**: 135–137.
48. Nelson DL, Blaese RM, Strober W et al. Constrictive pericarditis, intestinal lymphangiectasia, and reversible immunologic deficiency. *J Pediatr* 1975; **86**: 548–554.
49. Lee WS, John P, McKiernan P et al. Inferior vena cava occlusion and protein-losing enteropathy after liver transplantation in children. *J Pediatr Gastroenterol Nutr* 2002; **34**: 413–416.
50. Maki M, Harmoinen A, Vesikari T et al. Faecal excretion of alpha-1-antitrypsin in acute diarrhoea. *Arch Dis Child* 1982; **57**: 154–156.
51. Sutton DL, Kamath KR. Giardiasis with protein-losing enteropathy. *J Pediatr Gastroenterol Nutr* 1985 **4**: 56–59.
52. Bennish ML, Salam MA, Wahed MA. Enteric protein loss during shigellosis. *Am J Gastroenterol* 1993; **88**: 53–57.
53. Grill BB, Hillemeier AC, Gryboski JD. Fecal alpha 1-antitrypsin clearance in patients with inflammatory bowel disease. *J Pediatr Gastroenterol Nutr* 1984; **3**: 56–61.
54. Karbach U, Ewe K, Bodenstein H. Alpha 1-antitrypsin, a reliable endogenous marker for intestinal protein loss and its application in patients with Crohn's disease. *Gut* 1983; **24**: 718–723.
55. Dinari G, Rosenbach Y, Zahavi I et al. Random fecal alpha 1-antitrypsin excretion in children with intestinal disorders. *Am J Dis Child* 1984; **138**: 971–973.
56. Boccon-Gibod LA, Krichen HA, Carlier-Mercier LA et al. Digestive tract involvement with exudative enteropathy in Langerhans cell histiocytosis. *Pediatr Pathol* 1992; **12**: 515–524.
57. Santos-Machado TM, Cristofani LM, Almeida MT et al. Disseminated Langerhans' cell histiocytosis and massive protein-losing enteropathy. *Braz J Med Biol Res* 1999; **32**: 1095–1099.
58. Waldmann TA, Wochner RD, Laster L et al. Allergic gastroenteropathy. A cause of excessive gastrointestinal protein loss. *N Engl J Med* 1967; **276**: 762–769.
59. Dempsey PJ, Goldenring JR, Soroka CJ et al. Possible role of transforming growth factor alpha in the pathogenesis of Menetrier's disease: supportive evidence from humans and transgenic mice. *Gastroenterology* 1992; **103**: 1950–1963.
60. Sferra TJ, Pawel BR, Qualman SJ et al. Menetrier disease of childhood: role of cytomegalovirus and transforming growth factor alpha. *J Pediatr* 1996; **128**: 213–219.
61. Molina JF, Brown RF, Gedalia A et al. Protein losing enteropathy as the initial manifestation of childhood systemic lupus erythematosus. *J Rheumatol* 1996; **23**: 1269–1271.
62. Tsukahara M, Matsuo K, Kojima H. Protein-losing enteropathy in a boy with systemic lupus erythematosus. *J Pediatr* 1980; **97**: 778–780.
63. Edworthy SM, Fritzler MJ, Kelly JK et al. Protein-losing enteropathy in systemic lupus erythematosus associated with intestinal lymphangiectasia. *Am J Gastroenterol* 1990; **85**: 1398–1402.
64. Yazici Y, Erkan D, Levine DM et al. Protein-losing enteropathy in systemic lupus erythematosus: report of a severe, persistent case and review of pathophysiology. *Lupus* 2002; **11**: 119–123.
65. Lee CK, Han JM, Lee KN et al. Concurrent occurrence of chylothorax, chylous ascites, and protein-losing enteropathy in systemic lupus erythematosus. *J Rheumatol* 2002; **29**: 1330–1333.
66. Garcia-Consuegra J, Merino R, Alonso A et al. Systemic lupus erythematosus: a case report with unusual manifestations and favourable outcome after plasmapheresis. *Eur J Pediatr* 1992; **151**: 581–582.
67. Ossandon A, Bombardieri M, Coari G et al. Protein losing enteropathy in systemic lupus erythematosus: role of diet and octreotide. *Lupus* 2002; **11**: 465–466.
68. Reif S, Jain A, Santiago J et al Protein losing enteropathy as a manifestation of Henoch–Schonlein purpura, *Acta Paediatr Scand* 1991; **80**: 482–485.
69. Barajas DF, Bravo MB, Palomino UN et al. Familial hypouricemia due to an isolated tubular defect of urate reabsorption. *Pediatr Nephrol* 1993; **7**: 83–85.
70. Murch SH. Toward a molecular understanding of complex childhood enteropathies. *J Pediatr Gastroenterol Nutr* 2002; **34** (Suppl 1): S4–S10.
71. Murch SH, Winyard PJ, Koletzko S et al. Congenital enterocyte heparan sulphate deficiency with massive albumin loss, secretory diarrhoea, and malnutrition. *Lancet* 1996; **347**: 1299–1301.
72. Westphal V, Murch S, Kim S et al. Reduced heparan sulfate accumulation in enterocytes contributes to protein-losing enteropathy in a congenital disorder of glycosylation. *Am J Pathol* 2000; **157**: 1917–1925.
73. Vernier RL, Klein DJ, Sisson SP et al. Heparan sulfate-rich anionic sites in the human glomerular basement membrane. Decreased concentration in congenital nephrotic syndrome. *N Engl J Med* 1983; **309**: 1001–1009.
74. Powers MR, Blumenstock FA, Cooper JA et al. Role of albumin arginyl sites in albumin-induced reduction of endothelial hydraulic conductivity. *J Cell Physiol* 1989; **141**: 558-564.
75. Kanwar YS, Linker A, Farquhar MG. Increased permeability of the glomerular basement membrane to ferritin after removal of glycosaminoglycans (heparan sulfate) by enzyme digestion. *J Cell Biol* 1980; **86**: 688–693.

76. Aebi M, Hennet T. Congenital disorders of glycosylation: genetic model systems lead the way. *Trends Cell Biol* 2001; **11**: 136–141.
77. Helenius A, Aebi M. Intracellular functions of N-linked glycans. *Science* 2001; **291**: 2364–2369.
78. de Lonlay P, Seta N, Barrot S et al. A broad spectrum of clinical presentations in congenital disorders of glycosylation I: a series of 26 cases. *J Med Genet* 2001; **38**: 14–19.
79. Freeze HH. Disorders in protein glycosylation and potential therapy: tip of an iceberg? *J Pediatr* 1998; **133**: 593–600.
80. Harms HK, Zimmer KP, Kurnik K et al. Oral mannose therapy persistently corrects the severe clinical symptoms and biochemical abnormalities of phosphomannose isomerase deficiency. *Acta Paediatr* 2002; **91**: 1065–1072.

29 Short-bowel syndrome

Olivier Goulet

Introduction

Short-bowel syndrome is characterized by a state of malabsorption following extensive resection of the small bowel. It is a functional rather than an anatomical definition. The resection results in a state of insufficient nutritive supply requiring artificial nutrition. Until 20 years ago, the prognosis after extensive bowel resection was poor, especially in the neonatal period. The onset of parenteral nutrition (PN) and enteral feeding in the daily practice has transformed the outcome during the past two decades.[1–4] These methods allow infants and children with short-bowel syndrome to grow normally during the long period required for adaptation of the remaining small intestine. In addition to the requirement for PN, the child with intestinal failure from short-bowel syndrome may benefit from other established medical and surgical interventions, intended to improve the function of the remaining gut.[5] This chapter reviews the pathophysiology of short-bowel syndrome and describes the principles of its medical and surgical management.

Consequences of intestinal resection

The functional consequences of short-bowel syndrome depend on the length, surface and site of the resected small intestine (Table 29.1). The cause of resection and the age of the patient at the time at which surgery was carried out also influence the capacity of the remaining gut function and potential for adaptation. At birth, the small-bowel length is 250 ± 40 cm, and the increase in length is maximal during the first year of life.[6] The small-bowel length doubles during the last trimester of gestation, suggesting that a short-bowel remnant does not have the same prognosis in a preterm infant as in a full-term baby.[7,8] The same difference exists between neonates and older children. Despite this potential for growth and other factors determining the outcome, it is classical to consider three levels after small-bowel resection. According to the length of the small intestine measured along the anti-mesenteric border at surgery, short resection leaves more than 100–150 cm of small intestine, large resection leaves between 40 and 100 cm and massive resection less than 40 cm. In all cases, one should consider the age of the patient at the time or resection, the portion of small bowel resected and the functional integrity of the remaining small intestine.

Resection of the jejunum

Both the transit time and the direct contact of intraluminal nutrients with the jejunal epithelium determine the malabsorption syndrome following

Table 29.1 Consequences of intestinal resection

Malabsorption (nutrients, vitamins, minerals) 1–3
Gastric acid hypersecretion 4
Pancreatic insufficiency 4
Water and electrolyte losses 1–4
Hyperoxaluria 1–3
Biliary lithiasis 1, 3, 5
Liver disease 1, 3, 5
Bone disease 5

The numbers refer to the following: 1, disruption of the enterohepatic cycle; 2, reduction of the absorptive surface; 3, bacterial overgrowth; 4, gastric acid hypersecretion; 5, long-term parenteral nutrition extensive jejunal resection. The resulting malabsorption concerns all nutrients as well as minerals, electrolytes, trace elements and most of the vitamins. Severe diarrhea following extensive jejunal resection is associated with steatorrhea and creatorrhea. The degree of malabsorption is proportional to the length of jejunum resected and will be compensated, to some extent, by the ileum and/or by the process of adaptation in response to loss of intestinal surface.

Resection of the ileum

Despite the fact that, normally, most nutrients are absorbed in the proximal jejunum, the residual ileum is able to adapt and to assume the role of macronutrient absorption. However, the specialized cells of the terminal ileum, where vitamin B_{12}/intrinsic factor receptors are located and where bile salts are reabsorbed, cannot be replaced by jejunal hypertrophy. Thus, the ileum has specific functions which the jejunum cannot substitute. In addition, resection of the distal ileum usually includes the ileocecal valve (ICV). Finally, ileal resection impairs vitamin B_{12} absorption which can cause macrocytic anemia and neuropathy. Malabsorption of bile salts is responsible for specific complications:

(1) Secretory diarrhea may be severe and is related to the presence in excess of bile salts within the colon, causing injury to the colonic mucosa. The consequences are proportional to the concentration and dehydroxylation of bile salts into the lumen (deoxycholic and chenodeoxycholic acids).[9]

(2) The decrease of bile salt reabsorption by the ileum reduces their circulating pool and leads to lipid malabsorption and steatorrhea.[10] Unabsorbed fatty acids are then hydroxylated by colonic bacteria increasing mucosal injury and secretory diarrhea. Because of the decreased pool of bile salts, fat-soluble vitamins (A, D, E and K) are also prone to be malabsorbed.

(3) Cholelithiasis seems to be the direct consequence of the reduced concentration of bile salts in bile.[11,12] Resection of the terminal ileum, by disrupting the enterohepatic circulation of biliary acids, increases the *lithogenicity* of bile. Premature infants are especially exposed to cholelithiasis because of their low production of conjugated bile acids.[13]

(4) Hyperoxaluria with formation of renal stones results from loss of the ileum and subsequent lipid malabsorption.[14] This complication became rare with the increased use of diets rich in medium-chain triglycerides (MCTs) (see below).

Finally, extensive loss of the ileum reduces transit time by suppressing the so-called 'ileal brake'. It has been shown that the ileum has a greater potential for adaptation than the jejunum.[15] In addition, the ileum is the site of release of enteric hormones such as enteroglucagon, which are essential in the process of adaptation after extensive resection (see below).

Ileocecal valve resection

The resection of the ICV decreases transit time (ileocecal brake) and allows colonic bacteria to enter and populate the small intestine. Bacterial overgrowth may negatively impact on digestion and nutrient absorption, as bacteria compete for nutrients with enterocytes. Thus, ICV resection represents an additional major cause of malabsorption of nutrients, water and electrolytes, dehydroxylation of bile salts, mucosal injury and motility disorders.[16,17] The lack of the ICV appears greatly to influence the period required to achieve intestinal autonomy following efficient small-bowel adaptation.[18–20] In addition, ICV resection increases the risk for sepsis of intestinal origin. This occurred three times more frequently in infants without the ICV than in those with an intact cecum.[1]

Associated disorders

Beside the anatomical impairment and its consequences, massive small-bowel resection may be aggravated by several associated disorders.

(1) Gastric acid hypersecretion occurs in 50% or pediatric patients with short-bowel syndrome

while hypergastrinemia is inconstant.[21] Acid hypersecretion occurs early after resection and depends on the extent of the resection. Hypersecretion is transitory, but it increases with enteral feeding, leading to a larger amount or intestinal fluid loss. Gastric acid hypersecretion, by reducing the duodenal pH, decreases the activity of pancreatic enzymes such as amylase and lipase, which, in turn, increases fat malabsorption.

(2) Gastric emptying of liquids is more rapid following jejunal resection, although intestinal transit may still remain normal, because of the braking effect of the ileum.[22] The loss of inhibition on gastric emptying and intestinal transit in children without colon is related to a significant decrease in peptide YY, glucagon-like peptide I (GLP-I) and neurotensin.[23] Peptide YY is normally released from L cells in the ileum and colon when stimulated by fat or bile salts. These cells are missing in patients who have undergone distal ileal and colonic resection. Rapid gastric emptying may contribute to fluid losses in children with short-bowel syndrome.

(3) Alteration in gut motor activity may be observed, especially in case of prenatal small-bowel malformations (atresia) or severe postnatal pathology such as extensive necrotizing enterocolitis. They contribute together with repeated surgical procedures, by increasing plastic peritonitis, to impair motor activity leading to bacterial overgrowth and the above-mentioned complications. These particular patients are at highest risk of developing rapid and severe liver disease that impairs the intestinal adaptation process and may require combined liver–intestine transplantation (see below).

(4) Colonic and/or gastric resection is sometimes associated with small-bowel resection. The former aggravates water and electrolyte losses while the latter, by altering duodenal contents, further decreases intestinal absorption.

Finally, the main factors determining the outcome of short-bowel syndrome are the length of the intestinal remnant, whether this includes the ileum or not, the conservation of the ICV and the degree of injury or the functional integrity of the remaining small intestine.

Small-bowel adaptation after extensive intestinal resection

The goal of intestinal adaptation after massive small-bowel resection is to develop the ability to withdraw artificial nutrition thanks to a compensatory increase in the mucosal surface area and absorption capacity. Adaptation is a slow process accompanied by a gradual increase in the absorption capacity of nutrients, electrolytes and minerals.[24,25] Soon after resection, the physiological process of adaptation of the remaining small-bowel develops.[26] This comprises muscular hypertrophy (increased bowel diameter and wall thickness) and hyperplasia of the intestinal mucosa. This mucosal hyperplasia is characterized by an increased number of enterocytes per unit of small-bowel length, an increased rate of enterocyte proliferation and an increased villous height and crypt depth.[27] In animals, it was demonstrated that epithelial hyperplasia following gut resection resulted in increased mucosal mass, including higher mucosal wet weight, higher protein content as well as higher DNA and RNA content per unit of bowel length.[28] The complex regulation of gut mucosal growth involves a multitude of factors including hormonal mediators such as enteroglucagon, glucagon-like peptides, neurotensin, peptide YY, growth hormone and insulin-like growth factor (IGF).[28–32] Additionally, oral or enteral feeding stimulates the release of enterotrophic hormones such as gastrin, cholecystokinin (CCK) and neurotensin, which may further improve the process of gut adaptation.[29–32]

Intraluminal substrates and nutrients, provided by oral or enteral feeding, are essential for achieving intestinal adaptation after extensive resection. Intraluminal nutrients stimulate the adaptation of the intestinal mucosa through several mechanisms:

(1) Direct contact of intraluminal nutrients with intestinal cells;[33,34]

(2) Trophic effects of gastrointestinal secretions enhanced by food;[35,36]

(3) Release of several trophic hormones secreted by the gastrointestinal tract, mainly enteroglucagon.[37]

The postulated influence of CCK and secretin might be an indirect action via the stimulation of pancreatic secretions that could lead to the release of enteroglucagon.[38] In turn, enteroglucagon stimulates the cell turnover, motility and absorptive capacity of the small intestine.[39]

Glutamine (Gln) is the most important circulating amino acid. Many findings have emphasized the role of Gln for the metabolism of enterocytes suggesting the importance of Gln as a substrate during PN in patients with short-bowel syndrome.[40–43]

Ornithine-α-ketoglutarate has been shown to improve mucosal trophicity and to enhance intestinal adaptation in a rat model of extensive intestinal resection.[44] Ornithine-α-ketoglutarate is a precursor of glutamine and could also act by an increased production of polyamines by the enterocytes.

Short-chain fatty acids (SCFA) are produced from the fermentation of fibers by the colonic microflora. SCFA could be energetic substrates for the topical nutrition of intestinal cells.[45,46] In rats with short-bowel syndrome, pectin, a water-soluble, non-cellulose dietary fiber, was shown to enhance jejunal and colonic mucosal adaptation when added to the enteral diet[47] or PN mixture.[48] The question as to whether patients with short-bowel syndrome would benefit from diets enriched in pectin remains unanswered.

Besides nutrients, other factors seem to play an important role in the mucosal adaptation process:

(1) Growth-stimulating peptide has been shown to be synthesized in the rat proximal intestine after small-bowel resection;[49]

(2) Epidermal growth factor (EGF), produced in the salivary glands and duodenal cells, is a trophic substance for the gastrointestinal tract.[50–52] EGF is a polypeptide able to stimulate [^{3}H] thymidine incorporation into intestinal DNA when given at pharmacological doses to mice.[53] In addition, EGF infusion in rats is associated with a rise in galactose as well as in glycine absorption;[54]

(3) Polyamines (spermine, spermidine), whose synthesis is dependent on ornithine decarboxylase activity, greatly enhance intestinal cell turnover and protein synthesis;[55,56]

(4) Exogenous prostaglandin (16,16-dimethyl prostaglandin E_1) has been shown to stimulate mucosal hyperplasia in the gastric antrum and in the jejunum.[57,58]

Thus, adaptation of the remaining small bowel is dependent on exogenous and endogenous factors, emphasizing the usefulness of early enteral feeding after resection. It is hoped that in the future the utilization of exogenous trophic peptides will further enhance and optimize adaptation of the remaining intestine.

Clinical management of short-bowel syndrome

Initial surgery

Every time intestinal resection is performed for an acute event such as midgut volvulus, the initial surgery should aim at saving as much intestinal tissue as possible. In some situations, a so-called 'second-look procedure' can be performed 2–3 days later if the patient's condition permits it. The intestinal segments which have not recovered from the initial procedure can then be resected. In the case of intestinal atresia with a very dilated proximal loop, performing an enterostomy is indicated in order to avoid intestinal stasis and subsequent bacterial overgrowth. If an end-to-end anastomosis is performed, the proximal intestinal loop should undergo tapering anti-mesenteric enteroplasty.

When small-bowel resection includes the terminal ileum it is recommended that a gallbladder resection be performed.[12] We perform this whenever an extensive ileum resection is made in order to prevent the occurrence of cholelithiasis.

The question as to whether a gastrostomy should be performed at the initial phase depends on the experience of the team. Nevertheless, if long-term enteral nutrition is planned, a gastrostomy is better for the patient's comfort. Extensive small-bowel resection will require fluid replacement after surgery (see below) and, in a number of patients, long-term PN. Therefore, a permanent indwelling central venous catheter must be placed, such as a Broviac or Hickman catheter.

Medical therapy

Whatever the etiology of the short-bowel syndrome (Table 29.2), it is customary and informative to consider three phases in the clinical course after extensive resection.

The first phase follows small-bowel resection and is associated with massive losses of water and electrolytes. Severe diarrhea is increased by gastric hypersecretion. During this period, total PN is required in association with small amounts of substrates provided by the enteral route, orally or by continuous gastric infusion, as soon as intestinal transit has recovered. During the second phase, when intestinal transit is permanently re-established, intestinal function improves as a result of progressive adaptation of the remaining small bowel. PN allows the short bowel to develop and to become functional without exceeding its capacities. This period can take several months or years before the stage of maximal adaptation is reached. The third phase starts when intestinal function is sufficient to absorb nutrients, enabling PN to be withdrawn. All calories are provided by the oral route. Oral intake can then be further liberalized, both in volume and in variety, according to the tolerance of the patient. This long period requires special management and follow-up.

Phase 1

The major goals of medical therapy are to compensate for the intestinal losses while attempting to reduce them and to achieve nutritional repletion. Replacement solutions not uncommonly require a very high sodium concentration replacement, often as high as 80–100 mmol/l, in order to maintain fluid and electrolyte homeostasis. The requirements of massive intravenous fluids and the necessity to avoid multiple peripheral perfusions necessitate the early insertion of a central venous catheter. Such vascular access allows the safe replacement of volumes of fluid according to the evaluation of intestinal losses. Water, sodium and potassium requirements are also increased. When losses stabilize and the clinician becomes familiar with the management of the infant, fluid and electrolyte losses can be added to the PN solution and administered through a single infusion device. Patients with proximal enterostomy require special trace element supplementation. Zinc deficiency can lead to a decreased activity of zinc-dependent intestinal metalloenzymes such as alkaline phosphatase, leucine aminopeptidase and other intestinal disaccharidases.[59] On the other hand, PN provides adequate nutritional supply to the child, allowing optimal growth. Such nutritional support includes the use of 1.5–2.5 g/kg per day of amino acids through a pediatric solution, a caloric intake consisting of 70–80% of non-protein energy substrates such as dextrose and 20–30% energy provided by a 20% intravenous fat emulsion. Maintenance amounts of vitamins and trace elements are added to the PN solution by using commercially available preparations. Calcium, phosphate and magnesium are also added to the solution according to the patient's needs and the stability of the solution.

During the early phases of therapy, serum electrolytes, glucose, urea and calcium should be

Table 29.2 Etiology of short-bowel syndrome

Prenatal	Neonatal	Postnatal
Atresia (*unique or multiple*)	**Midgut volvulus** (*midgut* or *segmental*)	Midgut volvulus (*malrotation, bands or tumor*)
Apple peel syndrome	**Necrotizing enterocolitis**	**Complicated intussusception**
Midgut volvulus (*malrotation*)	**Arterial thrombosis**	**Arterial thrombosis**
Segmental volvulus (*with omphalomesenteric duct or intra-abdominal bands*)	**Venous thrombosis**	**Inflammatory bowel disease**
Abdominal wall defects	**Post-trauma resection**	
Gastroschisis > omphalocele	**Extensive angioma**	
Extensive Hirschsprung's disease		

measured daily. When the patient's condition and the intestinal losses become stable, blood monitoring can be less frequent. During the first stage after resection, H_2-receptor blocking agents (ranitidine) should be given intravenously to inhibit gastric hypersecretion: 15–20 mg/kg per day of ranitidine added to the PN solution, the drug being delivered as a continuous infusion. H_2-receptor-blocking agents, by increasing duodenal pH, also improve the digestion and absorption of nutrients.

The end of the phase of management is considered to be accomplished when the patient has recovered from the surgical procedure and is stable on PN with controlled intestinal losses and motility.

Phase 2

This phase of management is marked by the initiation of enteral and/or oral feeding and the gradual cycling of PN. As supported by the mechanisms of adaptation, there is a clear advantage in providing early gradual amounts of nutrients into the residual intestine. Indeed, intraluminal nutrition is mandatory for stimulating mucosal hyperplasia. The absence of luminal nutrients slows the intestinal hyperplasia process even when the appropriate amount of calories is given by PN.[60]

Phase 3

The transition between total PN and full enteral/oral feeding is achieved during phase 2 either in hospital or, better, on home PN when necessary. Phase 3 begins with the discontinuation of artificial nutrition. When the patient receives no more than two or three perfusions per week, PN discontinuation is attempted. If both protein–energy intake and intestinal function are adequate, normal weight gain and growth velocity must be achieved. If the weight gain remains correct after 3 months without PN, the central venous catheter is removed. If not, PN should be restarted for a few weeks or months. In about 80–90% of cases, the first attempt to stop PN completely is successful. When all the necessary calories are provided by oral feeding, oral intake can be further liberalized in both volume and variety. In a very small number of neonatal cases of short-bowel syndrome (less than 5% in our experience) eating *disorders* may be a serious problem. After eliminating all organic causes, reinforcement of psychological support is mandatory.

Mode of feeding

The mode of administration of feeding varies among different groups. Oral feeding seems to have several advantages, especially in neonates. Oral feeding is more physiological, by stimulating salivary secretion containing EGF, gallbladder motility and gastrointestinal secretions. In addition, oral feeding reduces PN-related liver disease. Early initiation of oral feeding, by allowing the infant to learn how to suck and swallow, is in addition the best way to prevent anorexia secondary to the absence of suckling and long-term hospitalization. The use of breast milk has the advantage of containing additional non-nutritive factors such as prostaglandins or EGF and it seems logical, despite the fact that it contains lactose. Oral feeding increases stool volume output and frequency even when a semi-elemental diet is used. Intestinal tolerance can be determined by the volume of the stools, their consistency, the number of bowel movements, the presence or absence of reducing substances and pH (<5). The amount of oral feeding should be started at 50–80 ml/day, divided into 6–8 meals. Thereafter, the amounts are progressively in-creased over several days or weeks. Depending on the remaining absorptive surface, diarrhea will develop when the amount of diet exceeds the digestive and absorptive capacities of the remaining small intestine.

Continuous enteral feeding (CEF) allows the enteral intake to be more rapidly increased. CEF can be achieved using either a nasogastric tube or a feeding gastrostomy. If a gastrostomy has not been placed during the initial surgical procedure, it is still possible to perform it afterwards percutaneously by upper gastrointestinal endoscopy. Whatever the gastric access, CEF allows gradual infusion of an appropriate liquid diet. The choice of nutrients depends on the capacity of digestion and absorption of the remaining small bowel, since there are alterations of gastric and pancreatic secretions, a disturbance of the intestinal flora and a reduced absorptive surface. Enteral nutrition is usually started slowly. The solution should contain no fiber, have an osmolality below 310 mOsm/kg, and contain substrates that are rapidly transferred across the intestine without leaving intraluminal residues. A dilute concentration is gradually increased from 0.6 to 1 kcal/ml according to digestive tolerance (stool losses, reducing substances). It is also important to avoid excessive fluid administration concurrently with PN which may overload the patient with fluid. CEF enhances absorption by permitting total saturation of the transporters in the gut 24 h a day. Bolus feeding through the nasogastric or gastrostomy tube is not tolerated and should be avoided. Adapted CEF subsequently decreases the PN requirements and reduces liver injury. The recent development of new portable infusion devices and backpacks permits older children, who are able to walk independently, to have reasonable mobility as they grow and develop physically. If the child is managed by using CEF, oral feeding should be maintained. Introduction of solid feedings by 6 months of age is also important to help the child learn to eat and swallow at an appropriate age, again to avoid feeding-aversion behavior.

Type of diet

The choice of an appropriate diet for CEF remains controversial. During the past decades, special diets were first used; each of the constituents could be modified independently. An important improvement has been the introduction of semi-elemental diets containing protein hydrolysates, oligosaccharides and a mixture of MCTs and long-chain triglycerides (LCTs).

Protein in the diet

It was demonstrated that the absorption of amino acids is more rapid and more efficient when given in the form of short peptides than in the form of free amino acids.[61–63] In addition to the quality of the protein, digestion and intestinal absorption of protein hydrolysates depends on the type of hydrolysate used: α-lactalbumin is better than casein.[64,65] Amino acid-based formulas have been used in pediatric patients with short-bowel syndrome and are well accepted by the infants.[65,66] Their beneficial effects have to be demonstrated by further studies.

Energetic substrates: carbohydrates and lipids

Because of the increased turnover of enterocytes in the small bowel, lactase activity appears to be depressed in patients with short-bowel syndrome. Oligosaccharides provide low osmolality and allow the amount of carbohydrates to be increased. The behavior of MCTs, their split products in the intestinal lumen and their absorption characteristics are mainly due to their greater water solubility.[67] MCTs are hydrolyzed more rapidly than LCTs in the small intestine by pancreatic lipase; they are converted almost exclusively into free fatty acids and glycerol and reach the liver directly via the portal circulation. Thus, even in the case of pancreatic insufficiency, MCTs may be absorbed intact. Moreover, MCTs have been shown to be absorbed, to some extent, within the stomach and duodenum. The unabsorbed fraction is then absorbed within the proximal part of the jejunum. The excessive content in the diet of MCTs can lead to osmotic diarrhea as a result of rapid hydrolysis of the MCTs' bulk.[68] Studies in animals with enterectomy have shown that MCTs are not as effective as LCTs in stimulating mucosal hyperplasia.[69] LCTs appear to be potentially more trophic than other nutrients for the mucosal mass. LCTs stimulate biliary and pancreatic secretions, which are themselves trophic factors. In addition, LCTs are a substantial source of linolenic and linoleic acids, which are essential substrates for endogenous prostaglandin synthesis.[70,71] Most of the formulas containing MCTs also include up to 50% of lipid in the form of LCTs. LCTs stimulate biliary and pancreatic secretions, which promote increased intestinal motility; when LCTs are in excess in the intestinal lumen, they may be hydroxylated by bacteria and reverse the rate of water and electrolyte absorption, resulting in aggravation of malabsorption. Under these conditions, oral therapy with cholestyramine (0.5–2 g/kg per day) may be helpful, and supplementation with essential fatty acids is crucial. Thus, an intake of 2–4 g/kg per day of lipids is recommended, depending on the absorption capacity and digestive tolerance.

Dietary fibers

It is possible for an intact colon to absorb daily energy from dietary fiber.[45,46] The role of SCFAs has been demonstrated in animals.[47,48] In patients with a preserved colon, a reasonable amount of dietary fiber may be progressively included in oral feeding. Because SCFAs are supposed to stimulate sodium and water absorption, infants and children might be expected to have a decreased stool output and sodium losses. However, this is not always observed in clinical practice. Therefore, soluble non-starch polysaccharides and some starches should be given, according to digestive tolerance and especially stool output as well as abdominal distension due to intracolonic fermentation of fiber by an abundant and modified intestinal bacterial microflora. In patients without a colon or with reduced colon length without an ICV, dietary fiber should be reduced or even avoided.

Bacterial overgrowth

Bacterial overgrowth is a frequent complication, causing mucosal injury, malabsorption and bacterial translocation. In addition, bacterial overgrowth exacerbates hepatotoxicity related to PN.[72–80] Indeed, deconjugation of bile acids by bacteria facilitates their reabsorption, leading to hepatotoxicity. Bacterial overgrowth is likely to occur in the case of ICV resection, poor motility of a dilated small-bowel segment, or when a tight anastomosis is present. After bacterial overgrowth has been confirmed by intestinal flora analysis (fecal and duodenal) and the hydrogen breath test, it is mandatory to stop it. Antimicrobial therapy as the combination of metronidazole and colimycin three times a day may be helpful. The efficiency of the antimicrobial therapy can be assessed by the clinical improvement or by the intestinal tolerance to food and mainly by performing stool balance studies. The use of broad-spectrum antimicrobial therapy is, in our opinion, contraindicated, because of the high risk of emergence of multiresistant bacteria and the anti-physiological effect on colonic flora. In the case of bacterial overgrowth, the administration of *Saccharomyces boulardii* may be effective. Whenever possible, performing an intestinal tapering procedure or resecting a tight anastomosis may be required to obtain the disappearance of bacterial overgrowth (see below). The use of prokinetic drugs for enhancing gut motor activity is strictly contraindicated in these conditions.

Parenteral nutrition cycling

Besides enteral feeding, phase 2 is characterized by the cycling of PN. As soon as the metabolic and nutritional status or the patient permits it, cyclic PN should be started. Cyclic infusion of nutrients allows the periods of feeding and fasting to be alternated, which induces a more physiological regulation of metabolism by insulin and glucagon; it prevents hyperinsulinism which is responsible for fat accumulation within the liver and adipose tissue.[81,82] Furthermore, cyclic PN favors a more normal physical activity whose importance in terms of nutrition and psychology has been demonstrated. The tolerance of this mode of nutrient delivery has been well documented in children. In addition, cyclic PN is the most appropriate condition for home PN whose development, since 1980, has dramatically improved the well-being and quality of life of patients requiring long-term PN.[83,84] Cyclic PN can be progressively achieved by slowly decreasing the infusion rate, followed by complete discontinuation of nutrient infusion for several hours per day. Long-term PN has to be adapted in order to avoid complications related to excessive or insufficient intakes.[85–88]

Adaptation to fluid losses

Extensive small-bowel resection is associated with gastric hypersecretion. The H_2 antagonists and proton pump inhibitors are useful in reducing gastric fluid secretion, and therefore will also reduce fluid losses. However, absorption of orally dosed medications may be impaired, and either large doses, oral medication, or intravenous delivery may be required. Although fluid losses are decreased, macronutrient and electrolyte absorption are not affected by H_2 antagonists and proton pump inhibitors.

Reduction of fluid loss

Fluid losses may require chronic control with hypomotility agents. Synthetic opiate derivatives such as loperamide may be beneficial in delaying gastric emptying and decreasing gastrointestinal motor activity. They allow the transit time to decrease and enhance intestinal transport. Nevertheless, loperamide must be used very carefully and should be avoided whenever a motility disorder leads to intestinal distension with subsequent bacterial overgrowth. In patients with ileal resection and watery stools, cholestyramine may bind bile acids and reduce biliary colitis and diarrhea. However, cholestyramine causes fat malabsorption and increases the risk of fat-soluble vitamin deficiency. Somatostatin analogs may be helpful for short-term use.[89] The mechanism of action is unclear, but octreotide may be useful in slowing intestinal transit time and increasing water and sodium absorption. However, octreotide reduces splanchnic protein synthesis, thereby reducing mucosal protein incorporation and villous growth rate, and may impair post-resectional intestinal adaptation. There is also an increased risk for cholelithiasis in the patient group already predisposed to this problem. Use in children has not been well studied and there are some concerns regarding the suppression of growth hormone in this population already at risk of poor growth.

Prevention of dehydration

In a child on cyclic PN, because of reduced water intake and persistence of intestinal losses, one should be careful when restarting PN. It is important to increase the infusion rate progressively during the first hour of PN, because the child may be mildly dehydrated. Especially infants with an extremely short-bowel or with a small-bowel stoma have obligatory losses of water and electrolytes even when fasting. The volume of effluent rises in proportion to the amount of distal intestine removed. Since the sodium concentration of the effluent is almost constant at about 90 mEq/l or greater, the sodium losses correlate directly with the volume of effluent and are increased by oral feeding. Despite large amounts of sodium given parenterally, fasting periods of cyclic PN should be carefully adapted. Patients with less than 60 cm of jejunum remaining between the duodenojejunal flexure and the stoma lose more fluid and sodium from the stoma than they can take in orally and may be at risk for developing negative water and sodium balance. Those patients with severe diarrhea are also subject to magnesium deficiency. Oral rehydration solutions with adequate sodium concentration can be given to maximize water and salt absorption. Such patients should be discouraged from drinking large quantities of water or diluted sodium solutions.

Complications of short-bowel syndrome and parenteral nutrition

Long-term PN exposes the patient to several complications, including catheter-related sepsis and thrombosis, bone disease and liver impairment.[72–80] Daily catheter care and prevention of septic complications are essential (see Chapter 33). Liver function tests should be performed on a regular basis because of the risk of cholestasis and liver injury. If initial surgery did not include a gall-bladder resection, ultrasonography aiming to look for sludge or cholelithiasis should be repeated every 3 months. In addition, the phosphorus and calcium status should be assessed and, if necessary, supplies should be given to prevent PN-related bone disease.

Liver disease is certainly the most frequent and the most severe complication in patients with short-bowel syndrome. Premature babies and/or small-for-gestational-age babies with severe necrotizing enterocolitis are at specially high risk of developing liver disease and, rapidly, end-stage liver failure, because of the combination of prematurity, sub-occlusion, Gram-negative sepsis and repeated catheter-related sepsis. In general, liver disease is mostly related to the impaired small intestine and is further aggravated by inadequate PN.

The main factors related to liver disease

These are thought to be:

(1) Disruption of the enterohepatic cycle (ileal disease or resection);

(2) Intestinal stasis with consecutive intraluminal bacterial overgrowth and/or translocation (endotoxinemia);[74–76]

(3) Recurrent catheter-related sepsis;[90]

(4) Prematurity itself, which might be an associated factor;[78]

(5) Inadequate PN intakes such as continuous PN infusion with excessive glucose intake (hyper-

insulinism) and subsequent steatosis or inadequate amino acid supply.[81]

Management for prevention or resolution of liver injury

This should include:

(1) Stimulation of the enterobiliary axis by ingestion of LCTs or breast milk, or by injection of CCK analogs;[38]

(2) Suppression of intraluminal bacterial overgrowth caused by intestinal stasis, by giving metronidazole and/or performing tapering enteroplasty;[91]

(3) The use of ursodesoxycholic acid (10–20 mg/kg per day) which might contribute to the decrease of liver injury;[92]

(4) PN intake, which should be adapted in terms of:

  (a) limiting glucose intakes to reduce hepatic fat accumulation;[93]

  (b) decreasing aluminium content of parenteral nutrition solution;[94]

  (c) using appropriate type and amount of intravenous fat emulsion which provides essential fatty acids and reduces glucose load;[95]

  (d) using the new pediatric adapted amino acid solutions which provide appropriate amino acids as well as taurine;[96]

  (e) performing cyclic parenteral nutrition that contributes towards reducing hyperinsulinism and reducing liver steatosis.[81]

Transition to parenteral nutrition weaning

When oral feeding and home PN are commenced in combination, the amounts and/or rate of PN infusion are progressively decreased. In our experience, the combination of oral feeding and cyclic PN allows home PN to be achieved in the best conditions. The combination of CEF and cyclic PN seems to us less logical, since nutritional support would take place only during the nocturnal period. If not, the patient would be dependent on artificial nutritional support for 24 h a day. In the past 20 years we have treated, in hospital and/or by home PN, over 200 patients, mainly infants, with short-bowel syndrome. The duration of stage 2 depends on several factors, which include: the length of the remaining total intestine, conservation of the ICV and the functional capacity of the remaining small intestine. The slow transition from total PN to full oral feeding requires time, during which the nutritional status has to be maintained at the optimal level. In this regard, home PN is the best tool both to maintain nutritional status and to achieve bowel adaptation. This is a physiological anabolic process which requires optimal nutritional status and liver function. The delay in achieving intestinal autonomy (PN weaning) depends on residual small-bowel length and ICV preservation (see below).[1–3] By using stool balance analysis we have shown that most patients who have been weaned from PN remain with a certain degree of malabsorption that is compensated by relative hyperphagia.[97] Conversely, trying to wean an infant with short-bowel syndrome from PN too rapidly leads to the risk of metabolic complications and failure to thrive.[97,98]

Long-term complications

The loss of ileum can lead to hyperoxaluria and subsequent renal stone formation. Oxaluria evaluation, as well as ultrasonography of the kidney, must be repeated every 6 months. Prevention of oxalic lithiasis includes a restricted diet containing LCTS, the addition of calcium to the diet and elimination from the diet of foods containing large amounts of oxalic acid.[99,100]

In the case of resection of the terminal ileum, vitamin B_{12} supplementation is required. An intramuscular dose of 1 mg every 6 months is recommended. Because of poor absorption of fat-soluble vitamins (A, D, E and K) follow-up and supplementation are necessary. Nutritional evaluation must also include research of zinc and biotin deficiency. After an extensive small-bowel resection and even after adaptation, one must take into account the possibility that the medications administered orally will not be absorbed at optimal levels. This becomes particularly important in the case of pediatric infections requiring antibiotics. On the other hand, unjustified use of antibiotics may lead to severe and protracted intestinal microflora impairment. Thus, antibiotic therapy should whenever possible be avoided, and if necessary be performed by a pediatric gastroenterologist.

D-Lactic acidosis

D-Lactic acidosis is a classical disorder following extensive small-bowel resection with preservation of the colon. Lactobacilli and other bacteria, including *Clostridium perfringens* and *Streptococcus bovis*, when present, ferment non-absorbed carbohydrate to D-lactic acid, which cannot be metabolized by D-lactate dehydrogenase. These organisms may proliferate in an acidic environment that may be promoted by the metabolism of unabsorbed carbohydrate to SCFAs. A metabolic acidosis may develop in the absence of hepatic dysfunction if significant absorption of D-lactic acid occurs.[101] Clinical symptoms include, in the rare and severe form, encephalopathy, headache, ataxia and dysarthria. D-Lactate concentrations will be increased in blood and urine (L-lactate concentration, is usually measured when serum lactate concentration is normal). The mechanism for the neurological symptoms is unknown. Thiamine deficiency should be excluded.[102,103] Spontaneous resolution is possible while treatments include oral metronidazole, neomycin, vancomycin (for 10–14 days) and avoidance of 'refined' carbohydrates.[104,105] *Saccharomyces boulardii* may be used in these circumstances.[106] Finally, chronic metabolic acidosis may cause impaired growth in some children with short-bowel syndrome.

Long-term follow-up and growth monitoring

During the long-term follow-up, weight gain and growth velocity must be regularly monitored. Dietary intake should be adapted to digestive tolerance, the child's preference and growth. Whenever failure to thrive occurs, it is important to perform a dietetic evaluation of the nutrient intake, stool balance studies and investigations for bacterial overgrowth.[80] Bone mineral mass has to be assessed by dual X-ray absorptiometry.[107] At this point one should discuss the opportunity for restarting artificial nutrition by enteral feeding or in some cases PN. We performed a retrospective study to analyze the outcome, the prognosis factors and the long-term growth of children after extensive small-bowel resection in the neonatal period.[108] The study included 87 children who had undergone extensive neonatal small-bowel resection, followed up over a mean 15-year period. The overall survival was 89.7%, depending on the date of birth. The duration of PN dependency varies according to the intestinal length and the presence of the ICV (Figure 29.1). All patients who remained PN dependent had less than 40 cm of small bowel and/or the absence of the ICV. A group of patients with a mean smal-bowel length of 35 ± 19 cm, resection of the ICV in 50% of cases and a PN duration of 47.4 ± 23.8 months had significant decrease in height and weight gain within the 4 years after cessation of PN, requiring a new period of enteral or parenteral feeding. Finally, the largest group included patients with a mean small-bowel length of 57 ± 19 cm, the presence of the ICV in 81% of cases and a PN duration of 16.1 ± 11.4 months. After PN weaning, they grew normally with normal puberty and final height as expected from genetic target height. PN duration is clearly influenced by the length of residual small bowel and the absence of the ICV. With good anatomic prognosis factors and short duration of initial PN, normal long-term growth may be predicted. Conversely, poor anatomical factors and protracted initial PN require careful monitoring of growth and may sometimes require nutritional support to be restarted. Patients permanently dependent on PN might be candidates for intestinal transplantation.

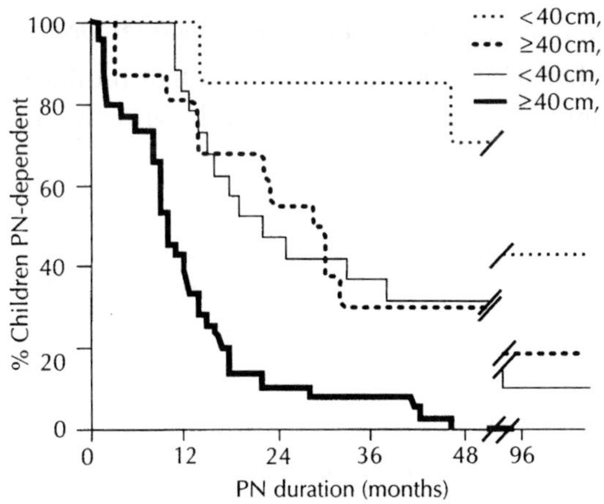

Figure 29.1 Parenteral nutrition (PN) duration according to anatomical factors. Note that 100% of children with small-bowel length 40–80 cm and the presence of ileocecal valve (ICV) are weaned from PN within 1 year. Conversely, a large percentage of children with <40 cm without the ICV remain dependent on long-term PN.

Long-term outcome and management of 'unadapted' short small bowel

Since the review published in 1972 by Wilmore, the prognosis of neonatal short-bowel syndrome has dramatically changed.[108–113] More than 90% of infants and children now survive after extensive small-bowel resection.[1–3] After neonatal extensive resection, the residual small intestine can adapt, even when its remaining length below the ligament or Treitz is shorter than 15 cm, the ICV being left intact. In older children having undergone extensive resection, the criterion for length is different. Adequate adaptation to ensure normal growth without artificial nutrition requires at least 40 cm below the Treitz angle measured at the time of resection.[114,115] In neonatal short-bowel syndrome, by separating our series of patients into two groups according to PN duration (< 48 months and > 48 months), assessments of factors such as functional capacity of the remaining short bowel or bacterial overgrowth emerge as being essential (Table 29.3).[116] Thus, a small number of patients, because of motility disorders or an especially short small bowel, will adapt only very slowly, if at all. In such patients, different medical and/or surgical approaches have been proposed.

Pharmacological enhancement of intestinal adaptation

Growth hormone and insulin-like growth factor-I

A number of studies have indicated that pituitary hormones modulate small-bowel growth in rodents.[117–119] In hypophysectomized rat pups, the rate of growth of the small intestine was decreased.[117] Administration of growth hormone (GH) to hypophysectomized rats restored the growth deficit of the small bowel. GH also stimulated small-bowel growth in intact animals.[120–122] Although GH receptors have been detected in rat intestinal mucosal cells,[123] the effects of GH on the gut may be mediated through IGF-I, since both type I and type II receptors for IGF have been demonstrated in rat[124] and rabbit gastrointestinal epithelium.[125] IGF-I is synthesized in the rat small intestine in a GH-dependent manner.[126] IGF-I treatment increased small-bowel mass in rats after 80% small-bowel resection or in rats with mucosal atrophy due to glucocorticoid treatment.[127]

In humans, it was shown that GH enhanced amino acid uptake by the small intestine *ex vivo*[128] and promoted crypt cell proliferation in cultured explants of duodenal mucosa.[129] Both open and randomized clinical trials have now been conducted in humans.[130–134] Their results are controversial and do not allow conclusions to be drawn on a long-term benefit in patients with short-bowel syndrome. GH administration (0.5 IU/kg per day or 0.024 mg/kg per day) alone for 8 weeks had no effect on the absorptive capacity of energy, protein, or fluid in ten patients (four with colon in continuity).[134]

In infants with short-bowel syndrome, recombinant human GH (rhGH) has been used for a 10-day period at a dose of 0.3 IU/kg per day. Reported data include only significant weight gain during rhGH treatment and a tendency to increase polyamine

Table 29.3 Factors predicting parental nutrition duration to be >48 months in infants with neonatal short-bowel syndrome, by univariate analysis

Parenteral nutrition duration	>48 months (n=10)	<48 months (n=43)	p Value
Intestinal atresia	80%	30%	<0.05
Small-bowel length <40 cm*	70%	32%	<0.05
Absence of ileocecal valve	80%	32%	<0.05
Associated colon resection	80%	21%	<0.01
Occurrence of Gram-negative sepsis	70%	16%	<0.01

*Anti-mesenteric small-bowel length measured from the Treitz angle

concentration in the small-bowel mucosa.[135] Recently, we performed a small, pilot, open-labeled trial in eight children with short-bowel syndrome with more than 3 years of PN dependency, still receiving >50% of their protein–energy requirements from PN. After 3 months of rhGH treatment (0.6 IU/kg per day) all the patients were weaned from PN. One-year follow-up indicated that 25% had been definitively PN weaned, 50% had decreased PN requirements and 25% did not change their PN dependency.[136] More prolonged and perhaps earlier use of rhGH in infants or children with short-bowel syndrome might be helpful for future management.

Glucagon-like-peptide-2

Glucagon-like peptide-2 (GLP-2) has been proposed for enhancing intestinal adaptation in patients with short-bowel syndrome.[137,138] GLP-2 is secreted from L cells of the ileum as well as from pancreatic A cells. It was shown that postprandial serum GLP-2 concentration was not unexpectedly depressed in patients who have had extensive small-bowel resection, especially including the ileum.[139] The relative lack of jejunal hypertrophy following ileal resection might be partly related to the resection of GLP-2-producing L cells. GLP-2 was used in a clinical setting (400 μg subcutaneously, twice a day for 35 days) was administered in a small, pilot, open-labeled trial to four patients with short-bowel syndrome without residual colon who required total PN and in four patients with sufficient residual jejunum where total PN was not required.[140] Jejunal villous height and crypt depth tended to increase, energy absorption tended to increase and fecal wet weight decreased, indicating increased fluid absorption. Regarding its origin (ileum) and its physiological effect, GLP-2 might be the most logical medical approach for early management of the patient with short-bowel syndrome with ileal resection. GLP-2 is not commercially available, but might be helpful in the near future if a genetically engineered analog of GLP-2 is developed.

Surgical treatment of the short-bowel syndrome

Under some circumstances, surgical procedures can slow down intestinal transit or increase the area of absorption. Several surgical procedures have been proposed for decreasing intestinal transit time. The construction of a valve or a sphincter with sutures and synthetic material, the denervation segments of the intestine, and the intussusception of intestinal loops have all been experimentally assessed.[141–145] The clinical experience is, however, more limited. Reversing segments of intestine aims at creating an antiperistaltic segment acting as a 'physiological valve' by causing retrograde peristalsis. Experimental results are conflicting, because the ideal length of the antiperistaltic segment has not been clearly established.[146,147] Pediatric patients having undergone such a procedure have been reported.[148] Most of the time, transit time is slowed down and absorption increased. A serious limitation of this procedure is that patients with very short remaining small bowel may not be able to afford the sacrifice of a 10-cm segment for reversal. Therefore, this procedure has never been used by our team. Interposition of a colonic segment has also been proposed both in isoperistaltic and in antiperistaltic fashions. Clinical results are poor, and show little benefit.[149–151] Intestinal tapering and lengthening have been performed in selected patients with dilated bowel segments.[152–157] Marked dilatation of the proximal intestine may occur secondary to chronic obstruction or adaptation. This situation leads to stasis and bacterial overgrowth which further aggravates malabsorption. Intestinal tapering and lengthening has the theoretical interest of not only tapering the dilated segment but also of using the divided intestine to increase in length. The procedure should be applied with caution, since there is a risk or 'jeopardizing' the divided segments. Long-term patency and function have been shown to occur in some patients.[158–160] Finally, in cases or non-adapted small bowel despite long-term trials, the only alternative is a small-bowel transplantation.

Conclusion

Infants with short-bowel syndrome from birth or early life should adapt, thanks to the physiological process of adaptation. Everything has to be done to promote intestinal adaptation and digestive autonomy, especially by using the digestive tract and the oral route as soon and as much as possible.

Unfortunately, too many infants have complications related to unadapted PN and become cholestatic with a course of end-stage liver disease requiring liver transplant. Some pediatric patients were reported to have received an isolated liver transplantation for end-stage liver disease complicating short-bowel syndrome.[161,162] By *using* appropriate long-term PN and home PN, only a few patients with an extremely short bowel will not become autonomous and will require isolated intestinal transplantation.[163–167]

REFERENCES

1. Goulet OJ, Revillon Y, Jan D et al. Neonatal short bowel syndrome. *J Pediatr* 1991; **119**: 18–23.
2. Georgeson KE, Breaux CW Jr. Outcome and intestinal adaptation in neonatal short-bowel syndrome. J Pediatr Surg 1992; **27**: 344–350.
3. Sondheimer JM, Cadnapaphornchai M, Sontag M, Zerbe GO. Predicting the duration of dependence on parenteral nutrition after neonatal intestinal resection. *J Pediatr* 1998; **132**: 80–84.
4. Warner BW, Chaet MS. Non transplant surgical options for the management of the short bowel syndrome. *J Pediatr Gastroenterol Nutr* 1993; **17**: 1–12.
5. Bianchi A. Autologous gastro-intestinal reconstruction. *Semin Pediatr Surg* 1995; **4**: 54–59.
6. Bryant J. Observations upon the growth and length of the human intestine. *Am J Med Sci* 1924; **167**: 499–520.
7. Siebert JR. Small intestine length in infants and children. *Am J Dis Child* 1980; **134**: 593–595.
8. Touloukian RJ, Smith GJW. Normal intestinal length in preterm infants. *J Pediatr Surg* 1983; **18**; 720–723.
9. Mitchell JE, Breuer RI, Zuckerman L. The colon influences ileal resection diarrhea. *Dig Dis Sci* 1980; **25**: 33–41.
10. Cosnes J, Gendre JP, Le Quintrec Y. Role of the ileocaecal valve and site of intestinal resection in malabsorption after extensive small-bowel resection. *Digestion* 1978; **18**: 329–336.
11. Mashako MNK, Cezard JP, Boige N et al. The effect of artificial feeding on cholestasis, gallbladder sludge and lithiasis in infants: correlation with plasma cholecystokinin levels. *Clin Nutr* 1991; **10**: 320–327.
12. Pellerin D, Bertin P, Nihoul-Fekete C, Ricour C. Cholelithiasis and ileal pathology in children. *J Pediatr Surg* 1975; **10**: 35–41.
13. Ohkohchi N, Andoh T, Izumi U et al. Disorder of bile acid metabolism in children with short bowel syndrome. *J Gastroenterol* 1997; **32**: 472–479.
14. Modigliani R, Labayle D, Aymes C et al. Evidence for excessive absorption of oxalate by the colon in enteric hyperoxaluria. *Scand J Gastroenterol* 1978; **13**: 187–192.
15. Dowling RH, Booth CC. Structural and functional changes following small intestinal resection in the rat. *Clin Sci* 1967; **32**: 139–149.
16. Gracey M. Intestinal microflora and bacterial overgrowth in early life. *J Pediatr Gastroenterol Nutr* 1982; **1**: 13–22.
17. King CE, Toskes PP. Small intestine bacterial overgrowth. *Gastroenterology* 1979; **76**: 1035–1055.
18. Carbonnel F, Cosnes J, Chevret et al. The role of anatomic factors in nutritional autonomy after extensive small bowel resection. *J Parenter Enteral Nutr* 1996; **20**: 275–280.
19. Nightingale JMD, Lennard-Jones JE, Gertner DJ et al. Colonic preservation reduces need for parenteral therapy, increases incidence of renal stones, but does not change high prevalence of gallstones in patients with a short bowel. *Gut* 1992; **33**: 1493–1497.
20. Nordgaard I, Hansen BS, Mortensen PB. Importance of colonic support for energy absorption as small-bowel failure proceeds. *Am J Clin Nutr* 1996; **64**: 222–231.
21. Strauss E, Gerson CD, Yalow RS. Hypersecretion of gastrin associated with short bowel syndrome. *Gastroenterology* 1974; **66**: 175–180.
22. Nightingale JMD, Kamm MA, van der Sijp JRM et al. Disturbed gastric emptying in the short bowel syndrome. Evidence for a colonic brake. *Gut* 1993; **34**: 1171–1176.
23. Nightingale JMD, Kamm MA, van der Sijp JRM. Gastrointestinal hormones in short bowel syndrome. Peptide YY may be the colonic brake to gastric emptying. *Gut* 1996; **39**: 267–272.
24. Bury KD. Carbohydrate digestion and absorption after massive resection of the small intestine. *Surg Gynecol Obstet* 1972; **135**: 177–187.
25. Urban E, Pena M. *In vivo* calcium transport by rat small intestine after massive small bowel resection. *Am J Physiol* 1974; **226**. 1304–1308.
26. Kurkchubasche AG, Rowe MI, Smith SD. Adaptation in short-bowel syndrome: reassessing old limits. *J Pediatr Surg* 1993; **28**: 1069–1071.
27. Sacks AI, Warwick GJ, Barnard JA. Early proliferative events following intestinal resection in the rat. *J Pediatr Gastroenterol Nutr* 1995; **21**: 158–164.
28. Sukhotnik I, Siplovich L, Shiloni E et al. Intestinal adaptation in short-bowel syndrome in infants and children: a collective review. *Pediatr Surg Int* 2002; **18**: 258–263.
29. Booth IW, Lander AD. Short bowel syndrome. *Baillière's Clin Gastroenterol* 1998; **12**: 739–773.
30. Jeppesen PB, Mortensen AP. Enhancing bowel adaptation in short bowel syndrome. *Curr Gastroenterol Rep* 2002; **4**: 338–347.

31. Wilmore DW. Growth factors and nutrients in the short bowel syndrome. *J Parenter Enteral Nutr* 1999; **23**: 117–120.
32. Ziegler TR, Mantell MP, Chow JC et al. Gut adaptation and the insulin growth factor system: regulation by glutamine and IGF-1 administration. *Am J Physiol* 1996; **277**: G866–875.
33. Dowling RH. The influence of luminal nutrition on intestinal adaptation after small bowel resection and bypass. In Dowling RH, Riecken EO, eds. *Intestinal Adaptation*. New York: Schattauer Verlag, 1974: 35–46.
34. Weser E, Heller R, Taxil T. Stimulation of mucosal growth in the rat ileum by bile and pancreatic secretions after jejunal resection. *Gastroenterology* 1977; **73**: 524–529.
35. Feldman El, Dowling RH, McNaughton J et al. Effects of oral versus intravenous nutrition on intestinal adaptation after small bowel resection in the dog. *Gastroenterology* 1976; **70**: 712–719.
36. Williamson RCN. Intestinal adaptation mechanisms of control. *N Engl J Med* 1978; **298**: 1444–1450.
37. Drucker DJ. Biological actions and therapeutic potential of the glucagon-like peptides. *Gastroenterology* 2002; **122**: 531–44.
38. Ling PR, Sheikh M, Boyce P et al. Cholecystokinin (CCK) secretion in patients with severe short bowel syndrome (SSBS). *Dig Dis Sci* 2001; **46**: 859–864.
39. Sigalet DL, Martin GR. Hormonal therapy for short bowel syndrome. *J Pediatr Surg* 2000; **35**: 360–64.
40. Souba W, Klimberg S, Plumley D et al. The role of glutamine in maintaining a healthy gut and supporting the metabolic response to injury and infection. *J Surg Res* 1990; **48**: 383–391.
41. Byrne TA, Morrissey TB, Nattakom TV et al. Growth hormone, glutamine, and a modified diet enhance nutrient absorption in patients with severe short bowel syndrome. *J Parenter Enteral Nutr* 1995; **19**: 296–302.
42. Beaugerie L, Carbonnel F, Hecketsweiler B et al. Effects of an isotonic oral rehydration solution, enriched with glutamine, on fluid and sodium absorption in patients with a short-bowel. *Aliment Pharmacol Ther* 1997; **11**: 741–746.
43. Scolapio JS. Effect of growth hormone, glutamine, and diet on body composition in short bowel syndrome: a randomized, controlled study. *J Parenter Enteral Nutr* 1999; **23**: 309–312.
44. Dumas F, De Bandt JP, Colomb V et al. Enteral ornithine alpha-ketoglutarate enhances intestinal adaptation to massive resection in rats. *Metabolism* 1998; **47**: 1366–1371.
45. Nordgaard I, Hansen BS, Mortensen PB. Colon as a digestive organ in patients with short bowel. *Lancet* 1994; **343**: 373–376.
46. Briet F, Flourie B, Achour L et al. Bacterial adaptation in patients with short bowel and colon in continuity. *Gastroenterology* 1995; **109**: 1446–1453.
47. Koruda MJ, Rolandelli RH, Settle RG et al. The effect of a pectin-supplemented elemental diet on intestinal adaptation to massive small bowel resection. *J Parenter Enteral Nutr* 1986; **10**: 343–350.
48. Koruda MJ, Rolandelli RH, Settle RG et al. Effect of parenteral nutrition supplemented with short-chain fatty acids on adaptation to massive small bowel resection. *Gastroenterology* 1988; **95**: 715–720.
49. Grey VL, Morin CL. Evidence for a growth-stimulating fraction in the rat after small bowel resection. *Gastroenterology* 1985; **89**: 1305–1312.
50. Weawer LT, Walker WA. Epidermal growth factor and the developing human gut. *Gastroenterology* 1988; **94**: 845–847.
51. Menard D, Arsenault P, Pothier P. Biologic effects or epidermal growth factor in human fetal jejunum. *Gastroenterology* 1988; **94**: 656–663.
52. Sham J, Martin G, Meddings JB, Sigalet DL. Epidermal growth factor improves nutritional outcome in a rat model of short bowel syndrome. *J Pediatric Surg* 2002; **37**: 765–769.
53. Schwartz MZ, Storozuk RB. Epidermal growth factor enhances small intestine function. *Gastroenterology* 1985; **88**: 158–60.
54. Malo C, Ménard D. Influence of epidermal growth factor on the development or suckling mouse intestinal mucosa. *Gastroenterology* 1982; **83**: 28–35.
55. Luk GD, Yang P. Distribution or polyamines and their biosynthetic enzymes in intestinal adaptation. *Am J Physiol* 1988; **254**: G194–G200.
56. Buts JP, De Keyser N, Kolanowski J et al. Maturation of villus and crypt cell functions in rat small intestine: role or dietary polyamines. *Dig Dis Sciences* 1993; **38**: 1091–1098.
57. Helander HF, Johansson C, Blom H, Uribe A. Trophic actions of E_2 prostaglandins in the rat gastrointestinal mucosa. A quantitative morphologic study. *Gastroenterology* 1985; **89**: 1393–1399.
58. Vanderhoof JA, Euler AR, Park JHY, Grandjean CJ. Augmentation of mucosal adaptation following massive small bowel resection by 16,16-dimethyl-PG E_2 in the rat. *Digestion* 1987; **36**: 213–219.
59. Vanderhoof JA, Park JHY, Grandjean CJ. Effect of zinc deficiency on mucosal hyperplasia following 70% resection. *Am J Clin Nutr* 1986; **44**: 670–677.
60. Ford WDA, Boelhouwer RU, King WWK et al. Total parenteral nutrition inhibits intestinal adaptive hyperplasia in young rats reversal by feeding. *Surgery* 1983; **96**: 527–534.
61. Grimble GK. Rees RG, Keohane PP et al. Effects of peptide chain length on absorption of egg protein hydrolysates in the normal human jejunum. *Gastroenterology* 1987; **92**: 136–142.
62. Silk DBA, Fairclough PD, Clark ML et al. Uses of a peptide rather than a free amino-acid nitrogen source in chemically defined elemental diets. *J Parenter Enteral Nutr* 1980; **4**: 548–553.
63. Fairelough PD, Hegarty JE, Silk DBA, Clark ML. Comparison of the absorption of two protein hydrolysates and their effects on water and electrolyte movements in the human jejunum. *Gut* 1980: **21**: 829–834.
64. Poullain MG, Cezard JP, Roger l, Mendy F. Effect of whey proteins, their oligopeptide hydrolysates and free amino acid mixtures on growth and nitrogen in fed and starved rats. *J Parenter Enteral Nutr* 1989; **13**: 382–386.
65. Bines J, Francis D, Hill D. Reducing parenteral requirement in children with short bowel syndrome: impact of an amino acid-based complete infant formula. *J Pediatr Gastroenterol Nutr* 1998; **26**: 123–128.
66. Andorsky DJ, Lund DP, Lillehei CW et al. Nutritional and other postoperative management of neonates with short bowel syndrome correlates with clinical outcomes. *J Pediatr* 2001; **139**: 27–33.
67. Bach AC, Babayan VK. Medium-chain triglycerides: an update. *Am J Clin Nutr* 1982; **36**: 950–962.
68. Jeppesen PB, Mortensen PB. The influence of a preserved colon on the absorption of medium chain fat in patients with small bowel resection. *Gut* 1998; **43**: 478–483.
69. Vanderhoof JA, Grandjean CJ, Burkley KT et al. Effect of high-percentage medium-chain triglyceride diet on mucosal adaptation following massive bowel resection in rats. *J Parenter Enteral Nutr* 1984; **8**: 685–689.

70. Grey VL, Garofalo C, Greenberg GR, Morin CL. The adaptation of the small intestine after resection in response to free fatty acids. *Am J Clin Nutr* 1984; **40**: 1235–1242.
71. Hart MH, Grandjean CL, Park JHY et al. Essential fatty acid deficiency and post-resection mucosal adaptation in the rat. *Gastroenterology* 1987; **94**: 682–687.
72. Goulet O, Richard S, Nezelof C et al. Parenteral nutrition associated liver disease in children with massive loss or intestine. *Clin Nutr* 1989; **8**: 24 (abstr).
73. Stanko RT, Nathan G, Mendelow H, Adibi SA. Development of hepatic cholestasis and fibrosis in patients with massive loss of intestine supported by prolonged parenteral nutrition. *Gastroenterology* 1987; **92**: 197–202.
74. Wolf A, Pohlandt F. Bacterial infection: the main cause of acute cholestasis in newborn infants receiving short-term parenteral nutrition. *J Pediatr Gastroenterol Nutr* 1989; **8**: 297–303.
75. Sondheimer JM, Asturias E, Cadnapaphornchai M. Infection and cholestasis in neonates with intestinal resection and long-term parenteral nutrition. *J Pediatr Gastroenterol Nutr* 1998; **27**: 131–137.
76. Braxton C, Lowry SF. Editorial: parenteral nutrition and liver dysfunction – new insight? *J Parenter Enteral Nutr* 1995; **19**: 3–4.
77. Kaufman SS. Prevention of parenteral nutrition-associated liver disease in children. *Pediatr Transplant* 2002; **6**: 37–42.
78. Merritt RJ. Medical progress: cholestasis associated with total parenteral nutrition. *J Pediatr Gastroenterol Nutr* 1986; **5**: 9–22.
79. Colomb V, Jobert-Giraud A, Lacaille F et al. Role of lipid emulsions in cholestasis associated with long-term parenteral nutrition in children. *J Parenter Enteral Nutr* 2000; **24**: 345–350.
80. Kaufman SS, Loseke CA, Lupo JV et al. Influence of bacterial overgrowth and intestinal inflammation on duration of parenteral nutrition in children with short bowel syndrome. *J Pediatr* 1997; **131**: 356–361.
81. Goulet O. Parenteral nutrition in pediatrics – indications and perspectives. *Acta Gastroenterol Belg* 1999; **62**: 210–215.
82. Salas JS, Dozio E, Goulet O et al. Energy expenditure and substrate utilization in the course of renutrition of malnourished children. *J Parenter Enteral Nutr* 1991; **15**: 288–293.
83. Vargas JH, Ament ME, Berquist WE. Long-term home parenteral nutrition in pediatrics: ten years of experience in 102 patients. *J Pediatr Gastroenterol Nutr* 1987; **6**: 24–32.
84. Colomb V, Goulet O, Ricour C. Home enteral and parenteral nutrition. *Baillière's Clin Gastroenterol* 1998; **122**: 877–894.
85. Moukarzel A, Song MK, Buchman AL et al. Excessive chromium intake in children receiving total parenteral nutrition. *Lancet* 1992; **339**: 385–388.
86. Buchman AL, Moukarzel AA. Metabolic bone disease associated with total parenteral nutrition. *Clin Nutr* 2000; **19**: 217–231.
87. Schiano TD, Klang MG, Quesada E et al. Thiamine status in patients receiving long-term home parenteral nutrition. *Am J Gastroenterol* 1996; **91**: 2555–2559.
88. Edes TE, Walk BE, Thorton WH, Fritsche KL. Essential fatty acid sufficiency does not preclude fat-soluble-vitamin deficiency in short-bowel syndrome. *Am J Clin Nutr* 1991; **53**: 499–502.
89. Niv Y, Charash B, Sperber AD, Oren M. Effect of octreotide on gastrostomy, duodenostomy, and cholecystostomy effluents: a physiologic study of fluid and electrolyte balance. *Am J Gastroenterol* 1997; **92**: 2107–2111.
90. Colomb V, Fabeiro M, Dabbas M et al. Central venous catheter-related infections in children on long-term home parenteral nutrition: incidence and risk factors. *Clin Nutr* 2000; **19**: 355–359.
91. Capron JP, Gineston JL, Herve MA. Metronidazole in prevention of cholestasis associated with total parenteral nutrition. *Lancet* 1983; **1**: 446–447.
92. Spagnuolo MI, Iorio R, Vegnente A, Guarino A. Ursodeoxycholic acid for treatment of cholestasis in children on long-term total parenteral nutrition: a pilot study. *Gastroenterology* 1996; **111**: 716–719.
93. Goulet O, Duhamel JF. Ricour C. Nutritional problems. In Tinker J, Rapin M, eds. *Care of the Critically Ill Patient*. New York: Springer Verlag, 1992: 1415–1436.
94. Advenier E, Landry C, Colomb V et al. Aluminium contamination of parenteral nutrition and aluminium in children on long-term parenteral nutrition. *J Pediatr Gastroenterol Nutr* 2003; **36**: 448–453.
95. Goulet O, de Potter S, Antebi H et al. Long-term efficacy and safety of a new olive oil-based intravenous fat emulsion in pediatric patients: a double-blind randomized study. *Am J Clin Nutr* 1999; **70**: 338–345.
96. Forchielli ML, Gura KM, Sandler R, Lo C. Aminosyn PF or Trophamine: which provides more protection from cholestasis associated with total parenteral nutrition? *J Pediatr Gastroenterol Nutr* 1995; **21**: 374–382.
97. Dabbas M, Jobert-Giraud A, Colomb V et al. Intestinal absorption in children with short bowel syndrome. *Clin Nutr* 1998; **17** (Suppl 1): 45 (abstr).
98. Liefaard G, Heineman E, Molenaar JC, Tibboel D. Prospective evaluation of the absorptive capacity of the bowel after major and minor resections in the neonates. *J Pediatr Surg* 1995; **30**: 388–391.
99. Barilla DE, Notz C, Kennedy D, Pak CYC. Renal oxalate excretion following oral oxalate loads in patients with ileal disease and with renal and absorptive hypercalciurias. Effect of calcium and magnesium. *Am J Med* 1978; **64**: 579–585.
100. Rockwell GF, Campfield T, Nelson BC, Uden PC. Oxalogenesis in parenteral nutrition solution components. *Nutrition* 1999; **14**: 836–839.
101. Hudson M, Pocknee R, Mowat NAG. D-lactic acidosis in short bowel syndrome – an examination of possible mechanisms. *Q J Med* 1990; **74**: 157–163.
102. From the Centers for Disease Control and Prevention. Lactic acidosis traced to thiamine deficiency related to nation wide shortage of multivitamins for total parenteral nutrition – United States 1997. *JAMA* 1997; **278**: 109, 111.
103. Kadakia SC. D-Lactic acidosis in a patient with jejunoileal bypass. *J Clin Gastroenterol* 1995; **20**: 154–156.
104. Marteau P, Messing B, Arrigoni E et al. Do patients with short-bowel syndrome need a lactose-free diet? *Nutrition* 1997; **13**: 13–16.
105. Scolapio JS, Nguyen JH, Steers J, Ukleja A. Success with intestinal failure: from adaptation to transplantation. *Dig Dis* 1999; **17**: 107–112.
106. Herek O. *Saccaromyces boulardii*: a possible addition to the standard treatment and prophylaxis of enterocolitis in Hirschsprung's disease? *Pediatr Surg Int* 2002; **18**: 567.
107. Dellert SF, Farrell MK, Specker BL, Heubi JE. Bone mineral content in children with short bowel syndrome after discontinuation of parenteral nutrition. *J Pediatr* 1998; **132**: 516–519.

108. Goulet O, Baglin-Gobet S, Jais JP et al. Outcome and long-term growth after extensive small bowel resection in the neonatal period: a survey of 87 children. *Eur J Pediatr Surg* 2004; in press

109. Leonberg BL, Chuang E, Eicher P et al. Long-term growth and development in children after home parenteral nutrition. *J Pediatr* 1998; **132**: 461–466.

110. Festen S, Brevoord JC, Goldhoorn GA et al. Excellent long-term outcome for survivors of apple peel atresia. *J Pediatr Surg* 2002; **37**: 61–65.

111. Dorney SFA, Ament MA, Berquist WE et al. Improved survival in very short small bowel of infancy with use of long-term parenteral nutrition. *J Pediatr* 1985; **107**: 521–525.

112. Surana R, Quinn FMJ, Puri P. Short-gut syndrome: intestinal adaptation in a patient with 12 cm of jejunum. *J Pediatr Gastroenterol Nutr* 1994; **19**: 246–249.

113. Hancock BJ, Wiseman NE. Lethal short-bowel syndrome. *J Pediatr Surg* 1990; **25**: 1131–1134.

114. Ricour C, Duhamel JF, Arnaud-Battandier F et al. Enteral and parenteral nutrition in the short bowel syndrome in children. *World J Surg* 1985; **9**: 310–315.

115. Goulet O, Ricour C. The short bowel syndrome. In Buts JP, Sokal E, eds. *Management of Digestive and Liver Disorders in Infants and Children*. Elsevier, 1993: 307–318.

116. Goulet O, Revillon Y, Jan D et al. Which patients need small bowel transplantation for neonatal short bowel syndrome? *Transplant Proc* 1992; **24**: 1058–1059.

117. Taylor B, Murphy GM, Dowling RH. Pituitary hormones and the small bowel: effect of hypophysectomy on intestinal adaptation to small bowel resection in the rat. *Eur J Clin Invest* 1979; **9**: 115–127.

118. Scow RO, Hagan SN. Effect of testosterone propionate and growth hormone on growth and chemical composition of muscle and other tissues in hypophysectomized male rats. *Endocrinology* 1965; **77**: 852–858.

119. Shulman DI, Shih Hu C, Duckett G, Lavallee-Grey M. Effects of short-term growth hormone therapy in rats undergoing 75% small intestinal resection. *J Pediatr Gastroenterol Nutr* 1992; **14**: 3–11.

120. Ulshen MA, Dowling RH, Fuller CR et al. Enhanced growth of small bowel in transgenic mice overexpressing bovine growth hormone. *Gastroenterology* 1993; **104**: 973–980.

121. Benhamou PH, Canarelli JP, Leroy C et al. Stimulation by recombinant human growth hormone of growth and development of remaining bowel after subtotal ileojejunectomy in rat. *J Pediatr Gastroenterol Nutr* 1994, **18**: 446–452.

122. Vanderhoof JA, Kollman KA, Griffin S, Adrian TE. Growth hormone and glutamine do not stimulate intestinal adaptation following massive small bowel resection in the rat. *J Pediatr Gastroenterol Nutr* 1997; **25**: 327–331.

123. Lobie PE, Briepohl S, Waters MJ. Growth hormone receptors in rat intestinal tract. *Endocrinology* 1990; **126**: 299–306.

124. Laburthe M, Rouyer-Fessard C, Gammeltoft S. Receptors for insulin-like growth factors I and II in rat gastro-intestinal epithelium. *Am J Physiol* 1988; **254**: G457–462.

125. Termanini B, Nardi RV, Finan TM. Insulin-like growth factor receptors in rabbit gastro-intestinal tract: characterization and autoradiographic localization. *Gastroenterology* 1990; **99**: 51–60.

126. Vanderhoof JA., McCusrer RH, Clark R et al. Truncated and native IGF-I enhance mucosal adaptation after jejunoileal resection. *Gastroenterology* 1992; **102**: 1949–1956.

127. Lemmey AB, Martin AA, Read LC et al. IGF-I and the truncated analogue des(1-3) 16F-I enhance growth in rats after gut resection. *Am J Physiol* 1991; **260**: E213–E219.

128. Inoue Y, Copeland EM, Souba WW. Growth hormone enhances amino-acid uptake by the human small intestine. *Ann Surg* 1994; **219**: 715–724.

129. Challacombe DN, Wheeler EE. The trophic action of human growth hormone duodenal mucosa cultured *in vitro*. *J Pediatr Gastroenterol Nutr* 1995; **21**: 50–53.

130. Byrne TA, Persiger RL, Young LS et al. A new treatment for patients with short bowel syndrome. *Ann Surg* 1995; **222**: 243–255.

131. Scolapio JS, Camilleri M, Fleming CR et al. Effect of growth hormone, glutamine, and diet on adaptation in short-bowel syndrome: a randomized, controlled study. *Gastroenterology* 1997; **113**: 1074–1081.

132. Seguy D, Vahedi K, Crenn P et al. Growth hormone benefit in very short bowel patients a randomized controlled trial. *Clin Nutr* 1999.

133. Szkudlarek J, Jeppesen P-B, Mortensen P-B. Effect of high dose growth hormone with glutamine and no change in diet on intestinal absoption in short bowel patients: a randomised, double blind, crossover, placebo controlled study. *Gut* 2000; **47**: 199–205.

134. Ellegard L, Bosaeus I, Nordgren S, Bengtsson BA. Low-dose recombinant human growth hormone increases body weight and lean body mass in patients with short bowel syndrome. *Ann Surg* 1997; **225**: 88–96.

135. Socha J, Ksiazyk J, Fogel WA et al. Is growth hormone a feasible adjuvant in the treatment of children after small bowel resection? *Clin Nutr* 1996; **15**: 185–188.

136. Dabbas-Tyan M, Colomb V, Rosilio M et al. Evaluation of the effect of recombinant human growth hormone (rhGH) treatment of children with short bowel syndrome. *J Pediatr Gastroenterol Nutr* 2000; **31**: 5165–5166.

137. Drucker DJ. Gut adaptation and the glucagon-like peptides. *Gut* 2002; **50**: 428–435.

138. L'Heureux MC, Brubaker PL. Therapeutic potential of the intestinotropic hormone, glucagon-like peptide-2. *Ann Med* 2001; **33**: 229–35.

139. Jeppesen PB, Hartmann B, Hansen BS et al. Impaired meal stimulated glucagon-like peptide 2 response in ileal resected short bowel patients with intestinal failure. *Gut* 1999; **45**: 559–563.

140. Jeppesen PB, Hartmann B, Thulesen J et al. Glucagon-like peptide 2 improves nutrient absorption in short-bowel patients with no colon. *Gastroenterology* 2001; **120**: 806–815.

141. Delaney HM, Parker JG, Gliedman ML. Experimental massive intestinal resection: comparison of surgical measures and spontaneous adaptation. *Arch Surg* 1970; **101**: 599–604.

142. Persemlidis D, Kark AE. Antiperistaltic segments for the treatment or short bowel syndrome. *Am J Gastroenterol* 1974; **62**: 526–530.

143. Stacchini A, Dido LJ, Primo ML et al. Artificial sphincter as surgical treatment for experimental massive resection of small intestine. *Am J Surg* 1982; **143**: 721–26.

144. Ricotta J, Zuidcma FD, Gadacz RT, Sadri D. Construction of an ileocaecal valve and its role in massive resection of the small intestine. *Surg Gynecol Obstet* 1981; **152**: 310–314.

145. Waddell WR, Kern F, Halgrimson CG, Woodbury JJ. A simple jejunocolic 'valve.' For relief of rapid transit and

the short bowel syndrome. *Arch Surg* 1970; **100**: 438–444.

146. Hakami M, Moslehy A, Mosavy SH. Reversed jejunal segment used to treat the short bowel syndrome. *Am Surg* 1975; **41**: 432–435.
147. Panis Y, Messing B, Rivet P et al. Segmental reversal of the small bowel as an alternative to intestinal transplantation in patients with short bowel syndrome. *Ann Surg* 1997; **225**: 401–407.
148. Trinkle JK, Bryant LR. Reversed colon segment in an infant with massive small bowel resection: a case report. *J Ky Med Assoc* 1967; **65**: 1090–1091.
149. Garcia VF, Templeton JM, Eichelberger MR et al. Colon interposition for the short bowel syndrome. *J Pediatr Surg* 1981; **16**: 994–995.
150. Glick PL, de Lorimier AA, Adzick NS, Harrison MR. Colon interposition: an adjuvant operation for short-gut syndrome. *J Pediatr Surg* 1984; **19**: 719–725.
151. Brolin RE. Colon interposition for extreme short bowel syndrome: a case report. *Surgery* 1986; **100**: 576–580.
152. Georgeson K, Halpin D, Figueroa R et al. Sequential intestinal lengthening procedures for refractory short bowel syndrome. *J Pediatr Surg* 1994; **29**: 316–320; discussion 320–311.
153. Thompson JS, Langnas AN, Pinch LW et al. Surgical approach to short-bowel syndrome. Experience in a population of 160 patients. *Ann Surg* 1995; **222**: 600–605; discussion 605–607.
154. Devine RM, Kelly KA. Surgical therapy of the short bowel syndrome. *Gastroenterol Clin North Am* 1989; **18**: 603–618.
155. Bianchi A. Intestinal loop lengthening a technique for increasing small intestinal length. *J Pediatr Surg* 1980; **15**: 145–151.
156. Bianchi A. Longitudinal intestinal lengthening and tailoring: results in 20 children. *J R Soc Med* 1997; **90**: 429–432.
157. Weber TR. Isoperistaltic bowel lengthening for short bowel syndrome in children. *Am J Surg* 1999; **178**: 600–604.
158. Thompson JS, Pinch LW, Young R, Vanderhoof JA. Long-term outcome of intestinal lengthening. *Transplant Proc* 2000; **32**: 1242–1243.
159. Waag KL, Hosie S, Wessel L. What do children look like after longitudinal intestinal lengthening? *Eur J Pediatr Surg* 1999; **9**: 260–262.
160. Figueroa-Colon R, Harris PR, Birdsong E et al. Impact of intestinal lengthening on the nutritional outcome for children with short bowel syndrome. *J Pediatr Surg* 1996; **31**: 912–916.
161. Lawrence JP, Dun SP, Billmire DF et al. Isolated liver transplantation for liver failure in patients with short bowel syndrome. *J Pediatr Surg* 1994; **29**: 751–753.
162. Horslen SP, Sudan DL, Iyer KR et al. Isolated liver transplantation in infants with end-stage liver disease associated with short bowel syndrome. *Ann Surg* 2002; **235**: 435–439.
163. Vanderhoof JA. Short bowel syndrome in children and small intestinal transplantation. *Pediatr Clin North Am* 1996; **43**: 533.
164. Grant D. Intestinal transplantation: 1997 Report of the International Registry. *Transplantation* 1999; **15**: 1061–1064.
165. Goulet O, Jan D, Lacaille F et al. Intestinal transplantation in children: preliminary experience in Paris. *J Parenter Enteral Nutr* 1999; **23**: S121–125.
166. Langnas AN, Sudan DL, Kaufman SS et al. Intestinal transplantation: a single center experience. *Transplant Proc* 2000; **32**: 1228.
167. Goulet O, Lacaille F, Jan D, Ricour C. Intestinal transplantation : indications, results and strategy. *Curr Opin Clin Nutr Metab Care* 2000; **3**: 329–333.

30 Lymphonodular hyperplasia

Jorma Kokkonen

Introduction

Small lymphoid nodules inside the mucosa lining the gastrointestinal tract are normal endoscopic findings among children.[1] However, greatly enlarged lymphoid nodules or a mass covering most of the view area and described as lymphoid nodular hyperplasia (LNH) may be considered abnormal. The most typical sites for LNH are the bulb of the duodenum, the colon and the terminal ileum, where small nodules are visible in nearly all subjects.[2,3] Assessment by videoendoscope has made LNH now perhaps the most common finding seen in pediatric examinations. During the era of X-ray examinations and fiberoscopes only heavy accumulations of lymphoid tissue were diagnosed, most cases with minor lesions remaining undiagnosed.[4] As we may examine only patients with long-term symptoms, for understandable reasons, we will never know the true prevalence of LNH in healthy subjects.

The clinical significance of LNH has long remained obscure. It was previously considered as normal or age-related in pediatric patients diagnosed as infants or small children.[2,4] Even now it may be considered as a finding peculiar to children, being only rarely diagnosed in adults.[5] In earlier literature, intestinal LNH was a rare finding, but was clearly associated with congenital or acquired immunodeficiency states, including IgA deficiency.[6–8] It has also been seen in HIV subjects even before the development of AIDS.[9] LNH may now be considered as a state indicating an ongoing or earlier up-regulated immune activity of the underlying mucosa.[10]

In a microscopic examination, a biopsy sample from the LNH site reveals follicles with or without germinal centers but usually no dense mononuclear or eosinophilic inflammation. LNH represents a multiplication of Peyer's patches, an accumulation of lymphoid cells specialized in handling antigens cross the mucosal barrier and regulation of the innate immune response. Recent evidence suggests that in subjects with LNH the local cytokine populations are skewed, showing similarities both with celiac disease and atopic allergy.

Assessment

To date there has been no objective method of measuring or evaluating the amount of intramural accumulations of lymphoid tissue downstream of the intestinal mucosa. Clusters of lymphoid nodules seen during an endoscopic examination may be considered significant. LNH may be considered as a hypernormal phenomenon, an enlargement and multiplication of normal lymphoid tissue (Figures 30.1a and b, 30.2a and b, 30.3a and b).

Wakefield et al used a four-step classification to describe the prominence of LNH at the terminal ileum.[11] We have also used this practical grading, using the following description: grade 0, no lymphoid follicles; grade 1, mild – lymphoid follicles dispersed on the walls; grade 2, moderate, lymphoid follicles filling the walls; and grade 3, severe – terminal ileum massed with lymphoid tissue, the valve protruding. However, in some patients there are segments where the one wall may be massed with lymphoid tissue while the other wall has no visible lymphoid accumulation. The same classification may also be applied to the bulb of the duodenum and colon, where mostly only grades 0–2 are usually seen.

A patchy and segmental appearance is a typical feature of LNH. In the foregut the nodules are most often seen in the bulb. Only in a quarter of cases

(a)

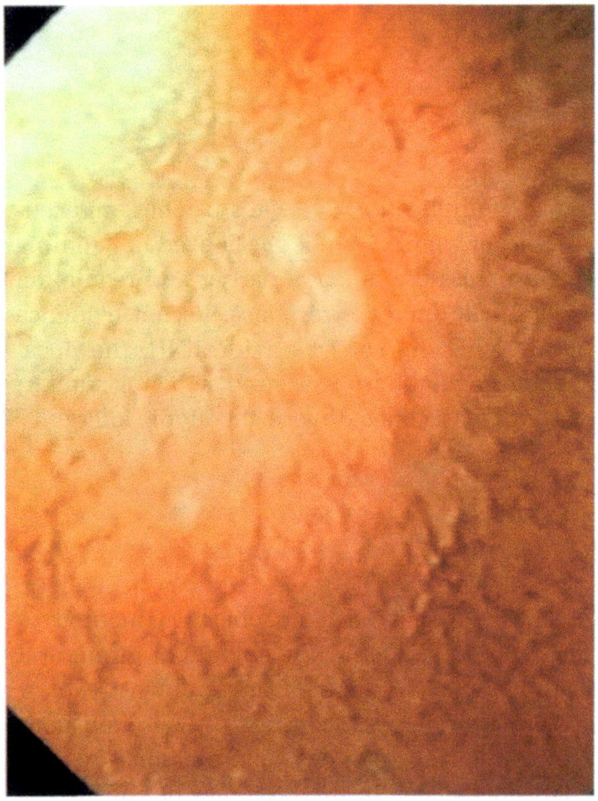

(b)

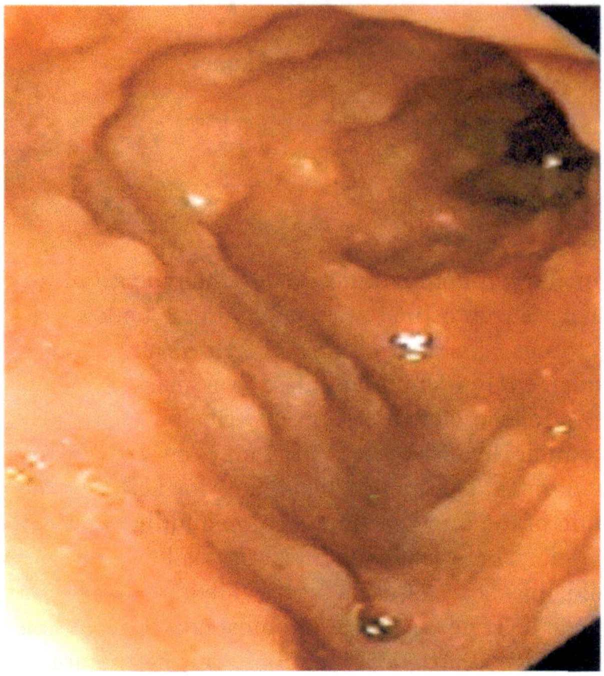

(c)

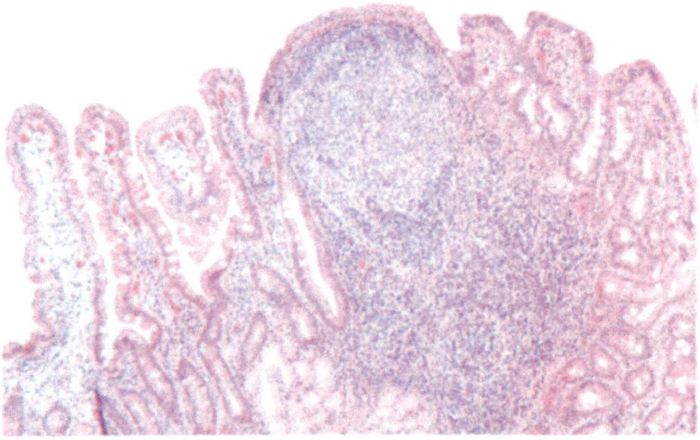

Figure 30.1 Normally in a close endoscopic view of the bulb of the duodenum, the villous architecture is visible on a plain mucosa (a). In lymphoid nodular hyperplasia (LNH) small bubbles are dispersed along the walls covering otherwise normal mucosa (b). A biopsy sample from the site of the LNH reveals a lymphoid nodule with a germinal center but surrounded by normal villi (c).

does the lesion continue to the descending duodenum. In the terminal ileum, LNH is usually restricted to an area of about 10–15 cm proximal to the valve. If massed just above the valve it usually becomes nodular and disappears entirely as it proceeds proximally in the ileum.

LNH must be actively sought during the examination. The underlying mucosa is healthy in that there is usually no inflammation. The visible LNH bubbles may be hidden between the folds. During the videoendoscopic examination the lesion is sought and assessed after the segments of the areas inspected are filled with air to the maximum possible and the nodularity is evaluated by sight. In the terminal ileum a protruding valve may reveal LNH inside the small intestine.

Histology and immunohistochemistry

A typical feature in the microscopic examination of a biopsy sample from a patient with LNH is an increased occurrence and enlargement of lymphoid follicles with or without germinal centers (Figures 30.1c, 30.2c, 30.3c). The centers are usually grossly enlarged and reactive as indicated by numerous tingle body macrophages. In advanced cases the outer margins of the T-cell zone may not be as well defined as in normal or mild cases, with the lymphoid compartment extending into the adjacent villi. There may also

(a)

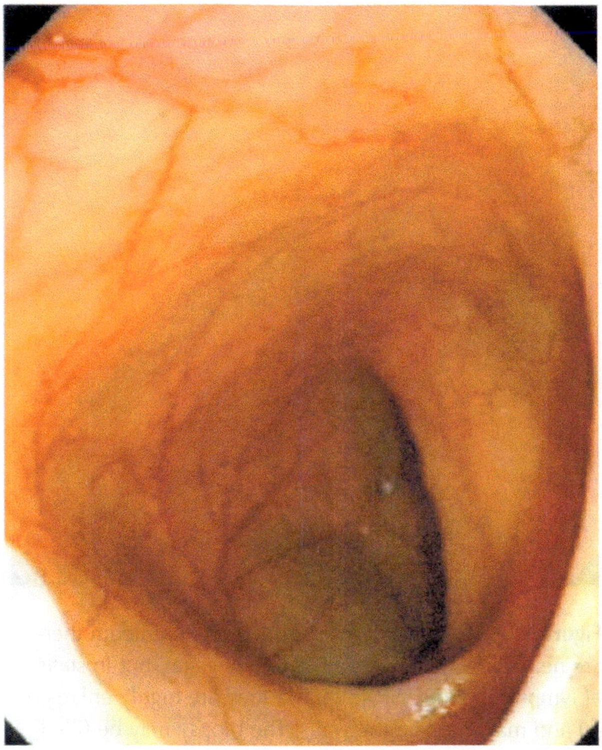

(b)

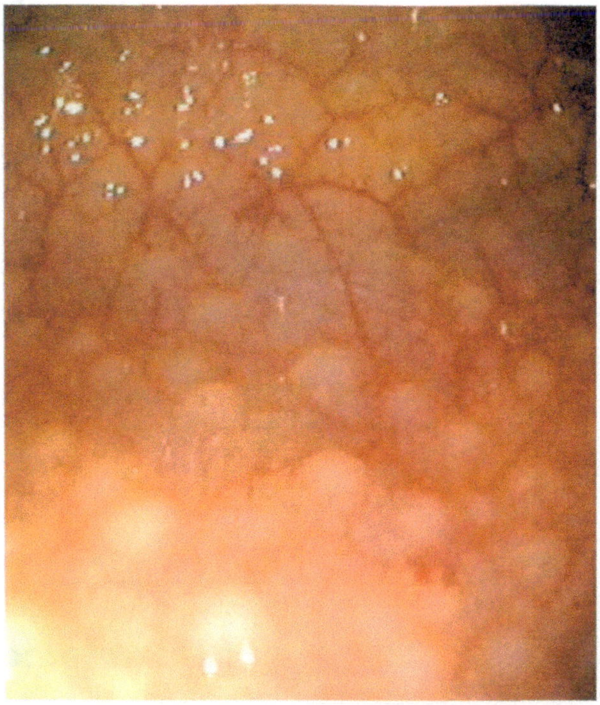

(c)

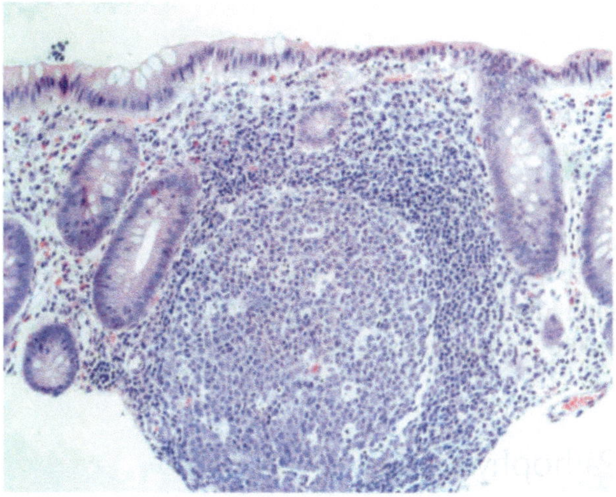

Figure 30.2 On the healthy mucosa of the colon the vascular pattern is clear (a). Lymphoid nodular hyperplasia may cover the mucosa as a dense madras (b) or be sparsely dispersed. A biopsy sample in a histological examination reveals accumulation of lymphoid tissue (c).

be disruption but not destruction of adjacent crypts, the number of which may be decreased. Typical cases have no villous atrophy, no slight villous abnormalities or mononuclear or even eosinophilic infiltration, as seen in celiac disease.[12] The histology of the colonic samples is quite similar, subepithelial apoptosis/debris being increased as well.

LNH may also be associated with other disorders such as celiac disease or colitis, which have their own characteristics. LNH seems to have a weak predilection for IgE-mediated diseases or IgE-prone subjects; these may have excessive eosinophilic cells in the histology of their samples.[13] These patients may also show markers of atopic food allergy, namely positive skin prick tests or food-specific IgE class antibodies. However, these patients are a minority.

An increased density of intraepithelial lymphocytes has been measured in the biopsy sample sites of LNH, especially $\gamma\delta^+$ T-cell receptor (TCR)-bearing T cells.[14,15] Accordingly, the proportion of $\gamma\delta^+$ T cells of the total amount of $CD3^+$ T cells, i.e. the $\gamma\delta^+/CD3^+$ ratio, is greater than in the controls. Another type of intraepithelial cell that is increased in LNH subjects is the cytotoxic TIA-1-expressing cell.[16]

The rise in both types of intraepithelial cell seems to be more associated with the underlying disorder than with the LNH itself. Indeed, in recent reports the numbers of intraepithelial $\gamma\delta^+$ cells as well as

(a)

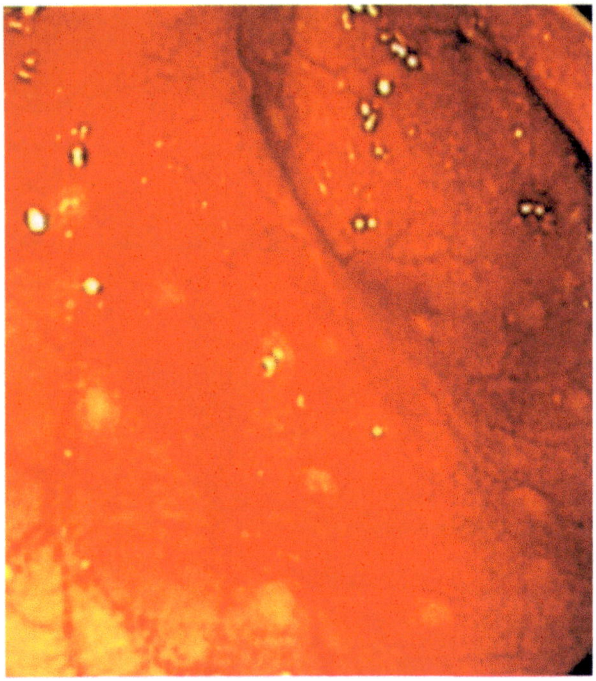

(b)

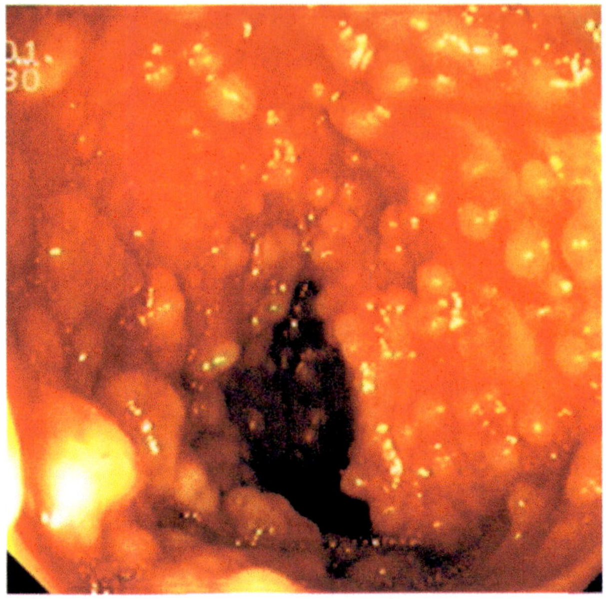

(c)

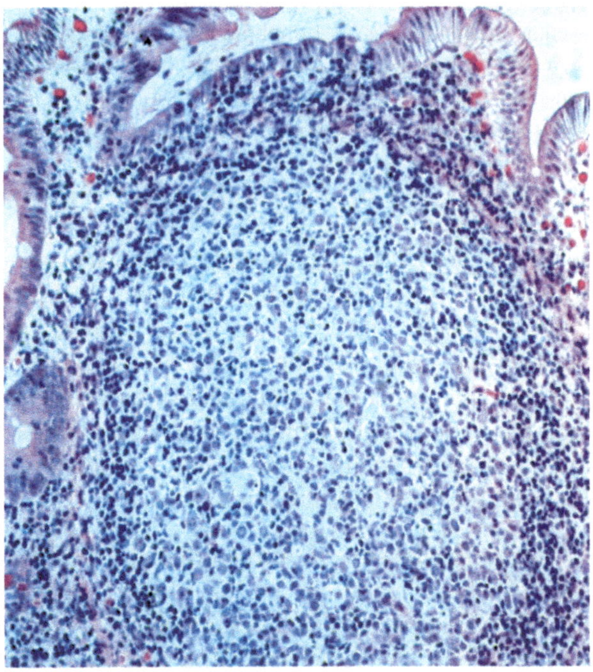

Figure 30.3 On the mucosa of the terminal ileum there are nearly always tiny lymphoid nodules (a), but in states of lymphoid nodular hyperplasia they are highly enlarged (b) and may mass on the walls. The biopsy may be filled with lymphoid tissue as large nodules (c) but interspersed normal villi may be found.

TIA-1 presenting T cells have been observed to be high in patients with food allergy.[13,15] However, we found the increased densities in untreated cases, but low densities in the subjects on an elimination diet. These findings indicate that in the delayed and local types of food allergy, as in celiac disease, the increment of γ/δ^+ T cells is associated with the activity of the disease.[17,18] However, even after an elimination diet, LNH seems to linger. Whether it is permanent or abates with time remains unknown.

To date, the exact pathogenetic significance of γ/δ^+ and TIA-1 T cells still remains obscure. Being typically increased in untreated celiac disease and food allergy, they may have profound significance in the pathogenesis of these disorders.

Pathophysiology

The segmental or patchy appearance of LNH probably underlines the fact that the lesion develops as an *in situ* activation of the innate immune response leading to multiplication of the lymphoid tissue. As hyper-reactivity to food-borne antigens is the most common state underlying LNH, this suggests that the lesion develops at the contact between luminal allergens and the immunologically activated cells inside the mucosa. Because of the passage of food juice and the timing of its contact with the mucosa, the most vulnerable places may be the bulb of the duodenum and the terminal ileum and colon, giving a reasonable explanation for the spread of the lesion in the gastrointestinal tract.

In a recent study we found evidence to suggest that, in food allergy as in celiac disease, cell-mediated immunity may be active and may cause the symptoms. However, we also found evidence showing that in LNH patients humoral immunity is also activated. The IgG and IgA class antibodies against milk proteins were increased in patients with LNH of the bulb of the duodenum.[19] These antibodies may have no pathogenetic significance in the process, their role being simply secondary, owing to the increment of B cells in and around the lymphoid follicles and through the interaction between B and T cells.[20,21] However, the humoral response relating to LNH may be dichotomous. We also found lower-than-normal levels of IgA and IgG class antibodies against milk allergens in subjects reacting rapidly in a blind challenge test.

Lacking villous atrophy and/or mononuclear inflammation, the symptoms in typical LNH cases may be due to an imbalance in cytokine cascades. LNH patients have more intraepithelial $\gamma\delta$-TCR$^+$ cells, which can produce a multiplicity of cytokines, including interleukin (IL)-2, interferon (IFN)-γ, tumor necrosis factor (TNF)-α, IL-4, IL-10 and transforming growth factor (TGF)-β, although to date there has been no detailed study of the subject. In infants with food allergy, Hauer et al showed an up-regulation of IFN-γ and, to a lesser extent, IL-4.[22] We found evidence in two experiments to show that, in patients with LNH and food allergy, the free secretion of IL-6 as measured in a biopsy sample was increased, as in celiac patients, but we failed to demonstrate any difference in the secretion of regulatory cytokines such as IL-10 and TGF-β. Examining the biopsy samples by a counter-polymerase chain reaction (PCR) method we found an up-regulation of chemokine receptor 4 (CCR-4) and IL-6 and down-regulation of IL-2 and IL-18 in LNH/food allergy cases (Paajanen et al, personal communication). Even in this study we saw no change in the regulatory cytokines as compared to the controls. At present, it seems possible that in LNH patients there is an imbalance in pre-allergic and pre-inflammatory cytokine function on the mucosa.

Unlike patients with celiac disease, subjects with LNH and food allergy display no increased prevalence of the HLA DQ-2 antigen (A0501/B0201).[14] HLA-DR seems to be only slightly up-regulated in the duodenal mucosa in these patients. There currently seems to be no evidence for genetic selection of LNH subjects. It seems clear that the process leading to an accumulation of lymphoid cells and tissue may take place in any subject with a temporary or permanent disorder in the protective mechanisms of the mucosal layer, leading to invasion of luminal antigens and up-regulation of the immune response *in situ* in any part of the gastrointestinal tract.

Differential diagnosis

In our series of 724 consecutive patients over 4 years, LNH was diagnosed in 135 (19%) in all (Table 30.1). The incidence was highest among the patients with food allergy, being found in more than 50% of the definitely diagnosed cases. It was found equally among the treated and untreated cases. As in the other centers regularly using endoscopic examinations to diagnose celiac disease, LNH was found in 10% of cases. The proportion was the same in both main types of inflammatory bowel disease (IBD) as well as in patients in whom we could make no definite diagnosis, even after rigorous examination.

LNH may be spread throughout the colon or as patches at any of the main segments. Among 301 consecutive subjects undergoing colonoscopy, we found 36 children with diffuse disease and 101 with segmental lesions. The transverse colon was the most common site for patchy lesions, followed by the cecum. Even in the colon the incidence of LNH was greatest among the patients with food allergy as diagnosed by history and a positive elimination–challenge test, rising to 77% of all cases. The patients also showed a 50% coincidence with diagnosed LNH in the foregut.

Within the spectrum of IBD, a quarter of patients with colitis showed LNH, but only a few presented with Crohn's disease. Colon et al found a similar association between LNH of the colon and IBD in 13 subjects in a 10-year retrospective study in which patients were examined mostly by radiographic methods, while 84 had no underlying disorder.[4]

Table 30.1 The presence of lymphoid nodular hyperplasia (LNH) on an endoscopic view in children examined for the first time with gastroduodenoscopy

	Number of subjects	LNH present	
		n	%
Esophagogastroduodenoscopy	724	135	19
untreated food allergy	96	47	49
celiac disease	138	9	7
IBD	76	10	13
Colonoscopy	301	137	46
untreated food allergy	71	55	77
IBD	83	28	34
Ileoscopy	204	105	51
untreated food allergy	51	38	74
IBD	64	20	31

IBD, inflammatory bowel disease

A new diagnostic entity showing LNH of the colon in half the patients is chronic constipation. Among these patients undergoing a challenge with cow's milk, a quarter showed a positive response during the succeeding 4 weeks. The other definite disorders occasionally showing LNH on the mucosa of the colon are diabetes, rheumatoid arthritis, vasculitis and chronic aggressive hepatitis. Finally, it could be demonstrated in about 10% of cases without any final diagnostic conclusions (Table 30.2).

In the colonoscopic examinations lymphoid mass or LNH of the terminal ileum was diagnosed in two-thirds of subjects in whom this end-point was reached. The valve of Bauchini was markedly protruded inside the colon in a quarter, all with an abundance of lymphoid tissue inside the ileum.

LNH of the terminal ileum was demonstrated in two-thirds of the subjects with defined food allergy, most having a mass of lymphoid tissue on the wall. It was seen in one in five with colitis,

Table 30.2 Clinical association of endoscopically visible lymphoid nodular hyperplasia (LNH) of the gastrointestinal tract

Level of gastrointestinal tract	LNH present
Foregut	
Stomach, normally no nodules	*Helicobacter pylori* infection
Upper small intestine, normally no nodules	food allergy and celiac disease
	autoimmune disorders: diabetes, chronic aggressive hepatitis, rheumatoid arthritis, vasculitis. IgA deficiency, unknown
Lower gastrointestinal tract	
Terminal ileum, normally small nodules dispersed evenly on the mucosa	food allergy inflammatory bowel disease: right-sided or pancolitis
Colon, normally small nodules seen in infants and small children	autoimmune disorders: chronic aggressive hepatitis, rehumatoid arthritis, unknown

while in subjects with Crohn's disease it was a surprisingly rare finding. In our series half the subjects with chronic constipation showed the lesion in the ileum. Wakefield et al reported an endoscopic LNH of the terminal ileum with histologically reactive follicular hyperplasia in 93% of children with developmental disorders, most having diarrhea and abdominal pains as well.[23] The same group also provoked a discussion about the coincidence of the measles virus and especially the measles vaccine and reactive follicular hyperplasia and/or ileocolitis.[24,25] In their original work they found virus antigens in 95% of the children with developmental disorders and LNH using the cell reverse transcriptase (RT) PCR method compared with 11% of the controls. However, the significance of finding virus particles with an extremely sensitive methods from the lymphoid tissue of the gastrintestinal tract remains open.[26]

As stated above, LNH can be seen in association with congenital or aquired immunodeficiency states including IgA deficiency and HIV infections.[7–10] It has also been seen in subjects even before the development of AIDS. Recently, the lesion has also been described also in patients with intestinal lymphomas.[27,28]

Food allergy

Food allergy may indeed be considered the most common disease underlying LNH.[29–33] However, in most cases the question is not about IgE-mediated disease but a local, T-cell mediated immune response, an immunological state close to celiac disease and a delayed immune response against food-borne allergens. In small children we may see infiltrations of eosinophils in biopsy samples, but most of the children of school age have no increment of eosinophils and mononuclear cells.

Two-thirds of subjects examined by both gastroduodenoscopy and colonoscopy, and shown by an elimination and challenge test to have food allergy, had LNH on the mucosa of the duodenum, ileum or colon. Only a few cases have had nodules spread all through the gastrointestinal tract. This finding confirms the view that food allergy in children may produce patchy or diffuse LNH in any part of the gastrointestinal tract.[34]

Symptoms

LNH in itself may not cause any symptoms, the underlying and altered immune response and skewing of the cytokine populations probably explaining the symptoms. As listed in Table 30.3, the most common symptoms in upper endoscopies have been abdominal pain, with or without 'from table to toilet' diarrhea. In the lower endoscopies the symptoms vary even more, from diarrhea/loose stools to constipation or blood in stools. A cascade of symptoms resembling irritable colon has perhaps been the most prominent seen in our patients. Indeed, at least in young adults with irritable colon, Simren et al found symptoms of food hypersensitivity but no general malabsorption in their patients, suggesting that some patients with this symptom cascade might have the same disease as we demonstrated in our subjects with LNH.[35] Examining a group of school children who had milk allergy in their infancy and half of the study group with abdominal symptoms, we also found no signs of general malabsorption, but the subjects had lactose intolerance three times more often and the height of the symptom group was lower than in the controls.[36] Our interpretation is that the ongoing immune activity might disturb the epithelial cell layer with the net result described above.

Table 30.3 Clinical symptoms of patients examined with gastroduodenoscopy and/or colonoscopy and having lymphoid nodular hyperplasia as an endoscopic finding

Upper instestinal symptoms
Recurrent abdominal pains
Nausea/vomiting
Eating disorders
Growth restricted
Anemia
Heartburn/regurgitation
Lower abdominal symptoms
Loose stools, intermittent diarrhea
From table-to-toilet diarrhea
Constipation
Blood in stool
Toiletting difficulties
Lactose intolerance

However, much investigation is still necessary to clarify the clinical significance of LNH.

Treatment and prognosis

As stated above LNH may be considered as an expression of an underlying immune response. There is no specific treatment. If the lesion is associated with another diagnosed disorder such as food allergy or IBD, these patients should be treated. In our clinical practice we have used budenoside in cases with LNH and a clinical picture of irritable colon but without definite association with food allergy. Most patients have shown a favorable response, but the approach still awaits controlled trials. Immunosupressive drugs in combination with other chemotherapy in patients with malignant lymphoma have been reported to diminish the nodules on the gut mucosa.[28]

LNH seems to be anatomic tissue in the sense that at least in subjects with food allergy, the nodules remain, even after avoiding the triggering foodstuff. This conclusion may be judged from the fact that the nodules are seen nearly as often in children with treated food allergy as in untreated cases. Moreover, we have re-examined a group of children with an abundance of LNH on the mucosa of the bulb or colon, and saw an equal amount of lymphoid tissue to that seen before the treatment. However, the immune activity as measured by γ/δ^+ intraepithelial lymphocytes seemed to diminish during the treatment.

In summary, LNH is a recently described condition. To date, there is only limited understanding of the phenomenon and its behavior.

REFERENCES

1. Bines JE, Winter HS. Lower endoscopy. In Walker WA, Durie PR, Hamilton JR, Walker-Smith J, Watkins JB, eds. *Pediatric Gastroenterology.* Philadelphia: Decker, 1991: 256–269.
2. Rossi T. Endoscopic examination of the colon in infancy and childhood. *Pediatr Clin North Am* 1988; **35**: 331–356.
3. Kaplan B, Benson J, Rothstein F et al. Lymphonodular hyperplasia of the colon as a pathologic finding in children with lower intestinal bleeding. *J Pediatr Gastroenterol Nutr* 1984; **3**: 704–708.
4. Colon A, DiPalma J, Leftridge C. Intestinal lymphonodular hyperplasia of childhood: patterns of presentation. *J Clin Gastroenterol* 1991; **13**: 163–166.
5. Fine KD, Seidel RH, Do K. The prevalence, anatomic distribution, and diagnosis of colonic causes of chronic diarrhea. *Gastrointest Endosc* 2000; **51**: 318–326.
6. Kohler PF, Cook RD, Brown WR et al. Common variable hypogammaglobulinemia with T-cell nodular lymphoid interstitial pneumonitis and B-cell nodular lymphoid hyperplasia: different lymphocyte populations with a similar response to prednisone therapy. *J Allergy Clin Immunol* 1982; **70**: 299–305.
7. Jacobson KW, de Shazo RD. Selective immunoglobulin A deficiency associated with nodular lymphoid hyperplasia. *J Allergy Clin Immunol* 1979; **64**: 516–521.
8. Lai Ping So A, Mayer L. Gastrointestinal manifestations of primary immunodeficiency disorders. *Semin Gastrointest Dis* 1997; **8**: 22–32.
9. Levendoglu H, Rosen Y. Nodular lymphoid hyperplasia of gut in HIV infection. *Am J Gastroenterol* 1992; **87**: 1200–1202.
10. Kokkonen J, Karttunen T. Lymphonodular hyperplasia on the mucosa of the lower gastrointestinal tract in children: an indication of enhanced immune response? *J Pediatr Gastroenterol Nutr* 2002; **34**: 42–46.
11. Wakefield AJ, Anthony A, Murch SH et al. Enterocolitis in children with developmental disorders. *Am J Gastroenterol* 2000; **95**: 2154–2156.
12. Kokkonen J, Haapalahti M, Laurila K et al. Cow's milk protein sensitive enteropathy at school age. *J Pediatr* 2001; **139**: 797–803.
13. Kokkonen J, Ruuska T, Karttunen T et al. Mucosal pathology of the foregut associating with food allergy and recurrent abdominal pains in children. *Acta Pediatr* 2001; **90**: 16–21.
14. Kokkonen J, Holm K, Karttunen T et al. Children with untreated food allergy express a relative increment in the density of duodenal g/d$^+$ T-cells. *Scand J Gastroenterol* 2000; **35**: 1137–1142.
15. Furlano RI, Anthony A, Day R et al. Colonic CD8 and gamma delta T-cell infiltration with epithelial damage in children with autism. *J Pediatr* 2001; **138**: 366–372.
16. Augustin M, Kokkonen J, Karttunen T. Increased densities of TIA-1 antigen bearing T-cells in duodenal samples of children with gastrointestinal food allergy. *J Pediatr Gastroenterol Nutr* 2001; **32**: 11–18.
17. Mäki M, Holm K, Collin P et al. Increase in gamma/delta T cell receptor bearing lymphocytes in normal small bowel mucosa in latent coeliac disease. *Gut* 1991; **32**: 1412–1414.
18. MacDonald T, Spencer J. Evidence for cell-mediated hypersensitivity as an important pathogenetic mechanism in food intolerance. *Clin Exp Allergy* 1995; **25** (Suppl 1): 10–13.

19. Kokkonen J, Tikkanen S, Karttunen TJ et al. Similar high level of immunoglobulin A and immunoglobulin G class milk antibodies and increment of local lymphoid tissue on the duodenal mucosa in subjects with cow's milk allergy and recurrent abdominal pains. *Pediatr Allergy Immunol* 2002; **13**: 129–136.
20. McGhee JR, Lamm ME, Strober W. Mucosal immune responses. An overview. In Ogra PL, Mestechy J, Lamm ME, Strober W, Bienenstock J, McGhee JR, eds. *Mucosal Immunology.* San Diego: Academic Press, 1999: 485–506.
21. Soothil JF, Stokes CR, Turner MW et al. Predisposing factors and development of reaginic allergy in infancy. *Clin Allergy* 1976; **6**: 305–319.
22. Hauer AC, Breese EJ, Walker-Smith JA et al. The frequency of cells secreting interferon-gamma and interleukin-4, -5, and -10 in the blood and duodenal mucosa of children with cow's milk hypersensitivity. *Pediatr Res* 1997; **42**: 629–638.
23. Wakefield AJ, Murch SH, Anthony A et al. Ileal–lymphoid–nodular hyperplasia, non-specific colitis, and pervasive developmental disorder in children. *Lancet* 1998; **351**: 637–641.
24. Ekbom A, Wakefield AJ, Zack M et al. Perinatal measles infection and subsequent Crohn's disease. *Lancet* 1994; **344**: 508–510.
25. Taylor B, Miller E, Farrington CP et al. Autism and measles, mumps, and rubella vaccine: no epidemiological evidence for a causal association. *Lancet* 1999; **353**: 2026–2029.
26. Madsen KM, Hviid A, Vestergaard M et al. A population-based study of measles, mumps, and rubella vaccination and autism. *N Engl J Med* 2002; **347**: 1477–1482.
27. Matuchansky C, Touchard G, Lemaire M et al. Malignant lymphoma of the small bowel associated with diffuse nodular lymphoid hyperplasia. *N Engl J Med* 1985; **313**: 166–171.
28. Jonsson OT, Birgisson S, Reykdal S. Resolution of nodular lymphoid hyperplasia of the gastrointestinal tract following chemotherapy for extraintestinal lymphoma. *Dig Dis Sci* 2002; **47**: 2463–2465.
29. Gottrand F, Erkan T, Fabriaux J-P et al. Food-induced bleeding from lymphonodular hyperplasia of the colon. *Am J Dis Child* 1993; **147**: 821–823.
30. Beaoui M, Guezmir M, Hamdi M et al. Lymphoid hyperplasia of the intestine in children. 15 cases. *Ann Pediatr (Paris)* 1992; **39**: 359–364.
31. Kokkonen J, Karttunen T, Niinimäki A. Lymphonodular hyperplasia as a sign of food allergy in children. *J Pediatr Gastroenterol Nutr* 1999; **29**: 57–62.
32. Kokkonen J, Tikkanen S, Savilahti E. Residual intestinal disease after milk allergy in infancy. *J Pediatr Gastroenterol Nutr* 2001; **32**: 156–161.
33. Kokkonen J. Lymphonodular hyperplasia of the duodenal bulb indicates food allergy in children. *Endoscopy* 1999; **31**: 464–468.
34. Crowe S, Perdue M. Gastrointestinal food hypersensitivity: basic mechanisms of pathophysiology. *Gastroenterology* 1992; **103**: 1075–1095.
35. Simren M, Mansson A, Langkilde AM et al. Food-related gastrointestinal symptoms in the irritable bowel syndrome. *Digestion* 2001; **63**: 108–115.
36. Tikkanen S, Kokkonen J, Juntti H et al. Status of children with cow's milk allergy in infancy by 10 years of age. *Acta Paediatr* 2000; **89**: 1–7.

31 Malnutrition

Michael H N Golden

Introduction

Nutrition is the process by which dietary constituents are converted into, maintain and sustain the body in health. Nutrition and genetic coding are the determinants of the body's development and composition; they modulate and control its function and enable it to resist disease. Nutrition is the major variable that determines the quality of the body – the 'soil' in which the 'seeds' of disease germinate. The battle between the nutritional 'soil' and the etiological 'seed' determines the course of most diseases. Both nutritional state and genetic endowment should be viewed separately from the agents of disease. They determine the internal environment in which the seeds of disease flourish or fail. Why should measles be a relatively minor exanthem in Europe and North America and a deadly killer in Africa, even in those with normal weight for age? Good nutrition gives 'positive health'. There is a whole spectrum of deteriorating nutrition that gradually compromises physiological reserve and function. In severe malnutrition there has been dietary inadequacy severe enough to compromise every function of the body including its ability to resist disease agents. Just as good nutrition leads to positive health and resistance to disease, poor nutrition leads to ill health and susceptibility to many diseases. If a patient has HIV and dies from pneumonia we conceive of this as a death from HIV. If a malnourished child dies from pneumonia we conceive of this death as being due to the pneumonia itself. This is wrong. The commonest cause of immunodeficiency is nutritional deprivation – the underlying cause of death is really malnutrition. The stark differences between the perception of HIV and malnutrition as causes of death illustrate the neglect of nutrition; academic kudos, research effort and funding interest hardly exist.

The nutritional state, by itself, alters the expression, course and response to treatment of all 'primary' diagnoses. Notwithstanding the diagnostic label attached to a patient, the accompanying malnutrition is often the main reason for morbidity and mortality; and yet, it is frequently the most amenable to treatment. A clinical history of severe weight loss or anorexia is not just a diagnostic pointer making a debilitating disease more probable; it is a signal calling for active treatment of the malnutrition and modification of treatment regimens for the primary diagnosis. The soil needs care and consideration equal to that given to the seed. Up to half of all patients admitted to hospital suffer from anthropometric malnutrition; many more suffer from micronutrient malnutrition.

If a malnourished patient with carcinoma is given radiotherapy, low antioxidant nutrient status often results in intolerable side-effects so that the treatment cannot continue and the patient dies – from carcinoma? Treatment has not just failed, it has been inadequate, if not wrong, because the nutrition of the patient has been neglected. Ensuring adequate nutrition of every patient is every pediatrician's duty.

Primary malnutrition is a condition of the dependent and vulnerable who rely on others for nourishment. It is seen most frequently in the young child, the elderly and groups such as prisoners and the mentally ill or disabled. Secondary malnutrition accompanies any disease that disturbs appetite, digestion, absorption or utilization of nutrients. In poor, technologically backward countries, malnutrition-associated disease is the major cause of death. More than half of all deaths have anthropometric malnutrition as the underlying cause;[1] many more are compromised by micronutrient malnutrition, not associated with weight loss. Malnutrition stunts the physical and mental development of the majority of the surviving population. Winston Churchill once said that he could think of 'no better investment than to put good food in the mouths of babies'; that statement is true today.

The term protein–energy malnutrition has been used to cover a number of clinical conditions in both adults and children, including: failure to thrive, marasmus, cachexia, phthisis, nutritional dwarfism, kwashiorkor and nutritional or famine edema. The large number of terms reflect the emphasis on particular clinical features. However, regardless of the clinical differences, most of the physiological, biochemical and body compositional features are common to all varieties of severe malnutrition. The principles of classification, investigation and management are the same for adults and children. The term protein–energy malnutrition is best avoided; it carries the false implication that protein and/or energy deficiencies are the direct cause of all these conditions.

Nature of nutritional deficiency

If a growing animal is given a diet devoid in folate there is a consumption of stores; the animal develops clinical signs characteristic of folate deficiency (and may die); and the concentration of folate in the tissues is markedly reduced. However, there is no effect upon growth or body weight until the illness is terminal.

If a growing animal is given a diet devoid of protein there is an immediate cessation of growth and then loss of weight. When such an animal dies from protein deficiency, the concentration of protein in its major tissues is absolutely normal; the animal will have died from a nutrient deficiency without any direct evidence of depletion of the nutrient except for failure to grow or loss of weight.

The absolute amount of the nutrient within the body in both folate and protein deficiency is less than normal, but with folate the reduced amount is contained within a normally sized body, whereas with protein the body size has contracted and the concentration maintained.

There is clearly a fundamental and distinct difference between these two responses to deprivation of a single nutrient. Most nutrients can be classified into those that give a folate-like (type I) or a protein-like (type II) response (Table 31.1). The characteristics of the two types of deficiency are summarized in Table 31.2.

Type I deficiency

When one thinks of deficiency of an essential nutrient, one automatically considers a type I deficiency. The diet is deficient. The low intake leads to a reduction in the tissue concentration. The metabolic pathways that depend upon this nutrient are compromised. Characteristic clinical signs and symptoms develop. The diagnosis is conceptually straightforward – measure the nutrient concentration in a tissue, test the metabolic pathway where the defect lies, demonstrate an

Table 31.1 Classification of nutrients according to whether the response to a deficiency is a reduced concentration in the tissues or a reduced growth rate. Energy does not fit into the classification. The type I can be looked upon as 'functional' nutrients, type II as the building blocks of tissue, and energy as the fuel that runs the system. The position of some essential nutrients, such as the essential fatty acids, is not clear

Type I	Type II
Iron	Nitrogen
Iodine	Sulfur
Selenium	Essential amino acids
Copper	Potassium
Calcium	Sodium
Manganese	Magnesium
Thiamine	Zinc
Riboflavine	Phosphorus
Pyridoxine	Chlorine
Niacin	Water
Ascorbic acid	
Retinol	
Tocopherol	
Calciferol	
Folic acid	
Cobalamine	
Vitamin K	

Table 31.2 Characteristics of the different types of nutritional deficiencies

Type 1	Type II
Tissue level variable	Tissue level fixed
Used in specific pathways	Ubiquitously used
Characteristic physical signs	No characteristic signs
Late or no growth response	Immediate growth response
Stored in the body	No body store
Buffered response	Responds to daily input
Not interdependent	Control each other's balance
Little excretory control	Sensitive physiological control
Variable in breast milk with maternal status	Fixed concentration in breast milk

effect of replacing the nutrient *in vitro* or *in vivo*, or recognize the specific clinical signs.

A critical feature of a type I deficiency is that there is no weight loss or growth failure. One cannot assume that all is well nutritionally from a growth chart. There may be one, several or multiple type I nutritional deficiencies and normal growth. Hence the devastation of measles in African children with a normal growth trajectory. Children in the West who exist on soft drinks, candy (sweets), crisps and other forms of 'empty calories' to become obese can have multiple micronutrient deficiencies. Obesity denotes only a chronic positive energy balance; it is a 'fat storage disease', not 'over-nutrition' – it is just as likely to be due to 'under-nutrition' from an unbalanced diet. Indeed, it is possible that nutritional deficiency is a cause of this fat storage disease. Recently in a besieged city in Angola there was a pellagra epidemic. Only the fat people developed pellagra (M.H. Golden, unpublished). To understand how this can occur is to understand the nature of nutritional deficiency.

Type II deficiency

The position with respect to the type II nutrients is different. Indeed, none of the strategies that can be used to diagnose a type I deficiency can be used to diagnose a deficiency of a type II nutrient. This gives rise to major difficulties, both conceptual and practical, when we try to understand, define, diagnose and treat these deficiencies. Much of the controversy that surrounds the definition of a deficiency, the signs and symptoms of deficiency, the requirements and the diagnosis of deficiency, of type II nutrients, stems from attempts to conceive of them as analogous to the type I nutrients.

The type II nutrients are the fundamental building blocks of the tissue itself. The tissue cannot be sustained without the normal complement of these nutrients, so, with deficiency, the whole tissue is catabolized and all the components of the tissue are excreted. When the tissue is to be resynthesized all the components have to be supplied in a balanced way. These nutrients can be thought about as being interdependent, just as the essential amino acids are usually considered together under the rubric protein. They have characteristic ratios that vary over quite a narrow range. They are required to be absorbed in approximately the same ratios as occur in the body. Some, such as phosphorus, zinc and magnesium, have a low availability from the diet, so they should be present in higher concentration and available in chemical form in any diet designed to promote convalescence.

As an understanding of these particular nutrients is integral to the problem of malnutrition, they will be considered in more detail.

Common response

The response to a deficiency – growth failure with a mild deficiency and weight loss with more profound deficiency – is the same for each type II nutrient. When nutritional growth failure or weight loss is seen, the particular nutrient that is lacking cannot be identified.

Every animal experiment in feeding a diet lacking a type II nutrient results in progressive diminution or cessation of growth, then weight loss. This response has been observed consistently and universally in all species studied, in both acute and chronic experiments, with each of the type II nutrients. The response to a habitual mild deficiency is progressive stunting (with the body in proportion). The extent of the stunting is a function of the degree of shortfall of the nutrient and time. With an acute deficiency, in either the child or the adult, there is a loss of tissue leading to wasting. The balance between the severity of the deficiency and its duration will determine the relative amounts of stunting and wasting produced. Mild, chronic deficiencies are more common than severe, acute deficiencies and stunting is consequently more common than wasting.

Type II nutrients are not stored in the body

There is a common repertoire of metabolic changes and 'reductive adaptations' that occur in response to each type II deficiency. However, because whole tissue is being broken down, or at least there is no net synthesis, all the nutrients released from the catabolized tissue and are in the diet in excess relative to the deficient nutrient have to be excreted. These nutrients are not stored in the body. The balance between the various type II nutrients in the diet is thus very important. In the face of a deficiency of any one of them there is a negative balance for them all. For example, if potassium is omitted from a parenteral feeding regimen, the patient will loose nitrogen, zinc, phosphorus and magnesium from the body. He will not necessarily be in negative balance for the type 1 nutrients such as calcium, iron or folate whist he is losing weight.

Dietary deficiency

When a deficient diet is given, the body has mechanisms to avidly conserve and recycle the deficient nutrient to maintain itself. For this reason, it is extremely difficult to produce clinical signs of a deficiency of these nutrients in the non-growing animal by dietary means alone. There usually has to be a pathological loss of the nutrient from the body. This is commonly by diarrhea. The loss can be sufficiently severe to compromise intestinal function so that the deficiency and diarrhea become persistent. The treatment has to be a change of diet to replace all type II nutrients that have been lost. Zinc, phosphorus and magnesium are frequently not replaced adequately.

Determinant of requirements

The rate of weight gain is the main determinant of the dietary requirement for a type II nutrient. For example, children given a diet that supplied just enough energy for them to maintain their body weight, without growing, are able to remain in zinc balance, and maintain their plasma zinc concentration, with an intake of only 0.08 mg Zn/kg per day. When the same children were gaining weight rapidly, their plasma zinc fell precipitously despite a ten-fold increase in the amount of zinc consumed (1 mg Zn/kg per day); this limited lean tissue synthesis so that the children became obese without regaining muscle. They required an amount that far exceeded the recommended dietary allowance to maintain synthesis of new lean tissue. During convalescence from illness the recommended daily allowance (RDA) for type II nutrients is not sufficient. RDAs are set for normal individuals. Of course an increased nutrient density must be supplied for all type II nutrients in the right balance to make the new tissue.

Children do not need a richer diet than adults

This contradicts what most pediatricians, nutritionists and lay people believe. A diet that has a sufficiently low concentration of a type II nutrient to give clinical signs, other than growth failure, will affect the elderly first, then adults and lastly children. This is a consequence of the higher relative energy requirement of the child. Thus, the protein requirement of the child, for maintenance of body weight, is about the same as for an adult (0.6 g/kg per day). However, the energy requirement for maintenance of the child is about 400 kJ/kg per day whilst that for the adult is about 160 kJ/kg per day. Hence, an adult must have a diet that supplies 6% of the energy as protein, whereas a child requires only about 2.4% of the energy as protein. Of course, for the child to grow normally, very much more protein is required. Interestingly, the increased requirement for normal growth brings the protein density up to that of the adult. We have evolved so that all the family can take the same diet. If the family has an adequate diet, it can be fed to the infant and child. It is not necessary to have special weaning foods. Nutritional requirements, when expressed as nutrient densities (per unit energy) are the same for infants, children, adolescents, adults, and the pregnant and lactating.

In a community, we do not expect to find anything other than growth failure in children, unless they have diseases which cause a pathological loss of the nutrient. If the local diet is sufficiently deficient to give rise to other clinical signs, these should be seen first in the elderly and last in children. However, there is such a wide gap between the concentration that gives growth failure and that which gives any other feature of deficiency, that even where growth failure is common other clinical signs are rare.

Anorexia

Anorexia is common to a deficiency of each type II nutrient; this is corrected if the nutrient is supplied. Thus, on supplementation of the single missing component a patient will regain his appetite and then have an increased intake of the newly balanced diet. Dietary intake data are often wrongly interpreted as indicating 'energy deficiency'. This is rarely the cause of a low dietary intake. Even in famine situations, the diet is normally so restricted that type II (and type I) deficiencies are usually present long before the total amount of food energy becomes limiting.

Of course, there are other causes of anorexia, in particular liver disease, infection and psychiatric abnormality, but type II nutrient deficiency is very common. This is one reason why most people with malabsorption do not increase their intake to compensate for the amounts being lost in the stools. Refusal to eat a diet that leads to disordered metabolism is defensive. There is a metabolic preference for 'consumption' of one's own tissues (a very good 'diet', to satisfy nutritional demands). This may have benefit in restoring metabolic balance, but in the long term it leads to severe malnutrition.

The anorexia is related to a balance of the type II nutrients. It is the relative surfeit of other nutrients, particularly amino acids, which need to be metabolized and excreted to prevent the toxicity that causes the anorexia. If the nutrient density of all the type II nutrients is low, but they are in balance, for example by adding lipid to the diet, the individual may not develop anorexia, but may become obese from the excess energy in the diet. They are still under-nourished.

When a supplementary diet is given to children which does not contain all the nutrients required for new tissue synthesis, it is possible to unbalance the diet and make the malnutrition worse, by diluting the marginal nutrients in the basic diet to a deficient level.

The type II nutrients have always given problems to clinicians and nutritionists because of the difficulty with diagnosis. Unfortunately, the non-specificity of weight loss and lack of confirmatory tests of an inadequate intake have led these nutrients to be largely ignored by clinicians, and their nutritional importance to be grossly underestimated. The phosphorus requirement is set as a function of calcium not as a critical nutrient in its own right. Textbooks of nutrition hardly mention potassium, magnesium, sodium, sulfur or chlorine deficiency. Yet, as a group, type II nutrient deficiency is responsible for malnutrition in half the World's children and for unrecognized problems of ill health in many others.

Classification of severe malnutrition

Any system of classification should have practical use, either to identify those individuals who require intervention or to examine the prevalence within a community so that preventive measures can be taken.

The rest of this chapter is devoted to severe wasting and edematous malnutrition.

Children

Weight-for-height and height-for-age

During childhood the most sensitive indicator of malnutrition (type II deficiency) is failure to achieve normal growth. The systems of classification compare the size of the child to a 'normal' reference; the reference recommended by the World Health Organization (WHO) is the American NCHS standard. Other standards have been used; however, standards derived from elite healthy populations from around the world are all very close to NCHS values. The NCHS standards are derived almost exclusively from artificially fed infants. They have a higher early weight gain than exclusively breast-fed children, much of the additional tissue being adipose. Thus, healthy normal breast-fed infants 'fall off' the present NCHS standards so that infants may appear to be more malnourished than they are. New standards are being prepared by WHO for infants and young children.

Normal growth is a continuous, balanced accretion of tissue in a predictable way that results in a steady, co-ordinated increase in height, weight and organ size. A mild insult which continues for a period of time results in slowing or cessation of growth. The child is normally proportioned but as time passes he falls further and further behind the actively growing child. Because of the shape of the normal growth curve the younger the child the more rapidly he will fall behind. If a normal child suddenly slows to half the normal growth rate, he will be twice his present age before he falls below 70% of normal height for his age and can be diagnosed as severely stunted.

A child who is exposed to a more severe insult will not only stop growing in height but will also lose weight. He becomes underweight for age much more quickly and is thin. The weight is low in relation to his height. Thus, within the group of children underweight for their age there are two conceptually different conditions: first, the stunted but normally proportioned (nutritional dwarfism); and second, the child of normal height who is thin and wasted (the original concept of marasmus). The two conditions can be differentiated by measuring the height as well as weight and age. Stunting is measured by the height of the child in relation to the height of a normal child of the same age (height-for-age) and wasting as the weight of the child in relation to a normal child of his same height, even though the normal child is usually chronologically younger (weight-for-height). The grades of stunting and wasting are shown in Table 31.3.

Two methods of expressing the data are in common use. The simplest is to express the weight/height of the child as a percentage of the normal. The second is to express the deficit in terms of multiples of the standard deviation of the normal (NCHS) population. The result is called a Z-score. The Z-score is much more difficult to calculate, but it is relatively age independent and expresses stunting and wasting in the same relative units. Clearly, any child who has a Z-score within ± 2 is, by definition, normal. Children who are more than three standard deviations from the normal have severe stunting or wasting. In children over 6 months of age, a deficit of 5% in height-for-age or 10% in weight-for-height is approximately equal to one Z-score. In terms of admission to feeding programs the weight-for-height percentage is preferred. This is because it

Table 31.3 The classification of severe malnutriton

	Normal	Mild*	Moderate*	Severe*
Weight-for-height deficit=wasting	90–120%† (+2 to -1 Z)‡	80–89% (-1 to -2 Z)	70–79% (-2 to -3 Z)	<70%** (-3 Z)
Height-for-age deficit=stunting	95–110% (+2 to -1 Z)	90–94% (-1 to -2 Z)	85–89% (-2 to -3 Z)	<85% (-3 Z)

* Without edema. The presence of edema denotes severe malnutrition (kwashiorkor), even without severe wasting

† Percentage of the median NCHS standard

‡ The Z-score is also used to define malnutrition. However, its use is largely confined to anthropometric surveys and academic analyses

more closely relates to prognosis, is easier to understand and can be extended to the adolescent (Figure 31.1).[2]

The wasted child presents an immediate clinical problem where rehabilitation can lead to restoration of lost tissue and function. Correction of stunting, on the other hand, is more likely to depend upon public health measures designed to improve the circumstances of the family. This system, together with the presence or absence of edema, anorexia and complicating illness is the most useful and appropriate for deciding which individuals require intensive treatment. Because stunting is much more common than wasting, systems based upon weight-for-age are no longer used (for example, these include the Gomez and Wellcome classifications).

Mid-upper-arm circumference

Between the ages of 1 and 5 years there is very little change in a normal child's arm circumference. This measurement thus gives a simple anthropometric measure of wasting which is almost age independent. Because stunting is common in most countries with a high prevalence of severe malnutrition a chronological age of more than 1 year is unreliable, so the cut-off point is usually 75 cm in height.

Adult

Body mass index

The assessment of malnutrition in adults is conceptually similar to weight-for-height in children. Stunting in adults usually represents chronic undernutrition in childhood. It is irreversible. This may have implications for the pathogenesis of adult disease. However, as there is no therapeutic action that can be taken, adult stunting is mainly of theoretical interest.

The object with adults is to classify their degree of 'thinness'. The most useful measure is the body mass index (BMI), defined as weight (kg) divided by the square of height (m): wt/(ht)^2. Exactly the same index is used to define grades of obesity.

Many sick adults cannot stand to have their height measured, and in those with kyphosis or scoliosis the measurement is not useful. In these patients there are several proxy measures for height that

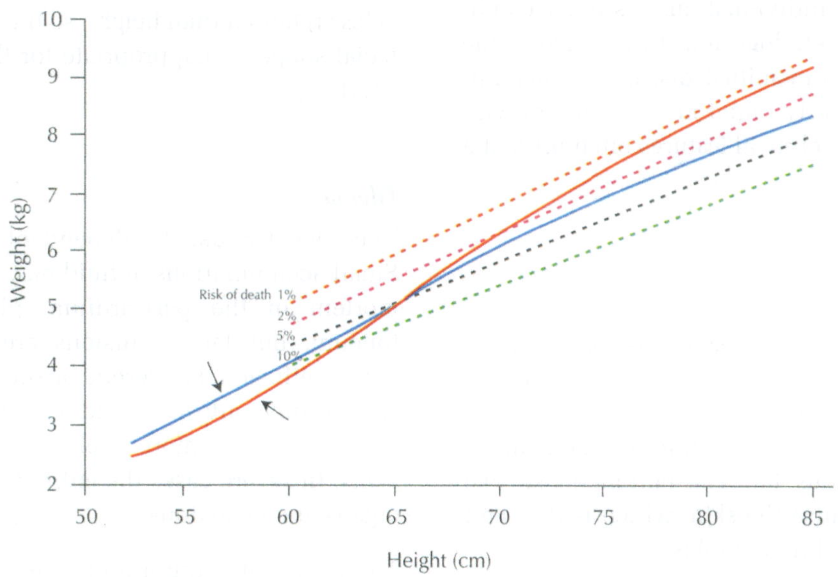

Figure 31.1 Weight-for-height curves for 70% of the NCHS (blue) standard and minus 3 Z-score units (red). The other lines are calculated as 'risk of death' cut-off points from the data of Prudhon et al.[2] Note that the 70% line is smooth and more closely parallel to the risk of death lines. The children admitted by Z-score but excluded by per cent of the median have a very low mortality (2%), whereas those admitted by per cent of the median and excluded by Z-score are young and have a high mortality (18%).

can be used. Although arm span is said to be equal to height, this is only so in those about 1.6 m tall. Clinically, the most useful measurement is demi-span. This is measured as the distance from the middle of the sternal notch to the tip of the middle finger in the coronal plane. Both sides should be measured; if there is a discrepancy the measurements should be repeated before taking the longest demi-span. Height (m) in both males and females can then be calculated from the formula:

Height = 0.73 * (2 x demi-span) + 0.43

Mid-upper-arm circumference

As with children, the mid-upper-arm circumference can be used to grade the degree of body wasting in adults. It is particularly used for pregnant women where the weight is higher than in the non-pregnant state.

Clinical features

Severe malnutrition can broadly be divided into three clinical syndromes: marasmus, kwashiorkor and nutritional dwarfism. In primary malnutrition each of these conditions is associated with poverty, deprivation and infection; therefore, they often co-exist in the same individual, just as other conditions which share etiological features (such as the various sexually transmitted diseases or helminthiasis) are frequently found in the same individual. Therefore, the clinical features often present a mixed picture.

Marasmus

The patient with classical marasmus has obviously lost weight with prominent ribs, zygoma and limb joints, gross loss of muscle mass particularly of the limb girdles – shoulders and buttocks – and almost absent subcutaneous fat. The bottom looks like 'baggy pants' because the skin, which is thin and atrophic, lies in redundant folds.

The textbooks describe the face as having a pinched look like an 'old man'. This does occur but is uncommon. It is much more common to have a relatively normal-looking face (Figure 31.2). This is important, because one cannot tell whether a person is severely wasted by just looking at the face. Many cases are missed in busy out-patient departments because the children are not stripped and examined properly, or screened with weight-for-height.

Kwashiorkor

The clinical syndrome of kwashiorkor was first described by Spanish doctors in the West Indies and then by the French in Vietnam; it did not enter the English literature until described by Williams in 1933.[3]

The *sine qua non* of kwashiorkor is bilateral pitting edema. Typically, a child of 1 to 2 years with fine friable discolored hair develops a typical skin rash, edema and hepatomegaly. Kwashiorkor is an acute illness which comes on abruptly. The history of swelling, loss of appetite and mood change is of a few days only (Figure 31.3).

Nutritional dwarfism

On casual observation the nutritional dwarf appears perfectly normal. It is only when the age of the patient is known that the short stature becomes apparent. However, dental development is less retarded than height, so that these children's facial shape is inappropriate for their size (Figure 31.4).

Edema

The edema is usually dependent and periorbital. Small accumulations of fluid may be found at post mortem in the pericardium, pleura and peritoneum, but large effusions are uncommon; if serous effusion is present, associated conditions such as tuberculosis should be sought. Adults with kwashiorkor are more likely to have serous effusions. In severe cases the entire body and internal organs are edematous.

The extent of sodium and water retention in the extracellular fluid is variable. It is almost always overestimated by clinicians. In mild edema of the feet only, the weight loss with resolution of edema is about 3% of body weight, with moderate edema 5% and with severe edema 10%. There are

(a) (b)

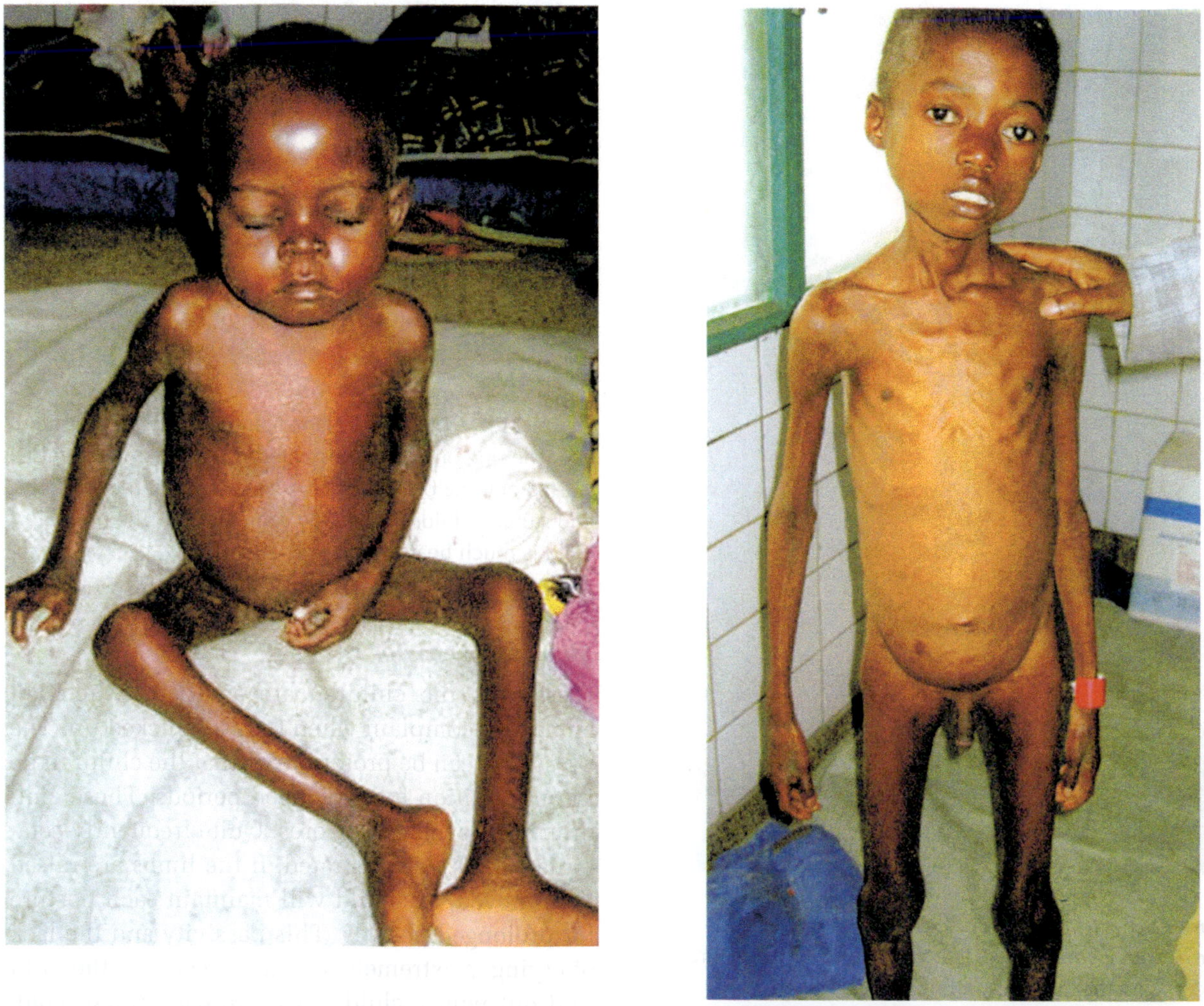

Figure 31.2 (a) A severely wasted child from the Democratic Republic of Congo (DRC). This child did not have edema. His face appears fat, not unlike the facial shape of many children with kwashiorkor. (b) A severely wasted youth from DRC. Note that he does not have an 'old man face' – if he were clothed, you would not realize that he was wasted. Note also the displacement of his cartilaginous rib forwards. This is a sign of a longstanding low intake of vitamin C or copper.

children with up to 30% or more recorded, but such cases are extremely rare.

Circulation

The retained sodium and water are not evenly distributed throughout the extracellular compartments. Depletion of the intravascular volume usually accompanies the enormous expansion of the interstitial space. This maldistribution gives rise to the anomalous statement that an edematous patient can be 'dehydrated'. This is semantically incorrect and we should use the adjective 'hypovolemic' to describe these patients. The use of the word 'dehydration' and the attendant concepts have led physicians to treat these patients, incorrectly, with rehydration solutions. In fact, the hypovolemia in edematous patients is a form of toxic shock and should not be treated with sodium-containing fluids.

Hepatomegaly

Hepatomegaly is frequently encountered in the West Indies. It is much less common in Africa or Asia, although it does occur. The liver may extend to the iliac brim. It is smooth, firm and not usually tender. The liver enlargement is due to fat accumulation, mainly as triglyceride. Up to half the wet weight of the liver can be fat, but it is usually

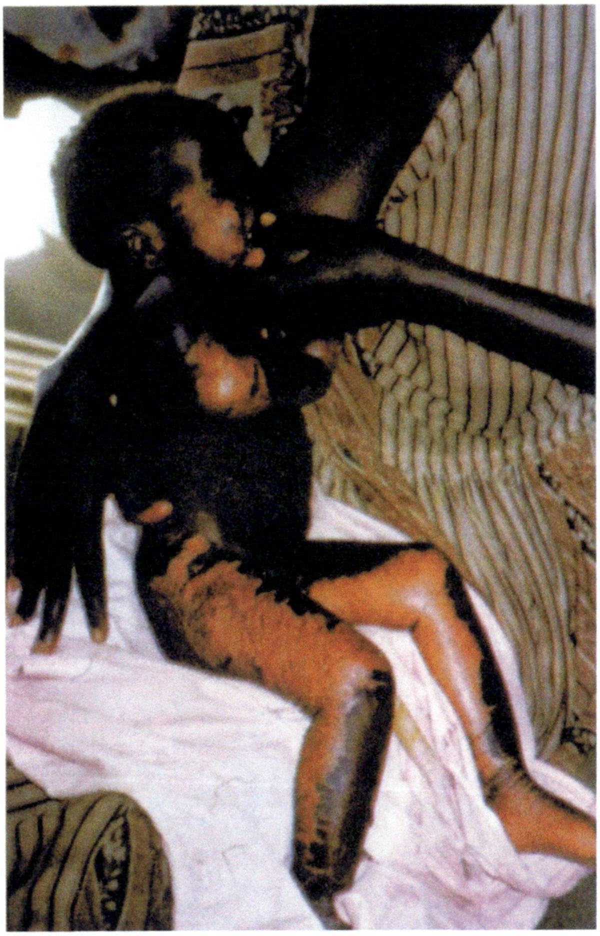

Figure 31.3 A child with extensive skin lesions and edema from Uganda. Note that this child is receiving breast milk. The mother appears anthropometrically normal.

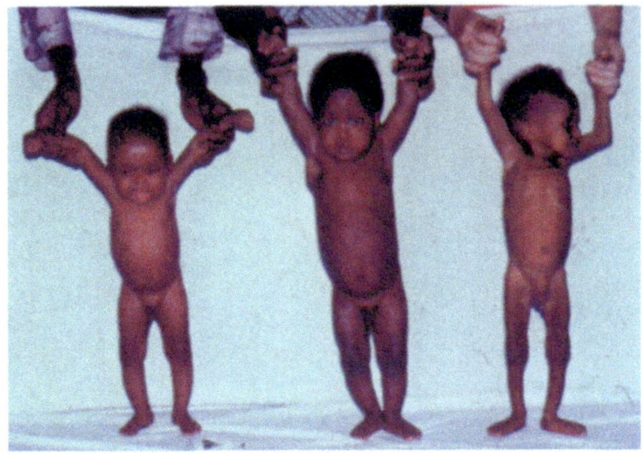

Figure 31.4 These three Jamaican children are the same age. The one on the left is stunted. The one on the right is wasted and the one in the middle is normal. The wasted and stunted children have the same weight. The normal child is much heavier.

much less than this. Signs of liver dysfunction such as petechiae or very slight hyperbilirubinemia are serious prognostic signs.

Splenomegaly

An enlarged spleen is very unusual in uncomplicated malnutrition. Where it occurs it is likely to be associated with particular infections such as malaria, kala azar or HIV, or a hemoglobinopathy.

Anorexia

Loss of appetite is a common feature of all forms of severe malnutrition. The most likely underlying causes are type II nutrient deficiency, infection and liver dysfunction. These patients nearly always have all three of these underlying causes compounding each other.

Mood and behavior

Classically the children are apathetic when left alone and complain when they are picked up. The passsivity can be profound, so that the children lie in one position for prolonged periods. These children can develop bed sores. Quite frequently catatonia can be demonstrated. If the limbs are raised then moved, the child will maintain each posture for prolonged periods. This passivity and the lack of crying is extremely serious. A good mother will find out why a child cries – hunger, thirst, cold, pain, unhappiness or being uncomfortable – and then put it right. If the child does not cry the mother thinks that none of these problems are affecting her child. The child is neglected. When a malnourished child is in the hospital the staff also neglect these children for the same reasons. This is why they should always be nursed together in a special unit.

A series of stereotyped, self-stimulating repetitive movements may occur; this is typical of psychosocial deprivation. One of the most damaging forms of self-stimulation is rumination. When alone, the child regurgitates the last meal, to re-taste it, then re-swallows it. Inevitably some is lost. In less severely deprived children intentional regurgitation may be the only way in which the child can get attention from a busy mother; it then becomes a learned habit that leads to malnutrition. Rumination and attention-seeking regurgitation are frequently confused with vomiting from a physical cause, so that many of these children undergo extensive gastrointestinal investigations.

Skin

In kwashiorkor there are skin changes that appear and progress like sunburn. The skin changes are acute, occurring over the course of a day or so. The skin first becomes darker in color, particularly over areas exposed to minor trauma or pressure. The superficial dermal layers then dry like thin parchment and split wherever they are stretched to reveal pale areas between the cracks (Figure 31.5). The dry cracked layer then peels off to leave hypopigmented extremely thin skin. If it is gently pinched between the fingers numerous small wrinkles appear, showing how thin and atrophic the epidermis is. The skin is very friable and ulcerates or macerates easily, particularly in the flexures, perineum and behind the ears. In severe cases it may appear as if the child has been burnt.

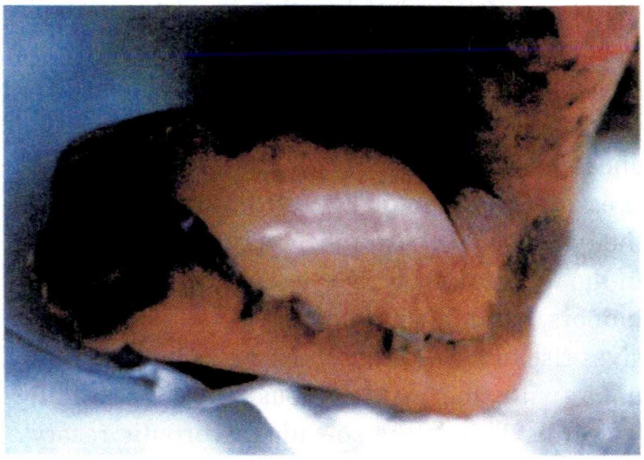

Figure 31.5 The stripping skin from this foot shows the different stages of the skin lesions of kwashiorkor.

Hair

There is atrophy of the hair roots of the scalp. They cease to synthesize protein, the bulb shrinks and the hair may be plucked out easily and painlessly. The patients may go completely bald. The reduction in synthesis is also seen in chemotherapy. When this sign is present there are also low levels of hepatic export proteins, such as albumin and transferrin showing that the slowing of synthesis is general throughout the body.

The hair itself becomes thin and straight and 'lifeless'. In patients with naturally curly hair the curls may be lifted up by the new straight hair to give the appearance of trees with straight trunks and a canopy – the 'forest sign'.

The hair may change color to red, brown, gray or blond. The basis for this change in color is unknown. Hair color changes bear no relation to prognosis and should not be used to classify these children.

Feminization

Unlike the hair on the scalp, the eyelashes grow long and luxuriant. There may also be excessive growth of lanugo hair. The face of little boys starts to look like girls. Breast enlargement is not uncommon; it occurs particularly in patients with gross hepatomegaly. The reason is not only the diminution of conjugation and excretion of steroid hormones by the liver. The small bowel bacterial overgrowth, that is almost universal in these children, deconjugate the conjugated steroids so that they are reabsorbed. These signs of feminization indicate longstanding chronic malnutrition with small-bowel overgrowth and fatty liver.

Cheeks

Fullness of the cheeks is commonly associated with edematous malnutrition (so-called jowls). The cause is unknown; it is not due to parotid enlargement.

Although there is usually marked parotid atrophy, in some patients, particularly malnourished adults, there is painless parotid enlargement. This seems to be associated with particular geographical locations. For example, it is common in one of the Comoro islands off the African coast but not on a neighboring island. The reason is unknown.

Bone

There is nearly always an enlargement of the costochondral junctions giving a 'rickety rosary'. The cause is not usually related to vitamin D deficiency. It is related to the very low available phosphorus and calcium in the diet. Harrison's sulci and other chest deformities are not only due to the pliability of the bone, but also to repeated chest infections. Smoke pollution from cooking fires is very common in the developing world – the reason why chest infections are more frequent in the wet seasons is that the cooking is then done indoors. Chronic vitamin C (or copper) deficiency gives rise to dislocation of the costochondral junctions with the cartilaginous chest protruding forwards. This is the so-called 'scorbutic rosary'. It is also common. Signs of acute scurvy are extremely uncommon. The sclera may be blue because the choroid pigment shows through, similar to that seen in congenital defects of collagen formation or structure. There is nearly always very marked osteopenia on X-ray. Despite the demineralization and collagen defects, and unlike osteitis fragilis, these children very rarely have fractures. The mothers must handle the children very gently indeed.

Abdominal swelling

The abdomen is usually protuberant. This is due to gas in the intestine rather than the enlarged liver. The gut gas is due to the very slow low-amplitude peristaltic waves. This is the main cause of the bacterial overgrowth. Frequently the abdominal wall is sufficiently thin for peristalsis to be easily visible. Bowel sounds are infrequent. In newly admitted patients there may be a succussion splash from the stomach or bowel.

Inflammation

The tympanic membranes are white and thickened (tympanosclerosis), usually without signs of inflammation. The tonsils are atrophic. It is unusual to find lymphadenopathy. When it occurs symmetrically it is usually associated with HIV disease. When asymmetrical it is usually tuberculosis. There is frequently oral, esophageal, gastric, colonic and perineal candidiasis.

Pus does not form, even on open skin lesions. There is almost no inflammatory response. This is why fever is uncommon; when it occurs, it is usually due to a high environmental temperature. Similarly, lobar pneumonia does not usually occur in the absence of inhalation.

Anemia

Anemia is almost universal to some degree. It is due to multi-micronutrient deficiency and infection. Thus, there is frequent evidence of deficiencies of folic acid, copper, vitamin E, pyridoxine, riboflavin and vitamin C, all of which can cause anemia. Schistocytosis is not uncommon because of the fragility of the red cells. Malaria is also a common cause of anemia. In urban areas the blood content of lead is often high. The iron stores are normally replete and iron deficiency is not usually the cause of anemia in severe malnutrition.

Other signs

Angular stomatitis, lingual atrophy, follicular hyperkeratosis, vitamin A-deficient eye signs and other signs of specific type 1 nutrient deficiencies frequently occur.

Pathophysiology

The sequence of events that occur in any malnourished individual is shown in Figure 31.6. Although the defects reinforce each other in a cyclical way, the best starting point is the reduction in dietary intake. This can be due to psychiatric illness, the anorexia associated with liver disease, infection, neoplasia, drug intoxication or a type II nutrient deficiency, to famine or starvation, upper intestinal disease, malabsorption or other losses of nutrients from the body.

Reduced mass

A reduction in body mass is the most obvious abnormality clinically, and forms the basis for the various anthropometric classifications of malnutrition. As weight is lost, the absolute nutritional requirements are reduced simply on the basis of the decreased mass. There is also a relative reduction in requirement so that each gram of body tissue requires less energy. This reduces

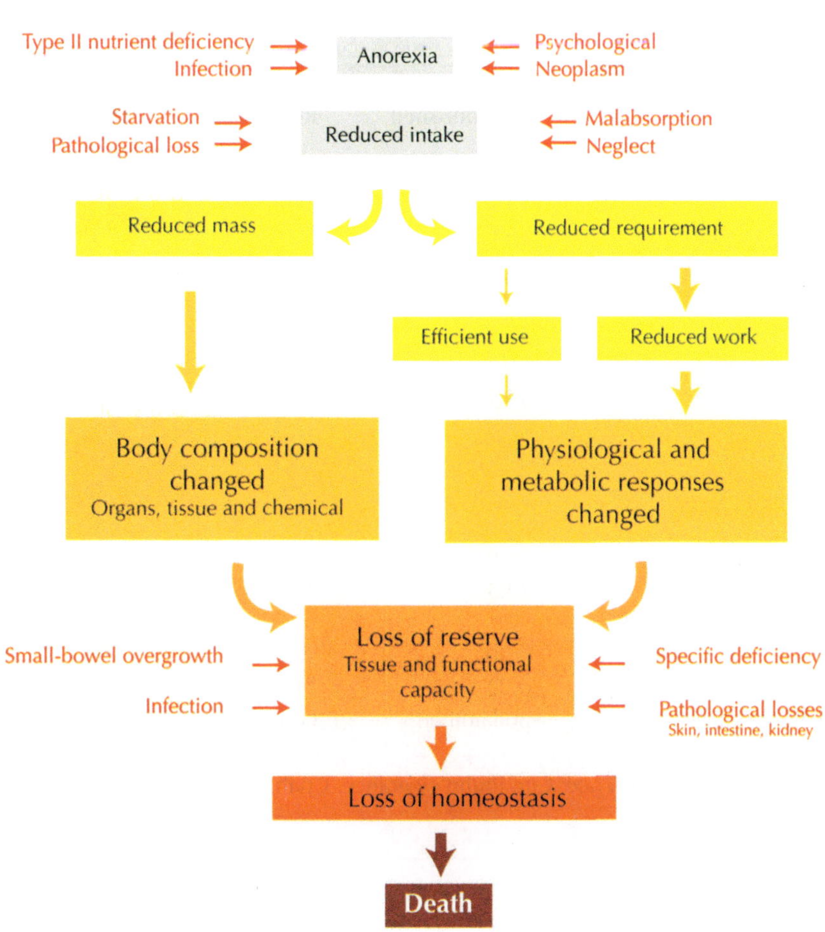

Figure 31.6 Schematic representation of the sequence of events in marasmus.

requirement by about one-third and is achieved over weeks or months by metabolic adaptation.

Efficient use and reduced work

The reduction in requirement comes about in two ways. First, nutrients are used more efficiently. However, we normally use our food quite efficiently, so that there is a relatively small absolute saving possible from increased efficiency. By far the most important adaptation is in the actual work performed by the whole body, its organs, tissues, cells, organelles and enzymatic machinery.

In the well-nourished individual the metabolic capacity far exceeds the demand. Energy is used to maintain this excess capacity for metabolic work. The excess allows us to cope with rapid increases in demand for activity or imposed stress. Thus, we can run at 30 km/h achieving a cardiac output of 20 l/min, eat 70 g protein and 10 g sodium at one sitting, then fast for several days without untoward effects. In health, we maintain all the digestive, absorptive, hepatic and renal capacity to deal with feast or famine. This 'physiological redundancy' is why 'unphysiological' stress tests need to be used to diagnose disordered function at an early stage. These 'reserves' of tissue and functional capacity are nutritionally expensive to synthesize, replace and maintain; they are sacrificed in malnutrition (Table 31.4).

Physiological and metabolic changes

The reduction in work of the cells of the body leads to major changes in the physiological and metabolic responses of the body. Indeed, no physiological function has so far been studied in severe

Table 31.4 Some changes in physiological function in malnourished children

	Malnourished	Recovered	Difference (%recovered)
Metabolic rate (kJ/kg$^{0.75}$ per day)	315	417	-24
Sodium pump activity (/h)	3.62	4.94	-27
Intracellular sodium (mM/kg DS)	169	109	+55
Intracellular potassium (mM/kg DS)	341	387	-12
Protein synthesis (g/kg per day)	4.0	6.3	-37
Protein breakdown (g/kg per day)	3.7	6.4	-42
Cardiac output (l/min per m^2)	4.77	6.90	-31
Stroke volume (ml/beat per m^2)	44.1	53.0	-22
Circulation time (s)	13.7	10.5	+30
GFR (Cin – ml/min per m^2)	47.1	92.4	-41
Renal blood flow (Cpah – ml/min per m^3)	249	321	-22
H^+ excretion after NH_4Cl (μEq/min)	10.4	28.4	-63
Osmolal clearance rate (ml/min)	0.20	0.66	-70
% Infused sodium excreted	22.3	48.7	-54
Sodium excreted (% of sodium filtered)			
Normal ECF	0.50	1.23	-59
Expanded ECF	0.82	11.07	-93
Response to temperature change	poikilotherm	homeotherm	—

DS, dry stool; GFR, glomerular filtration rate; Cin, inulin clearance; Cpah, *p*-aminohippurate clearance; ECF, extracellular fluid

undernutrition and found to be 'normal'. Some of the changes are listed in Table 31.5.

At the level of the whole body, spontaneous activity is severely curtailed – apathy and passivity. Children no longer play or explore, and adults sit in a state of suspended animation, only moving when absolutely necessary.

At the other end of the organizational spectrum is a fundamental adaptation: slowing of the sodium pump. Normally about one-third of basal energy requirements is consumed, pumping sodium out of cells and potassium back into the cells. This adaptation is at the cost of allowing the intracellular sodium concentration to rise and potassium to fall. The potassium lost from the cell cannot be accommodated in the extracellular fluid and is excreted. Slowing of the sodium pump also leads to a reduction in cellular electrical potential and delay in its restoration, hence there is a reduction in neuromuscular function and muscle rapidly fatigues. Other processes that depend upon a sodium gradient, such as amino acid and glucose transport, have a reduced capacity in malnutrition. A further one-third of basal energy requirement is used for the continual cycle of protein synthesis and breakdown in a process known as protein turnover. This is reduced by about 40%.

There is a reduction in cardiac output due to both a lowered heart rate and a lowered stroke volume. The ventricular function curves (stroke work/pressure) are altered so that the point of maximum performance occurs at a lower mean pressure; these patients are very easily precipitated into heart failure.

The maximum concentrating ability of the kidney is severely restricted. This means that one has to be very careful not to give a diet with a high renal solute load, and to ensure that sufficient water is taken. There is a very limited capacity to excrete free hydrogen ions, titratable acid and ammonia in response to an acid load. A common acid load comes from giving magnesium chloride as a dietary supplement. However, the most important renal abnormality is a particular and severe limitation of the ability to excrete sodium, particularly in response to an expanded extracellular fluid volume. These abnormalities are shown in Figure 31.7 and 31.8. With an expanded circulation it takes 10h for a malnourished child to excrete the sodium that a normal child can excrete in 20min.

The motility of the whole intestine is reduced and small-intestinal transit time increased. This leads directly to small-bowel bacterial overgrowth and a distended abdomen. However, it also affects the pharyngeus and esophagus. These children very readily inhale food because of these neuromuscular abnormalities. They should never be force-fed or held recumbent whilst they are fed. Inhalation of the liquid diet, insufficient to obstruct the main bronchi, is probably the most common reason for pneumonia in the malnourished child. It is preventable.

There is a reduction in gastric acid, bile and pancreatic enzyme production. The cellular enzymes and transport systems for nutrient absorption are compromised and the mucosa becomes flattened, but rarely to the degree found in primary intestinal disease such as gluten enteropathy; mitotic figures in the crypts become rare. That the defect is one of capacity and not a specific abnormality is demonstrated by absorption at low rates of presentation (perfusion) being relatively normal, whereas at high rates the digestive and absorptive capacity is overwhelmed.

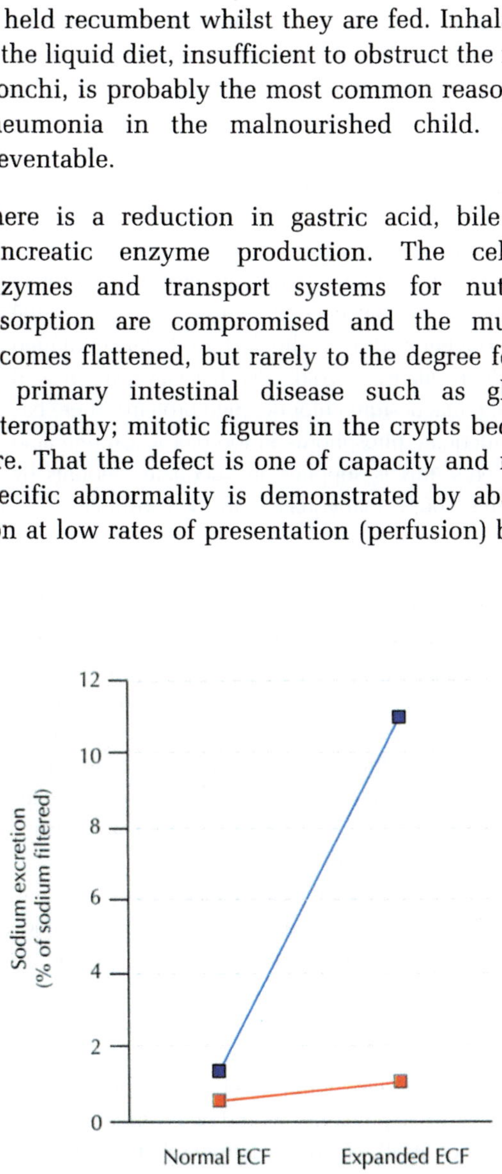

Figure 31.7 The fractional excretion rate of sodium (expressed as a per cent of filtered sodium) of malnourished (red) and normal patients (blue) who have a normal circulating volume and after expansion with a saline infusion. ECF, extracellular fluid.

The malnourished patient becomes poikilothermic. Even a modest reduction to 21°C or elevation to 33°C in environmental temperature may lead to hypothermia or pyrexia, respectively. It is not unusual for malnourished children in the tropics to develop hypothermia; in temperate climates hypothermia is common in the elderly. They are qualitatively different from normal. Normal individuals increase their oxygen consumption in response to a cool environment to maintain body heat; malnourished patients reduce their oxygen consumption in response to a cool environment (Figure 31.9). They never shiver. Once they become cold the slowing metabolism means that they will not recover without some form of external heat.

There are marked changes in the hormonal balance in malnutrition. Growth hormone levels are elevated with a low insulin concentration and a reduced insulin response to a test meal. Insulin-like growth factor (IGF)-I and II, catecholamine, glucagons, thyroxine and tri-iodothyronine, both free and bound, are all low; cortisol tends to be high. The response to injected hormones is diminished, with down-regulation of most receptors. Although there is glucose intolerance, glucose levels are generally lower than normal. The intolerance is partly due to liver dysfunction (thought to be due to slow initial phosphorylation of the monosaccharide) as the degree of galactose intolerance is similar to the degree of glucose intolerance. There is a very marked reduction in gluconeogenesis.

The febrile, acute phase and inflammatory responses, and the immune system also partake in the reductive adaptation; they are either absent or severely blunted in seriously malnourished patients. Infection is normally recognized by the body's response in terms of a fever, leukocytosis, pus formation, tachypnea, etc. When these responses do not occur, life-threatening infection may go completely unrecognized.

Body composition

There are changes in body composition. Most tissues contribute to the loss of weight, but, they

Table 31.5 The main physiological changes in severe malnutrition and their implications for management

Physiological change	Diagnostic and therapeutic implication
Cardiovascular system	
The heart is smaller and thinner than normal. The cardiac output and stroke volume are reduced. Saline infusion leads to greatly increased venous pressure. Overload of the heart readily leads to heart failure. Blood pressure is low. Renal perfusion is reduced. The circulation time is reduced. Plasma volume is usually normal and red cell volume reduced.	The children are vulnerable to both an increase and decrease in blood volume. Any decrease will further compromise tissue perfusion; an increase can easily produce acute heart failure. If dehydrated give restricted amounts of ReSoMal: do not give intravenous fluid unless in severe shock. Restrict blood transfusion to 10 ml/kg per day and cover with diuretic. Restrict the sodium intake from the diet and drugs. Give additional potassium, magnesium and phosphorus.
Genitourinary system	
Glomerular filtration is reduced. The excretion of acid or of an osmolar load is greatly reduced. Urinary phosphate output is low. Sodium excretion is lower than normal. The kidney is physiologically unresponsive. An expanded intravascular or extracellular volume does not lead to increased sodium excretion. Urinary tract infection is common.	Treat with diets that have a low renal solute load. Ensure that there is sufficient water in the diet. Do not overconcentrate the diet. Prevent further tissue breakdown (treat infection and give adequate energy – 80–100 kcal/kg per day) and do not give excess protein over and above that needed to restore tissue, to limit urea production. Protein should have balanced amino acids (high quality). Avoid salts that can give an acid load (e.g. magnesium chloride, high protein). There has to be adequate phosphorus in the diet to excrete acid equivalents (this is supplied in adequate amounts by cow's milk, but is inadequate with soy substitutes).
Gastrointestinal system	
The stomach produces much less acid than normal. The motility of the whole intestine is reduced. The pancreas is atrophied and produces a reduced amount of digestive enzymes. The small-intestinal mucosa is atrophic with reduced levels of digestive enzymes. Absorption is reduced when a lot of substrate is given either from a high concentration or from large amounts of more dilute solutions.	Only use diets in phase 1 that are hypo- or isotonic. Feed small amounts of diet often, to remain within absorptive capacity. If food is malabsorbed the first step is to increase the frequency and reduce the size of each feed (do not dilute the diet and give the same volume). The food is necessary to stimulate the intestine to regrow. Use antibiotics active against small-bowel bacterial overgrowth. Occasionally addition of pancreatic enzymes is useful. Persistent diarrhea nearly always responds to the diet alone.
Liver	
There is a reduction in the synthesis of all hepatic export proteins. Abnormal metabolites of amino acids are produced. The ability of the liver to take up, metabolize and excrete toxins is severely limited. The energy production from substrates (such as galactose, fructose) is much slower than normal. The capacity for gluconeogensis is limited, leading to hypoglycemia with stress of infection. Biliary secretion is reduced. Limited output of bile salts. Jaundice is uncommon. Liver function tests unreliable, because intracellular enzyme levels very low. Indocyanine green uptake very abnormal.	The child should not be given a large meal to metabolize at one time. The amount of protein should be within the capacity of the liver to metabolize it, but sufficient to stimulate synthesis of export proteins. This is much lower than the RDA. Prevention of catabolism is important. Drugs which depend upon hepatic disposal or are hepatotoxic should be given in reduced doses or not at all. Adequate carbohydrate should be given to prevent the necessity for gluconeogensis.

continued

Table 31.5 Continued

Immune system All aspects of immunity are diminished. Lymph glands, tonsils and the thymus are atrophic. Cell-mediated (T cell) immunity is particularly depressed. There is very little IgA in secretions. Complement components are low. Phagocytes do not kill ingested bacteria efficiently.	Assume all malnourished children have infections and overgrowth of mucosal surfaces. Blind antibiotic treatment should be given on admission to all children. Treatment will have to continue until the improved nutritional state leads to improvement of the immune system. Physically separate acute admissions from recovering children. Give measles vaccine and vitamin A. Treat with an antifungal agent.
Inflammatory response Tissue damage is not associated with inflammation; white cells do not migrate into areas of damage. The acute phase response is diminished.	Signs of infection are often absent even after careful examination. Localized infection such as lobar pneumonia is uncommon, generalized infection (bronchopneumonia) is common and may be present with no radiographic or other signs. Assessments of raised white cell count and fever are not necessary. Otitis usually does not give an inflamed or bulging ear. Urinary tract infection is normally symptomless. Hypoglycemia and hypothermia are both signs of severe infection.
Endocrine system Insulin is reduced and there is glucose intolerance. IGF-I is very low, although growth hormone is high. Cortisol is usually high.	The endocrine system may not be able to respond appropriately to large meals. Give small frequent meals. Do not give steroids; they are already high.
Temperature regulation The children are poikilothermic. Both heat generation in the cold and sweating in the heat are impaired. The children become hypothermic in a cold environment and pyrexial in a hot environment.	Maintain environment between 25 and 30°C. Put a max–min thermometer in the ward. Cover the children with clothes and blankets. Children to sleep with their mothers. Keep windows closed at night. Dry children quickly and well after washing and clothe them. Cool fevered children with tepid (not cold) water.
Cellular function The activity of the sodium pump is reduced (marasmus). The cell membranes are more leaky than normal (kwashiorkor). This leads to an increase in intracellular sodium and a decrease in intracellular potassium and magnesium. Protein synthesis is reduced.	All the children need large doses of potassium and magnesium. Sodium intake should be restricted. During recovery the sodium has to come out of the cells and potassium has to go in; this easily leads to cardiac overload and hypokalemia. Reversal of the electrolyte abnormality should be gradual and should occur after the kidney has recovered. If used at all digoxin doses should be halved.
Metabolic rate The basal metabolic rate is reduced by about 30%. The energy expenditure due to activity of these children is very low.	Internal heat production is limited. Most metabolic processes are sluggish.
Body composition There is particular atrophy of skin, subcutaneous fat and muscle. Fat is lost from the orbit. There is atrophy of many glands including the sweat, lachrymal and salivary glands.	Most signs of dehydration are unreliable: eyes may be sunken with loss of orbital fat. Atrophy leads to folds of skin. Skin, mouth and eyes are dry owing to gland atrophy. The children have limited reserves of energy. The respiratory muscles are easily exhausted.

ReSoMal; IGF, insulin-like growth receptor

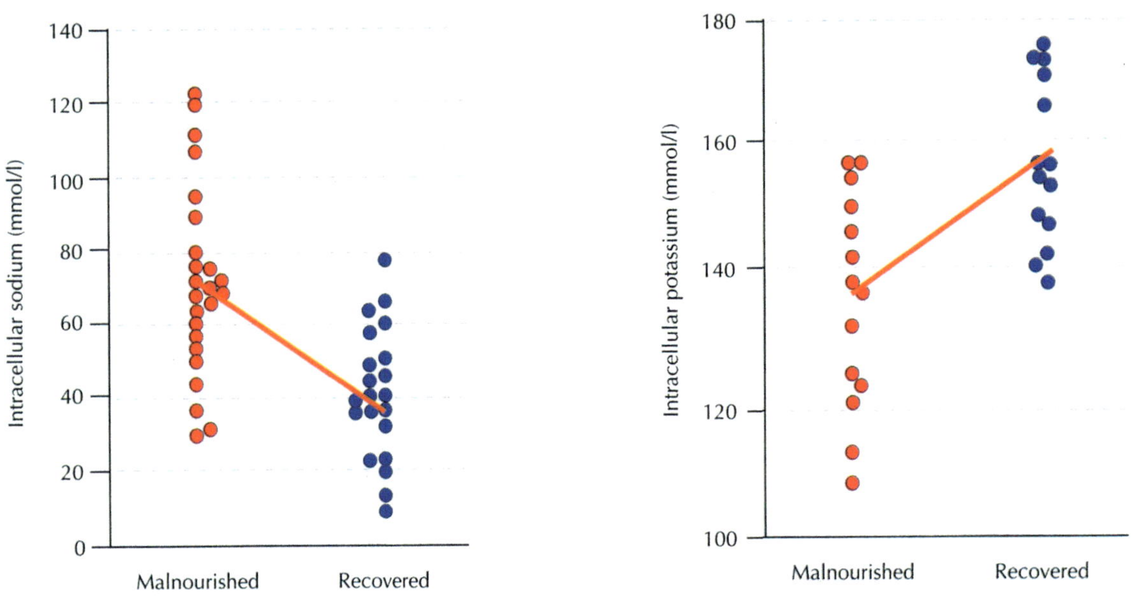

Figure 31.8 The intracellular sodium (a) and potassium (b) before and after recovery from marasmus.

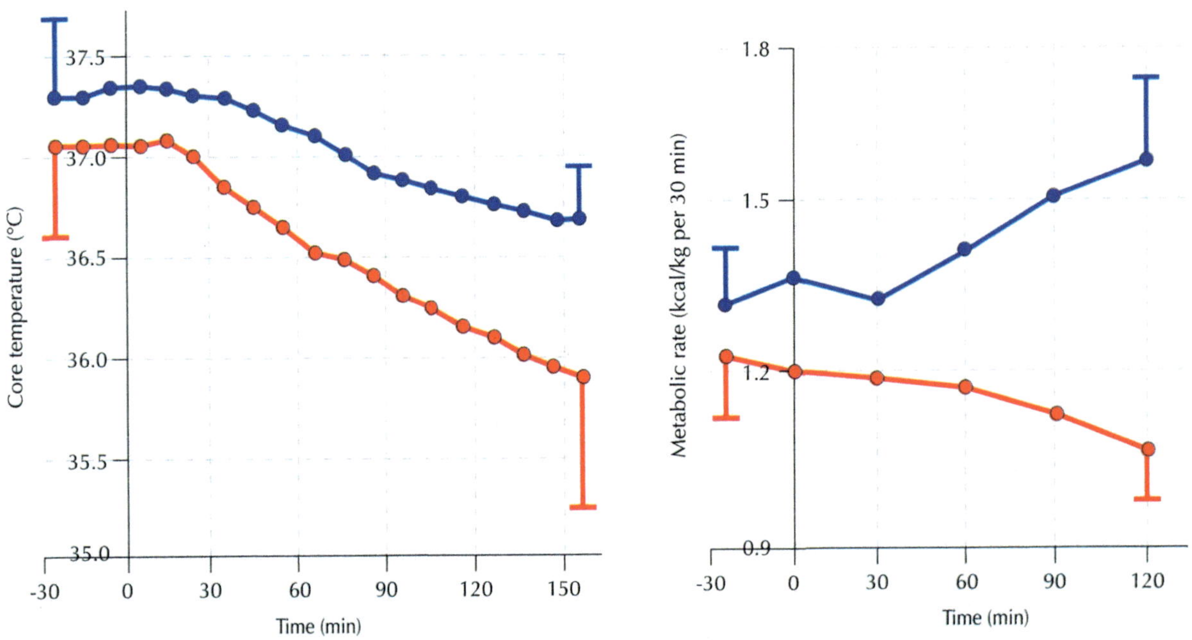

Figure 31.9 The body temperature response of exposure of malnourished (red) and recovered children (blue) to a low environmental temperature (a). The oxygen consumption (b) corresponding to (a). Note that, as the body temperature falls in the normal child, there is an increase in oxygen consumption, whereas in the malnourished child the oxygen consumption falls.

do not contribute equally. Subcutaneous fat may virtually disappear and muscle mass is often reduced by more than half. Skin and intestine are also disproportionately affected, whereas the viscera and the central nervous system are relatively well preserved.

The chemical composition of the whole body is altered because of the changes in the relative size of the organs. Those that are most atrophic are those that are used least. Thus, although the gluteus muscle may shrivel, the external ocular muscles are almost normal. The viscera are preserved at the expense of muscle, fat and skin. However, where loss would be critical to survival, it is much less marked. For example, malnourished children in Tchad, in the Sahara desert, have good skin. In this environment if the skin lost its function the children would rapidly desiccate.

However, there are also changes as a consequence of the reductive adaptations themselves. Critically, the reduction in activity of the sodium pump invariably leads to an increased total body sodium and reduced total body potassium, irrespective of the patient's state of hydration or the serum electrolyte concentrations. When there is also edema, the malnourished patient also has an increased extracellular as well as intracellular sodium concentration. The reduction in the enzyme, soluble protein and RNA complement, with relative increase in structural protein, is accompanied by reduction in those trace elements and vitamins used as enzymatic co-factors. They are not retained in the tissues without the parent proteins. The proportionate reduction in each of these components of soft tissue is about the same. Of course, during reversal of the adaptation the deficits of all these components has to be made good before any weight gain could occur. Iron is an exception. There is an increased concentration of tissue iron in most forms of severe malnutrition (but not in patients with chronic blood loss from, say, intestinal helminthiasis).

Loss of reserve

The cost of both the reductive adaptations and the reduction in functional tissue mass is to dispense, to a greater or lesser extent, with the reserve capacity. The malnourished individual has a reduced capacity to respond appropriately to the metabolic, environmental or infective stresses that do little harm to a well-nourished individual.

Vicious cycles

Superimposed upon the reduced ability to respond to metabolic and environmental changes are the pathological effects of the stresses themselves. The curtailment of the inflammatory and immune responses make infections ubiquitous. The atonic gut, achlorhydria, and poor secretion of IgA and bile salts combine to allow normal intestinal flora. Both bacteria and fungi overgrow the small intestine and stomach. These organisms directly damage the intestine, deconjugate bile salts and exacerbate any malabsorption. Unless they are suppressed, diarrhea may worsen when additional food is given. The gas produced and the intestinal stasis is the reason for abdominal swelling in malnutrition; such swelling is characteristic of small-bowel overgrowth.

The diarrhea and repeated infections give rise, in turn, to specific nutrient deficiencies, particularly of mineral elements. When the integrity of the skin is breached from the burn-like lesions of severe childhood malnutrition, bed sores, fistulae and traumatic or surgical lesions which become indolent, blood, serum and heat can be lost in considerable amounts.

The effect of the infections, small-bowel overgrowth, malabsorption, nutrient losses and thermal stress in the patient already adapted to malnutrition, is to exacerbate the anorexia and further reduce the intake. The cycle is now complete. The adaptations are reinforced and physiological function increasingly compromised. The debilitated patient reaches a self-perpetuating stage where increasing anorexia and organ dysfunction lead to rapid deterioration and death.

Loss of homeostasis

As the physiological and tissue reserve is whittled away and the effects of chronic infection and diarrhea deplete the patient, he becomes more and more 'brittle', like a diabetic patient losing homeostatic control of his blood sugar. However, unlike the diabetic, in the severely malnourished patient it is not just one organ or system that is functionally deranged but all of them. Finally, the patient simply cannot control his 'milieu interieur', everything slows down and stops.

When treatment regimens are planned they must always work within the patient's limited metabolic capacity whilst the reductive adaptations are reversed dietetically. Disequilibrium syndromes can occur during this reversal and lead to sudden unexpected death during early refeeding, even in previously obese patients who have been undergoing a prolonged period of energy restriction.

Although the classification of marasmus is based entirely upon anthropometric criteria, sickness and death are related to the disordered physiology rather than the precise degree of wasting. There is not a close correspondence between the two. There are usually accompanying type I nutrient deficiencies and pathological losses. The difficulty of relying solely on anthropometry is illustrated by the patient with anorexia nervosa. She normally has had a very restricted amount of a high-quality diet and is abnormally active. Even though the anthropometry is similar, many of the physiological changes are different, and these patients can tolerate a much lower body mass before they become dysfunctional. Bulemic patients are more like those with severe malnutrition.

Edematous malnutrition

In community surveys about 80% of patients with edematous malnutrition are not wasted, and most are not stunted. Ecologically the condition is 'over-dispersed' following a negative binomial distribution, whereas marasmus follows a normal Poisson distribution. That means that kwashiorkor occurs in geographical pockets; one village may have no cases whereas another in the same region has more cases than would be expected. Marasmus and kwashiorkor do not share a distribution, even when they are prevalent in the same area. Some villages have predominantly marasmus and others kwashiorkor.

Contrary to what is generally believed, about 25% of children with kwashiorkor are being breast fed, some exclusively. The type II nutrient concentration in breast milk is defended by the mother. In contrast, the concentration of type I nutrients in breast milk varies with the mother's intake and status. Samples of the breast milk, from mothers feeding children with kwashiorkor, are very low in antioxidants. These are all type I nutrients.

Edematous malnutrition, unlike other forms of malnutrition, is an acute illness. A patient who appears quite well may, over the course of a few days, become extremely irritable, progress through the various stages of the skin lesions and suddenly 'blow up' with edema. When they present they have almost complete retention of ingested sodium. Although they have a low blood pressure and signs of hypovolemia the sodium retention appears to be renal in origin, as it often does not recover with restoration of blood pressure and even over-expansion of the vascular volume. Although the level of aldosterone is high, it is unlikely to be the cause of the sodium retention, as it paradoxically increases when these patients commence diuresis to lose edema. Natriuretic peptides and their receptors have not been measured in kwashiorkor.

Kwashiorkor belongs to the family of diseases that includes toxic shock syndrome, adult respiratory distress syndrome, multiple organ failure and sick-cell syndrome. It also has similarities to patients with radiation injury, cytotoxic drug overdose and HIV infection in that they all lead to profound immuno-incompetence and abnormal glutathione metabolism.

In edematous malnutrition, in contrast to marasmus, there is an increased excretion of urinary nitrate. Nitrate is the end product of nitric oxide metabolism and a measure of the whole body nitric oxide production rate. The circulating levels and urinary excretion of the leukotrienes are also specifically increased. There is always a reduction in cellular glutathione concentration, a key intermediate in protection of the body from free radicals. Measurement of the ratio of NADPH/NADP in cells from these children shows that they have a marked deficit in reducing equivalents. Furthermore, examination of the sulfhydryl groups on proteins shows that an unusually large proportion of them are oxidized. Incubation of normal red cells *in vitro* with peroxides reproduces the profile of membrane lipids found in kwashiorkor.

Although they also have a high intracellular sodium and a low potassium concentration, as in marasmus, this comes about by quite a different mechanism. Their cell membranes become leaky to sodium and potassium; it is this membrane leakiness that leads to the loss of intracellular potassium and an increase in intracellular sodium. In fact, the sodium pump is quite the opposite to that in marasmus; in kwashiorkor it is more active than normal and their cells have an increased complement of Na^+K^+ATPase. When cellular glutathione is reduced in normal cells experimentally, to the levels seen in edematous malnutrition, the leakiness of the membrane is reproduced and the same electrolyte abnormalities that are seen in kwashiorkor arise. In kwashiorkor, the cell membranes have been damaged by oxidation.

In kwashiorkor there is also effacement of the podocytes of the glomerulus to resemble minimal-change nephrotic syndrome. However, there is no proteinuria. This is a morphological expression of a change in the surface anionic charge on the cell membranes. The defect can be corrected, *in vitro*, by perfusion with strongly anionic substances such as heparin. The loss of surface charge is due to the disruption of the glycosaminoglycans (GAGs) on the cell surface. Interestingly, these children do not get infections such as cholera which depend upon the organism attaching to surface complex carbohydrate receptors. Such receptor dysfunction may account for the abnormal renal sodium homeostasis, but at present there is no direct evidence for this speculation. The blood–brain barrier is dependent upon the integrity of surface GAGs. This may account for the fact that meningitis is uncommon in kwashiorkor (but not in marasmus). It also means that drugs that are neurotoxic if they enter the cerebrospinal fluid, but are normally excluded, should be used with extreme caution in edematous malnutrition. Ivermectin would be in this category.

Protein synthesis is disrupted. Electron microscopy of various tissues shows a marked reduction of the protein synthetic machinery. Hepatic export proteins are not made at a sufficient rate to maintain their circulating concentrations. Reduction in lipoprotein synthesis may be sufficient to account for the vast accumulation of triglyceride in the liver although it is likely that other mechanisms are involved. For example, there are very few peroxisomes seen in the cells and the abnormalities of NADPH biochemistry are likely to affect lipid metabolism profoundly.

Most textbooks ascribe kwashiorkor to protein deficiency. However, this theory is now untenable. Protein deficiency would not account for the physiological and biochemical abnormalities. Further, experimental protein deficiency does not reproduce the clinical features of kwashiorkor in any species of animal. Being a type II nutrient, protein deficiency does give stunting and wasting. The edema can resolve completely on a very low protein diet with no change in plasma albumin level. In the community, no differences have been found in the protein contents of the diets of those who develop kwashiorkor and those who develop marasmus.

How might poverty lead to kwashiorkor? First, poor people live crowded together, in a highly contaminated environment. They get many severe infections and small-bowel overgrowth. Indeed, epidemics of kwashiorkor follow epidemics of measles in the tropics, but not in the rich countries. Second, their diets are lacking in many of the type I nutrients that are crucial to protection from free radical damage, particularly: selenium, vitamin E, carotene, vitamin C, riboflavin, thiamine and nicotinic acid. From this list special mention should be made of selenium. Red cells become more dense as they age. Thus, by separating cells by their density, it is possible to look back in time to observe the selenium status during the evolution of the illness. Examination of the selenoenzyme, glutathione peroxidase, in age-fractionated cells shows that the children with kwashiorkor have become selenium deficient in the recent past. The areas of the world where kwashiorkor is common have mostly selenium-deficient soils.

When an infection, toxin or drug gives rise to tissue damage, cytokine release, leukotriene synthesis and free radical production, these patients lack the ability to protect and repair their liver, skin and vessels from acute damage. These defenses depend upon an orchestra of type I nutrients collectively referred to as antioxidants. It is this acute oxidative damage that both causes the syndrome of kwashiorkor and accounts for its similarity to several other serious conditions usually found in intensive care units.

Changes that occur during treatment

During successful treatment the physiological and body compositional changes reverse. Unfortunately, the order in which normal function returns can endanger the patient. With increased intake of antioxidants the leak in the cell membrane of kwashiorkor is repaired. With the increase in dietary intake the slow pump of marasmus regains its function. The sodium inside the cell is exported. In malnutrition the intracellular sodium is about 70 mmol/l cell water; the normal is about 30 mmol/l cell water. If 40 mmol/l were to be suddenly exported from the cell to be retained in the extracellular fluid at a concentration of 135 mmol/l, then there would be an increase of about 30% in the extracellular fluid volume. If this fluid were retained in the circulation it would precipitate volume overload and acute heart failure. In kwashiorkor, if the defect in the interstitial space is corrected, then edema fluid moves from the interstitial space to the vascular compartment; again, this leads to an additional expansion of the circulating volume in kwashiorkor.

Although the children often present with hypovolemia, during early treatment the situation is completely reversed to a situation of hypervolemia. This is always associated with a fall in hemoglobin concentration. Indeed, the red cells function as a 'marker' of blood volume. The expansion of the total blood volume can be assessed by the magnitude of the fall in hemoglobin concentration. The liver enlarges with the expansion of the blood volume and there may be an increase in respiratory rate, distension of the neck veins, increased vascular shadows on chest X-ray and signs of pulmonary edema.

The movement of sodium and water, to accumulate potentially in the vascular compartment, needs to take place after the kidney recovers its ability to excrete sodium. Where this does not happen the child is in great danger.

The determining factors are thus:

(1) The initial amount of edema fluid and increase in intracellular sodium;

(2) The rate and degree of recovery of the tissue and cellular lesions;

(3) The rate and degree of recovery of the renal lesions;

(4) Sodium intake from the diet, oral rehydration fluid and intravenous fluid;

(5) The additional expansion of the blood volume from a transfusion.

Children with edema are more susceptible than those without edema, children with severe edema are much more susceptible than those with minimal edema, and children with marasmus from areas where kwashiorkor is also common are much more susceptible than marasmic children from areas where the dietary deficiencies that give rise to kwashiorkor are uncommon. This electrolytic dysequilibrium, leading to heart failure, accounts for the majority of deaths after admission and for the differences in mortality rates between different regions of the developing world.

How can this be avoided? Even though antioxidant deficiency may be the immediate etiology of kwashiorkor, we should not treat the children with large amounts of antioxidants acutely. Modern diets (F75 and F100) contain significant amounts of the antioxidants, and the pathological changes reverse quite quickly in comparison to the diets that used to be used. If the staff do not understand the dangers of rapid reversal of the condition, fail to follow the protocol for the management of complications faithfully and do not guard against giving additional sodium or blood at this time, they should not use these treatments.

As we do not understand the renal lesions, it is unclear how to ensure that they are corrected at an early stage. During the early phase of treatment, when the sodium pump is recovering and the excess intracellular sodium is being exported to the extracellular compartment, acute circulatory overload and sudden death can easily occur when the kidney recovers more slowly than the sodium pump.

A low-sodium diet should always be used in the early stages. On admission the edge of the liver should be marked upon the skin with an indelible marker. Expansion and contraction of the liver is the easiest clinical way of assessing changes in blood volume (or changes in hematocrit, provided no one on the team will misinterpret this as anemia that requires transfusion).

After admission diarrhea should be ignored unless it is associated with significant weight loss that is not accounted for by resolution of edema, and contraction of the liver if it was initially enlarged. With treatment, great care should be taken that the weight, the respiratory rate or liver size does not increase excessively. If a blood transfusion is to be given, it must be given in the first 24 h after admission and the diets should not be given simultaneously. After this window is passed a blood transfusion should not be given (unless the staff have the capacity to do a small exchange transfusion) for at least 2 weeks. A hemoglobin level that falls after admission should not be treated. Intravenous lines should not be established to give drugs. Quinine infusions should be avoided. Indwelling canulae are also dangerous because of the need to administer anticoagulants. Large doses of the sodium salts of drugs (antibiotics, antacids, etc.) should not be used.

Heart failure is not easy to diagnose in this situation and many children are incorrectly diagnosed as having pneumonia. Persistent diarrhea, with which the child has already survived for several weeks, should not be treated acutely with rehydration fluids.

Investigations

A careful history and examination usually provide all the information required to treat these patients. The laboratory has a relatively minor role to play and is used for the identification and characterization of infection.

Tuberculosis is common; its diagnosis presents special difficulties as the mantoux test is usually negative irrespective of the presence or absence of active disease. Acid-fast bacilli can sometimes be recovered from laryngeal aspirate obtained with a mucus extractor. A chest X-ray should be scrutinized carefully for small tuberculous lesions. Children with tuberculosis should not be transferred to a tuberculosis ward where the staff have not been trained and organized to manage malnutrition. The management of the malnutrition takes precedence (over the course of a few weeks, malnutrition has a much worse prognosis and higher mortality rate than tuberculosis); tuberculosis treatment can be given in the malnutrition unit.

On the chest X-ray, infection causes much less shadowing than in well-nourished children and may even be absent in the presence of bronchopneumonia. The blood should be examined for malarial parasites if routine treatment is not being given to all severely malnourished patients. Testing for sickle cell disease is important in many communities. Hematocrit or hemoglobin may be helpful immediately on admission, although anemia is usually clinically obvious. Measurement of plasma constituents is unhelpful in management. Plasma concentrations bear no necessary relationship to whole body content. This is particularly true for potassium and sodium. Hyponatremia is frequently found and is a poor prognostic sign.

Therapy should be based upon clinical criteria; it should be guided by frequent reappraisal of the direction of clinical progress and does not require laboratory data. Investigations are used for help with diagnosis, not to control treatment.

Management

The aims of treatment are to identify and treat all the life-threatening problems whilst reversing the pathological and physiological abnormalities and deficiencies safely, then to feed the patient so that weight is gained at an accelerated rate to 'catch up' towards normal. In children the aim is to start to stimulate mental development, to protect the patient from relapse and to secure continued normal development after discharge.

There are two main criteria for admission to residential care: first, the presence of anorexia of more than a few days' duration; and second, any child who does not respond immediately to a trial of out-patient management, and who has either edema, regardless of weight, or $< 70\%$ weight-for-height.

The treatment is divided into several phases: an initial acute phase where the immediate threats to life are managed and treatment is initiated, a transition phase and a rehabilitation phase of intense feeding to return the child to a normal body composition and function and prepare for discharge. Then there is follow-up.

The acute phase

The mothers have often visited traditional healers, waited until it is clear that help is needed and the expense justified, and then traveled long distances. The ill children have to be triaged and 'fast tracked' through registration and out-patient clinics. They should all be given 10% sugar water as soon as they arrive. They should then have their weight and height measured, have a brief history and examination taken and be admitted. They should not be washed or manipulated excessively. The caretaker (mother) should be admitted with the child. There should be low adult beds for the child and the mother to sleep together.

We need to treat infections and start to reverse the physiological changes without the treatment overloading the limited capacity of the heart, kidney, intestine or liver. The therapeutic implications of the reductive physiological adaptations are given in Table 31.5.

Dehydration

Marasmus itself emulates all the signs of dehydration. It is almost impossible to make the diagnosis by examination. For this reason diagnoses of dehydration in the malnourished are always provisional. Only significant acute diarrhea needs treatment; children with persistent diarrhea should not be 'rehydrated'. A history of recent sinking of the eyes with significant watery diarrhea should be present. If the patient has true dehydration then this has to be treated with rehydration fluid. The patients are very vulnerable to over-hydration and fatal heart failure is common during the early stages of treatment. Additionally, there is nearly always some element of 'toxic shock' arising from their infections and small-bowel overgrowth. These patients are quite different from 'normal' persons with diarrhea or other types of dehydration. The management of diarrhea in the normal child intentionally and correctly gives excess fluid to ensure that all children receive adequate amounts. The kidney will readily excrete any excess that is given. This situation does not apply to the malnourished child. They are sensitive to sodium. For these reasons, oral rehydration fluids are given for a only short time in limited amounts. The normal solution used, ReSoMal, has a lower sodium (45 mmol/l) and higher potassium (40 mmol/l) content than that used for normally nourished patients (Table 31.6). The patients are also depleted in magnesium, zinc and phosphorus – solutions that contain these ions as well as the major electrolytes are particularly useful. Because of their difficulty with homeostasis, intravenous treatment is particularly dangerous and should be used only for unconscious patients with severe shock from dehydration.

Rehydration is managed by taking serial weights. This gives an accurate, quick and reliable way of assessing rehydration. On admission, with even small amounts of weight gain, there should be definite and obvious clinical improvement if the diagnosis was correct. If there is weight gain without clinical improvement then the diagnosis was incorrect. Daily weights are taken from all patients under care; the dehydrating effect of diarrhea occurring after admission can then be assessed accurately from the weight change. Rehydration should never be given that increases the weight more than the pre-diarrheal weight.

Dehydration denotes a lower than normal electrolyte and water content of the body. Edema denotes a higher than normal electrolyte and water content of the body. To say that an *edematous* patient is dehydrated is like diagnosing fever in a hypothermic patient – they are mutually exclusive diagnoses. That is not to say that a patient with kwashiorkor cannot be hypovolemic, indeed many are; but they are not dehydrated. The signs of 'dehydration' are nearly always related to toxic (or cardiogenic) shock in the edematous patient.

Shock

There are three common types of shock in the severely malnourished: dehydration, toxic shock due to sepsis and cardiogenic shock. There are frequently elements of all three in the moribund malnourished child. They are very difficult to differentiate. Toxic shock is difficult to treat successfully. In toxic shock, the stress of endotoxemia is superimposed upon the other problems of severe malnutrition. The veins and capillaries dilate, the cardiac muscle is weakened and the blood pressure falls. The combined effects of the toxin, the metabolic changes produced by cytokines and low perfusion of the organs leads to increasing shock. Renal perfusion is reduced to a

Table 31.6 Composition of an oral rehydration solution suitable from malnourished children

Component	Concentration per liter
Sodium	45 mmol (45 mEq)
Potassium	40 mmol (40 mEq)
Magnesium	3 mmol (6 mEq)
Glucose	10 g
Sucrose	25 g
Osmolality	291 mOsm
Zinc	300 µmol (19.5 mg)
Copper	45 µmol (2.9 mg)
Selenium	0.6 µmol (47 µg)

level where the kidney cannot excrete the end-products of metabolism; the intestine fails to absorb and then secretes fluid, bowel movement diminishes and petechial bleeding occurs throughout the intestine; liver perfusion is reduced, gluconeogenesis becomes ineffective and the blood sugar falls; even the metabolic stress of processing dietary protein can give liver failure, and high-protein diets are dangerous; there is a progressive decrease of awareness because of poor cerebral perfusion, anoxia, electrolyte disturbance and hypoglycemia. The low perfusion of the tissues reduces the metabolic rate to a stage where there is insufficient heat to maintain body temperature. Incipient toxic shock needs to be recognized in its early stages and this progression prevented. Management depends upon the maintenance of cardiac output, the removal of the source of the toxin by treating infection, the prevention of hypoglycemia and hypothermia, the strict avoidance of any stress such as giving excess fluid or protein, the provision of nutrition and the correction of deficiencies. If the circulation is compromised, treatment is by plasma expansion.

Diet

The principle of dietary management in the acute stage is to give enough to prevent hypoglycemia and hypothermia, to prevent any further tissue catabolism and to allow the patient to begin to reassemble his cellular enzymes; this must be done within the capacity of the intestine, liver and other organs. However, at this stage, not only may the functional capacity be easily exceeded, but deficiencies and nutrient imbalances may be aggravated if the patient is given too much food. It is as important for the patient not to gain new tissue when he is in this state as it is to prevent the further loss of existing tissue. This is done by carefully controlling the amount of food that is given. Children are given not less than 80 kcal/kg per day and not more than 100 kcal/kg per day; infants can be given somewhat higher levels; in adults the intake should be 30–40 kcal/kg per day. If less than 80 kcal/kg per day is given to a child, he will continue to use his own tissues for food and will deteriorate; if more than 100 kcal/kg per day is given, the child may develop a metabolic imbalance.

Because the amount of food that the intestine, liver and kidney can handle is limited, to keep within the capacity of the organs the diet is divided into small portions given at frequent intervals (normally eight feeds per day). The more 'brittle' the patient, the more restricted is his capacity and, thus, the smaller each feed has to be and the more frequently they are given. In the extremely ill patient, the diet is put into a nasogastric drip and given continuously; intravenous feeding can be used in specialized centers in rich countries, but the principles of management are exactly the same with these patients as with orally fed children in the tropics.

In the less severely ill patient, the diet is given less frequently. Recently the success of day-care treatment has shown that uncomplicated cases can be fed during the day and allowed home at night.

The diet should contain every essential nutrient (all the minerals, particularly potassium and magnesium, vitamins, protein and energy) the child needs to repair his tissues. If any one of the nutrients is not given in adequate amounts the child will not recover. He will suffer an acute deficiency of this nutrient as the energy intake increases. On the other hand, the diet should not contain a great excess of any nutrient as the excess will again cause a metabolic stress. The amounts of each of the nutrients that should be

Table 31.7 The desirable nutrient intake (per kg body weight) from the diet during the catch-up phase of treatment. The diet is most easily formulated as a single diet of 1 kcal/ml for transition phase and phase 2

Nutrient	Per kg body weight	Per kg body weight/ 100 kcal
Water	120–140 ml	120–140 ml
Energy	420 kJ	100 kcal
Protein	1–2 g	1–2 g
Electrolytes		
Sodium	<1.0 mmol	<23 mg
Potassium	>4.0 mmol	>160 mg
Magnesium	>0.6 mmol	>10 mg
Phosphorus	2.0 mmol	60 mg
Calcium	2.0 mmol	80 mg
Trace minerals		
Zinc	30 μmol	2.0 mg
Copper	4.5 μmol	0.3 mg
Selenium	60 nmol	4.7 μg
Iodine	100 nmol	12 μg
Water-soluble vitamins		
Thiamine	70 μg	70 μg
Riboflavin	200 μg	200 μg
Niacin	1000 μg	1000 μg
Pyridoxine	70 μg	70 μg
Cobalamin	100 ng	100 ng
Folic acid	100 μg	100 μg
Ascorbic acid	10 mg	10 mg
Pantothenic acid	300 μg	300 μg
Biotin	10 μg	10 μg
Fat-soluble vitamins		
Retinol	150 μg	150 μg
Calciferol	3 μg	3 μg
Tocopherol	2.2 mg	2.2 mg
Vitamin K	4 μg	4 μg
Lipids		
Total lipid	25–55% energy	
N-6 fatty acids	4.5% energy	
N-3 fatty acids	0.5% energy	

used for treating malnourished patients are given in Table 31.7.

Infections

Because of the poor inflammatory response, the usual physical signs of infection in the malnourished are unobtrusive or absent; infection expresses itself as apathy, drowsiness, hypothermia, hypoglycemia and death. Nearly all malnourished children have infections; many have multiple infections. They have overgrowth of their small intestines with organisms normally present in the colon, and normally commensal organisms, such as *Staphylococcus epidermidis*, become invasive. Infections are frequently the immediate cause of death.

Early, effective treatment with antibiotics is critical in suppressing small-bowel overgrowth, pre-venting toxic shock, improving the nutritional response to feeding and preventing mortality. For these reasons blind unselective wide-spectrum antibiotic treatment is recommended for all patients with severe malnutrition. Oral amoxicillin is a good choice. It effectively suppresses the bowel overgrowth (this disturbance of the flora is why it sometimes provokes diarrhea in normal children) and is also active against most of the common organisms. Some clinicians believe that antibiotics should be prescribed only for clearly defined infection. This is to confuse prophylaxis with blind treatment. Often microbiologists advocate specific treatment of the organisms they manage to isolate and recognize as pathogenic; this can be dangerous in malnourished patients because of the multiple organisms, the need to suppress commensals and failure to sample most of the potential sites of infection.

Measles

This involves herpes and other systemic viral infections. The mortality rate of severely malnourished patients with measles is very high. To reduce the risk of cross-infection from a newly admitted patient who is incubating measles, it is recommended that measles vaccine be given to all malnourished children on admission. Children with severe malnutrition often have vitamin A deficiency. This is particularly associated with death from measles.

Vitamin deficiency

In regions where measles or vitamin A deficiency is known to occur, even if clinical vitamin A deficiency is uncommon, vitamin A should be routinely given to all malnourished children on admission. They should receive three doses: one each on the 1st, 2nd and 14th day. The patients are normally also folic acid deficient. All patients should receive a single dose of 5 mg folic acid orally, on admission. It should not be repeated, as large doses of folic acid interfere with malaria treatment. Many patients are also deficient in riboflavin, ascorbic acid, pyridoxine, thiamine and the fat-soluble vitamins D, E and K. Where specific deficiencies are known to be common, the amounts can be increased in the therapeutic diet. However, for patients with clinical signs, therapeutic doses of the nutrients should be given. The commercial preparations of F75 and F100 have ample micronutrients and none need be given individually.

Hypoglycemia

All malnourished patients can develop hypoglycemia when they are fasted. However, this complication has been overemphasized in the past. In one series, one case of asymptomatic low blood sugar was found in 200 patients. The success of home, out-patient and day-care programs has confirmed that this is an uncommon complication. If there is concern about hypoglycemia then it can be prevented by giving frequent feeds throughout the day and night.

Eyelid retraction is a sign of sympathetic overactivity that is frequently present in children who are actively attempting to maintain their blood sugar (or circulating volume in dehydration). If a child sleeps with its eyes open, that child should be awoken and given sugar water (10%). A low body temperature, lethargy, limpness and clouding of consciousness are other features of hypoglycemia; unlike normal persons, sweating and pallor do not usually occur. If hypoglycemia is suspected, treatment should be given immediately.

If the patient is conscious or can be roused and will drink, give sugar in water or a formula feed by mouth, whichever is most quickly available, and stay beside the patient until he is alert.

If the patient is losing consciousness, is unrousable or has convulsions, a bolus injection of 1 ml/kg body weight of sterile 10% glucose should be given intravenously followed by nasogastric 10% sucrose to prevent recurrence.

When the patient regains consciousness, an oral feed of a milk preparation or of sugar water is given immediately. This patient should then be given frequent oral feeds to prevent recurrence.

Hypothermia

The neutral temperature for malnourished patients is 25–30°C. Staff, who are active and fully clothed, often find this temperature uncomfortably warm. They do not realize that a room temperature that is comfortable for themselves (20–24°C) is too cold for malnourished patients, particularly small, immobile, malnourished children. Young infants, those with marasmus, those with large areas of weeping skin and infected patients are particularly susceptible to hypothermia. Newly admitted patients should not be nursed near windows or other drafts. At night the mother should sleep in the same bed as the child. Little cages (cots or cribs) are used in many pediatric wards – they promote hypothermia, inhibit breast feeding and cause psychological stress for the child. The mother does not get adequate rest and this compromises her care of her child. Cots are for the benefit of the staff. The patients should be properly covered with hats, clothes and blankets. Washing should be kept to a minimum and done during the day; when patients are washed they must be immediately and carefully dried and not left wet. Hypothermia is a consequence of a low metabolic rate.

When rectal temperature is below 35.5°C (94.9°F) or underarm temperature below 35°C (95°F) the patient should be warmed. This is best done by using the 'kangaroo' technique. The carer is the 'incubator'. The child is put on the mother's bare chest and both are covered with a blanket; the mother is then given a hot drink to increase her skin blood flow. All hypothermic patients must also be treated for hypoglycemia.

Severe anemia

Deficiencies of the hematinics, folate, copper, vitamin E, ascorbic acid, pyridoxine and riboflavin are common. In urban areas blood levels of lead can be high. Malaria, hemoglobinopathies, favism and hookworm are regionally common. However, iron deficiency is not common, except in patients with chronic blood loss from intestinal helminths. The hemoglobin level usually increases rapidly during catch-up growth. Iron is added to the treatment only after transferrin has been resynthesized and bacteria are adequately treated. Moderately severe anemia is not otherwise treated.

If the hemoglobin concentration is less than 40 g/l on admission, then the patient can have a slow blood transfusion: 10 ml/kg body weight of whole blood or packed cells over at least 3 h. Anemia that is recognized after admission should not be treated. If the patient has heart failure secondary to anemia then the blood should be given as an exchange transfusion (an equal volume of blood is taken to that transfused; this is done by taking 2.5 ml/kg before transfusion and then at hourly intervals during the transfusion). It should be noted that anemia and heart failure often coexist. Heart failure that is due to the anemia is a high-output failure, similar to beriberi, with warm peripheries and a wide pulse pressure. It is dangerous to transfuse a patient with anemia in heart failure, if the heart failure is due to other causes.

Congestive heart failure and acute left heart failure

These are common complications and causes of death. They occur as a complication of overhydration (especially when intravenous fluids are given), blood transfusion, plasma transfusion, or with formulae or drugs that have a high sodium content. It can also occur during early recovery when sodium effluxes from the cells and edema fluid is resorbed into the circulation at a faster rate than can be excreted by the kidney. Heart failure may be more common in areas where the diet is low in selenium.

The important signs to look for are clinical deterioration with a gain in weight, an increasing respiratory rate or a rapid enlargement of the liver (Figure 31.10). Treatment should be started at this stage. However, heart failure has to be differentiated from inhalation, respiratory infection and toxic shock. The simplest way to make this differentiation is to examine the weight change. Respiratory distress with weight loss should be treated as pneumonia; with weight gain it should be treated as heart failure. The patient must be re-examined at very frequent intervals after any treatment is started so that, if there is not a rapid improvement, the diagnosis can be revised. The most useful signs are liver size and respiratory rate. Later signs are respiratory distress, rapid pulse, venous engorgement, cold hands and feet and a purple discoloration under the fingernails and tongue. Left heart failure often presents as sudden unexpected death.

When heart failure is diagnosed, *all* oral intake and intravenous fluids should be stopped (the treatment of heart failure takes precedence over feeding); the patient is fasted. This will ensure a negative fluid balance. If there is a danger of hypoglycemia then small amounts of 10% sugar water should be given orally. The fasting may also have the effect of allowing some sodium to return to the intracellular or interstitial compartments. It should be continued until the weight gained (a measure of the amount of fluid retention) since the start of symptoms has been re-lost, the respiratory rate has settled and the liver has returned to its admission size. A diuretic is given intravenously; the most appropriate diuretic is 1 mg/kg of frusemide. Most malnourished patients do not respond to this diuretic; it is given because some patients do respond and this cannot be predicted. As these patients have a low total body potassium level, frequently hypokalemia, full doses of digitalis are never given; however, digitalis inhibits the sodium pump and allows sodium to re-enter the cell. A single dose of 5 μg/kg digoxin should be given.

If the patient continues to deteriorate, the physician is certain of the diagnosis of heart failure and heroic measures are definitely called for. The patient can then be given a 5 ml/kg venesection. The blood should be kept sterile in the syringe, and the patient's condition carefully watched. If he deteriorates, then the blood should be slowly returned; if there is marked improvement over the next 10 min then the diagnosis was correct. No more than 10 ml/kg should ever be taken. Although, in the right circumstances this is a highly effective treatment, it should be used only by those with considerable experience. In practice, unless the parent fully understands and trusts the staff, such treatment opens the staff to being accused of causing the death by bleeding the child.

Experience with using agents that are used in other forms of heart failure have not been reported in heart failure associated with malnutrition. When heart failure is due to severe anemia then the treatment is by exchange transfusion, which is effectively transfusion and venesection combined. The amount of anemic blood withdrawn should exceed the amount of normal blood given.

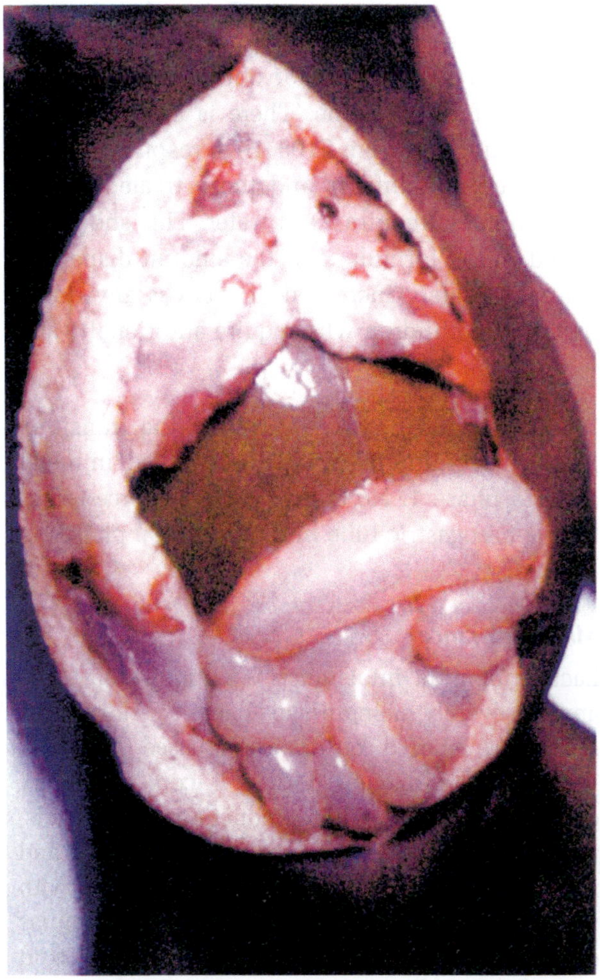

Figure 31.10 An autopsy of a child with marasmic-kwashiorkor. Note the fatty liver, the presence of some subcutaneous fat, the greatly distended loops of bowel and the thinned transparent nature of the bowel wall.

Transition phase

By the end of the acute phase the patients should have all their complications treated, edema should be resolving and treatment for infections started. A return of appetite is the sign that the patient is ready to progress to the transition phase. The appetite is used as a barometer of progress. Loss of appetite occurs when the patient's metabolic processes cannot cope with the dietary intake. Great care must be taken not to overload the patient whilst he has a poor appetite – this is a warning that something is wrong metabolically. The diet is changed to a high-energy diet called F100, but it is given in restricted amounts (Table 31.8). The volume given is the same as the diet given during the acute phase (F75), but as it is more concentrated the intake is increased by 25%. One would anticipate a weight gain on this diet of about 6 g/kg per day. No other changes are made to the regimen.

Because these patients may not be able to express thirst, their requirement for water may not be met from the formula alone. There is a considerable renal solute load from F100. High respiratory rates and fever, and infants and those treated in dry environments require extra water. This should be added to the formula, and the amount dispensed commensurately increased, if there is any doubt that all the children who require additional water will receive it.

If any complications arise during the transition phase the children should be returned immediately to phase 1. No child should be force-fed or have a nasogastric tube in the transition phase.

Table 31.8 A formula for use in malnourished children (F100)

Ingredients	Amount
Dried skim milk	80 g
Sugar	50 g
Oil	60 g
Mineral mix	to give the concentrations in Table 31.7
Vitamin mix	to give the concentrations in Table 31.7
Water	to 1000 ml

Milk intolerance

Lactose or milk intolerance is seldom seen, even among severely malnourished patients. All patients should be started on the milk-based formulas. Intolerance is diagnosed only if copious watery diarrhea occurs with the introduction of milk feeds, it clearly improves when milk intake is reduced and it recurs again when the patient is challenged with milk a second time. In such cases, milk formulas can be partially or totally substituted by other liquid foods. Milk feeds should be reintroduced and their effects noted before a patient is discharged with a 'diagnosis' of milk intolerance.

Very occasionally other strategies are needed. The simplest is to ferment the milk to yoghurt. This is highly effective. Lactose- and milk-free formulas can be used but they are rarely available where severe malnutrition is common. Sometimes the addition of pancreatic enzymes (such as Pancrex V®) to the diet is beneficial, particularly in cases of severe kwashiorkor.

Rehabilitation phase

Together the acute and transition phases of treatment usually take about 7 days, but this is quite variable. The features that determine whether the patient has entered the rehabilitation phase are the complete loss of edema and a good appetite. In older patients with primary intestinal disease who require intravenous or nasogastric drip feeding, feelings of hunger and 'well-being' denote this phase of management.

There is a great deal of flexibility in the way in which the rehabilitation phase of treatment is managed. There are now safe ready-to-use therapeutic formulas that can be used to continue the treatment at home. When well organized, with a home visitor and a good home environment, this approach is preferable.

The return of appetite means that infections are under control and there is no major electrolyte imbalance or deficiency, even though the patient's physiological responses are still abnormal and his capacity may be limited. At this stage the patient has resynthesized the cellular components needed to absorb and metabolize more food than is necessary for mere maintenance; he is ready to make new tissue. The single most important thing that determines the rate of recovery is the amount of the diet taken by the patient. The overriding principle of this phase is to feed the patient to appetite and to actively encourage him to eat.

Moving from the transition and the rehabilitation phases is achieved simply by increasing the amount of the same diet that is given until the patient starts to refuse to finish the feed. Sufficient time must be spent with the patient to enable him to try to finish each feed; the attitude of the caretaker is crucial to success. The patient should never be left alone to 'take what he wants' by himself – this is not what is meant by feeding to appetite.

As the patient gains weight, his appetite and requirement steadily increase. Each day the weight, the record of intake and the amount refused are plotted on a specially designed treatment chart. During rehabilitation most children and even adults take between 150 and 200 kcal/kg per day.

The formula should not be discontinued if visible fat appears in the stools, as a high proportion of fat is still absorbed. Fat malabsorption is, however, a frequent cause of the patient's failing to gain weight at the expected rate. Fat content should be decreased only if it clearly produces watery diarrhea.

It is appropriate to maintain the patients on the formula until they have achieved about 85% weight-for-height (children) or a BMI of 18 kg/m^2 (adults). At this time they usually signal their individual needs by reducing their appetites somewhat. They are then ready for discharge.

With adults the general principles of giving sufficiently high intakes of energy, protein and all minerals and vitamins to enable them to gain weight rapidly must still be followed, despite the fact that a mixed diet is given. Many normal diets have a low energy density (in the tropics), and have insufficient protein, minerals and vitamins to sustain the rapid rates of growth. Further, the mixed diets often contain phytic acid and other anti-nutrients that markedly reduce the absorption of phosphorus, zinc, iron and calcium. To counter these effects, F100 should be given between meals of the mixed diet. For example, if a mixed diet is given three times daily the formula feed should also be given three times daily to make six 'meals' each day.

Severely malnourished patients have a reduced iron-binding capacity; they are neither able to withhold iron from invading organisms nor to prevent the toxic effects of free iron itself. During the acute and intermediate phases of treatment iron should not be given, even in the presence of severe anemia. In the rehabilitation phase an iron supplement should be given.

Assessing progress

The patients should be weighed daily and their weight plotted on the special chart. It is useful to mark the target weight (BMI for adults) on the graph. They should gain weight at 5–20 g/kg per day, usually about 10–15 g/kg per day.

Emotional and psychological stimulation

At home patients, particularly children, are surrounded by familiar places and people. It is a major psychological trauma for a child to be separated from its mother, family and surroundings and to be closed into a cot with bars. The child needs to be with its mother and there should be adult beds for even very young patients so that the mother can sleep with the child. When the child is acutely ill the mother will sit by the bed. As he recovers he should be actively encouraged to interact with the other children. This is often discouraged by hospital staff on the grounds that it increases cross-infection and makes their job more difficult. This attitude, usually from senior staff, retards recovery and is much more damaging than the risk of cross-infection.

The malnourished child needs affection and tender care from the very start of treatment, and interaction with other children when he becomes active. This requires patience and understanding by the hospital staff and the caretaker. When the children are over the acute and intermediate phases, they can be up and about for prolonged periods on large play mats. The risk of cross-infection is not increased substantially and the benefit for the children is much more important than the convenience of the staff.

In hospital, it is not infrequent for ten different adults to interact with a patient over the course of a day, each one manipulating but rarely talking to or 'cuddling' the patient. This is not good. It is particularly bad if the mother is not with the child. Each adult should talk, smile and laugh with the patient affectionately.

Provision of child-oriented care, with affection and tenderness, is, of itself, insufficient. Severely malnourished children have delayed mental and behavioral development that requires treatment just as much as their delayed physical development. If such delays persist untreated they become the most serious long-term result of malnutrition. Psychological stimulation through play programs that start in hospital and continue after discharge can substantially reduce the mental retardation.

The austerity of the traditional hospital should not be used for children in phase 2. Traditional buildings such as the child lives in at home are much more appropriate. They can often be erected in the grounds of a hospital or health center.

There should be a large, safe, fenced area, with mats on the floor, where the children can play. Either mosquito nets or brightly colored mobiles should be over every bed. Hospital rooms should be brightly colored, with cheerful decorations that the children can relate to. Where possible the staff should not wear uniforms, or at least, have uniforms similar in design to standard maternal dress. Care is to be taken to avoid sensory deprivation; the child's face should not be covered, they must be able to see and hear what is going on around them; they should not be wrapped or tied to prevent them moving around in the bed or on the floor.

Toys must always be available. The mothers should be taught the importance of play and shown how to make the play materials. The toys should be safe, washable and appropriate for the child's level of development.

In hospital, one person should be in charge of organizing and running a play program. The play therapist should introduce new activities and play materials regularly; the activities should develop motor and language skills. It is useful to have a curriculum of activities and to play with each child in a structured way for 15–30 min each day. This is in addition to the informal mixing of the children. The mothers should be taught the elements of the curriculum, at the appropriate level. It must be emphasized that the family should continue to make toys and play with their children after discharge, and indeed, throughout the whole period of development of their child. For this reason, teaching the mother is even more important than teaching the child. The mother should be intimately involved in the play therapy.

Not only does increased physical activity encourage the development of the motor skills needed to explore the environment and play effectively but it may also enhance growth during nutritional rehabilitation. In immobile children, passive limb movements and allowing them to splash in a warm bath are helpful.

Preparation for discharge

There is not a sharp dividing line between the end of the rehabilitation phase and the preparation for discharge. The latter should be started during rehabilitation and completed after discharge.

By the time of actual discharge the child needs to be ready for full integration into the family and community. As this is the environment that led to malnutrition in the first place, the family has to be equipped to cope with the patient to prevent recurrence.

A child is usually considered ready for discharge when he reaches 85% of weight-for-height. Although these children are often referred to as 'recovered', this is not usually true. Many have the underlying effects of chronic malnutrition with stunting in height and delayed mental development; these defects also require attention. However, management of these conditions depends upon long-term changes aimed at improving the resources, diet, hygiene, knowledge and skills of the family as a whole, and not upon care directed at the child alone.

Attaining normal weight-for-height, of itself, is insufficient to discharge a child from the program. One of the problems with traditional hospital management is that anthropometric criteria alone are used for discharge, and follow-up is inadequate.

Whenever possible, a home visit should be made. The child should be enrolled in a supplementary feeding program and followed there *with regular* weighing for 4–6 months after 'recovery'. If there is no supplementary feeding program then community health workers or the local health clinic should follow these patients particularly. Where the patient is abandoned or the social and economic conditions at the home are hopeless, often because of absence of a caretaker, appeals should be made for foster homes or other forms of community support.

The patient and caretaker have much to achieve and learn while they are in contact with the health staff. Education cannot be left to the last few days before the patient is discharged. Parents or caretakers should be taught about the causes of the patient's malnutrition and how to prevent it in the future, whether the malnourished person is a child or infirm and elderly. For children, the parents need to know the consequences of malnutrition on future development and the steps that need to be taken, over a considerable time, to reverse any mental impairment and stunting in height. Practical instructions should be given on how to feed the child and continue nutritional rehabilitation at home. As these families are the most vulnerable within a community, the opportunity can usefully be taken to give instruction on child feeding and rearing practices, family planning, personal hygiene, methods of income generation, sexually transmitted diseases and many other topics.

Before discharge, children must be vaccinated in accordance with the local health regimen and provision made for booster doses to be given at the appropriate time.

General considerations

A child with severe malnutrition may indicate a serious problem in his household; the other children are also at risk. Therefore, nutritional and health education is not restricted to avoiding a recurrence of the index case, but should include the prevention or correction of nutritional problems of all the family members, especially young children, pregnant and lactating women and the elderly.

The presence of children with severe malnutrition also suggests a high prevalence of malnutrition in that community. Perhaps a survey should be conducted. Most relief agencies determine where the malnourished live in order to plan their surveys and programs. Health promotion can include education and promotional programs for community leaders, local action groups and the community as a whole. Such programs focus on the psychological needs of vulnerable groups, promotion of breast feeding, appropriate use of weaning foods, nutritional alternatives using traditional foods, the absolute importance of dietary variety in order to get all the essential nutrients, personal and environmental hygiene, water management, adequate feeding practices during illness and convalescence, immunizations, early treatment of diarrhea, pneumonia and other diseases, income-generating strategies and adult literacy classes.

Additional problems with management of malnourished patients

Staff attitudes

Sometimes a patient fails to respond because staff have a 'feeling' that their efforts for a particular patient are unlikely to succeed. This is particularly acute if they think that the child has HIV. In some places all failures are put down to HIV without any justification. Where such attitudes exist, the progress for the patient is poor; this in turn falsely confirms the 'correctness' of the original attitude and efforts are not made for future similar patients. This cause of failure-to-respond is among the most difficult to address, because it is usually based on the 'experience' of a long-serving senior staff. The dependence of each patient's well-being and survival on the attitudes of staff should be earnestly reviewed with them.

Infections

Atypical clinical manifestations of common infections occur in malnourished children. Infections with organisms that are not pathogenic in the well nourished are also common. The infections that are most commonly overlooked and interfere with a good nutritional response include: urinary tract infection, otitis media, tuberculosis, congenital syphilis, cytomegalovirus infection, hepatitis, AIDS, dengue, giardiasis, cryptosporidiosis and small-bowel bacterial overgrowth with secondary malabsorption.

HIV is often thought to be a major factor in centers that have poor results. This is a false assumption. In one center in Burundi, patients with HIV had a 6% mortality whilst those without had a 5% mortality (difference not significant; Y. Grellety, personal communication). The length of phase 1 and total stay was only 1 day longer in the HIV-positive patients. A high prevalence of HIV is not a reason for failure; these children and adults should not be abandoned. Treating the malnutrition is one very positive thing that can be done for these patients. In retrospect, this result should not surprise, because the state of the immune system and infection is very similar in HIV disease and severe malnutrition.

Specific nutrient deficiencies

Many specific nutrient deficiencies impair the immune response. They can be the underlying cause of an infection that does not respond as expected to antibiotics. Occasionally patients may have a profound deficiency of one or more specific nutrients that are not adequately replaced by the therapeutic diet or nutrient supplements. Many commercial multivitamin-and-mineral preparations lack particular nutrients or do not contain sufficient amounts to treat a deficiency. They are generally designed for use as supplements by healthy individuals. Use of such preparations leads to overlooking a deficiency assumed to be 'covered' by the treatment. The most frequently overlooked specific deficiencies include those of zinc, magnesium, copper, selenium, folic acid and vitamin E, although other micronutrients may be involved. Insufficient amounts of potassium, magnesium and phosphorus in the diet are common errors.

Associated pathological conditions

Malnutrition accompanies many congenital abnormalities, inborn errors of metabolism, tumors, immunological diseases and diseases of the major organs. All these conditions occur in areas where primary malnutrition is frequent, just as in rich countries, although they are less frequently recognized. Where primary malnutrition is prevalent children with secondary malnutrition are usually misdiagnosed as having primary malnutrition. As the prevalence of primary malnutrition falls the proportion of malnourished children who have an associated pathology rises. Failure to respond to treatment should lead to investigation of the major organ systems for primary pathology.

Specific dermatosis of kwashiorkor

Spontaneous resolution can be expected with improved nutrition. Atrophy of the skin in the perineum leads to severe napkin dermatitis, especially in children or the elderly with diarrhea or incontinence. The perineum should be left exposed to dry without napkins. A barrier such as zinc and castor oil ointment, petroleum jelly or paraffin gauze dressing (tulle gras) to raw areas helps to relieve pain and prevent infection. The management should be the same as that used for burns. The zinc supplement contained in the diet may be insufficient in these patients, as zinc deficiency almost always accompanies severe skin lesions. These patients should always be given systemic antibiotics.

Candidiasis

Most malnourished children have candidiasis. In the mouth it can be seen as whitish plaques. However, even when the mouth is free of lesions, it may occur in the esophagus, stomach and rectum as well as on any damp moist skin. In severe malnutrition systemic candidiasis with growth in the respiratory tract and blood also occurs. Oral nystatin suspension should be given to all patients with candidiasis. In addition, nystatin cream should be applied to any cutaneous lesions. Systemic candidiasis should be treated with drugs such as ketoconazole.

Drug metabolism in malnourished patients

Clearly the physiological and body compositional changes in the malnourished patient will alter the pharmocokinetics of many drugs. There has been very little research on this aspect of either primary malnutrition or even the malnutrition associated with neoplasia or intestinal disease. A patient with 7% of body weight as fat will have a very different response to a fat-soluble drug from one with 40% of body weight as fat, and yet this is rarely taken into consideration in prescribing. Poor absorption from the intestine, disordered hepatic conversion of drugs, reduced renal clearance, increased bacterial deconjugation of drugs excreted in the bile, and alterations in receptors and enzyme targets for drugs each affect their efficacy and potential toxicity. The changes are sufficiently complex for the result of giving a new drug to be unpredictable. Nevertheless, these factors should be considered in the treatment of all malnourished patients and, where available, therapeutic drug monitoring should be used. Clearly the variables are potentially extremely important. For example, if a patient with malnutrition, secondary to neoplasm, has features of kwashiorkor, is depleted in antioxidant nutrients and has a low cellular glutathione level, then giving cytotoxic drugs or radiotherapy may damage the patient irretrievably.

Unnecessary drugs should never be given during the acute stage. Unwanted toxic effects are more likely for most drugs. The list of drugs that do not need to be used is long. In particular, fever should be treated with tepid sponging, not with paracetamol. Vomiting should not be treated with the usual antiemetics (promethazine, etc.) and diarrhea should never be treated with an antispasmodic.

Many of the drugs used to treat tuberculosis are hepatotoxic. It is wise to use these drugs carefully during the first few days after admission.

Conclusions

The problems raised by malnutrition affect not only the individual but society as a whole, at medical, social, ethical, moral and political levels. Malnutrition in its numerous guises, especially amongst children and the elderly, is the most common serious illness in the world today. Lessons learnt from the study and management of these children have relevance for malnourished individuals of all ages and with a wide variety of disorders. A clear understanding of the etiology and pathogenesis is a prerequisite for designing effective intervention and prevention programs. The legacy of childhood malnutrition is to be seen in adults who are stunted physically and mentally; it may lay the seeds for many of the chronic diseases of unknown etiology in adult life.

REFERENCES

1. Pelletier DL. The relationship between child anthropometry and mortality in developing countries: implications for policy, programs and future research. *J Nutr* 1994; **124** (10 Suppl): 2047S–2081S.
2. Prudhon C, Briend A, Laurier D et al. Comparison of weight- and height-based indices for assessing risk of death in severely malnourished children. *Am J Epidemiol* 1996; **144**: 116–123.
3. Williams CD. A nutritional disease of childhood associated with a maize diet. *Arch Dis Child* 1933; **8**: 423–428.

32 Biotherapeutic and nutraceutical agents

Kirsi Laiho and Erika Isolauri

The science of nutrition: from basic needs to specific health effects

The role of the diet in health has changed as scientific knowledge has increased (Figure 32.1). The basic foundation lies in a healthy, balanced diet that follows the dietary recommendations and guidelines appropriate for age and life-stage with the aim of meeting the metabolic requirements and the needs for growth and development in children. The first goal of nutritional management is directed towards the prevention of direct diet-related deficiencies, such as scurvy caused by low vitamin C intake. The second target is the prevention of nutrition-related chronic diseases. For example, an unbalanced diet containing excessive amounts of saturated fatty acids has been shown to be associated with an increased risk of coronary heart disease. Furthermore, specific requirements for nutritional management are set by a variety of diseases necessitating carefully planned diets or usage of clinical dietary products. The current research interest is directed towards the invention of novel dietary compounds with specific effects in health promotion and management of diseases beyond the nutritional impact of food.

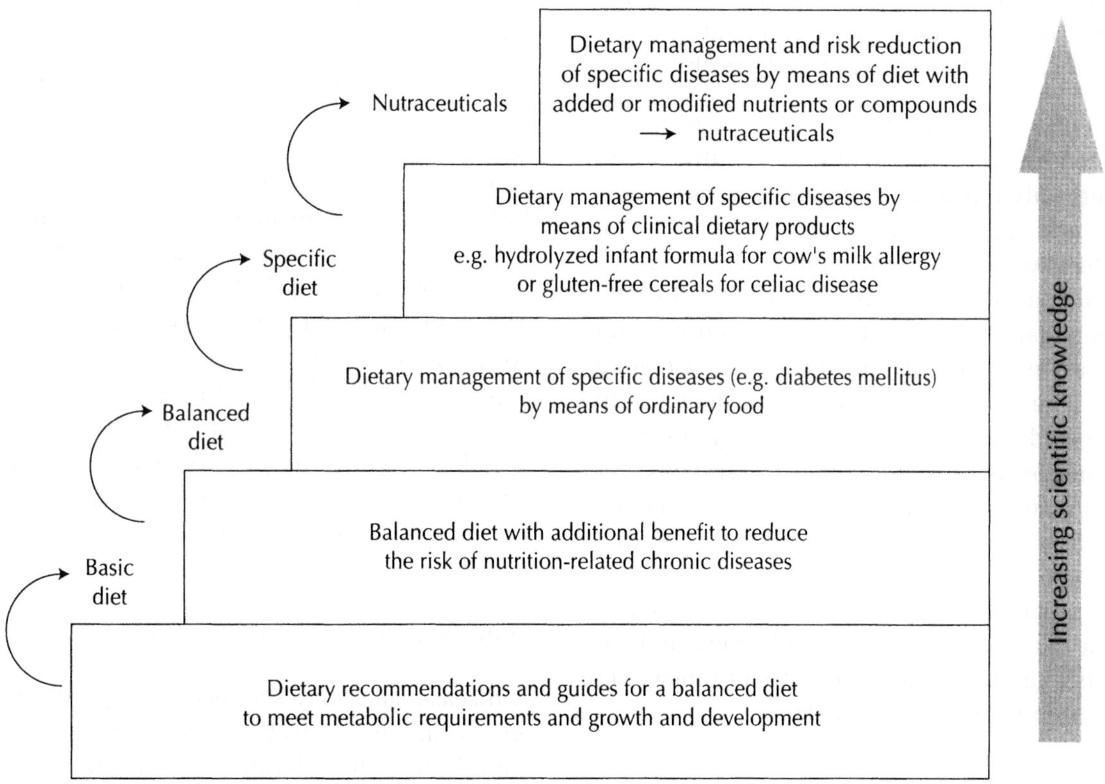

Figure 32.1 The steps of nutrition management.

Dietary recommendations and guidelines appropriate for age and life-stage

Dietary recommendations and guidelines are set to direct dietary food and nutrient intake for maintenance of health. Specifically, dietary recommendations aim at prevention of nutrient deficiencies but also at reducing the risk of developing nutrition-related chronic diseases.

The dietary recommendations vary amongst regions so that many countries have formed their own recommendations. However, major international health-related organizations such as the Food and Agriculture Organization (FAO) and World Health Organization (WHO) have searched for more uniform recommendations.[1–3] The reader is advised to refer to these or national original reports for detailed description of the recommendations. Dietary guidelines for populations have been given both as recommended daily intakes (recommended daily allowances, recommended nutrient intakes, dietary reference values/intakes) of certain nutrients and as food guides (e.g. food pyramid) that direct the consumption of foods and food groups. Food guides may also include recommendations on eating behavior and food habits.

The recommended nutrient intake is generally understood as the level of nutrients sufficient to meet the daily nutrient requirements of most individuals of a specific age and gender, based on an estimated average nutrient requirement plus two standard deviations above the mean. Specific recommendations are given for children and adults as well as for pregnant and lactating women. The recommendations can be deployed to provide guidance on appropriate dietary composition, for the assessment of dietary surveys, for outlining food policies or for food labeling purposes. The food guides, such as the well-known food pyramid, are more comprehensible and particularly helpful in nutrition counseling. The guides direct the use of foods or food products and aim to meet the nutrient intakes set by the recommended daily intake.

Early nutrition and later consequences

It is understood that dietary intake that satisfies nutritional demands and maintains a good nutritional status is important for the growth and development of children. However, the nutrition of the infant begins before birth, *in utero*, when the nutrition of the mother and also placental function regulate the growth and development of the fetus. The nutrition of the mother even before pregnancy may be important for the well-being of the fetus and child, as the nutrient stores that are being utilized during pregnancy and breast feeding are accumulated at an early stage.[4] As a good example, a sufficient availability of folic acid and the prophylactic supplementation of folic acid to the mother reduce the incidence of birth complications and neural tube defects.[5] Indication of an unbalanced nutrient intake (maternal hypercholesterolemia during pregnancy) induces changes in the fetus that determine the susceptibility of children to fatty-streak formation and subsequent atherosclerosis.[6]

Both epidemiological[7–9] and experimental[10,11] studies suggest that several chronic diseases of later life, including coronary heart disease, hypertension and type 2 diabetes, are programmed during the fetal period. This theory on the fetal origins of adult disease suggests that alterations in fetal nutrition and endocrine status result in developmental adaptations that predispose individuals to cardiovascular, metabolic and endocrine disease in adult life. One of the first reports showed that those individuals who had had low birth weights had relatively high death rates from coronary heart disease in adult life.[9] The results have since been replicated in other populations and with other chronic lifestyle-related diseases. Also, the mechanisms have been searched for in experimental studies and the specific causal relations are actively being explored. The research is also directed towards identifying critical phases in which the impact of nutrition is most important for the risk of chronic diseases.

Specific dietary requirements of disease

A disease state may set specific requirements for energy and nutrients, the deficiency of which may contribute to the deterioration of nutritional status and growth failure in children (Figure 32.2). The reduced energy availability may originate from three main sources: reduced food intake due to poor appetite or symptoms of disease such as gastrointestinal complaints or poor utilization of nutrients; increased losses, e.g. due to steatorrhea; or increased requirements, e.g. due to infections. On the other hand, physical activity may be reduced, owing to ill health, and compensates for increased energy requirements. Although cause–consequence relationships are difficult to prove, such events may result in exacerbation of the disease or in reduced survival. A careful monitoring of diet and nutritional status and intervention at an early stage are vital for the prevention, or halting the development, of this vicious cycle with possibly deleterious effects.

Nutritional intervention includes provision of sufficient amounts of energy and nutrients, by increasing the amount of food eaten or the nutrient density of the diet, or by using clinical nutritional products to enhance the nutrient density, or by providing an additional source of energy, for example as snacks. In a range of diseases with known nutritional management, the specific products, such as hydrolyzed infant formulas for cow's milk allergy,[12] low-protein and special amino acid products for phenylketonuria[13] or gluten-free products for celiac disease[14] are critical in the management of these patients. The next step might be the dietary management and risk reduction of specific diseases by means of diet with added or modified nutrients or compounds, i.e. nutraceuticals.

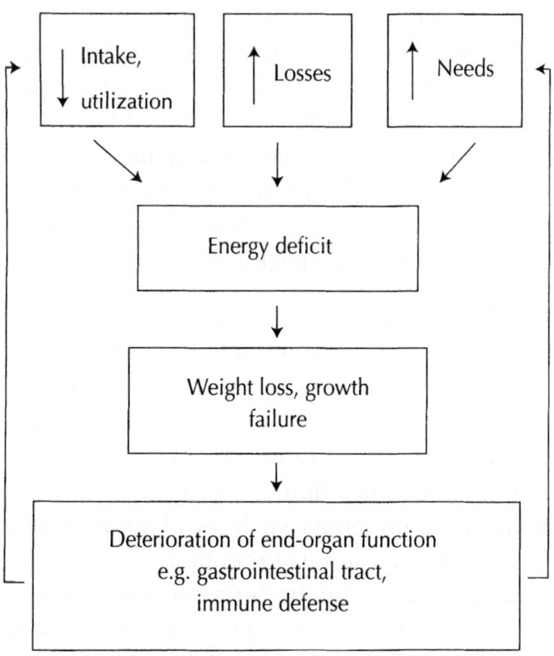

Figure 32.2 Possible causes for deterioration of nutritional status and growth failure in children.

Food consumption and risk of chronic diseases

The diet in Western societies has faced changes that reflect industrialization, urbanization, economic development and market globalization[15]. The availability of a more diverse selection of foods has improved the nutritional status of populations. However, not all the changes in food consumption have led to beneficial effects with regard to health status. The impacts of changes in the diet are further enforced by alterations in lifestyle such as decreased physical activity and increased tobacco use. In a recent report by expert panels in WHO and FAO, the global and regional food consumption patterns and estimated trends from 1960 to 2030 and their impact upon the prevalence of chronic, non-communicable, diseases were discussed.[15] According to the report, it may be possible to reduce the risk of cardiovascular diseases, cancer, diabetes and obesity by changing dietary habits. Particularly important targets contributing to deaths from chronic diseases are obesity, high blood pressure, high cholesterol concentrations and low levels of physical activity. According to the WHO/FAO expert panel, the key changes in food consumption in recent decades and also in the next 15–30 years, are increased energy intake and increased consumption of fat and added sugar, greater saturated fat intake and reduced intakes of complex carbohydrates and fiber.[15] Intakes of fruits and vegetables have increased in some areas, whilst the recommended high average intakes have been reached only in a minority of the world's population.[15]

In light of the link between early nutrition with later consequences, the importance of pediatric nutrition is further emphasized. Furthermore, dietary habits are established at an early age, by the number and type of experiences with various foods and also by model learning from parents, friends, day-care centers and schools.[16]

A population study comparing data on serum cholesterol, anthropometric indices and dietary intakes in children aged 1–18 years of age from Japan, Spain and the USA showed the effects of

Westernization on blood cholesterol concentration.[17] Both in Japan and in Spain the intake of total and saturated fat had increased substantially. In studies from Northern Europe, changes in food consumption and consequently in nutrient intakes towards the recommended intakes seemed to explain the serum cholesterol concentration which was reflected in a decline in coronary heart disease mortality.[18] It has also been shown that the unfavorable dietary habits, reflected in high intake of fat and saturated fatty acids contributing to the risk of coronary heart disease, may be adopted already in childhood.[19]

Cardiovascular diseases are a good example of diseases in which associations between food consumption, nutrient intake, biological markers of disease (serum cholesterol concentration) and risk of disease have been documented. It has also been shown that dietary interventions modifying food intake in adults[18] or in children[20] to resemble that recommended for healthy eating, result in beneficial changes in anthropometry and serum cholesterol concentration that are reflected in reduced risk of chronic Western diseases. Although fat intake in accordance with the recommended intake has been shown to be safe in terms of growth and neurological development,[21,22] concerns have been raised over low fat intake (< 22% or energy) during childhood and its effect on growth and development.[23]

Recently, novel dietary compounds have been identified that may promote the well-being of the host and reduce the risk of chronic disease. Concern over the impact of lifestyle changes upon the risk of diseases other than the traditional cardiovascular disease, obesity and diabetes, has also been raised and will be discussed in more detail in the chapter.

The model for infant feeding is the healthy, breast-fed infant

A healthy breast-fed infant is considered the model for optimal growth and development of infants. Apart from essential nutrients, human milk provides several types of bioactive compounds that support infant growth and contribute to the development of the host defense mechanisms, particularly in the gastrointestinal tract, where the major load of new antigens is encountered. Breast milk-derived immunomodulative and protective properties have been linked to several components: immunoglobulins, of which 90% are secretory IgA; cell-surface homologs (glycoconjugates and oligosaccharides); nutrients such as antioxidants and fatty acids, glutamine and dietary nucleotides; lactoferrin; and other bioactive agents such as hormones, growth factors and cytokines. Breast milk-derived secretory IgA contributes to immune exclusion of antigens in neonates, whose endogenous intestinal IgA production is immature.[24] Breast feeding not only confers passive protection but also actively stimulates the development of the infant's own immune system.

Several prospective clinical studies have suggested that breast milk may provide the infant with protection, possibly extending beyond childhood. A long duration of breast feeding, particularly the length of exclusive breast feeding, may reduce the risk of certain diseases including atopic dermatitis,[25] asthma[26] and obesity.[27,28] In contrast, short-term breast feeding (less than 3 months) or formula feeding has been associated with the risk of some chronic diseases including type 1 diabetes, celiac disease and inflammatory bowel disease.[29]

Breast milk composition is known to vary among lactating women.[30] One reason for the variability arises from differences in maternal dietary composition and nutrient stores accumulated before and during pregnancy. However, it may be possible to enforce the properties of breast milk, particularly the immune-protective properties, by modifying the maternal diet in a specific manner.[31,32]

When breast milk is not available in sufficient amounts for the infant, infant formulas that endeavor to mimic the breast milk composition provide undeniably the best replacement. Product development of infant formulas aims to imitate the breast milk composition by supplementation of innovative components such as oligosaccharides with prebiotic properties to promote the growth of lactobacilli and bifidobacteria in the intestinal microbiota. These evince powerful antipathogenic capabilities and are mainly responsible for colonization resistance in the intestine. Indeed, many breast-milk components including long-chain polyunsaturated fatty acids, oligosaccharides and nucleotides have since been used in immunonutrition beyond formula-age. Even the pre-milk provided by the cow after delivery – bovine colostrum – has been suggested to be used in humans for modulation of the immune system, as reviewed by Solomons.[33]

At weaning, the infant gradually transfers to adult-type feeding. The transition period may be significant in terms of adopting dietary habits. Intakes of some nutrients, particularly vitamin E and zinc, may be low during dietary transition in early childhood and may actually decrease, despite increases in energy intake.[34]

The integrity of the gut barrier function – the target of protective nutrients

The primary role of the gastrointestinal tract is digestion and absorption of nutrients to meet the metabolic requirements and the demands of normal growth and development. In addition to this, the intestinal mucosa provides a protective host defense against the constant presence in the gut lumen of antigens from food and micro-organisms. An abrupt change in gut barrier function occurs at birth, when it is switched from processing amniotic fluid to digesting milk and when the intestinal colonization commences.

Gut barrier

Protection against potentially harmful agents is ensured by a number of factors, including saliva, gastric acid, peristalsis, mucus, intestinal proteolysis, intestinal microbiota and epithelial cell membranes with intercellular junctional complexes.[35] The surface of mucosal membranes is protected by a local adaptive immune system. The gut-associated lymphoid tissue represents the largest mass of lymphoid tissue in the human body. Consequently, it comprises an important element of the total immunological capacity of the host. The regulatory events of the intestinal immune response take place in different compartments: aggregated in follicles and Peyer's patches, distributed within the mucosa and in the intestinal epithelium, as well as in secretory sites (reviewed in reference 24). IgA antibody production is abundant at mucosal surfaces. In contrast to IgA in serum, secretory IgA is present in dimeric or polymeric form. Secretory IgA is resistant to intraluminal proteolysis and does not activate inflammatory responses, which makes secretory IgA ideal for protecting mucosal surfaces. These elements in the gut are part of the common mucosal immune system, including the respiratory tract and lacrimal, salivary and mammary glands, and thereby an immune response initiated in the gut-associated lymphoid tissue can affect immune responses at other mucosal surfaces.

There are specialized antigen transport mechanisms in the villous epithelium and particularly in Peyer's patches, which are crucial in determining the subsequent immune responses to the antigen.[35] In addition to the first line of gut defense – immune exclusion – there are specialized antigen transport mechanisms in the villous epithelium. Antigens are absorbed across the epithelial layer by transcytosis, and here the main degradative pathway entails lysosomal processing of the antigen.[36,37] A minor pathway allows the transport of unprocessed antigens. Peyer's patches are covered by a unique epithelium. Antigen transport across this epithelium is characterized by rapid uptake and reduced degradation. In health, paracellular transfer of macromolecules is controlled by intact intercellular tight junctions, which prevent aberrant antigen absorption. The second line of host defense – immune elimination – is directed towards antigenic compounds penetrating the mucosa. Antigens are presented to subjacent T cells; these differentiate into various effector cells that mediate active immune regulation and promote the differentiation of IgA-secreting B cells.[38]

Initial signals for the maturation of the gut barrier functions are considered to stem from components of the innate immunity, which generates the necessary initial step for the targeted and specific function of the adaptive immune system.

Gut microbiota

The human gastrointestinal tract harbors a complex collection of micro-organisms, a specific microbiota for each person.[39] The generation of the immunophysical regulation in the gut depends on the establishment of the indigenous microbiota.

At birth the gastrointestinal tract of the newborn is sterile. The maternal intestinal microbiota is the first source of colonizing bacteria. Subsequently, the feeding practice and the home environment of the child influence the composition. Breast feeding encourages the growth of bifidobacteria, while formula-fed infants have a more complex microbiota with bifidobacteria, enterobacteria, lactobacilli, bacteroides, clostridia and streptococci.[40] New molecular methods indicate that bifidobacteria can reach up to 90% of the total fecal microbiota in breast-fed infants. After weaning, the composition of the microbiota resembles that of the adult. Although bacteria are distributed throughout the intestine, the major concentration of microbes and metabolic activity can be found in the large intestine. From culture-based data, it is thought that at least 500 different microbial species exist, although on a quantitative basis 10–20 genera probably predominate: *Bacteroides*, *Lactobacillus*, *Clostridium*, *Fusobacterium*, *Bifidobacterium*, *Eubacterium*, *Peptococcus*, *Peptostreptococcus*, *Escherichia* and *Veillonella*.[39]

The composition of the microbiota is associated with several disease states within the intestine and also beyond the gastrointestinal tract. Inflammation is accompanied by imbalance in the intestinal microbiota in such a way that the host–microbe interaction is disturbed and an immune response may be induced by resident bacteria.[41,42]

Modification of intestinal microbiota to increase the predominance of specific non-pathogenic bacteria and thereby to alter the intestinal milieu has been taken as an alternative to attain prophylactic or therapeutic effects in intestinal infectious conditions in childhood. Recent clinical and nutritional studies and characterization of the immunomodulatory potential of specific strains of the gut microbiota, beyond the effect on the composition of the microbiota, may lead to future applications also for allergic and inflammatory diseases. Such probiotics, acting as nutraceutical agents, need their mechanisms to be thoroughly clarified, either to control specific physiological processes in the evolution of disease in populations at-risk or to manage of specific diseases.

Protective nutrients for the gastrointestinal tract

The integrity of the intestinal mucosa and the structure of the villi are crucial for assimilation of nutrients from the gastrointestinal tract and for intestinal defense against invading pathogens and antigens. This is obvious in diseases such as celiac disease, where the structure of the intestinal villi is disturbed by dietary gluten thereby affecting nutrient assimilation and the nutritional status of the patients if an appropriate diet is not followed. However, despite an apparently normal histological presentation of the mucosa, the functionality of the enterocytes may be altered. It has been shown in malnourished patients that, despite a normal villous structure of the small intestine, the intestinal permeability may be increased.[43] Reduced integrity of the mucosa could even result in an outward diffusion of nutrients towards the lumen which would further prevent the absorption of nutrients.

Increased permeability of the intestinal mucosa may also result in increased susceptibility to infections. Infections may further cause deterioration of the intestinal integrity, owing to increased cell turnover, and therefore increase nutrient requirements. Turnover of cells in the gastrointestinal mucosa is rapid and its integrity mainly depends on the production of new cells at a rate equal to that at which cells are lost.[44] Therefore, even a short-term deficit in the nutrient supply to the mucosa may affect the mucosal integrity and result in villous atrophy. Nutrition through the gastrointestinal tract is important in maintaining the mucosal structure and function; lack of nutrients may result in decreased villous height, increased permeability and decreased immunity.

Probably the single most important nutrient to the mucosa is glutamine (both from luminal and vascular sides), which is consumed by replicating cells and affects the structure and function of the cells. Glutamine may be required in increased amounts by patients suffering from a catabolic insult such as injury or severe infection. In parenteral nutrition, glutamine improves nitrogen balance, supports gut function and alleviates catabolic demands upon muscle mass. However, whether glutamine is necessary for the preservation of normal intestinal morphology and function in humans during parenteral nutrition is not clear, as reviewed by Buchman.[45] In another systematic review, in enteral feeding of critically ill patients, the immune-enhancing nutrients including glutamine, arginine, neucleotides and n-3 fatty acids reduced the appearance of infectious complications, but not the overall mortality.[46]

Vitamin A is also important for the differentiation of cells and may have a central role in mucosal function. Deficiency impairs innate immunity by diminishing the function of neutrophils, macrophages and natural killer cells as well as antibody-mediated responses by T helper (Th) cells.[47] Vitamin A deficiency compromises mucosal epithelial barriers in the gastrointestinal tract, particularly when complicated by infection. Most data concerning the effects of nutrients on the structure and function of the epithelium are derived from experimental studies, but it has also been shown in children that recovering from diarrhea may be faster when vitamin A supplement is received compared to placebo.[48]

Probiotics and prebiotics

Recent demonstration that the gut microbiota is an important constituent of the intestine's mucosal barrier has introduced new therapeutic strategies for fighting enteric infections and possibly other intestinal inflammatory conditions (Figure 32.3). Three approaches for improving intestinal integrity include the use of probiotics, prebiotics and symbiotics. Probiotics are 'a live microbial food ingredient that is beneficial to health'. The prerequisites for probiotic action include survival in and adhesion to specific areas of the gastrointestinal tract and competitive exclusion of pathogens or harmful antigens. The application of probiotics has since been supplemented with the concept of prebiotics. A prebiotic is a 'nondigestible food ingredient that beneficially affects the host by selectively stimulating the growth and/or activity of one or a limited number of bacteria in the colon that have the potential to improve host health'. The most commonly used prebiotics are carbohydrate substrates with the ability to promote the components of the normal intestinal microbiota that may evince a health benefit to the host. However, prebiotics can also be nonabsorbable substrates which stimulate the growth

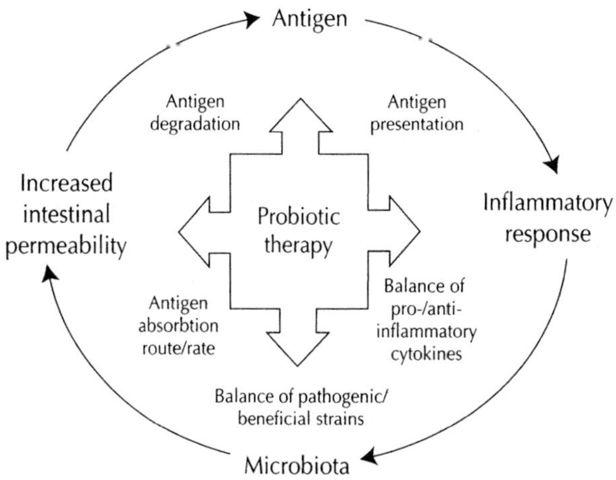

Figure 32.3 Potential targets for probiotic therapy (adapted from reference 42).

of probiotics. When the two are applied together, the concept is defined as symbiotic.

Recent research has expanded the definition of probiotics, by demonstrating that genetically engineered microbes and non-viable microbes may equally possess such potential.[42] However, normalization of the properties of unbalanced indigenous microbiota by specific strains forms the rationale of probiotic therapy. Oral introduction of probiotics has been shown to reinforce the various lines of gut defense: immune exclusion, immune elimination and immune regulation. Probiotics also stimulate non-specific host resistance to microbial pathogens and thereby aid in their eradication.

So far, the best-documented clinical application is the treatment of acute diarrhea by specific probiotic bacteria.[49] The beneficial clinical effect in infantile diarrhea by probiotic therapy has been explained by stabilization of the indigenous microbiota, reduction in the duration of rotavirus shedding and reduction in increased gut permeability caused by rotavirus infection, together with a significant increase in cells secreting IgA against rotavirus. The probiotic performance of strains is such that different probiotic strains, even strains belonging to the same species, have different immunomodulatory effects. Hence, current probiotic research is directed towards identification of specific strains with potential to reduce the risk of diseases associated with gut barrier dysfunction.

Modern nutrition for children – allergic disease

Allergic diseases, manifesting as atopic eczema, allergic rhinitis and asthma, are on the increase in industrialized countries, currently constituting the most common chronic diseases of childhood. Despite the pronounced hereditary element in allergic disease, genetic factors are unlikely to explain the increased emergence of the atopic-type immune responsiveness to environmental antigens. In contrast, changes in nutrition along with general environmental changes appear to shape the immune responder type of the host during a critical period of life. Specifically, the changes associated with Western lifestyle tend to favor the atopic Th 2-biased immune responder type.

The specific processes that initiate the vicious cycle of allergic inflammation, remain unresolved. Recent advances, however, call into question a causal cascade of exposure to antigenic proteins, sensitization and hypersensitivity; the exposure to allergens sensitizing the host immune system may not necessarily induce allergic disease. Indeed, sensitization to indoor allergens such as house dust mite, as assessed by specific IgE, but not the level of exposure to these allergens, has been associated with asthma, wheeze and increased bronchial responsiveness.[50] In like manner, exposure to cow's milk antigen during 3 days after birth, in 1533 breast-fed neonates, did not carry a risk of atopic disease during the first 5 years of age.[51,52] These data would imply that eradication of potential allergenic proteins from the early environment, including the diet, may not apply in allergy-prevention strategies.

In contrast, one justifiable strategy against allergic disease may be based on the administration of tolerogenic gut-processed peptide fragments of a specific protein, and the use of specific dietary compounds such as fatty acids and antioxidants, or on providing a microbial stimulus for the immature immune system by means of cultures of beneficial live micro-organisms characteristic of the healthy human gut microbiota.[53] However, before such strategies can be developed, a better understanding will be necessary of the processes initiating and regulating the allergic inflammatory response. Further, a better understanding of the interaction between nutrients is required. Consequently, the properties of specific dietary compounds and their combinations, in an optimal food matrix, might be exploited in the development of specific prophylactic and therapeutic interventions.

Elimination diets

Elimination of potentially allergenic foods, e.g. cow's milk, egg, wheat and fish, from the pregnant or breast-feeding mother's or the infant's diet has been a common approach in attempts to prevent allergic disease in high-risk infants. The approach of eliminating foods from the diet is perplexing, for two reasons. First, the benefits of elimination diets in prevention of allergic disease have been inconclusive.[54] Especially in long-term prevention of allergic disease, elimination diets have proved unsuccessful. Dietary antigens may actually be protective from allergic disease as they may induce tolerance to antigens rather than sensitization.[52,55] Second, besides allergenic proteins in the diet, other dietary factors might be associated with the development of allergic disease.

Recent studies on the immunomodulatory properties of fatty acids and the antioxidant properties of certain nutrients including ascorbic acid, α-tocopherol, β-carotene, selenium and zinc, have shown that food is not only a source of dietary antigens causing sensitization, but may also contain protective factors. Thus, elimination diets, i.e. eliminating specific offending antigens, should be reserved only to the management of proven food allergy. A better approach in the prevention of allergic disease might be to search for protective nutrients in the diet that may reinforce the immature immune defense of the infant.

Modification of allergenic proteins

The nutritional theories attracting current research interest relate to identification of active compounds which reinforce an anti-inflammatory, potentially tolerogenic type of immune response to assimilate allergenic challenges. Factors that influence the allergenicity of a protein include molecular complexity, solubility and stability, and its concentration. Heat treatment of cow's milk proteins can affect the conformational epitopes of allergens and facilitate their hydrolysis. To produce the least allergenic formulas for patients with documented cow's milk allergy, cow's milk proteins are modified by multiple enzymatic hydrolyses with progressive destruction of sequential epitopes. Such products are classified as partially hydrolyzed or extensively hydrolyzed formulas. However, enzymatic hydrolysis does not render the formula non-allergenic, as the optimal extent of hydrolysis is not known and traces of the original protein are detected in the hydrolysate.[56]

The approach may also be used in an attempt to reduce the risk of allergic disease.[57] Degradation of antigens is a necessary initial step in controlling inflammatory responsiveness to dietary antigens.[55,58,59] Such processing has been linked to the potential to generate peptides with suppressive effects on lymphocyte proliferation in healthy subjects; systemic immune responses to gut-processed antigens are preferentially directed towards suppression. The mechanisms of the preventive potential of specifically modified dietary proteins remain still poorly understood.

Dietary lipids

Increasing evidence has been provided to suggest that dietary lipids, especially long-chain polyunsaturated fatty acids (PUFA), and mediators synthesized from PUFA, regulate immune function and therefore contribute to the development and severity of the symptoms of allergic disease. Polyunsaturated n-6-series fatty acids derived from dietary linoleic acid (18:2, n-6) result in the production of eicosanoids, which are considered to have proinflammatory properties, whilst n-3-series fatty acids derived from dietary α-linolenic acid (18:3, n-3) appear to have less potent biological functions, even anti-inflammatory properties.[60] Owing to the typically higher dietary intake of linoleic acid than α-linolenic acid in developed countries, it is thought that the metabolism of linoleic acid predominates.

The most notable of the PUFA-derived mediators is arachidonic acid (20:4, n-6)-derived eicosanoid prostaglandin (PG)E_2. PGE_2 results in elevated IgE synthesis, owing to the induction of B-cell differentiation in the presence of interleukin IL-4.[61] Indeed, the most frequently reported abnormality in cell fatty acid composition of atopic patients has been an imbalance between series n-6 and n 3 fatty acids,[62–64] predisposing the patients to the adverse effects of PGE_2. Nevertheless, whether the observed alterations in the fatty acid composition of cells in the patients with atopic disease result from a primary defect that contributes to the onset of atopic disease or are a consequence of the atopic disease itself is currently poorly understood. This is especially intriguing as, despite their apparent proinflammatory role, n-6 fatty acids may also contribute to an anti-inflammatory intestinal environment, as antigen stimulation up-regulates PGE_2 production from arachidonic acid with ensuing suppression of antigen-specific T-cell proliferation in gut-associated lymphoid tissue.[65] However, the effects on dietary n-6 fatty acids may be counteracted by n-3 series fatty acids derived from dietary α-linolenic acid (18:3, n-3) or directly from marine food sources (eicosapentaenoic acid; 20:5, n-3 and docosahexaenoic acid; 22:6, n-3). Eicosanoids derived from α-linolenic acid appear to have a less potent biological, even anti-inflammatory, function compared to n-6-series fatty acids. The anti-inflammatory properties of n-3 fatty acids arise from their capacity to inhibit the release of arachidonic acid from membrane phospholipids, thereby reducing the production of arachidonic acid-derived eicosanoids whilst the synthesis of n-3 fatty acid-derived eicosanoids increases.[66] Owing to the likely interactions between the nutrients, the overall fatty acid composition and the quantity of fat within the diet with respect to other nutrients may be crucial in the search for the optimal diet for prevention and management of allergic disease.

Dietary antioxidants

In atopic disease, inflammatory processes result in endogenously generated oxidative stress which dietary antioxidants, such as ascorbic acid, β-carotene, α-tocopherol, selenium and zinc may counteract.[67] Both cellular enzyme-based antioxidants and diet-derived antioxidants counteract oxidative stress and dampen the inflammatory response.[67] Dietary antioxidants may thus be important in implementing the ability of the individual to restrain the inflammatory response and in avoiding injury to tissues. Low concentrations of β-carotene, ascorbate and α-tocopherol have been measured in plasma in wheezing illness, suggesting that antioxidant deficiencies may be associated with symptoms of allergic disease.[68] However, at present the role of antioxidants in the onset of allergic disease remains obscure. Moreover, data accumulated to date on the specific antioxidant agents and their dose and mechanisms are insufficient to provide any recommendation on their use, either in the prevention or in the management of allergic disease.

Probiotics in allergic diseases

Probiotics represent one example of immunomodulatory compounds for the allergic host. The immunomodulatory potential of the healthy gastrointestinal microbiota, the source of specific probiotic strains, is possibly associated with two structural components of bacteria, the lipopolysaccharide portion of Gram-negative bacteria (endotoxin) and a specified CpG motif in bacterial DNA.[69,70] These structures activate immunomodulatory genes via Toll-like receptors present, for example on macrophages, and dendritic and intestinal epithelial cells. The net effect on intestinal epithelial cells is immunosuppressive by way of inhibition of the transcription factor NF-κB pathway.[71] In addition, specific strains of the gut microbiota have been shown to contribute to a Th cell population promoting oral tolerance induction, and to counter allergy by generation of anti-inflammatory IL-10 and transforming growth factor (TGF)-β (reviewed in reference 41). The importance of the immunoregulatory potential of the gut microbiota is emphasized in the recent demonstration of cross-talk between the innate and the adaptive immune system; the nature of the initial immune response governs the homeostasis of the adaptive immune response.

The compositional development of the gut microbiota differs between infants developing and those not developing atopic manifestations. Healthy infants harbor a natural predominance of bifidobacteria with specific strains present, while those later manifesting atopy present with a reduced ratio of bifidobacteria to clostridia[72] and with distinct bifidobacterial microbiota.[73] Further, intestinal *Bifidobacterium* species from allergic infants induce proinflammatory cytokine production, in contrast to those from healthy infants.[74] Thus, the antiallergic potential of *Bifidobacterium* biota may be strain-specific.

Probiotics may aid in degradation/structural modification of enteral antigens, normalization of the properties of aberrant indigenous microbiota and of gut barrier functions, regulation of the secretion of inflammatory mediators and direction of the development of the immune system during the critical period of life when the risk of allergic disease is heightened.

Preliminary studies have revealed that cow's milk casein, a common allergen in cow's milk allergy, hydrolyzed with probiotic-derived enzymes suppresses lymphocyte proliferation and, more specifically, production of allergen-specific Th2 cytokins.[58,75] In experiments conducted by von der Weid et al,[59] probiotics inhibited proliferation of T cells and reduced secretion of both Th1 and Th2 cytokines whilst inducing the development of a population of T cells producing TGF-β and IL-10, reminiscent of tolerogenic Th3 cells. Furthermore, a specific probiotic strain has been demonstrated to suppress IgE responses and systemic anaphylaxis in a murine model of food allergy.[76]

Different probiotic strains appear to induce distinct and even opposing responses in murine dendritic cells and thus specific strains of the gut microbiota and probiotics may play a crucial role in determining the Th1/Th2/Th3-driving capacity of intestinal dendritic cells.[42] So far, clinical effects have been seen as a significant improvement in the clinical course of atopic eczema in infants given probiotic-supplemented elimination diets. The preventive potential of probiotics in atopic disease has been demonstrated in a double-blind, placebo-controlled study.[77] Probiotics administered pre- and postnatally for 6 months to children at high risk of atopic diseases succeeded in reducing the prevalence of atopic eczema by half, as compared with that in infants receiving placebo, and the effect was recently shown to extend beyond infancy.[78]

The challenge in terms of prevention and management of allergic disease is to identify and clarify the mechanisms of action of the dietary factors that may be protective. Well-controlled intervention studies are required to address the potential effects of different dietary modifications and supplementation to prevent and treat allergic disease or other chronic, mostly immunoinflammatory, diseases. In future, the most likely option may be the incorporation of probiotics and specific nutrients into the same products (nutraceuticals) to provide an optimal diet for individuals at risk. Unquestionably, the interactions between probiotics and nutrients need to be studied. However, nutraceuticals alone cannot resolve the challenge of atopic disease if the crucial role of the total composition of the overall diet is neglected.

Taken together, the direction of research should be focused towards searching for such dietary compounds that may have properties beyond the traditional nutritional effects, i.e. health promotion and risk reduction of a range of diseases. The research in allergic disease is achieving this extention by exploring novel prevention and management strategies. Consequently, research into allergic disease can be taken as a model for the development of nutritional management for other chronic immunoinflammatory diseases as well.

REFERENCES

1. World Health Organization. *Diet, Nutrition and the Prevention of Chronic Diseases*, a report of a WHO study group. Technical report series no. 797. Geneva: World Health Organization, 1990.
2. Food and Agriculture Organization. *Fats and Oils in Human Nutrition*. FAO food and nutrition paper no 57. Rome: Food and Agriculture Organization of the United Nations, 1993.
3. World Health Organization. *Trace Elements in Human Nutrition and Health*. Geneva: World Health Organization, 1996.
4. King JC. Physiology of pregnancy and nutrient metabolism. *Am J Clin Nutr* 2000; **71**: 1218–1225.
5. Scholl TO, Johnson WG. Folic acid: influence on the outcome of pregnancy. *Am J Clin Nutr* 2000; **71**: S1295–S1303.
6. Napoli C, Glass CK, Witztum JL et al. Influence of maternal hypercholesterolaemia during pregnancy on progression of early atherosclerotic lesions in childhood: Fate of Early Lesions in Children (FELIC) study. *Lancet* 1999; **354**: 1234–1241.
7. Forsdahl A. Are poor living conditions in childhood and adolescence an important risk factor for arteriosclerotic heart disease? *Br J Prev Soc Med* 1977; **31**: 91-95.
8. Barker DJP, Osmond C. Early growth and death from cardiovascular disease in women. *Br Med J* 1993; **1**: 1077–1081.
9. Osmond C, Barker DJP, Winter PD et al. Early growth and death from cardiovascular disease in women. *Br Med J* 1993; **307**: 519–524.
10. Langley SC, Jackson AA. Increased systolic blood pressure in adult rats induced by fetal exposure to maternal low protein diets. *Clin Sci* 1994; **86**: 217–222.
11. Desai M, Crowther N, Ozanne SE et al. Adult glucose and lipid metabolism may be programmed during fetal life. *Biochem Soc Trans* 1995; **23**: 331–335.
12. Isolauri E, Sütas Y, Mäkinen-Kiljunen S et al. Efficacy and safety of hydrolyzed cow milk and amino acid-derived formulas in infants with cow milk allergy. *J Pediatr* 1995; **127**: 550–557.
13. Smith I, Beasley MG, Ades AE. Intelligence and quality of dietary treatment in phenylketonuria. *Arch Dis Child* 1990; **65**: 472–478.
14. Sategna-Guidetti C, Grosso SB, Grosso S et al. The effects of 1-year gluten withdrawal on bone mass, bone metabolism and nutritional status in newly-diagnosed adult coeliac disease patients. *Aliment Pharmacol Ther* 2000; **14**: 35–43.
15. World Health Organization. *Diet, Nutrition and the Prevention of Chronic Diseases*, a report of a joint WHO/FAO expert consultation, 28 January–1 February 2002. WHO technical report series, 916. Geneva: World Health Organization, 2003.
16. Birch LL. Development of food preferences. *Annu Rev Nutr* 1999; **19**: 41–62.
17. Couch SC, Cross AT, Kida K et al. Rapid westernization of children's blood cholesterol in 3 countries: evidence for nutrient–gene interactions? *Am J Clin Nutr* 2000; **72**: 1266–1274.
18. Pietinen P, Vartiainen E, Seppänen R et al. Changes in diet in Finland from 1972 to 1992: impact on coronary heart disease risk. *Prev Med* 1996; **25**: 243–250.
19. Räsänen L, Ahola M, Kara R et al. Atherosclerosis precursors in Finnish children and adolescents. VIII. Food consumption and nutrient intakes. *Acta Paediatr Scand Suppl* 1985; **318**: 135–153.
20. Simell O, Niinikoski H, Rönnemaa T et al. Special Turku coronary risk factor intervention project for babies (STRIP). *Am J Clin Nutr* 2000; **72**: 1316–1331.
21. Lagström H, Seppänen R, Jokinen E et al. Influence of dietary fat on the nutrient intake and growth of children from 1 to 5 years of age: the Special Turku Coronary Risk Factor Intervention Project. *Am J Clin Nutr* 1999; **69**: 516–523.
22. Rask-Nissilä L, Jokinen E, Terho P et al. Effects of diet on the neurologic development of children at 5 years of age: the STRIP project. *J Pediatr* 2002; **140**: 328–333.
23. Uauy R, Mize CE, Castillo-Duran C. Fat intake during childhood: metabolic responses and effects on growth. *Am J Clin Nutr* 2000; **72**: 1354–1360.
24. Brandtzaeg P. Development of the mucosal immune system in humans. In Bindels JG, Goedhart AC, Visser HKA, eds. *Recent Developments in Infant Nutrition*. London: Kluwer Academic Publishers, 1996; 349–376.
25. Gdalevich M, Mimouni D, David M et al. Breast-feeding and the onset of atopic dermatitis in childhood: a

systematic review and meta-analysis of prospective studies. *J Am Acad Dermatol* 2001; **45**: 520–527.
26. Gdalevich M, Mimouni D, Mimouni M. Breast-feeding and the risk of bronchial asthma in childhood: a systematic review with meta-analysis of prospective studies. *J Pediatr* 2001; **139**: 261–266.
27. Gillman MW, Rifas-Shiman SL, Camargo CAJ et al. Risk of overweight among adolescents who were breastfed as infants. *JAMA* 2001; **16**: 2461–2467.
28. von Kries R, Koletzko B, Sauerwald T et al. Does breast-feeding protect against childhood obesity? *Adv Exp Med Biol* 2000; **478**: 29–39.
29. Davis MK. Breastfeeding and chronic disease in childhood and adolescence. *Pediatr Clin North Am* 2001; **48**: 125–141.
30. Michaelsen KM, Skafte L, Badsberg JH et al. Variation in macronutrients in human bank milk: influencing factors and implications for human milk banking. *J Pediatr Gastroenterol Nutr* 1990; **11**: 229–239.
31. Laiho K, Lampi A-M, Moilanen E et al. Breast milk fatty acids, eicosanoids and cytokines in mothers with and without allergic disease. *Pediatr Res* 2003; **53**: 642–647.
32. Rautava S, Kalliomäki M, Isolauri E. Probiotics during pregnancy and breastfeeding may confer immunomodulatory protection against atopic disease in the infant. *J Allergy Clin Immunol* 2002; **109**: 119–121.
33. Solomons NW. Modulation of the immune system and the response against pathogens with bovine colostrum concentrates. *Eur J Clin Nutr* 2002; **56**: S24–S28.
34. Picciano MF, Smiciklas-Wright H, Birch LL et al. Nutritional guidance is needed during dietary transition in early childhood. *Pediatr* 2000; **106**: 109–114.
35. Sanderson IR, Walker WA. Uptake and transport of macromolecules by the intestine: possible role in clinical disorders (an update). *Gastroenterology* 1993; **104**: 622–639.
36. Ducroc R, Heyman M, Beaufrere B et al. Horseradish peroxidase transport across rabbit jejunum and Peyer's patches *in vitro*. *Am J Physiol* 1983; **245**: G54–G58.
37. Isolauri E, Majamaa H, Arvola T et al. *Lactobacillus casei* strain GG reverses increased intestinal permeability induced by cow milk in suckling rats. *Gastroenterology* 1993; **105**: 1643–1650.
38. Brandtzaeg P. Development and basic mechanisms of human gut immunity. *Nutr Rev* 1998; **56**: S5–S18.
39. Salminen S, Bouley C, Boutron-Ruault M-C et al. Functional food science and gastrointestinal physiology and function. *Br J Nutr* 1998; **80**: 47–71.
40. Favier C, Vaughan E, de Vos W et al. Molecular monitoring of succession of bacterial communities in human neonates. *Appl Environ Microbiol* 2002; **68**: 219–226.
41. Isolauri E, Rautava S, Kalliomäki M et al. Role of probiotics in food hypersensitivity, *Curr Opin Allergy Clin Immunol* 2002; **2**: 263–271.
42. Isolauri E, Kirjavainen PV, Salminen S. Probiotics – a role in the treatment of intestinal infection and inflammation? *Gut* 2002; **50** (Suppl iii): 54–59.
43. Welsh FKS, Farmery SM, MacLennan K et al. Gut barrier function in malnourished patients. *Gut* 1998; **42**: 396–401.
44. Mathers JC. Nutrient regulation of intestinal proliferation and apoptosis. *Proc Nutr Soc* 1998; **57**: 219–223.
45. Buchman AL. Glutamine: commercially essential or conditionally essential? A critical appraisal of the human data. *Am J Clin Nutr* 2001; **74**: 25–32.
46. Heyland DK, Novak F, Drover JW et al. Should immunonutrition become routine in critically ill patients? A systematic review of the evidence. *J Am Med Assoc* 2001; **286**: 944–953.
47. Stephensen CB. Vitamin A, infection, and immune function. *Annu Rev Nutr* 2001; **21**: 167–192.
48. Thurnham DI, Northrop-Clewes CA, McCullough FS et al. Innate immunity, gut integrity, and vitamin A in Gambian and Indian infants. *J Infec Dis* 2000; **182**: S23–2S8.
49. Isolauri E. Probiotics for infectious diarrhoea. *Gut* 2003; **52**: 436–437.
50. Lau S, Illi S, Sommerfeld C et al. Early exposure to house-dust mite and cat allergens and development of childhood asthma: a cohort study. *Lancet* 2000; **356**: 1392–1397.
51. de Jong MH, Scharp-van der Linden VTM, Aalberse RC et al. Randomised controlled trial of brief neonatal exposure to cows' milk on the development of atopy. *Arch Dis Child* 1998; **79**: 126–130.
52. de Jong MH, Scharp-van der Linden VETM, Aalberse RC et al. The effect of brief neonatal exposure to cows' milk on atopic symptoms up to age 5. *Arch Dis Child* 2002; **86**: 365–369.
53. Laiho K, Hoppu U, Ouwehand A et al. Probiotics–on-going research on atopic individuals. *Br J Nutr* 2002; **88**: S19–S27.
54. Zeiger RS. Dietary manipulations in infants and their mothers and the natural course of atopic disease. *Pediatr Allergy Immunol* 1994; **5**: 33–43.
55. Barone KS, Reilly MR, Flanangan MP et al. Abrogation of oral tolerance by feeding encapsulated antigen. *Cell Immunol* 2000; **199**: 65–72.
56. Mäkinen-Kiljunen S, Sorva R. Bovine beta-lactoglobulin levels in hydrolysed protein formulas for infant feeding. *Clin Exp Allergy* 1993; **23**: 287–291.
57. Von Berg A, Koletzko S, Grubl A. The effect of hydrolyzed cow's milk formula for allergy prevention in the first year of life: the German Infant Nutritional Intervention Study, a randomized double-blind trial. *J Allergy Clin Immunol* 2003; **111**: 533–540.
58. Sütas Y, Soppi E, Korhonen H. Suppression of lymphocyte proliferation *in vitro* by bovine caseins hydrolysed with *Lactobacillus* GG-derived enzymes. *J Allergy Clin Immunol* 1996; **98**: 216–224.
59. von der Weid T, Bulliard C, Schiffrin EJ. Induction by a lactic acid bacterium of a population of CD4+ T cells with low proliferative capacity that produce transforming growth factor beta and interleukin-10. *Clin Diagn Lab Immunol* 2001; **8**: 695–701.
60. Sellmayer A, Koletzko B. Long-chain polyunsaturated fatty acids and eicosanoids in infants–physiological and pathophysiological aspects and open questions. *Lipids* 1999; **34**: 199–205.
61. Roper RL, Brown DM, Phipps P. Prostaglandin E2 promotes B lymphocyte Ig isotype switching to IgE. *J Immunol* 1995; **154**: 162–170.
62. Biagi PL, Hrelia S, Celadon M et al. Erythrocyte membrane fatty acid composition in children with atopic dermatitis compared to age-matched controls. *Acta Paediatr* 1993; **82**: 789–790.
63. Leichsenring M, Kochsiek U, Paul K. (n-6)-Fatty acids in plasma lipids of children with atopic bronchial asthma. *Pediatr Allergy Immunol* 1995; **6**: 209–212.
64. Yu G, Duchén K, Björkstén B. Fatty acid composition in colostrum and mature milk from non-atopic and atopic mothers during the first 6 months of lactation. *Acta Paediatr* 1998; **87**: 729–736.
65. Newberry RD, Stenson WF, Lorenz RG. Cyclooxygenase-2-dependent arachidonic acid metabolites are essential modulators of the intestinal immune response to dietary antigen. *Nature Med* 1999; **5**: 900–906.

66. Whelan J. Antagonistic effects of dietary arachidonic acid and n-3 polyunsaturated fatty acids. *J Nutr* 1996; **126**: 1086–1091.
67. Greene LS. Asthma, oxidant stress, and diet. *Nutrition* 1999; **15**: 899–907.
68. Bodner C, Godden D, Brown K et al. Antioxidant intake and adult-onset wheeze: a case–control study. *Eur Respir J* 1999; **13**: 22–30.
69. Hartmann G, Weiner GJ, Krieg AM. CpG DNA: a potent signal for growth, activation, and maturation of human dendritic cells. *Proc Natl Sci USA* 1999; **96**: 9305–9319.
70. Kranzer K, Bauer M, Lipford GB et al. CpG-oligodeoxynucleotides enhance T-cell receptor-triggered interferon-gamma production and up-regulation of CD69 via induction of antigen-presenting cell-derived interferon type I and interleukin-12. *Immunology* 2000; **99**: 170–178.
71. Neish AS, Gewirtz AT, Zeng H et al. Prokaryotic regulation of epithelial responses by inhibition of IkappaB-alpha ubiquitination. *Science* 2000; **289**: 1560–1563.
72. Kalliomäki M, Kirjavainen P, Eerola E et al. Distinct patterns of neonatal gut microflora in infants in whom atopy was and was not developing. *J Allergy Clin Immunol* 2001; **107**: 129–134.
73. Ouwehand AC, Isolauri E, He F et al. Differences in *Bifidobacterium* flora composition in allergic and healthy infants. *J Allergy Clin Immunol* 2001; **108**: 144–145.
74. He F, Morita H, Hashimoto H. Intestinal *Bifidobacterium* species induce varying cytokine production. *J Allergy Clin Immunol* 2002; **109**: 1035–1036.
75. Pochard P, Gosset P, Grangette C. Lactic acid bacteria inhibit TH2 cytokine production by mononuclear cells from allergic patients. *J Allergy Clin Immunol* 2002; **110**: 617–623.
76. Shida K, Takahashi R, Iwadate E. *Lactobacillus casei* strain Shirota suppresses serum immunoglobulin E and immunoglobulin G1 responses and systemic anaphylaxis in a food allergy model. *Clin Exp Allergy* 2002; **32**: 563–570.
77. Kalliomäki M, Salminen S, Arvilommi H et al. Probiotics in primary prevention of atopic disease: a randomised, placebo-controlled trial. *Lancet* 2001; **357**: 1076–1079.
78. Kalliomäki M, Salminen S, Poussa T et al. Probiotics and prevention of atopic disease – a 4-year follow-up of a randomised placebo-controlled trial. *Lancet* 2003; **361**: 1869–1871.

33 Enteral nutrition

Olivier Goulet and Virginie Colomb

Introduction

Enteral nutrition (EN) or enteral feeding is a technique for nutritional support which delivers a homogeneous, liquid nutritional admixture into the digestive tract by tube, into the stomach, or, more rarely in children, into the duodenum or the proximal jejunum. EN, has been used in pediatric patients for more than 30 years, in order to preserve nutritional status and normal growth, or to treat malnutrition when oral feedings cannot fill the protein–energy demand. EN is more physiological, usually safer, easier to administrate and less expensive than parenteral nutrition (PN). Therefore, EN should be preferred to PN in infants and children with malnutrition and/or nutritional risk,[1] when the intestinal tract is usable to provide nutrients. The physiological basis of continuous EN make it of great interest in pediatric patients with gastrointestinal (GI) disorders.[2,3] Nevertheless, this therapy is now widely used in a variety of extradigestive conditions.

EN, like PN, is always initiated in the hospital, but may be performed at home in case of chronic disease, leading to long-term dependency. Home EN has enlarged the field of indications and improved the psychological tolerance to long-term nutritional therapy.

Physiological basis of continuous enteral feeding

Gastrointestinal motility

In case of gastric administration of continuous enteral nutrition (CEN), a continuous gastric emptying related to infusion rate can be achieved, if the infusion rate, the caloric load and the osmolarity of the mixture are not excessive. When the infusion rate is below 3 kcal/min, the gastric emptying rate increases with increasing caloric load, up to the same level as that of the infusion rate.[4] Thus, a steady state is achieved between the amount of nutrients delivered into the stomach, the gastric secretion volume and the gastric emptying rate.

When the infusion rate is excessive and higher than the gastric emptying rate, the risk of vomiting increases. As the caloric load and/or osmolarity of the formula increase, the gastric emptying rate is reduced, to maintain a constant caloric load delivered to the duodenum; therefore, formulas with a concentration above 1 kcal/ml should be used with caution.[5] The nature of the energy supply does not seem to play a role in gastric function, except for the type of triglyceride (long-chain triglycerides (LCTs) or medium-chain triglycerides (MCTs)).[6]

The effects of CEN on intestinal motility can be analyzed by manometry. Migrating complexes are observed in adult patients during CEN, as during the fasting state.[7] The type of formula influences jejunal motility according to the nature of triglycerides and/or the molecular weight of peptides and proteins.[8] Infusion of MCTs or short peptides within the duodenal lumen is associated with the persistence of migrating complexes, as during fasting.[9] Very few data are available about the changes of colonic motility induced by CEN; the continuous gastric infusion of the nutritive formula modifies the gastrocolic reflex.

Gallbladder motility is maintained during EN, as assessed by ultrasonography.[10] The type of infused lipids (MCTs versus LCTs) influences gallbladder motility.[11] Biliary complications, such as sludge or cholelithiasis, are very rare during long-term CEN.

Digestive secretion and hormonal response

Gastric secretion depends mostly on protein intake, and in case of elemental diet, on amino acid composition.[12] The secretory response is not influenced by carbohydrates, but is reduced by lipids. It has not been demonstrated whether or not the type of diet (i.e. elemental, semi-elemental or polymeric) modifies gastric acid secretion.[6] Cholecystokinin secretion as well as pancreatic secretion are maintained during CEN. The amount of nitrogen infused within the jejunum correlates with the secretion of chymotrypsin and lipase.[13] Secretory responses do not differ between an elemental or polymeric nitrogen supply.[14]

Gastrin secretion is also maintained during CEN, but its response to protein load is decreased. Gastric or duodenal CEN stimulate insulin secretion, depending on the type of infused nutrients. The lack of steatosis during CEN suggests that the insulin response is lower when carbohydrates are infused enterally as compared to parenterally.[15]

Effects of continuous enteral nutrition on mucosal trophism

The effects of artificial nutrition on small-bowel mucosal trophism remain controversial. In experimental animal systems, CEN has been shown not to modify the absorption capacity of the proximal small bowel. In the distal small bowel and colon, however, enzymatic and functional capacity are decreased, despite a normal mucosal architecture; in addition, DNA as well as protein content are reduced.[16] These changes could be the consequence of the almost complete absorption of nutrients within the proximal part of the small bowel, leading to lack of stimulation of the distal segment. This suggests an ability of CEN to achieve bowel rest in the distal part of the bowel, providing efficient treatment for ileocolic inflammatory diseases.

Effects of continuous enteral nutrition on energy expenditure

The thermogenic effect of feeding is related to the increase of energy expenditure following ingestion of food. The increase in energy expenditure induced by CEN in normal subjects is lower than that for the same nutrient load as a bolus.[17,18] Thus, the constant administration of energy substrates might reduce the energy storage and maintain homeostasis at a lower energy expenditure.[19]

Finally, CEN by the slow and continuous administration of nutrients into the GI tract enables their optimal utilization to be achieved, despite intestinal illness. By changing the conditions of flow and of contact between the nutritive formula and the digestive tract, CEN may increase the capacity for intraluminal digestion and intestinal absorption. This feeding technique seems logical and efficient when the absorptive surface is reduced, e.g. in short-bowel syndrome, villous atrophy, enterocutaneous fistula or proximal enterostomy.

Indications

Indications for EN are different from indications for PN, since the use of EN as nutritional support is based on normal or at least partially preserved gut functions (Table 33.1).

Digestive indications

Since EN has a trophic effect on the intestinal mucosa, and helps maintain mucosal integrity, it plays an important role in the treatment of many digestive diseases, either replacing or completing oral feeding. Digestive diseases leading to an anatomical or functional reduction of the absorption capacity of the small bowel represent the first group; they include short-bowel syndrome, protracted diarrhea with villous atrophy and inflammatory bowel disease.

Short-bowel syndrome

Short-bowel syndrome (see Chapter 29) can be defined as malabsorption following small-intestinal resection. Prognosis after extensive intestinal resection has improved with the expanded use of PN over the past 20 years.[20–24] Following massive resection of the small intestine, the remaining small bowel undergoes an adaptative process characterized by epithelial hyperplasia (see Chapter

Table 33.1 Indications for enteral nutrition

Digestive indications
Short-bowel syndrome
Protracted diarrhea of infancy
Immunodeficiency
Graft-versus-host disease
Crohn's disease
Neonatal abdominal surgery
gastroschisis
omphalocele
meconial ileus
distal intestinal fistulae
small-bowel resection
necrotizing enterocolitis
complicated Hirschsprung's disease
chronic intestinal pseudo-obstruction syndrome
Other malabsorption syndromes
cystic fibrosis
cholestatic liver disease
In children with normal intestinal function
Eating disorders
disorders of sucking and swallowing
neurological impairment
Esophageal diseases
Hypermetabolic states
head injury
extensive burns
cancer, AIDS, bone marrow transplantation
renal failure
congenital heart diseases
chronic pulmonary diseases
Inborn errors of metabolism
glycogen storage diseases
deficiencies of urea cycle
Neonatology and prematurity
Abnormal eating behavior
anorexia nervosa
failure to thrive

29).[25] An early and optimal use of the enteral route is the condition of small-bowel adaptation. However, in children with short-bowel syndrome, oral feeding rarely permits a rapid reduction of the PN supply, because numerous patients have eating disorders instead of hyperphagia. In such conditions, CEN enables the delivery of nutrient to be increased to the digestive tract independently of the feeding behavior, with a known benefit on so-called intestinal adaptation, and added benefits on the prevention of PN-associated liver disease.[25] The delay for postoperative adaptation to occur depends on the length and quality of the residual bowel and on the presence of the ileocecal valve and colon.[21]

Severe protracted diarrhea of infancy

A syndrome of intractable diarrhea of infancy was first described by Avery et al in 1968. Its definition, presentation and outcome have considerably changed during the past two decades.[26] This syndrome could now be defined as persistent diarrhea despite prolonged bowel rest requiring long-term total PN in children when no effective treatment is available.[27,28] According to that definition, EN in this circumstance is indicated and often effective.[29,30] In fact, the reduction of digestive secretions, villous atrophy and acquired brush-border disaccharidase deficiency lead to malabsorption and malnutrition. Most of the time, a short course of PN followed by protracted CEN provides control of the disease within 6–8 weeks.[31,32] In a prospective study of CEN versus PN, Orenstein showed that the resolution of diarrhea was faster in the enterally fed group.[32]

The use of CEN in children and mainly infants with protracted diarrhea also presenting severe malnutrition may prove difficult. If the response to CEN is not good enough to provide rapidly adequate caloric supplies with resolution of diarrhea, PN should be started. Such decisions must be taken by experienced teams in specialized and well-staffed units.

Severely malnourished infants with some types of particularly severe celiac disease, intolerance to cow's milk proteins, protein hydrolysates, or specific malabsorption syndromes such as Anderson's disease, may also benefit from CEN.[33]

Inflammatory bowel diseases

Enteral feeding has been used for many years, particularly in Europe, not only to improve nutritional status and growth, but also to influence disease activity in patients with Crohn's disease.[34–43] It has been shown that CEN using an elemental diet is as effective as a high dose of steroids in inducing remission in pediatric patients with Crohn's disease involving the small intestine. The meta-analysis by Griffiths et al suggested that EN was inferior to steroid therapy.[44] This was largely an analysis of adult studies and excluded several pediatric studies showing striking efficacy. More recent meta-analyses have shown an equivalent effect of EN and steroids in achieving remission.[45,46] In addition, it is clear that EN is advantageous in preserving growth while remission is achieved. There are no relevant data in children. However, in adults, studies on the comparative effect of elemental diets, protein hydrolysates and intact protein formulas have shown induced remission of polymeric diets in controlling Crohn's disease involving the small bowel. How such treatment works in children with Crohn's disease is not clear. Certainly, the increased energy intake provided by EN must be one factor. However, there is evidence that such treatment may have a specific anti-inflammatory effect. A reduction of cytokine production by isolated lamina propria lymphocytes following EN with a polymeric casein-based formula was shown to an extent equivalent to that produced by steroids or cyclosporin.[43] In addition, Fell et al have shown a massive reduction in mRNA transcripts for interleukin (IL)-1β using its derivative CT3211.[47] Removal of antigenic material, alteration in intestinal microflora, changes in gut hormone levels and the presence of bioactive transforming growth factor (TGF) β-1 in casein-based formulas may all play a role in the clinical success of EN.[48,49] A glutamine-enriched polymeric diet offered no advantage over a standard low-glutamine polymeric diet in the treatment of active Crohn's disease.[50] EN may also be helpful in correction or maintenance of the nutritional state, especially during a relapse of Crohn's disease.[45] EN is part of the preparation for a surgical procedure and may be useful during recovery, especially after intestinal resections or enterostomies.

In case of severe digestive involvement during Schönlein–Henoch purpura, CEN can be used as nutritional support in the absence of occlusion.[51]

Neonatal abdominal surgery

In neonatal abdominal surgery for congenital or acquired disease, CEN, usually combined with PN, offers prolonged nutritional support. This has transformed the prognosis in many conditions and is particularly important in the following situations: reduction of the absorptive surface with enterocutaneous fistulae or extensive intestinal resection; and functional disorders of gut motility, such as malfunctions of a duodenojejunal anastomosis, 'plastic' peritonitis after repeated interventions, gastroschisis and omphalocele.

Chronic intestinal pseudo-obstruction syndrome, with neonatal onset, is a special condition in which EN is rarely tolerated and usually does not allow PN and/or a surgical procedure such as ileostomy to be avoided.[52–54]

Other malabsorption syndromes

Cystic fibrosis

Failure to thrive is common in children with cystic fibrosis (CF), and results from several factors, including malabsorption from pancreatic insufficiency, bile salt abnormalities, anorexia, increased energy expenditure, protein catabolism from pulmonary infections and/or fever.[55] Even with an optimal approach to oral feeding, some patients fail to respond to conservative nutritional therapy. EN is proposed as a second-stage intervention and can help to restore and maintain nutritional status.[56–58] EN is in most cases easily performed at home. It is generally performed during the night over 8–10 h; CF patients are asked to eat and drink as much as possible during the day. Nasogastric tube feeding is generally used as a first step. The tube is passed every night, 1–2 h after dinner, and removed in the early morning before physical therapy so that patients are not disturbed during the day for school attendance. In some children, a nasogastric tube becomes increasingly uncomfortable because of nausea, vomiting and nasal discomfort as a result of nasal polyposis or dislodgement during coughing in cases of pulmonary exacerbation. Thus, percutaneous endoscopic gastrostomy (PEG) has become the method of choice for performing long-term home nocturnal EN. A button device can be placed 2–3 months after PEG tube placement, thus improving the physical and psychological tolerance of EN.

It is important to look for glucose tolerance as well as for gastroesophageal reflux before starting EN. Psychological support of the patient is essential, since body image and self-esteem are frequently altered in CF patients, especially in cases of weight loss and/or failure to thrive. Nutritional support by EN, even recognized as necessary, is rightly considered by patients and/or parents as a new constraint.

Thus, the usefulness of EN must be precisely explained in order for it to become part of clear global therapeutic management. EN is required in malnourished children with decreased growth velocity, especially when transplantation is planned. Adequate EN, using either an intact formula with pancreatic enzyme extract or a semi-elemental diet can be achieved through either nasogastric or PEG tubes. Finally, it should be stressed that in CF nutritional supplementation improves not only nutritional status but also respiratory function.[58–60]

Cholestatic liver disease

Mechanisms leading to protein–energy malnutrition in infants and children with chronic liver disease are incompletely known.[61–63] They include reduced biliary secretion and intraluminal bile concentration resulting in malabsorption of lipid and fat-soluble vitamins. Energy requirements are increased by different mechanisms including portosystemic shunting and ascites, abnormal intermediary metabolism and the energy demands of complications such as sepsis or variceal bleeding. Anorexia is common in children with chronic liver disease resulting from organomegaly, abdominal pressure effects of ascites, congested gastric mucosa, reduced motility from portal hypertension, central effects of unidentified toxins, dietary manipulations such as fluid restriction or use of unpalatable feeds. Several factors contribute to long-chain polyunsaturated fatty acid (PUFA) deficiency including low PUFA intake, malabsorption and disturbed metabolism of long-chain PUFAs. Finally, the interaction of growth hormone with insulin-like growth factor (IGF)-I and its binding proteins constitute an important mechanism linking nutrition and growth.

The most common cause of cirrhosis in infants is biliary atresia. Since orthotopic liver transplantation (OLT) is the only effective treatment, the role of nutritional support preceding transplantation is of importance.[63,64] Nutritional support has a direct impact on survival and suitability as candidates for OLT, while the effect of preoperative nutritional support on outcome after OLT is a matter of debate.[65,66]

Oral food intake is most of the time insufficient in these children. EN providing MCT-rich feeds is recommended and should be associated with an adequate fat-soluble vitamin supply.[67,68] Many currently available commercial nutritional products are suitable for infants with chronic liver disease but none are ideal for all situations. Additives are usually necessary in infants and children with persistent failure to thrive. Ordinarily, nutritional management can be carried out at home. However, two issues remain controversial. First, children with portal hypertension may have esophagal varices with the risk of bleeding due to the nasogastric tube; in this circumstance, the use of a silicone tube is mandatory and home EN is contraindicated. Second, the use of branched-chain amino acids to feed children with chronic encephalopathy is debated.[69]

Indications in children with normal intestinal function

Eating disorders

EN is required in cases of inability to eat normally, i.e. in those situations that are secondary to structural or functional abnormalities of the upper GI tract or neurological impairment of the processes involved in sucking and/or swallowing (see also Chapter 15).

Esophageal diseases including esophageal atresia, fistula or stenosis, can result from sequelae of epidermolysis bullosa. These conditions often need EN, usually through gastrostomy or duodenal tubes.[70] The choice of feeding through a gastrostomy or a transpyloric tube must be assessed according to the patient's age, disease and condition.

Children with chronic diseases inducing immaturity or inability to feed orally, especially with sucking and swallowing troubles as seen in neurologically impaired children, with neuromuscular chronic diseases or cerebral palsy also require EN, using gastrostomy tubes.[71–73]

Other indications

Indications for EN have been extended in recent years to include several extraintestinal conditions.

Hypermetabolic states

Patients with acute hypermetabolic conditions, such as those resulting from head injury or burns, should receive an adequate nutrient supply, which should be given enterally in most cases.[74] EN has been used successfully in children with cancer, bone marrow transplantation or AIDS.[75–78]

All chronic diseases inducing both an increase in protein–caloric needs and anorexia, such as chronic renal failure[79,80] with or without hemodialysis awaiting transplantation, or congenital heart disease,[81,82] often induce malnutrition and failure to thrive. Children with these disorders benefit from EN, since improvement of nutritional status is expected to influence the outcome positively after transplantation.

Inborn errors of metabolism

EN is part of the treatment of numerous inherited metabolic diseases, which induce hypoglycemia (glycogen storage disease)[83–85] or increase protein catabolism, e.g. enzymatic deficiencies of the urea cycle.[86,87] CEN is required to avoid neurological consequences of these metabolic disorders.

Premature infants

EN is commonly used in premature infants, and in small-for-gestational age neonates with sucking and swallowing troubles. Mother's milk can be given, sometimes into the duodenum rather than into the stomach in low-birth-weight infants (less than 1000 g). All the factors discussed earlier must be carefully monitored in this high-risk group. Some physicians prefer to stop CEN in infants with respiratory disease, and to use total PN (see also Chapter 34).

Miscellaneous conditions

Miscellaneous indications for EN include primitive difficulties of eating behavior, including anorexia nervosa,[88–91] and chronic idiopathic failure to thrive. Failure to thrive may be due to a poor parent–child relationship leading to insufficient food intake. In such circumstances, tube feeding can be used to demonstrate that growth can be achieved if adequate nutrients are provided.[88,89] In older children and adolescents with anorexia nervosa, EN can be used according to the opinion and experience of the psychiatric team.[90,91]

Techniques

Material

Nasogastric tubes

The route of EN administration should be individually tailored, depending on the underlying condition. The intragastric route of administration is the more used in children, since it is the more physiological route. It permits the action of salivary and gastric enzymes, the bactericidal action of gastric acid and better mixing with biliary and pancreatic juice. Therefore, the duodenal or jejunal route is used in few circumstances in children. For intragastric EN, nasogastric tubes or gastrostomy tubes may be used. Nasogastric tube feeding is the best initial approach to EN, to evaluate the tolerance of EN before placing a permanent gastrostomy tube, and/or when a brief period of EN support is anticipated. The nasogastric tube may be made of polyvinylchloride (PVC), polyurethane or silicone. The tube size is chosen according to the weight and age of the child, with an external diameter as small as possible. The nasogastric tube is inserted nasogastrically by using the nose–umbilicus distance as a reference point. Its position is routinely checked by epigastric auscultation during the injection of air and the aspiration of fluid with a pH less than 3. Duodenal or jejunal tube placement is more difficult; the patient should be placed in the right lateral position and, if necessary, after intramuscular injection of metoclopramide. The position of the distal end of the tube is then checked by X-rays. Careful nasal fixation of the tube is used to avoid displacement; it is taped to the upper lip, the ipsilateral cheek and the external ear. In some particular indications for EN, the feeding tube may also be introduced through the mouth, especially in premature babies. The placement of the nasogastric tube made of PVC is easier, but these tubes should be changed every 2–4 days. Indeed, the tube becomes rigid if left longer, whereas the silicone or polyurethane tube may be used over 3-week periods or more. On the other hand, silicone and polyurethane tubes are more flexible and are more easily displaced by vomiting; they are preferentially used for transpyloric and long-term EN. When the child requires prolonged EN (more than 2 or 3 months) and when EN is well tolerated, a gastrostomy should be considered.

Percutaneous gastrostromy

The PEG technique has revolutionized the placement of enteric feeding tubes in children. It is now a widely used and well-tolerated technique in children.[92–95] This relatively simple and fast procedure can be performed during upper-GI endoscopy in an endoscopy suite with the use of conscious sedation and local anesthesia or under general anesthesia. Several techniques have been developed with the common basic principle that the endoscope locates the site of tube placement from within the stomach. The transillumination of the light from the endoscope through the abdominal wall identifies the site of skin incision. The ideal site is on the greater curvature of the stomach with the stoma sited on the anterior abdominal wall, below the costal margin with consideration to the axis of bending and to the clothing. To reduce the risk of infection at the stoma site, perioperative antibiotic prophylaxis is recommended. The tube can be used within 12–24 h, while post-insertion edema at the stoma site is closely monitored. Care should be taken not to pull the bolster too high. The initial PEG tube is changed after 2–3 months, by which time a good tract has formed. Button-replacement gastrostomy devices provide patients a cosmetic advantage in case of long-term EN. PEG is contraindicated only in a few patients with previous abdominal surgery, abnormal abdominal anatomy, or severe deformities of the chest and spine that modify the position of the stomach. In such cases, a surgical gastrostomy tube should be placed. The implantation of a jejunal feeding tube, via PEG, is a possible method for the treatment of inadequate oral feeding in patients who are affected by gastroesophageal reflux and is thus an alternative to fundoplication and drugs.[96,97] Special PEG techniques have also been developed for ICU patients.[98]

EN may be delivered by bolus or pump-controlled techniques, but should not be administered by gravity in children. Pumps recommended for pediatric use have to provide clear flow rate display and alarms. Miniaturized and battery-powered pumps are specially designed for home and ambulatory EN.

Nutrients

Nitrogen The absorption of amino acids is more rapid and efficient when given in the form of short peptides rather than free amino acids.[99,100] In addition, the quality, in terms of digestion and intestinal absorption of protein hydrolysates, depends on the type of hydrolysate; for example, lactalbumin is superior to casein.[101,102] Thus, the initial formula should be based on polypeptides, with a lower osmolality, rather than on a mixture of free amino acids. Nitrogen needs vary depending on tolerance, and range from 350 to 500 mg/kg per day, or even more in some highly catabolic situations. The nitrogen/calorie ratio must be considered; protein intakes should represent 10% of the energy intake, especially for premature infants.[103]

Carbohydrates Disaccharidase enzymatic activities are depressed in disease involving the small-intestine mucosa. Lactase appears to be the most sensitive to injury and the last of the disaccharidases to recover. In addition, certain drugs such as neomycin or colchicine depress the intestinal disaccharidases. Therefore, it is important to avoid dietary sources of lactose. Other disaccharides should also be omitted from the solution used for initial feeding, as their corresponding brush-border enzymatic activities are reduced. The only carbohydrate allowed during the initial days of EN should be glucose, but its high osmolality (5.5 mOsmol/g) limits the rate of infusion, and thus the total amount given. The later addition of fructose may lead to an increase of disaccharidase activity, so making it easier to substitute maltose and sucrose for glucose. The subsequent introduction of low-osmolality oligosaccharides may allow the intake to reach 20 or even 24 g/kg per day, especially in infants, without resulting in a final solution osmolality higher than 350 mOsm/l.

Lipids The behavior of MCTs within the intestinal lumen and their absorption characteristics are primarily due to their greater water solubility.[104,105] MCTs are hydrolyzed faster than LCTs in the small intestine by pancreatic lipase; they are converted almost exclusively into free fatty acids and glycerol and directly reach the portal circulation and the liver. Nevertheless, in case of pancreatic insufficiency, MCTs may be absorbed intact. The excessive use of a MCT-containing diet can lead to osmotic diarrhea as a result of their rapid hydrolysis. Dicarboxylic aciduria has been described in infants supplemented with MCT-rich formulas without any evidence of a deleterious effect.[106] The provision of essential fatty acids (EFA) must be considered since MCTs contain no EFA. Furthermore, MCTs decrease the absorption of LCTs; therefore, supplementation with linoleic acid must be provided. However, its addition to a formula based on MCTs may be insufficient to prevent EFA deficiency, thus making it necessary to provide EFA parenterally. Nevertheless, most formulas containing MCTs include up to 50% of lipid as LCTs. By stimulating biliary and pancreatic secretions, LCTs promote increased intestinal motility; LCTs in excess in the intestinal lumen, especially if they are hydroxylated by bacteria, reverse the rate of water and electrolyte absorption and increase malabsorption. In those conditions, the addition of cholestyramine associated with EFA supplementation may be appropriate. Finally, a lipid intake of 3–4 g/kg per day may be achieved, depending on the absorption capacity and digestive tolerance.

Other components In infants and children, the recommended energy intake varies from 70 to 100 kcal/kg per day, and water rarely exceeds 80 ml/kg per day. The recommendations for average supplies of vitamins and trace elements are shown in Tables 33.2 and 33.3. Competition between trace elements such as copper and zinc has been taken into account in these recommendations; the daily supplement should be higher in premature than in full-term infants.

Table 33.2 Vitamin requirements

	Infants	Children
Vitamin A (μg)	300–750	450–1000
Vitamin D (IU)	400–1000	200–2500
Vitamin E (mg)	3–10	10–15
Vitamin K (μg)	50–75	50–70
Vitamin B_1 (mg)	0.4–0.5	1.5–3
Vitamin B_2 (mg)	0.4–0.6	1.1–3.6
Vitamin B_5 (mg)	2–5	0.5–5
Vitamin B_6 (mg)	0.1–1.0	1.5–2
Vitamin B_{12} (μg)	0.3–3	3–100
Vitamin C (mg)	25–35	20–100
Folic acid (μg)	20–80	100–500
Biotin (μg)	35–50	150–300
Niacin (mg)	6–8	5–40

Table 33.3 Trace element requirements

Element	Infants (/kg/day)	Children (/day)
Iron (mg)	50	100–2500
Zinc (mg)	100–250	1000–5000
Copper (mg)	20–30	200–300
Selenium (μg)	2–3	30–60
Manganese (μg)	1–10	50–250
Molybdenum (μg)	0.25–3	50–70
Chrome (μg)	0.25–2	10–20
Iodine (μg)	1–5	50–100
Fluoride (μg)	20	500–1000

Choice of a formula

Enteral feeding formulas are divided into several families. The choice of a formula is made according to numerous parameters, such as protein–caloric needs, digestive function and tolerance to fluid intake – all obviously dependent on the age and on the underlying disease.

(1) In newborns and young infants with normal or nearly normal intestinal function, breast or humanized milk may be used, while commercial polymeric diets are available for older children. Blenderized diets can be prepared using food from the kitchen, but are usually replaced by polymeric formulas containing 'intact' proteins with or without fibers, which are commercially available; they are indicated in most non-stressed patients, with normal gut function. These formulas contain 1 kcal/ml (standard) to 1.5 kcal/ml (calorically dense).

(2) In case of GI disease, the choice of the nutritive solution must take into account not only the child's age and nutritional status but also the underlying digestive disease, e.g. the presence of anatomical and functional changes in the

intestine, whether due to an extensive reduction of the absorptive surface, to enteropathy or to pancreatic insufficiency. Limiting factors in such cases are impairment of gastric, biliary and pancreatic secretions, disturbances of the intestinal flora and malabsorption. The osmolarity of enteral formulas should be kept below 320 mOsmol/kg, nutrients should be rapidly transferred across the intestine and they should not leave an intraluminal residue. Substrates requiring intraluminal hydrolysis (proteins, starches, LCTs) should be excluded, as should potentially highly antigenic substrates (cow's milk proteins, gluten and soy). Oligomeric or 'semi-elemental' diets are designed for use in patients with malabsorption, such as in short-bowel syndrome, CF, cholestasis or food allergy. These diets include dipeptides, tripeptides and a few free amino acids, combined with LCTs and MCTs, and carbohydrates including glucose polymers and maltodextrins. Powder formulas enable progressive adaptation of the concentration to the clinical condition (for example, to increase the concentration progressively from 0.65 kcal/ml up to 1 kcal/ml or more). Ready-to-use formulas usually contain 1 kcal/ml.

(3) Free amino acid-based formulas tend to have a higher osmolality. For instance, the amino acid-based formula Neocate® specifically designed for infants under 1 year of age, has an osmolality of 360 mOsm. The lipid component is a mixture of safflower, coconut and soy oils to provide essential and non-essential fatty acids. The carbohydrates are from corn syrup solids or maltodextrins, both derived from corn starch and differing in the size of glucose polymers. They are indicated especially in children with severe food allergy who do not tolerate even the peptide-based formulas. Children with severe malabsorption or short-bowel syndrome unable to tolerate peptide-based formulas (protein hydrolysates) might benefit from the free amino acid-based formulas.[107,108]

(4) Special formulas are proposed for some indications such as renal failure, liver failure, pulmonary disease, diabetes and metabolic diseases. On the other hand, special formulas have been developed for preterm infants, who are characterized by the following factors: decreased energy and glycogen stores, limited gastric capacity, reduced intestinal peristalsis, reduced bile salt pool and delayed enzymatic development. The main differences in the composition of premature and term infant formulas include: partial substitution of oligosaccharides for lactose; increased protein content to support rapid growth; 60:40 whey/casein ratio to increase essential amino acid intakes and protein digestibility; partial substitution of LCTs by MCTs; and adapted concentrations of vitamin E, calcium, phosphorus and iron.

(5) Nutritional formulas in which each of the constituents is modified independently are mostly used in special conditions, e.g. selective malabsorption. In that case, glucose may be given initially as the calorie source, the amount being increased progressively and controlled according to the stool volume, pH and absence of reducing substances in the stools. In the first days of feeding, at least, a molar ratio of glucose and so-dium is maintained. Then, protein hydrolysates are gradually introduced according to digestive tolerance. The caloric enteral intake usually increases from 10–15 to 70–80 kcal/kg per day over the first week. In a second step, qualitative and quantitative changes are gradually made: fructose is added to the glucose, and then disaccharides are introduced, starting with maltose. Nitrogen and lipids are simultaneously increased. During this period, the introduction of oligosaccharides precede that of a commercially available semi-elemental diet.

Regulation of intakes and rhythm of enteral nutritional delivery

EN should be progressively introduced, depending on the child's nutritional status and the indications for EN. In case of digestive disease, CEN can be used after a prolonged period of PN or simply after a brief phase of peripheral venous infusion. The first step includes the progressive reduction of the parenteral intake and the stepwise increase of EN according to the digestive tolerance. The semi-elemental diet (protein hydrolysates) can be used early, by progressively increasing the volume as well as the concentration, according to digestive tolerance and until optimal energy and nitrogen intakes are achieved. The water and sodium supply should be increased to compensate for the intestinal losses generally induced by the start of EN; the tolerance is estimated from the weight of the child, from the volume and osmolality of urine samples and from the plasma osmolality. The tolerance and needs are estimated from 24-h urine analysis, while attempting to maintain natriuresis of 2–3 mmol/kg per day. At the same time, potassium intake is adjusted as a function of the nitrogen and energy intakes.

The rhythm of EN delivery depends on the underlying disease. Intermittent feeding using a bolus is more physiological and well tolerated when the digestive function is normal. Continuous cyclic nocturnal EN is better tolerated in some patients who do not tolerate bolus feeding, and provides less interference with daytime oral intake. However, a continuous 24/24 h rhythm of delivery is indicated in case of impaired digestive function.

The weaning period varies from a few days to several weeks or months. Eating disorders can be avoided by the maintenance of sucking and swallowing functions during the period of CEN. It has also been demonstrated that non-nutritive sucking during CEN enhances growth and intestinal maturation in premature babies.[109,110] Weaning includes a period of continuous night-time feeding supplemented by several meals in the daytime until the latter account for 50% of the total intake. Oral feeding must be carefully increased because of the relatively low intestinal activity due to long-term CEN.

Complications of enteral therapy

These are rare but serious. Strict adherence to the procedure indicated and careful supervision are essential to prevent them.[111,112]

Gastrointestinal complications

Vomiting and aspiration are the most threatening complications associated with tube feeding, at home as well as in the hospital, while its incidence seems to be low in children on home EN.[113] Irregular flow rate of infusion, delayed gastric emptying due to the underlying disease or to the drugs, gastroesophageal reflux and tube placement or migration into the distal esophagus, behavioral vomiting and formula intolerance are risk factors for vomiting and aspiration. The possible preventive effect of a semirecumbent position has been discussed.[114]

Diarrhea is the most common complication of EN, and can occur in about 30% of patients. It might result in dehydration and hypoglycemia. It may be due to multiple causes, especially intraduodenal infusion, high osmolarity, excess or irregular infusion rate and bacterial contamination of the formula. Increased stool losses occur when the combined absorptive capacity of the small bowel and the salvaging capacity of the colon are exceeded.

Mechanical complications

Tube-related complications such as nasal trauma due to placement of a nasogastric tube, laryngeal ulceration or stenosis, esophageal stricture or perforation mainly if an introducer is used, gastric or duodenal perforation, intestinal bleeding and bowel intussusception are exceptional in children, but have been described with PVC tubes left for 8 days or more.[115–117] Pyloric stenosis has been reported after prolonged duodenal feeding in premature babies; this is probably due both to the presence of the transpyloric tube and to spasm of the pylorus caused by the direct infusion of lipid into the duodenum.

Ear, nose and throat complications are frequent in children who receive EN through a nasogastric tube. The incidence of these complications must be taken into account when making a decision for a gastrostomy.

Complications from PEG placement include worsening of gastroesophageal reflux, dumping syndrome (if the PEG is to close to the pylorus) and gastrocolic fistula. Local skin problems include infection, cellulitis, granulomas and leaking. Leaking of formula, which may be the consequence of lack of adequate inflation of the balloon, or to malfunction of the antireflux valve, induces a vicious cycle with enlarging stoma and skin problems.

Infectious complications

EN tubes have been associated with outbreaks of antimicrobial-resistant organisms. The enteral feed administration sets become colonized externally by microbes grown from the enteral tube hub, and therefore serve as a reservoir of organisms that can be cross-transmitted.[118–125] Adherence to standard precautions is critical when handling enteral feeding apparatuses. Bacterial contamination of the nutritive solution with enterotoxin-producing bacteria such as coliforms or *Enterobacter cloacae*,[122] at the time of preparation, storage or delivery to the patient, leads to gastroenteritis and/or septicemia.[123–125] The relationship between bacterial contamination of enteral formula and diarrhea may be a matter of debate when EN is delivered into the stomach, because of the protective role of gastric acid, the risk of bowel contamination being theoretically higher when EN is delivered below the pylorus. Furthermore, in hospitalized patients, bacteriological monitoring of formula samples is mandatory; manipulation of the tubing and feed reservoirs must be careful. Ready-to-use commercial formulas are therefore recommended for home EN and in hospitals.

Since necrotizing enterocolitis may occur in premature infants and neonates suffering from hypoxia and infections, the abdomen must be checked daily very carefully. Because of the risk of infectious complications and necrotizing enterocolitis, some teams prefer PN to this technique for premature babies weighing less than 1500 g, who require respiratory assistance. Prevention of such complications requires the use of the gastric route as far as possible, strict limitation of duodenal infusions and safe preparation of solutions.

Metabolic complications

Metabolic complications of EN are rare when compared to those of PN. However, especially in severely malnourished children, water overload or electrolyte imbalance should be avoided by careful monitoring. In those particular patients, phosphatemia should be monitored and phosphate supplementation provided.

Dehydration and hypernatremia may occur in case of diarrhea or vomiting, which may result from a formula that is hyperosmolar or too concentrated. Hypoglycemia may be due to sudden discontinuation of infusion, especially in infants, in malnourished children or when EN is used to prevent hypoglycemia in metabolic diseases such as glycogenosis. In children on cyclic EN who do not eat orally, a progressive decrease in infusion rate is recommended to prevent hypoglycemia.

Home enteral nutrition

Indications

Home EN is a logical alternative to long-term hospitalization when long-term EN support is necessary (more than 1 month) in a patient in stable clinical condition. Home EN has been shown to be an effective and safe method, compatible with the best possible quality of life.[126–129] Major cost savings induced by home EN as compared to hospitalization have been demonstrated. The importance of families' teaching and medical follow-up to prevent somatic and psychological complications should not be underestimated.

Prevalence and incidence

The origins of home EN are much older than those of home PN. In North America, 20 000 patients received home EN in 1985 and 150 000 in 1992 (about 500 per million population). Based on an estimated growth rate of 25% per year, about 500 000 patients may have been on home EN in the USA in 1997.[130,131] The British Association of Enteral and Parenteral Nutrition estimated that the number of patients on home EN was about 40 per million population, about ten-fold the number of home PN patients in the same country at the same time. Children accounted for 30–40% of home EN patients in Britain, compared to about 20% in the USA.[130,132,133] However, the lack of national registers in most European countries makes estimation difficult.

Organization

The quality of home EN programs depends on the organization of multidisciplinary nutrition support teams, based on a tight collaboration between the different professionals including physicians, home care nurses, dietitians, pharmacists and social workers. In some countries, pumps, disposable equipment and nutrients for home EN are mainly delivered by hospitals, while in others, such as the USA, where they are the most developed, home care companies participate in patients' training and provide a delivery service and a 24-h emergency phone contact. With expansion of the home care industry, it is important to ensure that adequate standards of care are provided. The American Society of Parenteral and Enteral Nutrition and the British Association of Parenteral and Enteral Nutrition have produced such standards.[132,133]

Parents' teaching

Tolerance and efficacy of EN have to be demonstrated at the hospital before home EN is organized. As for home PN, home EN in children is feasible only when the family is highly motivated and able to deal with technical aspects. Parents' teaching is based on a nutrition multidisciplinary hospital team including a physician, nurse, dietitian and pharmacist. Parents are taught not only about technical aspects but also about risks, complications and their prevention. The hospital team ensures a 24/24h phone contact and regular follow-up, in close co-operation with the general practitioner. The help of a community nurse may be required, especially in case of placement of a nasogastric tube.

Results

Quality of life

Although home EN, like home PN, is usually considered by children and families as an improvement of their quality of life, psychological consequences of this technique have to be carefully estimated and prevented. The placement of a nasogastric tube is distressing to parents and children. A tube *in situ* for continuous 24/24h infusion is a major problem, particularly in older children and adolescents, because it induces an unwelcome public interest. These problems are solved by the use of gastrostomy. Children and families may also suffer from the suppression of meals taken together, which are usually considered as an important time in family life. Adequate psychological preparation and follow-up improve the tolerance in children and parents of home EN.[134,135]

Outcome

Outcome studies in home EN patients have been fewer than those in patients on home PN. Improvement of the nutritional status and low mortality rate (always related to major underlying diseases) are usually described in children on home EN.[136–138] However, few data have been given about the outcome of such pediatric patients in the long term.

Cost and funding

Home EN is far from being as expensive as home PN. The total cost per day of home EN was about $35 in the USA in 1992, when the cost per day of home PN was about $300.[131] The cost savings associated with providing home EN estimated by the British Association for Parenteral and Enteral Nutrition in 1994 were about 70%.[126] In most countries, patients on home EN are funded by the National Health Service, although in the USA they are mostly paid for by insurance companies.[130,139]

REFERENCES

1. Sermet-Gaudelus I, Poisson-Salomon AS, Colomb V et al. Simple pediatric nutritional risk score to identify children at risk of malnutrition. *Am J Clin Nutr* 2000; **72**: 64–70.
2. Ricour C, Duhamel JF, Nihoul-Fekete C. Nutrition entérale à débit constant chez l'enfant – techniques et indications dans 170 cas de 1969 à 1975. *Arch Fr Pediatr* 1977; **34**: 154–170.
3. American Society for Parenteral and Enteral Nutrition (ASPEN). Board of Directors. Guidelines for the use of enteral nutrition in the adult patient. *J Enteral Parent Nutr* 1987; **11**: 435–439.
4. Sogni P, Vidon N, Huchet B, Bernier JP. Gastric and duodeno-pancreatic functions during naso-gastric feeding in man: effect of infusion rate. *Gastroenterology* 1991; **98**: 344 (abstr).
5. Meyer JE. Motility of the stomach and gastroduodenal function. In Johnson LR, ed. *Physiology of the Gastrointestinal Tract*. New York: Raven Press, 1987: 613–629.
6. Hunt JN, Knox MT. A relation between the chain length of fatty acids and the slowing of gastric emptying. *J Physiol* 1968; **194**: 327–336.
7. Montoya ML, Carriere D, Hebuterne X et al. Motricité duodénale au cours de l'alimentation entérale à débit constant. *Gastroenterol Clin Biol* 1988; **12**: 143 (abstr).
8. Ducrotte P. Motricité digestive au cours de la nutrition entérale. *Ann Gastroenterol Hepatol* 1988; **24**: 277–280.
9. Ducrotte P, Chayvialle JA, Lerebours E et al. Effects of intravenous and intraduodenal fat on jejunal motility and on plasma cholecystokinin in man. *Dig Dis Sci* 1988; **33**: 558–564.
10. Douard H, Cosnes J, Sebog A et al. Etude échographique de la motricité vésiculaire au cours de l'alimentation entérale continue exclusive. *Gastroenterol Clin Biol* 1987; **11**: 643–647.
11. Pet I, Ladas S, Forgacs IC et al. Comparison of effects of ingested medium- and long-chain triglyceride on gall-bladder volume and release of cholecystokinin and other gut peptides. *Dig Dis Sci* 1987; **32**: 481–486.
12. Taylor IL, Byrne WJ, Christie DL et al. Effect of individual L-amino acids on gastric acid secretion and serum gastric and pancreatic polypeptide release in humans. *Gastroenterology* 1982; **83**: 273–275.
13. Grant JP, Dabey MC, Crae J, Snyder PJ. Effect of enteral nutrition on human pancreatic secretions. *J Parenter Enteral Nutr* 1987; **11**: 302–308.
14. Vidon N, Chaussade S, Merite F et al. Inhibitory effect of high caloric load of carbohydrates or lipids on human pancreatic secretions: a jejunal brake. *Am J Clin Nutr* 1989; **50**: 231–236.
15. Freeman JB, Fairfull-Smith RJ. Current concepts of enteral feeding. In *Advances in Enteral Feeding*. Kingsport, TN: Year Book Medical Publishers, 1983; **16**: 75–112.
16. Monn CL, Ling V, Bourassa D. Small intestinal and colonic changes induced by a chemically defined diet. *Dig Dis Sci* 1980; **25**: 123–128.
17. Heymsfield SB, Casper K, Grossman GD. Bioenergetic and metabolic response to continuous versus intermittent nasoenteric feeding. *Metabolism* 1987; **36**: 570–575.
18. Nacht CA, Schutz Y, Vernet O et al. Continuous versus single bolus enteral nutrition: comparison of energy metabolism in humans. *Am J Physiol* 1986; **251**: E524–E529.
19. Leblanc J, Cabanac M, Samson P. Reduced post prandial heat production with gavage as compared with meal feeding in human subjects. *Am J Physiol* 1984; **246**: E95–E101.
20. Ricour C, Duhamel JF, Arnaud-Battandier F et al. Enteral and parenteral nutrition in the short bowel syndrome in children. *World J Surg* 1985; **9**: 310–315.
21. Goulet O, Revillon Y, Jan D et al. Neonatal short bowel syndrome. *J Pediatr* 1991; **119**: 18–23.
22. Galea MH, Holliday H, Carachi R, Kapila L. Short bowel syndrome: a collective review. *J Pediatr Surg* 1992; **27**: 592–596.
23. Vanderhoof JA, Langnas A, Pinch L et al. Short bowel syndrome. *J Pediatr Gastroenterol Nutr* 1992; **14**: 359–370.
24. Sondheimer J, Cadnapaphornchai M, Sontag M, Zerbe GO. Predicting the duration of dependence on parenteral nutrition after neonatal intestinal resection. *J Pediatr* 1998; **132**: 80–84.
25. Kaufman SS. Prevention of parenteral nutrition-associated liver disease in children. *Pediatr Transplant* 2002; **6**: 37–42.
26. Avery GB, Villavicencio O, Lilly JR, Randolph JG. Intractable diarrhea of infancy. *Pediatrics* 1968; **41**: 712–722.
27. Goulet O, Brousse N, Canioni D et al. Syndrome of intractable diarrhea with persistent villous atrophy in early childhood: a clinicopathological survey of 47 cases. *J Pediatr Gastroenterol Nutr* 1998; **26**: 151–161.
28. Guarino A, Spagnulo MI, Russo S et al. Etiology and risk factors of severe and protracted diarrhea. *J Pediatr Gastroenterol Nutr* 1995; **20**: 173–178.
29. Brasseur D, Goyens P. Enteral nutrition for therapy of chronic diarrhea. *Diarrheal Dis* 1997; **38**: 289–316.
30. Guandalini S. Prolonged diarrhea: etiology and pathogenesis. *Diarrheal Dis* 1997; **38**: 153–170.
31. Weizman Z, Schmueli A, Deckelbaum RJ. Continuous nasogastric drip elemental feeding: alternative for prolonged parenteral nutrition in severe prolonged diarrhea. *Am J Dis Child* 1983; **137**: 253–255.
32. Orenstein SR. Enteral versus parenteral therapy for intractable diarrhea of infancy: a prospective, randomized trial. *J Pediatr* 1986; **109**: 277–286.
33. Vanderhoof J, Murray ND, Kaufman SS et al. Intolerance to protein hydrolysate infant formulas: an under recognized cause of gastrointestinal symptoms in infants. *J Pediatr* 1997; **131**: 741–744.
34. Morin CL, Roulet M, Roy CC, Lapointe N. Continuous elemental enteral alimentation in the treatment of children and adolescents with Crohn's disease. *J Parenter Enteral Nutr* 1982; **6**: 194–199.
35. O'Morain C, Segal AW, Levi AJ. Elemental diet as primary treatment of acute Crohn's disease: a controlled trial. *BMJ* 1984; **288**: 1859–1862.
36. Seidman EG, Roy CC, Weber AM, Morin CL. Nutritional therapy of Crohn's disease in childhood. *Dig Dis Sci* 1987; **32** (Suppl): 82S–88S.
37. Sanderson IR, Udeen S, Davies PSW et al. Remission induced by an elemental diet in small bowel Crohn's disease. *Arch Dis Child* 1987; **61**: 123–127.
38. Rigaud D, Cosnes J, Le Quintrec Y et al. Controlled trial comparing two types of enteral nutrition in treatment of active Crohn's disease: elemental vs polymeric diet. *Gut* 1991; **32**: 1492–1497.
39. Belli DC, Seidman E, Bouthillier L et al. Chronic intermittent elemental diet improves growth failure in children with Crohn's disease. *Gastroenterology* 1988; **94**: 603–610.

40. Thomas AG, Taylor F, Miller V. Dietary intake and nutritional treatment in childhood Crohn's disease. *J Pediatr Gastroenterol Nutr* 1993; **17**: 75–81.
41. Ruuska T, Savilahti E, Maki M et al. Exclusive whole protein enteral diet versus prednisolone in the treatment of active Crohn's disease in children. *J Pediatr Gastroenterol Nutr* 1994; **19**: 175–180.
42. Beattie RM, Schiffin EJS, Donnet-Hughes A et al. Polymeric nutrition as the primary therapy in children with small bowel Crohn's disease. *Aliment Pharmacol Ther* 1994; **8**: 609–615.
43. Breese EJ, Michie CA, Nicholls SW et al. The effect of treatment of lymphokine-secreting cells in the intestinal mucosa of children with Crohn's disease. *Aliment Pharmacol Ther* 1995; **9**: 547–553.
44. Griffiths AM, Ohlsson A, Sherrnan PM, Sutherland LR. Meta-analysis of enteral nutrition as a primary treatment of active Crohn's disease. *Gastroenterology* 1995; **108**: 1056–1067.
45. Heuschkel RB, Menache CC, Megerian JT, Baird AE. Enteral nutrition and corticosteroids in the treatment of active Crohn's disease in children. *J Pediatr Gastroenterol Nutr* 2000; **31**: 8–15.
46. Zachos M, Tondeur M, Griffiths AM. Enteral nutritional therapy for inducing remission of Crohn's disease. *Cochrane Database Syst Rev* 2001; **3**: CD000542.
47. Fell JM, Paintin M, Arnaud-Battandier F et al. Mucosal healing and a fall in mucosal pro-inflammatory cytokine mRNA induced by a specific oral polymeric diet in paediatric Crohn's disease. *Aliment Pharmacol Ther* 2000; **14**: 281–289.
48. Murch S, Walker-Smith JW. Nutrition in inflammatory bowel disease. *Baillière's Clin Gastroenterol* 1998; **122**: 719–738.
49. Akobeng AK, Miller V, Stanton J et al. Double-blind randomized controlled trial of glutamine-enriched polymeric diet in the treatment of active Crohn's disease. *J Pediatr Gastroenterol Nutr* 2000; **30**: 78–84.
50. Ruemmele FM, Roy CC, Levy E, Seidman EG. Nutrition as primary therapy in pediatric Crohn's disease: fact or fantasy? *J Pediatr* 2000; **136**: 285–291.
51. Colomb V, Goulet O, Gorski AM et al. Forme digestive sévère de purpura rhumatoïde. Etude rétrospective de 19 observations chez l'enfant. *Arch Fr Pediatr* 1990; **47**: 9–12.
52. Goulet O, Jobert-Giraud A, Michel JL et al. Chronic intestinal pseudoobstruction syndrome in pediatric patients. *Eur J Pediatr Surg* 1999; **9**: 83–89.
53. Faure C, Goulet O, Ategbo S et al. Chronic intestinal pseudoobstruction syndrome: clinical analysis, outcome and prognosis in 105 children. *Dig Dis Sci* 1999; **44**: 953–959.
54. Heneyke S, Smith VV, Spitz L, Milla PJ. Chronic intestinal pseudo-obstruction : treatment and long term follow up of 44 patients. *Arch Dis Child* 1999; **81**: 21–27.
55. Turck D, Michaud L. Cystic fibrosis: nutritional consequences and management. *Baillières Clin Gastroenterol* 1998; **12**: 805–822.
56. Bertrand JM, Morin CL, Lasalle R et al. Short term clinical, nutritional and functional effect of continuous elemental enteral alimentation in children with cystic fibrosis. *J Pediatr* 1984; **104**: 41–46.
57. Boland MP, Stoski D, Macdonald N et al. Chronic jejunostomy feeding with a non-elemental formula in undernourished patients with cystic fibrosis. *Lancet* 1986; **1**: 232–234.
58. Shephard RW, Holt TL, Thomas BJ et al. Nutritional rehabilitation in cystic fibrosis, controlled studies of effects on nutritional and growth retardation, body protein turnover and course of pulmonary disease. *J Pediatr* 1986; **109**: 788–794.
59. Gaskin K, Allen J. Exocrine pancreatic disease including cystic fibrosis. In Walker A, Watkins J, Duggan C, eds. *Nutrition in Pediatrics. Basic Science and Clinical Applications.* London: BC Decker, 2003: 671–685.
60. Steinkamp G, Von Der Hardt H. Improvement of nutritional status and lung function after long-term nocturnal gastrostomy feeding in cystic fibrosis. *J Pediatr* 1994; **124**: 244–249.
61. Goulet OJ, De Ville De Goyet J, Otte JB, Ricour C. Preoperative nutritional evaluation and support for liver transplantation in children. *Transplant Proc* 1987; **19**: 3249–3255.
62. Kaufmann SS, Murray ND, Wood RP et al. Nutritional support for the infant with extra hepatic biliary atresia. *J Pediatr* 1987; **110**: 679–686.
63. Protheroe SM, Kelly DA. Cholestasis and end-stage liver disease. *Baillières Clin Gastroenterol* 1998; **12**: 823–841.
64. Moreno LA, Gottrand F, Hoden S et al. Improvement of nutritional status in cholestatic children with supplemental nocturnal enteral nutrition. *J Pediatr Gastroenterol Nutr* 1991; **2**: 213–216.
65. Moukarzel AA, Najm I, Vargas J et al. Effect of nutritional status on outcome of orthotopic liver transplantation in pediatric patients. *Transplant Proc* 1990; **22**: 1560–1563.
66. Campos AC, Matias JE, Coelho JC. Nutritional aspects of liver transplantation. *Curr Opin Clin Nutr Metab Care* 2002; **5**: 297–307.
67. Sokal EM. Nutritional and medical care in chronic cholestasis. In Buts JP, Sokal EM, eds. *Management of Digestive and Liver Disorders in Infants and Children.* Amsterdam: Elsevier, 1993: 537–542.
68. Kaufmann SS, Scrivner DJ, Murray ND et al. Influence of Portagen and Pregestimil on essential fatty acid status in infantile liver disease. *Pediatrics* 1992; **89**: 151–154.
69. Sokal EM, Baudoux MC, Collette E et al. Branched chain amino acids improve body composition and nitrogen balance in a rat model of extra-hepatic biliary atresia. *Pediatr Res* 1996; **40**: 66–71.
70. Haynes L, Atherton DJ, Ade-Ajayi N et al. Gastrostomy and growth in dystrophic epidermolysis bullosa. *Br J Dermatol* 1996; **134**: 872–879.
71. Fung EB, Samson-Fang L, Stallings VA et al. Feeding dysfunction is associated with poor growth and health status in children with cerebral palsy. *J Am Diet Assoc* 2002; **102**: 361–373.
72. Samson-Fang L, Butler C, O'Donnell M. Effects of gastrostomy feeding in children with cerebral palsy: an AACPDM evidence report. *Dev Med Child Neurol* 2003; **45**: 415–426.
73. Wales PW, Diamond IR, Dutta S et al. Fundoplication and gastrostomy versus image-guided gastrojejunal tube for enteral feeding in neurologically impaired children with gastresophageal reflux. *J Pediatr Surg* 2002; **37**: 407–412.
74. Briassoulis G, Zavras N, Hatzis T. Malnutrition, nutritional indices, and early enteral feeding in critically ill children. *Nutrition* 2001; **17**: 548–557.
75. Donaldson SS, Jundt S, Ricour C et al. Radiation enteritis in children. *Cancer* 1975; **35**: 1167–1178.
76. Mauer AM, Burgess JB, Donaldson SS et al. Special nutrition needs of children with malignancies: a review. *J Parenter Enteral Nutr* 1990; **14**: 315–324.
77. Deswarte-Wallace J, Firouzbakhsh S, Finklestein JZ. Using research to change practice: enteral feedings for pediatric oncology patients. *J Pediatr Oncol Nurs* 2001;**18**: 217–223.

78. Pietsch JB, Ford C, Whitlock JA. Nasogastric tube feedings in children with high-risk cancer: a pilot study. *J Pediatr Hematol Oncol* 1999; **21**: 111–114, Comment 88–90.
79. Wasmer SJ, Abitbol C, Alexander S et al. Nutritional requirements for infants with renal failure. *Am J Kidney Dis* 1986, **7**: 300–305.
80. Kleinknecht C, Laouari D, Burtin M et al. Contribution of experimental studies on the nutritional management of children with chronic renal failure. *Pediatr Nephrol* 1991; **5**: 487–491.
81. Salzer HR, Haschke F, Wimmer M et al. Growth and nutritional intake of infants with congenital heart disease. *Pediatr Cardiol* 1989; **10**: 17–23.
82. Bougle D, Iselin M, Kahyat A, Duhamel JF. Nutritional treatment of congenital heart disease. *Arch Dis Child* 1986; **61**: 799–801.
83. Jouvet P, Jugie M, Rabier D et al. Combined nutritional support and continuous extracorporeal removal therapy in the severe acute phase of maple syrup urine disease. *Intensive Care Med* 2001; **27**: 1798–1806.
84. Greene HL, Slonim AE, Barr IA, Moran JR. Type 1 glycogen storage disease. Five years of management with nocturnal intragastric feeding. *J Pediatr* 1980; **96**: 590–595.
85. Fernandes J, Alaupovic P, Wit JM. Gastric drip feeding in patients with glycogen storage disease type I: its effects on growth and plasma lipids and apolipoproteins. *Pediatric Res* 1989; **25**: 327–331.
86. Collins JE, Leornard JV. The dietary management of inborn errors of metabolism. *Hum Nutr Appl Nutr* 1985, **39A**: 255–272.
87. Stanbury JB, Wyngaarden JB, Fredrickson DS et al. *The Metabolic Basis of Inherited Disease*, 5th edn. New York: McGraw Hill.
88. Franck DA, Ziesel SH. Failure to thrive. *Pediatr Clin North Am* 1988; **35**: 1187–1206.
89. Bithoney WG, McJunkin JJ, Michalek J et al. The effect of a multidisciplinary team approach on weight gain in monoorganic failure-to-thrive children. *J Dev Behav Pediatr* 1991; **12**: 254–258.
90. Fosson A, Knibbs J, Bryant-Waugh R, Lask B. Early onset anorexia nervosa. *Arch Dis Child* 1987; **62**: 114–118.
91. de Tournemire R, Alvin P. Anorexia nervosa and severe malnutrition: nutritional practice guidelines in pediatrics. *Arch Pediatr* 2002; **9**: 429–433.
92. Mamel JJ. Percutaneous endoscopic gastrostomy. *Am J Gastroenterol* 1989; **84**: 703–710.
93. Ho CS, Yee ACN, McPherson R. Complications of surgical and percutaneous non endoscopic gastrostomy: review of 233 patients. *Gastroenterology* 1988, **95**: 1206–1210.
94. Anderson C. Enteral feeding: a change in practice. *J Child Health Care* 2000; **4**: 160–162.
95. Segal D, Michaud L, Guimber D et al. Late-onset complications of percutaneous endoscopic gastrostomy in children. *J Pediatr Gastroenterol Nutr* 2001; **33**: 495–500.
96. Gauderer MW. Percutaneous endoscopic gastrostomy and the evolution of contemporary long-term enteral access. *Clin Nutr* 2002; **21**: 103–110.
97. Doede T, Faiss S, Schier F. Jejunal feeding tubes via gastrostomy in children. *Endoscopy* 2002; **34**: 539–542.
98. Carrillo EH, Heniford BT, Osborne DL et al. Bedside percutaneous endoscopic gastrostomy. A safe alternative for early nutritional support in critically ill trauma patients. *Surg Endosc* 1997; **11**: 1068–1071.
99. Grimble GK, Rees RG, Keohane PP et al. Effect of peptide chain length on absorption of egg protein hydrolysates in the normal human jejunum. *Gastroenterology* 1987; **92**: 136–142.
100. Silk DBA, Fairclough PO, Clark ML et al Uses of a peptide rather than a free amino-acid nitrogen source in chemically defined elemental diets. *J Parenter Enteral Nutr* 1980; 4: 548–553.
101. Fairclough PD, Hegarty JE, Silk DBA, Clark ML. Comparison of the absorption of two protein hydrolysates and their effects on water and electrolyte movements in the human jejunum. *Gut* 1980; **21**: 829–834.
102. Poullain MG, Cezard JP, Roger L, Mendy F. Effect of whey proteins, their oligopeptide hydrolysates and free amino acid mixtures on growth and nitrogen in fed and starved rats. *J Parenter Enteral Nutr* 1989; **13**: 382–386.
103. Burrin DG, Stoll B. Key nutrients and growth factors for the neonatal gastrointestinal tract. *Clin Perinatol* 2002; **29**: 65–96.
104. Bach AC, Babayan VK. Medium-chain triglycerides: an update. *Am J Clin Nutr* 1982; **36**: 950–962.
105. Ingenbleek Y. Les triglycérides à chaînes moyennes en nutrition clinique. *Nutr Clin Metab* 1989; **3**: 3–15.
106. Lima LAM, Gray OP, Losty H. Excretion of dicarboxylic acids following administration of medium chain triglycérides. *J Parenter Enteral Nutr* 1987; **11**: 600–601.
107. Bines J, Francis D, Hill D. Reducing parenteral requirement in children with short bowel syndrome: impact of an amino acid-based complete infant formula. *J Pediatr Gastroenterol Nutr* 1998; **26**: 123–128.
108. Andorsky DJ, Lund DP, Lillehei CW et al. Nutritional and other postoperative management of neonates with short bowel syndrome correlates with clinical outcomes. *J Pediatr* 2001; **139**: 27–33.
109. Berbaum JC, Pereira GR, Watkins JB, Peckham GJ. Non nutritive sucking during gavage feeding enhances growth and maturation in premature infants. *Pediatrics* 1983; **71**: 41–45.
110. Widstrom AM, Marchini G, Matthiesen AS et al. Non nutritive sucking in tube-fed preterm infants: effects on gastric motility and gastric contents of somatostatin. *J Pediatr* 1988; **7**: 517–523.
111. American Gastroenterological Association Patient Care Committee. American Gastroenterological Association technical review on tube feeding for enteral nutrition. *Gastroenterology* 1995; **108**: 1282–1301.
112. Aspen Board of Directors and the Clinical Guidelines Task Force. Guidelines for the use of parenteral and enteral nutrition in adult and pediatric patients. *J Parenter Enteral Nutr* 2002; **26**(1 Suppl): 1SA–138SA.
113. Iyer PU. Nutritional support in the critically ill child. *Indian J Pediatr* 2002; **69**: 405–410.
114. Gorman SR, Armstrong G, Allen KR et al. Scarcity in the midst of plenty: enteral tube feeding complicated by scurvy. *J Pediatr Gastroenterol Nutr* 2002; **35**: 93–95.
115. Perez-Rodriguez J, Quero J, Frias EG, Omenaca F. Duodenal perforation in a neonate by a tube of silicone rubber during transpyloric feeding. *J Pediatr* 1978; **92**: 113–114.
116. Hand RW, Kempster M, Levy JH et al. Inadvertent transbronchial insertion of narrow bore feeding tubes into the pleural space. *JAMA* 1984; **251**: 2396–2397.
117. Boros SJ, Reynolds JW. Duodenal perforation: a complication of neonatal nasojejunal feeding. *J Pediatr* 1974; **85**: 107–108.
118. Anderson KR, Norris DJ, Godfrey LB et al. Bacterial contamination of tube-feeding formulas. *J Parenter Enteral Nutr* 1984; **8**: 673–678.
119. Casewell MW, Cooper JE, Webster M. Enteral feeds contaminated with *Enterobacter cloacae* as a cause of septicaemia. *BMJ* 1981; **282**: 973.
120. De Leeuw IH, Vandewoude MF. Bacterial contamination of enteral diets. *Gut* 1986; **27**: 56–57.

121. Goulet O, Duhamel JF, Ricour C. Nutritional problems. In Tinker J, Zapol WM, eds. *Care of the Critically Ill Patient*. Berlin: Springer Verlag, 1992: 1415–1436.
122. Patchell CJ, Anderton A, Macdonald A et al. Bacterial contamination of enteral feeds. *Arch Dis Child* 1994; **70**: 327–330.
123. Mehall JR, Kite CA, Gilliam CH et al. Enteral feeding tubes are a reservoir for nosocomial antibiotic-resistant pathogens. *J Pediatr Surg* 2002; **37**: 1011–1012.
124. Matlow A, Wray R, Goldman C et al. Microbial contamination of enteral feed administration sets in a pediatric institution. *Am J Infect Control* 2003; **31**: 49–53.
125. Mehall JR, Kite CA, Saltzman DA et al. Prospective study of the incidence and complications of bacterial contamination of enteral feeding in neonates. *J Pediatr Surg* 2002; **37**: 1177–1182.
126. Greene HL, Helinek GL, Folk CC et al. Nasogastric tube feeding at home: a method for adjunctive nutritional support of malnourished patients. *Am J Clin Nutr* 1981; **34**: 1131–1138.
127. Reeves-Garcia J, Heyman MB. A survey of complications of pediatric home enteral tube feedings and discussion of developmental and psychosocial issues. *Nutrition* 1988; **4**: 375–377.
128. Aiges H, Markowitz J, Rosa J, Daum F. Home nocturnal supplemental nasogastric feedings in growth-retarded adolescents with Crohn's disease. *Gastroenterology* 1989; **97**: 905–910.
129. Claris-Appiani A, Ardissino GL, Dacco V et al. Catch-up growth in children with chronic renal failure treated with long-term enteral nutrition. *J Parenter Enteral Nutr* 1995; **19**: 175–178.
130. Elia M. An international perspective on artificial nutritional support in the community. *Lancet* 1995; **345**: 1345–1349.
131. Howard L, Ament M, Fleming CR et al. Current use and clinical outcome of home parenteral and enteral nutrition therapies in the United States. *Gastroenterology* 1995; **109**: 355–365.
132. Elia M. Home enteral nutrition: some general aspects and comparison between the USA and Britain. *Nutrition* 1994; **10**: 1–9.
133. Parker T, Neale, Elia M. Home enteral tube feeding in East Anglia. *Eur J Clin Nutr* 1996; **50**: 47–53.
134. Holden CE, Puntis JWL, Charlton CPL, Booth IW. Nasogastric feeding at home: acceptability and safety. *Arch Dis Child* 1991; **66**: 148–151.
135. Holden CE, Macdonald A, Ward M et al. Psychological preparation for nasogastric feeding in children. *Br J Nurs* 1997; **6**: 376–385.
136. Ganga-Zanzou PS, Hankard R, Gottrand F et al. Nutrition entérale à domicile chez l'enfant et l'adolescent. Expérience à propos de 79 patients. *Ann Pediatr* 1995; **42**: 295–231.
137. Liptak GS. Home care for children who have chronic conditions. *Pediatr Rev* 1997; **18**: 271–273.
138. Marin OE, Glassman MS, Schoew BT, Caplan DB. Safety and efficacy of percutaneous endoscopic gastrostomy in children. *Am J Gastroenterol* 1994; **98**: 357–360.
139. Crocker KS. Current status of home infusion therapy. *Nutr Clin Pract* 1992; **7**: 256–263.

34 Parenteral nutrition in infants and children

Olivier Goulet and Virginie Colomb

Introduction

In the late 1960s in the USA, Dudrick and Wilmore demonstrated that long-term administration of hypertonic nutrient infusates through a catheter inserted into the superior vena cava was feasible, with immediate dilution of the hypertonic solution, preventing damage to the vein.[1,2] By infusing a hypertonic mixture of glucose, protein hydrolysate, electrolytes, minerals and vitamins, they proved that it was possible to achieve normal growth and development in an infant with multiple small-bowel atresia.[1,2] Indeed, parenteral nutrition (PN), since its introduction in clinical practice during the late 1960s has enabled many patients to survive and has reduced the incidence of malnutrition related to a variety of digestive and non-digestive diseases. With antibiotics, antitumoral chemotherapy and organ transplantation, PN can be considered as one of the most important therapeutic advances over the past 50 years since it has demonstrated its potential for changing the course of both medical and surgical patients.

Technical aspects, psychological consequences of feeding 'deprivation' and a high rate of complications led to suspicion of this therapeutic strategy at the early phase of its development. However, continuous clinical and basic research has allowed improvements in its efficiency and reduction in the rate of complications. PN is now widely used in a variety of indications as reviewed below. PN provides macro- and micronutrients and calories directly through the systemic circulation. Although such delivery short circuits the portal circulation, macronutrients such as lipids, glucose and amino acids, and micronutrients, can be infused in high concentrations without causing harmful effects and these are sufficient for nutritional maintenance and normal growth in children. Nevertheless, in some situations, such as those encountered in neonatology, gastroenterology or hematology, PN could be better adapted to the clinical condition by providing specific nutrients. This chapter will briefly review the indications, modalities, intakes and complications of PN for infants, children and adolescents. A specific chapter in this book is dedicated to parenteral nutrition in the newborn. Many references to reviews are provided and the reader is invited to refer to these for further details.

Indications of parenteral nutrition

Digestive and extradigestive indications

PN is indicated in children for prevention or treatment of malnutrition, whatever its cause, as soon as it becomes impossible to use the enteral route. The range of PN indications, related both to digestive and non-digestive diseases (Table 34.1), has greatly increased during the last few years. However, because of the iatrogenic risk of the technique, especially when its use is prolonged, each indication should be discussed while PN should be, as often as possible, performed in specialized units, such as intensive care, hematology–oncology or gastroenterology units.

Gastrointestinal (GI) indications for PN can be subdivided into three main situations: malabsorption syndromes,[3–5] indications of bowel rest (e.g. Crohn's disease),[6,7] and congenital or acquired neonatal pathology of the GI tract. Short-bowel syndrome is the oldest and one of the most classic indications for long-term PN.[8–13] Some congenital or acquired metabolic diseases, such as severe hepatic or renal failure with Gl complications may benefit from PN with appropriate amino acid solutions. An increasing area of use of PN is represented by the management of children with malignant disease.

Table 34.1 Indications for parenteral nutrition

Digestive indications
Malabsorption medical and/or surgical
Protracted and intractable diarrhea
Short-bowel syndrome
Enterocutaneous fistula
Proximal enterostomy
Intestinal bacterial overgrowth
Immune deficiency
Indication of bowel rest
Inflammatory bowel disease (Crohn's disease, ulcerative colitis, unidentified colitis)
Necrotizing enterocolitis
Intestinal lymphangiectasy
Acute pancreatitis
Systemic disease: Schönlein–Henoch, periarteritis
Radiation enteritis
Congenital or acquired neonatal pathology of the GI tract
Gastroschisis
Omphalocele
Meconial ileus
Extensive small-bowel resection
Necrotizing enterocolitis
Complicated Hirschsprung's disease
Chronic intestinal pseudo-obstruction syndrome
Extradigestive indications
Neonatology: premature baby <1200–1500g
Metabolic disease
End-stage liver disease
Congenital disorders of metabolism
Cystic fibrosis
Hematology and oncology
Solid tumors
Leukemia
Bone marrow transplantation
Nephrology
Severe renal disease
Severe tubulopathy
Renal failure
Hypercatabolism
Burned
Polytraumatism
Surgery

Due to both the treatment and the disease, these patients often suffer from anorexia and vomiting which may preclude adequate oral or enteral feeding.[14] In addition, chemotherapy and/or radiation may damage the intestinal mucosa and blood vessels including lymphatics and, thus, interfere with GI motility. Finally, PN has dramatically changed the management of oncological chemotherapy protocols.[14–16]

PN can also be indicated as a nutritional supplement in end-stage liver disease, during the waiting period before orthotopic liver transplantation.[17–20] The same is required in the severe phase of cystic fibrosis when lung transplantation is required.

Sometimes PN may be the only way of maintaining an adequate nutritional intake even when the GI tract is intact, for example after multiple trauma or extensive burns. In these situations, PN may also be necessary to maintain nutritional status despite increased nitrogen catabolism or excessive nitrogen losses.

Long-term parenteral nutrition

Cyclic parenteral nutrition

As soon as permitted by the metabolic and nutritional status, cyclic PN should be started. The term cyclic PN refers to the administration of intravenous fluids intermittently with regular breaks from infusion.[21–23] The metabolic, physical and psychological advantages of cyclic infusion are well known and the tolerance of such a mode of PN delivery has been documented in children.[24–30] Cyclic PN might lower the risk for the development of liver disease. Hwang et al carried out a prospective study in adults on PN who were exhibiting various degrees of presumed PN-associated liver disease.[31] Patients who developed hyperbilirubinemia were randomized to either remain on continuous PN or were placed on cyclic PN. Patients with initial serum bilirubin of less than 20mg/dl, who remained on continuous PN, had a significant rise in serum bilirubin compared with the cyclic PN group. There was no apparent advantage of cyclic PN in patients with serum bilirubin greater than 20mg/dl. Similar studies in pediatric patients are not available. Finally, cyclic PN offers the advantage of increasing the mobility of the patient and family, and cyclic PN is the only way in which PN can be delivered at home.

Home parenteral nutrition

Home PN is the only alternative to prolonged hospitalization for patients requiring long-term PN.[32–36] Such patients certainly need to be managed by a specialized center, from which a home PN program can be organized.[37] Nutrition is generally mixed parenteral and enteral, but it may be exclusively parenteral, lasting for months or years. Indications include total or subtotal resection of the small bowel; chronic intestinal pseudo-obstruction syndromes; intractable diarrhea caused by refractory atrophy of the intestinal mucosa with severe and persistent malabsorption, either alone or in association with an immune deficiency; and some cases of inflammatory bowel diseases (IBDs), especially severe Crohn's disease, either extensive and/or with multiple surgery, with growth retardation or that have not responded to other therapy. The objective of long-term PN in these cases is to ensure normal growth of the child while the inflammatory syndrome subsides or while waiting for the residual intestinal condition to become stable.

Whatever the duration of PN and the prognosis of the disease, home PN offers the patients and their families the best possible quality of life.[37] In addition, home PN reduces the cost of care, when compared to prolonged hospitalization.[36] Cyclic infusion, adequate and appropriate provision of macro- and micronutrients, and improvements in central venous catheters (CVCs) and nutritional mixtures have all played a major role in making home PN possible. The development of an infrastructure for patient training and follow-up, a PN-solution compounding unit, and an efficient domiciliary delivery service are required to organize home PN. Over the past 25 years, more than 300 children treated at Necker-Enfants Malades Hospital have been discharged on home PN. Most home PN indications were primary digestive diseases: short-bowel syndrome accounted for 47% of the indications, the other main indications being IBD (11%), chronic intestinal pseudo-obstruction syndrome (10%) and intractable diarrhea of infancy (8%). Fifty-four per cent of the patients have been weaned from PN, 26% are still on home PN, and 16% have died. Survival rates at 2 and 10 years were 97% and 81%, respectively. Most of the PN-related complications were from infection, with about two CVC-related infection for 1000 home PN days (Colomb et al. Submitted for publication). However, the most life-threatening home PN-related complication is liver disease. The French results, as well as those of other teams (Boston), suggest that home PN is the best option for children in need of long-term PN.

Ethical dilemmas may arise for children with extensive GI resection, microvillous atrophy or persistent villous atrophy who are never able to tolerate full enteral feeding. In such patients, in whom intestinal autonomy cannot be achieved, intestinal transplantation may represent the only alternative to lifelong PN.[38–41] Indications for intestinal transplantation are not only extreme short-bowel syndromes but also all situations in which the small intestine is unable to achieve nutritional requirements; this includes intractable diarrhea of infancy (chronic villous atrophy, microvillus inclusion disease) or severe motility disorders such as chronic intestinal pseudo-obstruction syndrome.

Parenteral nutrition in clinical practice

Vascular access

Central venous access for the purpose of supplying parenteral nutrition to the pediatric age group requires a careful definition of the patient's caloric need, estimated duration of therapy, and an assessment of available sites. Peripheral venous administration is the easiest and least hazardous method, requiring rigorous asepsis, especially in malnourished children. However, only iso-osmolar solutes, providing insufficient protein-energy intake, can be used because of the risk of superficial phlebitis. In some cases, a further limiting factor can be that access to superficial veins is restricted or impossible. Peripherally inserted central catheters offer a new technology for accessing central veins while obviating the risk of central vein access.[42]

Infusion into the superior vena cava with a CVC is often necessary.[43] However, the use of a CVC is accompanied by specific complications, such as thrombosis or sepsis. There are several routes of central vein access and there are a variety of catheters available for placement. Tunneled percutaneous placement of silicone rubber-cuffed catheters via the subclavian vein approach is the most commonly used technique, the size of the catheter being selected according to the child's weight and age.[44–46] A CVC with a Dacron® cuff, ensuring efficient anchoring, may be inserted either percutaneously or surgically. In each case the cutaneous and venous entry sites should be separated by a 5–10-cm subcutaneous tunnel; one must be careful since subcutaneous tissue is particularly thin in severely malnourished children.[43] The risks of such access catheters include the mechanical risks of placement, venous thrombosis of the access sites and, most importantly, catheter-related infections, either at the exit site or at the subcutaneous tunnel or pouch, or even generalized sepsis. The cutaneous exit site should be given meticulous daily care using iodinized disinfectants and be protected by an occlusive dressing, which is changed every day. Implantable devices for long-term vascular access are also used in children, especially in those with cancer requiring intravenous chemotherapy.[47] The exclusive use of these devices for long-term home PN is rare and, in our experience, not well accepted by the children. In long-term home PN patients who have received many CVCs, we create an arteriovenous fistula.[48] With a full knowledge of the spectrum of access techniques, access materials and risks, safe total parenteral nutrition can be safely delivered to the children in need.

The use of a 0.22-mm antibacterial membrane filter between the catheter and the administration tubing during perfusion remains recommended. The choice of pump is important, satisfying three criteria: reliability at low flow rates; ease of use; and fitted with a safety alarm capable of signaling a change in flow rate, an air bubble or a blockage leading to increased pressure. Solutions for parenteral nutrition must be prepared under strict asepsis by using antibacterial filters under a laminar flow hood.

Parenteral nutrition supplies

After a period of development of the technique and of improvement in prevention of complications, PN is now widely used in a variety of indications in pediatric patients. Macro- and micronutrients given exclusively through the central vein for prolonged periods are sufficient for nutritional recovery and maintenance as well as long-term growth in children. One of the current objectives is to adapt the PN intakes to the clinical and nutritional situation. Indeed, it is essential that the composition of the intravenous feeding solution be adjusted according to age and disease as well as to the clinical and biological criteria and as a function of the progressive transition from parenteral to enteral feeding.

Energy requirements

Defining energy requirements is mandatory to achieve adequate energy intake and to avoid overfeeding or underfeeding. Basal metabolic rate (BMR) and resting energy expenditure (EE) may be used for achieving adequate energy intake. BMR is the EE of a recumbent patient in a thermoneutral environment after a 12–18 h fast just when the individual has awakened, but before starting daily activities. BMR reflects the EE required for vital processes. Resting EE refers to the EE of a person at rest in a thermoneutral environment. BMR and resting EE do not usually differ by more than 10%. Equations may be used for calculating BMR or resting EE.[49–51] Most of them are based on body weight, height, age and sex. None of them will predict energy requirements with acceptable precision for daily clinical use.[49] The resting EE of a stable hospitalized child requiring PN may be measured by using indirect calorimetry.[52] However, energy intake must cover total EE, that is the sum of requirements for basal metabolism, thermic effect of food, thermoregulation and physical activity. In older children, physical activity may account for a large proportion of total EE, especially when he is able to be on cyclic PN. On the other hand, requirements for a malnourished child who requires catch-up growth, or the requirements for a critically ill patient are a matter of debate. Some data are available in infants or children after surgery[53–55] or in an ICU.[56–60] It has been thought that aggression, such as surgery, inflammation state or sepsis, increases energy requirements proportionally to the severity of the illness. However, the increased EE is short-lived. Newborns have a 20% increase in resting EE after major surgery, but this elevation returns to baseline within 12–24 h.[53] Another study performed by Jaksic et al failed to show any difference in EE between non-ventilated surgical neonates (gastro-schisis, atresia, volvulus) on postoperative day 16 (±12 SD) compared with infants on extracorporeal life support studied at 7 ± 3 days of age.[54]

Finally, these studies suggest that postoperative or critically ill infants and children do not require much more than their resting EE. Overestimation of the energy requirements for the entire postoperative period, or for any protracted period of time, may result in overfeeding and subsequent metabolic impairment. In addition, there may be significant interindividual variations in EE.

Measuring resting EE in critically ill infants and children is difficult because of the expensive equipment and the expertise required. Nevertheless, Pierro et al and White et al proposed formulas for estimating EE in intensive care patients.[61,62] On a daily clinical practice, energy intake may be adapted and monitored according to the patient's weight gain, the absence of water overload and evidence of overfeeding. In premature babies and infants, supplies vary from 150 kcal/kg per day to 100 kcal/kg per day, and are reduced to 60–80 kcal/kg per day in older children and adolescents.

Energy sources

Glucose

Glucose is the unique carbohydrate used during total PN. Few data are available for establishing the optimal glucose intake for children receiving PN and thus avoiding overfeeding from glucose. From the estimation of glucose utilization by the brain, which varies according to age, it is possible to discuss two issues: the contribution of gluconeogenesis in the glucose supply; and the glucose oxidation capacity on total body level.[63] Gluconeogenesis provides a significant amount of glucose (even in preterm infants) and suggests that not all the glucose has to be provided exogenously.[64,65]

The rate of parenteral glucose delivery must be kept constant without exceeding the maximum rate of glucose oxidation (RGO), which differs strongly among patients according to age and clinical status. In critically burned children, the maximal RGO has been found to be 5 mg/kg per min.[66] In appropriate-for-gestational-age preterm infants, the RGO does not exceed 6–7 mg/kg per min (9.5 g/kg per day),[67] while in term surgical infants or infants on long-term total PN, the maximal RGO is about 12 mg/kg per min (18 g/kg per day).[68–70] Data collected in stable adult patients on long-term PN show a maximal RGO much lower than in children and infants.[71,72] By excluding the preterm infants and by taking into account the brain to total body weight ratio, and according to glucose brain consumption, one could consider that maximal RGO is continuously decreasing from birth to adulthood. Thus, the rate of glucose administration should be adapted to age and clinical situation, e.g. premature babies, critically ill patients, severe malnutrition (Table 34.2).

Consequences of excessive glucose intake (Table 34.3)

When glucose is administered in excess of the amount that can be directly oxidized for energy and glycogen production, the excess is directed to lipogenesis[73,74] and promotes fat deposition, which may be a nutritional goal in some clinical situations. This conversion probably accounts, in part, for the increase in EE observed with high rates of glucose infusion.[71] Excessive glucose intake is thought to increase CO_2 production and minute ventilation but few relevant data are available to support this evidence.[75–77] Total energy delivery, as well as amino acid intake, are responsible for increased CO_2 production and minute ventilation.[76,77] Excessive glucose intake may also impair liver function, especially by inducing steatosis, while its

Table 34.2 Recommended range of glucose intake for infants and children

Glucose/kg body weight per 24 h	Day 1	Day 2	Day 3	Day 4
Infant < 10 kg	8	12	14	16–18
Child < 15 kg	6	8	10	12–14
15–20 kg	4	6	8	10–12
20–30 kg	4	6	8	< 12
>30 kg	3	5	8	< 10

Intakes have to be adapted to clinical situations (i.e. severe malnutrition, sepsis); use of drugs (i.e. steroids, somatostatin, tacrolimus, etc.); expected weight gain for normal or catch-up growth; oral and/or enteral energy simultaneous intake

Table 34.3 Consequences of excessive glucose intake

Hyperglycemia
Increased CO_2 production and minute ventilation
Increased energy expenditure
Lipogenesis and fat tissue deposition
Steatosis and liver dysfunction (increased transaminases)
Increased production of VLDL triglycerides

VLDL, very low-density lipoprotein

contribution to the development of cholestasis is not clearly established.[78,79] Studies in normal adult volunteers suggest that high carbohydrate feeding leads to an increase in total very low-density lipoprotein (VLDL) triglyceride secretion rate from *de novo* synthesis primarily due to stimulation of the secretion of preformed fatty acids.[80] The results imply that the liver derives all its energy from carbohydrate oxidation as opposed to fatty acid oxidation, such that fatty acids taken up by the liver are channeled into VLDL triglycerides.[80] Hepatic steatosis results when export of the VLDL triglycerides does not keep pace with production.[80,81]

It is obvious that PN is associated with an increased risk of infectious complications compared with enteral feeding or no nutritional support.[82–85] Nevertheless, data suggest that hyperglycemia might be a risk factor for infection,[86–88] especially in critically ill patients.[89] These data have to be confirmed. Total PN may be associated with insulin resistance, due to both the substrate infusion and the underlying disease.[32] Therefore, particular attention must be paid to glucose tolerance (hyperglycemia, glucosuria) at the time of starting cyclic PN, when decreasing the duration of infusion may lead to excessive increase in the glucose rate of delivery. In patients on stable long-term total PN, glucosuria may reveal a stressful event, particularly infection, which impairs sensitivity to insulin. Recommendations for glucose administration during cyclic PN are provided in Table 34.4.

Table 34.4 Cyclic parenteral nutrition (PN)

Cyclic PN is well tolerated and may be used from 3–6 months of age
Advantages of cyclic PN
achieves insulin/glucagon balance
improves protein synthesis
prevention of liver disease
physical and psychological
home parenteral nutrition
Hyperinsulinic response prevents hyperglycemia even with a rate of glucose infusion as high as 1.4 g/kg/h
Safety recommendations
use maximum rate of infusion <1.2 g/kg/h
slow increase and decrease of infusion to avoid hyper/hypoglycemia or osmotic load

Lipids

Intravenous fat emulsions (IVFEs) are usually added to the PN regimen because they provide essential fatty acids and a concentrated source of calories with a relatively low osmotic load. IVFEs enable the physician to provide a highly concentrated source: 2.2 kcal/ml for the 20% emulsion, compared to 0.68 kcal/ml for a 20% dextrose solution. The concentrated calories and low osmolality of IVFEs make them ideal for peripheral parenteral nutrition. The use of IVFEs also allows the energy input to be diversified, with a reduction in the consequences of excessive glucose supply. In addition, it was well demonstrated in adults, as well as in pediatric patients, that the use of IVFEs improves net nitrogen balance.[69,90–92]

The most widely used IVFEs in infants and children, derived from soybean oil, provide 100% long-chain triglycerides. Since essential fatty acids are required for a variety of physiological functions, prolonged lipid-free total PN is likely to produce essential fatty acid deficiency,[93–96] when glucose infusion stimulates insulin secretion, which reduces lipolytic activity and prevents release of tissue linoleic acid stores. The onset of essential fatty acid deficiency is even more rapid when there is a pre-existing nutritional lack, such as in small-for-gestational-age neonates and premature babies or malnourished infants. Newborns and pre-weanlings have very limited essential fatty acid stores; therefore, 70% of infants less than 1 year old on lipid-free total PN develop essential fatty acid deficiency within 1–2 weeks.[97] The restart of

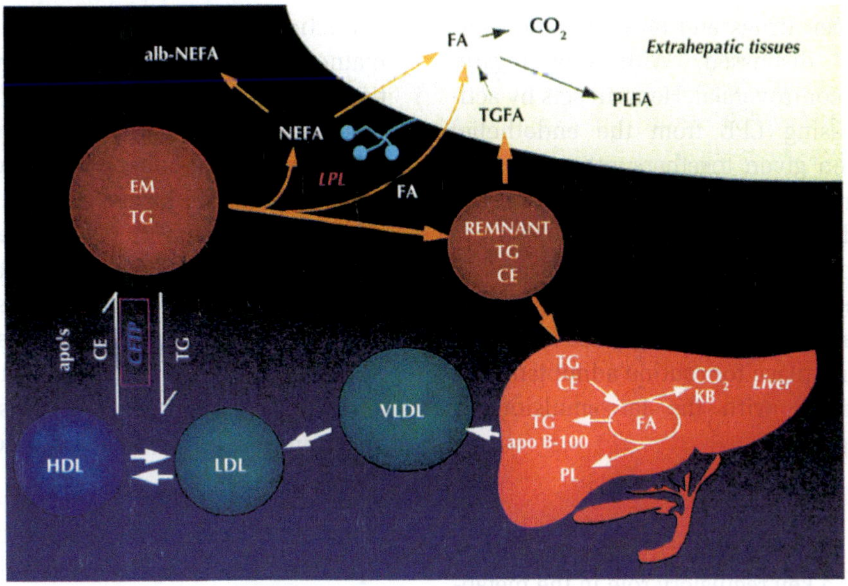

Figure 34.1 Metabolism of intravenous fat emulsions. NEFA, non-essential fatty acids; TG, triglycerides; PL, phospholipids; LPL, lipoprotein lipase; CETP, cholesterol ester transferase.

anabolism, because of adequate energy and nitrogen intakes, can lead to onset of essential fatty acid deficiency. A linoleic acid supply of about 2–3% of the total energy input is recommended in children on total PN.[98] A daily supply of 4% or 450mg of linoleic acid per 100kcal is often necessary to correct a pre-existing deficiency. IVFEs also include α-linolenic acid (C18:3 n-3). Although its function and requirements are still poorly defined, an intake of about 40–50mg/kg per 24h, equal to about 0.5% of the total energy intake, is normally provided.

Administration of IVFEs is required as soon as possible in a patient on total PN, according to the clinical status. Two important issues have to be considered for IVFE administration: the rate of IVFE delivery is a major determinant of the rate of fat clearance from the bloodstream and the optimal glucose/lipid ratio for optimal energetic substrate utilization (oxidation) and avoidance of fat overload.

Intravascular metabolism of lipids

Clearance of lipid emulsions

The composition of IVFEs results in a mixture of artificial chylomicrons having physicochemical characteristics very similar to those of the natural chylomicrons produced by enterocytes. They are hydrolyzed by lipoprotein lipase (LPL) in capillaries of adipose tissue and muscle. This step determines the rate at which fatty acids from the emulsion are transported into the tissue for storage or oxidation. Like many other key enzymes, LPL can be regulated both in amount and in activity. The amount of LPL at the capillary endothelium is under hormonal control, while its activity is regulated by the specific activator apo CII[99] (Figure 34.1).

Lipid clearance tests have been developed in the past but are not used routinely in clinical practice. They allow understanding of the factors determining the elimination of exogenous fat emulsions from the circulation.[100] Patients with moderate trauma, for example after cholecystectomy, have an increased fractional elimination rate in comparison with healthy controls. Critically ill patients on the other hand have an elimination rate which is lower or close to that of healthy controls.[101]

The composition of an exogenous fat emulsion is also important in determining its elimination from the circulation. The emulsifying agent is one important factor in this respect. The egg yolk phospholipids that are mostly used, give emulsions that are eliminated very rapidly. IVFEs with high concentrations of phospholipids, i.e. 10% emulsions, should be avoided as they carry a higher risk of producing high serum levels of triglycerides, cholesterol and phospholipids than other emulsions, i.e. 20% and 30% emulsions.[102,103]

Interaction between drugs and fat elimination has frequently been discussed. With this regard, heparin remains controversial. Heparin acts by activating and releasing LPL from the endothelial surface and, when given together with exogenous fat emulsions, causes a sharp increase in circulating LPL activity and free fatty acid levels. Sometimes this might be a positive effect, but in patients with already high free fatty acid levels an increase in lipolysis may lead to extremely high free fatty acid values. There is no place for routine administration of heparin together with the fat emulsion as proposed in the past.[104]

Interactions with lipoproteins

Lipoproteins play a key regulatory role in the metabolism and elimination of exogenous lipids. Endogenous VLDL particles undergo degradation to LDL in plasma under the action of LPL. These particles contain apo CII which acts as an activator of LPL. Exogenous triglyceride particles are hand-led in the same way but have to acquire apo CII mainly from the high-density lipoprotein (HDL) fraction before they can be hydrolyzed. During the degradation of VLDL particles there is a continuous exchange of apolipoproteins and surface material. The serum HDL concentration is positively correlated to the fractional elimination rate of exogenous fat emulsions.

Routine assessment of patients receiving IVFEs should include, before and during the course of treatment: fasting plasma triglycerides, total cholesterol, and plasma LDL and HDL cholesterol. A normal plasma triglyceride level does not mean that exogenous triglycerides are adequately used (oxidation) or stored (adipose tissue). Indeed, part of the exogenous lipid may be cleared by other mechanisms, especially capture by the reticuloendothelial system (RES). In contrast, high plasma triglyceride levels suggest impaired clearance related to excessive infusion rate and/or decreased LPL activity. Reduced LPL activity may be due to prematurity, malnutrition, acidosis, hyponatremia, hypoalbuminemia-related high free fatty acid plasma levels, high plasma phospholipid levels, or cytokines such as tumor necrosis factor-α (TNF-α).

Contraindictions to the use of IVFEs

Despite the advantages of IVFEs and the need to correct any essential fatty acid deficiency, there are restrictions to the administration of lipids to malnourished patients. The lower the capillary tissue mass (a situation found in preterm infants and malnourished patients), the slower is the rate of intravenous fat emulsion clearance. Therefore, the longer the infusion time, the less is the risk for the patient to develop hypertriglyceridemia.[105,106] In very malnourished patients, LPL activity reappears rapidly with the onset of anabolism. The substrate itself also stimulates LPL synthesis. It is therefore recommended that IVFEs should not be administered until a few days after the start of parenteral nutrition in severely malnourished patients.

There may also be several classic contraindications to the use of IVFEs during the initial phase, such as sepsis, thrombocytopenia, disseminated intravascular coagulation, respiratory distress syndrome or metabolic acidosis. Furthermore, administration of IVFEs during neonatal jaundice must be handled carefully as there is a risk of displacing non-conjugated bilirubin from albumin with free fatty acids. Finally, inadequate clearance of IVFEs may result in RES overload as suggested by the so-called 'fat overload syndrome' (see below).

Optimal glucose/fat ratio

In the past, total PN for adults, children and infants provided most of the energy as glucose, although it was not precisely known how much of the intravenously administered glucose was oxidized. Glucose-based total PN has been shown to cause adverse effects related to glucose storage, particularly as fat. This might account for the extensive lipid deposition reported both in liver and adipose tissue.[107,108] In these conditions, fat infusion further increases fat deposition and may result in fat overloading. Thus, substitution of part of the glucose calories avoids the undesirable effects reported with glucose-based total PN. Studies performed in infants or neonates have assessed glucose and fat utilization.[109] By using five isocaloric total PN regimens differing in their glucose/lipid ratio, it was possible to assess for the optimal glucose infusion rate.[110] Fat infusion aiming at a significant contribution to the coverage of energy expenditure requires that glucose oxidation be equal to or lower than maximal oxidative glucose disposal. Hence, glucose infusion rates should not exceed 18 g/kg per day. A study in malnourished infants and young children showed that the amount of infused lipid mmust be adapted to lipid oxidation capacity.[110] There is a maximal lipid utilization rate of about 3.3–3.6 g/kg per day. Above these values there is an increased risk of fat deposition secondary to the incomplete metabolic utilization of infused lipid. Pierro et al showed similar results in a short-term study performed in surgical neonates on total PN.[111]

Fat overload syndrome

Clinical expression

IVFEs have been thought to impair immune function, but no relevant data are available suggesting an impairment.[112] Acute clinical and biological expression was described as mimicking septic syndrome but related to macrophage activation. Symptoms include high fever, hepatosplenomegaly, jaundice, respiratory distress syndrome, bleeding, thrombocytopenia, disseminated intra-vascular coagulation, metabolic acidosis and hypoalbuminemia.[113] This so-called 'fat overload syndrome' is thought to be related to the capture of exogenous particles by the RES. Cessation of lipid administration is insufficient most of the time for improving a patient's condition. Steroids may stop the process of macrophage activation. More recently we reported several cases of severe cholestasis apparently related to long-term administration of intravenous lipids.[114]

Mechanisms of lipid toxicity

Although lipids are necessary in patients on PN, they are strongly suspected to be toxic in some cases. The metabolism of their oxidized fraction is relatively well known; far less is known about the destiny of the non-oxidized fraction, which is captured by the RES in the liver and also by the spleen, bone marrow and lungs. Chronic administration of lipid emulsions might overload reticuloendothelial cells and induce their acute or chronic activation. It must be noticed, however, that an excess of liver macrophages and portal infiltration with eosinophils has previously been described in PN-dependent patients, although not attributed to lipid toxicity.[115] Accumulation of exogenous lipids in the liver Kupffer cells may also impair the clearance of endotoxins and increase their deleterious effect on the liver. Moreover, the peroxidation of exogenous lipids could produce toxic metabolites despite the simultaneous infusion of vitamin E.[116] Phytosterols contained in lipid emulsions may also have a deleterious effect on biliary secretion.[117]

Short-term as well as long-term lipid use must be included in all total PN programs in infants and children. However, there is a relationship between lipid emulsions, macrophage activation syndrome, thrombocytopenia and cholestasis in a pediatric population homogeneous for liver disease risk factors. Since lipids are indispensable in PN-dependent children, we recommend prevention through limitation of lipid supply and infusion rhythm to the patient's theoretical oxidizing capacity (Table 34.5). The preventive role of long-term use of emulsions containing a low proportion of polyunsaturated fatty acids needs to be explored in further studies.

Table 34.5 Recommendations for lipid administration

Use of 20% lipid emulsion
Maximal daily amount of 2–2.5 g/kg (<30% of non-protein energy intake)
Slow infusion rate, such as 0.10–0.15 g/kg per h
Addition of α-tocopherol 0.6 mg/g of long-chain triglycerides
Routine monitoring of triglyceride plasma levels, liver function tests and platelet count

Other types of intravenous fat emulsion

Non-protein energy is provided by glucose and lipids. The oxidation rate of these two components is dependent on the glucose/lipid ratio, type and quality of fat emulsion, and the clinical, nutritional, and metabolic state of the patient. Most of the knowledge comes from studies performed in children of different age groups and by using the reference 20% soybean oil emulsion. Concerns have been raised about providing infants and children with soy oil-based emulsions as their sole lipid intake. New intravenous fat emulsions are now used and others are currently under development.

Medium-chain triglycerides

Emulsions containing 50% of their triglycerides as medium-chain triglycerides (MCTs) have been shown to be cleared more rapidly and are now widely used in adult and pediatric patients.[118–120] Fatty acids from the hydrolysis of MCTs are the primary substrate for ketogenesis. Carnitine is needed to transport long-chain fatty acids into the mitochondria, but malnourished and seriously ill patients may be carnitine-depleted. An energy source able to bypass this route into the mitochondria would in theory, be useful for such patients. The MCT/long-chain triglyceride (LCT) lipid emulsion (B. Braun, Germany) contains 50% LCTs to avoid any possible side-effects from excessive amounts of MCTs and to provide essential fatty acids. Medium-chain fatty acids can enter the mitochondria by simple diffusion, independent of the carnitine enzyme, and produce an elevation of plasma ketones.[118,119] MCTs have been shown to improve nitrogen balance in postoperative patients but this positive effect remains controversial according to several other studies.[120–122] There have been several published studies in children using MCTs.[123–126] Their use in malnourished infants after 15 days on total PN indicates that they are well tolerated and could provide advantages in terms of nitrogen metabolism by supplying the equivalent of 25% non-protein energy intake.[124] MCT emulsions have also been used in home PN pediatric patients with beneficial effect in reducing cholestasis.[125]

Structured triglyceride emulsion

To improve the safety and the efficiency of MCT-containing fat emulsions, a structured triglyceride emulsion, containing both long-chain and medium-chain fatty acids bound to the same carbon skeleton, has been synthesized. Such structured triglyceride emulsions have been shown to improve nitrogen retention and muscle protein synthesis in animal models and in humans.[127,128] There is is no study currently available in pediatric patients.

Fish oil-based emulsions

Fish oil triglycerides are also now being considered for PN either as pure fish oil particles or incorporated into MCT/LCT emulsions. Fish oil is now proposed as a component of lipid emulsions. By providing a high amount of long-chain polyunsaturated fatty acids (PUFAs), they are reported to have anti-inflammatory effects.[129,130] There is a study currently being carried out in pediatric patients.

Olive oil-based IVFEs

It is well known that a high intake of monounsaturated fatty acids in the form of olive oil is associated with a lower incidence of cardiovascular morbidity.[131] In patients dependent on long-term PN, the availability of intravenous fat emulsions containing lower amounts of unsaturated fatty acids could be of interest.[132,133] New 20% fat emulsions containing 17% olive oil and only 3% soybean oil are now available.[133] It has been shown in a long-term pediatric study that olive oil-based emulsion preserves essential fatty acid status and fatty acid elongation and decreases total cholesterol.[133] The olive oil group showed better measurements of antioxidant activity against lipid peroxidation. The same olive oil- and vitamin E-enriched emulsion was recently reported as a valuable alternative for PN of preterm infants who are often exposed to oxidative stress, while their antioxidative defense is weak.[134]

Carnitine and α-tocopherol

Carnitine plays a central role in metabolism especially for optimal oxidation of fatty acids.[135] Carnitine, in the form of acylcarnitine transfers free fatty acids into mitochondria, where they are recombined with co-enzyme A (CoA) to form acyl-CoA.[135] Plasma levels of carnitine decrease rapidly in premature newborns and small-for-gestational-age neonates during the first days of life if no exogenous carnitine is provided.[136] Available studies did not assess the use of carnitine during long-term PN, a situation that is more likely to result in carnitine deficiency. Some authors have raised the question of carnitine supplementation for children on total PN.[137] As yet, in the absence of specific recommendations, a supplement of 2 mg/kg per day may be advisable.[138] Supplementation with α-tocopherol as antioxidant, added to IVFEs at a dose of 0.6 mg/g of unsaturated fatty acids is also recommended.

Nitrogen intake

Energy supply should be closely correlated with that of nitrogen. Nitrogen intake obviously depends on the age and degree of malnutrition.[140] In premature babies the intake varies from 400–500 mg to 650 mg/kg per day.[141] In infants, the intake varies from 400 mg[142] to 800 mg/kg per day in the case of great nitrogen losses from the GI tract. In older children, 300mg/kg per day is usually sufficient. Such intakes, which are higher than the growth requirement, cover excessive nitrogen losses induced by catabolism. Greater amounts are unsuitable, because with a constant caloric intake there is a negative correlation between nitrogen intake and the amount retained and the subsequent danger of hyperaminoacidemia, metabolic acidosis or iso-osmolar coma. Such intakes may also be responsible for excessive urinary losses of calcium and phosphorus and subsequent bone mineralization impairment.[143] Finally, usual nitrogen/energy ratio varies around 1g of nitrogen for 200–250kcal.

Nitrogen sources

Nitrogen sources available for PN come from various mixtures of crystalline L-amino acids. They have been shown to be effective in clinical use, providing appropriate nitrogen utilization and retention. Amino acid solutions for use in PN are selected according to the following criteria:[144,145]

(1) Whether the solution contains all or only some of the naturally occurring amino acids;

(2) Total amino acid nitrogen content;

(3) Osmolality and electrolyte content;

(4) Amount of essential amino acids per gram of total nitrogen (E/T);

(5) Non-nitrogen nutrient content (glucose, fructose).

New pediatric solutions have been developed which appear to be better suited for use in newborns, premature babies or malnourished infants (Primene, Clintec®; Vaminolac, Pharmacia®). Such products have an E/T ratio greater than 3 and differ from standard solutions in having a higher percentage of branched-chain amino acids; modified aromatic amino acid content (a one-third reduction in phenylalanine); modified sulfur amino acid content, with methionine reduced by 50% and an increase in cysteine content (both solutions also contain taurine, which is absent from standard solutions); and increased lysine content.

Other sources of nitrogen

Protein-energy malnutrition secondary to chronic disease, as well as acute illness such as injury or infection, are associated with loss of body fat and skeletal muscle mass. The loss of body tissue may be minimal and of little consequence in patients with normal nutritional status and a brief, self-limiting illness lasting a few days. However, when the disease is prolonged and the patient is malnourished, a variety of clinical events may occur in association with the catabolic state. These alterations include immunosuppression, delayed wound healing and tissue repair, and loss of muscle strength.[146] The accelerated breakdown of body protein can be slowed by the administration of adequate quantities of energy, protein (amino acids) and other essential nutrients. However, measurements of body composition and substrate-flux studies indicate that it is extremely difficult to maintain or replenish body protein during catabolism.[146] Thus, reducing the debility associated with the catabolic process could potentially enhance recovery and decrease the consequences of illness on protein retention and height–growth velocity. Because the efficacy of nutrition cannot be improved easily by quantitative modifications, attention has focused in recent years on qualitative improvments. The addition of specific amino acids or other sources of nitrogen to the feeding formulas might be logical in critically ill children (sepsis, burns, trauma) or in patients with chronic inflammatory processes such as severe Crohn's disease.

Glutamine

Glutamine is the most abundant amino acid in the body.[147] However, glutamine is absent from the currently available amino acids solutions. Indeed, glutamine is considered as unstable in aqueous solutions and during heat sterilization with the formation of pyroglutamic acid and ammonia. Although glutamine is a non-essential amino acid, the nutritional requirement for this amino acid during catabolic illness may differ greatly from that during health.[147] During starvation or stress, the concentration of free glutamine in the intracellular amino acid pool of skeletal muscle rapidly decreases. Glutamine exported from the muscle is used primarily by visceral organs; in the kidney it serves as an ammonia donor; in the gastrointestinal tract it serves as a primary oxidizable fuel source for enterocytes and colonocytes.[148,149] Glutamine also supports other rapidly proliferating tissue, such as fibroblasts or lymphocytes. Glutamine-supplemented total PN has been shown to preserve gut structure and to improve gut immune function in animal models.[150] Studies have shown the clinical benefits of glutamine-supplemented total PN in adult patients undergoing bone marrow transplantation.[151–154] The use of glutamine-containing dipeptides is proposed because of the instability of free glutamine. Improved nitrogen balance has been shown in patients receiving alanyl-glutamine-supplemented total PN.[155] In addition, glutamine dipeptide-supplemented PN prevents intestinal atrophy and increased permeability in critically ill adult patients.[156]

Ornithine α-ketoglutarate

Another source of nitrogen for patients on PN is represented by ornithine α-ketoglutarate (OKG). This is a salt formed with two molecules of ornithine and one molecule of α-ketoglutarate. OKG has been successfully used by the enteral and parenteral route in burn, traumatized and surgical patients and in chronically malnourished patients.[159,160] According to the situation, OKG administration decreases muscle protein catabolism and/or increases protein synthesis. The mechanism of action of OKG is not fully understood, but it was clearly demonstrated that it is a precursor of glutamine.[162,163] In addition, the secretion of anabolic hormones (insulin, human growth hormone) and the synthesis of metabolites (polyamines, arginine, ketoacids) may be involved.[160,161] In prepubertal children on PN, administration of OKG (15 g/day) reversed growth retardation and increased insulin-like growth factor I (IGF-I) plasma levels.[161]

Finally, it seems likely that, in the near future a more specific therapeutic approach to protein metabolism might be achieved. This prospect is of great importance for children with regard to the consequences of inadequate protein metabolism on growth velocity.

Table 34.6 Vitamin requirements

	Infants	Children
Vitamin A (μg)	300–750	450–1000
Vitamin D (IU)	100-1000	200–2500
Vitamin E (mg)	3–10	10–15
Vitamin K (μg)	50–75	50–70
Vitamin B_1 (mg)	0.4–0.5	1.5–3
Vitamin B_2 (mg)	0.4–0.6	1.1–3.6
Vitamin B_5 (mg)	2–5	0.5–5
Vitamin B_6 (mg)	0.1–1.0	1.5–2
Vitamin B_{12} (μg)	0.3–3	3–100
Vitamin C (mg)	25–35	20–100
Folic acid (μg)	20–80	100–500
Biotin (μg)	35–50	150–300
Niacin (mg)	6–8	5–40

Table 34.7 Trace element requirements

Element	Infants (/kg/day)	Children (/day)
Iron (mg)	50	100–2500
Zinc (mg)	100–250	1000–5000
Copper (mg)	20–30	200–300
Selenium (μg)	2–3	30–60
Manganese (μg)	1–10	50–250
Molybdenum (μg)	0.25–10	50–70
Chrome (μg)	0.25–2	10–20
Iodine (μg)	1–5	50–100
Fluoride (μg)	20	500–1000

Other components of PN solutions

Water and electrolyte intake must be varied according to the age and condition of the child, needing adjustment, for example, if there are intestinal losses. Premature babies need 150–200 ml water per kilogram body weight daily to maintain equilibrium; infants require 120–140 ml/kg and older children 80–100 ml/kg per day. All normal babies and children need 3–5 mmol chloride, sodium and potassium per kilogram per day. When there are losses due to vomiting or gastric aspiration 8 mmol sodium, 1 mmol potassium, 6 mmol H^+ ions and 12 mmol chloride should be added to each 100 ml of water. In the case of an enterostomy, 15 mmol sodium, 1 mmol potassium, 10 mmol of chloride and 5 mmol bicarbonate should be added to each 100 ml of water.

With a nitrogen intake of 400 mg/kg per day and a calcium intake of 1.7 mmol/kg per day, the daily requirement of phosphorus is 2.3 mmol/kg for bone growth and nitrogen anabolism. If the phosphorus intake is lower or the intake of nitrogen and/or calcium is higher, severe phosphorus depletion results. Magnesium requirements are usually satisfied by 1 mmol/kg per day.

Vitamin and trace element intakes are provided as a function of the intake of the respective nutrients and their anabolism. For infants and older children, adherence to the recommendations in Tables 34.6 and 34.7 helps to prevent depletion or excess. These intakes should be adjusted in cases of catabolic stress, such as an infection or intestinal losses.

All-in-one mixture[162–168]

Administration of IVFEs together with the glucose amino acids in a three-in-one mixture is now widely used in children. There are a number of potential advantages to PN admixtures but also some drawbacks. In addition to reducing cost, use of a PN admixture simplifies the patient's life in that only a single infusion pump with less tubing and other accessories is needed.[162] There is also evidence that it reduces the risk of bacterial growth in intravenous fat emulsion even after 24 h.[163]

Stability is directly related to the concentration of the components, and is dependent on pH and temperature. If the mixture is not compatible, the fat emulsion will break, forming an oil–water interphase that can be seen floating on top of the mixture. Because the admixture is a physical mix of naturally incompatible substances (oil and water, calcium and phosphorus), their utilization requires strict attention to pharmaceutical guidelines for preparation, storage and use.[164,165] Particulate matter (mobile, undissolved substances such as precipitates of calcium and phosphorus that are unintentionally present in products) resulting from inappropriate preparation or storage can be life-threatening. To reduce the risk of precipitates reaching the patient an in-line filter should be used. This should be a 1.2 μm air-eliminating filter (in contrast to the 0.22 μm air-eliminating filter recommended for non-lipid-containing PN). A PN admixture is considered inappropriate for administration if $>0.4\%$ of the total fat contains particles $>5\,\mu m$ in size.[166] Some drugs are compatible with PN admixtures but not with traditional PN, and vice versa.[167]

It is possible to formulate total PN mixtures that have good short-term stability and that satisfy the nutritional requirements of most patients. Several companies produce a three-in-one mixture with good long-term stability. Retention of long-term stability in a mixture containing electrolytes is more difficult, although advances are being made in this area. The development of complete total PN mixtures with long-term stability will be assisted by advances in our understanding of the fundamental physical chemistry of colloid mixtures, particularly the interaction between emulsions and amino acids. Indeed such a ternary solution may lead to lipid instability, and/or catheter obstruction. PN admixtures should only be used in patients who are clinically stable. Solutions may be stable when refrigerated and become unstable at room temperature. Changes in the formulation of PN admixtures are more costly than changes in traditional (two-in-one) PN because of the wastage of both the dextrose amino acid and its components, and the intravenous fat emulsion. A number of questions remain about PN admixtures. These include the appropriate dosing of some vitamins, the true risks related to particulate matter and fat-droplet size, and drug compatibilities.

Refeeding syndrome

Pathophysiology

If PN is required because of severe malnutrition and inability of the GI tract to cover the protein-energy requirements, it has to be provided very carefully.[168] Indeed, refeeding syndrome may be observed in severely malnourished patients receiving concentrated calories via PN.[169] This syndrome includes the metabolic and physiological consequences of the depletion, repletion, compartmental shifts and inter-relationships of the following: phosphorus, potassium, magnesium, glucose metabolism, vitamin deficiency and fluid resuscitation.[170,171] The net effect of the hormonal and metabolic changes of starvation is to facilitate survival by a reduction in basal metabolic rate, conservation of protein and prolongation of organ function, despite the preferential catabolism of skeletal muscle tissue. Infants and children who have suffered from malnutrition for weeks or months will also experience a significant loss of visceral cell mass. Refeeding the malnourished child disrupts the adaptative state of semi-starvation.

As refeeding is initiated there is a rapid reversal in insulin, thyroid and adrenergic endocrine systems. Basal metabolic rate increases and glucose becomes the predominant cellular fuel. The body immediately begins the process of rebuilding lost tissue. Anabolism is accompanied by a positive balance of intracellular minerals. As minerals shift to intracellular spaces, serum levels may plummet. Body fluid compartments redistribute as intracellular fluid increases; extracellular fluid may increase or decrease depending on the previous intake, the persistent digestive losses and the refeeding regimen. These rapid changes in metabolic status can create life-threatening complications, so the nutritional regimen must be chosen wisely and monitored closely. Several potential metabolic complications of the refeeding syndrome are listed in the Table 34.8.

To reduce the risk of refeeding complications, several conditions are required at the initial phase of renutrition of severely malnourished infants and children.

Prevention of water and sodium overload

It is necessary to reduce the patient's water and sodium intake, depending on the hydration state, to prevent water and sodium overload resulting from their excessive retention, accentuated by increased secretions of vasopressin and aldosterone. Early weight gain may be the consequence of fluid retention. The monitoring of water and electrolyte intake must include uncontrolled losses as well as those from the GI tract. One of the difficulties in such situations is the need to take into account a third factor, such as intraperitoneal or intestinal fluid retention. Monitoring of body weight changes, urine collection, and assessment of blood and urinary electrolytes are essential.

Oncotic pressure restoration

The infusion of macromolecules aims to restore oncotic pressure and to minimize hemodynamic problems, worsened by a water–electrolyte imbalance. Albumin is the best infusate, but fresh-frozen

Table 34.8 Metabolic disorders associated with refeeding syndrome

Hypophosphatemia
Cardiac: altered myocardial function, arrhythmia, congestive heart failure, sudden death
Hematological: altered red blood cell morphology, hemolytic anemia, white blood cell dysfunction, thrombocytopenia, depressed platelet function, bleeding
Hepatic: liver dysfunction
Neuromuscular: acute areflexic paralysis, confusion, coma, cranial nerve palsies, diffuse sensory loss, Guillain–Barré-like syndrome, lethargy, paresthesias, rhabdomyolysis, seizures, weakness
Respiratory: acute ventilatory failure

Hypokalemia
Cardiac: arrhythmias, cardiac arrest, increased digitalis sensitivity, orthostatic hypotension, ECG changes (T-wave flattening or inversion, U waves, ST segment depression)
Gastrointestinal: constipation, ileus, exacerbation of hepatic encephalopathy
Metabolic: glucose intolerance, hyporeftexia, paralysis, paresthesias, respiratory depression, rhabdomyolysis, weakness
Renal: decreased urinary concentrating ability, polyuria and polydypsia, nephropathy with decreased glomerular filtration rate, myoglobinuria (secondary to rhabdomyolysis)

Hypomagnesemia
Cardiac: arrhythmias, tachycardia, torsade de pointes
Gastrointestinal: abdominal pain, anorexia, diarrhea, constipation
Neuromuscular: ataxia, confusion, fasciculations, hyporeftexia, irritability, muscle tremors, painful paresthesias, personality changes, positive Trousseau's sign, seizures, tetany, vertigo, weakness

plasma or blood may be required in cases of anemia and/or coagulation disorders. Artificial ventilation may be required in those, generally few, cases having a poor cardiorespiratory status.

Intake of carbohydrates

Constant administration of carbohydrate is required to maintain blood glucose homeostasis as the reserves are very low; parenteral administration of glucose requires care because of the risk of hyperglycemia with osmotic diuresis and hyperosmolar coma.

Potassium repletion

Correction of potassium depletion is of great importance, but should be achieved progressively with monitoring of renal and cardiac functions. It can be dangerous to try to correct the deficiency too rapidly at a stage where the capacity for fixing potassium remains low because of reduced protein mass; excessive intake leads to the cardiac risk of hyperkalemia.

Body temperature monitoring

It must be monitored, since protein-energy malnutrition (PEM) can lead to hypothermia, often associated with hypoglycemia and bradycardia. On the other hand, hyperthermia or excessive reheating increases water loss as well as energy expenditure. Maintenance of a stable body temperature between 36°C and 37°C by appropriate warming techniques is essential. Careful daily nursing to prevent cutaneous lesions and musculotendinous retractions is also very important.

Prevention of infection

The infective, metabolic and GI problems must be constantly borne in mind during treatment of pediatric patients with severe PEM. The risk of infection, an expression of both specific and non-specific immunity depression, may jeopardize the prognosis and aggravate nutritional problems at any time. Clinical and paraclinical investigations must be performed repeatedly, to look for widening foci of infection (respiratory, GI, skeletal and urinary) and for their systemic spread. When a localized or systemic infection is identified, specific treatment is urgently required. The routine use of antibiotics in the absence of bacteriological evidence in a malnourished child is inadvisable; antibiotics should only be given if sufficient indirect evidence points to the likelihood of infection. Active intestinal parasitosis should, of course, be vigorously treated. Evidence or suspicion of an infection is an essential factor in modifying water, electrolyte and nutrient intake and also in the choice of the feeding technique.

Protein and energy intake

It is difficult to suppress protein catabolism under these conditions of stress and low-energy intake. Excessive nitrogen intake may lead to hyperammonemia and/or acidosis by exceeding the renal clearance capacity for H^+ and phosphate ions. An intake of 0.5–1 g/kg of parenteral amino acids or oral peptide is sufficient to maintain the plasma amino acid pool. The protein-energy deficiency and other related disorders must be corrected during the days following the initial period of stress. This type of correction should be made carefully and gradually since the deficits are profound and of longstanding. It is essential to provide both nitrogen and calories simultaneously and in the correct ratio. The increase in energy intake, if progressive, avoids acute episodes of sodium and water retention accompanied by oliguria and a fall in urinary sodium and potassium output. It is likely that these changes are carbohydrate dependent, since their occurrence and equally rapid reversal develop with changes in glucose rate of glucose infusion. This antinatriuretic effect of glucose appears to be similar to the antinatriuresis observed during feeding after a phase of experimental fasting. The insulin secreted induces sodium tubular reabsorption, and the alkalosis that develops might be due to increased tubular absorption of bicarbonate.

Micronutrients

The provision of appropriate nutrient solutions requires an understanding of the nutritional relationships between nutrients electrolytes, vitamins and trace elements. It is during this initial phase that any deficit due to incorrect intake will become apparent through either clinical or laboratory signs. These deficits can usually be prevented by giving them in the following proportions: 200–250 kcal, nitrogen 1 g, calcium 1.8 mmol, phosphorus 2.9 mmol, magnesium 1.0 mmol, potassium 10 mmol, sodium and chloride 7 mmol, zinc 1.2 mg. Similarly, it is essential to adapt the intake of copper, manganese, chromium, iron, iodine, cobalt and fluoride, and the group B vitamins in particular; also, the intakes of essential fatty acids, tocopherol and selenium.

Adaptation of intake

After the initial phase of renutrition, most complications can be prevented by careful supervision and the provision of appropriate intakes. It is essential that the infusion rate, body temperature, cardiac and respiratory function, urinary volume, twice daily weight and digestive output are continuously monitored. During the first 5 days and also when the osmotic load is increased, urine should be checked for osmolality, pH, glucose and protein. The plasma and urinary ion data, plus the calcium, phosphorus, magnesium, glucose and hematocrits should be obtained twice during the first week, and then once weekly; plasma proteins, albumin, bilirubin, alkaline phosphatase and transaminase values should be assessed routinely. These data, and knowledge of the patient's state and age, should make it possible to progressively regulate and control the intake and avoid problems of overload or depletion.

Table 34.9 Complications during parenteral nutrition (PN)

Infectious
Local skin infections
Catheter-related sepsis
Complications of catheter-related sepsis: endocarditis, osteomyelitis
Metabolic
Water and/or sodium overload
Hyperosmolar coma
Excessive urinary losses
Hyperglycemia with glycosuria–hypoglycemia
Metabolic acidosis
Hyperazotemia–hyperammonemia
Hypokalemia
Hypophosphatemia
Hypercalcemia–hypercalciuria
Hypertriglyceridemia–hypercholesterolemia
Nutritional deficiencies
Essential fatty acid deficiency
Carnitine deficiency
Trace element deficiency: Fe, Zn, Cu, Se, Mo, etc.
Vitamin deficiency: A, E, B, B_{12}, folates, etc.
Long-term total PN
Total PN liver disease
Total PN bone disease
Hematological and coagulation disorders

Complications of parenteral nutrition (Table 34.9)

Catheter-related sepsis

In hospital as well as at home, catheter-related sepsis is one of the most serious complications which can arise during parenteral nutrition.[172–175] A 2-year prospective study of 185 CVCs showed a sepsis rate of 0.26%, with an overall incidence of one catheter-related sepsis per 278 days of total PN.[176] Systemic antibiotics provided sepsis control in 88% of the cases while CVC removal was required in the other cases. The factors significantly correlated with sepsis were: age (1–5 years); CVC type (surgically inserted CVCs were more frequently infected); local hemorrhage following CVC insertion; and local suppuration at the skin exit site.

Prevention of catheter-related sepsis requires strict asepsis during both CVC insertion and changes of filter and infusion sets. Daily care of the CVC skin exit site is of great importance. All PN solutions must be prepared under a laminar flow hood and filtered. The care of the child should be undertaken by physicians and nurses who have been specifically trained in this technique. Fever or clinical signs suggestive of catheter-related sepsis should lead to a thorough search for a source of sepsis, together with a white blood cell count, C-reactive protein and coagulation tests. Samples for blood culture should be taken via the catheter and from a peripheral vein. If fever persists, antibiotic therapy should be started early and include antibiotics against *Staphylococcus*. Coagulase-negative staphylococci (CoNS) is the most frequent blood culture isolate from neonates, infants and children with CVCs.[172,176] Clinicians vary in their management of suspected line sepsis, particularly that caused by CoNS. A vancomycin-containing regimen is widely used in infants and children suspected of having line sepsis. Procedures to prevent CoNS-positive blood cultures and to differentiate CoNS contaminants from pathogens are needed. For safely decreasing vancomycin use, clinical practice guidelines should be developed, implemented and evaluated. The guidelines should include optimal skin antisepsis and catheter disinfection before obtaining blood for culture, obtaining two blood cultures and using adjunctive tests and information to help differentiate contaminants from pathogens, and restriction on empiric vancomycin use.

Both catheter removal and infection dissemination may be avoided by starting antibiotics soon after onset of fever. However, removal of the catheter is systematically considered in case of fungal infection, infection due to *Staphylococcus aureus* with cutaneous infection, or if the patient continues to deteriorate even when appropriate antibiotic therapy had been started. In neonates who were infected with *Staphylococcus aureus* or with non-enteric Gram-negative rods, it was shown that delayed removal of the CVC was associated with complicated bacteremia.[174]

Otherwise, removal of the catheter is considered when blood cultures remain positive after several days of optimal antibiotic treatment, or when the PN program is close to completion. With good technique, displacement or obstruction of the catheter, or thrombosis of large vessels are rare. Careful technique should also help prevent superficial venous thrombophlebitis and the risk of dissemination of septic emboli.

Parenteral nutrition-related bone disease

The so-called PN-related bone disease resembles rickets, with fractures of the limbs which are sometimes asymptomatic and are only discovered after routine X-ray examination.[177] The most constant laboratory features are an elevated alkaline phosphatase activity and hypercalciuria, with normal or subnormal levels of vitamin D metabolites and parathyroid hormone. Bone histology shows osteomalacia-like changes with reduced mineralization and excess of osteoid tissue. The etiology of these bone lesions is probably multifactorial: excess vitamin D or disorders of its metabolism mean that it must be given very carefully on long-term parenteral nutrition. It is also possible to reduce the hypercalciuria by ensuring that the supplies of phosphorus, nitrogen and energy are properly balanced, while reducing the supply of amino acids, especially the sulfur-containing amino acids.[178] Finally, it is necessary to ensure that the solutions used for children during long-term PN are not contaminated with alum-inum.[179,180] Prevention of this 'bone disease' depends primarily on regular measurements of urinary calcium, which should not exceed 5 mg/kg per 24 h, and serum alkaline phosphatase activity. Measurement of bone mineral content is now widely performed using dual X-ray absorptiometry (DEXA) scan.[181]

Parenteral nutrition-related liver disease

Liver disease is a major side-effect of long-term PN. Fifteen years after the first reports its pathogeny is not completely understood.[182] Disruption of bile acid enterohepatic circulation in case of ileal amputation, impairment in choleresis in the absence of oral feeding, bacterial overgrowth due to bowel obstruction, stasis and lack of ileocecal valvula, are patient-dependent factors thought to contribute to PN-associated cholestasis.[183] One mechanism might be an increase in bile concentration of lithocholic acid.[184] Bacterial infections were also proposed as a co-factor in PN-related cholestasis, since the sepsis-associated cholestasis has been well described, both in human and animal models.[185–187] Duration of PN is also a known risk factor. Qualitative aspects of PN are also a matter of debate. It was experimentally demonstrated that an excess in total energy delivered induces liver lesions, reversible when decreasing the energy supply.[188] The role of amino acids was suspected, either an excess or a lack of them,[189,190] and an excessive glucose supply might induce steatosis through the increase in *de novo* lipogenesis.[191] Hepatobiliary complications of PN are now well recognized and documented. Such liver involvement may result in some cases in end-stage liver disease within a few months or years. Many PN-related and patient-related risk factors are involved in those hepatobiliary complications. Since the underlying digestive disease plays a prominent role, some pediatric patients requiring long-term PN are at high risk of developing liver disease. Short-bowel syndrome may be associated with disruption of bile acid enterohepatic circulation due to ileal amputation, impairment in choleresis when oral feeding is impossible, bacterial overgrowth due to bowel obstruction, stasis and lack of ileocecal valvula, which are all factors thought to contribute to PN-associated cholestasis. Recurrent septic episodes either catheter-related (Gram-positive bacteria) or digestive-related (Gram-negative sepsis from in-traluminal bacterial overgrowth) also contribute to liver injury.[192–197] Prematurity itself might be an associated factor. In addition, inadequate PN may have an additional deleterious effect on the liver because of metabolic disorders or micronutrient overload. Indeed, continuous PN infusion with excessive glucose intake is associated with hyperinsulinism and subsequent steatosis.[144] Inad-equate amino acid supply is thought to be responsible for metabolic dysfunction of the liver. Excessive aluminum, iron, or chromium intake might be responsible for liver injury.[179,180,198,199]

The earliest and most sensitive, but not specific laboratory markers are serum alkaline phosphatase and γ-glutamyl transferase activities, while hyperbilirubinemia is the latest marker of cholestasis to appear. Steatosis is the first non-specific histological abnormality. Steatosis may result either from excessive glucose supply leading to lipogenesis, or from the deposition of exogenous IVFE. Clinical liver enlargement, confirmed by ultrasonography, may appear within a few days after PN onset. Cholestasis together with portal and periportal cell infiltration leads to fibrosis. This indicates severe liver disease, which can lead to cirrhosis and liver failure, but is fortunately rare if PN is performed correctly. More recently, the association of cholestasis with thrombocytopenia has been described in patients on PN,[114] but the link between liver disease and the RES overload needs to be better understood.

Careful monitoring of hepatic function is extremely important in order to minimize factors responsible for liver disease. Some measures have been found to limit or reverse liver disease and may include:

(1) The stimulation of the entero-biliary axis by ingestion of LCTs or breast milk, or by injection of cholecystokinin analogs;[200]

(2) The reduction of intraluminal bacterial overgrowth caused by intestinal stasis by giving metronidazole and/or performing tapering enteroplasty;[201]

(3) The use of ursodesoxycholic acid (10–20 mg/kg per day) or tauroursodeoxycholic acid could contribute in decreasing liver injury;[202,203]

PN intake should be adapted by:

(1) Limiting glucose intakes to reduce hepatic fat accumulation;[204–207]

(2) Using the appropriate type and amount of intravenous fat emulsion, which provides essential fatty acids, reduces glucose load and limits peroxidation;[133,196,208]

(3) Controlling the lipid supply and rate of delivery and/or stopping IVFEs as soon as thrombocytopenia, hyperbilirubinemia and/or jaundice appear;[114]

(4) Using the new pediatric-adapted amino acid solutions which provide appropriate amino acids as well as taurine;[144,209]

(5) Performing cyclic PN, which helps to reduce hyperinsulinism and liver steatosis;[25–32]

(6) Adapting the iron intake and decreasing aluminum content of the PN solution.[210,211]

When cholestasis occurs, biliary obstruction, infection or drug toxicity should be ruled out by appropriate investigations. Decrease in platelet count below 150 000/mm^3 associated with an increase in plasma transaminases, and a further increase in plasma bilirubin, should lead to strong suspicion of lipid toxicity when all other explanations are ruled out. Bone marrow aspiration, liver biopsy and temporary suspension or decrease in lipid infusion should be discussed. Lipid infusion should be stopped until normalization of bilirubin level and platelet count. Essential fatty acid deficiency must be carefully checked. In case of persistent cholestasis after a 2-month suspension of lipid infusion, an irreversible course of the liver disease should be suspected. Reintroduction of lipid emulsions should be attempted under strict supervision, below the previous dosage, beginning with 1 or 2 perfusions per week. Medium-chain-based emulsions (50% MCT) might help to minimize the LCT load and theoretically their hepatic deposition and long-term toxicity, but neither the current study nor other clinical data have demonstrated any effects of MCT-based emulsions to prevent or to reverse long-term PN-associated cholestasis or hematological complications. Emulsions based on olive oil might also reduce the risk of lipid toxicity due to peroxidation, by decreasing the amount of linoleic acid.

Conclusions

Parenteral nutrition has become a widely used therapeutic option in clinical nutrition. One of the goals of PN is to have the same nutritional efficacy as that of normal oral feeding. Clinical research in the field of PN is necessary. This research has three main objectives: the reduction of PN-related complications; the study of the tolerance and efficacy of new substrates (lipids, amino acids, growth factors, etc); and the study of energy and/or protein metabolism during PN, especially in children in whom growth is the main goal of nutritional support.

Parenteral nutrition should be reserved for appropriate indications and avoided each time the enteral route is able to ensure adequate nutritional intakes for correction of malnutrition and/or normal growth. The successful deployment of a multidisciplinary nutrition support team minimizes inappropriate prescription of parenteral nutrition.

REFERENCES

1. Dudrick SJ, Wilmore DW, Vars HM, Rhoads JE. Long-term total parenteral nutrition with growth, development and positive nitrogen balance. *Surgery* 1968; **64**: 134–142.
2. Wilmore DM, Dudrick SJ. Growth and development of an infant receiving all nutrients by vein. *JAMA* 1968; **203**: 860–864.
3. Goulet O, Brousse N, Canioni D et al. Syndrome of intractable diarrhoea with persistent villus atrophy in early childhood: a clinicopathological survey of 47 cases. *J Pediatr Gastroenterol Nutr* 1998; **26**: 151–161.
4. Goulet O. Intractable diarrhea of infancy. In Walker A et al., eds. *Pediatric Gastrointestinal Disease*. Decker, 2000: 762–772.
5. Guarino A, Immacolata Spagnulo M, Russo S et al. Etiology and risk factors of severe and protracted diarrhea. *J Pediatr Gastroenterol Nutr* 1995; **20**: 173–178.
6. Lerebours E, Messing B, Chevalier B et al. An evaluation of total parenteral nutrition in the management of steroid-dependent and steroidresistant patients with Crohn's disease. *J Parent Ent Nutr* 1988; **10**: 274–278.
7. Tsujikawa T, Andoh A, Fujiyama Y. Enteral and parenteral nutrition therapy for Crohn's disease. *Curr Pharm Des* 2003; **9**: 323–332.
8. Goulet O, Ricour C. The short bowel syndrome. In Buts E, Sokal JP, eds. *Management of Digestive and Liver Disorders in Infants and Children*. Elsevier Sciences Publisher, 1993: 307–318.
9. Goulet O, Revillon Y, Jan D et al. Neonatal short bowel syndrome. *J Pediatr* 1991; **119**: 18–23.
10. Sondheimer JM, Cadnapaphornchai M, Sontag M, Zerbe GO. Predicting the duration of dependence on parenteral nutrition after neonatal intestinal resection. *J Pediatr* 1998; **132**: 80–84.
11. Leonberg BL, Chuang E, Eicher P et al. Long-term growth and development in children after home parenteral nutrition. *J Pediatr* 1998; **132**: 461–466.
12. Dellert SF, Farrell MK, Specker BL, Heubi JE. Bone mineral content in children with short bowel syndrome after discontinuation of parenteral nutrition. *J Pediatr* 1998; **132**: 516–519.
13. Festen S, Brevoord JC, Goldhoorn GA et al. Excellent long-term outcome for survivors of apple peel atresia. *J Pediatr Surg* 2002; **37**: 61–65.
14. Rickard KA, Godshall B, Loghmani ES. Integration of nutrition support into oncology treatment protocols for high and low nutritional risk children with Wilm's tumor. *Cancer* 1989; **64**: 491–509.
15. Gomez-Almaguer D, Montemayor J, Gonzales-Llano O et al. Improvement in the nutritional status of children with standard-risk acute lymphoblastic leukemia is associated with better tolerance to continuation chemotherapy. *Int J Pediatr Hematol Oncol* 1995; **2**: 53–56.
16. Colomb V. Nutrition en cancérologie : aspects pédiatriques. *Nutr Clin Metabol* 2001; **15**: 325–334.
17. Goulet O, De Ville De Goyet J, Otte JB, Ricour C. Preoperative nutritional evaluation and support for liver transplantation in children. *Transplant Proc* 1987; **19**: 3249–3255.
18. Moukarzel AA, Najm I, Vargas J et al. Effect of nutritional status on outcome of orthotopic liver transplantation in pediatric patients. *Transplant Proc* 1990; **22**: 1560–1563.
19. Sheperd RW, Chin SE, Cleghorn GJ et al. Malnutrition in children with chronic liver disease accepted for liver transplantation: clinical profile and effect in outcome. *J Pediatr Health* 1991; **27**: 295–299.
20. Roggero P, Catalotti E, Ulla L et al. Factors influencing malnutrition in children waiting for liver transplantation. *Am J Clin Nutr* 1997; **65**: 1852–1857.
21. Matuchansky C, Messing B, Jeejeebhoy et al. Cyclical parenteral nutrition. *Lancet* 1992; **340**: 588–592.

22. Just B, Messing B, Darmaun D et al. Comparison of substrate utilization by indirect calorimetry during cyclic and continuous total parenteral nutrition. *Am J Clin Nutr* 1990; **51**: 107–111.
23. Gramlich LM. Cyclic parenteral nutrition: considerations of carbohydrate and lipid metabolism. *Nutr Clin Pract* 1994; **9**: 49–50.
24. Colomb V, Charbit M, Goulet O et al. Renal function in young patients on long-term cyclic parenteral nutrition. *Transplant Proc* 1996; **28**: 2785.
25. MacFie J. Cyclic parenteral nutrition. *Nutrition* 1997; **13**: 46–48.
26. Nicol JJ, Hoagland RL, Heitlinger LA. The prevalence of nausea and vomiting in pediatric patients receiving home parenteral nutrition. *Nutr Clin Pract* 1995; **10**: 189–192.
27. Collier S, Crough J, Hendricks K, Caballero B. Use of cyclic parenteral nutrition in infants less than 6 months of age. *Nutr Clin Pract* 1994; **9**: 65–68.
28. Lienhardt A, Rakotoambinina B, Colomb V et al. Insulin secretion and sensitivity in children on cyclic total parenteral nutrition. *JPEN J Parenter Enteral Nutr* 1998; **22**: 382–386.
29. Colomb V, Dabbas M, Goulet O et al. Prepubertal growth in children with long-term parenteral nutrition. *Horm Res* 2002; **58** (Suppl 1): 2–6.
30. Beghin L, Michaud L, Hankard R et al. Total energy expenditure and physical activity in children treated with home parenteral nutrition. *Pediatr Res* 2003; **53**: 684–690.
31. Hwang TL, Lue MC, Chen LL. Early use of cyclic TPN prevents further deterioration of liver functions for the TPN patients with impaired liver function. *Hepatogastroenterology* 2000; **47**: 1347–1350.
32. Vargas JH, Ament ME, Berquist WE et al. Long-term home parenteral nutrition in pediatrics: ten years of experience in 102 patients. *J Pediatr Gastroenterol Nutr* 1987; **6**: 24–32.
33. Ricour C, Gorski AM, Goulet O et al. Home parenteral nutrition in children: 8 years of experience with 112 patients. *Clin Nutr* 1990; **9**: 65–71.
34. Messing B, Lemann M, Landais P et al. Prognosis of patients with chronic intestinal failure receiving long-term home parenteral nutrition in France and Belgium. *Gastroenterology* 1995; **108**: 1005–1010.
35. Howard L, Ament M, Fleming R et al. Current use and clinical outcome of home parenteral and enteral nutrition therapies in the United States. *Gastroenterology* 1995; **109**: 355–365.
36. Howard L, Hassan N. Home parenteral nutrition: 25 years later. *Clin Nutr* 1998; **27**: 418–512.
37. Colomb V, Goulet O, Ricour C. Home enteral and parenteral nutrition. *Baillière's Clin Gastroenterol* 1998; **122**: 877–894.
38. Grant D. Intestinal transplantation: 1997 Report of the International Registry. *Transplantation* 1999; **15**: 1061–1064.
39. Goulet O, Jan D, Lacaille F et al. Intestinal transplantation in children: preliminary experience in Paris. *JPEN J Parenter Enteral Nutr* 1999; **23**: S121–S125.
40. Goulet O, Lacaille F, Jan D, Ricour C. Intestinal transplantation: indications, results and strategy. *Curr Opin Clin Nutr Metab Care* 2000; **3**: 329–333.
41. Goulet O, Ruemmele F, Lacaille F, Colomb V. Intestinal failure. *J Pediatr Gastroenterol Nutr* 2003; (in press).
42. Chung DH, Ziegler MM. Central venous catheter access. *Nutrition* 1998; **14**: 119–123.
43. Jan D, Goulet O. Accès vasculaires. In Ricour C, Ghisolfi J, Putet G, Goulet O, eds. *Traité de Nutrition Pédiatrique*. Paris: Maloine Editeur, 1993: 831–838.
44. Shulman R, Pokorny W, Martin CG et al. Comparison of percutaneous and surgical placement of central venous catheter in neonates. *J Pediatr Surg* 1986; **21**:348–350.
45. Ahn WS, Kang JS. An easy technique for long term central venous catheterization and subcutaneous tunneling of the silastic catheter in neonates and infants. *J Pediatr Surg* 1986; **21**: 344–347.
46. Weber TR, West KW, Grosfeld JL. Broviac central venous catheterization in infants and children. *Am J Surg* 1983; **145**: 202–204.
47. Reinberg O, Beck D. A new implantable device for long-term vascular access in children. *Eur J Pediatr Surg* 1992; **2**: 183–185.
48. Ricour C, Revillon Y, Bougle D et al. Nutrition parentérale par fistule artérioveineuse. *Arch Fr Pediatr* 1983; **40**: 457–460.
49. Schofield W. Predicting basal metabolic rate, new standards and review of previous work. *Hum Nutr Clin Nutr* 1985; **39 (Suppl 1)**; 5–41.
50. Goulet O. Assessment of nutritional status in clinical practice. *Baillière's Clin Gastroenterol* 1998; **12**: 645–669.
51. Duro D, Rising R, Cole C et al. New equations for calculating the components of energy expenditure in infants. *J Pediatr* 2002; **140**: 534–539.
52. Goran MI, Shewchuk R, Gower BA. Longitudinal changes in fatness in white children: no effect of childhood energy expenditure. *Am J Clin Nutr* 1998; **67**: 309–316.
53. Pierro A, Jones MO, Donnell SC. Total parenteral nutrition in surgical infants. *Biochem Soc Trans* 1998; **26**: 131–136.
54. Jaksic T, Shew SB, Keshen TH et al. Do critically ill surgical neonates have increased energy expenditure? *J Pediatr Surg* 2001; **36**: 63–67.
55. Lloyd DA. Energy requirements of surgical newborn infants receiving parenteral nutrition. *Nutrition* 1998; **14**: 101–104.
56. Garza JJ, Shew SB, Keshen TH et al. Energy expenditure in ill premature neonates. *J Pediatr Surg* 2002; **37**: 289–293.
57. Coss-Bu JA, Klish WJ, Walding D et al. Energy metabolism, nitrogen balance, and substrate utilization in critically ill children 1–3. *Am J Clin Nutr* 2001; **74**: 664–669.
58. Koen FM, Joosten KFM, Verhoeven JJ, Hazelzet JA. Energy expenditure and substrate utilization in mechanically ventilated children. *Nutrition* 1999; **15**: 444–448.
59. Turi RA, Petros AJ, Eaton S et al. Energy metabolism of infants and children with systemic inflammatory response syndrome and sepsis. *Ann Surg* 2001; **233**: 581–587.
60. White MS, Shepherd RW, McEniery JA. Energy expenditure measurements in ventilated critically ill children: within- and between-day variability. *J Parenter Enteral Nutr* 1999; **23**: 300–304.
61. Pierro A, Jones MO, Hammond P et al. A new equation to predict the resting energy expenditure of surgical infants. *J Pediatr Surg* 1994; **29**: 1103–1108.
62. White MS, Shepherd RW, McEniery JA. Energy expenditure in 100 ventilated, critically ill children: improving the accuracy of predictive equations. *Crit Care Med* 2000; **28**: 2307–2312.
63. Kalhan SC, Kilic I. Carbohydrate as nutrient in the infant and child: range of acceptable intake. *Europ J Clin Nutr* 1999; **53**: S94–S100.
64. Denne SC, Karn CA, Wang J, Liechty EA. Effect of intravenous glucose and lipid on proteolysis and glucose production in normal newborns. *Am J Physiol* 1995; **269**: E361–E367.

65. Sunehag AL, Haymond MW, Schanler RJ et al. Gluconeogenesis in very low birth weight infants receiving total parenteral nutrition. *Diabetes* 1999; **48**: 791–800.
66. Sheridan RL, Yu YM, Prelack K et al. Maximal parenteral glucose oxidation in hypermetabolic young children: a stable isotope study. *J Parenter Enteral Nutr* 1998; **22**: 212–216.
67. Lafeber HN, Sulkers EJ, Chapman TE, Sauer PJ. Glucose production and oxidation in preterm infants during total parenteral nutrition. *Pediatr Res* 1990; **28**: 153–157.
68. Jones MO, Pierro A, Hammond P et al. Glucose utilization in the surgical newborn infant receiving total parenteral nutrition. *J Pediatr Surg* 1993; **28**: 1121–1125.
69. Nose O, Tipton JR, Ament ME. Effect of the energy source on changes in energy expenditure, respiratory quotient, and nitrogen balance during total parenteral nutrition in children. *Pediatr Res* 1987; **21**: 538–541.
70. Bresson JL, Narcy P, Putet G, Ricour C. Energy substrate utilization in infants receiving total parenteral nutrition with different glucose to fat ratios. *Pediatr Res* 1989; **25**: 645–648.
71. Elwyn DH, Askanazi J, Kinney JM, Gump FE. Kinetics of energy substrates. *Acta Chir Scand* Suppl 1981; **507**: 209–219.
72. Koretz RL, Lipman TO, Klein S. AGA Technical review on parenteral nutrition. *Gastroenterology* 2001; **121**: 970–1001.
73. Robin AP, Carpentier YA, Askanazi J et al. Metabolic consequences of hypercaloric glucose infusions. *Acta Chir Belg* 1981; **80**: 133–140.
74. Bresson JL. Protein and energy requirements. *Baillière's Clin Gastroenterol* 1998; **12**: 631–646.
75. Talpers SS, Romberger DJ, Bunce SB, Pingleton SK. Nutritionally associated increased carbon dioxide production. Excess total calories vs high proportion of carbohydrate calories. *Chest* 1992; **102**: 551–555.
76. Askanazi J, Weissman C, LaSala PA et al. Effect of protein intake on ventilatory drive. *Anesthesiology* 1984; **60**: 106–10.
77. Rodriguez JL, Askanazi J, Weissman C et al. Ventilatory and metabolic effects of glucose infusions. *Chest* 1985; **88**: 512–518.
78. Burke JF, Wolfe RR, Mullany CJ et al. Glucose requirements following burn injury. Parameters of optimal glucose infusion and possible hepatic and respiratory abnormalities following excessive glucose intake. *Ann Surg* 1979; **190**: 274–285.
79. Tulikoura I, Huikuri K. Morphological fatty changes and function of the liver, serum free fatty acids, and triglycerides during parenteral nutrition. *Scand J Gastroenterol* 1982; **17**: 177–185.
80. Aarsland A, Chinkes D, Wolfe RR. Contributions of de novo synthesis of fatty acids to total VLDL-triglyceride secretion during prolonged hyperglycemia/hyperinsulinemia in normal man. *J Clin Invest* 1996; **98**: 2008–2017.
81. Klein CJ, Stanek GS, Wiles CE 3rd. Overfeeding macronutrients to critically ill adults: metabolic complications. *J Am Diet Assoc* 1998; **98**: 795–806.
82. The Veterans Affairs Total Parenteral Nutrition Cooperative Study group. Perioperative total parenteral nutrition in surgical patients. *N Engl J Med* 1991; **325**: 525–532.
83. Kudsk KA, Croce MA, Fabian TC et al. Enteral versus parenteral feeding. Effects on septic morbidity after blunt and penetrating abdominal trauma. *Ann Surg* 1992; **215**: 503–511.
84. Moore FA, Feliciano DV, Andrassy RJ et al. Early enteral feeding, compared with parenteral, reduces postoperative septic complications. The results of a meta-analysis. *Ann Surg* 1992; **216**: 172–183.
85. Cruccetti A, Pierro A, Uronen H, Klein N. Surgical infants on total parenteral nutrition have impaired cytokine responses to microbial challenge. *J Pediatr Surg* 2003; **38**: 138–142.
86. Khaodhiar L, McCowen K, Bistrian B. Perioperative hyperglycemia, infection or risk? *Curr Opin Clin Nutr Metab Care* 1999; **2**: 79–82.
87. Engelich G, Wright DG, Hartshorn KL. Acquired disorders of phagocyte function complicating medical and surgical illnesses. *Clin Infect Dis* 2001; **33**: 2040–2048.
88. Bistrian BR. Hyperglycemia and infection: which is the chicken and which is the egg? *J Parenter Enteral Nutr* 2001; **25**: 180–181.
89. Gore DC, Chinkes D, Heggers J. Association of hyperglycemia with increased mortality after severe burn injury. *J Trauma* 2001; **51**: 540–544.
90. Macfie J, Smith RC, Hill GL. Glucose or fat as a nonprotein energy source? A controlled clinical trial in gastroenterological patients requiring intravenous nutrition. *Gastroenterology* 1981; **80**: 103–107.
91. Pineault M, Chessex P, Bisaillon S, Brisson G. Total parenteral nutrition in the newborn: impact of the quality of infused energy on nitrogen metabolism. *Am J Clin Nutr* 1988; **47**: 298–304.
92. Bresson JL, Bader B, Rocchiccioli F et al. Protein-metabolism kinetics and energy-substrate utilization in infants fed parenteral solutions with different glucose-fat ratios. *Am J Clin Nutr* 1991; **54**: 370–376.
93. Lefkowitz JB, Evers AS, Elliott WJ, Needleman P. Essential fatty deficiency: a new look at an old problem. *Prostaglandins Leukot Med* 1986; **23**: 123–127.
94. Roesner M, Grant JP. Intravenous lipid emulsions. *Nutr Clin Pract* 1987; **1**: 96–107.
95. Goulet O, Duhamel JF, Ricour C. Nutritional problems. In Tinker J, Zapol W, eds. *Care in the Critically Ill Patients*, Berlin, Heidelberg, New York, Springer Verlag 1992: 1415–1436.
96. Adolph M. Lipid emulsions in parenteral nutrition. *Ann Nutr Metabol* 1999; **43**: 1–13.
97. Koletzko B. Lipid supply and metabolism in infancy. *Curr Opin Clin Nutr Metab Care* 1998; **1**: 171–177.
98. Bistrian BR. Clinical aspects of essential fatty acid metabolism: Jonathan Rhoads Lecture. *JPEN J Parenter Enteral Nutr* 2003; **27**: 168–175.
99. Olivecrona G, Olivecrona T. Clearance of artificial triacylglycerol particles. *Curr Opin Clin Nutr Metab Care* 1998; **1**: 143–151.
100. Carpentier YA. Intravascular metabolism of fat emulsions: the Arvid Wretling lecture ESPEN 1988. *Clin Nutr* 1989; **8**: 115–125.
101. Carpentier YA, Simoens C, Siderova V et al. Recent developments in lipid emulsions: relevance to intensive care. *Nutrition* 1997; **13**: 735–785.
102. Kao LC, Cheng MH, Warburton D. Triglycerides, free fatty acids, free fatty acids/albumin molar ratio, and cholesterol levels in serum of neonates receiving long-term lipid infusions: controlled trial of continuous and intermittent regimens. *J Pediatr* 1984; **104**: 429–435.
103. Haumont D, Deckelbaum RJ, Richelle M et al. Plasma lipid and plasma lipoprotein concentrations in low birth weight infants given parenteral nutrition with twenty or ten percent lipid emulsion. *J Pediatr* 1989; **115**: 787–793.
104. Spear ML, Stahl GE, Hamosh M et al. Effect of heparin dose and infusion rate on lipid clearance and bilirubin binding in premature infants receiving intravenous fat emulsions. *J Pediatr* 1988; **112**: 94–98.

105. Haumont D, Richelle M, Deckelbaum RJ et al. Effect of liposomal content of lipid emulsions on plasma lipid concentrations in low birth weight infants receiving parenteral nutrition. *J Pediatr* 1992; **121**: 759–763.
106. Putet G. Lipid metabolism of the micropremie. *Clin Perinatol* 2000; **27**: 57–69.
107. Defronzo RA, Jacot E, Jequier E et al. The effect of insulin on the disposal of intravenous glucose. *Diabetes* 1981; **30**: 1000–1007.
108. Stein PT, Mullen JL. Hepatic fat accumulation in man with excess parenteral glucose. *Nutr Res* 1985; **5**: 1347–1351.
109. Bresson JL, Narcy P, Putet G et al. Energy substrate utilization in infants receiving total parenteral nutrition with different glucose to fat ratios. *Pediatr Res* 1989; **25**: 645.
110. Salas J, Girardet JP, De Potter S et al. Glucose versus glucose-fat mixture in the course of total parenteral nutrition: effects on substrate utilization and energy metabolism in malnourished children. *Clin Nutr* 1991; **10**: 272–278.
111. Pierro A, Carnielli V, Filler RM et al. Metabolism of intravenous fat emulsion in the surgical newborn. *J Pediatr Surg* 1989; **24**: 95.
112. Palmblad J. Intravenous lipid emulsions and host defense a critical review. *Clin Nutr* 1991; **10**: 303–308.
113. Goulet O, Girot R, Maier-Redelsperger M et al. Hematologic disorders following prolonged use of intravenous fat in children. *JPEN* 1986; **10**: 284–288.
114. Colomb V, Jobert-Giraud A, Lacaille F et al. Role of lipid emulsions in cholestasis associated with long-term parenteral nutrition in children. *JPEN* 2000; **24**: 345–350.
115. Tanner A, Keyhani A, Reiner R et al. Proteolytic enzymes released by liver macrophages may promote hepatic injury in a rat model of hepatic damage. *Gastroenterology* 1981; **80**: 647–654.
116. Neuzil J, Darlow BA, Inder TE et al. Oxidation of parenteral lipid emulsion by ambient and phototherapy lights: potential toxicity of routine parenteral feeding. *J Pediatr* 1995; **126**: 785–790.
117. Clayton PT, Bowron A, Mills KA et al. Phytosterolemia in children with parenteral nutrition-cholestatic associated liver disease. *Gastroenterology* 1993; **105**: 1806–1813.
118. Bach AC, Frey A, Lutz O. Clinical and experimental effects of medium-chain triglyceride based fat emulsions – A review. *Clin Nutr* 1989; **8**: 223–235.
119. Dennison AR, Ball M, Crowe PJ et al. The metabolic consequences of infusing emulsions containing medium-chain triglycerides for parenteral nutrition: a comparative study with conventional lipid. *Ann Royal Coll Surg Engl* 1986; **68**: 119–122.
120. Dennison AR, Ball M, Hands LJ et al. Total parenteral nutrition using conventional and medium-chain triglycerides: effects on liver functions tests, complement and nitrogen balance. *JPEN* 1988; **12**: 15–19.
121. Bach AC, Guiraud M, Gibault JP et al. Medium-chain triglycerides in septic patients on total parenteral nutrition. *Clin Nutr* 1988; **7**: 157–163.
122. Beaufrère B, Chassard D, Broussolle C et al. Effects of D-β-hydrohyxybutyrate and long- and medium-chain triglycerides on leucine metabolim in humans. *Am J Physiol* 1992; **262**: E268–E274.
123. Lima LAM. Neonatal parenteral nutrition with medium chain triglycerides: rationale for research. *J Parenter Enteral Nutr* 1989; **l3**: 312–317.
124. Bresson JL, Narcy P, Sachs C et al. Energy substrate competition: comparative study of LCT and MCT utilization during continuous TPN in infants. *Clin Nutr* 1986; **5 (Suppl)**: 54(A).
125. Goulet O, De Potter S, Postaire M et al. Long term total parenteral nutrition in children: utilization of medium chain triglycerides. *Nutrition* 1992; **8**: 33–37.
126. Rubin M, Moser A, Naor N et al. Effect of three intravenously administered fat emulsions containing different concentrations of fatty acids on the plasma fatty acids composition of premature infants. *J Pediatr* 1994; **125**: 596–602.
127. Maiz A, Yamazaki K, Sobrado J et al. Protein metabolism during total parenteral nutrition in injured rats using medium-chain triglycerides. *Metabolism* 1984; **33**: 901–909.
128. Chambrier C, Guiraud M, Gibault JP et al. Medium- and long-chain triacylglycerols in postoperative patients: structured lipids versus a physical mixture. *Nutrition* 1999; **15**: 274–277.
129. Waitzberg DL, Lotierzo PH, Logullo AF et al. Parenteral lipid emulsions and phagocytic systems. *Br J Nutr* 2002; **87 (Suppl 1)**: S49–S57.
130. Mayer K, Gokorsch S, Fegbeutel C et al. Parenteral nutrition with fish oil modulates cytokine response in patients with sepsis. *Am J Respir Crit Care Med* 2003; **167**: 1321–1328.
131. Louheranta AM, Porkkala-Sarataho EK, Nyssönen MK et al. Linoleic acid intake and susceptibility of very-low-density and low-density lipoproteins to oxidation in man. *Am J Clin Nutr* 1996; **63**: 698–703.
132. Brouwer CB, de Bruin TWA, Jansen H, Erkelens DW. Different clearance of intravenously administered olive oil and soybean-oil emulsions: role of hepatic lipase. *Am J Clin Nutr* 1993; **57**: 533–539.
133. Goulet O, de Potter S, Antebi H et al. Long-term efficacy and safety of a new olive oil-based intravenous fat emulsion in pediatric patients: a double-blind randomized study. *Am J Clin Nutr* 1999; **70**: 338–345.
134. Göbel Y, Koletzko B, Böhles HJ et al. Parenteral fat emulsions based on olive and soybean oils: a randomized clinical trial in preterm infants. *J Pediatr Gastroenterol Nutr* 2003; **37**: 161–67.
135. Borum PR. Should carnitine be added to parenteral nutrition solutions? *Nutr Clin Prac* 2000; **15**: 153–154.
136. Penn D, Schmidt-Sommerfeld E, Pascu F. Decreased tissue carnitine concentrations in newborn infants receiving total parenteral nutrition. *J Pediatr* 1981; **98**: 976–978.
137. Rawcliffe PM, Giles P, Barlett S et al. Carnitine as a possible adjunct in parenteral feeding. *Clin Nutr* 1984; **3**: 141–145.
138. Penn D, Ludwigs B, Schmidt-Sommerfied E, Pascu F. Effect of nutrition on tissue carnitine concentrations in infants of different gestational ages. *Biol Neonate* 1985; **47**: 130–135.
139. Cairns PA, Stalker DJ. Carnitine supplementation of parenterally fed neonates. *Cochrane Database Syst Rev* 2000; **4**: CD000950.
140. Pellett PL. Protein requirements in humans. *Am J Clin Nutr* 1990; **51**: 723–737.
141. Eason LB, Halata MS, Dweck HS. Parenteral nutrition in the newborn: a practical guide. *Pediatr Clin North Am* 1982; **29**: 1171–1190.
142. Goulet O, De Potter S, Salas J et al. Leucine metabolism at graded amino-acid intakes in children receiving parenteral nutrition. *Am J Physiol* 1993; **265**: E540–E546.
143. Bengoa JM, Sitrin MD, Wood RJ, Rosenberg IH. Amino-acid induced hypercalciuria in patients on total parenteral nutrition. *Am J Clin Nutr* 1983; **38**: 264–269.

144. Coran AG, Drongowski RA. Studies on the toxicity and efficacy of a new amino acid solution in pediatric parenteral nutrition. *J Parenter Enter Nutr* 1987; **11**: 368–377.
145. Corriol. O. Les solutions injectables d'acides aminés pour nutrition parentérale. Critères de choix thérapeutiques. *Nutr Clin Metabol* 1987; **1**: 17–30.
146. Wolfe RR, Goodenough RD, Burke JF, Wolfe MM. Response of protein and urea kinetics in burn patients to different level of protein intake. *Ann Surg* 1983; **197**: 163–171.
147. Neu J, DeMarco V, Li N. Glutamine: clinical applications and mechanisms of action. *Curr Opin Clin Nutr Metab Care* 2002; **5**: 69–75.
148. Hartmann F, Plauth M. Intestinal glutamine metabolism. *Metabolism* 1989; **38**: 18–24.
149. Hankard R, Goulet O, Ricour C et al. Glutamine metabolism in children with short bowel syndrome: a stable isotope study. *Pediatr Res* 1994; **36**: 202–206.
150. Calder PC. Glutamine and the immune system. *Clin Nutr* 1994; **13**: 2–8.
151. Schloerb PR, Amare M. Total parenteral nutrition with glutamine in bone marrow transplantation and other clinical applications. *J Parent Enter Nutr* 1993; **17**: 407–413.
152. Young LS, Bye R, Scheltinga M et al. Patients receiving glutamine supplemented intravenous *J Parenter Enteral Nutr* 1993; **17**: 422–427.
153. Ziegler TR, Young LS, Benfell K et al. Clinical and metabolic efficacy of glutamine supplemented parenteral nutrition after bone marrow transplantation. *Ann Int Med* 1992; **116**: 821–828.
154. Furst P, Stehle P. The potential use of parenteral dipeptides in clinical nutrition. *Nutr Clin Pract* 1993; **8**: 106–114.
155. Tremel H, Kienle B, Weilemann LS et al. Glutamine dipeptide supplemented parenteral nutrition maintains intestinal function in the critically ill. *Gastroenterology* 1994; **107**: 1595–1601.
156. Jiang ZM, Cao JD, Zhu XG et al. The impact of glutamine dipeptide on nitrogen balance, intestinal permeability and clinical outcome of post operative patients. *JPEN* 1999; **23**: S62–S66.
157. Hammarqvist F, Wernerman J, Von Der Decken A, Vinnars E. Alpha ketoglutarate preserves protein synthesis and free glutamine in skeletal muscle after surgery. *Surgery* 1991; **109**: 28–31.
158. Wernerman J, Hammarkvist F, Ali MR, Vinnars E. Glutamine and ornithine a ketoglutarate but not branched chain amino acids reduce the loss of muscle glutamine after surgical trauma. *Metabolism* 1989; **38**: 63–66.
159. Cynober LA. The use of alpha-ketoglutarate salts in clinical nutrition and metabolic care. *Curr Opin Clin Nutr Metab Care* 1999; **2**: 33–37.
160. Dumas F, De Bandt JP, Colomb V et al. Enteral ornithine alpha-ketoglutarate enhances intestinal adaptation to massive resection in rats. *Metabolism* 1998; **47**: 1366–1371.
161. Moukarzel AA, Goulet O, Salas JS et al. Growth retardation in children receiving long-term total parenteral nutrition: effects of ornithine alpha-ketoglutarate. *Am J Clin Nutr* 1994; **60**: 408–413.
162. Rollins CJ, Elsberry VA, Pollack KA et al. Three-in-one parenteral nutrition: a safe and economical method of nutritional support for infants. *J Parenter Enteral Nutr* 1990; **14**: 290–294.
163. Didier ME, Fischer S, Maki DG. Total nutrient admixtures appear safer than lipid emulsion alone as regards microbial contamination: growth properties of microbial pathogens at room temperature. *J Parenter Enteral Nutr* 1990; **22**. 291–296.
164. Hardy G, Ball P, McElroy B. Basic principles for compounding all-in-one parenteral nutrition admixtures. *Curr Opin Clin Nutr Metab Care* 1998; **1**: 291–296.
165. McKinnon BT. FDA safety alert: hazards of precipitation associated with parenteral nutrition. *Nutr Clin Prac* 1996; **11**: 59–65.
166. Bethune K, Allwood M, Grainger C, Wormleighton C. Use of filters during the preparation and administration of parenteral nutrition: position paper and guidelines prepared by a British pharmaceutical nutrition group working party. *Nutrition* 2001; **17**: 403–408.
167. Trissel LA, Gilbert DL, Martinez JF et al. Compatibility of medications with 3-in-1 parenteral nutrition admixtures. *J Parenter Enteral Nutr* 1999; **23**: 67–74.
168. Havala T, Shronts E. Managing the complications associated with refeeding. *Nutr Clin Prac* 1990; **5**: 23–29.
169. SM, Kirby DF. The refeeding syndrome: a review. *J Parenter Enter Nutr* 1989; **14**: 90–97.
170. Crook MA, Hally V, Panteli J. The importance of the refeeding syndrome. *Nutrition* 2001; **17**: 632–637.
171. Alpers DH, Klein S. Refeeding the malnourished patient. *Curr Opin Gastroenterol* 1999; **15**: 151–153.
172. Colomb V, Fabeiro M, Dabbas M et al. Central venous catheter-related infections in children on long-term home parenteral nutrition: incidence and risk factors. *Clin Nutr* 2000; **19**: 355–359.
173. Rubin LG, Sanchez PJ, Siegel J et al. Pediatric Prevention Network. Evaluation and treatment of neonates with suspected late-onset sepsis: a survey of neonatologists' practices. *Pediatrics* 2002; **110**: 42.
174. Benjamin DK Jr, Miller W, Garges H et al. Bacteremia, central catheters, and neonates: when to pull the line. *Pediatrics* 2001; **107**: 1272–1276.
175. Moukarzel AA, Haddad I, Ament ME et al. 230 patient-years of experience with home long-term parenteral nutrition in childhood: natural history and life of central venous catheters. *J Pediatr Surg*. 1994; **29**: 1323–1327.
176. Goulet O, Larchet M, Gaillard JL et al. Catheter related sepsis during long-term parenteral nutrition in pediatric gastroenterology patients: a study of 185 consecutive central venous catheter. *Clin Nutr* 1990; **9**: 73–78.
177. Buchman AL, Moukarzel A. Metabolic bone disease associated with total parenteral nutrition. *Clin Nutr* 2000; **19**: 217–231.
178. Hicks W, Hardy G. Phosphate supplementation for hypophosphataemia and parenteral nutrition. *Curr Opin Clin Nutr Metabol Care* 2001; **4**: 227–233.
179. Klein GL, Leichtner AM, Heyman MB. Aluminium in large and small volume parenterals used in total parenteral nutrition: response to the Food and Drug Administration notice of proposed rule by the North American Society for Pediatric Gastroenterology and Nutrition. *J Pediatr Gastroenterol Nutr* 1998; **27**: 457–460.
180. Popinska K, Kierkus J, Lyszkowska M et al. Aluminium contamination of parenteral nutrition additives, amino acid solutions, and lipid emulsions. *Nutrition* 1999; **15**: 683–686.
181. Dellert SF, Farrell MK, Specker BL, Heubi JE. Bone mineral content in children with short bowel syndrome after discontinuation of parenteral nutrition. *J Pediatr* 1998; **132**: 516–519.
182. Quigley EMM, Marsh MN, Shaffer JL, Markin RS. Hepatobiliary complications of total parenteral nutrition. *Gastroenterology* 1993; **104**: 286–301.

183. Colomb V, Goulet O, Rambaud C et al. Long term parenteral nutrition in children: liver and gallbladder disease. *Transplant Proc* 1992; **24**: 1054–1055.
184. Fouin Fortunet H, Le Quernec L, Erlinger S et al. Hepatic alterations during total parenteral nutrition in patients with inflammatory bowel disease: a possible consequence of lithocholate toxicity. *Gastroenterology* 1982; **82**: 932–937.
185. Beath SV, Davies P, Papadopoulou A et al. Parenteral nutrition-related cholestasis in postsurgical neonates: multivariate analysis of risk factors. *J Pediatr Surg* 1996; **31**: 604–606.
186. Moseley RH. Sepsis-associated cholestasis. *Gastroenterology* 1997; **112**: 302–305.
187. Roelofsen H, Schoemaker B, Bakker C et al. Impaired hepatocanalicular organic anion transport in endotoxemic rats. *Am J Physiol* 1995; **269**: G427–G434.
188. Noel M, Chevenne D, Porquet D. Utility of insulin-like growth factor-I and its binding protein assays. *Curr Opin Clin Nutr Metab Care* 2001; **4**: 399–405.
189. Moss RL, Das JB, Ansari G, Raffensperger JG. Hepatobiliary dysfunction during total parenteral nutrition is caused by infusate, not the route of administration. *J Pediatr Surg* 1993; **28**: 391–397.
190. Belli DC, Fournier LA, Lepage G et al. Total parenteral nutrition-associated cholestasis in rats: comparison of different amino acid mixtures. *JPEN* 1987; **11**: 67–73.
191. Reif S, Tano M, Oliverio R. Total parenteral nutrition induced steatosis: reversal by parenteral lipid infusion. *JPEN* 1991; **15**: 102–104.
192. Wolf A, Pohlandt F. Bacterial infection: the main cause of acute cholestasis in newborn infants receiving short-term parenteral nutrition. *J Pediatr Gastroenterol Nutr* 1989; **8**: 297–303.
193. Moss RL, Das JB, Raffensperger JG. Total parenteral nurition-associated cholestasis: clinical and histopathological correlation. *J Pediatr Surg* 1993; **28**: 1270–1275.
194. Braxton C, Lowry SF. Editorial: parenteral nutrition and liver dysfunction-new insight? *JPEN* 1995; **19**: 3–4.
195. Kaufman SS, Loseke CA, Lupo JV et al. Influence of bacterial overgrowth and intestinal inflammation on duration of parenteral nutrition in children with short bowel syndrome. *J Pediatr* 1997; **131**: 356–361.
196. Sondheimer JM, Asturias E, Cadnapaphornchai M. Infection and cholestasis in neonates with intestinal resection and long-term parenteral nutrition. *J Pediatr Gastroenterol Nutr* 1998; **27**: 131–137.
197. Kaufman SS. Prevention of parenteral nutrition-associated liver disease in children. *Pediatr Transplant* 2002; **6**: 37–42.
198. Ben Hariz M, Goulet O, De Potter S et al. Iron overload in children receiving prolonged parenteral nutrition. *J Pediatr* 1993; **123**: 238–241.
199. Moukarzel A, Song MK, Buchman AL et al. Excessive chromium intake in children receiving total parenteral nutrition. *Lancet* 1992; **339**: 385–388.
200. Ling PR, Sheikh M, Boyce P et al. Cholecystokinin (CCK) secretion in patients with severe short bowel syndrome (SSBS). *Dig Dis Sci* 2001; **46**: 859–864.
201. Capron JP, Gineston JL. Herve MA. Metronidazole in prevention of cholestasis associated with total parenteral nutrition. *Lancet* 1983; **1**: 446–447.
202. Spagnuolo MI, Iorio R, Vegnente A, Guarino A. Ursodeoxycholic acid for treatment of cholestasis in children on long-term total parenteral nutrition: a pilot study. *Gastroenterology* 1996; **111**: 716–719.
203. Heubi JE, Wiechmann DA, Creutzinger V et al. Tauroursodeoxycholic acid (TUDCA) in the prevention of total parenteral nutrition-associated liver disease. *J Pediatr* 2002; **141**: 237–242.
204. Salas JS, Dozio E, Goulet O et al. Energy expenditure and substrate utilization in the course of renutrition of malnourished children. *J Parenter Enteral Nutr* 1991; **15**: 288–293.
205. Lienhardt A, Rakotoambinina B, Colomb V et al. Insulin secretion and sensitivity in children on cyclic total parenteral nutrition. *JPEN J Parenter Enteral Nutr* 1998; **22**: 382–386.
206. Beghin L, Michaud L, Hankard R et al. Total energy expenditure and physical activity in children treated with home parenteral nutrition. *Pediatr Res* 2003; **53**: 684–690.
207. Shulman RJ, Phillips S. Parenteral nutrition in infants and children. *J Pediatr Gastroenterol Nutr* 2003; **36**: 587–607.
208. Dahlstrom KA, Goulet O, Roberts RL et al. Lipid tolerance in children receiving long-term parenteral nutrition: a biochemical and immunologic study. *J Pediatr* 1988; **113**: 985–990.
209. Forchielli ML, Gura KM, Sandler R, Lo C. Aminosyn PF or Trophamine: which provides more protection from cholestasis associated with total parenteral nutrition? *J Pediatr Gastroenterol Nutr* 1995: **21**: 374–382.
210. Ben Hariz M, Goulet O, Colomb V et al. Inappropriate iron intake in children on long-term parenteral nutrition: outcome after iron withdrawal. *Clin Nutr* 1997; **16**: 251–255.
211. Advenier E, Landry C, Colomb V et al. Aluminum contamination of parenteral nutrition and aluminum loading in children on long-term parenteral nutrition. *J Pediatr Gastroenterol Nutr* 2003; **36**: 448–453.

35 Gastrointestinal problems of the newborn

Moti M Chowdhury and Agostino Pierro

Introduction

The birth of a newborn in most cases marks a joyous occasion for a family. However, occasionally it is dampened by the tragedy of a congenital anomaly or illness within the first few weeks of life, a period that accounts for most childhood fatalities. In this chapter we endeavor to outline some of the acquired problems relating to the gastrointestinal (GI) tract. Whilst it is acknowledged that almost all acquired GI problems of childhood may present within the neonatal period, most are rare events in newborns (e.g. appendicitis, intussusception, inflammatory bowel disease), and it would be beyond the scope of this chapter to discuss all such problems exhaustively. In this chapter we focus instead on the four common GI problems encountered in the first few weeks of life: necrotizing enterocolitis (NEC), gastroesophageal reflux (GER), infantile hypertrophic pyloric stenosis (IHPS) and inguinal hernia.

Necrotizing enterocolitis

NEC is a disease predominantly of premature infants characterized by a variable degree of intestinal necrosis, which may or may not be complicated by perforation and fulminant sepsis.

Epidemiology

NEC is the most common surgical emergency in the neonatal period,[1] affecting 0.5% of all live births and 3–5% of low-birth-weight live births. Although primarily a disease of the preterm infant, 6–13% are in full-term infants.[2–4] There is a male preponderance of 2 : 1.[3]

Etiology

Whilst the precise mechanism of NEC remains unclear, a number of predisposing risk factors have been identified: low birth weight, prematurity, enteral feeds and sepsis.

Low birth weight

Low birth weight (< 1500 g) is the single most important risk factor for NEC development.[5–10]

Prematurity

Approximately 90% of NEC cases are found in premature infants, with mean gestational age of 30–32 weeks, and mean gestational age in those undergoing surgery of 31–37 weeks.[11] The increased incidence of NEC in this group may be due to greater susceptibility of the premature gut to the stresses of hypoxia, ischemia and the mucosal damage of hyperosmolar feeds in this group.

Enteral feeds

Infants who are breast fed are 3–10 times less likely to develop NEC than those given formula feeds.[12–14] Breast milk contains immunoglobulins (IgA and IgG) and white cells which are thought to confer protection on the breast-fed infant[13,15] via two methods. First, breast milk induces colonization of the neonatal intestine with bifidobacteria, which reduces the risk of subsequent colonization by pathogens.[16,17] Second, inappropriate colonization with these pathogens is inhibited by the immunoglobulin and white cell content of breast milk. Furthermore, hyperosmolar formula feeds can induce mucosal damage,[18] whilst bacterial fermentation of the high carbohydrate content in hyperosmolar feeds has the potential to contribute large quantities of hydrogen gas to the pneumatosis intestinalis.

Sepsis

Although a number of organisms (see Pathophysiology below) have been cultured in pathological specimens of NEC, many are from the bowel flora, suggesting a mechanism involving an imbalance between the host and the organism rather than direct virulence of the organism.[14,19]

In addition to these recognized risk factors, a number of other weak associations have been reported with the development of NEC (Table 35.1).

Table 35.1 Risk factors for development of necrotizing enterocolitis
Low birth weight
Prematurity
Enteral feeds
Sepsis
Intrauterine growth restriction[11,188,189]
Fetal distress[190]
Exposure to antenatal or postnatal glucocorticoids[7]
Premature rupture of membranes[191,192]
Birth asphyxia[14]
Respiratory disease,[191] e.g. hyaline membrane disease
Congenital heart disease, e.g. coarctation, patent ductus arteriosis[193]
Maternal cocaine abuse[194,195]
Umbilical artery catheterization[196]

Pathophysiology

The precise pathophysiology of NEC remains unclear, but it is considered to be multifactorial in origin – the culmination of microbial colonization and inflammatory insult with mucosal injury to an intestine that is compromised by hypoxic ischemia and/or immaturity.[1,20] Hypoxia and circulatory ischemia result in preferential distribution of the limited blood supply to vital organs such as the heart, brain and kidney, at the expense of compromising blood flow away from non-vital regions including the splanchnic circulation of the intestinal tract (the Herring–Breur reflex). Intestinal ischemia and bacterial colonization stimulate pro-inflammatory mediators (including interferon-γ,[21,22] tumor necrosis factor (TNF)-α[23] and platelet activating factor (PAF)[24,25]), which through multiple cascades may lead to variable degrees of coagulative and ischemic necrosis of the bowel.[20]

Furthermore free radicals released from inflammatory cascades following ischemia and reperfusion contribute to the tissue necrosis by causing lipid peroxidative damage to cellular membranes.[26] Diffusion of free radicals and the effect of gas-forming organisms within the gut wall result in the pathognomonic pneumatosis intestinalis that is seen on radiographs in 90% of cases.[27]

Transmural necrosis with bacterial translocation across the gut wall may result in perforation with peritonitis, bacteremia or septicemia. Up to 35% of patients with NEC have positive cultures,[28] with the most common implicated pathogens being *Klebsiella*,[29] *Escherichia coli*,[29] *Clostridium difficile*[30,31] and *Streptococcus faecalis*.[32]

The increased propensity of premature infants to develop NEC injury is attributed to a number of additional factors. These include a deficient intestinal microbial host defense, poor development of the mucosal barrier,[33,34] an immature mucosa at greater susceptibility to hyperosmolar feeds[18] and an accentuated pro-inflammatory response.[35,36] If the intestinal injury is short-lived, the pathological course may be followed by healing with fibrosis, with or without a resulting stricture in the affected bowel. The disease most commonly involves the terminal ileum and ascending colon, but it may affect variable segments of the small and large intestine, being isolated (30%), multifocal (55%) or pan-intestinal (15%) (Figure 35.1).[37]

Clinical signs and symptoms

The clinical course of NEC is variable, with two-thirds of patients developing the condition within the first week of life.[38] The severity of the disease may be categorized clinically using the original Bell's staging system for NEC[39] outlined below, a classification later modified by Walsh and Kliegman.[40]

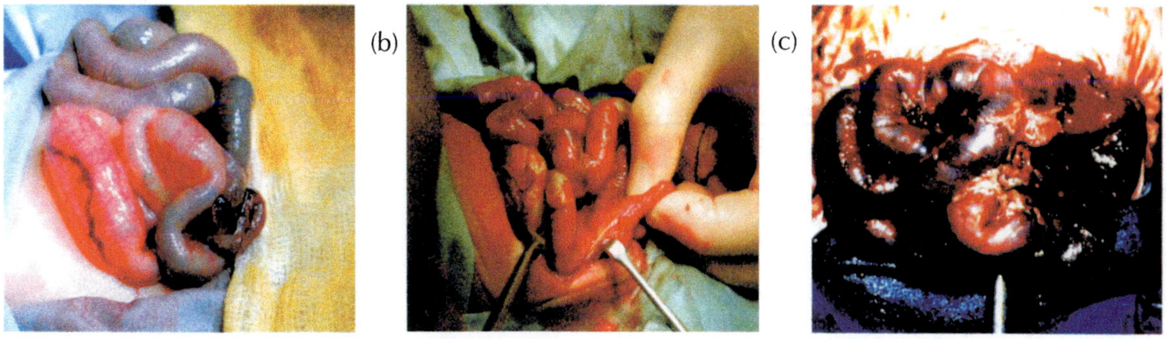

Figure 35.1 Intraoperative illustration of (a) isolated necrotizing enterocolitis (NEC), (b) multifocal NEC, (c) pan-intestinal NEC.

Stage I

Suspected NEC. At the early stage, symptoms and signs are usually non-specific, e.g. irritability, fever, apneas and bradycardias, and poor toleration of feeds. Many of these children are more likely to be suffering from feeding intolerance commonly associated with prematurity or low birth weight, but nonetheless they should be regarded as at risk of developing more fulminant disease.

Stage II

Established NEC. These babies will have established clinical and radiographic signs of NEC with moderate–profound systemic illness, including metabolic acidosis and thrombocytopenia. Vomiting/aspirates are usually bilious or blood-stained whilst stools are likely to be blood-stained. Abdominal distension, abdominal wall erythema and edema are usual, and there may or may not be evidence of perforation clinically and/or radiologically. A clinically palpable intra-abdominal mass (reported in 11%[38]) may indicate the presence of persistently dilated bowel loops or, if the disease is localized, an intraperitoneal abscess.

Stage III

Advanced NEC with systemic instability. As well as features of stage II disease, these babies have cardiovascular instability (hypotension), severe metabolic acidosis and coagulative derangements. There will usually be abdominal and radiological evidence of perforation, peritonitis and ascites with generalized sepsis.

Complications

At least 10%[41] of NEC cases develop one or more of the following complications, with their incidences being significantly more common in preterm infants.[37]

(1) Metabolic disorders including metabolic acidosis and disseminated intravascular coagulation (DIC);

(2) Perforation with peritonitis and septicemia;

(3) Localized intraperitoneal abscess formation;

(4) Healing by fibrosis with stricture formation (20% in term infants and 31% in preterm infants[37]);

(5) Massive gut involvement that requires resection may result in short-bowel syndrome,[42,43] with resultant failure to thrive or, worse still, pan-intestinal involvement that is incompatible with life;

(6) Recurrence of the disease (9–14%[37]);

(7) Infants with stage II or III disease are commonly at risk of developing psychomotor retardation,[44–49] although this may be more attributed to the high incidence of prematurity than a direct effect of NEC.

Diagnosis with differential

The differential diagnoses of NEC are outlined in Table 35.2. Investigations for diagnosis of NEC include the following.

Table 35.2 Differential diagnosis of necrotizing enterocolitis

Feeding intolerance of prematurity
Spontaneous intestinal perforation
Malrotation/volvulus
Neonatal sepsis with ileus
Congenital intestinal obstruction (intestinal atresia, Hirschsprung's disease)
Neonatal pseudomembranous colitis (rare)
Neonatal appendicitis (rare)

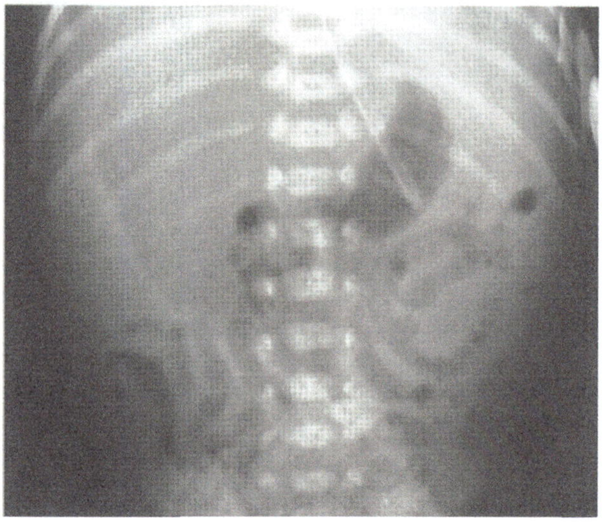

Figure 35.2 Abdominal X-ray demonstrating pneumoperitoneum from perforated necrotizing enterocolitis.

Abdominal X-ray (Figure 35.2) may demonstrate dilated bowel loops, edematous bowel wall, ascites, intramural gas (pneumatosis intestinalis), portal vein gas and free air in the peritoneal cavity (pneumoperitoneum). Signs of a pneumoperitoneum include the 'football sign' (central collection of free air outlining the falciform ligament and umbilical arteries), localized gas in the right upper quadrant (the 'right upper quadrant gas sign'), or gas on both sides of the bowel wall ('Rigler's sign'). The presence of a single/multiple loops of bowel retaining the same shape or position for 24–36 h ('fixed-loop sign') may suggest full-thickness bowel necrosis.

In metabolic acidosis, the hemoglobin level may fall, owing to hemorrhage and sepsis, whilst leukocyte and platelet counts[37,50] may be depressed, particularly in association with DIC.[37]

Bacteriological screening should include blood culture and collection of swabs from the nose, throat, umbilicus and rectum.

Treatment options

The initial management of NEC consists of stabilization of the infant and resting of the intestinal tract by means of discontinuation of enteral feeds for 10 days, total parenteral nutrition, decompression of the stomach by a nasogastric tube, fluid resuscitation, intravenous antibiotics for 7–14 days and correction of any metabolic derangement. However, up to 50% of neonates with NEC develop advanced disease that requires surgery.[51] Indications for surgery include:

(1) Clinical deterioration despite maximal medical treatment;

(2) A pneumoperitoneum, indicating perforated NEC;

(3) An abdominal mass with persistent intestinal obstruction or sepsis;

(4) The development of an intestinal stricture.

The options for surgery are between primary peritoneal drainage or laparotomy. However, the optimum choice between primary peritoneal drainage and laparotomy remains controversial, particularly in low-birth-weight infants (< 1000 g). Peritoneal drainage offers temporary decompression, drainage and stabilization of patients whilst awaiting surgery, or in patients too unstable to be able to tolerate surgery/anesthesia. Peritoneal drains, using either Penrose drains or an improvised finger of a latex glove, are inserted in the right and/or left iliac fossas, under local anesthesia (Figure 35.3). Those weighing > 1000 g who have no associated morbidities and are clinically stable, are preferentially treated by primary laparotomy.[52] The principal surgical objectives of laparotomy in acute NEC are to control sepsis, to remove gangrenous bowel and to preserve as much bowel length as possible.[53–55] Within these objectives, a

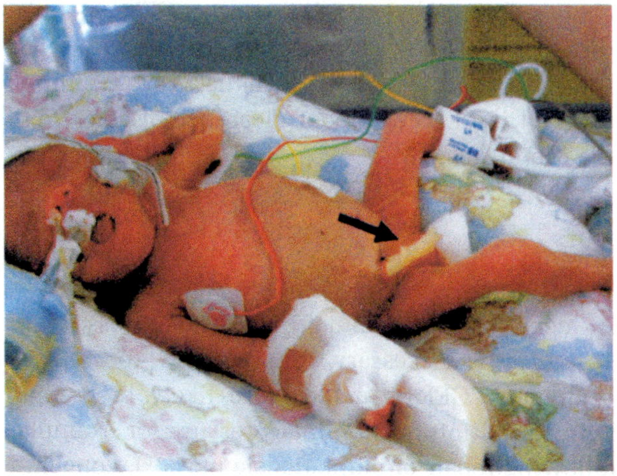

Figure 35.3 An infant with a peritoneal drain (arrow) inserted into the right iliac fossa.

number of options exist, including: resection with enterostomy; resection with primary anastomosis; proximal jejunostomy; the 'clip and drop' technique; or to 'patch, drain and wait'. The option exercised is highly variable between surgeons[9,56–59] and is often influenced by the site and extent of the disease. An algorithm of the authors' preferred surgical approach for the management of advanced NEC is illustrated in Figure 35.4.

Prognosis

The outcome from NEC is highly variable, with the postoperative complication and mortality rates ranging between 10 and 70%. These depend on:

(1) Stage of the disease;[14,49,60,61]

(2) Extent of disease involvement, with the lowest survival in pan-intestinal disease;[5,8,11,37,42,49,62–65]

(3) Birth weight;[5–10,14,49]

(4) Gestational age,[5,14,37,49,63,66,67] with 77% survival in term infants compared to 66% in preterm infants;

(5) Presence of associated medical co-morbidities;[7,49,68]

(6) Modality of operative treatment. This affects the postoperative complication rate for multifocal NEC (85% survival after resection and primary anastomosis compared to 50% with enterostomy alone) but not isolated NEC.[37]

Contrary to popular belief, the loss of the ileocecal valve is not associated with increased complication or mortality rates,[37,69,70] suggesting that these neonates adapt rapidly to the loss of the ileocecal valve.

Gastroesophageal reflux

GER is a physiological process characterized by the involuntary passage of gastric contents into the lower esophagus not induced by noxious stimuli. The phenomenon is considered as GER disease only when it causes the patient to be symptomatic or results in pathological complications.

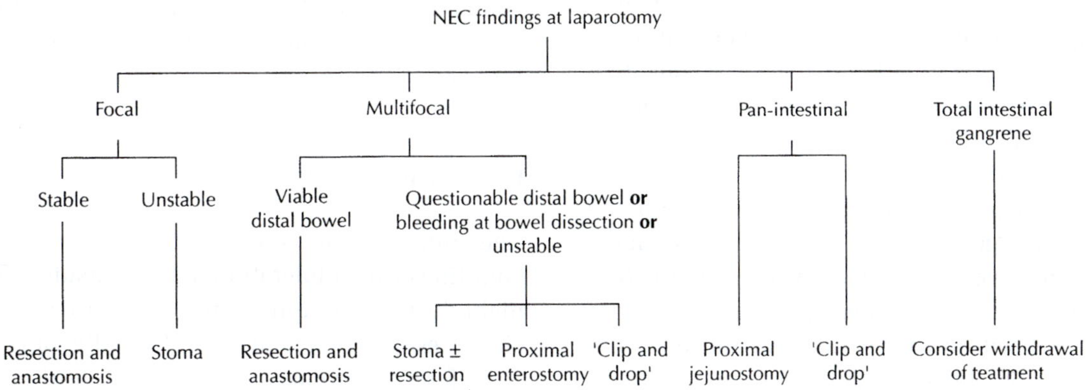

Figure 35.4 Algorithm of the authors' preferred operative management of advanced necrotizing enterocolitis (NEC) (reproduced with permission from *Seminars in Perinatology* 2003).

Epidemiology

Most newborns have some degree of GER, but the majority resolve spontaneously, with the prevalence decreasing to 18% in childhood.[71] The male/female ratio is 1.6.[72] The incidence of GER is highest in neurologically impaired children (70%), who comprise 44–67% of children undergoing anti-reflux surgery.[73–75]

Pathophysiology

A number of physiological and anatomical factors normally contribute to prevent chronic reflux of gastric contents into the lower esophagus. The combination of esophageal motility and gravity facilitates esophageal clearance of refluxed material as well as of saliva, which is rich in bicarbonate, that coats the esophagus. These esophageal clearance mechanisms are usually developed by 31 weeks' gestation.[76] Other physiological barriers to GER include antral contractions facilitating gastric emptying, and the production of mucus, prostaglandin and epithelial growth factors, which help to prevent damage to the esophageal mucosa.

Anatomically the length of the intra-abdominal esophagus, the phrenoesophageal ligaments, the gastric mucosal 'rosette' and the esophageal hiatus (which is a sling formed by the crura of the diaphragm causing a pinchcock effect) all contribute to a higher-pressure zone in the lower esophagus. This high-pressure zone forms the lower esophageal sphincter (LES), a physiological rather than a true anatomical sphincter. Pressures at this gastroesophageal junction (10–30 mmHg) are greater than gastric luminal pressure (5 mmHg), thereby preventing retrograde passage of gastric contents. In addition, the acute angle of His (made by the esophagus and the axis of the stomach) and the above physiological factors cumulatively contribute to limit the volume and frequency of gastric contents refluxing into the lower esophagus. Much of these anatomical features, however, are poorly developed in the first weeks of an infant's life, predisposing it to a higher risk of GER within this period. For instance, the angle of His is obtuse in newborns and decreases only as the infant grows; also, the length of the intra-abdominal esophagus is shorter, only 1 cm at birth, compared to 3 cm by 3 months of age. Other abnormalities that predispose to GER include disruption of the gastroesophageal junction (with resulting hiatus hernia), weakness or incompetence of the LES and poor clearance of acid from the esophagus.[77]

Etiology

A mean intra-abdominal pressure of less than 10 mmHg is necessary for the LES to remain competent. GER is made more likely in groups with raised intra-abdominal pressure for example following repair of omphalocele (43%[78]), congenital diaphragmatic hernia[79] and chronic respiratory infections.

Neurologically impaired children have the highest incidence of GER (65–70%[80]). This is due to a combination of poor esophageal and gastric motility (due to vagal nerve dysfunction), chronic supine positioning, abdominal spasticity, diaphragmatic flaccidity, scoliosis, retching and increased use of gastrostomy for feeding.

Insertion of gastrostomy tubes has been reported to be associated with the development or *worsening* of pre-existing GER. The gastrostomy, which fixes the stomach to the anterior abdominal wall, potentially opens the angle of His[81] and lowers the LES pressure[82] thereby predisposing to GER.

GER occurs in 30–80% of children treated for esophageal atresia, the incidence being related to the length of the atresia gap. The GER is attributed partly to poor esophageal motility in these patients and partly to a shortened esophagus. The shortened esophagus, from the original anomaly and compounded by the surgical repair, results in upward displacement of the gastroesophageal junction.

Clinical signs and symptoms

The infant with GER typically presents with vomiting or poor toleration of feeds, made worse at night during the supine position. Those with associated esophagitis may manifest clinically with Sandifer's syndrome, a voluntary dystonic contortion of the head, neck and trunk. These movements have been shown to improve peristalsis in the lower esophagus. If GER is left untreated, failure to thrive from calorie deprivation may ensue. Reflux of gastric contents into the airways may result in coughing and choking, and chronic aspiration may cause the infant to present with complications of GER, including laryngospasm with apneic and bradycardia spells (particularly during sleep), stridor or pneumonia.

Complications

(1) Failure to thrive secondary to calorie deprivation occurs in up to 20–52% of children.[83,84]

(2) Iron deficiency anemia, seen in 31%,[83] may indicate significant reflux esophagitis with blood loss.

(3) Aspiration of gastric contents may cause laryngospasm and subsequently obstructive apneas and bradycardias (17%[84]), particularly during sleep, or be complicated by pneumonia (in 31%[83]) or subglottic stenosis.

(4) Bronchopulmonary dysplasia (60%[84]), bronchiectasis, bronchitis and asthma. The mechanism of these complications is not clear. One hypothesis is that reflux of gastric contents may stimulate vagal afferents in the distal esophagus which may cause a reflex vagovagal bronchoconstriction.[85,86]

(5) Persistent GER may result in esophagitis, which in turn may lead to sticture with dysphagia or, in older children, Barrett's esophagus, a recognized pre-malignant condition.

Diagnosis with differential

The differential diagnoses of an infant with clinical features of GER are outlined in Table 35.3. Investigations used for diagnosis of GER include the following.

Twenty-four-hour pH monitoring is currently the most sensitive and specific test available for diagnosing GER. Monitoring is performed for 24 continuous hours, during which time the patient is fed only breast milk, formula or apple juice. The juice is preferable, as the alkaline content of milk feeds may neutralize the gastric acid reflux and thereby potentially produce a false-negative result.

Table 35.3 Differential diagnosis of gastroesophageal reflux

Infantile hypertrophic pyloric stenosis
Overfeeding/feeding disorders
Malrotation
Gastroenteritis
Neonatal sepsis
Neurological pathology (e.g. raised intracranial pressure from hydrocephalus)
Laryngeal cleft

Acid reflux is defined by pH <4.0 in the lower esophagus. Esophageal exposure to gastric acid is assessed in terms of the cumulative time during which the esophageal pH is below 4.0, expressed as the percentage of the total 24 h. A positive test for GER is indicated by a pH below 4.0 for more than 5% of the duration of the study.

Upper GI contrast studies (Figure 35.5) may diagnose active episodes of GER. However, they are more useful for detecting anatomical abnormalities, e.g. hiatus hernia, stricture and esophageal motility. They may rule out the presence of malrotation of the bowel or gastric outlet obstruction as a cause of vomiting.

A gastric isotope scintiscan is used if gastric emptying is not visualized on upper GI contrast studies. 99m-Technetium is added to the infant's formula followed by monitoring with a gamma counter. Retention of $>50\%$ of the radioisotope in the stomach after 90 min, in the absence of mechanical obstruction, indicates delayed gastric emptying.

Esophagoscopy allows visualization of the gastroesophageal mucosa. However, only 40% of cases of GER will demonstrate unequivocal esophagitis. Endoscopy is therefore a poor tool for diagnosis of GER, and is more useful in the assessment of complications of reflux (e.g. esophagitis or stricture) and in obtaining biopsies (e.g. *Helicobacter pylori* infections or development of Barrett's esophagus).

Esophageal manometry enables measurement of the LES tone. However, the LES tone is low at birth, rising to a mean pressure of 10–15 mmHg by

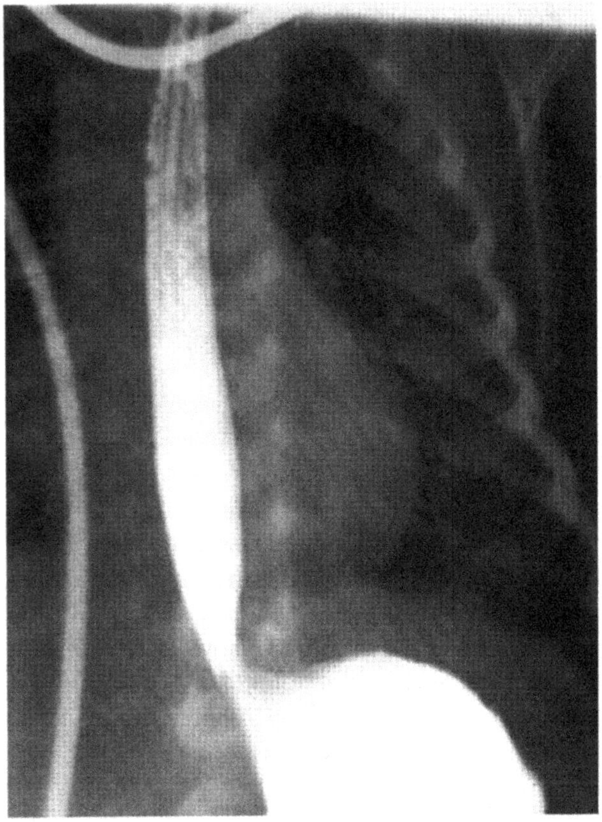

Figure 35.5 Upper gastrointestinal contrast study demonstrating gastroesophageal reflux.

6 months of age. Thus, sphincter tone will be physiologically low in neonates, and therefore has little application in diagnosing GER in this age group.

Chest X-ray may identify pulmonary complications of GER.

Lipid-laden alveolar macrophages in tracheal aspirates/bronchoalveolar lavage may indicate aspiration secondary to GER. However, the sensitivity and specificity for detecting GER are as low as 38% and 59%, respectively.[87] Furthermore, elevated levels of lipid-laden macrophages are found in a number of pulmonary disease without any evidence of aspiration.[88]

Treatment options

The two main aims of treatment are to prevent the respiratory complications of GER and to improve the nutritional status of the child from resumption of normal feeding.

Medical therapy

Conservative measures for GER in infants are frequently advocated. They include the avoidance of medications that reduce LES tone (caffeine, theophylline, anticholinergics), dietary modifications (changing the feed pattern with use of frequent, small-volume feeds) and positioning maneuvers. However, many of these have no confirmed efficacy. Thickening of formula feeds (e.g. with carob bean gum, or rice flour) may reduce frank emesis but does not reduce GER measurably compared to placebo.[89–92] Furthermore, there are no quality data to support the opinion that more frequent but smaller-volume feedings reduce GER.[93] With respect to positioning maneuvers, positioning at a 60° head elevation increases GER compared to the prone position.[94] However, the association of the prone position with sudden infant death syndrome has brought controversy with this maneuver. No significant difference has been found between the flat and head-elevation prone positions.[95]

Pharmacotherapy forms the main first-line treatment modality of GER. A wide spectrum of agents is now available (Table 35.4), aimed at decreasing acid secretion and increasing gastric emptying. Detailed descriptions of the pharmacological mechanisms of these agents can be found elsewhere.

Surgical treatment

Whilst medical therapy serves to decrease the acid content of the refluxate, other components of the refluxate (e.g. bile pepsin, trypsin) remain unaffected. Surgery therefore becomes indicated in infants who do not respond to medical treatment, or who experience apparent life-threatening events (e.g. laryngospasm and apneas), or have anatomical problems such as hiatus hernias or esophageal strictures. Operative options available for treatment of GER are Nissen's fundoplication (used in 64%[74]) and Thal (34%[74]), Toupet (1.5%[74]), Dor, Boerema, Boix–Ochoa, Collis–Belsey and Hill procedures. Nissen's fundoplication (Figure 35.6)[96] is the most popular method, and involves a 360° wrap of the fundus of the stomach, brought round the posterior aspect of the esophagus. It controls GER by increasing the acuteness of the angle of His and lengthening the intra-abdominal esophagus,

Table 35.4 Pharmacotherapy of gastroesophageal reflux (GER)

Antacids, e.g. Gaviscon®
H_2 blockers, e.g. ranitidine
Proton pump inhibitors, e.g. omeprazole
Prokinetic agents, e.g. dopamine antagonists (e.g. metoclopramide), postganglionic 5-HT4 agonist/acetylcholine agonists (e.g. cisapride), erythromycin, bethanecol or domperidone. Prokinetics increase LES tone and esophageal peristalsis thereby improving gastric emptying. However, concerns regarding the safety of cisapride on the myocardium, with reports of arrhythmias and prolonged QT interval, has restricted its clinical use
γ-Aminobutyric acid (GABA) agonists, e.g. baclofen, are agents that inhibit GER episodes by inhibition of transient relaxations of the LES,[197,198] and are currently being considered for clinical trials

LES, lower esophageal sphincter

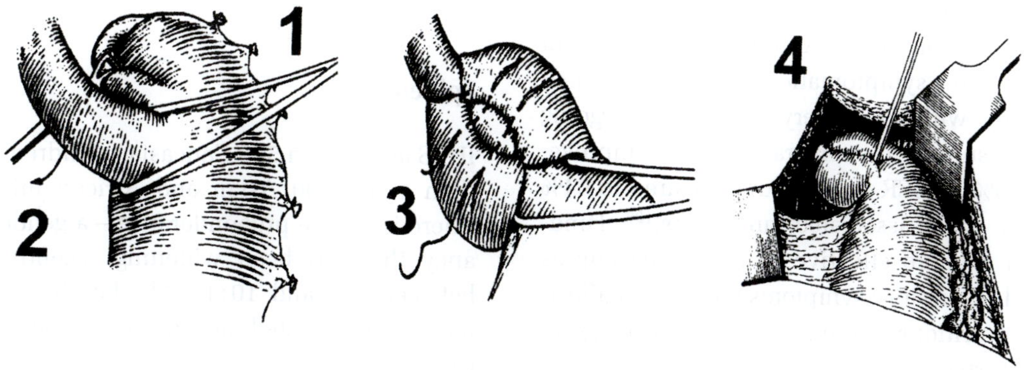

Figure 35.6 Nissen's fundoplication 1, Mobilization of the fundus of the stomach by division of short gastric vessels. 2, Fundus folded round the posterior aspect of the esophagus. 3, A loose wrap formed, using interrupted sutures. 4, The completed stomach wrap. (Adapted with permission from reference 187).

thereby increasing the high-pressure zone at the LES. A concurrent gastrostomy is frequently placed, particularly in neurologically impaired children, those with feeding difficulties and poor weight gain, or slow gastric emptying. The Thal procedure[97] is an anterior fundoplication with a partial (180–270°) wrap of the fundus of the stomach to the intra-abdominal esophagus. The benefit of the Thal procedure is that it allows the patient to belch and release any bloating, which is not feasible with Nissen's fundoplication. Fundoplication procedures may be performed by the open or laparoscopic method. Reliable data comparing outcomes between the two approaches are, however, limited in children. Non-randomized studies suggest that the laparoscopic approach offers better cosmesis and, if not favorable, is at least comparable with respect to operative time, postoperative pain, time to feeds and complication rate.[98–101]

Recently, two further endoscopic techniques have been described for the treatment of GER. The first is endoscopic radiofrequency energy delivery to the gastroesophageal junction around the LES. Early data suggest that this can achieve resolution of symptoms of GER in 87% of patients,[102] but is associated with significant mortality and morbidity, including aspiration, pleural effusion and atrial fibrillation.[103] The second is endoscopic gastroplication,[104] which involves internally plicating the stomach on itself approximately 1 cm below the gastroesophageal junction to alter the angle of His and thereby decrease reflux of gastric contents. Early results indicate poorer outcomes compared to fundoplications, with 75% still requiring adjuvant medical treatment and 6% undergoing fundoplication due to therapeutic failure.[105] Furthermore, the data reported with both these procedures have so far been limited to adult populations, and their application in pediatrics remains unclear.

Prognosis

The prognosis of infants with GER is highly variable, depending on the presence of associated anomalies (e.g. esophageal atresia, congenital diaphragmatic hernia, neurological disorders), anatomical problems (e.g. hiatus hernia), prematurity of the infant, or the presence of established complications of GER. Approximately 80% of patients with symptomatic GER are treated successfully without surgery. Infants undergoing anti-reflux surgery demonstrate clinical improvement in 90%, if GER is isolated, compared to 64% of infants with associated anomalies.[106] Fundoplication is more effective in improving emesis (76%) and respiratory symptoms (66%) than affecting the nutritional status, with persistence of failure to thrive in 62% of patients.

Complications following fundoplication repairs (Table 35.5) occur in up to 24%, with the neurologically impaired having up to six-fold increased incidence compared to those neurologically normal.[73–75,106–113] A repeat fundoplication is required in up to 24% of cases, due to either failure of the wrap (disruption, herniation or excessive tightness) or recurrence of GER. Recurrence of GER symptoms after fundoplication is more frequent in infants, particularly those with previous esophageal atresia repair (42%), with half of these requiring a second procedure.[106]

Table 35.5 Complications following fundoplication

Disruption of the wrap with recurrence of GER (8–12%)
Dysphagia from an excessively tight wrap (2–12%)
Herniation of the wrap (2–10%)
Gas bloating (4–10%) particularly with Nissen's fundoplications
Adhesive intestinal obstruction (2–10%)
Poor esophageal clearance (in patients with esophageal atresia)
Splenic injury (0.5%)
Mortality (0–13%)

GER, gastroesophageal reflux

Infantile hypertrophic pyloric stenosis

IHPS is the second most common condition in infancy that requires surgery. The treatment of pyloromyotomy was first described by Fredet in 1907, and then my Ramstedt 4 years later.[114]

Epidemiology

IHPS affects 1 in 500 Caucasian children and fewer than 1 in 1000 Asian and African infants.[115–118] There is a male preponderance – a gender discrepancy that has been widening recently, reported between 4:1 and 10:1.[119–125] Firstborn males are most often affected, accounting for 40–60% of all cases.

Etiology

In spite of IHPS being one of the most common and earliest recognized surgical problems in infants, its precise etiology remains unclear. Two proposed risk factors are breast feeding and a positive family history. Twenty per cent of infants with IHPS have a positive family history. Although more common in males, a positive family history is four times as common from affected mothers than fathers.[126] Overall, there is a 15–20-fold increase in risk of a child of an affected parent developing pyloric stenosis compared to the general population.[126,127] It is also more common in multiple births.[128,129] The incidence of Smith–Lemli–Opitz syndrome diagnosed in infants with IHPS is 150-fold higher than in the general population.[117] This, and other congenital gastrointestinal and urinary tract malformations that are more common with IHPS,[118] suggest a genetic role in its etiology. The mode of inheritance is likely to be multifactorial, although evidence of reduced expression of the neuronal nitric oxide synthase (nNOS) gene, which is responsible for the smooth-muscle relaxant nitric oxide (NO), has been found.[130,131] The influence of breast feeding on IHPS is more controversial. A number of groups have found that infants with IHPS were twice as likely to have been breast fed.[116,132,133] However, Hitchcock et al[134] found no such link whilst Pisacane et al[135] found a protective effect from breast feeding.

Pathophysiology

Whilst the precise mechanism of IHPS remains unclear, a number of causative factors have been reported.

First, is failure of relaxation of the pylorus. The circular layer of smooth muscle of the pylorus is stimulated by the myenteric plexus, whilst its relaxation is dependent on non-adrenergic, non-cholinergic (NANC) inhibitory motor neurons. Depletion of these nerves (either primary absence or degeneration) in pyloric muscle may be the cause of the excessively contracted hypertrophic circular pyloric muscle.[136] This hypothesis is further supported by the demonstration of reduced expression of the nNOS gene (responsible for NO synthesis, a mediator of NANC inhibitory nerves) in animals models[130] and depleted nNOS mRNA in the pyloric muscle of patients with IHPS.[131] The influence of uncompensated pylorus contractility may also explain why neonates receiving erythromycin, which induces the activity of migrating motor complexes in the stomach[137] and increases pyloric contraction,[138] have up to a seven-fold increased risk[139,140] of developing IHPS. It is suggested that this marked increase in motility may lead to hypertrophy of the pylorus.[139]

Increased expression of insulin-like growth factor-I[141,142] and transforming growth factor-β[143] found in hypertrophic pyloric muscle, may indicate a hormonal role in smooth-muscle hypertrophy in IHPS.

Increased amounts of extracellular matrix proteins, particularly collagen, have been reported within the circular muscle wall of the pylorus in IHPS. This may account for the hypertrophic wall of the pylorus.[144,145]

Hypertrophy of the circular smooth muscle wall of the pylorus up to four-fold results in pyloric luminal outflow obstruction. The infant vomits obstructed milk feeds and with it gastric acid contents (hydrochloric acid), resulting in dehydration with a hypochloremic, hypokalemic metabolic alkalosis.

Clinical signs and symptoms

The infant with IHPS typically presents with vomiting, usually at 3–6 weeks of age, although up to one-third start vomiting within the first week of life.[121,146] Vomiting may initially be effortless, but with time it becomes forceful, described as 'projectile'. The vomitus is usually milk feeds, practically never bilious, and if severe may contain some 'coffee-ground' flecks of altered blood from secondary gastritis in 15–20%.[133] The infant is frequently hungry for further feeds, despite the vomiting. Constipation is common. Jaundice may occur in 3%, and is attributed to the adverse effect of starvation on hepatic glucuronyl transferase activity.[133] Clinically, dehydration from severe vomiting, loss of weight and failure to thrive may ensue. Abdominal examination may reveal visible peristalsis of the obstructed pylorus (from left to right) in 75–95% of cases, and a pyloric 'tumor' mass, felt like an 'olive', representing the hypertrophic pylorus, usually in the epigastrium or upper quadrants of the abdomen. Successful palpation of the pyloric tumor can be achieved in up to 90% of cases,[147] and may be aided by maneuvers such as nasogastric decompression of the stomach (which is usually distended with gas swallowed by a hungry crying child), palpation through the midline gap between the two rectus muscles or at the lateral margins of the recti, flexing the hips, or allowing the child to suck on a passifier or a 'test feed' of dextrose solution (which should be aspirated back from the nasogastric tube).

Complications

(1) Dehydration and metabolic imbalance;

(2) Intraoperative duodenal perforation. This may occur in 3–4%;[148,149]

(3) Postoperative complications. These include transient persistence of vomiting in 3–19%[122,148]

(particularly those with a protracted preoperative history of vomiting); wound infection (1–4%);[148] or wound dehiscence (1.4%).[149] With experience and earlier diagnosis, mortality fell from 59% in 1925 to almost nil by 1975.[121,148,150]

Diagnosis with differential

The differential diagnosis of a vomiting child in this age group is usually an overfed child or GER. Less commonly, the following should be considered: incarcerated inguinal hernia, malrotation of the bowel (particularly if vomiting is bilious), congenital causes of gastric outlet obstruction (e.g. webs or duplications), or medical conditions (e.g. sepsis, raised intracranial pressure).

Over the past 30 years, increased reliance on imaging has decreased clinical diagnosis from up to 90% of cases[147,151,152] to as little as 23%.[152] Ultrasound diagnosis, which has a sensitivity and specificity for detecting IHPS of 95–100%,[153,154] is the most popular mode of imaging, but some groups continue to use upper GI contrast studies (Figure 35.7). At least one imaging study is now performed in 96%, with diagnosis by radiological means alone having increased to up to 65%.[155] The criteria for ultrasound diagnosis of IHPS (Figure 35.8) in a term infant include a pyloric diameter of >11 mm, muscle wall thickness of >3 mm and pyloric canal length of >16 mm. However, overreliance on imaging of a clinically obvious palpable tumor is cost-ineffective, and may delay treatment unnecessarily, particularly if a false-negative result is reported,[156] and should be discouraged.

Infants with suspected IHPS should routinely undergo analysis of serum electrolytes and acid–base status, which will typically demonstrate a hypokalemic, hypochloremic metabolic acidosis, secondary to loss of gastric acid and dehydration from vomiting.

Treatment options

Initial management of IHPS is rehydration and correction of biochemical derangements. Various fluid regimens are advocated; one such is an infusion of 0.45% saline with dextrose solution (10%

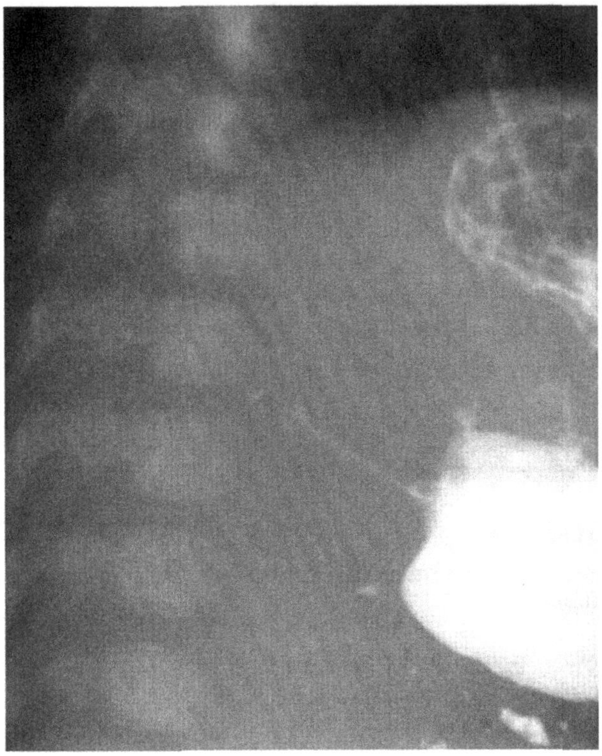

Figure 35.7 Upper gastrointestinal contrast study demonstrating narrowed gastric outlet from pyloric stenosis ('string sign').

for neonates and 4% for older infants) with 10 mmol potassium chloride. Only after correction and adequate rehydration is the definitive surgery performed. The operation, Fredet–Ramstedt's pyloromyotomy, may be performed by the open or laparoscopic method. Whilst the laparoscopic approach offers better cosmesis, clinical outcomes appear comparable.[157,158] The open method may be performed using a vertical midline, right upper quadrant transverse, or an umbilical incision. No difference in complications were found between the right upper quadrant and vertical incisions.[159] The hypertrophic pyloric muscle (Figure 35.9) is split longitudinally, releasing the mucosal tension within. The optimum timing of re-commencing feeding postoperatively following an uncomplicated pyloromyotomy remains controversial. Advocates of early feeding *ad libitum* immediately following recovery from anesthesia report shorter time to full feeds and shorter hospital stay.[160] Others, who report higher incidence of emesis from such

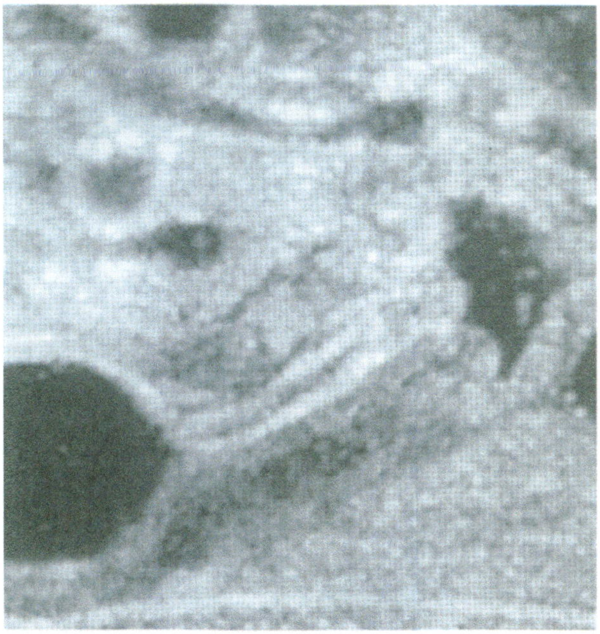

Figure 35.8 Ultrasound scan demonstrating pyloric stenosis.

a regimen, favor delaying feeding for 6–12 h.[161] Feeding is usually delayed for 24 h in those complicated with an intraoperative mucosal perforation.

Inguinal hernia

A hernia is defined as an abnormal protrusion of a viscus or part of a viscus through its coverings into an abnormal anatomical site. Inguinal hernia is the most common condition requiring surgery during childhood. Almost all are indirect, i.e. they pass through the internal inguinal ring and through the inguinal canal.

Epidemiology

Inguinal hernias affect one in 50 term male infants and up to 30% of premature infants.[162] There is a male preponderance, reported between 4:1 and 9:1.[163–169] In males, 60% of hernias occur on the right, 30% occur on the left and 10% are bilateral.[170] Bilateral herniais are more common in females and in premature infants (15–24%).[166,169,171,172] A contralateral hernia is found in 50–60% of infants under 6 months of age, although the majority of these are not manifested clinically.

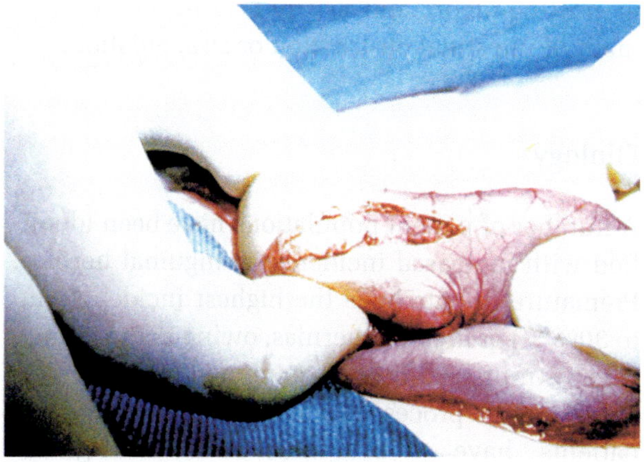

Figure 35.9 Ramstedt's pyloromyotomy.

Pathogenesis

The processus vaginalis is a peritoneal diverticulum that passes through the internal inguinal ring at 3 months *in utero*. During the 7th month *in utero*, the testis descends from its intra-abdominal position at the urogenital ridge, into the scrotum, and as it does so it takes part of the processus with it into the scrotum. The processus is usually obliterated shortly before birth, leaving only the portion of the processus surrounding the testis, which is now called the tunica vaginalis. In 10–20% of the population the processus remains patent throughout life.[173] Failure of obliteration of the processus leaves a potential communicating sac that allows passage of peritoneal fluid (hydrocele) or abdominal contents (hernia) into the groin or scrotum. The hernial sac may contain bowel or, additionally in girls, ovary or Fallopian tube. The descent of the right testis and the subsequent obliteration of its processus vaginalis occur later than the left. For this reason right-sided hernias are twice as common. In girls, the canal of Nuck undergoes the same obliteration as the processus vaginalis in boys, but the obliteration is more likely to be complete, explaining the lower incidence of inguinal hernias in girls. If the hernia becomes irreducible (incarceration), the sac contents are at risk of injury. Incarceration of bowel within the hernia is most common, and it may lead to the development of intestinal obstruction or strangulation.

Etiology

A number of patient populations have been identified with increased incidence of inguinal hernias. Premature infants have the highest incidence (up to 30%[162]) of inguinal hernias, owing to the premature birth preceding full completion of the obliteration of the processus vaginalis. Cystic fibrosis patients have a 15% incidence of inguinal hernias.[174] This increased risk is thought to be related to an altered embryogenesis of the Wolffian duct structures that also leads to an absent vas deferens in male infants with cystic fibrosis. Increased incidence is also found in patients with connective tissue disorders (e.g. Ehlers–Danlos syndrome[175,176]) and mucopolysaccharidosis (Hunter–Hurler syndrome[177]); children with ventriculoperitoneal shunt;[178] children receiving chronic peritoneal dialysis;[179,180] and children with congenital dislocation of the hips.[181]

Clinical signs and symptoms

The hernia is often noticed by parents, for example on changing the infant's diaper, as a swelling, either in the groin (inguinal hernia) or scrotum (inguinoscrotal hernia; Figure 35.10). In most cases the infant is asymptomatic. The hernia may become prominent on straining or crying. However, a child in discomfort, or who is vomiting, particularly bile, should alert to the possibility of an obstructed or strangulated inguinal hernia. Features of intestinal obstruction include bilious vomiting, constipation and abdominal distension. A strangulated hernia will cause severe discomfort from ischemic bowel or testis and tenderness of hernial contents. It may cause passage of blood in the stools, with or without features of obstruction. Occasionally the only clinical evidence of a hernial sac may be a thickened spermatic cord compared to the contralateral cord.

Complications

Of infants with an inguinal hernia, 20–50%[182,183] present with incarceration, the risk being highest in the first 6 months of life. The main complications associated with incarceration (most frequently bowel contents) are intestinal obstruction or strangulation with testicular necrosis and/or bowel necrosis.

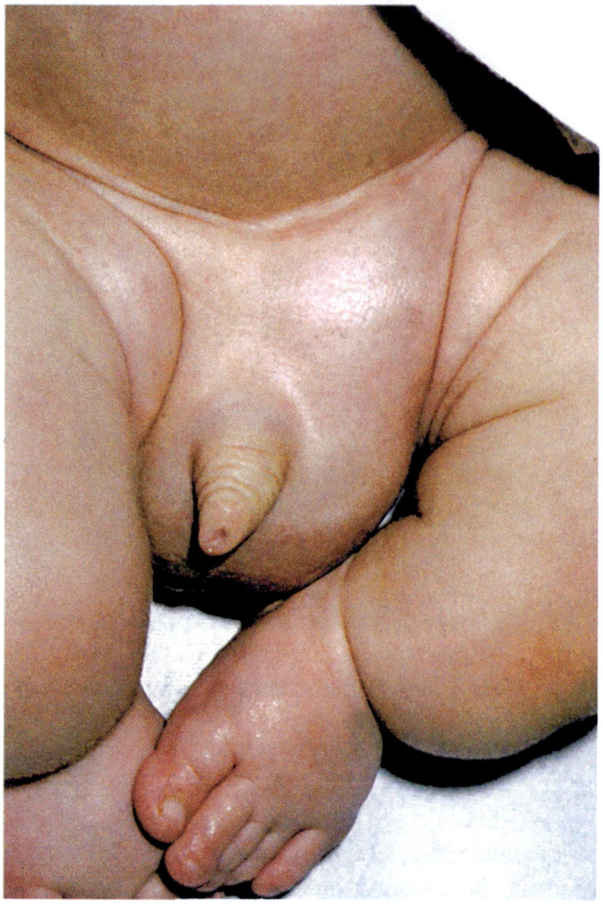

Figure 35.10 Bilateral inguinoscrotal hernias.

Diagnosis with differential

The primary differential diagnosis in boys is between a hernia and a hydrocele. The latter is cystic in consistency and easily transilluminates. Other differentials include an undescended or retractile testis, inguinal lymphadenopathy and rarely inguinal abscess. The ability to delineate the upper margin of the swelling distinguishes it from an inguinal hernia. The diagnosis is almost exclusively clinical; rarely, ultrasound confirmation may be used where there is reason for doubt. The presence of an intestinal obstruction complicating an incarcerated inguinal hernia may be confirmed by plain abdominal X-ray, which will demonstrate dilated loops of bowel.

Treatment options

Surgery is indicated in all cases, because of the danger of incarceration and strangulation of hernial sac contents. The timing of surgery is determined by three factors: the age of the child, its clinical condition, and whether the hernia has become complicated. In infants, in whom strangulation is most common, the hernia operation should be performed at the earliest possible date, even if the infant is asymptomatic, provided the infant's clinical status allows it. Premature, ventilated and critically ill infants with an uncomplicated hernia may have it repaired once they are stable. An irreducible hernia with or without strangulation or obstruction requires immediate surgery, irrespective of age. An incarcerated hernia that has been reduced successfully but with great difficulty may benefit from delayed repair of the hernia after 24–48 h, to allow edema of bowel contents that is usually present to settle preoperatively.

The hernia may be repaired by the open or laparoscopic method, although the optimal approach remains unproven. At surgery, if the hernia is uncomplicated, the PPV is mobilized and ligated at the internal ring. If the hernia is complicated by non-viable bowel within the sac, resection of the affected bowel with end-to-end anastomosis is performed. The decision as to whether the contralateral groin should be explored routinely under the same anesthetic remains controversial.[163,169,184] This practice is generally not favored, as it would lead to unnecessary surgery in about 80% and has the potential for damage to cord structures. However, the argument is less decisive in premature infants, who have a higher incidence of contralateral patent processus and risk of incarceration in the first 6 months of life. The laparoscopic approach to the repair of the hernia has the added benefit of allowing inspection of the abdominal exit of the contralateral internal inguinal ring during repair of the primary hernia, and avoids a potentially unnecessary contralateral groin exploration.

Postoperative complication rates from inguinal hernia repair are low, particularly with uncomplicated hernias. Reported complications include:

(1) Testicular atrophy by up to 25% volume, seen in 6% of cases.[185] The incidence of atrophy (15%) is highest after a period of incarceration and strangulation, and may be compounded by iatrogenic surgical trauma of testicular vessels;

(2) Wound infection/hematoma (1–4%[165–169]);

(3) Recurrence of the hernia (1–4%[165–168,182]);

(4) Ascending testis, which may occur in up to 2%,[167–169,186] owing to surgical adhesions restraining cord structures. These infants may require orchidopexy to return the testis to the scrotum;

(5) Iatrogenic damage to cord structures, e.g. vas deferens (0–2%).

REFERENCES

1. Kliegman RM, Fanaroff AA. Necrotizing enterocolitis. *N Engl J Med* 1984; **310**: 1093–1103.
2. Wiswell TE, Robertson CF, Jones TA, Tuttle DJ. Necrotizing enterocolitis in full-term infants. A case–control study. *Am J Dis Child* 1988; **142**: 532–535.
3. Kliegman RM, Fanaroff AA. Neonatal necrotizing enterocolitis: a nine-year experience. *Am J Dis Child* 1981; **135**: 603–607.
4. Leong GM, Drew JH. Necrotizing enterocolitis: a 15-year experience. *Aust NZ J Obstet Gynaecol* 1987; **27**: 40–44.
5. Cikrit D, Mastandrea J, West KW et al. Necrotizing enterocolitis: factors affecting mortality in 101 surgical cases. *Surgery* 1984; **96**: 648–655.
6. Llanos AR, Moss ME, Pinzon MC et al. Epidemiology of neonatal necrotising enterocolitis: a population-based study. *Paediatr Perinat Epidemiol* 2002; **16**: 342–349.
7. Guthrie SO, Gordon PV, Thomas V et al. Necrotizing enterocolitis among neonates in the United States. *J Perinatol* 2003; **23**: 278–285.

8. Kanto WP Jr, Wilson R, Ricketts RR. Management and outcome of necrotizing enterocolitis. *Clin Pediatr (Phila)* 1985; **24**: 79–82.
9. Ricketts RR, Jerles ML. Neonatal necrotizing enterocolitis: experience with 100 consecutive surgical patients. *World J Surg* 1990; **14**: 600–605.
10. Narang A, Rao R, Bhakoo ON. Neonatal necrotizing enterocolitis an epidemiological study. *Indian Pediatr* 1993; **30**: 1207–1214.
11. de Souza JC, da Motta UI, Ketzer CR. Prognostic factors of mortality in newborns with necrotizing enterocolitis submitted to exploratory laparotomy. *J Pediatr Surg* 2001; **36**: 482–486.
12. McGuire W, Anthony MY. Donor human milk versus formula for preventing necrotising enterocolitis in preterm infants: systematic review. *Arch Dis Child Fetal Neonatal Ed* 2003; **88**: F11–F14.
13. Lucas A, Cole TJ. Breast milk and neonatal necrotising enterocolitis. *Lancet* 1990; **336**: 1519–1523.
14. Buch NA, Ahmad SM, Ali SW, Hassan HM. An epidemiological study of neonatal necrotizing enterocolitis. *Saudi Med J* 2001; **22**: 231–237.
15. Barlow B, Santulli TV, Heird WC et al. An experimental study of acute neonatal enterocolitis – the importance of breast milk. *J Pediatr Surg* 1974; **9**: 587–595.
16. Yoshioka H, Iseki K, Fujita K. Development and differences of intestinal flora in the neonatal period in breast-fed and bottle-fed infants. *Pediatrics* 1983; **72**: 317–321.
17. Gibson GR, Wang X. Regulatory effects of bifidobacteria on the growth of other colonic bacteria. *J Appl Bacteriol* 1994; **77**: 412–420.
18. Book LS, Herbst JJ, Atherton SO, Jung AL. Necrotizing enterocolitis in low-birth-weight infants fed an elemental formula. *J Pediatr* 1975; **87**: 602–605.
19. Walther FJ, Verloove-Vanhorick SP, Brand R, Ruys JH. A prospective survey of necrotising enterocolitis in very low birthweight infants. *Paediatr Perinat Epidemiol* 1989; **3**: 53–61.
20. Kliegman RM. Models of the pathogenesis of necrotizing enterocolitis. *J Pediatr* 1990; **117**: S2–S5.
21. Ford H, Watkins S, Reblock K, Rowe M. The role of inflammatory cytokines and nitric oxide in the pathogenesis of necrotizing enterocolitis. *J Pediatr Surg* 1997; **32**: 275–282.
22. Ford HR, Sorrells DL, Knisely AS. Inflammatory cytokines, nitric oxide, and necrotizing enterocolitis. *Semin Pediatr Surg* 1996; **5**: 155–159.
23. Morecroft JA, Spitz L, Hamilton PA, Holmes SJ. Plasma cytokine levels in necrotizing enterocolitis. *Acta Paediatr Suppl* 1994; **396**: 18–20.
24. Caplan MS, Hedlund E, Adler L, Hsueh W. Role of asphyxia and feeding in a neonatal rat model of necrotizing enterocolitis. *Pediatr Pathol* 1994; **14**: 1017–1028.
25. Muguruma K, Gray PW, Tjoelker LW, Johnston JM. The central role of PAF in necrotizing enterocolitis development. *Adv Exp Med Biol* 1997; **407**: 379–382.
26. Vannucci RC. Current and potentially new management strategies for perinatal hypoxic–ischemic encephalopathy. *Pediatrics* 1990; **85**: 961–968.
27. Kliegman RM, Fanaroff AA. Neonatal necrotizing enterocolitis in the absence of pneumatosis intestinalis. *Am J Dis Child* 1982; **136**: 618–620.
28. Kliegman RM. Neonatal necrotizing enterocolitis: implications for an infectious disease. *Pediatr Clin North Am* 1979; **26**: 327–344.
29. Bell MJ, Shackelford P, Feigin RD et al. Epidemiologic and bacteriologic evaluation of neonatal necrotizing enterocolitis. *J Pediatr Surg* 1979; **14**: 1–4.
30. Lawrence G, Bates J, Gaul A. Pathogenesis of neonatal necrotising enterocolitis. *Lancet* 1982; **1**: 137–139.
31. Han VK, Sayed H, Chance GW et al. An outbreak of *Clostridium difficile* necrotizing enterocolitis: a case for oral vancomycin therapy? *Pediatrics* 1983; **71**: 935–941.
32. Dobson SR, Baker CJ. Enterococcal sepsis in neonates: features by age at onset and occurrence of focal infection. *Pediatrics* 1990; **85**: 165–171.
33. Shin CE, Falcone RA Jr, Stuart L et al. Diminished epidermal growth factor levels in infants with necrotizing enterocolitis. *J Pediatr Surg* 2000; **35**: 173–176.
34. Lawrence JP, Brevetti L, Obiso RJ et al. Effects of epidermal growth factor and *Clostridium difficile* toxin B in a model of mucosal injury. *J Pediatr Surg* 1997; **32**: 430–433.
35. Nanthakumar NN, Fusunyan RD, Sanderson I, Walker WA. Inflammation in the developing human intestine: a possible pathophysiologic contribution to necrotizing enterocolitis. *Proc Natl Acad Sci USA* 2000; **97**: 6043–6048.
36. Walker WA. Breast milk and the prevention of neonatal and preterm gastrointestinal disease states: a new perspective. *Zhonghua Min Guo Xiao Er Ke Yi Xue Hui Za Zhi* 1997; **38**: 321–331.
37. Fasoli L, Turi RA, Spitz L et al. Necrotizing enterocolitis: extent of disease and surgical treatment. *J Pediatr Surg* 1999; **34**: 1096–1099.
38. Yu VY, Tudehope DI, Gill GJ. Neonatal necrotizing enterocolitis: 1. Clinical aspects. *Med J Aust* 1977; **1**: 685–688.
39. Bell MJ, Ternberg JL, Feigin RD *et al.* Neonatal necrotizing enterocolitis. Therapeutic decisions based upon clinical staging. *Ann Surg* 1978; **187**: 1–7.
40. Walsh MC, Kliegman RM. Necrotizing enterocolitis: treatment based on staging criteria. *Pediatr Clin North Am* 1986; **33**: 179–201.
41. Stevenson DK, Kerner JA, Malachowski N, Sunshine P. Late morbidity among survivors of necrotizing enterocolitis. *Pediatrics* 1980; **66**: 925–927.
42. Ricketts RR. Surgical treatment of necrotizing enterocolitis and the short bowel syndrome. *Clin Perinatol* 1994; **21**: 365–387.
43. Grosfeld JL, Rescorla FJ, West KW. Short bowel syndrome in infancy and childhood. Analysis of survival in 60 patients. *Am J Surg* 1986; **151**: 41–46.
44. Chacko J, Ford WD, Haslam R. Growth and neurodevelopmental outcome in extremely-low-birth-weight infants after laparotomy. *Pediatr Surg Int* 1999; **15**: 496–499.
45. Vohr BR, Wright LL, Dusick AM et al. Neurodevelopmental and functional outcomes of extremely low birth weight infants in the National Institute of Child Health and Human Development Neonatal Research Network, 1993–1994. *Pediatrics* 2000; **105**: 1216–1226.
46. Simon NP, Brady NR, Stafford RL, Powell RW. The effect of abdominal incisions on early motor development of infants with necrotizing enterocolitis. *Dev Med Child Neurol* 1993; **35**: 49–53.
47. Voss M, Moore SW, van der Merwe, I, Pieper C. Fulminanting necrotising enterocolitis: outcome and prognostic factors. *Pediatr Surg Int* 1998; **13**: 576–580.
48. Grosfeld JL, Molinari F, Chaet M et al. Gastrointestinal perforation and peritonitis in infants and children: experience with 179 cases over ten years. *Surgery* 1996; **120**: 650–655.
49. Stanford A, Upperman JS, Boyle P et al. Long-term follow-up of patients with necrotizing enterocolitis. *J Pediatr Surg* 2002; **37**: 1048–1050.
50. Ververidis M, Kiely EM, Spitz L et al. The clinical significance of thrombocytopenia in neonates with

necrotizing enterocolitis. *J Pediatr Surg* 2001; **36**: 799–803.

51. Kosloske AM. Surgery of necrotizing enterocolitis. *World J Surg* 1985; **9**: 277–284.
52. Ein SH, Marshall DG, Girvan D. Peritoneal drainage under local anesthesia for perforations from necrotizing enterocolitis. *J Pediatr Surg* 1977; **12**: 963–967.
53. Albanese CT, Rowe MI. Necrotizing enterocolitis. In O'Neill JAJ, Rowe MI, Grosfeld JL et al., eds. *Pediatric Surgery*, vol 2. St Louis: Mosby, 1998: 1297–1332.
54. Pierro A. Necrotizing enterocolitis: pathogenesis and treatment. *Br J Hosp Med* 1997; **58**: 126–128.
55. Fasoli L, Turi RA, Spitz L et al. Necrotizing enterocolitis: extent of disease and surgical treatment. *J Pediatr Surg* 1999; **34**: 1096–1099.
56. Sparnon AL, Kiely EM. Resection and primary anastomosis for necrotizing enterocolitis. *Pediatr Surg Int* 1987; **2**: 101–104.
57. Cooper A, Ross AJ III, O'Neill JA Jr, Schnaufer L. Resection with primary anastomosis for necrotizing enterocolitis: a contrasting view. *J Pediatr Surg* 1988; **23**: 64–68.
58. Griffiths DM, Forbes DA, Pemberton PJ, Penn IA. Primary anastomosis for necrotising enterocolitis: a 12-year experience. *J Pediatr Surg* 1989; **24**: 515–518.
59. Harberg FJ, McGill CW, Saleem MM et al. Resection with primary anastomosis for necrotizing enterocolitis. *J Pediatr Surg* 1983; **18**: 743–746.
60. Yaseen H, Kamaledin K, Al Umran K et al. Epidemiology and outcome of 'early-onset' vs 'late-onset' necrotizing enterocolitis. *Indian J Pediatr* 2002; **69**: 481–484.
61. Narang A, Rao R, Bhakoo ON. Neonatal necrotizing enterocolitis: a clinical study. *Indian Pediatr* 1993; **30**: 1417–1422.
62. Kabeer A, Gunnlaugsson S, Coren C. Neonatal necrotizing enterocolitis. A 12-year review at a county hospital. *Dis Colon Rectum* 1995; **38**: 866–872.
63. Rowe MI, Reblock KK, Kurkchubasche AG, Healey PJ. Necrotizing enterocolitis in the extremely low birth weight infant. *J Pediatr Surg* 1994; **29**: 987–990.
64. Fasching G, Hollwarth ME, Schmidt B. Necrotizing enterocolitis in very-low-birth-weight infants. *Pediatr Surg Int* 1992; **7**: 428–430.
65. Beasley SW, Auldist AW, Ramanujan TM. The surgical management of neonatal necrotizing enterocolitis 1975–1984. *Pediatr Surg Int* 1994; **1**: 210–217.
66. Chan K, Ohlsson A, Synnes A et al. Survival, morbidity, and resource use of infants of 25 weeks' gestational age or less. *Am J Obstet Gynecol* 2001; **185**: 220–226.
67. Horwitz JR, Lally KP, Cheu HW et al. Complications after surgical intervention for necrotizing enterocolitis: a multicenter review. *J Pediatr Surg* 1995; **30**: 994–998.
68. Rivera-Moreno MA, Mercado-Arellano JA, Ulloa-Ricardez A, Franco-Gutierrez M. [Risk factors related to mortality in newborns with stage III necrosing enterocolitis]. *Gac Med Mex* 1999; **135**: 245–251.
69. Ladd AP, Rescorla FJ, West KW et al. Long-term follow-up after bowel resection for necrotizing enterocolitis: factors affecting outcome. *J Pediatr Surg* 1998; **33**: 967–972.
70. Georgeson KE, Breaux CW Jr. Outcome and intestinal adaptation in neonatal short-bowel syndrome. *J Pediatr Surg* 1992; **27**: 344–348.
71. Bagucka B, De Schepper J, Peelman M et al. Acid gastro–esophageal reflux in the 10 degrees-reversed-Trendelenburg-position in supine sleeping infants. *Acta Paediatr Taiwan* 1999; **40**: 298–301.
72. El Mouzan MI, Abdullah AM, Al Sanie AM, Al Khalifah SI. Pattern of gastroesophageal reflux in children. *Saudi Med J* 2001; **22**: 419–422.
73. Rice H, Seashore JH, Touloukian RJ. Evaluation of Nissen fundoplication in neurologically impaired children. *J Pediatr Surg* 1991; **26**: 697–701.
74. Fonkalsrud EW, Ashcraft KW, Coran AG *et al.* Surgical treatment of gastroesophageal reflux in children: a combined hospital study of 7467 patients. *Pediatrics* 1998; **101**: 419–422.
75. Inge TH, Carmeci C, Ohara LJ et al. Outcome of Nissen fundoplication using intraoperative manometry in children. *J Pediatr Surg* 1998; **33**: 1614–1617.
76. Omari TI, Barnett C, Snel A et al. Mechanisms of gastroesophageal reflux in healthy premature infants. *J Pediatr* 1998; **133**: 650–654.
77. Cadiot G, Bruhat A, Rigaud D et al. Multivariate analysis of pathophysiological factors in reflux oesophagitis. *Gut* 1997; **40**: 167–174.
78. Koivusalo A, Rintala R, Lindahl H. Gastroesophageal reflux in children with a congenital abdominal wall defect. *J Pediatr Surg* 1999; **34**: 1127–1129.
79. Rasheed K, Coughlan G, O'Donnell B. Congenital diaphragmatic hernia in the newborn. Outcome in 59 consecutive cases over a ten year period (1980–1989). *Ir J Med Sci* 1992; **161**: 16–17.
80. Mollitt DL, Golladay ES, Seibert JJ. Symptomatic gastroesophageal reflux following gastrostomy in neurologically impaired patients. *Pediatrics* 1985; **75**: 1124–1126.
81. Papaila JG, Vane DW, Colville C et al. The effect of various types of gastrostomy on the lower esophageal sphincter. *J Pediatr Surg* 1987; **22**: 1198–1202.
82. Jolley SG, Tunell WP, Hoelzer DJ et al. Lower esophageal pressure changes with tube gastrostomy: a causative factor of gastroesophageal reflux in children? *J Pediatr Surg* 1986; **21**: 624–627.
83. Reyes AL, Cash AJ, Green SH, Booth IW. Gastrooesophageal reflux in children with cerebral palsy. *Child Care Health Dev* 1993; **19**: 109–118.
84. St Cyr JA, Ferrara TB, Thompson TR et al. Nissen fundoplication for gastroesophageal reflux in infants. *J Thorac Cardiovasc Surg* 1986; **92**: 661–666.
85. Downing SE, Lee JC. Laryngeal chemosensitivity: a possible mechanism for sudden infant death. *Pediatrics* 1975; **55**: 640–649.
86. Harned HS, Myracle J Jr, Ferreiro J. Respiratory suppression and swallowing from introduction of fluids into the laryngeal region of the lamb. *Pediatr Res* 1978; **12**: 1003–1009.
87. Krishnan U, Mitchell JD, Tobias V et al. Fat laden macrophages in tracheal aspirates as a marker of reflux aspiration: a negative report. *J Pediatr Gastroenterol Nutr* 2002; **35**: 309–313.
88. Knauer-Fischer S, Ratjen F. Lipid-laden macrophages in bronchoalveolar lavage fluid as a marker for pulmonary aspiration. *Pediatr Pulmonol* 1999; **27**: 419–422.
89. Bailey DJ, Andres JM, Danek GD, Pineiro-Carrero VM. Lack of efficacy of thickened feeding as treatment for gastroesophageal reflux. *J Pediatr* 1987; **110**: 187–189.
90. Khoshoo V, Fried M, Pencharz P. Incidence of gastroesophageal reflux with casein and whey-based formulas. *J Pediatr Gastroenterol Nutr* 1993; **17**: 116–117.
91. Orenstein SR, Magill HL, Brooks P. Thickening of infant feedings for therapy of gastroesophageal reflux. *J Pediatr* 1987; **110**: 181–186.
92. Vandenplas Y, Hachimi-Idrissi S, Casteels A et al. A clinical trial with an 'anti-regurgitation' formula. *Eur J Pediatr* 1994; **153**: 419–423.

93. Carroll AE, Garrison MM, Christakis DA. A systematic review of nonpharmacological and nonsurgical therapies for gastroesophageal reflux in infants. *Arch Pediatr Adolesc Med* 2002; **156**: 109–113.
94. Orenstein SR, Whitington PF, Orenstein DM. The infant seat as treatment for gastroesophageal reflux. *N Engl J Med* 1983; **309**: 760–763.
95. Orenstein SR. Prone positioning in infant gastroesophageal reflux: is elevation of the head worth the trouble? *J Pediatr* 1990; **117**: 184–187.
96. Nissen R. Gastropexy and fundoplication in surgical treatment of hiatal hernia. *Am J Dig Dis* 1961; **6**: 959–961.
97. Thal AP. A unified approach to surgical problems of the esophagogastric junction. *Ann Surg* 1968; **168**: 542–550.
98. Martinez JM, Halverson A, Magnuson DK, Sackier JM. Laparoscopic versus open Nissen fundoplication: outcome of surgery in monozygotic twins. *J Laparoendosc Adv Surg Tech A* 1997; **7**: 323–326.
99. Esposito C, Garipoli V, De Pasquale M et al. Laparoscopic versus traditional fundoplication in the treatment of children with refractory gastro-oesophageal reflux. *Ital J Gastroenterol Hepatol* 1997; **29**: 399–402.
100. Mattioli G, Repetto P, Carlini C et al. Laparoscopic vs open approach for the treatment of gastroesophageal reflux in children. *Surg Endosc* 2002; **16**: 750–752.
101. Collins JB III, Georgeson KE, Vicente Y, Hardin WD Jr. Comparison of open and laparoscopic gastrostomy and fundoplication in 120 patients. *J Pediatr Surg* 1995; **30**: 1065–1070.
102. Triadafilopoulos G, Dibaise JK, Nostrant TT et al. Radiofrequency energy delivery to the gastroesophageal junction for the treatment of GERD. *Gastrointest Endosc* 2001; **53**: 407–415.
103. Katz PO. Gastroesophageal reflux disease: new treatments. *Rev Gastroenterol Disord* 2002; **2**: 66–74.
104. Filipi CJ, Lehman GA, Rothstein RI et al. Transoral, flexible endoscopic suturing for treatment of GERD: a multicenter trial. *Gastrointest Endosc* 2001; **53**: 416–422.
105. Rothestein RI, Pohl H Grove M et al. Endoscopic gastric plication for the treatment of GERD; two-year follow up results. *Am J Gastroenterol* 2001; **96**: 53 (abstr).
106. Kubiak R, Spitz L, Kiely EM et al. Effectiveness of fundoplication in early infancy. *J Pediatr Surg* 1999; **34**: 295–299.
107. Weber TR. A prospective analysis of factors influencing outcome after fundoplication. *J Pediatr Surg* 1995; **30**: 1061–1063.
108. Vane DW, Harmel RP Jr, King DR, Boles ET Jr. The effectiveness of Nissen fundoplication in neurologically impaired children with gastroesophageal reflux. *Surgery* 1985; **98**: 662–667.
109. Dedinsky GK, Vane DW, Black T et al. Complications and reoperation after Nissen fundoplication in childhood. *Am J Surg* 1987; **153**: 177–183.
110. Pearl RH, Robie DK, Ein SH et al. Complications of gastroesophageal antireflux surgery in neurologically impaired versus neurologically normal children. *J Pediatr Surg* 1990; **25**: 1169–1173.
111. Spillane AJ, Currie B, Shi E. Fundoplication in children: experience with 106 cases. *Aust NZ J Surg* 1996; **66**: 753–756.
112. Bensoussan AL, Yazbeck S, Carceller-Blanchard A. Results and complications of Toupet partial posterior wrap: 10 years' experience. *J Pediatr Surg* 1994; **29**: 1215–1217.
113. Dalla Vecchia LK, Grosfeld JL, West KW et al. Reoperation after Nissen fundoplication in children with gastroesophageal reflux: experience with 130 patients. *Ann Surg* 1997; **226**: 315–321.
114. Benson CD. Infantile pyloric stenosis. Historical aspects and current surgical concepts. *Prog Pediatr Surg* 1970; **1**: 63–88.
115. Kerr AM. Unprecedented rise in incidence of infantile hypertrophic pyloric stenosis. *BMJ* 1980; **281**: 714–715.
116. Webb AR, Lari J, Dodge JA. Infantile hypertrophic pyloric stenosis in South Glamorgan 1970–9. Effects of changes in feeding practice. *Arch Dis Child* 1983; **58**: 586–590.
117. Schechter R, Torfs CP, Bateson TF. The epidemiology of infantile hypertrophic pyloric stenosis. *Paediatr Perinat Epidemiol* 1997; **11**: 407–427.
118. Applegate MS, Druschel CM. The epidemiology of infantile hypertrophic pyloric stenosis in New York State, 1983 to 1990. *Arch Pediatr Adolesc Med* 1995; **149**: 1123–1129.
119. Stringer MD, Brereton RJ. Current management of infantile hypertrophic pyloric stenosis. *Br J Hosp Med* 1990; **43**: 266–272.
120. Habbick BF, Khanna C, To T. Infantile hypertrophic pyloric stenosis: a study of feeding practices and other possible causes. *CMAJ* 1989; **140**: 401–404.
121. Tandoh JF, Hesse AA. Infantile hypertrophic pyloric stenosis in Ghana. *West Afr J Med* 1992; **11**: 135–139.
122. Graham DA, Mogridge N, Abbott GD et al. Pyloric stenosis: the Christchurch experience. *NZ Med J* 1993; **106**: 57–59.
123. Haahr P, Nielsen JP. Infantile hypertrophic pyloric stenosis. A 25-year study from the county of Viborg. *Ugeskr Laeger* 2000; **162**: 3456–3459.
124. Tam PK, Chan J. Increasing incidence of hypertrophic pyloric stenosis. *Arch Dis Child* 1991; **66**: 530–531.
125. Jedd MB, Melton LJ III, Griffin MR et al. Trends in infantile hypertrophic pyloric stenosis in Olmsted County, Minnesota, 1950–1984. *Paediatr Perinat Epidemiol* 1988; **2**: 148–157.
126. Finsen VR. Infantile hypertrophic pyloric stenosis – unusual familial incidence. *Arch Dis Child* 1979; **54**: 720–721.
127. Mitchell LE, Risch N. The genetics of infantile hypertrophic pyloric stenosis. A reanalysis. *Am J Dis Child* 1993; **147**: 1203–1211.
128. Hicks LM, Morgan A, Anderson MR. Pyloric stenosis – a report of triplet females and notes on its inheritance. *J Pediatr Surg* 1981; **16**: 739–740.
129. Spitz L. Congenital hypertrophic pyloric stenosis in triplets. *Arch Dis Child* 1974; **49**: 325.
130. Huang PL, Dawson TM, Bredt DS et al. Targeted disruption of the neuronal nitric oxide synthase gene. *Cell* 1993; **75**: 1273–1286.
131. Kusafuka T, Puri P. Altered messenger RNA expression of the neuronal nitric oxide synthase gene in infantile hypertrophic pyloric stenosis. *Pediatr Surg Int* 1997; **12**: 576–579.
132. Jedd MB, Melton LJ III, Griffin MR et al. Factors associated with infantile hypertrophic pyloric stenosis. *Am J Dis Child* 1988; **142**: 334–337.
133. Dodge JA. Infantile hypertrophic pyloric stenosis in Belfast, 1957–1969. *Arch Dis Child* 1975; **50**: 171–178.
134. Hitchcock NE, Gilmour AI, Gracey M, Burke V. Pyloric stenosis in Western Australia, 1971–84. *Arch Dis Child* 1987; **62**: 512–513.
135. Pisacane A, de Luca U, Criscuolo L et al. Breast feeding and hypertrophic pyloric stenosis: population based case–control study. *BMJ* 1996; **312**: 745–746.
136. Wattchow DA, Furness JB, Costa M. Distribution and coexistence of peptides in nerve fibers of the external

muscle of the human gastrointestinal tract. *Gastroenterology* 1988; **95**: 32–41.

137. Jadcherla SR, Klee G, Berseth CL. Regulation of migrating motor complexes by motilin and pancreatic polypeptide in human infants. *Pediatr Res* 1997; **42**: 365–369.

138. Boiron M, Dorval E, Metman EH et al. Erythromycin elicits opposite effects on antro-bulbar and duodenal motility: analysis in diabetics by cineradiography. *Arch Physiol Biochem* 1997; **105**: 591–595.

139. Honein MA, Paulozzi LJ, Himelright IM et al. Infantile hypertrophic pyloric stenosis after pertussis prophylaxis with erythromcyin: a case review and cohort study. *Lancet* 1999; **354**: 2101–2105.

140. SanFilippo A. Infantile hypertrophic pyloric stenosis related to ingestion of erythromycine estolate: a report of five cases. *J Pediatr Surg* 1976; **11**: 177–180.

141. Ohshiro K, Puri P. Increased insulin-like growth factor-I mRNA expression in pyloric muscle in infantile hypertrophic pyloric stenosis. *Pediatr Surg Int* 1998; **13**: 253–255.

142. Ohshiro K, Puri P. Increased insulin-like growth factor and platelet-derived growth factor system in the pyloric muscle in infantile hypertrophic pyloric stenosis. *J Pediatr Surg* 1998; **33**: 378–381.

143. Pueyo C, Ohshiro K, Puri P. Increased transforming growth factor beta-11 in infantile hypertrophic pyloric stenosis. Presented at the international symposium *State of the Art in Pediatric Surgery*, Dublin, Ireland 1997.

144. Miyazaki E, Yamataka T, Ohshiro K et al. Active collagen synthesis in infantile hypertrophic pyloric stenosis. *Pediatr Surg Int* 1998; **13**: 237–239.

145. Cass DT, Zhang AL. Extracellular matrix changes in congenital hypertrophic pyloric stenosis. *Pediatr Surg Int* 1991; **6**: 190–194.

146. Andrassy RJ, Haff RC, Larsen GL. Infantile hypertrophic pyloric stenosis during the first week of life. Approaches to diagnosis, based on observations of a newborn whose vomiting began on the first day. *Clin Pediatr (Phila)* 1977; **16**: 475–476.

147. Sharma M, Jain SK, Pathania OP, Taneja SB. The Indian experience with hypertrophic pyloric stenosis. *Clin Pediatr (Phila)* 1990; **29**: 566–568.

148. Hulka F, Harrison MW, Campbell TJ, Campbell JR. Complications of pyloromyotomy for infantile hypertrophic pyloric stenosis. *Am J Surg* 1997; **173**: 450–452.

149. Zhang AL, Cass DT, Dubois RS, Cartmill T. Infantile hypertrophic pyloric stenosis: a clinical review from a general hospital. *J Paediatr Child Health* 1993; **29**: 372–378.

150. Mitchell KG, Cachia SM. Infantile hypertrophic pyloric stenosis. *Scott Med J* 1981; **26**: 245–249.

151. Macdessi J, Oates RK. Clinical diagnosis of pyloric stenosis: a declining art. *BMJ* 1993; **306**: 553–555.

152. Hulka F, Campbell TJ, Campbell JR, Harrison MW. Evolution in the recognition of infantile hypertrophic pyloric stenosis. *Pediatrics* 1997; **100**: E9.

153. Hernanz-Schulman M, Sells LL, Ambrosino MM et al. Hypertrophic pyloric stenosis in the infant without a palpable olive: accuracy of sonographic diagnosis. *Radiology* 1994; **193**: 771–776.

154. van der Schouw YT, van der Velden MT, Hitge-Boetes C et al. Diagnosis of hypertrophic pyloric stenosis: value of sonography when used in conjunction with clinical findings and laboratory data. *Am J Roentgenol* 1994; **163**: 905–909.

155. Poon TS, Zhang AL, Cartmill T, Cass DT. Changing patterns of diagnosis and treatment of infantile hypertrophic pyloric stenosis: a clinical audit of 303 patients. *J Pediatr Surg* 1996; **31**: 1611–1615.

156. Abbas AE, Weiss SM, Alvear DT. Infantile hypertrophic pyloric stenosis: delays in diagnosis and overutilization of imaging modalities. *Am Surg* 1999; **65**: 73–76.

157. Downey EC Jr. Laparoscopic pyloromyotomy. *Semin Pediatr Surg* 1998; **7**: 220–224.

158. Bufo AJ, Merry C, Shah R et al. Laparoscopic pyloromyotomy: a safer technique. *Pediatr Surg Int* 1998; **13**: 240–242.

159. Hingston G. Ramstedt's pyloromyotomy – what is the correct incision? *NZ Med J* 1996; **109**: 276–278.

160. Garza JJ, Morash D, Dzakovic A et al. *Ad libitum* feeding decreases hospital stay for neonates after pyloromyotomy. *J Pediatr Surg* 2002; **37**: 493–495.

161. Golladay ES, Broadwater JR, Mollitt DL. Pyloric stenosis – a timed perspective. *Arch.Surg* 1987; **122**: 825–826.

162. Harper RG, Garcia A, Sia C. Inguinal hernia: a common problem of premature infants weighing 1,000 grams or less at birth. *Pediatrics* 1975; **56**: 112–115.

163. Surana R, Puri P. Is contralateral exploration necessary in infants with unilateral inguinal hernia? *J Pediatr Surg* 1993; **28**: 1026–1027.

164. Misra D, Hewitt G, Potts SR et al. Inguinal herniotomy in young infants, with emphasis on premature neonates. *J Pediatr Surg* 1994; **29**: 1496–1498.

165. Fung A, Barsoum G, Bentley TM et al. Inguinal herniotomy in young infants. *Br J Surg* 1992; **79**: 1071–1072.

166. Harvey MH, Johnstone MJ, Fossard DP. Inguinal herniotomy in children: a five year survey. *Br J Surg* 1985; **72**: 485–487.

167. Tam PK, Tsang TM, Saing H. Inguinal hernia in Chinese children. *Aust NZ J Surg* 1988; **58**: 403–406.

168. Yeung YP, Cheng MS, Ho KL, Yip AW. Day-case inguinal herniotomy in Chinese children: retrospective study. *Hong Kong Med J* 2002; **8**: 245–248.

169. Morecroft JA, Stringer MD, Higgins M et al. Follow-up after inguinal herniotomy or surgery for hydrocele in boys. *Br J Surg* 1993; **80**: 1613–1614.

170. Momoh JT. External hernia in Nigerian children. *Ann Trop Paediatr* 1985; **5**: 197–200.

171. Tackett LD, Breuer CK, Luks FI et al. Incidence of contralateral inguinal hernia: a prospective analysis. *J Pediatr Surg* 1999; **34**: 684–687.

172. Peevy KJ, Speed FA, Hoff CJ. Epidemiology of inguinal hernia in preterm neonates. *Pediatrics* 1986; **77**: 246–247.

173. Devlin HB. *Management of Abdominal Hernias*. London: Butterworths, 1988: 75.

174. Holsclaw DS, Shwachman H. Increased incidence of inguinal hernia, hydrocele, and undescended testicle in males with cystic fibrosis. *Pediatrics* 1971; **48**: 442–445.

175. Liem MS, van der GY, Beemer FA, van Vroonhoven TJ. Increased risk for inguinal hernia in patients with Ehlers–Danlos syndrome. *Surgery* 1997; **122**: 114–115.

176. McEntyre RL, Raffensperger JG. Surgical complications of Ehlers–Danlos syndrome in children. *J Pediatr Surg* 1977; **12**: 531–535.

177. Coran AG, Eraklis AJ. Inguinal hernia in the Hurler–Hunter syndrome. *Surgery* 1967; **61**: 302–304.

178. Moazam F, Glenn JD, Kaplan BJ et al. Inguinal hernias after ventriculoperitoneal shunt procedures in pediatric patients. *Surg Gynecol Obstet* 1984; **159**: 570–572.

179. Tank ES, Hatch DA. Hernias complicating chronic ambulatory peritoneal dialysis in children. *J Pediatr Surg* 1986; **21**: 41–42.

180. Tsai TC, Huang FY, Hsu JC et al. Continuous ambulatory peritoneal dialysis complicating with abdominal

hernias in children. *Zhonghua Min Guo Xiao Er Ke Yi Xue Hui Za Zhi* 1996; **37**: 263–265.
181. Uden A, Lindhagen T. Inguinal hernia in patients with congenital dislocation of the hip. A sign of general connective tissue disorder. *Acta Orthop Scand* 1988; **59**: 667–668.
182. Carneiro PM. Inguinal herniotomy in children. *East Afr Med J* 1990; **67**: 359–364.
183. Palmer BV. Incarcerated inguinal hernia in children. *Ann R Coll Surg Engl* 1978; **60**: 121–124.
184. McGregor DB, Halverson K, McVay CB. The unilateral pediatric inguinal hernia: should the contralateral side by explored? *J Pediatr Surg* 1980; **15**: 313–317.
185. Leung WY, Poon M, Fan TW et al. Testicular volume of boys after inguinal herniotomy: combined clinical and radiological follow–up. *Pediatr Surg Int* 1999; **15**: 40–41.
186. Surana R, Puri P. Iatrogenic ascent of the testis: an under–recognized complication of inguinal hernia operation in children. *Br J Urol* 1994; **73**: 580–581.
187. Spitz L. Nissen fundoplication. In Dudley H, Carter D, Russell RCG et al., eds. *Rob and Smith's Operative Surgery*. London: Buttersworth, 1988: 240–246.
188. Bell MJ. Peritonitis in the newborn – current concepts. *Pediatr Clin North Am* 1985; **32**: 1181–1201.
189. Dykes EH, Fitzgerald RJ, O'Donnell B. Surgery for neonatal necrotising enterocolitis in Ireland 1980–1985. *Intensive Care Med* 1989; **15 Suppl 1**: S24–S26.
190. Flores-Nava G, Joachin-Roy H, Rodriguez-Cueto G. [Risk factors in neonatal necrotizing enterocolitis]. *Biol Med Hosp Infant Mex* 1993; **50**: 645–649.
191. Martinez-Tallo E, Claure N, Bancalari E. Necrotizing enterocolitis in full-term or near-term infants: risk factors. *Biol Neonate* 1997; **71**: 292–298.
192. Kadalraja R, Patole SK, Muller R, Whitehall JS. Comparison of clinical characteristics and high-risk factors in Australian aboriginal and non-aboriginal neonates with necrotising enterocolitis. *Int J Clin Pract* 2001; **55**: 251–254.
193. Leung MP, Chau KT, Hui PW et al. Necrotizing enterocolitis in neonates with symptomatic congenital heart disease. *J Pediatr* 1988; **113**: 1044–1046.
194. Sehgal S, Ewing C, Waring P et al. Morbidity of low-birthweight infants with intrauterine cocaine exposure. *J Natl Med Assoc* 1993; **85**: 20–24.
195. Lopez SL, Taeusch HW, Findlay RD, Walther FJ. Time of onset of necrotizing enterocolitis in newborn infants with known prenatal cocaine exposure. *Clin Pediatr (Phila)* 1995; **34**: 424–429.
196. Rand T, Weninger M, Kohlhauser C et al. Effects of umbilical arterial catheterization on mesenteric hemodynamics. *Pediatr Radiol* 1996; **26**: 435–438.
197. Lidums I, Lehmann A, Checklin H et al. Control of transient lower esophageal sphincter relaxations and reflux by the GABA(B) agonist baclofen in normal subjects. *Gastroenterology* 2000; **118**: 7–13.
198. Zhang Q, Lehmann A, Rigda R et al. Control of transient lower oesophageal sphincter relaxations and reflux by the GABA(B) agonist baclofen in patients with gastro-oesophageal reflux disease. *Gut* 2002; **50**: 19–24.

36 Enteral nutrition in preterm infants

Mario De Curtis and Jacques Rigo

Introduction

Currently, there is little consensus among neonatologists on the optimal way to initiate, proceed with or maintain enteral feeding in preterm infants. Most routines in neonatal intensive care units derive more from an empirical approach than from controlled studies. Nevertheless, the enormous number of studies conducted in this field over the past few years have greatly contributed to our knowledge of the nutrition of preterm infants, even if many doubts still remain.

The gastrointestinal tract of preterm infants and especially of very-low-birth-weight (VLBW) infants is immature at birth and initially incapable of performing full digestion and absorption. Immature gastrointestinal motility manifests itself in so-called 'feeding intolerance', which is characterized by delayed gastric emptying, abdominal distension, water stool passage or constipation.[1]

The advent of intensive care and the increased survival of premature infants led to the problem of necrotizing enterocolitis (NEC), which almost always occurred in infants who were fed. Consequently, enteral feeding was avoided as a strategy to prevent NEC. The introduction of enteral feeding was delayed, often for prolonged periods and parenteral nutritional was considered as the best nutrition route for VLBW infants in the first period of life.

Enteral nutrition during the early adaptive period

More recent studies have suggested that associating parenteral nutrition and early postnatal enteral feeding with small amounts of human milk or formula (called 'minimal enteral feeding', 'gastrointestinal priming', 'trophic feeding' and 'hypocaloric feeding') could help improve the development of the gastrointestinal tract, gut hormone release and gut motility.[2] Results of clinical trials in premature infants support the opinion that minimal enteral feeding has some clinical benefits, such as reducing the time to start full enteral feeding and length of hospitalization without increasing the risk of NEC.[3] The precise impact of minimal enteral feedings is still difficult to evaluate, because the studies carried out, aside from being based on a limited number of infants, considered different criteria of inclusion, feeding protocols and outcome measures. Thus, the meta-analysis is a less effective tool for reaching clear conclusions, whereas a larger trial with a single uniform protocol could clarify many of these issues.

In VLBW infants, the preferred early feeding regimen is human milk, which can be initiated, according to clinical conditions, even on the day of birth, or the following days, in small quantities, e.g. 1–2 ml colostrum every 6 h, progressively increasing the volume and frequency. Feeds should be given with a continuous infusion pump or by gavage. A recent review showed that there was no significant difference in somatic growth, days to discharge or the incidence of NEC for infants fed by continuous versus intermittent bolus tube feeding.[4] In any case the tube should be aspirated regularly in order to determine feeding tolerance. Gastric residues are usually measured every 3 h in infants aged less than 32 weeks and even more frequently in smaller and sick infants. The aspirate is reinfused to reduce the loss of enzymes and electrolytes. There is little rationale for the practice of diluting milk; the dilution does not promote maturation of gut motility.[5]

The ideal rate of progression of milk volume given to VLBW infants is controversial. While a Cochrane Review has concluded that a rapid rate of advancing feeds was not associated with a higher risk of NEC,[6] a recent study suggested that rapid advancement of enteral feeding might increase the risk of NEC.[7] Although additional studies are needed, a small progressive increment of 10 ml/kg per day after a few days of stabilization can be recommended.

Nutrition during the intermediate and stable growth period

Transition from the early adaptive to an intermediate and stable growing period is related to stable clinical and metabolic conditions and tolerance of minimal enteral feeding. During this period enteral feeding can be slightly increased, up to 140–180 ml/kg per day, whereas the amount of parenteral fluid is progressively reduced and interrupted as soon as 100–120 ml/kg per day is well tolerated.

Nutrient needs during enteral feeding

Water

Total fluid intake is related to ingested calorie and protein intake as well as to the renal solute load. During the early phase there is a progressive cornification of the epidermidis causing a significant reduction of perspiratio insensibilis and an improvement of renal function.[8] The goal of fluid administration is to replace water loss, maintain water and electrolyte homeostasis and provide extra water and electrolytes to build up new tissues. Renal solute load (RSL) plays a major role in the water balance of enterally fed preterm infants. It can be defined as water-soluble waste products excreted through the kidney. The excretion of these products requires a given amount of water, which affects the net water balance. As the RSL increases, the minimal urinary water excretion increases, owing to the relative immaturity of the premature kidney to concentrate urine. The RSL is closely related to the nitrogen and electrolyte content of the diet, and its potential RSL can be estimated according to the following formula, expressed in millimoles (mmol, or milliosmoles, mOsm): Potential RSL = N/28 + Na + Cl + K + P, where N/28 indicates the excretion, in mg, of nitrogenous substances such as urea (urea contains two nitrogen atoms, atomic weight 14), Na is sodium, Cl is chloride, K is potassium and P is available phosphorus which is the same as total phosphorus in milk-based formulas.[9] The potential RSL of mature human milk is 14 mOsm/100 kcal,[10] whereas that of currently available premature infant formulas is about 26 mOsm/100 kcal,[11] Maximum amounts of solutes in a formula providing 81 kcal/100 ml has been estimated in non-growing preterm infants as 32 mOsm/100 kcal,[12] taking into account a formula intake of 150 ml/kg per day, skin and lung water loss of 75 ml/kg per day and stool loss of 8–11 ml/kg per day.[13] In such conditions, at least 64 ml/kg per day are available for urinary excretion, considering that the great majority of preterm infants without renal disease can concentrate urine to 600 mOsm/l.[14]

Because the growing infant incorporates into new tissue a portion of the substances present in the diet (protein, potassium, phosphate, etc.), which in the non-growing subject would be presented to the kidney for excretion, an 'osmolar equivalent of weight gain' was removed from the calculated potential renal solute load. A theoretical estimate of the size of this sparing effect, based on the body composition of the newborn infant, in a study on relatively large premature infants (mean birth weight 1787 g and gestational age 33 weeks), suggested an osmolar equivalent of 0.9 mmol/g weight gain and half the expected true osmolar load of adapted formulas.[15] In the stable growing period, the water requirement, accounting for security levels, is 130–160 ml/kg per day.

Protein

The goal in estimating the protein requirements of preterm infants is to provide the quantity and quality of protein needed to obtain a growth similar to that observed in the fetus during the third trimester of intrauterine life, and to obtain an early postnatal catch-up growth, keeping in mind that the accretion of lean body mass needs to be considered more than absolute weight gain.[16]

Protein utilization is influenced by several factors such as quality and quantity of the protein supply, dietary protein energy ratio, gut immaturity and nutritional status. Dietary protein needs for preterm infants have been estimated by two different methods. The first, the empirical approach, measures biochemical or physiological responses to graded intakes. The second method, the factorial approach, considers the requirements as the sum of the essential losses (e.g. urine, feces, skin), plus the amount incorporated into newly formed tissues.

The empirical approach evaluates physiological and biochemical variables to determine minimum and maximum protein needs in the growing preterm infant. The measures used in these types of study are: anthropometry (weight, length, head circumference, skinfold thickness); nitrogen balance or retention; metabolic or chemical indices (plasma and urinary amino acids, serum albumin, total protein, immunoglobulin, retinal binding protein and transthyretin – most of which provide an indirect reflection of protein synthesis); indirect calorimetry, to evaluate energy balance and – in combination with nitrogen balance – the composition of weight gain; isotope studies of whole-body nitrogen kinetics (used as indirect measures of protein synthesis rates); body composition, by dual energy X-ray absorptiometry; and development assessment, studying the effect of quality and quantity of protein on neurological development through various neurometric tests such as the Neonatal Behavioral Assessment scale and the Bayley Scales of Infant Development.[17]

In the factorial approach, compositional analysis of fetal tissues has been a valuable source of data for our understanding of the nutrient needs of the fetus and, by extension, those of the growing preterm infant. Fetal accretion rates have been obtained from compositional analyses of aborted fetuses or stillborn infants.[18] From these data, the protein increment for growth has been estimated as approximatly 2.3 g/kg per day,[19] but more recent data seem to indicate a value closer to 2.5 g/kg per day. Protein requirement is thus calculated by adding to this value the obligatory losses, and the amount needed for the additional catch-up growth. In a large population of preterm infants receiving a controlled energy intake, the minimal protein supply necessary to obtain a zero nitrogen balance (to cover all nitrogen losses) was calculated to be 0.74 g/kg per day.[20] A similar value was estimated to cover the need for catch-up growth.[21] Thus, the protein requirements in VLBW infants, so calculated, reach 3.8–4 g/kg per day. The recommended dietary protein allowance needs to be adapted to the fractional absorption rate and protein efficiency as well as to individual variations.

Nitrogen absorption and utilization were recently reviewed on 226 metabolic balances performed in recent years in preterm infants fed human milk, human milk fortifiers and various preterm formulas.[22] Data are summarized in Table 36.1.

Nitrogen absorption rate (absorbed/intake) differs significantly according to the feeding regimen. It was higher with powder whey-predominant protein preterm formulas (90.7%) than with human milk supplemented with fortifiers (82.7%), powder protein hydrolyzed formulas (84.3%) or ready-to-use liquid whey-predominant preterm formulas (86.0 %) (Table 36.1). Those differences result from the nature of the various types of protein supply. In human milk, non-nutritional protein content (lactoferrin, sIgA, lysozyme) or non-protein nitrogen content (oligosaccharides) are absorbed less than the nutritional protein content (whey proteins, caseins) and contribute to a significant part of fecal excretion. An interesting observation is the relatively lower absorption rate of ready-to-use liquid preterm formulas or protein hydrolyzed preterm formulas, where the technical process seems to impair nitrogen absorption in relation to heat treatment – inducing some Maillard reaction – or to preliminary hydrolysis, altering the physiological absorption process in the lumen or at the border of the gastrointestinal tract.[23]

The efficiency of protein gain, estimated by the ratio between retained and metabolizable nitrogen (absorbed), differs also according to the feeding regimen (Table 36.1). The highest values were obtained in preterm infants fed powder (77.7%) and liquid (77.5%) preterm formulas. It was significantly lower in those fed protein-hydrolyzed formulas (74.0%) and fortified human milk (72.1%).[22] The lower value obtained with fortified human milk may be related to non-protein nitrogen, which represents 20–25% of total nitrogen content of human milk, but still 13.5–17% of total nitrogen content of fortified human milk. As

Table 36.1 Nitrogen balances according to feeding regimen in preterm infants (from reference 22)

Amount (mg/kg per day)	Fortified human milk[a] (n=88)	Powder whey-predominant preterm formulas[b] (n=49)	Liquid whey-predominant preterm formulas[c] (n=58)	Powder protein-hydrolyzed formulas[d] (n=31)
Intake	517±86[d]	522 ± 70[d]	506 ± 58	553 ± 56[ab]
Fecal excretion	90±28[bc]	49±19[acd]	71±28[abd]	87±26[bc]
Absorbed	428±76[bd]	474±75[ac]	434±52[bd]	466±51[ac]
Urinary excretion	121±45[c]	106±36	98±21[ad]	122±39[c]
Retained	307±56[bcd]	368±57[acd]	337±46[ab]	343±42[ab]
Absorption (%)	82.7±4.8[bc]	90.7±3.3[acd]	86.0±5.0[ab]	84.3±4.0[b]
Net protein utilization* (%)	59.7±7.7[bc]	71.5±6.5[acd]	66.6±5.8[abd]	62.4±6.5[bc]
Protein efficiency† (%)	72.1±7.6[bc]	77.7±6.4[ad]	77.5±4.4[ad]	74.0 ± 6.9[bc]

* Nitrogen retention/nitrogen intake
†† Nitrogen retention/nitrogen absorption
abcd Values with like letters $p < 0.05$

demonstrated for urea nitrogen, the contribution of this metabolizable non-protein nitrogen fraction to protein gain is lower than that of the α-lactalbumin or the casein content of human milk. Therefore, regarding the net protein utilization (N retained/N intake), preterm formulas appear to be more efficient than human milk with or without protein supplementation. However, the net protein utilization of formulas can be altered by some technical processes, such as those required for hydrolysis.[23] Thus, adapted for fractional absorption rate and protein efficiency, the recommended protein allowance could reach 4.5 g/kg per day in extremely-low-birth-weight (ELBW) infants with significant catch-up growth requirements.[16]

The potential risk of such an aggressive nutritional strategy is a metabolic stress resulting from protein overload or unbalanced amino acid supply. Therefore, the most recent technologies will be necessary to improve nitrogen bioavailability, reduce Maillard reactions and provide the most balanced amino acid composition.

The whey/casein ratio significantly influences individual amino acid intakes and plasma amino acid concentrations. Plasma threonine is increased and tryptophan relatively decreased in infants fed a whey-predominant formula, whereas methionine and aromatic amino acids are increased in those fed a casein-predominant formula.[24,25] The high plasma threonine concentration, observed in preterm infants fed whey-predominant formulas, is related to the glycomacropeptide obtained from casein by enzymatic casein precipitation of cow's milk proteins. Acidic precipitation, by contrast, removes the glycomacropeptide rich in threonine from the soluble phase.[26] Today it is possible to design whey-predominant formulas with a lower threonine content.[27–29] In 14 preterm infants receiving either an enzymatic or an acidic whey-predominant formula, a significant reduction in plasma threonine concentration was observed in acidic whey-protein formula-fed infants (27.9 ± 8.5 μmol/dl), compared to those receiving conventional enzymatic whey-protein formula (37.5 ± 8.4 μmol/dl). All other plasma amino acid concentrations were similar, with the exception of valine, which was slightly reduced in acidic whey protein formula-fed infants.[27]

In addition to these technological treatments, performed to remove the glycomacropeptide and reduce the threonine content, the ratio between different cow's milk protein contents was modified to increase the relative percentage of α-lactoalbumin. Indeed, this protein fraction is naturally rich in tryptophan and helps normalize the low levels of this amino acid frequently observed in whey-predominant formula-fed infants.[30,31]

Formulas based on hydrolyzed proteins have been recently proposed for the feeding of preterm infants to reduce gastrointestinal problems such as delayed gastric emptying, abdominal distension, hard stools and feeding intolerance.[32,33] The technological processes necessary to perform hydrolysis and reduce protein antigenicity may, however, modify the amino acid content and/or amino acid bioavailability.[34] The use of a higher percentage of whey in protein-hydrolyzed formulas further worsens the plasma amino acid pattern previously observed with the use of whey-predominant formulas by increasing threonine and decreasing aromatic amino acid concentrations.[32] Moreover, a significant decrease of plasma histidine and tryptophan concentrations, probably due to a relative reduction in amino acid bioavailability, was also observed. Using a more appropriate technology, these formulas have been corrected for the threonine content and supplemented with histidine and tryptophan.[35–37]

Formulas do not contain any of the biologically active immune substances, nor enzymes, hormones or growth factors found in human milk. The long-term implications of this deficiency has not been determined. Several studies have been performed to evaluate the functional properties of non-nutritional compounds, such as nucleotides, polyamines, growth factors or prebiotics, which could potentially improve the quality of these new formulas, although no definitive conclusions are currently available.[17]

Considering the revised protein recommendations, large multicenter randomized studies need to evaluate the improvement in growth and in body composition, as well as the reduction in incidence of postnatal growth restriction expected from an aggressive nutritional policy in preterm infants. Further studies are also needed to identify more sensitive markers of protein toxicity, to determine the safety and efficacy of such a high protein supply and to evaluate the beneficial impact on short- and long-term growth and development.

Energy

The energy demands for preterm infants depend on many factors including fetal and neonatal development, genetically determined metabolic rate, thermal environment, activity, sleep status, nutritional status, nutrient intake, body composition and occurrence of illness. Energy intake recommendation for preterm infants, calculated for 150 ml/kg per day of formula, by different nutrition committees, range between 98 and 139 kcal/kg per day, while the more recent recommendations range between 110 and 135 kcal/kg per day.[11,17,38,39]

Energy retention, in premature infants, after the first 2–3 days of life, is about 85–90% of energy intake. The remainder is lost in stool and a small quantity as urea in the urine. Energy retained is in part stored in tissues as protein and mainly as fat, and in part lost as energy expenditure. After birth, fat deposition represents a higher proportion of weight gain than *in utero*.[40] Rapid accretion of body fat appears to be unavoidable, although it can be altered considerably by dietary manipulation of the protein/energy ratio.[40,41] A fat deposition of 20–25% of weight gain has been proposed as a reasonable goal for preterm infants but there are, however, no long-term data to justify this limit.[42]

Protein/energy ratio

Protein and energy needs are reciprocally limiting, the intake of one affecting the ability of the infant to assimilate the other. A suboptimal range of the protein/energy ratio leads to untoward consequences.[43] If energy intake is inadequate, protein is used as an energy source and the nitrogen balance becomes less positive. Increasing the caloric intake will spare protein loss and improve nitrogen retention. If there is a surfeit of energy with limited protein intake, the protein retention reaches a plateau and the energy excess is used only for fat deposition.[43] Nevertheless, when the protein supply is satisfactory (close to 4.0 g/kg per day), the effect of energy increase from 130 to 155 kcal/kg per day on protein retention appears to be minimal – about 0.1 g of protein/kg per day.[44] An additional issue concerns the partition of energy intake between fat and carbohydrates. It seems that carbohydrates are slightly more effective than fat in sparing protein oxidation. At the same two levels of energy supply the advantage of a diet containing 65% of non-protein energy as carbohydrate versus 35% on nitrogen retention represented about 0.15g of protein/kg per day in enterally fed low-birth-weight (LBW) infants.[44]

Analysis of various studies in preterm infants fed human milk,[45–51] human milk fortifiers[46,49,52–57] and various preterm formulas[45,47,50–52,55,56,58–61] allows the evaluation of the main determinant of weight gain, nitrogen retention and fat mass deposition. From these data, the major determinants of weight gain, lean body mass gain, fat accretion and protein retention may be determined using stepwise regression analysis. Protein intake and protein/energy ratio are the main determinants of weight gain. Protein intake is the only determinant of lean body mass gain in contrast to fat mass gain, which is positively related to energy intake and negatively to protein/energy ratio.[16] Protein gain and lean body mass gain increase significantly with protein intake without any additional significant influence of energy intake and protein/energy ratio. According to these data, as well as to the factorial approach, new recommendations for protein and protein/energy ratio can be suggested (Table 36.2) in relation to post-conceptional age and the need for catch-up growth.[16] Thus, according to this calculation, recommended intakes for preterm infants at 26–30 weeks' postconceptional age should have 3.8–4.4g of protein/kg per day with a protein/energy ratio between 3.0 and 3.3g/100kcal, according to their relative postnatal growth restriction. These values are in the range of the recent suggestion from an Expert Panel of the Life Sciences Research Office and the American Society for Nutritional Sciences who suggested 3.4–4.3g of protein/kg per day with an energy intake of 120kcal/kg per day and a protein/energy ratio between 2.5 and 3.6g/100kcal.[17]

Fat

Fat provides the major source of energy in growing preterm infants, representing approximately 50% of the non-protein energy content of human milk and current infant formulas. Although a mainly carbohydrate-based diet appears beneficial in terms of sparing protein oxidation, enhancing growth and protein accretion as well as to improve quiet sleep and influence the distribution of behavior activity states in VLBW infants, it is generally accepted that metabolizable long-chain fat should be at least equal to the fat deposition in growing tissues.[62] Accordingly, a fat intake of 5.4–7.2g/kg per day (or 40–54% of energy content) has been recommended.[38]

The newborn's capability of digesting triglycerides is not fully developed in premature infants. Lipid malabsorption is the result of low levels of pancreatic lipase and bile salts. The bile acid pool is only half the size of that of a full-term infant. In premature infants there is an alternative mechanism for digestion of dietary fat, represented by intragastric lipolysis, due to lingual and gastric lipases, secreted by the 25th week of gestation, that compensate for the low concentration of pancreatic lipase. Human milk provides additional

Table 36.2 Revised recommended protein intake and protein/energy ratio for preterm infants according to post-conceptional age (PCA) and need for catch-up growth (from reference 16)

	Without need for catch-up growth	With need for catch-up growth
26–30 weeks' PCA: 16–18g/kg per day LBM 14% protein retention	3.8–4.2g/kg per day PER: ±3.0	4.4g/kg per day PER: ±3.3
30–36 weeks' PCA: 14–15g/kg per day LBM 15% protein retention	3.4–3.6g/kg per day PER: ±2.8	3.6–4.0g/kg per day PER: ±3.0
36–40 weeks' PCA: 13g/kg per day LBM 17% protein retention	2.8–3.2g/kg per day PER: 2.4–2.6	3.0–3.4g/kg per day PER: 2.6–2.8

LBM, lean body mass; PER, protein/energy ratio

lipases: lipoprotein lipase, bile salt-stimulated esterase and non-activated lipase, which improves intestinal lipolysis.[63]

Lipid digestion and absorption are also affected by fatty acid composition, the triglyceride structure and the calcium content of the milk. Fatty acid absorption is related to chain length and degree of unsaturation. Thus, medium-chain triglycerides (MCTs) with 8–10 carbon atoms are hydrolyzed more readily than long-chain triglycerides (LCTs), and fatty acids with more double bonds are absorbed more efficiently. In order to improve fat absorption, commercial formulas contain a significant quantity of MCTs that are more easily absorbed than LCTs and transported directly to the liver via the portal vein as non-esterified fatty acids. The use of MCTs instead of LCTs in preterm infant formulas can reduce the formation of calcium and magnesium soaps with unabsorbed long-chain saturated fatty acids and, thereby, increase calcium and magnesium absorption. However, it needs to be stressed that the energy content of MCTs corresponds to about 85% of that of LCTs. In addition, the use of MCTs in formulas induces an increase in plasma ketones as well as in urinary excretion of dicarboxylic acids, suggesting that MCT metabolism could be slightly limited.[64] Moreover, since MCTs do not contain essential fatty acids, a high MCT intake can reduce the availability of the essential long-chain fatty acids necessary for normal growth and development. It is recommended that the maximum MCT intake in preterm formula be limited to 40–50% of total fat content.[17,38]

In human milk, long-chain fatty acids are preferentially positioned in the sn-2 position on the glycerol and are thus directly absorbed as monoglyceride. The use of formulas with palmitic acid with preferential esterification in the sn-2 position (β-palmitate) induces a minimal positive effect on energy balance but increases mineral absorption, leading to a significant reduction of insoluble calcium soap formation with free palmitic acid (16:0) and stearic acid (18:0). In preterm infants the rate of calcium absorption was markedly increased from 42% in a control formula to 57% in a formula containing 74% of palmitate esterified in the triglyceride sn-2 position (as β-palmitate).[65] It is noteworthy, however, that for commercial reasons, some preterm infant formulas available today with β-palmitate contain lower proportions of this structured triglyceride than those evaluated in previous clinical trials.

A fraction of fat must be provided as essential fatty acids; these are necessary to ensure optimal fatty acid composition and function of growing tissue and for normal eicosanoid synthesis. In preterm infants linoleic acid intakes of 3.2–12.8% energy intake have been recommended.[17]

Because humans cannot insert double bonds at the n-3 and n-6 positions, fatty acids with double bonds in these positions cannot be synthesized endogenously. Therefore, either specific n-3 and n-6 fatty acids or the precursor of each series such as linoleic acid (18:3n-3) and α-linolenic acid (18:2n-6) must be provided as a component of the diet. Both linoleic and α-linolenic acid are metabolized by a series of desaturation and elongation reactions to more unsaturated longer-chain fatty acids. Important metabolites of these two fatty acids include 20:5n-3 eicosapentaenoic acid (EPA), 22:6n-3 docosahexaenoic acid (DHA) and 20:4n-6 arachidonic acid (AA).

The biochemistry and metabolism of the essential fatty acids is complex, involving differences in metabolism and competition between the various n-6 and n-3 fatty acids. The desaturase enzymes show substrate preference in the order n-3 > n-6 > n-9, and are inhibited by products of either the n-6 or n-3 fatty-acid series.[66,67] Consequently, the rate of desaturation of linoleic acid (18:2n-6) to arachidonic acid (20:4n-6) and of α-linolenic acid (18:3n-3) to docosahexaenoic acid (22:6n-3) depends on the quantities of linoleic acid (18:2n-6) and α-linolenic acid (18:3n-3) substrate and preformed arachidonic acid (20:4n-6, AA) and/or docosahexaenoic acid (22:6n-3, DHA) in the diet. Accordingly, a linoleic/α-linolenic acid ratio of 5-16 : 1 wt/wt is currently recommended.[17]

Eicosapentaenoic acid (20:5n-3, EPA), which is found predominantly in fish oil, may also inhibit synthesis of arachidonic acid (20:4n-6). Thus, the infant's ability to maintain tissue arachidonic acid (20:4n-6, AA) levels may be lost if inappropriately high amounts of eicosapentaenoic acid (20:5n-3, EPA) or a high ratio of 22:6n-3 and 20:5n-3 to 20:4n-6 are provided by the diet.[68] In addition, the rate of precursors and long-chain polyunsaturated fatty acids (PUFAs) oxidation for energy production differs for each fatty acid and may influence biological activities and their multiple interactions.[68]

Considering that endogenous synthesis of long-chain PUFAs is limited in preterm infants, these fatty acids were considered as semi-essential or essential for preterm infants, and numerous studies evaluated the consequences of early neonatal deficiencies as well as the need of formula supplementation. Available sources of essential fatty acids are vegetal oils, whereas those of long-chain PUFAs include egg yolk lipid, phospholipid and triglyceride, fish oils and oils produced by single-celled organisms (microalgal and fungal oils).

Several studies have suggested that the long-chain PUFAs supply in preterm infants has a beneficial effect on growth, visual and cognitive function, as well as on the immune system. Although some methodological limits of these studies do not allow definitive conclusions to be drawn, most of the formulas in Europe and the USA are currently supplemented with long-chain PUFAs. However, as membranes enriched with PUFAs are particularly susceptible to oxidative damage, concern over the use of long-chain PUFAs in infant formulas might suggest the need for a higher vitamin E intake.

Several expert groups have recommended the routine addition of DHA and AA to LBW infant formulas.[17,38,69] Based on biochemical analyses, comparison with estimated intrauterine accretion rates, and the ranges of intakes with human milk feeding, a consensus group of experts on perinatal fatty-acid metabolism recently recommended the supplementation of formulas for preterm infants with DHA in the range of 0.35–0.5% of the fatty acids, and with AA in an AA/DHA ratio of 1.2–2 wt/wt.[14,63]

Carbohydrates

Carbohydrates represent approximately 40% of the energy intake of infants ingesting human milk or infant formulas. By virtue of their important biological effects, they improve nutritional status and function of the intestine and colon via the stimulatory effects of short-chain fatty acids on cell proliferation and ion absorption, stimulate insulin secretion and metabolism and growth and enhance the metabolic response to growth hormone and calcium absorption. Thus, they are essential to the overall health of the gastrointestinal tract and the fulfillment of energy requirements.

The predominant carbohydrate in mammalian milk and in term infant formula is lactose; after digestion by lactase, lactose is absorbed as glucose and galactose, which utilize the same carrier mechanism. In the human fetus, intestinal lactase activity is measurable by 10–12 weeks of gestation. There is a gradual increase in lactase activity with advancing gestation, although the activity remains low until about 36 weeks of gestation, when it reaches the levels seen in full-term neonates.[70]

Based on the low lactase activity in early gestation and the estimated length of the bowel, it was calculated that a preterm infant weighing 1300–1400 g might be expected to have nearly 50–70% of the lactose ingested passing unabsorbed into the colon[71] where, under the action of bacterial flora, it is transformed into short fatty acids and then absorbed. No difference in fecal carbohydrate loss was found in preterm infants fed formulas containing either 100% lactose or 50% lactose and 50% glucose.[72] Lactose not fully digested in many preterm and term infants could serve as a source of nutrition for beneficial bacterial flora in the colon. Through the process of fermentation, this not only facilitates colonic water and electrolyte absorption but also stimulates cell turnover of both the colon and the small intestine. In premature infants early exposure to lactose seems to induce intestinal lactase.[73] Regarding the relationship between lactose intake and calcium absorption, data in human adults seem to indicate that, in lactose-tolerant subjects, lactose does not appear to have any beneficial effect on calcium bioavailability.[74] In lactose-intolerant subjects, such as preterm infants, there is a significant level of uncertainty. Whether lactose in the distal bowel increases or impairs calcium absorption in preterm infants has yet to be defined.[17]

Quantitatively, other than lactose, oligosaccharides are the largest carbohydrate component in mature human milk and represent the third largest solute load after lactose and fat.[75,76] The concentration of oligosaccharides in human milk has been observed to change with the duration of lactation, being highest in the colostrum (about 20–23 g/l), about 20 g/l on day 4 and about 13 g/l on day 120 of lactation.[77] Many of the protective effects of human milk against diarrheal diseases, respiratory and ear infections, documented from a number of clinical epidemiological studies in developed and developing countries have been attributed to oligosaccharides.

In preterm formula a significant part of the carbohydrate is given as glucose polymers. These sugars have the advantage of providing a higher caloric intake without a corresponding rise in osmolarity. Glucose polymers are pure carbohydrates prepared by controlled acid/enzyme hydrolysis of cornstarch. They consist of polymers of glucose of varying chain length, although the majority are of medium (6–10 glucose units) chain length with a small amount (usually < 2%) of free glucose. Glucose polymers are mainly linear, with the glucose residue attached by α-1,4 glucosidic bonds. They have been used as nutritional supplements for adults and infants because of their lower osmolality (as compared with glucose or other hexose solutions) and therefore their possible rapid gastric emptying, and for being less sweet than fructose or sucrose.[78]

Glucose polymers are hydrolyzed by salivary, pancreatic and intestinal amylase and maltases to free glucose, which is rapidly absorbed. The efficiency of the absorption has been examined only in preterm babies at relatively older postnatal age and not in VLBW infants in the first few weeks after birth. A further advantage of glucose polymers for preterm infant formulas includes the possibility of faster gastric empting than after feeding either glucose or lactose.[79] Despite the importance of carbohydrate and the wide agreement that some lactose intake may be beneficial, there are no precise requirements for carbohydrate, glucose and galactose with respect to the preterm infant. The level of carbohydrate present in mature human milk or bovine milk formulas is accepted as sufficient to support glucose needs as well as normal growth and development. Optimal carbohydrate intakes in VLBW infants, estimated as (Energy intake−protein intake*4−fat intake*9)/4, corresponds to 7–20 g/kg per day. Nevertheless, it is also recommended that the carbohydrate intake in preterm infants represents 50–60% of the non-protein energy and that lactose accounts for at least 40% of the carbohydrate intake.[17]

Calcium and phosphorus

After birth, the use of the gastrointestinal tract to provide all nutrients for growth causes a large reduction in calcium bioavailability. Various factors affect calcium absorption: vitamin D status, solubility of calcium salts, and the quality and quantity of fat intake. In preterm infants, the vitamin D requirements are influenced by body stores at birth which in turn are related to the length of gestation and maternal stores. Therefore, the daily requirement could differ according to country.[80] In the USA, where dairy products are routinely supplemented with vitamin D, a daily additional intake of 400 IU in the formula appears sufficient to maintain an adequate plasma concentration of 25-OH and 1-25$(OH)_2$ vitamin D. By contrast, in some parts of Europe, cord blood concentration of 25-OH vitamin D of premature infants is frequently less than 10 μg/ml; in this case up to 1000 IU/day of vitamin D are recommended.[81] The increased needs of premature infants could be partly due to a relative malabsorption of vitamin D, resulting from a low secretion of bile acids.

Numerous mineral balance studies have been performed in preterm infants fed human milk or formula (Table 36.3).[32,80,82–85] In preterm infants fed human milk, calcium absorption ranged from 60 to 70% depending on the calcium intake whereas calcium retention was related to the phosphorus supply. Supplementation of human milk with phosphorus alone improved calcium retention from 25 to 35 mg/kg per day. When calcium and phosphorus were provided together or as human milk fortifiers, calcium retention reached 60 mg/kg per day and the recent use of human milk fortifiers containing highly soluble calcium glycerophosphate improved calcium retention up to 90 mg/kg per day (Table 36.3).

In formula-fed infants, calcium absorption is usually less than with human milk, ranging from 35 to 60% of intake. Calcium absorption is related to calcium, fat intakes and techniques of milk preparation. With ready-to-use liquid formulas,

Table 36.3 Mineral balance in very-low-birth-weight infants fed human milk or preterm formulas

Diet	Reference	Calcium intake (mg/kg per day)	Calcium absorption (%)	Calcium retention (mg/kg per day)	Phosphorus intake (mg/kg per day)	Phosphorus absorption (%)	Phosphorus retention (mg/kg per day)
HM (*n*=10)	80	58±11	71±14	25±12	24±6	92±4	21±5
HM + Ca+P (*n*=8)	80	90±11	73±13	63±12	62±5	93±2	53±4
HM + HMF (*n*=7)	80	101±19	66±7	65±14	78±13	94±2	62±9
HM + HMF2 (*n*=9)	*	170±13	57±17	91±27	87±6	94±2	61±12
PTF1 (*n*=39)	32	91±14	51±17	45±18	63±9	89±6	42±8
PTF2 (*n*=12)	*	103±16	43±18	41±22	64±8	92±3	40±7
PTF3 (*n*=7)	80	118±10	65±14	68±11	72±3	92±2	60±6
PTF4 (*n*=19)	32	120±21	44±16	48±22	70±9	78±12	43±11
PTF5(*n*=8)	*	120±19	46±18	50±20	75±12	88±6	45±10
PTF6 (*n*=7)	83	135±4	46±13	59±17	88±3	91±5	53±7
PTF7 (*n*=7)	*	161±11	41±13	58±22	90±5	59±8	50±8
PTF8 (*n*=6)	84	162±5	49±6	78±11	78±2	92±2	49±3
PTF9 (*n*=6)	84	162±5	64±5	100±8	75±2	92±2	58±3
PTF10 (*n*=9)	83	164±13	55±13	85±18	93±4	90±4	63±8
PTF11 (*n*=8)	*	172±11	34±12	54±25	95±6	60±6	51±10
PTF12 (*n*=11)	85	225±6	36±6	76±13	120±4	64±5	64±5

HM, human milk; HMF, human milk fortifier; PTF, preterm formula
* Unpublished data

calcium absorption is usually lower than with powder formulas. With the use of formulas with a well-absorbed fat blend of about 85%, the formation of a calcium soap is of minimal interest in clinical practice. Owing to the poor solubility of calcium salts, especially calcium phosphate, the calcium content measured in the formula could be significantly lower than the claimed value, and additional loss due to precipitation may occur before feeding. Therefore, the actual amount of calcium provided by feeding needs to be chemically measured in each infant during metabolic balance studies. As shown in Table 34.3, a calcium retention close to 90 mg/kg per day could currently be expected in preterm infants fed preterm formula with a highly soluble calcium content. Nevertheless, these values are still lower than the values estimated during the last trimester of gestation (100–120 mg/kg per day) and still considered as the target mineral accretion for VLBW infants.

Accordingly, it could be recommended that the calcium intake in preterm infants range between 130 and 170 mg/kg per day with a calcium/phosphorus ratio close to 1.8, as long as the calcium absorption rate is 45–60%.

Iron

Preterm infants require iron for erythropoiesis, brain development, muscle function and cardiac function. The symptoms of iron deficiency are due to tissue-level losses of iron containing enzymes and iron–sulfur proteins, not just to anemia. Oski has estimated that, in the absence of iron supplementation and blood loss, the VLBW preterm infant has enough iron stores to last 2 months and becomes anemic before liver stores are completely depleted.[86]

Table 36.4 Recommended enteral micro-mineral intakes (μg/kg per day) for preterm infants (from reference 87)

	Transitional period (0–14 days)	Stable/post-discharge periods
Iron	0	2000–4000
Zinc	500–800	1000–2000*
Copper	120	120–150
Selenium	1.3	1.3–4.5
Chromium	0.5	0.1–2.25
Molybdenum	0.3	0.3–4.0
Manganese	0.75	0.75–7.5
Iodine	11–27	10–60

*Post-discharge supplement of 0.5 mg/kg per day for infants fed human milk

Preterm infants need supplemental iron after 2 weeks of age. The enteral route appears safest. Iron can be supplied by preterm formula, human milk fortifier or medicinal iron drops. The enteral dose for the preterm infant not receiving erythropoietin ranges from 2 to 4 mg/kg per day depending on the degree of prematurity and the amount of uncompensated phlebotomy. The recent introduction of erythropoietin puts a greater stress on iron balance, forcing the infant to mobilize endogenous iron stores at a faster rate. For infants receiving this medication, an enteral dose of 6 mg/kg per day is recommended. No study has demonstrated oxidative toxicity from enteral iron given at conventional doses in preterm infants.

Studies are currently addressing the need for iron after discharge in preterm infants. Their iron needs will probably remain greater than those of term infants because of their more rapid relative rate of growth and therefore blood volume expansion. Given their lower endogenous iron stores, it would be prudent to screen these infants earlier (e.g. 2 months post-discharge) than term infants.

Other trace elements

Trace elements contribute less than 0.01% of total body weight. They function as constituents of metalloenzymes, cofactors for metal ion-activated enzymes, or components of vitamins, hormones and proteins. Because the fetus accumulates stores of trace elements, especially during the third trimester of pregnancy, premature infants have low stores at birth and are at risk of developing mineral deficiencies if intakes are inadequate for their growth requirements.

Trace minerals with established physiological importance in humans include zinc, copper, selenium, manganese, chromium, molybdenum, fluoride and iodine. The recommended oral intakes for infants are listed in Table 36.4.[87] Potentially toxic trace minerals for pediatric patients are lead and aluminum.

Oral vitamin requirements

Vitamins are organic compounds that are essential for metabolic reactions but are not synthesized by the body. Vitamins are classified as water soluble or fat soluble, based on the biochemical structure and function of the compound. The recommended oral intakes of vitamins for infants are shown in Table 36.5.[11]

Water-soluble vitamins that cannot be formed by precursors (with the exception of niacin from tryptophan) and do not accumulate in the body (with the exception of vitamin B_{12}) include B complex vitamins and vitamin C. They serve as prosthetic groups for enzymes involved in amino acid metabolism, energy production and nucleic acid synthesis. A daily intake is required to prevent deficiency. Excretion occurs in the urine and bile. Altered urinary losses due to renal immaturity during the first week of life predispose a preterm infant to vitamin deficiency or excess.

Fat-soluble vitamins include vitamin A, D, E and K. These vitamins function physiologically in the conformation and function of complex molecules and membranes and are important for the development and function of highly specialized tissues. They can be built from precursors, are excreted with difficulty and accumulate in the body, and therefore they can produce toxicity. They are not required daily and deficient states develop slowly. Fat-soluble vitamins require carrier systems, usually lipoproteins, for solubility in blood, and intestinal absorption depends on fat absorption.

Table 36.5 Recommended oral intake of vitamins for preterm infants (from reference 11, American Academy of Pediatrics, Committee on Nutrition, 1998)

Vitamin (amount per 100 kcal)	AAPCON Recommendations for premature infants (1998)	Consensus Recommendations for infants with VLBW (1993)
Fat soluble		
Vitamin A (IU)	75–225	583–1250
Vitamin D (IU)	270	125–333
Vitamin E (IU)	>1.1	5–10
Vitamin K (μg)	4	6.66–8.33
Water soluble		
Vitamin B_6 (μg)	>35	125–175
Vitamin B_{12} (μg)	>0.35	0.25
Vitamin C (mg)	35	15–20
Biotin (μg)	>1.5	3–5
Folic acid (μg)	33	21–42
Niacin (mg)	>0.25	3–4
Pantothenate (mg)	0.3	1–1.5
Riboflavin (μg)	>60	200–300
Thiamine (μg)	>40	150–200

AAPCON, American Academy of Pediatrics Committee on Nutrition; VLBW, very low birth weight

Practical aspects of enteral nutrition

Breast milk

Benefit of human milk

The American Academy of Pediatrics has acknowledged the advantages of human milk feeding with the statement that it is the preferred feeding for all infants, including those born preterm.[88] The benefits of human milk for gastrointestinal function, host defense and neurodevelopmental outcome are well known. The amino acid composition of human milk is suitable for the nutritional requirements of preterm infants who are, because of incomplete development of some amino acid metabolic pathways, at risk of developing a deficit or an overload of essential and semi-essential amino acids.

Clinical studies performed in various parts of the world have shown that preterm infants fed human milk have fewer infections than those fed on formula.[89] This effect has been observed with both fresh and pasteurised human milk. There are studies showing a protective effect of breast milk on the incidence of NEC. A meta-analysis of randomized controlled trials was performed to determine whether enteral feeding with donor human milk, compared with formula, reduced the incidence of NEC in preterm infants. They found that feeding with donor human milk was also associated with a significantly reduced risk of NEC; infants who received donor human milk were three times less likely to develop NEC and four times less likely to have confirmed NEC.[90]

The protective effect of human milk has been attributed to several factors, such as macrophages, lymphocytes, sIgA, lysozyme, lactoferrin, oligosaccharides, nucleotides, cytokines, growth factors and enzymes. Immune defense can be provided by an interaction between these factors. Human milk can play a protective role through the enteromammary immune system. The mother's presence in the neonatal nursery, particularly the premature infant's skin-to-skin contact with the mother, may induce the production of specific antibodies against the nosocomial pathogens present in the nursery.[88] Breast milk enhances the growth, motility and maturity of the gastrointestinal tract; compared to formulas it induces faster gastric emptying.[91]

Preterm infants with a birth weight below 1850g, fed human milk during hospitalization, showed better neurological development. At 7.5–8 years they showed a higher intelligence quotient compared to those fed formula, even after controlling for the mother's education and social class.[92] Higher mental developmental index scores were reported in VLBW (< 1250g) infants at 18 months of age who received human milk, compared to those who never received human milk in hospital.

In premature infants, visual function may also be improved by the feeding of human milk.[93] This positive effect of human milk on neurodevelopment and visual function has been attributed to the high quantity of the very long-chain PUFA present in human milk. Other potential factors of human milk that might contribute to neurodevelopment are cholesterol, antioxidants, taurine growth factors and micronutrients.

Limits of human milk

Despite the potential benefits, nutrients of human milk are not sufficient to cover the greater needs of VLBW infants and to ensure a growth similar to that of the fetus during the last period of gestation. Breast milk composition is different depending on the gestational age of the infant at birth, collection methods (e.g. drip method versus expression with a pump), and whether pooled milk or the infant's own mother's milk is used.[94] Greater concentrations of nitrogen, immune proteins, total lipids, medium-chain fatty acids, energy, vitamins, some minerals (calcium and phosphorus) and trace elements in milk from mothers who give birth prematurely (preterm milk) compared with milk of mothers giving birth at term (term milk) have been observed.[95] The higher concentrations of these nutrients tend to decline as lactation progresses, so exclusive feeding of mature preterm milk from 2 weeks postnatally may lead to nutrient deficiencies in the rapidly growing preterm infant.

The reason for the difference in nutrient density between preterm and term milk is not well known. Early interruption of pregnancy might induce an incomplete maturation of mammary glands to support normal lactation. There may be a paracellular leakage of serum proteins and ions through junctions that have not completely closed.[96] Also, a different hormonal profile in women who deliver prematurely compared with those who deliver at term could be responsible for a different milk composition.[96] It has also been suggested that the greater nutrient density in preterm milk could be related to the higher concentration of nutrients in a lower volume of milk.[97]

One of the main limits of human milk is its production. Mothers of preterm infants, for several reasons (stress, poor maternal health, delayed initiation of lactation) produce an inadequate quantity of milk. Moreover a restriction of fluid intake in VLBW infants could reduce the volume of human milk given, and thus not offer a sufficient quantity of nutrients.

Fortification of human milk

In order to meet the unique nutritional requirements of VLBW infants and to preserve the singular benefit of human milk, human milk fortifiers which increase the nutritional content of human milk, have been produced. In fact, the protein content of human milk may be too low to permit adequate growth, the low sodium level may lead to hyponatremia, and the amounts of calcium and phosphorus could be below the intake needed to achieve fetal rates of bone mineral accretion.

Through a process of human milk lacto-engineering, human milk can be fortified with skim and cream components derived from heat-treated, lyophilized mature donor human milk to produce a 'human milk formula'.[98] This method of fortification avoids cow's milk proteins but it is impractical for most neonatal units, since it involves a complex process and requires a large supply of donor milk.

Preterm human milk, fortified with protein of bovine origin, has become the standard practice in most neonatal units. As shown in Table 36.6, the composition of several fortifiers expressed per gram of protein varies both qualitatively and quan-

Table 36.6 Composition of various human milk fortifiers (expressed per gram of protein)

	Eoprotin (Milupa) powder	FM-85 (Nestlé) powder	BMF (Nutricia) bag 1.5 g	EHMF1 (M-J) bag 0.9 g	SHMF (Abbott) bag 0.9 g	WHMF (Wyeth) bag 2 g	EHMF2 (M-J) bag 0.8 g	EHMF3 (M-J) bag 0.8 g
Protein (g)	1	1	1	1	1	1	1	1
Fat (g)	0	0	0	0	0.36	0	0.58	0.91
Carbohydrate (g)	3.48	4.3	2.86	3.9*	1.8	2.0	1.0	0.2
Sodium (mg)	3.3	32.3	8.7	10.3	15.0	15.0	1.0	15.0
Potassium (mg)	4.0	13.8	5.7	23.0	62.9	20.0	18.2	26.0
Calcium (mg)	62	61	87	136	117	80	82	82
Magnesium (mg)	3.5	2.4	8.6	1.5	7.0	2.0	0.9	0.9
Phosphorus (mg)	42.3	40.7	58.4	66.8	67.2	40.0	41.0	45.0
Chloride (mg)	24.9	22.2	10.1	26.0	37.9	14.0	8.2	12.0
Energy (kcal)	31.7	21.4	14.3	20.7	14.0	13.0	12.7	12.7
Osmolality (mOsm)	90	96	85	177	90	136	59—	

* Including the carbohydrate content of calcium glycerophosphate

titatively. In general, they contain bovine whey protein (intact or hydrolyzed), carbohydrates (mainly or exclusively glucose polymers or maltodextrins), minerals and electrolytes such as sodium, calcium, phosphorus and magnesium and some also contain micronutrients (zinc and copper) and vitamins.

The properties of human milk may be changed by nutrient fortification. For example, the addition of human milk fortifiers induces a rapid and clinically significant increase in osmolality, frequently above 400 mOsm/kg H_2O, a value at least 40% higher than that of human milk.[99] This is the result of the osmotic content of the fortifier but also of the rapid and continuous activity of human milk amylase on the dextrin content of fortifiers. Such an increase in osmolality may at least partly explain some minimal clinical disturbances, such as abdominal discomfort and delayed gastric emptying, but in some cases it might increase the risk of NEC in preterm infants.[100] Recently, in order to avoid these problems, fortifiers with whole proteins, reduced carbohydrate content and fat supplementation have been proposed.[101] The presence of fat in fortifiers has the advantage of increasing the energy intake of human milk without increasing osmolality values. However, this needs further technological studies, because the action of human milk lipase on triglycerides of fortifiers could produce instability in human milk.

Many studies have evaluated growth, metabolic balance and weight gain composition in preterm infants fed fortified human milk.[49,98,102–108] The addition of multinutrient fortifiers to human milk resulted in short-term improvements in weight gain and increments in both length and head circumference growth during hospital stay. For ethical reasons, it is now unlikely that further studies evaluating fortification of human milk in comparison with no fortification will be conducted. Although the fortification of human milk improves the growth of preterm infants, growth both in general and referred to specific parameters (such as lean body mass, fat mass and bone mineral content) is significantly lower in fortified human milk-fed infants than in those fed preterm formula (Table 36.7). These differences could be related to the lower protein content but also to the reduction in metabolizable protein and energy available for new tissues synthesis.

Questions have been raised as to whether the addition of bovine-derived human milk fortifiers can

Table 36.7 Nutritional intake, growth and weight gain in preterm infants fed fortified human milk (HMF) and preterm formula (PTF) (from reference 16)

Amount (/kg per day)	HMF (n=48)	PTF (n=86)	p Value
Volume intake (ml)	164±12	152±12	<0.001
Energy (kcal)	118±10	119±12	0.57
Protein (g)	2.9±0.3	3.3±0.4	<0.001
Weight gain (g)	15.7±2.3	19.6±3.1	<0.001
Length gain (cm/week)	0.95±0.34	1.07±0.35	0.06
Head circumference gain (cm/week)	0.97±0.25	1.05±0.30	0.010
Lean body mass (g)	12.4±2.3	14.7±3.0	<0.001
Fat mass (g)	3.2±1.6	4.7±1.8	<0.001
Bone mineral content (mg)	215±86	263±83	0.002
Bone area (cm^2)	1.18±0.41	1.51±0.39	<0.001

affect feeding tolerance in premature infants. No differences in feeding tolerance were reported in a meta-analysis comparing premature infants fed fortified human milk or unfortified human milk.[109] In contrast, fortifiers have recently been considered as risk factors for NEC in VLBW infants.[100] When compared with premature infants fed preterm formula, infants fed exclusively fortified human milk had a significantly lower incidence of NEC and/or sepsis, had fewer positive blood cultures and required less antibiotic administration.[89]

The effect of nutrient fortification on some of the general host defense properties of milk have been evaluated. Fortification did not affect the concentration of IgA in milk.[110] When fortified human milk was evaluated under simulated nursery conditions, bacterial colony counts were not significantly different after 20h of storage at refrigerator temperature, but increased from 20 to 24h when maintained at incubator temperature.[110]

Early use of a human milk fortifier up to 1.3g of protein/100ml is recommended for more immature or smaller preterm infants, beginning from the time when they are able to tolerate 50–70ml/kg per day of milk. Preference should be given to fortifiers with higher protein density and lower osmotic load. Additional studies are required to define the optimal delay in commencing fortification, the safe daily increment in enteral feeding and the beneficial effects on growth and development of the more recent human milk fortifiers in VLBW infants.

Preterm formulas

When human milk is not available or extremely limited, cow's-milk-based formulas for preterm infants must be used. Over the past 20 years, there has been a significant improvement in the nutrient composition of preterm formulas in order to meet the nutritional needs of growing preterm infants. VLBW infants fed these formulas showed an improvement of fat absorption, nitrogen retention, bone mineralization and weight gain, when compared to VLBW infants fed standard term formulas or pooled human milk. Although numerous consensus conferences have been organized, the optimal formula for VLBW infants has not yet been designed. European preterm formulas present several differences in the nutrient composition when compared to American formulas. The latter have a higher MCT and a lower long-chain PUFA content, provide less lactose, and have a higher mineral intake.

Nevertheless, according to more recent data, a general profile in macronutrients could probably be suggested. Energy content could be slightly higher than at present (80–90 kcal/100 ml in order to provide 130–135 kcal/kg per day with a volume intake close to 160 ml/kg per day). According to the protein requirements, the protein content would represent 3.3 g/100 kcal, i.e. 2.6–3.0 g/100 ml. Whey-predominant protein with reduced glycomacropeptide and α-lactalbumin enrichment could be used to optimize the amino acid profile. Up to now the use of protein-hydrolyzed formulas have not been recommended. Their amino acid pattern is relatively unbalanced and the net protein utilization and protein efficiency are relatively impaired in comparison to whole protein, in contrast to the minimal clinical advantages observed, such as an improvement in gastric emptying or a reduced transit time.[32,111] The partition of the non-protein energy supply would favor the carbohydrate content up to 50–60% in view of its suggested benefits in sparing protein oxidation, enhancing growth and protein accretion as well as improving quiet sleep and influencing the distribution of behavioral activity states in VLBW infants. According to the relatively reduced intestinal lactase activity, the lactose content could be relatively reduced and substituted with glucose polymers with the characteristic of maintaining the low osmolality of the formulas. The remaining energy supply would be covered by fat with a fat blend carefully designed to reduce the long-chain saturated fatty acid content, and provide the essential fatty acids (linoleic and α-linolenic acid) in an appropriate ratio as well as the long-chain PUFA such as DHA and AA. In order to improve fat absorption, an important quota of fat could be given as MCT with a maximum of 30–40%. Highly metabolizable (50–60% absorption rate) calcium content would be limited to 100–120 mg/100 ml. A higher calcium supply does not seem useful. According to the expected nitrogen and calcium retention, the phosphorus content of this formula would represent 55–65 mg/100 ml, considering a phosphorus absorption close to 90%.

Additional components of human milk, such as nucleotides, polyamine prebiotics and glutamine, are currently under investigation, and the results need to be available before their use in preterm formulas.[17]

Preterm formulas are available as powder or liquid in glass bottles or cans. Liquid formulas have the advantage that they provide sterile feeding thereby reducing possible infections reported in pre-term infants fed powder formulas such as the *Enterobacter sakazakii.*[112] Nevertheless, it worth remembering that with liquid formulas, there is frequent discordance between claimed and available content of several nutrients. For instance, part of the calcium content of liquid formula may precipitate on the wall of the container reducing the calcium truly available to the preterm infants. In addition, the heat treatment necessary to sterilize the liquid formulas reduces the bioavailability of various nutrients such as proteins, calcium or copper. The impaired bioavailability is directly related to the importance of heat treatment and is probably lower in the ultra heat treated (UHT) brickpack formula. In summary, powder formulas allowing adaptation of nutrient density and being of higher nutritional value, remain the formulas of choice for the feeding of VLBW infants when human milk is not available.

Post-discharge nutrition in preterm infants

Protein- and mineral-enriched formulas have been proposed to feed preterm infants after discharge with the aim of minimizing as much as possible, postnatal growth restriction during the early weeks of life, inducing early catch-up growth and reducing the adult adverse effects of early malnutrition. In most neonatal units, the discharge of VLBW infants usually occurs usually when premature infants reach a corrected gestational age of 35–36 weeks and a weight of about 1800–2100 g. By that time, they have accumulated energy, protein and mineral deficits and still present higher nutrient requirements than healthy infants appropriate for gestational term. The potential benefits of enriched formula on growth have been investigated following the first study of Lucas et al in 1992 who introduced the concept of the post-discharge formula.[113]

Although the various studies differed in design and reported conflicting results, they allow a global analysis to be made. Comments follow:

(1) Among the VLBW infants, not all preterm infants are at similar risk of later growth

failure. Small-for-gestational-age infants and those appropriate for gestational age developing postnatal growth restriction seem to be the population at higher risk, while infants appropriate for corrected age at the time of discharge from the hospital subsequently continue to maintain appropriate growth.[114]

(2) Energy intakes were the main determinant of milk volume intakes. Compared to regular (standard) formula, an increase in energy density had no influence on energy supply, in contrast to the increase in protein density that influences protein intake, and protein metabolism.

(3) A positive effect of growth parameters was not observed in all studies, but the benefit of the nutrient-enriched formula on growth, when observed, was mainly seen during the early post-discharge period (between discharge and term), in infants with very low birth weights.[115,116] In addition, the growth benefit could be related to the preterm infants without a postnatal growth deficit at the time of discharge.[117]

(4) There is a strong gender influence on the result of diet manipulation during the post-discharge period. The main positive results are limited to boys.

(5) The safety of prolonged high-protein intake during the early period of life in preterm infants after discharge has not been established, in contrast to the minimal benefits suggested by the various studies. High-protein intake, by inducing an increase in biochemical parameters of nitrogen metabolism (urea, amino acids, ammonia), could enhance the development of several diseases, such as obesity and hypertension later in life.[118]

Since early nutrition should not be considered simply in terms of providing immediate nutritional needs but also for the biological effects with possibly lasting or lifelong significance, it seems prudent to suggest an enriched formula only in infants at risk of future growth failure.[119]

Mothers of infants at low risk of longitudinal growth restriction should be encouraged to feed them their own milk. Careful attention is necessary to evaluate the appropriateness of intakes and growth just before and in the first week after discharge. In early discharge a supplementation with fortified human milk or formula might be necessary in order to improve the nutrient supply in relation to the remaining state of prematurity.

In infants with a low risk of longitudinal growth restriction, fed on formula at the time of discharge, a regular formula with relatively low protein density (2.2 g/100 kcal) should be provided with particular attention to its long-chain PUFAs, mineral and trace element content.

Infants at high risk of longitudinal growth restriction, should be breast fed or should receive human milk supplemented with fortified human milk or formula, in order to improve the nutrient supply and promote catch-up growth. An evaluation of nutrient intakes and growth should be done frequently to optimize growth and biological parameters.

In infants at high risk of longitudinal growth restriction, on formula at the time of discharge, a specific post-discharge formula with higher protein and mineral density but also adapted in long-chain PUFAs and trace elements should be provided. Intakes and growth would also be recorded weekly and thereafter monthly to ensure that nutrient supplementation is in agreement with growth and biological results.

Further research should be initiated in order to determine the specific nutritional needs of growth-restricted preterm infants in order to design more specific post-discharge formulas and evaluate their effect on the long-term incidence of growth restriction as well as somatic and neurodevelopmental outcomes.

REFERENCES

1. Ziegler EE, Thureen PJ, Carlson SJ. Aggressive nutrition of the very low birthweight infant. *Clin Perinatol* 2002; **29**: 225–244.
2. Lucas A, Bloom SR, Aynsley-Green A. Gut hormones and 'minimal enteral feeding'. *Acta Paediatr Scand* 1986; **75**: 719–723.
3. Tyson JE, Kennedy K. Minimal enteral nutrition in parenterally fed neonates. 1997. *http://www.nichd.nih.gov/cochraneonatal/tyson//tyson.htm.*
4. Premji S, Chessel L. Continuous nasogastric milk feeding versus intermittent bolus milk feeding for premature infants less than 1500 grams, *Cochrane Database Syst Rev* 2003; **1**: CD001819.
5. Currao WJ, Cox C, Shapiro DL. Diluted formula for beginning the feeding of premature infants. *Am J Dis Child* 1988; **142**: 730–731.
6. Kennedy KA, Tyson JE, Chamnanvanakij S. Rapid versus slow rate of advancement of feedings for promoting growth and preventing necrotizing enterocolitis in parenterally fed low birthweight infants. *Cochrane Database Syst Rev* 2000; **2**: CD001241.
7. Berseth CL, Bisquera JA, Paje VU. Prolonging small feeding volumes early in life decreases the incidence of necrotizing enterocolitis in very low birth weight infants. *Pediatrics* 2003; **111**: 529–534.
8. Davies ID, Avner ED. Fluid and electrolyte management. In Fanaroff AA, Martin RJ, eds. *Neonatal–Perinatal Medicine.* 7th edn. St Louis, MO: Mosby, 2002: 619–627.
9. Fomon SJ, Ziegler EE. Renal solute load and potential solute load in infancy. *J Pediatr* 1999; **134**: 11–14.
10. Fomon SJ, Ziegler EE. Renal solute load. In *Nutrition of Normal Infants.* St. Louis, MO: Mosby-Year Book, 1993: 91–102.
11. American Academy of Pediatrics, Committee on Nutrition. Nutritional needs of preterm infants. In Kleinman RE, ed. *Pediatric Nutrition Handbook*, 4th edn. Elk Grove Village, Il: American Academy of Pediatrics, 1998: 55–87.
12. Raiten DJ, Talbot JM, Waters JH. Assessment of nutrient requirements for infant formulas. Prepared by the Life Sciences Research Office, 9650 Rockville Pike, Bethesda MD. *J Nutr* 1998; **128** (Suppl 11S).
13. Parmar V, Abdulrazzaq YM, Brooke OG. Stool water in preterm neonates. *Arch Dis Child* 1986; **61**: 1136–1137.
14. Chevalier RL. Developmental renal physiology of the low birth weight pre-term newborn. *J Urol* 1996; **156**: 714–719.
15. De Curtis M, Senterre J, Rigo J. Renal solute load in preterm infants. *Arch Dis Child* 1990; **65**: 357–360.
16. Rigo J. Protein, amino acid and other nitrogen compounds. In Tsang RC, Uauy R, Koletzko et al., eds. *Nutritional Needs of the Preterm Infant.* Cincinnati, OH: Digital Educational Publishing, 2004: 43–76 (in press).
17. Klein CJ. Nutrient requirements for preterm infant formulas. *J Nutr* 2002; **132**: 1395S–1577S.
18. Sparks JW. Human intrauterine growth and nutrient accretion. *Semin Perinatol* 1984; **8**: 74–93.
19. Nutrition Committee CPS. Nutrient needs and feeding of premature infants. *Can Med Assoc J* 1995; **152**: 1765–1785.
20. Zello GA, Menendez CE, Rafii M et al. Minimum protein intake for the preterm neonate determined by protein and amino acid kinetics *Pediatric Res* 2003; **53**: 338–344.
21. Embleton NE, Pang N, Cooke RJ. Postnatal malnutrition and growth retardation: an inevitable consequence of current recommendations in preterm infants? *Pediatrics* 2001; **107**: 270–273.
22. Rigo J, Putet G, Picaud JC et al Nitrogen balance and plasma amino acids in the evaluation of protein sources for extremely low birthweight infants. In Ziegler EE, Lucas A, Moro GE, eds. *Nutrition of the Very Low Birthweight Infant.* 43rd Nestlè Nutrition Workshop, Nestec Ltd. Philadelphia: Vevey/Lippincott Williams & Wilkins, 1999: 139–153.
23. Rudloff S, Lonnerdal B. Solubility and digestibility of milk proteins in infant formula exposed to different heat treatments. *J Pediatr Gastroenterol Nutr* 1992; **15**: 25–33.
24. Cooke R, Watson D, Werkman S et al. Effects of type of dietary protein on acid–base status, protein nutritional status, plasma levels of amino acids, and nutrient balance in the very low birth weight infant. *J Pediatr* 1992; **121**: 444–451.
25. Rigo J, Senterre J. Optimal threonine intake for preterm infants fed on oral or parenteral nutrition. *J Parenter Enteral Nutr* 1980; **4**: 15–17.
26. Boehm G, Cervantes H, Georgi G et al. Effect of increasing dietary threonine intakes on amino acid metabolism of central nervous system and peripheral tissues in growing rats. *Pediatr Res* 1998; **44**: 900–906.
27. Rigo J, Boehm G, Georgi G et al. An infant formula free of glycomacropeptide prevents hyperthreoninemia in formula-fed preterm infants. *J Pediatr Gastroenterol Nutr* 2001; **32**: 127–130.
28. Picaud JC, Rigo J, Normand S et al. Nutritional efficacy of preterm formula with a partially hydrolyzed protein source: a randomized pilot study. *J Pediatr Gastroenterol Nutr* 2001; **32**: 555–561.
29. Raïhïa NCR, Nesci AF, Cajozzo C et al. Protein quantity and quality in infant formula: closer to the reference. In Raïhä NCR, Rubaltelli FF, eds. *Infant Formula: Closer to the Reference.* Nestlé Nutrition Workshop Series, Nestec Ltd. Philadelphia: Vevey/Lippincott Williams & Wilkins, 2002; **47**: 53–69.
30. Heine WE, Klein PD, Reeds PJ. The importance of alpha-lactoalbumin in infant nutrition. *J Nutr* 1991; **121**: 277–283.
31. Heine WE, Radke M, Wutzke KD et al. Alfa-lactalbumin-enriched low-protein infant formulas: a comparison to breast milk feeding. *Acta Paediatr* 1996; **85**: 1024–1028.
32. Rigo J, Salle BL, Picaud J-C et al. Nutritional evaluation of protein hydrolysate formulas. *Eur J Clin Nutr* 1995; **49**: S26–S38.
33. Mihatsh WA, Hogel J, Pohlandt F. Hydrolysed protein accelerates the gastrointestinal transport of formula in preterm infants. *Acta Paediatr* 2001; **90**: 196–198.
34. Lee YH. Food-processing approaches to altering allergenic potential of milk-based formula. *J Pediatr* 1992; **121**: S47–S50.
35. Picaud JC, Rigo J, Normand S et al. Nutritional efficacy of preterm formula with a partially hydrolyzed protein source: a randomized pilot study. *J Pediatr Gastroenterol Nutr* 2001; **32**: 555–561.
36. Lajoie N, Gauthier SF, Pouliot Y. Improved storage stability of model infant formula by whey peptides fractions. *J Agric Food Chem* 2001; **49**: 1999–2007.
37. Mihatsh WA, Pohlandt F. Protein hydrolysate formula maintains homeostasis of plasma amino acids in preterm infants. *J Pediatr Gastroenterol Nutr* 1999; **29**: 406–410.
38. ESPGAN Committee on Nutrition. Comment on the content and composition of lipids in infant formulas. *Acta Paediatr Scand* 1991; **80**: 887–896.
39. Health Canada Health Protection Branch of Canada, *Guidelines for the Composition and Clinical Testing of Formulas for Preterm Infants.* Report of an *Ad Hoc* Expert Consultation to the Health Protection Branch, Health Canada. Ottawa, Ontario: Canadian Government Publishing Center, 1995.
40. Bell EF. Diet and body composition of preterm infants. *Acta Paediatr* 1994; **405** (Suppl): 25–28.

41. Kashyap S, Heird WC. Protein requirements of low birth weight, very low birth weight and small for gestational age infants. In Raiha NCR ed. *Protein Metabolism During Infancy*. 33rd edn. Nestlé Nutrition Workshop Series, vol 33. New York: Raven Press, 1994: 133–155.
42. Putet G. Energy. In Tsang RC, Lucas A, Uauy R, Zlotkin S, eds. *Nutritional Needs of the Preterm Infant*. New York: Williams & Wilkins, 1993: 15–28.
43. Micheli JL, Schutz T. Protein. In Tsang RC, Lucas A, Uauy R, Zlotkin S, eds. *Nutritional Needs of the Preterm Infant: Scientific Basis and Practical Guidelines*. Baltimore, MD: Williams and Wilkins, 1993: 29–46.
44. Kashyap S, Towers HM, Sahni R et al. Effects of quality of energy on substrate oxidation in enterally fed, low-birth-weight infants. *Am J Clin Nutr* 2001; **74**: 374–380.
45. Pencharz PB, Farri L, Papageorgiou A. The effect of human milk and low-protein formulae on the rates of total body protein turnover and urinary 3-methyl-histidine excretion of preterm infants. *Clin Sci* 1983; **64**: 611–616.
46. Putet G, Picaud JC, Salle BL et al. Utilization and storage of energy. In Salle BL, Swyer PR, eds. *Nutrition of the Low-Birthweight Infant*. Nestlé Nutrition Workshop Series. Nestec Ltd., New York: Vevey/Raven Press, 1993; **32**: 61–69.
47. Whyte RK, Haslam R, Vlainic C et al. Energy balance and nitrogen balance in growing low-birthweight infants fed human milk or formula. *Pediatr Res* 1983; **17**: 891–898.
48. Kashyap S, Forsyth M, Zucker C et al. Effect of varying protein and energy intakes on growth and metabolic response in low birth weight infants. *J Pediatr* 1986; **108**: 955–963.
49. Kashyap S, Schulze KF, Forsyth M et al. Growth, nutrient retention and metabolic response of low-birthweight infants fed supplemented and unsupplemented preterm human milk. *Am J Clin Nutr* 1990; **52**: 254–262.
50. Roberts SB, Lucas A. Energetic efficiency and nutrient accretion in preterm infants fed extremes of dietary intake. *Clin Nutr* 1987; **416**: 105–113.
51. Schultze KF, Stefanski M, Masterson J et al. Energy expenditure, energy balance and composition of weight gain in low birth weight infants fed diets of different protein and energy content. *J Pediatr* 1987; **110**: 753–759.
52. Reichman B, Chessex P, Verellen G et al. Dietary composition and macronutrient storage in preterm infants. *Pediatrics* 1983; **72**: 322–328.
53. Boehm G, Muller DM, Senger H et al. Nitrogen and fat balances in very low birth weight infants fed formula fortifier with human milk or bovine milk protein. *Eur J Pediatr* 1993; **152**: 236–239.
54. Schanler RJ, Abrams SA. Postnatal attainment of intrauterine macromineral accretion rate birth weight infants fed fortified human milk. *J Pediatr* 1995; **126**: 441–447.
55. Polberger S, Raihä NC, Juvonen P et al. Individualised protein fortification of human milk for preterm infants: comparison of ultrafiltrated human milk protein and a bovine whey fortifier. *J Pediatr Gastroenterol Nutr* 1999; **29**: 332–338.
56. Reiss BB, Hall RT, Schanler RJ et al. Enhanced growth of preterm infants fed a new powdered human milk fortifier: a randomized, controlled trial. *Pediatrics* 2000; **106**: 581–588.
57. Porcelli P, Schanler R, Greer F et al. Growth in human milk-fed very low birth weight infants receiving a new human milk fortifier. *Ann Nutr Metab* 2000; **44**: 2–10.
58. Putet G, Senterre J, Rigo G et al. Nutrient balance, energy utilization and composition of weight gain in very-low-birth-weight-infants fed pooled human milk or preterm formula. *J Pediatr* 1984; **105**: 79–85.
59. De Curtis M, Brooke OG. Energy and nitrogen balances in very low birth weight infants. *Arch Dis Child* 1987; **62**: 830–832.
60. Kashyap S, Schuylze KF, Ramakrishan R et al. Evaluation of a mathematical model for predicting the relationship between protein and energy intakes of low-birth-weight infants and the rate and composition of weight gain. *Pediatr Res* 1994; **35**: 704–712.
61. Putet G, Senterre J, Rigo J et al. Energy balance and composition of body weight. *Biol Neonate* 1987; **52** (Suppl 1): 17–24.
62. Rodriguez M, Funkes S, Fink M et al. Plasma fatty acids and the [13C] linoleic acid metabolism in preterm infants fed a formula with medium-chain triglycerides. *J Lipid Res* 2003; **44**: 41–48.
63. Hamosh M, Henderson TR, Ellis LA et al. Digestive enzymes in human milk: stability at suboptimal storage temperatures. *J Pediatr Gastroenterol Nutr* 1997; **24**: 38–43.
64. Henderson MJ, Dear PRF. Dicarboxylic aciduria and medium chain triglyceride supplemented milk. *Arch Dis Child* 1990; **61**: 610–611.
65. Lucas A, Quinlan P, Abrams S et al. Randomised controlled trial of a synthetic triglyceride milk formula for preterm infants. *Arch Dis Child Fetal Neonatal Ed.* 1997; **77**: F178–F184.
66. Koletzko B. Lipid supply and metabolism in infancy. *Curr Opin Clin Nutr Metab Care* 1998; **1**: 171–177.
67. Innis SM. The role of dietary n-6 and n-3 fatty acids in the developing brain. *Dev Neurosci* 2000; **22**: 474–480.
68. Koletzko BV, Innis SM. Lipids. In Tsang RC, Uauy R, Koletzko et al. eds. *Nutritional Needs of the Preterm Infant*. Cincinnati, OH: Digital Educational Publishing, 2004: 43–76 (in press).
69. Koletzko B, Agostoni C, Carlson SE et al. Long chain polyunsaturated fatty acids (LC-PUFA) and perinatal development. *Acta Paediatr* 2001; **90**: 460–464.
70. Auricchio S, Rubino A, Murset G. Intestinal glucosidase activity in the human embryo, fetus and newborn. *Pediatrics* 1965; **35**: 944–954.
71. Watkins JB. Developmental aspects of carbohydrate malabsorption in the premature infant. In Lifshitz F, ed. *Carbohydrate Intolerance in Infancy*. New York: Marcel Dekker, 1982: 61–73.
72. Murray RD, Boutton TW, Klein PD et al. Comparative absorption of [^{13}C]glucose and [^{13}C]lactose by premature infants. *Am J Clin Nutr* 1990; **51**: 59–66.
73. Shulman RJ, Schanler RJ, Lau C et al. Early feeding, feeding intolerance, and lactase activity in preterm infants. *J Pediatr* 1998; **133**: 645–659.
74. Zittermann A, Bock P, Drummer C et al. Lactose does not enhance calcium bioavailability in lactose-tolerant, healthy adults. *Am J Clin Nutr* 2000; **71**: 931–936.
75. Brand Miller J, McVeagh P. Human milk oligosaccharides: 130 reasons to breast-feed. *Br J Nutr* 1999; **82**: 333–335.
76. Coppa GV, Pierani P, Zampini L et al. Oligosaccharides in human milk during different phases of lactation. *Acta Paediatr Suppl* 1999; **430**: 89–94.
77. Coppa GV, Gabrielli O, Pierani P et al, Changes in carbohydrate composition in human milk over 4 months of lactation. *Pediatrics* 1993; **91**: 637–641.
78. Shulman RJ, Feste A, Ou C. Absorption of lactose, glucose polymers, or combination in premature infants. *J Pediatr* 1995; **127**: 626–631.
79. Siegel M, Kranz B, Lebenthal E. Effect of fat and carbohydrate composition on the gastric emptying of isocaloric feedings in premature infants. *Gastroenterology* 1985; **89**: 785–790.
80. Salle BL, Senterre J, Putet G. Calcium, phosphorus, magnesium and vitamin D requirements in premature infants. In Salle BL, Swyer PR, eds. *Nutrition of the Low Birthweight Infant*. Nestlé Nutrition Workshop Series, vol. 32, Nestec Ltd., New York: Vevey/Raven Press, 1993: 125–134.

81. Salle B, Senterre J, Glorieux FH et al. Vitamin D metabolism in preterm infants. *Biol Neonate* 1987; **52**: 119–130.
82. Rigo J, De Curtis M, Salle BL et al. Bone mineral metabolism in the micropremie. *Clin Perinatol* 2000; **27**: 147–170.
83. Rigo J, Picaud JC, Lapillonne A et al. Metabolic balance and plasma AA concentrations in VLBW infants fed a new acidic whey hydrolysate preterm formula. *J Pediatr Gastroenterol Nutr* 1997; **24**: 491A.
84. Carnielli VP, Luijendijk IH, Goudoever JB et al. Feeding premature newborn infants palmitic acid in amounts and stereoisomeric position similar to that of human milk: effects on fat and mineral balance. *Am J Clin Nutr* 1995; **61**: 1037–1042.
85. Cooke R, Hollis B, Conner C et al. Vitamin D and mineral metabolism in the very low birth weight infant receiving 400 IU of vitamin D. *J Pediatr* 1990; **116**: 423–428.
86. Oski FA. Iron requirements of the premature infant. In Tsang RC, ed. *Vitamin and Mineral Requirements in Preterm Infants*. New York: Marcel Dekker, 1985; 9–21.
87. Rao R, Georgieff M. Microminerals. In Tsang RC, Uauy R, Koletzko et al. eds. *Nutritional Needs of the Preterm Infant*. Cincinnati, OH: Digital Educational Publishing, 2004: 43–76 (in press).
88. American Academy of Pediatrics, Work Group on Breastfeeding. Breastfeeding and the use of human milk. *Pediatrics* 1997; **100**: 1035–1039.
89. Schanler RJ, Shulman RJ, Lau C. Feeding strategies for premature infants: beneficial outcomes of feeding fortified human milk vs preterm formula. *Pediatrics* 1998; **103**: 1150–1157.
90. McGuire W, Antont MY. Donor human milk versus formula for preventing necrotising enterocolitis in preterm infants: systematic review. *Arch Dis Child Fetal Neonatal Ed* 2003; **88**: F11–F14.
91. Schanler RJ, Hurst NM, Lau C. The use of human milk and breastfeeding in premature infants. *Clin Perinatol* 1999; **26**: 379–398.
92. Lucas A, Morley R, Cole J et al. A randomized multicentre study of human milk versus formula and later development in preterm infants. *Arch Dis Child* 1994; **70**: F141–F146.
93. Carlson SE, Werkman SH, Rhodes PG et al. Visual-acuity development in healthy preterm infants: effect of marine-oil supplementation. *Am J Clin Nutr* 1993; **58**: 35–42.
94. Atkinson SA, Bryan MH. The effect of gestational stage at delivery on human milk components. In Jensen RG, ed. *Handbook of Milk Composition*. San Diego: Academic Press, 1995: 222–237.
95. Atkinson SA. Human milk feeding of the micropremie. *Clin Perinatol* 2000; **27**: 235–247.
96. Linzell JL, Peaker M. Changes in colostrums composition and in permeability of mammary epithelium at about the time of parturition in the goat. *J Physiol* 1974; **243**: 129–151.
97. Anderson GH. The effect of prematurity on milk composition and its physiological basis. *Fed Proc* 1984; **43**: 2438–2442.
98. Senterre J, Voyer M, Putet G et al. Nitrogen, fat and mineral balance studies in preterm infants fed bank human milk, a human milk formula, or a low-birth-weight infant formula. In Baum JD, ed. *Human Milk Processing, Fractionation, and the Nutrition of the Low Birth-Weight Baby*. Nestlé Nutrition Workshop series, New York: Raven Press, 1983; **3**: 102–111.
99. De Curtis M, Candusso M, Pieltain C et al. Effect of fortification on the osmolality of human milk. *Arch Dis Child Fetal Neonatal Ed* 1999; **81**: F141–F143.
100. Hallstrom M, Koivisto AM, Janas M et al. Frequency of and risk factors for necrotizing enterocolitis in infants born before 33 weeks of gestation. *Acta Paediatr* 2003; **92**: 111–113.
101. Porcelli P, Schanler R, Greer F et al. Growth in human milk-fed very low birth weight infants receiving a new human milk fortifier. *Ann Nutr Metab* 2000; **44**: 2–10.
102. Pieltain C, De Curtis M, Gerard P et al. Weight gain composition in preterm infants fed fortified human milk or preterm formula. *Pediatr Res* 2001; **49**: 120–124.
103. Putet G, Rigo J, Salle B et al. Supplementation of pooled human milk with casein hydrolysate: energy and nitrogen balance and weight gain composition in very-low-birth-weight-infants. *Pediatr Res* 1987; **21**: 458–461.
104. Picaud JC, Putet G, Rigo J et al. Metabolic and energy balance in small-and-appropriate for gestational age in very low-birth-weight infants, *Acta Paediatr Suppl* 1994; **405**: 54–59.
105. Rigo J, Senterre J, Putet G et al. Various human milk fortifiers in low birth weight infants fed pooled human milk: plasma and urinary amino acid concentrations. In Koletzko B, Okken A, Rey J, Salle B, Van Biervliet JP, eds. *Recent Advances in Infant Feeding*. New York: Georg Thiem Verlag, 1992: 164–170.
106. Boehm G, Muller DM, Senger H et al. Nitrogen and fat balances in very low birth weight infants fed formula fortifier with human milk or bovine milk protein. *Eur J Pediatr* 1993; **152**: 236–239.
107. Schanler RJ, Abrams SA. Postnatal attainment of intrauterine macromineral accretion rate birth weight infants fed fortified human milk. *J Pediatr* 1995; **126**: 441–447.
108. Moody GJ, Schanler RJ, Lau C et al. Feeding tolerance in premature infants fed fortified human milk. *J Pediatr Gastroenterol Nutr* 2000; **30**: 408–412.
109. Kuschel CA, Harding JE. Multicomponent fortified human milk for promoting growth in preterm infants. *Cochrane Review* 2001; **3**: http://www.cochranelibrary.com/enter
110. Jocson MAL, Mason EO, Schanler RJ. The effects of nutrient fortification and varying storage conditions on host defense properties of human milk. *Pediatrics* 1997; **100**: 240–243.
111. Mihatsch WA, Hogel J, Pohlandt F. Hydrolysed protein accelerates the gastrointestinal transport of formula in preterm infants. *Acta Paediatr* 2001; **90**: 1–3.
112. Bar-Oz B, Preminger A, Peleg O et al. *Enterobacter sakazakii* infection in the newborn. *Acta Paediatr* 2001; **90**: 356–358.
113. Lucas A, Bishop NJ, King FJ et al. Randomised trial of nutrition for preterm infants after discharge. *Arch Dis Child* 1992; **67**: 324–327.
114. Rigo J, Boboli H, Franckart G et al. Surveillance de l'ancien prematuré: croissance et nutrition. *Arch Pédiatr* 1998; **5**: 449–453.
115. Brunton JA, Saigal S, Atkinson SA. Growth and body composition in infants with bronchopulmonary dysplasia up to 3 months corrected age: a randomized trial of a high-energy nutrient-enriched formula fed after hospital discharge. *J Pediatr* 1998; **133**: 340–345.
116. Cooke RJ, McCormick K, Griffin IJ et al. Feeding preterm infants after hospital discharge: effect of dietary manipulation on nutrient intake and growth. *Pediatr Res* 1998; **43**: 355–360.
117. De Curtis M, Pieltain C, Rigo J. Body composition in preterm infants fed standard or enriched formula after hospital discharge. *Eur J Nutr* 2002; **41**: 177–182.
118. Rolland-Cachera MF. Early adiposity rebound is not associated with energy or fat intake in infancy. *Pediatrics* 2001; **108**: 218–219.
119. De Curtis M, Pieltain C, Rigo J. Nutrition of preterm infants on discharge from hospital. In Raiha NCR, Rubaltelli FF, eds. *Infant Formula: Closer to the Reference*. Nestlè Nutrition Workshop Series, Nestec Ltd. Vevey/Lippincott Williams & Wilkins Philadelphia, 2002; **47** (Suppl): 149–163.

37 Parenteral nutrition in premature infants

Jacques Rigo and Mario De Curtis

Introduction

Over the past decades there has been a dramatic increase in the survival of preterm infants, especially very-low-birth-weight (VLBW) infants. Prenatal steroids to enhance pulmonary maturation, the use of exogenous surfactant for the treatment of the respiratory distress syndrome, and better prenatal obstetric and postnatal neonatal intensive care have all played a major role in improving survival rate in these infants.[1–3]

With the major advances in life-support measures, nutrition has become one the most debated issues in the care of low-birth-weight infants; in this regard, several reports have shown the important effect of nutrition during the first period of life on early and late outcome.[4]

Although the general objective of a nutritional regimen for preterm infants is to support life and achieve a growth rate sufficient to fulfill the individual's genetic potential, there are many controversies on how to attain this goal. In this chapter we discuss the most important features regarding the nutrition of preterm, and particularly VLBW infants, outlining the main aspects of parenteral nutrition.

Nutritional requirements

While the nutritional reference standard for full-term newborns is an exclusively breast-fed infant, no similar standard is available for preterm infants. In the neonatal period, preterm infants and especially VLBW infants have greater nutritional needs in order to achieve optimal growth than at any other time in their life. Preterm birth is associated with decreased nutrient storage, and the clinical conditions after birth may increase nutrient needs.

The recommended nutrient intakes of preterm infants are still a matter of debate, arising from the lack of consensus on the short- and long-term objectives for early nutrition. Current nutritional recommendations from various international committees (American Academy of Pediatrics, European Society for Pediatric Gastroenterology, Hepatology and Nutrition, Canadian Academy of Pediatrics) are based on healthy preterm infants and designed to provide postnatal nutrient retention during the 'stable-growing' period equivalent to the intrauterine gain of a normal fetus. They do not take into consideration the relatively long transitional period that induces the cumulative nutritional deficit and the need to obtain an early catch-up growth.[5–7]

The postnatal use of the gastrointestinal tract, instead of placental transfer, and the metabolic changes that occur immediately after birth, do not allow provision of the quantitative or qualitative supply of all the nutrients needed to approximate fetal growth of the comparable corrected age. Additional nutritional deprivations can also arise from neonatal illnesses such as metabolic stress, infectious diseases, necrotizing enterocolitis or bronchopulmonary dysplasia, which often further decrease nutrient supply.

In practice, the shorter the gestation of a neonate the more challenging are the influences of immaturity and the accompanying morbidity on nutritional supply during the early weeks of life. As a result of this cumulative nutritional deficit during early life, most growth parameters remain subnormal by the time the preterm infant reaches a corrected age of 40 weeks (Figure 37.1); this phenomenon worsens in the case of VLBW and

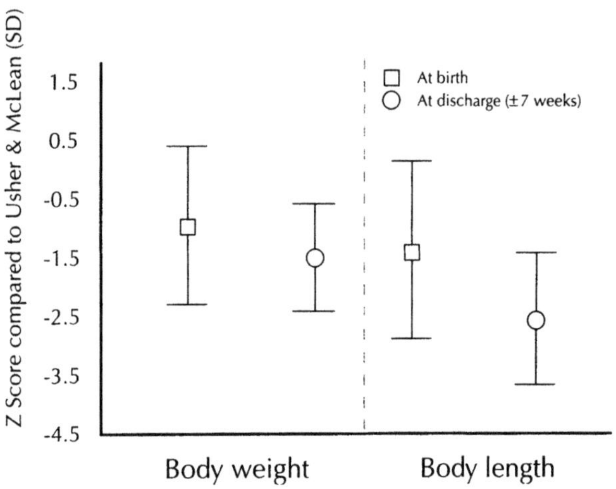

Figure 37.1 Z score of body weight, body length determined in healthy very-low-birth-weight infants (birth weight <1500g; $n = 96$) at the time of discharge. Anthropometric parameters compared to intrauterine reference values.[9]

extremely-low-birth-weight (ELBW) infants suggesting that the current nutritional recommendations need to be re-evaluated taking into account this early nutritional gap and the need for an early catch-up growth.[8–10]

Taking into consideration that in VLBW infants, severe postnatal growth restriction has potentially long-term deleterious effects on growth, neurodevelopmental outcome and adult health, several recent papers have focused on the early nutritional gap and the need for a catch-up growth during the first weeks of life with the aim of reducing growth restriction at the time of discharge.[8–10]

Nutritional program in VLBW infants at birth

Nutrition of preterm infants may be divided into two subsequent periods: the early adaptive or 'transition' period from birth to the 2nd week of life, followed by the 'stable-growing' period, up to discharge from the neonatal unit. Depending on birth weight and gestational age the transition period may be prolonged, particularly in ELBW infants with major clinical disorders.

Immediately after birth, due to multiple medical problems, most VLBW infants are unable to start enteral feeding and thus require parenteral supplies for immaturity, severe illness, limited body stores or increased energy expenditure. Parenteral nutrition (PN), consisting of intravenous glucose, amino acids, lipids, electrolytes, minerals, trace elements and vitamins, is presently proposed from the first days of life and, if appropriately designed, this can promote early positive nitrogen retention and growth. Minimal enteral nutrition will be added as early as possible to provide a small quantity of milk to stimulate the enterocytes. As the infant matures and the medical conditions stabilize, PN can be slowly replaced by enteral nutrition.

Nutrition of VLBW infants during the transition period should cover as much as possible the nutritional needs, to limit the inevitable cumulative nutritional deficit, induce a positive nitrogen balance and reinitiate weight gain and longitudinal growth. To date, early nutritional strategies vary dramatically among centers and there are no definitive and well-accepted regimens demonstrating long-term benefits in ELBW and VLBW infants. To reduce the temporary interruption of the transfer of nutrients, a so-called 'aggressive' nutrition has recently been proposed by several nutritionists, consisting of a high-protein supply (>2g amino acids/kg per day) and the use of intravenous lipids (0.5–1.0g lipid/kg per day), from the first day of life, associated when necessary, with the use of insulin to improve carbohydrate tolerance during the early adaptive period.[10,11]

Nutrition during the 'stable-growth' period on PN, is given exceptionally, when preterm infants are recovering from severe gastrointestinal problems, to prevent or limit the use of the gastrointestinal tract. In most preterm infants, nutritional supplies are provided using the mother's milk supplemented with human milk fortifiers or preterm formulas specially designed for VLBW infants. The objective of nutrition in this period is to minimize postnatal growth deficit, maximize longitudinal growth and induce catch-up growth. Although the optimal nutritional supply is still controversial, more recent studies suggest that, in order specifically to enhance lean mass growth and improve the early catch-up growth in preterm infants, the use of a high-protein regimen combined with a high protein-energy density regimen (4.0–4.4g of protein/kg per day with a protein/energy ratio up to 3.3g/100kcal) promotes growth without metabolic stress in VLBW infants.[12,13]

Parenteral nutrition

PN provides the infant's requirements for growth and development when the infant's size or clinical conditions preclude enteral feeding. PN in preterm infants is prescribed especially for those with respiratory distress, before starting enteral feeding, and can be increased slowly to avoid overloading the immature gastrointestinal tract while continuing to satisfy nutritional requirements.

A recent report indicates that in the USA, even though over the last 15 years, there has been a decrease in the length of days of PN in VLBW infants, most of these VLBW infants receive parenterally delivered nutrients as their major source of nutrition for the first few days to weeks of life.[14]

Today PN is seen by many neonatologists as a means of achieving rapid nutrition and administering nutrients that could be delayed and/or insufficiently absorbed via the enteral route, especially in the presence of conditions considered to be hazardous to the intestine and thus increasing the risk for necrotizing enterocolitis. PN allows infusion of concentrated hypertonic nutrient solutions without excessive fluid intake (which is not well tolerated by most VLBW infants), through an indwelling catheter, the tip of which is in the superior vena cava just above the right atrium. This technique was first described by Wilmore and Dudrick in 1968.[15]

Nowadays, in ELBW infants, PN is usually administered through the umbilical vessels for a limited number of days, followed by the use of a silastic catheter introduced percutaneously from a peripheral vein. Less frequently, in bigger preterm infants, a catheter is inserted surgically into either the internal or external jugular vein and tunneled subcutaneously. Currently, the use of direct infusion via peripheral veins has become less common because of the relatively high osmolarity of the solution that can lead to endothelial damage, frequent interruption of continuous feeding and relative reduction of the nutritional supplies.

Fluids

A number of physiological changes and adaptive processes that occur at birth, immediately or subsequently affect water and electrolyte metabolism. In particular, placental clearance and placental supply of fluids, electrolytes and nutrients are discontinued, and a considerable insensible water loss and infant thermoregulation begin to occur. Compensatory regulative processes (such as renal adaptation, start of oral intake) need time to counteract these effects on body water pools.

Just after the birth, there is a fall in urinary output due to a decreased glomerular filtration rate. This relative oliguria, which may last for a variable period (hours or days), is mainly determined by the presence of conditions and diseases, such as respiratory distress syndrome. Oliguria is then followed by a diuretic phase, during which a contraction of extracellular fluid volume occurs. The end of this transitional period is usually characterized by a urine volume < 2.0 ml/kg per h, urine osmolarity greater than serum osmolarity, fractional sodium excretion diminishing from $> 3\%$ to $< 1\%$ and specific gravity above 1012. In preterm infants, these changes are completed after 3–5 days.

Fluid and electrolyte administration during this period allows contraction of the extracellular fluid space without compromising intravascular fluid volume and cardiovascular function, maintains normal serum electrolyte concentrations, allows sufficient urinary output to excrete waste products and prevents oliguria (< 0.5–1.0 ml/kg per h) for more than 12 h. It also important to ensure regulation of body temperature by providing enough fluid for transepidermal evaporation, and to give enough caloric supply to meet energy maintenance needs during this period.

If extremely preterm infants are nursed in maximally humidified incubators their fluid requirements are similar to those of more mature infants. The infant's weight must be monitored, at the same time of day, at least once daily, and in infants < 1000 g even twice a day in the first 2 weeks of life.

The practical determinants of fluid requirements are weight, urine volume and osmolarity. Insensible fluid losses in VLBW infants can be enormous, especially when the baby is under a radiant warmer and is undergoing phototherapy. A reduction of insensible water loss can be obtained by increasing the humidity of incubators. Increased fluid loss occurs when the infant is placed under radiant warmers or undergoes phototherapy.[16] Fluid requirements are decreased with the use of double-walled incubators, heat shields or plastic blankets and high-ambient humidity.[17,18]

The following intermediate phase is characterized by a decrease in insensible water loss from the skin, the increasing maturation of the epidermis, and improved renal function. In this period fluid and electrolytes have to be increased in order to cover the requirements (120–150 ml/kg per day) and to allow adequate growth. During this period the amount of parenteral fluid can be reduced and enteral feeding can be augmented. Infants with bronchopulmonary dysplasia, patent ductus arteriosus, renal failure and respiratory distress syndrome, are very vulnerable to fluid overload.

Energy

Energy must be supplied by nutrient intake to cover two major components, energy expenditure and growth. A caloric intake of 40–60 kcal/kg per day approximates energy expenditure and is a reasonable goal for the maintenance requirements of premature infants for the first days after birth. The energy cost of gaining 1 g of new tissue is about 5 kcal. This value is influenced largely by quantity of fat deposition ranging between 20 and 40% of postnatal weight gain in premature infants, according to the feeding regimen.[19] The lower the fat deposition, the lower is the cost of growth; thus, energy cost of weight gain during the third trimester of intrauterine life, 16–20 g/kg per day, with 15% fat, is lower than that for postnatal weight gain accounting for a higher fat deposition, up to 40%.

In contrast to what is generally proposed, the energy requirement in PN approximates to that of enteral nutrition. In fact, the energy content of amino acid solutions in PN is lower than that provided by the protein in enteral nutrition (human milk or formulas). The gross energy, measured by calorimetric bomb, provided by glucose used in PN is less than that provided by the carbohydrate content of formulas. In contrast, while the metabolizable energy of amino acid solutions and glucose, given by the parenteral route, is identical to total intake, the metabolizable energy of dietary protein and carbohydrates represents about 90% of the intake.[20,21] Consequently, the recommendation for energy intake during the stable-growing period in VLBW infants on PN corresponds to 110–135 kcal/kg per day.

Carbohydrates

Glucose is the most widely used intravenous carbohydrate for neonates, because it is readily available to the brain. The monohydrate form of dextrose is used for intravenous solutions; each gram provides 3.7 kcal upon complete oxidation.[20] As the solution concentration increases, so does osmolarity, ranging from approximately 255 mOsm/l for a 5% solution to 1020 mOsm/l for a 20% solution. Many other non-glucose carbohydrates have been tried, but with limited success.

The newborn infant is often in a transitional stage of glucose homeostasis and is, therefore, subject to hyper- or hypoglycemia. Although the definition and the long-term consequences of neonatal hypoglycemia remain controversial, plasma glucose concentration should be monitored and corrected if it falls below 35 mg/dl (1.9 mmol/l) during the first days of life.[22] In the first few days of life, VLBW infants are more susceptible to hyperglycemia often associated with glucosuria, which seems to be caused by a persistent endogenous hepatic glucose production secondary to an insensitivity of hepatocytes to insulin.[23–25] The definition of hyperglycemia varies but is generally set at a plasma level above 150 mg/dl (8.3 mmol/l). However the upper 'safe' limit of blood glucose concentration in the neonate is not well defined and, as for hypoglycemia, there is a great variation in terms of the diagnosis and management of hyperglycemia. The increase in serum osmolarity induced by the increase in blood glucose has been associated with higher mortality and a higher rate of intracranial hemorrhage. Glycosuria associated with hyperglycemia results from the relatively low renal threshold for glucose excretion in the preterm infant compared with the adult and may increase the risk of dehydration. Risks for hyperglycemia and glycosuria increase with decreasing gestation and birth weight, and is estimated to be between 20% and 86% during the first few days of life in preterm infants who survive their first week.[26,27]

If hyperglycemia is detected early through frequent glucose monitoring, plasma glucose levels can be decreased by reducing insensible water loss, glucose infusion rate and by providing exogenous insulin supply. Decreasing volume intake and glucose concentration reduces energy supply and consequently growth and nitrogen retention. Insulin administration helps control plasma glucose concentration, achieve increased energy intake and promote nitrogen retention and growth, although there is need for more data on its safety and long-term consequences as a growth-promoting agent. More recently, it has been proposed that high amino acid intake, 2–3 g/kg per day from the first day, in addition to preventing catabolism and promoting anabolism, may have several other beneficial effects including decreasing the frequency and severity of neonatal hyperglycemia by stimulating endogenous insulin secretion and stimulating growth by enhancing the secretion of insulin and insulin-like growth factors.[28]

In practice, 6 g/kg per day of intravenous glucose are generally well tolerated (4–5 mg/kg per min) even on the first day of life in VLBW infants. If this intake is tolerated, it may be increased to 8, 10 and up to 12–18 g/kg per day. If it is not tolerated, progression of glucose intake will be stopped and insulin perfusion will be considered according to clinical and nutritional status with an initial dose of 0.05 IU/kg per h.[29]

Protein

In order to define the protein requirements for preterm infants more precisely, it has been suggested that lean body mass be taken into account instead of weight gain, also considering that preterm infants present a high fat deposition in the postnatal period. Table 37.1 shows the revised recommended protein intake and protein/energy ratio for preterm infants according to postconceptional age and the need for catch-up growth.[12] It should be stressed that these recommendations derive especially from studies on preterm infants greater than 1000 g rather than on ELBW infants (< 750 g). Estimates for these ELBW infants are extrapolated from data involving larger premature infants.

During the early transitional period, approximately 1.0–1.5 g/kg per day of protein prevent breakdown of endogenous tissue. Recently, several studies have underlined the importance of an early introduction of higher protein/amino acid supply (2.5–3 g/kg per day) in VLBW infants even on the first day of life.[30] No significant changes in blood pH, ammonia, urea and creatinine concentrations were observed with such a regimen.[30] Such high-protein supply could also be beneficial in preterm infants with increased protein breakdown, induced by prenatal maternal corticosteroid

Table 37.1 Revised recommended protein intake and protein/energy ratio for preterm infants according to postconceptional age (PCA) and the need for catch-up growth[12]

	Without need for catch-up growth	With need for catch-up growth
26–30 weeks PCA: 16–18 g/kg per day LBM 14% protein retention	3.8–4.2 g/kg per day PER: ±3.0	4.4 g/kg per day PER: ±3.3
30–36 weeks PCA: 14–15 g/kg per day LBM 15% protein retention	3.4–3.6 g/kg per day PER: ±2.8	3.6-4.0 g/kg per day PER: ± 3.0
36–40 weeks PCA: 13 g/kg per day LBM 17% protein retention	2.8–3.2 g/kg per day PER: 2.4–2.6	3.0-3.4 g/kg per day PER: 2.6–2.8

LBM, lean body mass; PER, protein/energy ratio

therapy and by catabolic stress due to diseases or early neonatal surgery.

Amino acid composition of solutions for parenteral nutrition

Considerable improvements in parenteral amino acid solutions have been made since the 1960s when the source of intravenous protein was casein hydrolysate. The use of a crystalline amino acid mixture in the early 1980s helped to improve the nitrogen utilization whereas, more specific pediatric amino acid solutions were designed in the early 1990s with a high essential/non-essential amino acid ratio and conditionally essential amino acid content for use in preterm infants. Despite the new evidence, the reference optimal solution for PN has not yet been well defined because the optimal value for plasma amino acid concentrations in preterm infants is still a matter of debate.

At least three different 'gold standards' have been proposed for premature infants: first, the amino acid concentrations from the umbilical cord obtained following fetal cord puncture or after birth; second, the amino acid concentrations of rapidly growing preterm infants receiving their mother's milk or human milk supplemented with human milk proteins; and third, the amino acid concentrations of healthy breast-fed term infants.

The amino acid concentrations observed in VLBW infants during the last trimester of gestation or in well-growing preterm infants fed an optimal intake of human milk protein appear to be safe. However, considering the large differences observed between fetal and postnatal values of some amino acids (THR, VAL, TYR, PHE, LYS and HIS), a combined reference has been proposed taking into account the mean ± 1 SD of the values obtained in cord blood and in the postprandial serum of preterm infants fed human milk supplemented with human milk proteins (Figure 37.2).[31]

Nevertheless, despite the diverse composition of parenteral amino acid solutions used in pediatric care, nitrogen utilization does not change signifi-

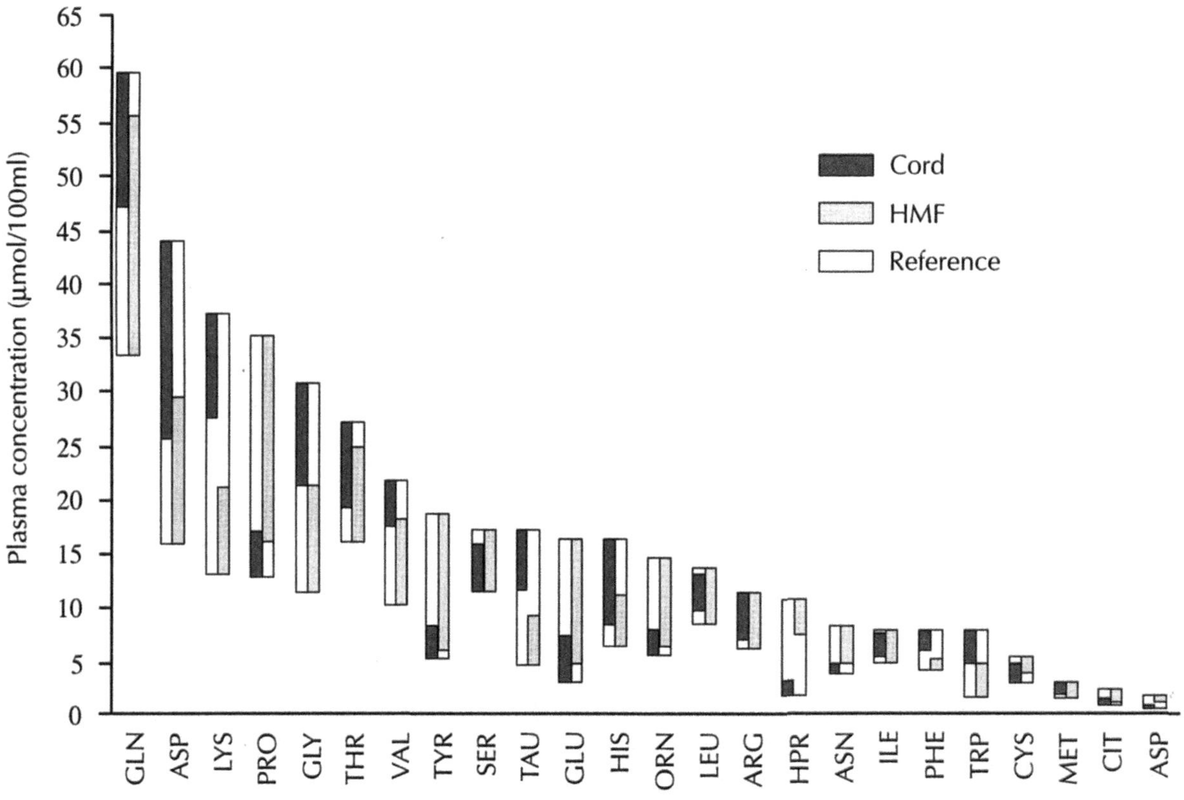

Figure 37.2 Plasma amino acid reference (adapted from reference 31). HMF, human milk fortified with human milk protein; Cord, cord blood concentrations.

cantly.[32,33] Nitrogen amino acid content is related to the amino acid composition and varies according to the solution, and is frequently lower than in enteral nutrition (160 mg/g of protein). Therefore, it is probably preferable to consider nitrogen rather than amino acid intake in total PN.

Analysis of a large number of nitrogen balances in preterm infants shows that a nitrogen retention of 380 mg/kg per day can be obtained with a nitrogen intake of 530 mg/kg per day (Figure 37.3),[33–43] which corresponds to a net protein utilization (nitrogen retention/nitrogen intake) of 70%, a value quite similar to that recorded in oral nutrition (60–72%).[44] These data indicate that the nitrogen requirement in PN is close to 95% of the enteral requirement, but corresponds to a similar amino acid versus protein requirement in parenteral and enteral nutrition.

Parenterally fed preterm infants are at risk of toxicity from excessive amino acid intake, immature metabolic pathways, absence of first hepatic crossing and lack of small-intestinal metabolism. Therefore, optimal amino acid pattern for parenteral amino acid solutions in preterm infants still needs to be determined, and new solutions should be developed keeping in mind the following principles:

(1) The requirement of essential amino acids in VLBW infants is greater than in term neonates or older infants;[45]

(2) The activity of phenylalanine hydroxylase as well as tyrosine aminotransferase and 4-dioxyphenylpyruvate dioxygenase is considered to be immature during the neonatal period;[46]

(3) The activity of cystathionase in neonates is low and cysteine synthesis from methionine is reduced;[47]

(4) Nutritional supply of taurine is probably necessary during the neonatal period. Although cysteine sulphinic activity has been demonstrated in preterm infants, taurine is probably considered as a conditionally essential amino acid in neonates;[48]

(5) In addition to cysteine and tyrosine, histidine and arginine are categorized as semi-essential amino acids in neonates;[49]

(6) Organ dysfunction tends to occur when some amino acids are administered in high (methionine) or low (arginine, glutamine) amounts.[50,51]

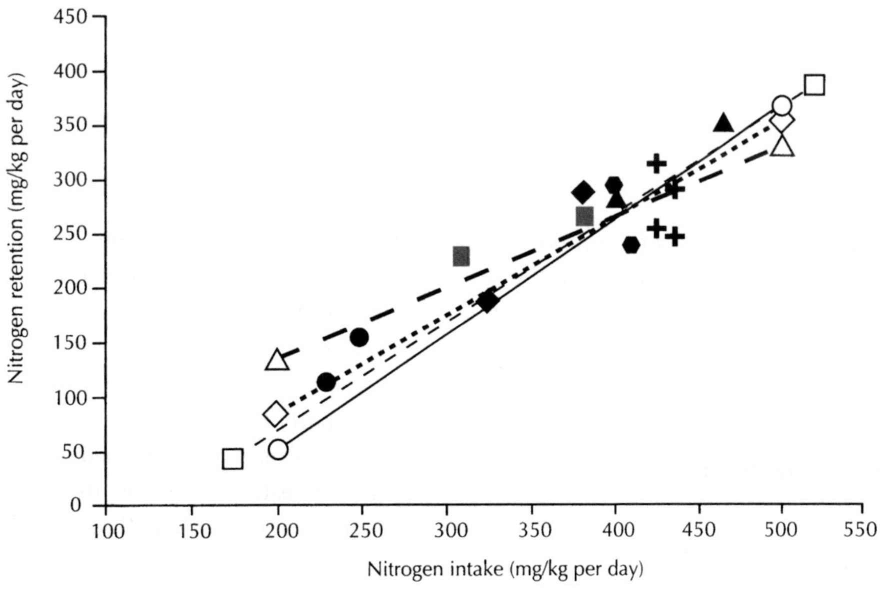

Figure 37.3 Relationship between nitrogen retention and nitrogen intake in parenterally fed preterm infants.[12,33–43]

Table 37.2 Composition of commercially available parenteral amino acid solutions[12]

	Aminoplasmal-Aminoped (Pfrimmer-kabi)	Aminosyn (Abbott)	Aminosyn-PF (Abbott)	Aminovemos N-Pad (Fresenios)	FreAmine III (McGaw)	Neophan (Cutter)	MPF (FAO/WHO) General use
Trp	4	1.6	1.8	1.8	1.5	2.1	1.3
Ile	5.1	7.2	7.6	6.4	6.9	4.7	5.6
Leu	7.6	9.4	11.9	10.7	9.1	10.7	12.5
Val	6.1	8	6.5	7.1	6.6	5.5	4.5
Lys	8.8	7.2	6.8	7.1	7.3	8.6	8.8
Met	2	4	1.8	4.3	5.3	2	3.5
Phe	3.1	4.4	4.3	4.6	5.6	4.1	9.4
Thr	5.1	5.2	5.1	5.1	4	5.5	6.5
His	4.6	3	3.1	4.1	2.8	3.2	6
Arg	9.1	9.8	12.3	6.4	9.5	6.3	7.9
Orn	0	0	0	0	0	0	0
Gly	2	12.8	3.9	4.1	14	3.2	10.7
Ala	15.9	12.8	7	7.1	7.1	9.7	6.2
Glu	9.3	0	8.2	0	0	10.9	6.5
Asp	6.6	0	5.3	0	0	6.3	3.8
Pro	6.1	8.6	8.1	16.1	11.2	8.6	3.3
Ser	2	4.2	5	9	5.9	5.8	2.2
Tyr	1.1*	0.4	0.6	1.6*		0.7	0.3
Cys	1	0		0.6	0.2	1.5	1
Tau	0.3	0	0.7	0	0		0
AAA	46%	50%	49%	51%	49%	46%	58%
BCAA	19%	25%	26%	24%	23%	21%	23%
Nitrogen	160	167	165	152	162	153	165

Continued

To date, the normalization of plasma amnio acid concentrations in PN has never been achieved due to the poor solubility of free tyrosine and cystine and the absence of an adequate and safe metabolic substitute.[52]

Table 37.2 shows some commercially available parenteral amino acid solutions.

Amino acids for special purposes

Arginine

Arginine is a precursor of nitric oxide; inadequate availability has been implicated in various neonatal diseases, such as persistent pulmonary hypertension and necrotizing enterocolitis. Recent evidence suggests that the *de novo* arginine synthesis in the neonate relies on small-intestinal metabolism, and that dietary arginine requirements could be higher in the parentally fed infants.[53] Currently, arginine content varies widely in pediatric parenteral solutions suggesting that the dietary requirement in parenteral and oral nutrition must be elucidated.

Glutamine

Glutamine is the most abundant amino acid in the human body and the main one supplied to the fetus

Table 37.2 Continued

	PED (B. Braun)	Pleamine-P (Fuso, Japan)	Primene (Baxter)	Travasol (Clintec)	Trophamine (Kendall–McGaw)	VAMIN Infant (Kabivitrun)
Trp	1	1.6	2	1.8	2	2.2
Ile	2.8	10.5	6.7	6	8.2	4.8
Leu	5	21	10	7.3	14	10.8
Val	3.2	7.9	7.6	5.8	7.8	5.5
Lys	9	6.3	11	5.8	8.2	8.6
Met	1.6	2	2.4	4	3.3	2
Phe	3.8	3.3	4.2	5.6	4.8	4.2
Thr	6	3.2	3.7	4.2	4.2	5.5
His	6	3.3	3.8	4.8	4.8	3.2
Arg	4.4	13.2	8.4	11.5	12.1	6.3
Orn	0	0	2.2	0	0	0
Gly	9.8	2.6	4	10.3	3.7	3.2
Ala	11.6	6.8	8	20.7	5.3	9.7
Glu	19.6	1.1	10	0	5	10.9
Asp	3.8	1.1	6	0	3.2	6.3
Pro	5.4	7.9	3	6.8	6.8	8.6
Ser	2	5.3	4	5	3.8	5.9
Tyr	0.6	0.8	0.5	0.4	0.7*	0.8
Cys	1.7	2	1.7	0	0.2	1.5
Tau	0	0.2	0.6	0	0.3	0
AAA	38%	59%	51%	45%	57%	47%
BCAA	11%	39%	24%	19%	30%	21%
Nitrogen	149	177	161	173	168	154

All amino acid mixtures are in % amino acid content. Nitrogen expressed as mg/100 ml
AAA, aromatic amino acid; BCAA, branched chain amino acid
* Mixture of L-tyrosine and *N*-acetyl-L-tyrosine

through the placenta. Glutamine is thought to be an important fuel for rapidly dividing cells such as enterocytes and lymphocytes. It is a regulator of acid–base balance via ammonium, as well as an important precursor of nucleic acids, nucleotides amino sugars and protein. There is, however, little information on the role of glutamine in children and infants or as to whether glutamine supplementation is beneficial in preterm babies. In ELBW infants and during critical illnesses glutamine could be a conditionally essential amino acid.[54]

Reviewing the available studies in preterm infants for the Cochrane database, Tubman and Thompson[55] did not find evidence to support the routine use of parenteral or enteral glutamine supplementation in preterm infants. A more recent, multicentric study on ELBW infants showed that parenteral glutamine supplementation can increase plasma glutamine concentrations, but the potential clinical effects of such glutamine supplementation remain to be elucidated.[56]

Intravenous lipids

Intravenous lipid emulsions are important constituents of total PN as they provide energy and essential fatty acids to VLBW infants. Lipid emulsions consist of different oils, egg yolk phospholipids and glycerol. The fat particles in the emulsions resemble endogenously produced chylomicrons in terms of size, physicochemical properties and metabolism, and are hydrolyzed by lipoprotein lipase. The rate of infused triglyceride clearance is determined by the available lipase activity and by the uptake of unesterified fatty acid products related to the adipose tissue mass and/or fatty acid oxidation in muscles. Intravenous lipid emulsions provide high caloric, isotonic solutions of linoleic acid (18:2n-6) and linolenic acid (18:3n-3), as well as other fatty acids, and can also be given through peripheral lines. Traditionally, lipid infusions are prepared from soybean oil triglycerides emulsified with egg yolk phospholipids. Typical soybean oil contains about 45–55% linoleic acid (18:2n-6) and 6–9% linolenic acid (18:3n-3), but very little saturated or monounsaturated fat (Table 37.3).[57] There are considerable concerns over the effect of these emulsions on the composition of the fatty acids deposited in the developing tissues of preterm infants.

Intravenous lipids play two separate roles in the PN of VLBW infants. One is the role of intravenous lipids as an energy substrate to be readily utilized by VLBW infants. There is some evidence that the supply of some of the energy as lipids is preferable over carbohydrate as the sole energy substrate.[58] Amino acid oxidation and protein breakdown were significantly lower when lipids provided 50% of the non-protein calories than when glucose alone served as the energy substrate. Advantages of lipids emulsions over concentrated glucose solutions also include their isotonicity and greater energy density, the latter meaning that less volume is required per calorie. This is particularly true for 20% lipid emulsion, which is preferred over the 10% emulsion because it leads to a more normal pattern of plasma phospholipid and cholesterol than the 10% intralipid.[59] This beneficial effect of the 20% emulsion is attributed to the lower phospholipid content (per gram of triglyceride), although for the lower phospholipid content, the 20% emulsion delivers less long-chain polyunsat-

Table 37.3 Commercial intravenous lipid emulsions currently used in preterm infants[57]

	Soybean	Soybean/MCT	Olive/soybean	Soybean/fish
Product names	Intralipid (Pharmacia) Ivelip (Clintec) Lipofundin (Braun) Lipovenös (Fresenius) Liposyn III (Abbott)	Lipofundin MCT(Braun)	ClinOleic (Clintec)	Lipovenous + Omegavenös, 9+1 parts mix (Fresenius)
Triglycerides (%)	10, 20 & 30	20	20	10
Ratio of phospholipids/ triglycerides (mg/g)	120, 60 & 40	60	60	66
Glycerol (%)	2.5	2.5	2.25	2.5
kcal/ml	1.1–2.0	1.9	2.0	—
Fatty acid composition (% wt/wt)				
Medium chain (8:0+10:0)	n.d.	50	n.d.	n.d.
Palmitic (16:0)	9–11.2	5	13.5	10.8
Stearic (18:0)	4–4.2	2	2.9	3.7
Oleic (18:1n9)	20.4–26	12	59.5	19.9
Linoleic (18:2n6)	52.4–54.5	27	18.5	49.7
linolenic (18:3n3)	8–8.5	4	2	6.5
linolenic (18:3n6)				
Arachidonic (20:4n6)	n.d.–0.2	n.d.	0.2	0.2
Eicosapentaenoic (20:5n3)	n.d.	n.d.	n.d.	2.4
Docosahexaenoic (22:6n3)	n.d.–0.1	n.d.	0.1	2.3

MCT, medium-chain triglyceride, n.d. not determined

urated fatty acids (PUFAs) (contained in the phospholipid fraction) than the 10% emulsion. For this reason, it seems that, at least in the first days of life, until the lipid dose reaches 2.0 g/kg per day, the 10% emulsion could be preferable over the 20% emulsion.[10] The other role is as a source of essential fatty acids as well as long-chain PUFAs. It is well known that when preterm infants are maintained on lipid-free PN there is a rapid essential fatty acid deficiency. An essential fatty acid deficiency is known to interfere with normal lung surfactant synthesis, possibly further impairing pulmonary function in infants already at risk for respiratory problems.[60] Abnormalities in platelet function, which could have implications for clinical bleeding, have also been described.[61] Essential fatty acid deficiency is avoided by infusions of 0.5–1.0 g lipid per kg per day.[62] The importance of long-chain PUFAs for the development of the brain and the retina has also been recognized. Preterm infants are unable to form sufficient quantities of long-chain PUFAs from the respective precursor fatty acids (linoleic and α-linolenic acids) and thus depend on an exogenous source of long-chain PUFAs.[63,64] Intravenous lipid emulsions contain small amounts of these fatty acids as part of the egg phospholipid used as a stabilizer.

More recently, new lipids emulsions containing a mixture of medium-chain and long-chain triglycerides (MCTs and LCTs), a mixture of MCTs, LCTs and fish oil, or based on olive and soybean oil, are receiving increasing attention.[65–70] All these solutions are designed to reduce the high linoleic and α-linolenic acid supplies provided by the classic soybean oil, improve the fatty acid composition of plasma lipids, reduce the risk of peroxidation and provide additional long-chain PUFAs with the use of fish oil. Infused MCTs are rapidly cleared,[65] although studies of parenterally fed newborn infants have not confirmed a benefit of mixed MCT–long-chain fatty acid emulsions on protein accretion[66] and plasma fatty acid pattern.[67] The addition of fish oil to MCT and LCT solutions has not led to adverse effects, although a significant increase in plasma α-tocopherol and eicosapentaenoic acid in the high-density lipoprotein phospholipid[68] was seen. The most promising appears to be the lipid emulsion based on olive and soybean oil. In preterm infants, it produces more physiological levels of linoleic and oleic acid and a better antioxidant status than the conventional soybean oil emulsion.[69,70]

Concerns had been raised in some retrospective studies, about the potentially adverse effects of early lipid infusion in preterm infants on later outcomes, such as increased rates of chronic lung disease and mortality.[71,72] However, a meta-analysis of the five prospective controlled trials in low-birth-weight infants on this issue has shown that early lipid infusion within the first 5 days of life is not associated with an increased risk of adverse outcomes.[73] There is no credible evidence of potentially adverse effects of intravenous lipid emulsions when these are properly used. Proper use includes slow and continuous infusion rate (< 150 mg/kg per h), slow increase in dosage and avoidance of high dose (i.e. > 3 g/kg per day).[74] It has been suggested that triglyceride concentrations should be maintained at around 150–200 mg/dl as an upper limit in VLBW infants, especially in unstable clinical situations.

Considering that even a short delay in adding fat to the PN of preterm infants leads to biochemical essential fatty acid deficiency, infusion of lipids should commence within 24 h of birth for infants > 28 weeks' gestation and > 1000 g. The dose should be increased, as tolerated, at a rate of 0.5 g every 1–2 days to a maximum of 3 g/kg per day. In all cases, the triglyceride infusion dose should be adjusted to maintain a serum lipid level not exceeding 200 mg/dl. Infants < 28 weeks' gestation or < 1000 g may have low lipase activity or limited adipose mass for clearance of free fatty acids. A more cautious approach should be taken by assessing serum lipid clearance in these infants throughout the infusion period. Lipid clearance should also be monitored in all infants as the infusion approaches and exceeds 3 g/kg per day. In infants with sepsis, or in those with severely impaired oxygenation, the lipid infusion should be restricted to 0.5–1.0 g/kg per day, which is sufficient to prevent essential fatty acid deficiency.

Because carnitine synthesis and storage are not sufficiently developed at birth, particularly in preterm infants, and because no commercial intravenous solution contains carnitine, infants parenterally fed present low plasma and tissue carnitine levels that decline with postnatal age. Although more studies are needed to define the role of L-carnitine during the first days of life in VLBW infants, a carnitine supplementation of 15 μmol/100 kcal is advised for infants on total PN for more than 4 weeks.

Electrolytes, minerals and trace elements

Sodium

Sodium exists predominantly as an extracellular ion, and its requirements are unaltered by PN. The normal sodium requirement is assumed to be 3 mmol/kg per day. During the first week of life, infants of less than 28 weeks' gestation often receive additional sodium supply from sources other than the parenteral solution, i.e. blood transfusion, bicarbonate or drugs, and lose more water than sodium. Therefore, to prevent hyperosmolar hypernatremia, some authors suggest very close monitoring of sodium intake during the first week of life, while others recommend the complete exclusion of sodium during the first few days in ELBW infants. Frequent monitoring and customization of serum sodium and water/sodium is mandatory especially in infants with congestive heart failure, acute renal failure or chronic diuretic therapy.

Potassium

The normal requirement for potassium for growing preterm infants is assumed to be 1–2 mmol/kg per day. It should be withheld in the first 3 days after birth in those who are extremely preterm because of the risk of developing non-oliguric hyperkalemia from immature distal tubular function. An adjustment of potassium intake is required if the infant is on diuretics or has poor urine output.

Chloride

The recommended intake is 2–3 mmol/kg per day and the chloride maintenance intake must not be lower than 1 mmol/kg per day.

Calcium, phosphorus and magnesium

Inadequate calcium and phosphorus intake has been associated with diminished bone mineralization in parenterally fed premature infants. This occurs when protein and energy are adequate for growth, but calcium and phosphorus are insufficient to sustain appropriate skeletal mineralization.[75–78] Calcium and phosphorus cannot be provided through the same parenteral solution at concentrations needed to support *in utero* accretion, because of precipitation. The solubility of calcium and phosphorus in parenteral solutions depends on temperature, type and concentration of amino acid, dextrose concentration, pH of the calcium salt, the sequence of addition of calcium and phosphorus to the solution, calcium/phosphorus ratio and the presence of lipids.[79] More acidic pediatric amino acid solutions improve calcium and phosphorus solubility. With a range of fluid intake of 120–150 ml/kg per day, it is advisable to supply a calcium content of 50–60 mg/dl (1.25–1.5 mmol/l), a phosphorus content of 40–45 mg/dl (1.25–1.5 mmol/l) and a magnesium content of 5–7 mg/dl (2.1–2.9 mmol/l) corresponding to a calcium phosphorus ratio of 1.3:1 by weight and 1:1 by molar ratio in the total PN solution. It must be underlined that this quantity of calcium provided by the parenteral route is about 60–75% of that deposited by the fetus during the last trimester of gestation (100–120 mg/kg per day) but similar or higher than that obtained in enteral nutrition with the available preterm formulas. Administering sufficient amounts of calcium and phosphorus in PN solutions is no longer a problem in countries where organic phosphate preparations are available and the amounts of calcium and phosphorus available with PN could be theoretically higher than that absorbed using the enteral route.[80] However, information on bone mineralization of ELBW infants receiving what appears to be an adequate calcium and phosphate intake is still limited.

The usual dose of magnesium is about 6 mg/kg per day (2.5 mmol/kg per day), delivered as sulfate. This dose is rarely adjusted unless the infant has persistent hypocalcemia secondary to hypomagnesemia, or the infant has abnormally high magnesium levels due to maternal treatment with magnesium sulfate. Serum magnesium levels before magnesium supplementation with a PN solution should be checked in any small infant whose mother was treated for hypertension or pre-eclampsia.

Trace elements

Nine trace elements (or trace minerals) are nutritionally essential for humans: iron, zinc, copper, selenium, molybdenum, chromium, manganese and iodine. Although trace elements make up a small fraction of the total mineral content of the human body, they play an important role in numerous metabolic pathways. The infant born prematurely is at increased risk of developing trace mineral deficiencies. Premature birth is associated with low stores at birth, because accretion of trace minerals takes place during the last trimester of pregnancy. Rapid postnatal growth, unknown requirements, and variable intake of trace minerals also put the preterm infant at risk for deficiencies.[79]

During the early years of PN, it was thought that frequent plasma and/or blood transfusions provided the necessary trace minerals. Reports of zinc and copper deficiencies, even in infants who had received these transfusions, demonstrated the inadequacy of this approach and led to the availability of zinc and copper additives. The exact requirements of premature infants for most of the microminerals remain poorly defined because of the paucity of randomized controlled trials assessing their efficacy and safety. Recent studies have better delineated the range of suggested micromineral delivery to this population and Table 37.4 shows the recommended enteral and parenteral intake of trace elements for preterm infants for the transition period from the first 2 weeks of life to the following stable and post-discharge period.[81]

Research concerning the parenteral requirements of these nutrients by infants is, of course, hindered by the difficulties in both measuring plasma concentrations of the nutrients using small volumes of plasma, and interpreting the physiological significance of plasma concentrations. Accurate studies on the retention of these nutrients are also notoriously difficult.

Intravenous vitamins

Table 37.5 shows the recommended parenteral intake of vitamins for preterm infants. These guidelines, suggested in the past years by different committees provide a theoretical recommendation to obtain the optimal intake which is, however, unachievable with current commercial preparations. The delivery of vitamins from parenteral solutions can be lower than intended. Fat-soluble vitamins may be adsorbed into the storage bag and delivering tubing and may alter when exposed to light, oxygen or heat. As much as 80% of available vitamin A and 30% of vitamins D and E are lost during administration due to adherence to tubing and photodegradation especially during phototherapy[82].

Therefore, significant destruction may occur within the newborn intensive care unit environment, where higher environmental temperatures and light levels are commonplace. Vitalipid®

Table 37.4 Recommended micromineral intakes for preterm infants on total parenteral nutrition[81]

	Transitional period (0–14 days) (µg/kg per day)	Stable/post-discharge periods (>14 days) (µg/kg per day)
Iron	0	100–200
Zinc	150	400
Copper	0, 20*	20*
Selenium	0–1.3	1.5–4.5
Chromium	0–0.05	0.05–0.3
Molybdenum	0	0.25–1.0†
Manganese	0, 0.75*	1.0*
Iodine	0–1.0	1.0

* Should be withheld when hepatic cholestasis is present
† For long-term total parenteral nutrition only

Table 37.5 Recommended parenteral intake of vitamins for preterm infants (dose/kg per day)[81]

Vitamins	Consensus recommendations
Fat Soluble	
Vitamin A (IU)	700–1500
with lung disease	1500–2800
Vitamin D (IU)	40–160
Vitamin E (IU)	3.5 (max = 7)
Vitamin K (μg)	8–10 (300 at birth)
Water soluble	
Vitamin B_6 (μg)	150–200
Vitamin B_{12} (μg)	0.3
Vitamin C (mg)	15–25
Biotin (μg)	5–8
Folic acid (μg)	56
Niacin (mg)	4–6.8
Pantothenate (mg)	1–2
Riboflavin (μg)	150–200
Thiamin (μg)	200–350

(Kabivitrum, Stockholm), a lipid preparation available in Europe, is an intravenous soybean oil emulsion that contains vitamins A, D, E and K, thus reducing adsorption into the plastic tubing. Further clinical studies are needed to assess the vitamin status of VLBW and ill infants who receive parenteral solutions for prolonged periods and to evaluate the effects of the peroxide load induced by photo-exposed intravenous multivitamin solutions.[83]

Complications of parenteral nutrition

The main complications of PN, as shown in Table 37.6, can be metabolic, infective or catheter-related. Several complications (e.g. electrolyte imbalance, hypoglycemia, hyperglycemia, hypo/hypercalcemia, hypophosphatemia) can be corrected and prevented by manipulating the components of the solution. Other potentially more serious complications (e.g. cholestasis) are less easily corrected.

Table 37.6 Possible complications of parenteral nutrition

Metabolic complications
Cholestasis
Electrolyte imbalance
Essential fatty acid deficiency
Hyperammonemia
Hypertriglyceridemia
Hypocalcemia/hypercalcemia
Hypoglycemia/hyperglycemia
Metabolic acidosis
Metabolic bone disease
Prerenal nitrogen
Vitamin, mineral and trace elements deficiencies

Infectious complications
Bacterial
Fungal

Catheter-related complications
Vascular perforation
Embolism
Improper insertion resulting in extravasation, pneumothorax, hemorrhage, pleural effusion or pericardial tamponade
Local irritation, infiltration
Thromboses

Cholestasis

Cholestasis is a well-known complication associated with PN.[84,85] The initial lesion seen histologically is intracellular and intracanicular cholestasis, followed by portal inflammation. With prolonged administration, portal fibrosis and ultimately cirrhosis may develop. Cholestasis induced by PN is associated, initially with the elevation of serum bile acids and γ-glutamyl-transpeptidase (GGTP) and then with direct hyperbilirubinemia and jaundice. Elevation of hepatic transaminases, SGOT and SGPT is a late finding. Premature infants receiving PN for prolonged periods are at high risk of developing cholestasis.[86]

Incidence of cholestasis represents about 50% in infants with a birth weight < 1000g after 2 months of total PN. The etiology of cholestasis seems to be multifactorial and the main suspected factors are hypoxia, hemodynamic instability, sepsis and some components of the solutions.[87–89] It has also been suggested that hepatic dysfunction may be caused by the overgrowth of the intestinal flora in static gut. Fasting is also linked to development of cholestasis. This complication is less frequent when enteral feeding, even hypocaloric, is started. Abnormal amino acid pattern and taurine deficiency in some amino acid mixtures used as part of PN have been considered as possible etiological factors, but currently used solutions contain amino acids (including taurine), designed to maintain normal infant serum amino acid profiles.[89] Usually cholestasis resolves with discontinuation of PN but there are some reports of advanced liver disease in infants parenterally fed for several months.

Several measures have been suggested to prevent cholestasis induced by total PN such as: use of minimal enteral feeding, early introduction of enteral feeds to stimulate bile flow, use of balanced parenteral solutions, and reducing lipid infusion. In newborns and young infants with total PN-associated cholestasis who require continued PN, limiting the protein intake to 2 g/kg per day may help minimize amino acid-related hepatic toxicity. Ursodeoxycholic acid treatment seems to improve the course of PN-associated cholestasis not only in children and adults but also in premature infants, leading to an early sustained decrease in bilirubin levels after 2 weeks of therapy.[90]

Infection

Bacterial and/or fungal infection is another complication of PN. The most common isolated agents are *Staphylococcus epidermidis*, *Staphylococcus aureus* and *Candida albicans*. The incidence of sepsis as a complication of PN increases as gestational age decreases and the duration of PN increases. Even if infection is often a catheter-related complication it seems that the composition of solutions may predispose to sepsis. Intravenous lipid have been associated with coagulase-negative staphylococcal bacteremia and *Malessezia furfur* fungemia.[91] Table 37.7 shows the main precautions that should be taken to minimize the risk of sepsis.

Catheter-related complications

The main complications associated with venous catheter are usually the result of: improper insertion or placement; bacterial or fungal colonization of the catheter; and vessel irritation and/or thrombosis. Peripheral Teflon® catheters are prone to infiltration in a short time and to be colonized with bacteria at a rate of over 30% when they have been in place for more than 3 days.

Central venous catheters have a lower incidence of infiltration and deliver higher concentrations of the solution, but can be associated with severe complications. Broviac® catheters are associated with a higher incidence of infection (5–60%) and/or thrombosis in the neonatal period. At present, with the small silastic catheters introduced percutaneously, the incidence of sepsis and/or thrombosis is lower than with Broviac catheters. Thrombosis in these small-bore catheters can be minimized by adding heparin to the solution. In order to obtain a correct intravenous nutrition and avoid the high risks of complications, the patient must be closely monitored. Table 37.8 shows the main parameters that need to be checked.

Table 37.7 Precautions taken to minimize the risk of sepsis
Preparation of individual aliquots of parenteral nutrition solutions in the pharmacy
Manipulations carried out in the ward to be avoided
Central venous silastic catheters must be placed under strict aseptic conditions
Skin exit side for catheter placed in area which can be meticulously cleansed
Proper care of the site and all the connectors and essential tubings
Addition of heparin (1 unit/ml) to the infusate for peripheral/central venous catheters

Table 37.8 Monitoring during parenteral nutrition

Measurement of body weight daily and body length and head circumference weekly
Initially, during grading up of parenteral nutrients or during periods of metabolic instability:
- strict fluid balance
- 6–12 hourly urine/blood glucose
- daily plasma sodium, potassium, calcium, urea and acid–base

When on full parenteral nutrition and during metabolic steady state:
- strict fluid balance
- 12–24 hourly urine/blood glucose
- plasma sodium, potassium, calcium, urea and acid–base once/twice weekly

Plasma magnesium, phosphorus, alkaline phosphatase, albumin, transaminases and bilirubin weekly

Plasma triglycerides, amino acids, trace elements and ammonia not usually routinely monitored

Screening for infection or coagulation defects as indicated

Practical aspects of parenteral nutrition in VLBW infants

Tailored or standard parenteral solutions

Parenteral solutions can be prescribed using either of two formats: tailored or standard.[92] Tailored solutions are formulated specifically to meet the daily nutritional requirements of the individual patient, whereas standard solutions are designed to provide a formulation that meets most of the nutritional needs of the stable biochemical and metabolic parameters. Both of these methods have advantages and disadvantages associated with their use.

Tailored solutions are based on the principle that no single parenteral regimen can be ideal for all patients, for a wide variety of pathological processes, all age groups, or for the same patient during a single disease. The main advantage of tailored solutions is flexibility. Each solution is formulated for an individual patient and can be modified when the patient's nutritional needs and metabolic, electrolyte or clinical status changes.

The disadvantage of these solutions is linked to the time involved in calculation and label preparation, which today is nevertheless diminished with the use of specific computer programs. These solutions should be prepared with strict aseptic techniques, possibly in the pharmacy, not in the ward, and stored in a refrigerator at 4°C. The solutions thus prepared are stable for 96h and should be allowed to reach room temperature slowly and not warmed before infusion.

Standard solutions contain fixed amounts of each component per unit volume. In some hospitals there are several types of fixed solutions to cover the nutritional requirements of premature infants more adequately. The advantages of these solutions is that they include all the essential nutrients in fixed amounts, which eliminates the chances of inadvertent omission or overload. The major disadvantage of standard solutions is their lack of patient specificity and the need of minimal adjustment particularly during the first days of life.[92]

Nutrient intake

Table 37.9 shows the composition of a ready-to-use parenteral solution for VLBW infants and Table 37.10 the daily nutrient intake (kg/day) given by total PN according to the new practice of 'aggressive nutrition' proposed to minimize the interruption of nutrient intake induced by premature birth. In any case, nutrient intakes are always indicative and have to be modified according to each patient, his/her clinical picture, biochemical data and tolerance to nutrient intake. Thus, this standard solution could be diluted with free water according to fluid requirement and natrium chloride could be adapted after a few days of life.

The following suggestions could be useful in the management of a parenterally fed VLBW infant.

(1) In the first days of life fluid intake should be increased if daily weight loss is >5%, total weight loss is >12–15%, serum sodium is >150 mmol/l, urinary osmolality is >350 mOsm/l and if the infant is under phototherapy or managed in a radian incubator. In contrast, fluid intakes should be reduced if daily weight loss is <2% or there is a weight gain and serum sodium is <130 mmol/l.

(2) Glucose should be routinely administered after birth and progressively increased with the objective of increasing energy intake. When a glucose infusion rate of 6 mg/kg per min or less leads to hyperglycemia, the use of insulin is advised. Insulin should be discontinued as soon as glucose tolerance is established *and* the energy supply necessary for growth can be delivered without hyperglycemia. If insulin is used, strict blood glucose monitoring is mandatory to avoid hypoglycemia.

(3) The starting dose of amino acids in the first day of life should be higher than that currently advised. Intake should never be less than 1.0 g/kg per day and the starting dose should preferably be 2.5–3 g/kg per day. When

Table 37.9 Composition of a ready-to-use binary parenteral solution (per 100 ml) adapted for very-low-birth-weight infants

Glucose (g)	12.0
Amino acid (g)	2.7
Calcium (mg)	56
Phosphorus (mg)	43
Magnesium (mg)	4
Sodium (mmol)	1.6
Potassium (mmol)	1.5
Chloride (mmol)	2.0
Energy (kcal)*	55

* Energy (kcal) = amino acids (g)x3.75+glucose x 3.75

Table 37.10 Daily nutrient intake (kg/day) of very-low-birth-weight infants (<1500 g) in total parenteral nutrition according the 'aggressive approach'

	Day 1	Day 2	Day 3	Day 4	Day 5	Day 6	Day 7
Parenteral solution (ml)	50	70	100	120	140	150	150
Amino acid solution 10% (ml)	10	7	—	—	—	—	—
Lipid emulsion 20% (ml)	4	6	9	12	14	14	15
Glucose (g)	6.0	8.4	12.0	14.4	16.8	18.0	18.0
Amino acid (g)	2.4	2.6	2.7	3.2	3.8	4.1	4.1
Lipid (g)	0.8	1.2	1.8	2.4	2.8	2.8	3.0
Calcium (mg)	28	39	56	67	78	84	84
Phosphorus (mg)	22	30	43	52	60	65	65
Magnesium (mg)	2.0	2.8	4.0	4.8	5.6	6.4	6.4
Sodium (mmol)	0.8	1.1	1.6	1.9	2.2	2.4	2.4
Potassium (mmol)	0.8	1.1	1.5	1.8	2.1	2.3	2.3
Chloride (mmol)	1.0	1.4	2.0	2.4	2.8	3.0	3.0
Energy (kcal)*	39	52	72	88	103	109	111
Fluid (ml)	64	83	109	132	154	164	165

*Energy (kcal) = amino acids (g) x 3.75+glucose (g) x 3.75 + lipids(g) x 9.3
These nutrient intakes are a mere indication and have to be modified according to the characteristics, clinical picture and biochemical data of the individual patient

energy intakes reach about 70 kcal/kg per day and there is no enteral protein intake, the dose should be increased progressively to 3.5–4.4 g/kg per day.

(4) Although many neonatal intensive care units start lipid infusion only after the first few days, it seems logical to start parenteral lipids during the first day in order to avoid a prolonged interruption of essential fatty acids and long-chain PUFAs. The starting dose of 0.5–1 g/kg per day should gradually be increased to 3–3.5 g/kg per day. The lipid infusion should be adjusted to maintain a serum lipid level < 200 mg/dl.

REFERENCES

1. Jobe A. Pulmonary surfactant therapy. *N Engl J Med* 1993; **328**: 861–868.
2. NIH Consensus Conference. Effect of corticosteroids for fetal maturation on perinatal outcomes. *J Assoc Med Assoc* 1995; **273**: 413–417.
3. Hauth JC, Goldenberg RL, Andrews WW et al. Reduced incidence of preterm delivery with metronidazole and erythromycin in women with bacterial vaginosis. *N Engl J Med* 1995; **333**: 1732–1736.
4. Lucas A. Programming by early nutrition in man. In Bock GR, Whelan J, eds. *The Childhood Environment and Adult Disease*. Ciba Foundation Symposium 156. Chichester: *Wiley* 1991: 38–55.
5. American Academy of Pediatrics. Nutritional needs of preterm infants. In Kleinman RE, ed. *Pediatric Nutrition Handbook*, 4th edn. Elk Grove Village: American Academy of Pediatrics 1998: 55–87.
6. Committee on Nutrition of the preterm infant, European Society for Paediatric Gastroenterology and Nutrition. Nutrition and feeding of preterm infants. *Acta Paediatr Scand* 1987; **336 (Suppl)**: 1–14.
7. Nutrition Committee CPS. Nutrient needs and feeding of premature infants. *Can Med Assoc J* 1995; **152:** 1765–1785.
8. Embleton NE, Pang N, Cooke RJ. Postnatal malnutrition and growth retardation: an inevitable consequence of current recommendations in preterm infants? *Pediatrics* 2001; **107**: 270–273.
9. Rigo J, De Curtis M, Pieltain C. Nutritional assessment and body composition of preterm infants. *Semin Neonatol* 2002; **6**: 383–391.
10. Ziegler EE, Thureen PJ, Carlson SJ. Aggressive nutrition of the very low birthweight infant. *Clin Perinatol* 2002; **29**: 225–244.
11. Wilson DC, Cairns P, Halliday HL et al. Randomised controlled trial of an aggressive nutritional regimen in sick very low birthweight infants. *Arch Dis Child* 1997; **77**: 4F–11F.
12. Rigo J. Protein, amino acid and other nitrogen compounds. In Tsang RC, Uauy R, Koletzko B, Zlotkin SH, Hansen JW. *Nutritional Needs for the Preterm Infant*. Digital Educational Publishing, Ohio Cincinnati, 2004: in press.
13. Cooke RJ, Rigo J, Embleton ND, Ziegler EE. Nutrient balance and metabolic status in preterm infants fed two levels of dietary protein. *Pediatr Res* 2002; **4**: 318A.
14. Ehrenkranz RA, Younes N, Lemons JA et al. Longitudinal growth of hospitalized very low birth weight infants. *Pediatrics* 1999; **104:** 280–289.
15. Wilmore DW, Dudrick SJ. Growth and development of an infant receiving all nutrients exclusively by vein. *JAMA* 1968; **203**: 860–864.
16. Bell EF, Neidich GA, Cashore WJ et al. Combined effect of radiant warmer and phototherapy on insensible water loss in low-birth-weight infants. *J Pediatr* 1979; **94**: 810–813.
17. Yek TF, Voora S, Lilien LD et al. Oxygen consumption and insensible water loss in premature infants in single versus double walled incubators. *J Pediatr* 1980; **97**: 967–971.
18. Harpin VA, Rutter N. Humidification of incubators. *Arch Dis Child* 1985; **60**: 219–224.
19. Putet G. Energy. In Tsang RC, Lucas A, Uauy R, Zlotkin S, eds. *Nutritional Needs of the Preterm Infant*. New York, Williams & Wilkins, 1993: 15–28.
20. De Curtis M, Senterre J, Rigo J. Estimated and measured energy content of infant formulas. *J Pediatr Gastroenterol Nutr* 1986; **5**: 746–749.
21. Putet G, Senterre J, Rigo et al. Nutrient balance, energy utilization and composition of weight gain in very low birth weight infants fed pooled human milk or preterm formula. *J Pediatr* 1984; **105**: 79–105.
22. Pildes R. Hypoglycemia and hyperglycemia in tiny infants. *Clin Perinatol* 1986; **13**: 351–375.
23. Farrag HM, Cowett RM. Glucose homeostasis in the micropremie. *Clin Perinatol* 1986; **27**: 1–22.
24. Farrag, HM, Nawrath LM, Healey J et al. Persistent glucose production and greater peripheral sensitivity to insulin in the neonate vs. the adult. *Am J Physiol* 1997; **272**: E86–E93.
25. Cowett RM, Andersen GE, Maguire CA et al. Ontogeny of glucose homeostasis in low birth weight infants. *J Pediatr* 1988; **112**: 462–465.
26. Dweck HS, Cassady G. Glucose intolerance in infants of very low birth weight. I. Incidence of hyperglycemia in infants of birth weights 1,100 grams or less. *Pediatrics* 1974; **53**: 189–195.
27. Louik C, Mitchell AA, Epstein MF et al. Risk factors for neonatal hyperglycemia associated with 10% dextrose infusion. *Am J Dis Child* 1985; **139**: 783–786.
28. Thureen PJ, Scheer B, Anderson SM et al. Effect of hyperinsulinemia on amino acid utilization in the ovine fetus. *Am J Physiol* 2000; **279**: E1294–E1302.
29. Binder ND, Raschko PK, Benda GI et al. Insulin infusion with parenteral nutrition in extremely low birth weight infants with hyperglycemia. *J Pediatr* 1989; **114**: 273–80.

30. Thureen PJ, Melara D, Fennessey V et al. Effect of low *versus* high intravenous amino acid intake on very low birth weight infants in the early neonatal period. *Pediatr Res* 2003; **53**: 24–32.
31. Rigo J. Azote et acides aminés. In Ricour C, Ghisolfi J, Putet G, Goulet O. eds. *Traité de Nutrition Pédiatrique*, Paris: Maloine, 1993: 852–866.
32. Rigo J, Senterre J. Significance of plasma amino acid pattern in preterm infants. *Biol Neonate* 1987; **52**: 41–49.
33. Duffy B, Gunn T, Collinge J et al, The effect of varying protein quality and energy intake on the nitrogen metabolism of parenterally fed very low birthweight (<600g) infants, *Pediatr Res* 1981; **15**: 1040–1044.
34. Heird WC, Hay W, Helms RA et al. Pediatric parenteral amino acid mixture in low birth weight infants. *Pediatrics* 1988; **81**: 41–50.
35. Rigo J, Senterre J, Putet G et al. A new amino acid solution specially adapted to preterm infants. *Clin Nutr* 1987; **6**: 105–109.
36. Bell EF, Filer LJ Jr, Pon Wong A et al. Effects of a parenteral nutrition regimen containing dicarboxylic amino acids on plasma, erythrocyte, and urinary amino acid concentrations of young infants. *Am J Clin Nutr* 1983; **37**: 99–107.
37. Rigo J, Senterre J. Parenteral nutrition in the very-low-birth-weight infant. In Kretchmer N, Minkowski A, eds. *Nutritional Adaptation of the Gastrointestinal Tract of the Newborn*. New York: Raven Press 1983: 191–207.
38. Zlotkin SH, Bryan MH, Anderson GH. Cysteine supplementation to cysteine free intravenous feeding regimens in newborn infants. *Am J Clin Nutr* 1981; **34**: 914–923.
39. Malloy MH, Rassin DK, Richardson JC. Total parenteral nutrition in sick preterm infants: effects of cysteine supplementation with nitrogen intakes of 240 and 400 mg/kg/day. *J Pediatr Gastroenterol Nutr* 1984; **3**: 239–244.
40. Chessex P, Zebiche H, Pineault M et al. Effect of amino acid composition of parenteral solutions on nitrogen retention and metabolic response in very-low-birth weight infants. *J Pediatr* 1985; **106**: 111–117.
41. Pineault M, Chessex P, Bisaillon S et al. Total parenteral nutrition in the newborn: impact of the quality of infused energy on nitrogen metabolism. *Am J Clin Nutr* 1988; **47**: 298–304.
42. Kovar IZ, Saini J, Morgan JB. The sick very low birth-weight infant fed by parenteral nutrition: studies of nitrogen and energy. *Eur J Clin Nutr* 1989; **43**: 339–346.
43. Coran AG, Drongowski RA. Studies on the toxicity and efficacity of a new amino acid solution in pediatric parenteral nutrition. *J Parenter Enter Nutr* 1987; **11**: 368–377.
44. Rigo J, Putet G, Picaud JC et al. Nitrogen balance and plasma amino acids in the evaluation of protein sources for extremely low birthweight infants. In Ziegler EE, Lucas A, Moro GE, eds. *Nutrition of the Very Low Birthweight Infant*. 43°Nestlè Nutrition Workshop, Nestec Ltd, Philadelphia: Vevey/Lippincott Williams & Wilkins, 1999: 139–153.
45. Munro HN. Amino acid requirements and metabolism and their relevance to parenteral nutrition. In Wilkinson AW. ed. *Parenteral Nutrition*. London: Churchill Livingstone, 1972: 34.
46. Raiha NC. Biochemical basis for nutritional management of preterm infants. *Pediatrics* 1974; **53**: 147–156.
47. Gaull G, Sturman JA, Raïha NCR. Development of mammalian sulfur metabolism: absence of cystathionase in human fetal tissues. *Pediatr Res* 1972; **6**: 538–547.
48. Rigo J, Senterre J. Is taurine essential for the neonate? *Biol Neonate* 1977; **32**: 73–76.
49. Holt LE, Snyderman SE. The amino acid requirement of infants. *JAMA* 1961; **174**: 100–104.
50. Olney JW, Ho Ol, Rhee V. Brain-damaging potential of protein hydrolysates. *N Engl J Med* 1973; **289**: 391–395.
51. Becker RM, Wu G, Galanko JA et al. Reduced serum amino acid concentrations in infants with necrotizing enterocolitis. *J Pediatr* 2000; **137**: 785–793.
52. Van Goudoever JB, Sulkers EJ, Timmermans M et al. Aminoacid solutions for premature infants during the first week of life: The role of N-acetyl-L-cysteine and N-acetyl-L-tyrosine. *Parenter Enteral Nutr* 1994; **18**: 404–408.
53. Brunton JA, Ball RO, Pencharz PB. Current total parenteral nutrition solutions for the neonate are inadequate. *Curr Opin Clin Nutr Metab Care* 2000; **3**: 299–304.
54. Lacey JM, Wilmore DW. Is glutamine a conditionally essential amino acid? *Nutr Rev* 1990; **48**: 297-309.
55. Tubman TR, Thompson SW. Glutamine supplementation for prevention of morbidity in preterm infants. *Cochrane Database Syst Rev* 2001; **4**: CD001457.
56. Poindexter BB, Ehrenhranz RA, Stoll BJ et al. Effect of parenteral glutamine supplementation on plasma amino acid concentrations in extremely low-birth-weight infants. *Am J Clin Nutr* 2003; **77**: 737–743.
57. Koletzko B. Importance of dietary lipids. In Tsang R, Zlotkin SH, Nichols B, Hansen JW, eds. *Nutrition During infancy. Principles and Practice*, 1st edn. Cincinnati: Digital Educational Publishing, 1997: 123–153.
58. Van Aerde JE, Sauer PJ, Pencharz PB et al. Metabolic consequences of increasing energy intake by adding lipid to parenteral nutrition in full-term infants. *Am J Clin Nutr* 1994; **59**: 659–662.
59. Haumont D, Deckelbaum RJ, Richelle M et al. Plasma lipid and plasma lipoprotein concentrations in low birth weight infants given parenteral nutrition with twenty or ten percent lipid emulsion. *J Pediatr* 1989; **115**: 787–793.
60. Fidler N, Sauerwald T, Pohl A et al. Docosahexaenoic acid transfer into human milk after dietary supplementation: a randomised clinical trial. *J Lipid Res* 2000; **41**: 1376–1383.
61. Jensen CL, Maude M, Anderson RE et al. Effect of docosahexaenoic acid supplementation of lactating women on the fatty acid composition of breast milk lipids and maternal and infant plasma phospholipids. *Am J Clin Nutr* 2000; **71 (Suppl 1)**: 292S–299S.
62. Koletzko B, Sinclair A. Long-chain polyunsaturated fatty acids in diets for infants: choices for recommending and regulating bodies and for manufacturers of dietary products. *Lipids* 1999; **34**: 215–220.
63. Uauy R, Birch DG, Birch EE et al. Effect of dietary omega-3 fatty acids on retinal function of very-low-birth-weight neonates. *Pediatr Res* 1990; **28**: 485–492.
64. Carlson SE, Werkman SH. A randomized trial of visual attention of preterm infants fed docosahexaenoic acid until two months. *Lipids* 1996; **31**: 85–90.
65. Rubin M, Harell D, Naor N et al. Lipid infusion with different triglyceride cores (long-chain vs.medium-chain/long-chain triglycerides): effect on plasma lipids and bilirubin binding in premature infants. *J Parenter Enteral Nutr* 1991; **15**: 642–646.
66. Liet JM, Piloquet H, Marchini JS et al. Leucine metabolism in preterm infants receiving parenteral nutrition with medium chain compared with long chain triacylglycerol emulsions. *Am J Clin Nutr* 1999; **69**: 539–543.
67. Angsten G, Boberg M, Cederblad G et al. Metabolic effects in neonates receiving intravenous medium chain triglycerides. *Acta Paediatr* 2002; **91**: 188–197.
68. Van Herreweghe I, Dupont I, Hansen V et al. New perspectives in lipid emulsions for preterm infants: a

mixture of medium chain, (MCT), soybean oil (LCT), and fish oil (FO). *Pediatr Res* 2002; **51**: 1853A.

69. Putet G. Lipid metabolism of the micropremie *Clin Perinatol* 2000; **27**: 57–69.
70. Gobel Y, Koletzko B, Bohles HJ et al, Parenteral fat emulsions based on olive and soybean oils: a randomised clinical trial in preterm infants. *J Pediatr Gastroenterol Nutr* 2003; **37**:161–167.
71. Hammerman C, Aramburo MJ. Decreased lipid intake reduces morbidity in sick premature neonates. *J Pediatr* 1988; **113**: 1083–1088.
72. Cooke RWI. Factors associated with chronic lung disease in preterm infants. *Arch Dis Child* 1991; **66**: 776–779.
73. Wilson DC, Fox GF, Ohlsson A. Meta-analyses of effects of early or late introduction of intravenous lipids to preterm infants on mortality and chronic lung disease [abstract]. *J Pediatr Gastroenterol Nutr* 1998; **26**: 599.
74. Kao LC, Cheng MH, Warburton D. Triglycerides, free fatty acids, free fatty acids/albumin molar ratio, and cholesterol levels in serum of neonates receiving long-term lipid infusions: controlled trial of continuous and intermittent regimens. *J Pediatr* 1984; **104**: 429–435.
75. Rigo J, De Curtis M, Salle BL et al. Bone mineral metabolism in the micropremie. *Clin Perinatol* 2000; **27**: 147–170.
76. Rigo J, De Curtis M, Nyamugabo K et al. Premature Bone. In Tzang and Bonjour, eds. *Nutrition and Bone Development.* 42° Nestlé Nutrition Workshop. Puebla, 1997; **41**: 83–97.
77. Rigo J, De Curtis M, Nyamugabo K et al. Whole body calcium content in term and preterm neonates. *Eur J Pediatr* 1998; **157**: 259–264.
78. Rigo J, Nyamugabo K, De Curtis M et al. Bone mineralization during the first year of life. In Bindels JG, Goedhardt AC, Visser HKA, eds. *Recent Development in Infant Nutrition.* Tenth Nutricia Simposium Scheveningen, The Hague, The Nederlands, 1995: 98–111.
79. Aggett PJ. Trace elements of the micropremie. *Clin Perinatol* 2000; **27**: 119–129.
80. Prinzivalli M, Ceccarelli S. Sodium D-fructose-1,6-diphosphate vs. sodium monohydrogen phosphate in total parenteral nutrition: a comparative in vitro assessment of calcium phosphate compatibility. *J Parenter Enteral Nutr* 1999; **23**: 326–332.
81. Raghavendra R, Georgieff M. Microminerals. In Tsang RC, Uauy R, Koletzko B et al, eds. *Nutritional Needs for the Preterm Infant.* Cincinnati, Ohio: Digital Educational Publishing 2004: in press.
82. Gilles J, Jones G, Penchaarz P. Delivery of vitamins A, D and E in parenteral nutrition solutions. *J Parenter Enteral Nutr* 1983; **7**: 11–14.
83. Laborie S, Lavoie JC, Chessex P. Increased urinary peroxides in newborn infants receiving parenteral nutrition exposed to light. *J Pediatr* 2000; **136**: 628–632.
84. Merritt RJ. Cholestasis associated with total parenteral nutrition. *J Pediatr Gastroenterol Nutr* 1986; **5**: 9–22.
85. Whitington P. Cholestasis associated with total parenteral nutrition in infants. *Hepatology* 1986; **5**: 693–696.
86. Beale EF, Nelson RM, Bucciarelli RL et al. Intrahepatic cholestasis associated with parenteral nutrition in premature infants. *Pediatrics* 1979; **64**: 342–347.
87. Beath SV, Davies P, Papadopoulou A et al. Parenteral nutrition-related cholestasis in postsurgical neonates: multivariate analysis of risk factors. *J Pediatr Surg* 1996; **31**: 604–606.
88. Brown MR, Thunberg BJ, Golub L et al. Decreased cholestasis with enteral instead of intravenous protein in the very low-birth-weight infant. *J Pediatr Gastroenterol Nutr* 1989; **9**: 21–27.
89. Heird WC, Dell RB, Helms RA et al. Amino acid mixture designed to maintain normal plasma amino acid patterns in infants and children requiring parenteral nutrition. *Pediatrics* 1987; **80**: 401–408.
90. Levine A, Maayan A, Shamir R et al. Parenteral nutrition-associated cholestasis in preterm neonates: evaluation of ursodeoxycholic acid treatment. *J Pediatr Endocrinol Metab* 1999; **12**: 549–553.
91. Long JB, Keyserling HL. Catheter-related infection in infants due to an unusual yeast-*Malessezia furfur. Pediatrics* 1985; **76**: 896–900.
92. Poole RL, Kerner JA. Practical steps in prescribing intravenous feeding. In Yu VYH, MacMahon RA, eds. *Intravenous Feeding of the Neonate.* Edward Arnold 1992: 259–264.

38 Approach to gastrointestinal bleeding

Samy Cadranel and Michèle Scaillon

Introduction

Gastrointestinal (GI) bleeding, an uncommon phenomenon in infants and children, is most often felt, by parents and caregivers, as very dramatic, needing emergency treatment, regardless of the importance of the bleeding. Adequate management of the situation – which can obviously be life-threatening – requires experience, common sense and good co-ordination from the nursing staff and physicians in charge.

Epidemiology

In the general population, bleeding from the upper GI tract occurs with a prevalence of 100 in 100 000 adults per year, whereas lower GI bleeding is five times less frequent. The vast majority of hospitalizations occur in patients with concurrent illness and advanced age.[1] The overall incidence seems lower in Europe, for instance 45 in 100 000 as reported in a Dutch study.[2] In childhood, bleeding is less frequent but potentially serious, and the proportion of upper and lower intestinal bleeding appears to be roughly similar to that reported in the adult literature.[3] However, the etiology can be different, largely depending on the age of the child. There are no reliable quantitative data about the epidemiology of GI bleeding in ambulatory pediatric patients.[4] Children are usually in better condition, with the notable exception of the newborn period, the critically ill child in an intensive care unit (ICU) and children with portal hypertension and end-stage liver failure.[5] Many medications used in adults have not been standardized in children and the devices available for emergency endoscopic treatment may sometimes be too large for the child's limited GI tract caliber.

Despite important technical and training improvements in the management of acute bleeding in the adult patient, occurring during the past 30 years, the morbidity and mortality has remained unchanged, at around 6–7%.[6]

This finding is probably biased, reflecting only a considerable decrease of the less dramatic bleedings related to relapsing gastroduodenal ulcers due to the active eradication of *Helicobacter pylori.* During the same period, the systematic use of medications that control gastric acidity (such as anti-H_2 blockers or protein pump inhibitors (PPIs)) has succeeded in considerably reducing acute bleeding episodes in ICU patients (adults and children alike).[7]

Presentations and definitions

GI hemorrhage may present in different fashions. Acute GI bleeding is obvious GI blood loss, and is often associated with hemodynamic compromise. Gross GI bleeding that occurs intermittently is defined as acute-recurrent bleeding. Occult blood loss is a chronic source of GI blood loss usually detected by either a positive fecal occult blood test or iron deficiency anemia.

Regurgitations or vomiting of large quantities of red or digested brownish 'coffee ground' blood by mouth is called 'hematemesis'; the source of the bleeding is located between the esophagus and the ligament of Treitz. This is not always a sign of GI bleeding, since it may sometimes be confused with 'hemoptysia' which is triggered by cough, or with a bleeding from a nasopharyngeal origin. The brownish aspect of regurgitations can also be due to other causes such as cola or coffee drinks, sometimes misinterpreted by the family as blood.

'Melena' describes black, tarry, foul-smelling stool, and its presence usually indicates an upper intestinal source. Rarely, a proximal colonic bleeding may present as melena. Melena associated with hematemesis again implies a voluminous upper GI source.

'Hematochezia' (red blood passed per rectum) usually indicates a lower GI source, although voluminous blood loss from any location may present in this manner. In the unstable patient, presumption of an upper GI source dictates management, regardless of the color of blood per rectum.

Streaks of fresh blood on the feces or after defecation are not a sign of a severe hemorrhage but of a benign light bleeding often overestimated by the family. In the pediatric patient, 'occult' bleeding is usually discovered during a work-up of side-ropenic anemia together with clinical manifestations of chronic blood loss: fatigue, pallor or lightheadedness.

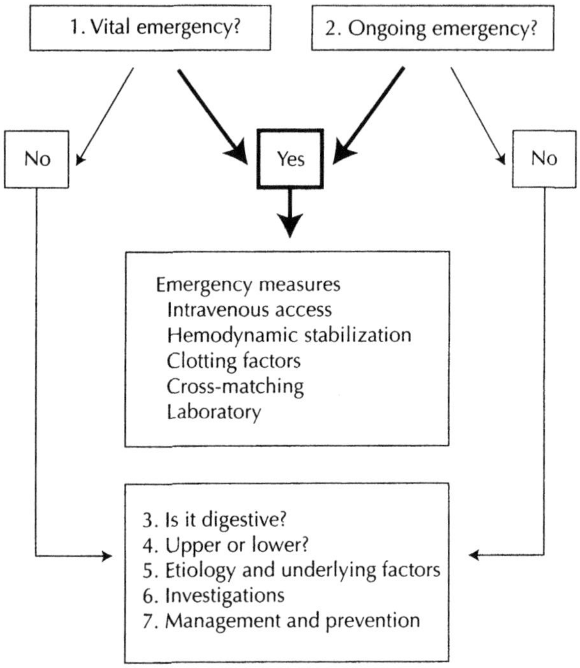

Figure 38.1 Practical approach to gastrointestinal bleeding in children.

Practical approach

Extensive and comprehensive descriptions of all possible situations generating GI bleeding (some of them very rare in childhood) and of the different causes, diagnostic procedures and treatments have been published elsewhere and especially in classical textbooks.[8–11] The purpose of the present chapter is to focus on a practical approach to GI bleeding in children and we have arbitrarily organized it in seven gradual steps (Figure 38.1).

Is it a life-threatening emergency due to the blood loss?

The symptoms such as pallor, agitation, sweating, tachycardia or low blood pressure (this is a severe but late complication) are usually very clear and should be evaluated accurately in order to initiate adequate resuscitation measures. Treating or preventing hypovolemia is the first step in stabilization. A secure large-bore intravenous access – or a central line for the monitoring of central venous pressure – is mandatory, since shock can develop at any time if uncontrolled bleeding persists. Blood should be drawn for blood typing and cross-matching. At this stage, extra blood samples for hematocrit, hemoglobin, coagulation, and red and white blood cell and platelet counts are necessary. A low mean corpuscular volume (MCV) suggests a chronic blood loss and an elevated blood urea nitrogen (BUN) due to the absorption of intestinal blood points mainly to upper GI bleeding.[12,13] It is also advisable, whenever possible, to initiate investigations for etiological factors (such as liver function tests) by drawing extra blood samples. Management by fluid and/or colloid infusion can then be started.

Once the stabilization has been obtained these children must be admitted to an ICU, ideally connected with a pediatric surgery department.

Is the bleeding still ongoing?

Relevant familial or personal surgical or medical histories should be taken as soon as possible. Every effort should be made to obtain a complete list of all medications administered to the child. This may prove difficult to obtain from upset parents: it is strongly recommended to use a locally adapted checklist of drugs, which should be available and ready in the emergency room.

Invasive monitoring is not always necessary and should be reserved for such situations where an ongoing bleeding is obvious or whenever history or physical examination suggests a potential for re-bleeding. Early insertion of a large-bore nasogastric tube is helpful for assessing possible continuing bleeding from the upper GI tract. We use a double-lumen tube (e.g. Salem sump™, Sherwood Medical, St Louis, MO, USA), which enables decompression, aspiration and also lavage using saline as preparation for a diagnostic endoscopic procedure. Attempts to stop an ongoing bleeding with iced saline lavage, a classical technique[14,15] once considered as helpful is no longer recommended, since it is rarely useful and potentially harmful.[16–18]

Is it a gastrointestinal tract bleeding?

Hemoptysis is rare in children and usually associated with respiratory symptoms. Blood swallowed during an unrecognized epistaxis can mimic GI bleeding and present as hematemesis but also as melena. Previous episodes of epistaxis should be recorded. A rapid examination of the nasal cavity can easily diagnose the source of the bleeding.

Not all vomiting or stools stained in red are blood. Additives coloring food, drink mixes or medicines can be mistaken for blood. Tomatoes, beets, cherries and cranberries may look like blood when vomited or passed per rectum by a child with diarrhea. Bismuth, iron supplements, spinach and dark chocolate can give a dark coloration to stools, which may be mistaken for melena. The very dark feces of constipated children are usually easy to distinguish from melena. Diapers can acquire a pink discoloration if some time elapses prior to their disposal.

The testing for occult blood is usually performed on a stool specimen by a Guaiac reaction. Guaiac is a colorless compound that turns blue in contact with substances with peroxidase activity (e.g. hemoglobin) and hydrogen peroxide. This test is easy, inexpensive and convenient, but the reaction is not specific for blood. Many substances with peroxidase activity may yield a false-positive result. Ingested red meat, certain fruits and vegetables such as cantaloupes, radishes, bean sprouts, cauliflower, broccoli and grapes have enough peroxidase activity to cause a positive reaction. Oral iron preparations may also cause false-positive reactions.

In the newborn, suspected GI bleeding can be due to swallowed maternal blood and should be ruled out by the Apt test. The test is based on the denaturation, in an alkaline milieu, of adult hemoglobin to a yellow-brown solution of alkaline globin hematin whereas fetal hemoglobin, resists and is colored to a pink solution.

Is it an upper or a lower gastrointestinal bleeding?

Logically, hematemesis or melena indicates bleeding from the upper GI tract, while hematochezia indicates bleeding from a colonic source. However, this simple distinction can be confusing in the newborn and in infants. The transit time can be very quick and undigested red blood hematochezia (instead of digested melena) may be the only symptom of a hemorrhage occurring in the upper segment of the GI tract.

Similarly, in some instances, melena is the only manifestation of colonic blood trapped during sufficient time to permit the degradation of hemoglobin by the intestinal flora. Small-intestinal bleeding manifests as either melena or hematochezia. Simultaneous mixed digested black and undigested fresh red blood suggests a Meckel's diverticulum or a large upper GI bleeding.

The nasogastric tube, used as a tool for monitoring the continuity of bleeding, can also be used as a first-step investigation to distinguish between an upper or a lower GI bleeding origin; blood-stained gastric fluid indicates an upper GI source. However, a clear or bilious stained fluid does not exclude a duodenal origin of the bleeding.

Guaiac testing for occult bleeding from gastric aspirates is not reliable. Needless to say, a complete and oriented history taking can provide useful clues, such as recent medication with non-steroidal anti-inflammatory drugs (NSAIDs), previous ulcer, familial history of polyposis, or liver disease. Associated symptoms such as bloody mucous diarrhea suggest a colonic or terminal small-bowel source.

A careful physical examination looking for signs of portal hypertension, splenic or liver enlargement, cutaneous stigma of Peutz–Jeghers polyposis or syndromes associated with vascular abnormalities is essential. A thorough examination of the oral and nasal cavity as well as the anal region can rule out simple diagnoses.

What are the etiology and underlying factors?

GI bleeding occurs at all ages with similar etiologies and mechanisms. However, the frequency and presentation varies according to age (Table 38.1) and underlying factors.

Neonatal period

Bleeding from coagulation abnormalities due to vitamin K deficiency is becoming rare since this condition is corrected by systematic vitamin K supplementation at birth.[19,20]

The most frequent cause of upper GI bleeding in the neonatal period is the poorly understood 'neonatal esophagogastritis' which affects acutely distressed newborns. The course is most often benign and self-limited. The availability of miniaturized fiberscopes has enabled the recognition of this condition as a cause of GI bleeding in a series of 14 out of 32 newborns published in 1989.[21] The same group reviewed their series of endoscopies performed in the neonatal period; 158 out of 219 newborns presented with esophagitis.[22] Other authors reported findings in 17 full-term newborns and attributed the lesions to a traumatic origin, because of the distribution of the lesions (more severe in the upper esophagus), of the early onset (almost at birth) and the very rapid healing.[23] Finnish authors drew attention to the presence of gastric lesions, highly prevalent in preterm infants in the ICU[24] and claimed that mechanical ventilation has the main risk factor, but factors included also the mode of delivery and hypotension after birth, which increase the risk of stress-induced gastric lesions.[25] Other French groups insisted on the extension of the lesions involving the esopha-

Table 38.1 Main sources of gastrointestinal (GI) bleeding according to age and frequency

Newborn	1 month to 2 years	2–16 years
Upper GI bleeding		
Maternal blood (Apt test)	esophagitis	esophagitis
Coagulation factors	gastritis	gastritis
Esophagitis	acute ulcer	acute ulcer
Gastritis	Mallory–Weiss syndrome	Mallory–Weiss syndrome
Duodenitis	varices	varices
Vascular malformation	vascular abnormalities	vascular abnormalities
	GI duplications	GI duplications
Lower GI bleeding		
Maternal blood (Apt test)	anal fissures	anal fissures
Coagulopathy	infectious colitis	infectious colitis
NEC	vascular anomalies	vascular anomalies
Other enterocolitides	allergic colitis	polyp(s)
Volvulus	Meckel's diverticulum	IBD
		vasculitis
		Henoch–Schönlein purpura
		hemolytic uremic syndrome
		hemorrhoids

IBD, inflammatory bowel disease

gus and the stomach, or the stomach and the duodenum, or the whole upper GI tract.[26]

A case–control study concluded that there was a possible protection by breast feeding.[27] A recent case–control multicenter study in France pointed out the possible role of antacid drugs used by mothers during the last month of pregnancy, and emphasized the possible protective role of early breast feeding against severe lesions.[28]

In the neonatal period, rectal bleeding (sometimes from an upper GI source) is infrequent and differs little from rectal bleeding in older infants. However, necrotizing enterocolitis occurs early, especially in the preterm infant and after the first oral feedings.[29] Besides bloody stools, symptomatology includes abdominal distension, decreased activity and feeding difficulties. Radiological signs such as pneumatosis intestinalis and air in the biliary system are pathognomonic. The condition is severe and may result in sepsis.

Infancy

In infants, esophagitis due to gastroesophageal reflux disease is the most frequent cause of upper GI bleeding. In addition, although infrequent, it is sometimes an early complication of hypertrophic pyloric stenosis.[30] Gastroduodenal ulcers are rare, since *Helicobacter pylori* infection, an etiological factor in peptic ulceration, is not a common finding in this age group, at least in industrialized regions. Furthermore, interferon (IFN)-γ secretion in the stomach of *H. pylori*-infected patients is lower in children than in adults, and this could protect children from development of severe gastroduodenal diseases such as ulcer disease.[31]

Rectal red blood mixed with mucus and loose stools suggests an infectious cause. Viral infection is seldom the cause of rectal bleeding. However, many known pathogenic bacteria such as *Salmonella, Shigella, Campylobacter jejuni* and some strains of *Escherichia coli* can cause acute rectal bleeding through invasive colonic lesions. The role of *Clostridium difficile* is more debated[32,33] whereas we have observed *Yersinia enterocolitica*-associated colonic lesions that closely resemble those observed in inflammatory bowel diseases (S. Cadranel, personal communication).[34] Rectal bleeding can also occur through colonic parasitic infections with *Entamoeba histolytica* and *Dientamoeba fragilis*. In this age group, cow's milk is the most frequent cause of food allergy producing occult or even frank blood loss. It occurs mostly in formula-fed infants, although the same allergy can be induced indirectly through breast milk. Resolution of the symptoms usually occurs shortly after recognition of this condition and further avoidance of dairy products by the breast-feeding mother or switching to a non-allergenic formula.

In this age group, because of potential severe complications and sequelae, intussusception needs early recognition and adequate management.[34] It occurs more frequently in male infants (3 : 1) aged 3–24 months presenting with acute paroxysmal abdominal pain alternating with symptom-free periods and, later on, passage of 'currant jelly' stools. An association between antibiotic use and primary idiopathic intussusception has been reported recently.[35]

Hirschsprung's related enterocolitis may affect undiagnosed constipated infants, but also patients of any age who had undergone complicated operations.[36]

Childhood

In older children upper GI bleeding suggests an acid-related disease such as peptic esophagitis or gastritis.

The Mallory–Weiss tear is a mucosal laceration at the level of the cardia following vomiting with or without symptoms of epigastric pain.[37–39] The bleeding is usually self-limited. Retching can also cause mild-to-moderate bleeding through superficial ecchymotic traumatic lesions of the fundic mucosa.

In industrialized regions, upper GI bleeding due to *Helicobacter pylori*-associated gastritis or ulcer is seldom observed in children younger than 5 years.[40] Nevertheless, systematic antral and fundic biopsies are recommended for histological study and microbiological culture.[41] Esophagitis is the most frequent cause of acute upper GI bleeding in children with brain damage. The complaints of these neurologically impaired children are often unrecognized during long periods of time resulting in chronic occult blood losses and esophageal stenosis.[42]

In children mentally retarded or with behavioral abnormalities, the possibility of ingesting foreign bodies as a source of upper GI bleeding should be considered.

Portal hypertension and deficient coagulation factors complicating liver diseases are the most dramatic causes of upper GI bleeding. The adequate management of esophageal varices and preventive treatment of portal hypertension need close collaboration between a skilled pediatric gastroenterology staff and a well-equipped ICU. A common complication of portal hypertension is the typical gastropathy in which the gastric mucosa from portal hypertensive patients exhibits a typical vascular dilatation and congestion that seems more extensive after endoscopic sclerotherapy of varices.[43]

In pediatric ICUs the systematic prophylaxis with H_2-receptor blockers and, more recently PPIs, has resulted in a dramatic decrease of peptic stress ulcers affecting mainly children with severe burns, with acute neurological diseases or undergoing major surgical procedures. Ventilator-associated pneumonia and upper airway colonization with Gram-negative bacilli does not seem to be aggravated by these drugs.[44]

The Dieulafoy's lesion is an unusually large mucosal ulcer eroding a submucosal artery. This unusual lesion is observed in children who present with massive hematemesis (sometimes hematochezia) without the usually associated symptoms of ulcer. In most cases the lesion is found in the proximal stomach, but it can occur at any site of the GI tract.[45]

One of the most frequent causes of upper GI bleeding in young children used to be acetylsalicylic compounds. These can cause acute gastric erosions but also deep extensive ulcers.[46] Stenotic scarring may develop in the pyloric region as a result of the healing of such 'kissing ulcers'. Recently, ibuprofen has become widely used in children in the USA and also in continental Europe as an analgesic and antipyretic drug.[47,48] Its innocuousness is controversial and, along with all NSAIDs, should be avoided in children with portal hypertension.[49]

Other drugs potentially causing upper GI bleeding include anticoagulants and antimitotics used in oncological patients and inducing esophageal and gastric mucitis.

Hematemesis was the main symptom reported in an epidemic of dengue hemorrhagic fever in children in India.[50]

Juvenile polyps are the most common cause of rectal bleeding in this age group and affect 3–4% of the population in Mexico.[51] Rectal bleeding from juvenile polyps is usually mild and self-limited, although the relapsing episodes can cause emotional trouble in the child and family. Polyps are to be found mainly in the rectum and sigmoid.[52] However, in our personal series, 20% of all juvenile polyps occurred in other parts of the colon, including the cecum. Retrieval of polyps for histological study is strongly recommended, especially in case of multiple polyps (10% in our series).

Meckel's diverticulum is a congenital anomaly occurring in 2% of the population. While it commonly remains clinically silent, it may also present at any age, typically with intermittent, painless frank hematochezia in children. In a series of 164 children undergoing laparotomy between 1970 and 1989, a Meckel's diverticulum was discovered at laparotomy. There were 120 boys and 44 girls with a mean age of 5.2 years (range 0–18 years). Forty-seven cases were asymptomatic, representing an incidental finding at laparotomy, 25 were resected and ectopic gastric mucosa was present in seven specimens (28%). Of the 117 symptomatic patients, 49 (42%) presented with bowel obstruction, 45 (38%) had rectal bleeding, 16 (14%) had diverticulitis and seven (6%) had umbilical pathology.[53] In another more recent review, no sex ratio differences were observed.[54]

Duplication cysts containing gastric mucosa that may ulcerate and bleed represent other causes of bleeding from the small intestine. Of special interest are antral duplications that cause hypergastrinemia, with consequent ulceration and bleeding.[55] Other lesions as a source of bleeding from the small bowel include infectious enteritis, lymphonodular hyperplasia,[56] typhlitis,[57] Crohn's disease and several vasculitides.

In Henoch–Schönlein purpura, gastrointestinal bleeding has been reported in 33% of cases.[58] Hemolytic uromic syndrome is another vascular complication following several strains of Shiga-toxin producing *Escherichia coli*.[59–61] Other causes of GI bleeding have been described, such as cytomegalovirus (CMV)-associated hematochezia in HIV-infected children[62] and also complications of graft-versus-host disease after bone marrow transplant[59–63] and post-chemotherapy neutro-penic enterocolitis in children with cancer.[64] Acute major gastrointestinal hemorrhage is uncommon in inflammatory bowel disease and most cases are due to Crohn's disease without a predilection for site of involvement.[65] Although rare, bacterial overgrowth may present as a cause of lower GI bleeding.[66]

Vascular anomalies are a rare cause of bleeding in children. The symptoms vary according to the site and size of the bleeding lesion. Hemangiomas are proliferative lesions with a tendency to regress spontaneously, whereas vascular malformations are non-proliferative and do not regress. These rare causes of GI bleeding include Osler–Rendu–Weber disease and Klippel –Trenaunay, Turner's and blue-rubber bleb nevus syndromes.

How should diagnostic investigations be used?

The introduction in pediatrics of fiberoptic endoscopes, some 30 years ago,[67–69] has progressively but radically changed the investigation of GI bleeding. GI bleeding implies a mucosal lesion that will always be better detected by endoscopy than by any other 'indirect visualization' means. Biopsies for further study of microscopic lesions and, more recently, endoscopic treatment has become possible; endoscopy has logically become the first diagnostic step (see below). Consequently, contrast radiology is seldom – if ever – used in upper GI bleeding, since barium contrast, even with double contrast, is too insensitive to detect superficial mucosal lesions.

Imaging

Has the plain abdominal X-ray film become obsolete? The main advantage of this simple procedure is that it is available almost everywhere. Plain abdominal radiographs may provide useful information in children with upper GI or rectal bleeding when pain or vomiting is present, and can clearly show bowel obstruction or perforation.

Echography, with Doppler ultrasound, is one of the best diagnostic tools for visualizing the vascular system and evaluating the blood flow when portal hypertension is suspected. It can provide valuable information about vascular abnormalities. Echography is also able to detect bowel wall thickening, intussusceptions or, on some occasions, intraluminal masses. However, it can seldom be used as the first step in the investigation and has probably no utility as a first approach to a massive hematemesis.

Computed tomography (CT) and magnetic resonance imaging (MRI) can be helpful for the detection of mass lesions or vascular malformations. An important limitation to these investigations is the fact that they require adequate sedation, in order to avoid unwanted movements of the child.

The most popular form of scintigraphy is the 'Meckel's scan' using technetium-99m pertechnetate, which accumulates in functional gastric mucosa such as Meckel's diverticulum; but also in other ectopic gastric mucosa, for instance in duplication cysts. However, this test is far from being accurate in all instances and as many as 20% false-positive and 20% false-negative results are observed.[70]

The 'bleeding scan' is another scintigraphic technique that can be used to identify a bleeding site that cannot be reached by endoscopy. Technetium-99m-labeled red blood cells from a sample of the patient's blood are re-injected into the bloodstream. Bleeding rates of 0.1 ml/min are detectable through gamma camera images of the abdomen every 5 min for the first hour and then at regular intervals for as long as 24 h if needed. A minimum bleeding of 500 ml is necessary to obtain a positive scan in cases of lower GI hemorrhage.[71–73]

Angiography detects active bleeding lesions or chronic recurrent blood losses if the estimated rate of bleeding exceeds 0.5 ml/min. The disadvantages of this technique, besides its invasiveness requiring general anesthesia, are frequent false-negative results. Its main advantages are the correct identification of the bleeding site – for further surgery – and the possibility of using the catheter for therapy either with selective infusion of vasopressin or embolization.[74,75]

Endoscopy

The considerable progress achieved in the miniaturization of endoscopes and also in the field of sedation and anesthesia has substantially changed the role of endoscopy in the handling of GI bleeding in children.

The availability of instruments that can be used at any age, ranging from the slimmest 6 mm outer diameter 'neonatoscopes' to the standard 9 mm gastroscopes, has enabled pediatric gastroenterology to deal more easily with the diagnosis of GI bleeding. Also, modern video-endoscopes facilitate teamwork and training. However, the use of therapeutic probes usually requires the 2.8 mm operating channel diameter of the standard adult endoscope which is difficult to employ in children younger than 2 years, even under general anesthesia.

Prompt upper endoscopy guarantees a more accurate result, since identification of the bleeding site can vary from 82% when endoscopy is performed within 24 h to 48% if done over 72 h of an upper GI bleeding.[8]

For bleeding of the lower GI tract, rigid endoscopes are seldom used and are replaced by the most 'user-friendly' flexible instruments. Miniaturized colonoscopes of 10 mm in outer diameter can be easily used in children older than 5 years, properly sedated, and under the control of a trained pediatric anesthesiologist. In younger children the various pediatric gastroscopes can be used, taking into account that they are not designed with the same characteristics of colonoscopes (more stiff and less handy). Colonoscopy is not always an easy procedure and a clean intestinal lumen is sometimes difficult to obtain. In non-emergency conditions, a plain abdominal X-ray film permits assessment of the degree of stool retention and starting with the necessary steps to void the colon from its fecal contents. We recommend, when possible, a strict diet without residues for 4–5 days prior to the colonoscopy and a semi-liquid diet on the last day. Many preparations combining enemas with large quantities of oral polyethyleneglycol (PEG) solution (sometimes administered through a nasogastric tube) have proved disappointing and poorly tolerated. We prefer, at least in children older than 6 years, an oral preparation consisting of the combination of sodium phosphate (acting as an osmotic laxative within 2 h), and bisacodyl (acting within 6–8 h) (Prepacol® Delpharm, Bretigny-sur-Orge, France).

Enteroscopy and wireless capsule video-endoscopy

Modern video-endoscopes have a working length of 100 cm, enabling, in experienced hands, a thorough and accurate investigation of the upper GI tract as far as the ligament of Treitz. From the opposite side, investigation of the entire colon and 10–20 cm of the terminal ileum is also possible. However, bleeding originating from the small bowel is not accessible to conventional endoscopic instruments. The development of a long 'enteroscope' with easy maneuverability in order to explore the entire small bowel seems a futuristic dream; on some occasions peroperative endoscopy with the surgeon directing the progress of the instrument can be helpful.

The wireless capsule endoscopy is currently the outstanding technical innovation in diagnostic gastrointestinal endoscopy.[76,77] Especially for small-bowel diseases, this new technique offers several potential advantages compared to traditional diagnostic tools. Capsule endoscopy is a painless procedure that can be performed as an ambulatory endoscopic examination. The first experimental studies showed good tolerance of the capsule endoscopy and the possibility of a complete visual investigation of the small bowel. Clinical studies have demonstrated possible fields of application in obscure chronic or intermittent GI blood loss and inflammatory bowel disease, with better results than with classical push-enteroscopy or radiological imaging.[78–80] The major risk of the procedure – intestinal obstruction by the capsule – may hinder its use in the diagnosis of polyps or tumors in the small bowel. It will probably progressively replace the cumbersome and disappointing push-enteroscopy. The capsule is relatively large but can be swallowed by children older than 8 years.[81,82]

Management and prevention

Most GI bleedings are self-limited and need only close observation; others require medications or even aggressive and invasive endoscopic management. Many treatments and techniques are theoretically possible, extrapolated from adult studies to the pediatric patient. The regimen implemented for a child should be individualized, taking into account the supposed or confirmed origin and etiology of the bleeding, the underlying medical condition and the age. Guidelines for pediatric situations need controlled trials in order to provide an evidence-based approach; thus, they are currently based on local competence and equipment. A local protocol should be available in order to improve the quality and efficacy of the management.[83]

The two main and serious origins of clear upper GI bleeding are peptic and variceal.

Peptic lesions

Medical treatment is based on acid suppression and is often started empirically because a peptic origin is frequent in pediatrics (40% of the moderate or severe hematemesis in the series reported by Mougenot and Balquet).[84] Currently, H_2-receptor antagonists and PPIs are widely used, and ranitidine and omeprazole are the most extensively studied molecules in each class, respectively. They can be given either intravenously or orally. The multiple-unit pellet system enables dispersion in water and an easier use in small children unable to swallow tablets. In bleeding peptic ulcers, the pharmacotherapy is aimed at improving the environment of the bleeding point by keeping the gastric pH above the proteolytic range for pepsin and curing the initial lesion. This kind of treatment is also indicated for preventing stress ulcers.

Ranitidine Serum concentrations of ranitidine necessary to inhibit gastric acid secretion by at least 90% ranged between 40 and 60 ng/ml in children aged 3–16 years.[85] The pharmacokinetics of ranitidine in critically ill children is variable. In a study in mechanically ventilated, critically ill children weighing at least 10 kg, the proposed doses of ranitidine, needed to reach a gastric pH of >4 for stress ulcer prophylaxis, depended on the regimen by bolus or continuous infusion. The recommended bolus regimen is 1.5 mg/kg administered every 8 h. In continuous infusion, the recommended intravenous loading dose is 0.45 mg/kg, followed by a continuous infusion of 0.15 mg/kg per hour. Thereafter, gastric pH should be monitored and the dose of ranitidine adjusted accordingly.[86] Children with acute central nervous system injury or pediatric risk of mortality (PRISM) scores of >20 show a poor control of gastric pH.[87] In another study, no significant differences were observed, regarding the raising of gastric pH values above 4, between a bolus regimen with 1 mg/kg in two doses 6 h apart or a continuous infusion regimen of ranitidine bolus of 0.15 mg/kg followed by continuous infusion at 0.15 mg/kg per hour for 12 h. Proposed doses are shown in Table 38.2. There was no correlation between illness severity scores and gastric pH values.[88] Smaller volumes can be perfused with bolus infusions, whereas continuous infusions of ranitidine often need a second line, since many drugs are incompatible with ranitidine; however, continuous infusion decreases the variability of gastric pH in children in an ICU.[87] Critically ill children with normal renal and hepatic function should be treated with a minimum 3 mg/kg per day of intravenous ranitidine and the dose should be titrated to a gastric pH of ≥ 4.[89]

In full-term newborns, with a stable renal and hepatic function treated with extracorporeal membrane oxygenation, ranitidine administered as a single 2 mg/kg dose over 10 min is able, within 90 min after administration, to increase the intragastric pH to >5 and to maintain it at >4 for a minimum of 15 h.[90]

In a study in 30 full-term newborns treated for bleeding erosions during the first 2 days of life, a rate of less than 0.2 mg/kg per hour seemed to be advisable for continuous ranitidine infusion, whereas the 5 mg/kg twice a day regimen could be considered adequate for oral therapy.[91] Preterm infants need significantly smaller doses of ranitidine to keep their intraluminal gastric pH over 4. The required optimal dose of ranitidine is 0.5 mg/kg body weight twice a day and that for full-term infants 1.5 mg/kg body weight three times a day.[92] In premature infants with bronchopulmonary dysplasia, infusion of 0.0625 mg/kg per hour of ranitidine during dexamethasone administration is sufficient to increase and maintain the gastric pH above 4.[93] The doses of ranitidine should be adjusted in patients with severe renal failure even when undergoing regular hemodialysis.[94,95] The bolus injections ought to be slow

Table 38.2 Proposed doses of ranitidine for critically ill newborns, infants and children

	References	Bolus IV	Continuous infusion	Orally
Children				
	Lugo (2001)[86]	1.5 mg/kg tid	loading dose 0.45 mg/kg, followed by 0.15 mg/kg/ per h	
Adults	Marchant (1988)[139]		loading dose 50 mg, followed by 0.15 mg/kg per h or 0.25 mg/kg per h (high risk)	
Infants				
Full-term	Kuusela (1998)[92]	1.5 mg/kg tid		
	Fontana (1993)[91]	0.2 mg/kg per h		5 mg/kg bid
	Wells (1998)[90]	2 mg/kg bid		
Preterm	Kuusela (1998)[92]	0.5 mg/kg bid		

IV, intravenous; tid, three times a day; bid, twice a day

because of the risk of bradycardia. The tolerance effect of ranitidine could lead, as reported in adults, to a rapid loss of antisecretory activity on days 2 and 3.[96]

Oral doses reported in the literature vary from to 6–10 mg/kg per day, twice or three times a day during 8 weeks to cure esophagitis to 2.5–10 mg/kg per day during 4–8 weeks for ulcers.

Omeprazole The oral dose range of omeprazole for management of gastroesophageal reflux disease and acid-related diseases is 0.3–3.5 mg/kg with a maximum of 80 mg/day). Orally, 1 mg/kg per day every 12 or 24 h or simply tablets of 10 mg under and 20 mg above 20 kg of weight are most often prescribed.

In children aged 3 months to 19 years, the pharmacokinetics of intravenous doses from 36.9 to 139 mg/1.73 m^2 were: systemic clearance of 0.23 l/kg per hour; volume of distribution of 0.45 l/kg; elimination half-life of 0.86 h with a high individual variability.[97]

In adults, after an initial bolus of 80 mg of omeprazole, the infusion rate of 8 mg/h is significantly superior to 40 mg/6 h.[96–98]

In nine adult patients with duodenal ulcers, a daily intravenous dose of 40 mg omeprazole was not sufficient to keep the intragastric pH above 4 in all patients during the first day of treatment. After 5 days, 1 single daily low dose of 10 mg intravenously and 20 mg orally were effective and dependable in reducing 24-h intragastric acidity.[99] In adults, the best regimen to raise the intragastric pH above levels alleged to allow hemostasis in patients with peptic ulcer bleeding (and subsequent healing of the ulcer) seems to be an initial bolus of omeprazole followed by a continuous infusion for 72 h and then switching to a single oral dose.[100]

Prevention of stress ulcers or re-bleeding An evidence-based medicine review of published trials yields sufficient evidence to support the use of prophylactic acid suppression in critically ill patients with coagulopathies or in those who are receiving prolonged mechanical ventilation. Not enough data have accumulated to prove the superiority of intravenous PPIs to intravenous H_2-receptor antagonists for the prophylaxis of clinically important stress ulcer bleeding. With respect to acute GI bleeding, intravenous PPI is significantly more effective than an intravenous H_2-receptor antagonist in reducing the rate of re-bleeding after hemostasis in patients with bleeding peptic ulcer.[101] In adult patients, a recent placebo-controlled trial of high-dose parenteral omeprazole after an initial endoscopic treatment of bleeding peptic ulcers demonstrated a substantial reduction in the risk of re-bleeding[102] and a meta-analysis showed a significant beneficial effect of acid-decreasing agents in lowering re-bleeding and surgery rates, but demonstrated no effect upon mortality.[103]

Portal hypertension

Esophageal variceal bleeding is one of the severe consequences of portal hypertension. However, the bleeding site may sometimes be otherwise than the cardiac regions, for instance at the level of a portoenterostomy anastomosis, in the rectal mucosa or in the gastric cavity as a consequence of a hypertensive gastropathy. The management becomes even more difficult, because of coagulation abnormalities, infection and cirrhotic encephalopathy needing their own specific treatments. Endotracheal intubation should be considered especially to protect against blood flow during hemesis.

Variceal bleeding is the most common cause of severe GI bleeding in childhood. Biliary atresia and portal venous obstruction are the most common causes. Hemorrhages due to portal hypertension from pre-hepatic obstruction carry a better prognosis but are more precocious than those from an intrahepatic origin, as observed in cirrhosis or liver fibrosis. Varices in patients with biliary atresia are at high risk of bleeding and need careful preventive monitoring.

A recent extensive literature search identified 13 randomized control trials with a clear indication of the number of adult patients with ongoing bleeding and their clinical outcomes. Treatment of esophageal varices with band ligation appeared to be the most effective approach (91%), significantly ($p < 0.02$) more successful than vasoconstrictive treatment with vasopressin/terlipressin (68%) or vasoactive treatment with somatostatin/octreotide (76%), although not statistically superior to sclerotherapy (81%). Sclerotherapy was not statistically better than medical treatments.[104] Somatostatin and octreotide were more effective than pitressin plus nitroglycerine in patients with acute variceal hemorrhage, with fewer side-effects.[105]

In the pediatric literature, studies are rare. Vasopressin has side-effects such as arrhythmias, hypertension, oliguria and seizures. The doses presented in the literature range from 0.1 to 0.4 U/1.73 m^2 per min. Data suggest that the use of intravenous vasopressin at doses greater than 0.01 U/kg per min to control GI bleeding will increase the incidence of complications but not improve the control of bleeding.[106]

Terlipressin (triglycyl lysine vasopressin) is a synthetic analog of vasopressin. It can be administered as intermittent slow bolus (20–30 min) injections at a dose of 20–30 μg/kg every 4–8 h (maximum 1 mg). In a critical analysis of the literature it was considered as the vasoactive agent of choice in acute variceal bleeding in adults.[107] The same group reported that terlipressin appears to be the only pharmacological agent, compared to placebo, that reduces the mortality rate in acute esophageal variceal and hypertensive gastropathy bleedings.[108]

Somatostatin and octreotide appear to be equivalent in terms of therapeutic efficacy but octreotide is the less expensive option. For suspected variceal bleeding, an octreotide infusion should be initiated immediately. In order to prevent further bleeding the drug should be continued for 2–5 days after an endoscopic variceal ligation.[109] Octreotide is indicated in pediatric patients for non-digestive (e.g. nesidioblastosis) or non-bleeding digestive diseases (secretory diarrhea, pancreatitis, motility disorders, fistulae). A wide range of well-tolerated doses has been prescribed, from 1.4 to 20 μg/kg per day, subcutaneously. Some cases of chronic GI bleeding are also reported and have been controlled by 4–8 μg per day during 24–52 months.[110] The potential of octreotide to treat children with different gastrointestinal diseases was assessed in a recent review.[111]

The circulating half-life of octreotide is prolonged in cirrhotics, suggesting that the dosage regimens should be modified in such patients and be administered by continuous intravenous infusion to have a therapeutic effect in the management of acute variceal bleeding.[112] Some results favor octreotide over vasopressin/terlipressin in the control of esophageal variceal bleeding and suggest that it is a safe and effective adjunctive therapy after variceal obliteration techniques.[113]

In pediatric indications, GI bleeding control has been obtained using an initial dose of 1 μg/kg as a bolus infusion given in 5 min, followed by a 1 μg/kg per hour continuous infusion in children ranging in age from 2 to 18 years. Once variceal bleeding is suspected, octreotide infusion should be started, and continued for 5–7 days.[114,115] In children with acute bleeding, immediate pharmacotherapy with octreotide is recommended together with endoscopic variceal band ligation or sclerotherapy; all children surviving variceal hemorrhage should undergo secondary prophylaxis with band ligation.[116]

A randomized controlled trial in cirrhotic adults has shown that a bolus injection of somatostatin caused an immediate and marked decrease of the hepatic venous pressure gradient and azygos blood flow. The decrease seemed more pronounced compared to the effect of octreotide, probably owing to a nitric oxide-induced mechanism.[117] Continuous somatostatin infusions of 500–250 μg per hour have no systemic effects, but a more pronounced effect on splanchnic hemodynamics than the recommended 250 μg/h.[118] In patients with active bleeding at endoscopy, the 500 μg/h infusion dose achieved a higher rate of control of bleeding (82 vs. 60%, $p < 0.05$), fewer transfusions (3.7 ± 2.7 vs. 2.5 ± 2.3 units of blood, $p = 0.07$)[119] and better survival (93 vs. 70%, $p < 0.05$) than expected. There are no recommendations for this adaptation of the doses in children classically proposed as 3.5 μg/kg per hour after a slow bolus of 3.5 μg/kg.

Prevention of bleeding from portal hypertension Meta-analysis of the adult literature has shown significant reductions in the incidence of the first bleeding in cirrhotic adults by a treatment with a β-blocker. A randomized controlled trial found that primary prophylaxis of variceal hemorrhage was equal in the comparison of band ligation to propranolol,[120] and superior to isosorbide mononitrate. The efficacy and safety[121] in a pediatric population is presented in limited series. The dose schedule ranges from 1.5 to 9 mg/kg per day in three doses to reach a 25% reduction of the heart rate. A preventive reduction of the portal blood flow could be an adjuvant medical treatment waiting for the complete eradication of the varices by endoscopic procedures. Propranolol is contraindicated in cases with asthma, obstructive lung or cardiac disease or diabetes type 1.

The transjugular intrahepatic portosystemic shunt (TIPS)[122] and surgical portosystemic shunts with an autologous vessel have specific indications in cases of liver disease. TIPS is useful in patients who are candidates for transplantation.[123]

The technique of mesenteric–left portal bypass (Rex shunt) offers an elegant solution when the vascular anatomy allows this liver revascularization.[124,125]

Endoscopic treatment Endoscopic treatment is indicated in emergency conditions in order to stop an uncontrolled ongoing focal lesion such as an ulcer or varix. It is also indicated as a preventive measure to reduce the possibility of re-bleeding from esophageal varices or from colonic polyps. Treatment of high-risk lesions, such as hemorrhage from an eroded duodenal vessel should be approached with caution and with an available surgical team back-up. Most hemostatic endoscopic techniques commonly used in adults, such as electrocoagulation, laser photocoagulation, injection of epinephrine (adrenaline) and of sclerosants, band ligation and mechanical clips, have been applied in children. However, the series are limited, since these conditions are not frequent in pediatrics.[126,127] Furthermore, the instruments require a large working channel (available only in conventional endoscopes). Therefore, many devices cannot be used in pediatric instruments with narrow channels (2.0 mm), and conventional endoscopes cannot be inserted in small children. However, the needles used for injection techniques are also used for sclerotherapy and fit easily into the channel of pediatric endoscopes. Epinephrine is injected around the bleeding site without causing tissue destruction. This is a simple, inexpensive method. Argon plasma coagulation, a non-contact electrocoagulation, can also be used through the same narrow pediatric working channels.

Portal hypertension can be treated endoscopically either by using classical sclerotherapy or, more recently, by elastic band ligation of varices. Pediatric gastroenterology units managing children with liver diseases require trained endoscopists capable of performing both techniques. On many occasions bleeding from esophageal varices is self-limited and the insertion of Sengstaken–Blackmore tubes is unnecessary, since it is always poorly tolerated by children and induces anxiety without a clearly demonstrated benefit. The technique of injection of sclerosants (50% aetoxysclerol is the most commonly used agent) is no different from that used in adults, except that the volumes injected must be considerably reduced since serious complications such as strictures and perforations are dose related. Injection of cyanoacrylate (Histoacryl®) glue has, occasionally, also been reported.[128]

Sclerotherapy is used in extrahepatic as well as in intrahepatic liver diseases with a reported efficacy of 90%.[129–131] Secondary esophageal strictures occur in 5–20%, whereas deep ulcerations and perforations are rare. We recommend a semi-liquid diet during 2 days following sclerotherapy or band ligation. Coughing and vomiting should also be prevented.

Elastic band ligation of varices is currently used in most pediatric gastroenterology centers with success. It is a quick procedure requiring greater endoscopic skill because of the relatively large device used to release the elastic band.[132–134] Recent devices allow multiple elastic ligations, although it seems difficult (and probably dangerous) to ligate more than two or three varices at the same time. Only large varices deserve band ligation and the complete cure of esophageal varices combines initial band ligation with subsequent sclerotherapy.[135,136]

Endoscopic treatment of the lower GI tract is primarily polypectomy. On rare occasions other hemostatic techniques such as laser, sclerotherapy, band ligation and electrocautery have been used for vascular colonic anomalies. The polypectomy technique is similar to that used in the adult with the same snares and electrocautery units. The main differences reside in the fact that it is advisable to perform these procedures under general anesthesia, not only for the sake of pain relief but also for safety reasons, unnecessary movements being most undesirable and potentially dangerous. Although the vast majority of polyps are of the benign juvenile type, every effort in order to retrieve the polyp for histology studies is strongly recommended.[137] It is also advisable to limit the number of polyps removed at the same procedure to a maximum of ten.

Aspirin and other NSAIDs have been used to reduce the number of polyps in patients with familial adenomatous polyposis. Cyclooxygenase-2 inhibitors have now been approved by the Food and Drug Administration for adjuvant treatment of familial adenomatous polyposis.[138]

REFERENCES

1. Longstreth GF. Epidemiology of hospitalization for acute upper gastrointestinal hemorrage: a population based study. *Am J Gastroenterol* 1995; **90**: 206–210.
2. Vreeburg EM, Snel P, de Bruijne JW et al. Acute upper gastrointestinal bleeding in the Amsterdam area: incidence, diagnosis, and clinical outcome. *Am J Gastroenterol* 1997; **92**: 236–243.
3. Stav K, Reif S. Gastrointestinal bleeding in children – etiology and diagnosis. Survey of patients in a Tel Aviv medical center, in the years 1990 to 1997. *Harefuah* 2000; **138**: 534–538.
4. Fox V. Gastrointestinal bleeding in infancy and childhood. *Gastroenterol Clin North Am* 2000; **29**: 37–67.
5. Chaibou M, Tucci M, Dugas MA et al. Clinically significant upper GI bleeding in a pediatric intensive care unit. *Pediatrics* 1998; **102**: 933–938.
6. Chalasani N, Kahi C, Francois F et al. Improved patient survival after acute variceal bleeding: a multicenter, cohort study. *Am J Gastroenterol* 2003; **98**: 653–659.
7. Lacroix J, Nadeau D, Laberge S et al. Frequency of upper gastrointestinal tract bleeding in a pediatric intensive careunit. *Crit Care Med* 1992; **20**: 35–42.
8. Mougenot JF, Duche M. Hemorragies digestives. In Navarro J, Schmitz J, eds. *Gastroenterologie Pediatrique*, 2nd edn. Paris: Flammarion, 2000: 612–621.
9. Faubion WA, Perrault J. Gastrointestinal bleeding. In Walker WA, Durie PR, Hamilton JR, Walker-Smith JA, Watkins JB, eds. *Pediatric Gastrointestinal Disease*, 3rd edn. Hamilton, Ontario: BC Decker, 2000: 164–178.
10. Bacchini PL, Ruspaggiari C, Fornaroli F, Torroni F. L'endocopia digestiva in Urgenza. In De Angelis GL, ed. *L'endoscopia digestiva in eta pediatrica e giovanile*. Rome: EMSI, 2002: 111–113.
11. Donatone JO, Ben R. Hemorragia Digestiva. In Morano J, ed. *Pediatría*. Buenos Aires: Atlante, 1997: 705–716.
12. Richards RJ, Donica MB, Grayer D. Can the blood urea nitrogen/creatinine ratio distinguish upper from lower gastrointestinal bleeding? *J Clin Gastroenterol* 1990; **12**: 500–504.
13. Stellato T, Rhodes RS, McDougal WS. Azotemia in upper gastrointestinal hemorrhage. A review. *Am J Gastroenterol* 1980; **73**: 486–489.
14. Moss G. Technique of iced saline lavage in upper GI hemorrhage. *Am J Surg* 1971; **122**: 565–566.

15. Dusek JL. Iced gastric lavage slows bleeding in gastric hemorrhage. *Crit Care Nurse* 1984; **4**: 8.
16. Rana S. Gastric lavage in upper GI hemorrhage: should iced saline solution be used? *J Assoc Physicians India* 1990; **38**: 377.
17. Andrus CH, Ponsky JL. The effects of irrigant temperature in upper GI hemorrhage: a requiem for iced saline lavage. *Am J Gastroenterol* 1987; **82**: 1062–1064.
18. Gilbert DA, Saunders DR. Iced saline lavage does not slow bleeding from experimental canine gastric ulcers. *Dig Dis Sci* 1981; **26**: 1065–1068.
19. Kelly D. Vitamin K-deficiency bleeding in neonates. *J Pediatr Gastroenterol Nutr* 1999; **29**: 532.
20. Cornelissen M, von Kries R, Loughnan P, Schubiger G. Prevention of vitamin K deficiency bleeding: efficacy of different multiple oral dose schedules of vitamin K. *Eur J Pediatr* 1997; **156**: 126–130.
21. de Boissieu D, Bargaoui K, Sakiroglu O et al. Esophagogastroduodenitis in the newborn. A propos of 32 cases. *Arch Fr Pediatr* 1989; **46**: 711–715.
22. de Boissieu D, Dupont C, Barbet JP et al. Distinct features of upper GI endoscopy in the newborn. *J Pediatr Gastroenterol Nutr* 1994; **18**: 334–338.
23. Deneyer M, Goossens A, Pipeleers-Marichal M et al. Esophagitis of likely traumatic origin in newborns. *J Pediatr Gastroenterol Nurtr* 1992; **15**: 81–84.
24. Maki M, Ruuska T, Kuusela AL et al. High prevalence of asymptomatic esophageal and gastric lesions in preterm infants in intensive care. *Crit Care Med* 1993; **21**: 1817–1819.
25. Kuusela AL, Maki M, Ruuska T, Laippala P. Stress-induced gastric findings in critically ill newborn infants: frequency and risk factors. *Intensive Care Med* 2000; **26**: 1501–1506.
26. Ganga-Zandzou PS, Ategbo S, Michaud L et al. Neonatal esophago-gastro-duodenoscopy. A propos of 123 examinations performed on 107 newborn infants. *Arch Pediatr* 1997; **4**: 320–324.
27. Benhamou PH, Cheikh A, Francoual C et al. Possible protection by breast-feeding against severe esophageal and gastric lesions in the neonate. A case–control study. *Biol Neonate* 1998; **73**: 337–339.
28. Benhamou PH, Francoual C, Glangeaud MC et al. Risk factors for severe esophageal and gastric lesions in term neonates: a case–control study. *J Pediatr Gastroenterol Nutr* 2000; **31**: 377–380.
29. Kliegman RM, Fanaroff AA. Necrotizing enterocolitis. *N Engl J Med* 1984; **310**: 1093–1103.
30. Takeuchi S, Tamate S, Nakahira M, Kadowaki H. Esophagitis in infants with hypertrophic pyloric stenosis: a source of hematemesis. *J Pediatr Surg* 1993; **28**: 59–62.
31. Bontems P, Robert F, Van Gossum A et al. *Helicobacter pylori* modulation of gastric and duodenal mucosal T cell cytokine secretions in children compared with adults. *Helicobacter* 2003; **8**: 216–226.
32. Donta ST, Myers MG. *Clostridium difficile* toxin in asymptomatic neonates. *J Pediatr* 1982; **15**: 431–434.
33. Sherertz RJ, Sarubbi FA. The prevalence of *Clostridium difficile* and toxin in a nursery population: a comparison between patients with necrotizing enterocolitis and an asymptomatic group. *J Pediatr* 1982; **100**: 435–439.
34. Ein SH, Alton D, Palder SB et al. Intussusception in the 1990s: has 25 years made a difference? *Pediatr Surg Int* 1997; **12**: 374–376.
35. Spiro DM, Arnold DH, Barone F. Association between antibiotic use and primary idiopathic intussusception. *Arch Pediatr Adolesc Med* 2003; **157**: 54–59.
36. Murthi GV, Raine PA. Preoperative enterocolitis is associated with poorer long-term bowel function after Soave–Boley endorectal pull-through for Hirschsprung disease. *J Pediatr Surg* 2003; **38**: 69–72.
37. Cannon RA, Lee G, Cox KL. Gastrointestinal hemorrhage due to Mallory–Weiss syndrome in an infant, *J Pediatr Gastroenterol Nutr* 1985; **4**: 323–324.
38. Lamiell JM, Weyandt TB. Mallory–Weiss syndrome in two children. *J Pediatr* 1978; **92**: 583–584.
39. Bak-Romaniszyn L, Malecka-Panas E, Czkwianianc E, Planeta-Malecka I. Mallory–Weiss syndrome in children. *Dis Esophagus* 1999; **12**: 65–67.
40. Rotenbacher D, Bode G, Brenner H. Dynamics of *Helicobacter pylori* infection in early childhood in a high-risk group living in Germany: loss of infection higher than acquisition. *Aliment Pharmacol Ther* 2002; **16**: 1663–1668.
41. De Giacomo C, Valdambrini V, Lizzoli F et al. A population-based survey on GI tract symptoms and *Helicobacter pylori* infection in children and adolescents. *Helicobacter* 2002; **7**: 356–363.
42. Norrashidah AW, Henry RL. Fundoplication in children with gastro-oesophageal reflux disease. *J Pediatr Child Health* 2002; **38**: 156–159.
43. Yachha SK, Ghoshal UC, Gupta R et al. Portal hypertensive gastropathy in children with extrahepatic portal venous obstruction: role of variceal obliteration by endoscopic sclerotherapy and *Helicobacter pylori*. *J Pediatr Gastroenterol Nutr* 1996; **23**: 20–23.
44. Lopriore E, Markhorst DG, Gemke RJ. Ventilator-associated pneumonia and upper airway colonisation with Gram negative bacilli: the role of stress ulcer prophylaxis in children. *Intensive Care Med* 2002; **28**: 763–767.
45. Stark ME, Gostout CJ, Balm RK. Clinical features and endoscopic management of Dieulafoy's disease. *Gastrointest Endosc* 1992; **38**: 545–550.
46. Descos B, Hermier M, Foasso MF. Comparative study of 4 groups of gastroduodenal ulcers in children. *Arch Fr Pediatr* 1984; **41**: 399–404.
47. Autret-Leca E. A general overview of the use of ibuprofen in paediatrics. *Int J Clin Pract* 2003; **135**: 9–12.
48. Lesko SM. The safety of ibuprofen suspension in children. *Int J Clin Pract* 2003; **135**: 50–53.
49. Litalien C, Jacqz-Aigrain E. Risks and benefits of nonsteroidal anti-inflammatory drugs in children: a comparison with paracetamol. *Paediatr Drugs* 2001; **3**: 817–858.
50. Aggarwal A, Chandra J, Aneja S et al. An epidemic of dengue hemorrhagic fever and dengue shock syndrome in children in Delhi. *Indian Pediatr* 1998; **35**: 727–732.
51. Cervantes-Bustamante R, Ramirez-Mayans J, Mata-Rivera N et al. Juvenile polyposis in Mexican children. *Rev Gastroenterol Mex* 2002; **67**: 150–154.
52. Mougenot JF, Baldassare ME, Mashako LM. Recto-colic polyps in the child. Analysis of183 cases. *Arch Fr Pediatr* 1989; **46**: 245–248.
53. St-Vil D, Brandt ML, Panic S et al. Meckel's diverticulum in children: a 20-year review. *J Pediatr Surg* 1991; **26**: 1289–1292.
54. Pinero A, Martinez-Barba E, Canteras M et al. Surgical management and complications of Meckel's diverticulum in 90 patients. *Eur J Surg* 2002; **168**: 8–12.
55. Stephen TC, Bendon RW, Nagaraj HS, Sachdeva R. Antral duplication cyst: a cause of hypergastrinemia, recurrent peptic ulceration, and hemorrhage. *J Pediatr Gastroenterol Nutr* 1998; **26**: 216–218.
56. Kaplan B, Benson J, Rothstein F et al. Lymphonodular hyperplasia of the colon as a pathologic finding in children with lower gastrointestinal bleeding. *J Pediatr Gastroenterol Nutr* 1984; **3**: 704–708.
57. Meyerovitz MF, Fellows KE. Typhlitis: a cause of gastrointestinal hemorrhage in children. *Am J Roentgenol* 1984; **143**: 833–835.
58. Saulsbury FT. Henoch–Schönlein purpura in children. Report of 100 patients and review of the literature. *Medicine (Baltimore)* 1999; **78**: 395–409.

59. Yoshioka K, Yagi K, Moriguchi N. Clinical features and treatment of children with hemolytic uremic syndrome caused by enterohemorrhagic *Escherichia coli* 0157:H7 infection: experience of an outbreak in Sakai City, 1996. *Pediatr Int* 1999; **41**: 223–227.
60. Elliott EJ, Robins-Browne RM, O'Loughlin EV et al. Nationwide study of haemolytic uraemic syndrome: clinical, microbiological and epidemiological features. *Arch Dis Child* 2001; **85**: 125–131.
61. Misselwitz J, Karch H, Bielazewska M et al. Cluster of haemolytic–uremic syndrome caused by Shiga toxin-producing *Escherichia coli* 026:H11. *Pediatr Infect Dis J* 2003; **22**: 349–354.
62. Ukarapol N, Chartapisak W, Lertprasertsuk N et al. Cytomegalovirus-associated manifestations involving the digestive tract in children with human immunodeficiency virus infection. *J Pediatr Gastroenterol Nutr* 2002; **35**: 669–673.
63. Chirletti P, Caronna R, Arcese W et al. Gastrointestinal emergencies in patients with acute intestinal graft-versus-host disease. *Leuk Lymphoma* 1998; **29**: 129–137.
64. Martinez Martinez L, Sastre Urgelles A, Ortega Martinez L et al. Neutropenic enterocolitis in children with cancer. *An Esp Pediatr* 1997; **46**: 367–371.
65. Pardi DS, Loftus EV Jr, Tremaine WJ et al. Acute major GI hemorrhage in inflammatory bowel disease. *Gastrointest Endosc* 1999; **49**: 153–157.
66. Gorski AM, Goulet O, Jehannin B et al. Digestive hemorrhage and bacterial overgrowth in children. *Arch Fr Pediatr* 1988; **45**: 569–571.
67. Cremer M, Rodesch P, Cadranel S. Fiberendoscopy of the GI tract in children. Experience with newly designed fiberscopes. *Endoscopy* 1974; **6**: 18–19.
68. Cadranel S, Rodesch P. Pediatric endoscopy in children: preparation and sedation. *Gastroenterology* 1977; **71**: 41–45.
69. Cadranel S, Rodesch P, Peeters JP, Cremer M. Fiberendoscopy of the gastrointestinal tract in children. A series of 100 examinations. *Am J Dis Child* 1977; **131**: 41–45.
70. Majd M. Radionuclide imaging in pediatrics. *Pediatr Clin North Am* 1985; **32**: 1559–1579.
71. Wesselhoeft CW, DeLuca FG, Luke M. Positive 99mTc-pertechnetate scan in a child with intestinal arteriovenous malformation. *Pediatr Surg* 1986; **21**: 71–72.
72. Smith R, Copely DJ, Bolen FH. 99mTc RBC scintigraphy: correlation of gastrointestinal bleeding rates with scintigraphic findings. *Am J Roentgenol* 1987; **148**: 869–874.
73. Maeda M, Yamashiro Y. Diagnostic red blood cell scintigraphy in GI tract bleeding from an intestinal hemangioma. *J Pediatr Gastroenterol Nutr* 1986; **5**: 987–989.
74. Afshani E, Berger PE. Gastrointestinal tract angiography in infants and children. *J Pediatr Gastroenterol Nutr* 1986; **5**: 173–186.
75. Meyerovitz MF, Fellows KE. Angiography in gastrointestinal bleeding in children. *Am J Roentgenol* 1984; **143**: 837–840.
76. Rabenstein T, Krauss N, Hahn EG, Konturek P. Wireless capsule endoscopy – beyond the frontiers of flexible gastrointestinal endoscopy. *Med Sci Monit* 2002; **8**: 128–132.
77. Fritscher-Ravens A, Swain CP. The wireless capsule: new light in the darkness. *Dig Dis* 2002; **20**: 127–133.
78. Costamagna G, Shah SK, Riccioni ME et al. A prospective trial comparing small bowel radiographs and video capsule endoscopy for suspected small bowel disease. *Gastroenterology* 2002; **123**: 999–1005.
79. Eliakim R, Fischer D, Suissa A et al. Wireless capsule video endoscopy is a superior diagnostic tool in comparison to barium follow-through and computerized tomography in patients with suspected Crohn's disease. *Eur J Gastroenterol Hepatol* 2003; **15**: 363–367.
80. Saurin JC, Delvaux M, Gaudin JL et al. Diagnostic value of endoscopic capsule in patients with obscure digestive bleeding: blinded comparison with video push-enteroscopy. *Endoscopy* 2003; **35**: 576–584.
81. Seidman EG. Wireless capsule video-endoscopy: an odyssey beyond the end of the scope. *J Pediatr Gastroenterol Nutr* 2002; **34**: 333–334.
82. Mallet E, Cron J, Stoller J. Wireless-capsule video-endoscopy: preliminary results in children. *Arch Pediatr* 2003; **10**: 244–245.
83. Anwar RM, Dhanji A, Fish A, Singh S. Impact of protocol-based guidelines on the management and outcome of acute upper gastrointestinal hemorrhage in a district general hospital. *Can J Gastroenterol* 2003; **17**: 97–100.
84. Mougenot JF, Balquet P. Les hématémèses de l'enfant. Approche diagnostique actuelle. *In Journées Parisiennes de Pédiatrie*. Paris: Flammarion Médecine-Sciences, 1978: 243–253.
85. Blumer JL, Rothstein FC, Kaplan BS et al. Pharmacokinetic determination of ranitidine pharmacodynamics in pediatric ulcer disease. *J Pediatr* 1986; **108**: 630.
86. Lugo RA, Harrison AM, Cash J et al. Pharmacokinetics and pharmacodynamics of ranitidine in critically ill children. *Crit Care Med* 2001; **29**: 759–764.
87. Gedeit RG, Weigle CG, Havens PL, Werlin SL. Control and variability of gastric pH in critically ill children. *Crit Care Med* 1993; **21**: 1850–1855.
88. Osteyee JL, Banner W Jr. Effects of two dosing regimens of intravenous ranitidine on gastric pH in critically ill children. *Am J Crit Care* 1994; **3**: 267–272.
89. Harrison AM, Lugo RA, Vernon DD. Gastric pH control in critically ill children receiving intravenous ranitidine. *Crit Care Med* 1998; **26**: 1433–1436.
90. Wells TG, Heulitt MJ, Taylor BJ et al. Pharmacokinetics and pharmacodynamics of ranitidine in neonates treated with extracorporeal membrane oxygenation. *J Clin Pharmacol* 1998; **38**: 402–407.
91. Fontana M, Tornaghi R, Petrillo M et al. Ranitidine treatment in newborn infants: effects on gastric acidity and serum prolactin levels. *J Pediatr Gastroenterol Nutr* 1993; **16**: 406–411.
92. Kuusela AL. Long-term gastric pH monitoring for determining optimal dose of ranitidine for critically ill preterm and term neonates. *Arch Dis Child Fetal Neonatal Ed* 1998; **78**: 151–153.
93. Kelly EJ, Chatfield SL, Brownlee KG et al. The effect of intravenous ranitidine on the intragastric pH of preterm infants receiving dexamethasone. *Arch Dis Child* 1993; **69**: 37–39.
94. Garg DC, Baltodano N, Jallad NS et al. Pharmacokinetics of ranitidine in patients with renal failure. *J Clin Pharmacol* 1986; **26**: 286–291.
95. Garg DC, Baltodano N, Perez GO et al. Pharmacokinetics of ranitidine after intravenous administration in hemodialysis patients. *Pharmacology* 1985; **31**: 189–193.
96. Netzer P, Gaia C, Sandoz M et al. Effect of repeated injection and continuous infusion of omeprazole and ranitidine on intragastric pH over 72 hours. *Am J Gastroenterol* 1999; **94**: 351–357.
97. Jacqz-Aigrain E, Bellaich M, Faure C et al. Pharmacokinetics of intravenous omeprazole in children. *Eur J Clin Pharmacol* 1994; **47**: 181–185.
98. Kiilerich S, Rannem T, Elsborg L. Effect of intravenous infusion of omeprazole and ranitidine on twenty-four-hour intragastric pH in patients with a history of duodenal ulcer. *Digestion* 1995; **56**: 25–30.
99. Cederberg C, Thomson AB, Mahachai V et al. Effect of intravenous and oral omeprazole on 24-hour intragastric

acidity in duodenal ulcer patients. *Gastroenterology* 1992; **103**: 913–918.

100. Hasselgren G, Keelan M, Kirdeikis P. Optimization of acid suppression for patients with peptic ulcer bleeding: an intragastric pH-metry study with omeprazole. *Eur J Gastroenterol Hepatol* 1998; **7**: 601–606.
101. Cash BD. Evidence-based medicine as it applies to acid suppression in the hospitalized patient. *Crit Care Med* 2002; **30**: S373–S378.
102. Fasseas P, Leybishkis B, Rocca G. Omeprazole versus ranitidine in the medical treatment of acute upper gastrointestinal bleeding: assessment by early repeat endoscopy. *Int J Clin Pract* 2001; **55**: 661–664.
103. Selby NM, Kubba AK, Hawkey CJ. Acid suppression in peptic ulcer haemorrhage: a 'meta-analysis'. *Aliment Pharmacol Ther* 2000; **14**: 1119–1126.
104. Gross M, Schiemann U, Muhlhofer A, Zoller WG. Meta-analysis: efficacy of therapeutic regimens in ongoing variceal bleeding. *Endoscopy* 2001; **33**: 737–746.
105. Zhang HB, Wong BC, Zhou XM. Effects of somatostatin, octreotide and pitressin plus nitroglycerine on systemic and portal haemodynamics in the control of acute variceal bleeding. *Int J Clin Pract* 2002; **56**: 447–451.
106. Tuggle DW, Bennett KG, Scott J, Tunell WP. Intravenous vaso-pressin gastrointestinal hemorrhage in children. *J Pediatr Surg* 1988; **23**: 627–629.
107. Ioannou GN, Doust J, Rockey DC. Systematic review: terlipressin in acute oesophageal variceal haemorrhage. *Aliment Pharmacol Ther* 2003; **17**: 53–64.
108. Ioannou G, Doust J, Rockey DC. Terlipressin for acute esophageal variceal hemorrhage. *Cochrane Database Syst Rev* 2003; CD002147
109. Sadowski DC. Use of octreotide in the acute management of bleeding esophageal varices. *Can J Gastroenterol* 1997; **11**: 339–343.
110. Zellos A, Schwarz KB. Efficacy of octreotide in children with chronic gastrointestinal bleeding. *J Pediatr Gastroenterol Nutr* 2000; **30**: 442–446.
111. Heikenen JB, Pohl JF, Werlin SL, Bucuvalas JC. Octreotide in pediatric patients. *J Pediatr Gastroenterol Nutr* 2002; **35**: 600–609.
112. Jenkins SA, Nott DM, Baxter JN. Pharmacokinetics of octreotide in patients with cirrhosis and portal hypertension; relationship between the plasma levels of the analogue and the magnitude and duration of the reduction in corrected wedged hepatic venous pressure. *HPB Surg* 1998; **11**: 13–21.
113 Corley DA, Cello JP, Adkisson W et al. Octreotide for acute esophageal variceal bleeding: a meta-analysis. *Gastroenterology* 2001; **120**: 946–954.
114. Siafakas C, Fox VL, Nurko S. Use of octreotide for the treatment of severe gastrointestinal bleeding in children. *J Pediatr Gastroenterol Nutr* 1998; **26**: 356–359.
115. Tauber MT, Harris AG, Rochiccioli P. Clinical use of the long acting somatostatin analogue octreotide in pediatrics. *Eur J Pediatr* 1994; **153**: 304–310.
116. McKiernan PJ. Treatment of variceal bleeding. *Gastrointest Endosc Clin North Am* 2001; **11**: 789–812.
117. Matrella E, Valatas V, Notas G et al. Bolus somatostatin but not octreotide reduces hepatic sinusoidal pressure by a NO-independent mechanism in chronic liver disease. *Aliment Pharmacol Ther* 2001; **15**: 857–864.
118. Cirera I, Feu F, Luca A et al. Effects of bolus injections and continuous infusions of somatostatin and placebo in patients with cirrhosis: a double-blind hemodynamic investigation. *Hepatology* 1995; **22**: 106–111.
119. Moitinho E, Planas R, Banares R et al. Variceal Bleeding Study Group. Multicenter randomized controlled trial comparing different schedules of somatostatin in the treatment of acute variceal bleeding. *J Hepatol* 2001; **35**: 712–718.
120. Lui HF, Stanley AJ, Forrest EH et al. Primary prophylaxis of variceal hemorrhage: a randomized controlled trial. *Gastroenterology* 2002; **123**: 735–744.
121. Shashidhar H, Langhans N, Grand RJ. Propranolol in prevention of portal hypertensive hemorrhage in children: a pilot study. *J Pediatr Gastroenterol Nutr* 1999; **29**: 12–17.
122. Rossle M, Haag K, Ochs A et al. The transjugular intrahepatic portosystemic stent–shunt procedure for variceal bleeding. *N Engl J Med* 1994; **330**: 165–171.
123. Heyman MB, LaBerge JM, Somberg KA et al. Transjugular intrahepatic portosystemic shunts (TIPS) in children. *J Pediatr* 1997; **131**: 914–919.
124. de Ville de Goyet J, Clapuyt P, Otte JB. Extrahilar mesenterico-left portal shunt to relieve extrahepatic portal hypertension after partial liver transplant. *Transplantation* 1992; **53**: 231-232.
125. Fuchs J, Warmann S, Kardorff R et al. Mesenterico-left portal vein bypass in children with congenital extrahepatic portal vein thrombosis: a unique curative approach. *J Pediatr Gastroenterol Nutr* 2003; **36**: 213–216.
126. Kato SG, Ozawa A, Ebina K et al. Endoscopic ethanol injection for treatment of bleeding peptic ulcer. *Eur J Pediatr* 1994; **153**: 873–875.
127. Noronha PA, Leist MH. Endoscopic laser therapy for GI bleeding from congenital lesions. *J Pediatr Gastroenterol Nutr* 1988; **7**: 375–378.
128. Fuster S, Costaguta A, Tobacco O. Treatment of bleeding gastric varices with tissue adhesive (Histoacryl) in children. *Endoscopy* 1998; **30**: S39–S40.
129. Hassall E, Berquist WE, Ament ME et al. Sclerotherapy for extrahepatic portal hypertension in childhood. *J Pediatr* 1989; **115**: 69–74.
130. Sokal EM, Van Hoorebeeck N, Van Obergh L et al. Upper GI tract bleeding in cirrhotic children candidates for liver transplantation. *Eur J Pediatr* 1992; **151**: 326–328.
131. Stringer MD, Howard ER. Longterm outcome after injection sclerotherapy for oesophageal varices in children with extrahepatic portal hypertension. *Gut* 1994; **35**: 257–259.
132. Yachha SK, Sharma BC, Kumar M et al. Endoscopic sclerotherapy for esophageal varices in children with extrahepatic portal venous obstruction: a follow up study. *J Pediatr Gastroenterol Nutr* 1997; **24**: 49–52.
133. Fox VL, Carr-Locke DL, Connors PJ et al. Endoscopic ligation of esophageal varices in children. *J Pediatr Gastroenterol Nutr* 1995; **20**: 202–208.
134. Cano J, Urruzuno P, Medinal E et al. Treatment of esophageal varices by endoscopic ligation in children. *Eur J Pediatr Surg* 1995; **5**: 299–302.
135. Saski T, Hasegawa T, Nakajima K et al. Endoscopic variceal ligation in the management of gastroesophageal varices in postoperative biliary atresia. *J Pediat Surg* 1998; **33**: 1628–1632.
136. Price MR, Sartorelli KH, Karrer FM et al. Management of esophageal varices in children by endoscopic variceal ligation. *J Pediatr Surg* 1996; **31**: 1056–1059.
137. Latt TT, Nicholl R, Domizio P et al. Rectal bleeding and polyps. *Arch Dis Child* 1993; **69**: 144–147.
138. Giercksky KE. COX-2 inhibition and prevention of cancer. *Best Pract Res Clin Gastroenterol* 2001; **15**: 821–833.
139. Marchant J, Summers K, McIsaac RL, Wood JR. A comparison of two ranitidine infusion regimens in critically ill patients. *Aliment Pharmacol Ther* 1988; **2**: 55–63.

39 Approach to the child with acute diarrhea

Hania Szajewska and Jacek Z Mrukowicz

Introduction

In this chapter we present a pragmatic, evidence-based approach to the child with acute diarrhea, which is a result of an extensive review of several diagnostic and treatment options that have been studied in children. We searched MEDLINE for relevant, good-quality observational studies on etiology, epidemiology, risk factors, clinical presentation, complications and diagnostic work-up. To evaluate treatments for acute diarrhea, we focused on data from meta-analyses, systematic reviews and randomized controlled clinical trials in MEDLINE, the Cochrane Library and the Cochrane Central Register of Controlled Trials. Finally, we searched MEDLINE for published evidence-based clinical practice guidelines developed by respected scientific societies or expert groups. We included conclusions from these documents in our chapter, because they contain recommendations based usually on a process of balancing benefit and harm of available approaches and interventions, and are commonly used to improve the quality of health care in many countries. In all cases the last search date was May 2003.

Background

Management of a child presenting with diarrhea is a logical chain of clinical decisions guided by answers to the following main questions.

(1) Does the patient have acute diarrhea?
(2) What is the presumed etiology of diarrhea (infectious vs. non-infectious)?
(3) Should the patient be treated in an ambulatory setting or in the hospital?
(4) Are stool cultures or any other laboratory tests required?
(5) How should the patient be rehydrated: orally or intravenously?
(6) How should the patient be managed nutritionally?
(7) Should the patient receive any antimicrobial drug, and – if yes – which one is the most suitable?
(8) Should the patient be treated with any other drug or preparation (antidiarrheal, antimotility, antiemetic)?
(9) Are there any complications or specific clinical situations that require modification of the recommended approach?

Below, we provide readers with the information required to answer those questions and make the best decisions for each patient.

Definitions

In published clinical practice guidelines and consensus documents, diarrhea is defined as a change in bowel movement for the individual child, characterized by an increase in the water content, volume and – usually – frequency of stools.[1,2] This definition also applies to exclusively breast-fed infants, in whom patterns of bowel habits vary widely from several soft or loose stools per day in one group of infants to one or two soft stools every 4–5 days in the other. For practical purposes and epidemiological investigations, diagnostic criteria in children – except for exclusively breast-fed infants – include a decrease in consistency (loose or liquid) and increase in frequency of bowel movements to ≥ 3 per 24 h.[1,3] Since the increased water content in stools is the most important criterion (frequent passage of formed stools is not diarrhea), some authors advise to diagnose diarrhea when the volume of loose stools exceeds 10 g/kg of body weight per 24 h in children and 200 g/24 h in adolescents and adults.[2] Although this definition is more precise and may be used in a research setting, it is impractical and difficult to incorporate into daily medical practice.

Depending on the duration of the diarrhea, the illness may be considered acute, persistent, or chronic. Acute diarrhea is an episode of less than 14 days in duration (usually a few days). Diarrhea lasting longer than 14 days is called persistent diarrhea, and longer than 30 days – chronic.[3] This categorization is somewhat arbitrary, but longer duration of diarrhea (> 14 days) significantly increases the probability that symptoms are caused by some specific pathogens (see below) or the etiology of the disease is non-infectious, and the risk of a poor outcome is greater. Therefore, a more detailed diagnostic work-up towards a different etiology and modification of management are required. Persistent diarrhea, often of presumed infectious etiology, complicated by malnutrition and a high risk of serious non-intestinal infections, is a significant problem in developing countries.[1] In this chapter we will discuss exclusively the management of acute diarrhea in immunocompetent children.

Prevalence, incidence and disease burden

Acute diarrhea is one of the most common diseases in children, and the second leading cause of morbidity and mortality worldwide. Every child encounters at least one diarrheal episode.[3–6] The attack rate in developed countries ranges from 1.2 to 1.9 illnesses per person annually in the general population, and is higher in the first 2–3 years of life (2.5 illnesses per child per year to even five in those attending day-care centers).[3] The incidence is greater in developing countries, and in some tropical areas may reach even 6–10 episodes per child annually in children aged < 3 years.[7,8] The estimated global number of deaths due to diarrheal diseases in children is 2.9–3.3 million annually (7945–9041 per day!), with most case fatalities taking place in infants and young children in the developing world.[9,10] However, the disease is not inconsequential in developed countries, leading to a great number of medical visit and hospital admissions. In the USA, for example, it was estimated that only for rotavirus – the leading cause of gastroenteritis in young children – by the age of 5 years one in eight children seeks medical attention, one in 78 is hospitalized and one in 100 000–200 000 die.[11]

Etiology

In the vast majority of cases acute diarrhea is a symptom of gut infection – mostly viral, or bacterial, less frequently parasitic (Table 39.1).[12–18] In immunocompetent, well-nourished children, yeasts (*Candida*) are not implicated as a cause of diarrhea.[19] The prevalence of specific intestinal pathogens differs between developed and developing countries and depends on age. In developed countries most episodes, especially in young children (< 5 years), result from enteric viral infections (mainly group A rotavirus). The second most prevalent group are bacterial infections: *Salmonella* spp., *Campylobacter* spp., *Shigella* spp. and *Escherichia coli* (enterotoxigenic, ETEC; enteropathogenic, EPEC; enterohemorrhagic, EHEC; enteroaggregative, EagEC; and diffusely adherent, DAEC).[15,16,20–23] The prevalence of bacterial pathogens in older children (> 5 years) is greater than in younger children.[16,24] In developing countries in young children (< 5 years) bacterial infections predominate slightly over viral causes (with group A rotavirus being the most common virus implicated). Bacterial pathogens most frequently isolated in this age group include: *E. coli*, *Shigella* spp., *Salmonella* spp. (including *S. typhi*) and *Vibrio cholerae*.[8,13,14,17,18] The prevalence of bacterial pathogens increases with age.[8]

Pathogenesis

From the practical point of view infectious acute diarrhea may be classified as *non-inflammatory* (watery) and *inflammatory* (invasive). In the first type the main symptoms include watery diarrhea, with or without vomiting, with little or no inflammatory response in the stool (no gross blood or red blood cells and leukocytes or lactoferrin). The etiologies of non-inflammatory infectious diarrhea include: enteric viruses, bacteria that do not invade the intestinal wall or bloodstream (EPEC, DAEC, EAggEC), bacteria that produce enterotoxin-mediated secretory diarrhea (ETEC, *Vibrio cholerae*) and some parasites (*Giardia*, *Cryptosporidium*).[3]

Table 39.1 Etiological agents of acute infectious diarrhea in immunocompetent children

Viruses*	Bacteria*	Bacterial enterotoxins*†	Parasites*
Group A rotavirus‡	*Salmonella* spp.†‡	*Staphylococcus aureus* (toxins A, B, C, D, E)	*Cryptosporidium parvum*
Caliciviruses and Norwalk virus	*Campylobacter jejuni,*‡ *Campylobacter coli*	*Clostridium perfringens* (toxins A, C)	*Giardia lamblia*
Astrovirus	*Shigella* spp.	*Bacillus cereus* (heat-labile and heat-stabile toxin)	*Blastocystis hominis*
Adenovirus (type 40/41)	*Escherichia coli*: EPEC,‡‡ EHEC, EIEC, ETEC,‡‡ EAggEC, DAEC		*Entamoeba histolytica*‡‡
Group B rotavirus** Group C rotavirus**	*Yersinia enterocolitica, Yersinia pseudotuberculosis*		*Balantidium coli*
Picobirnavirus**	*Clostridium difficile*		*Isospora belli***
Others (coronavirus, norovirus, parvovirus, torovirus, Breda virus)†† *Listeria monocytogenes*†**	*Vibrio cholerae*‡‡		*Cyclospora* spp.**
	*Vibrio parahaemolyticus*** *Plesiomonas shigelloides*** *Aeromonas hydrophila***		

EPEC, enteropathogenic *E. coli*, EHEC, enterohemorrhagic *E. coli* (also known as Shiga-toxin-producing *E. coli*); EIEC, enteroinvasive *E. coli*; ETEC, enterotoxigenic *E. coli*; EaggEC, enteroaggregative *E. coli*; DAEC, diffusely adherent *E. coli*

*In order of decreasing prevalence in the particular category in developed countries; †implicated in food-borne illness; ‡common in developed countries; ** rare cause; †† unknown role in children; ‡‡found in developing countries and endemic regions

Inflammatory diarrhea, characterized by gross (dysentery) or occult blood and/or an increased number of leukocytes (or increased level of their marker lactoferrin) in the stool, is the result of intestinal wall invasion by *Salmonella*, *Shigella*, *Campylobacter*, *Yersinia enterocolitica*, hemorrhagic *E. coli* (O157:H7), enteroinvasive *E. coli* (EIEC) or *Clostridium difficile*.[1,3] This classification is helpful in planning selective microbiological testing and selecting patients who may benefit from empirical antibacterial therapy.[3,25] For a more comprehensive and specific discussion of infectious diarrheas, see Chapters 9–12.

Complications

The main complications of acute diarrhea are dehydration (leading to hypovolemic shock in severe cases) and – especially in developing countries – malnutrition (particularly in persistent diarrhea).[1] The mainstay of management is therefore adequate rehydration and early resumed, appropriate feeding.[1,26–28] In more severe cases, especially in malnourished children and when clear fluids, broth or cow's milk were used instead of oral rehydration solution for initial treatment of dehydration, electrolyte abnormalities (hyper- or hyponatremia, hypokalemia) may be present.[28–30] Hyponatremia is especially common in children with shigellosis and in severly malnourished children with edema.[1] In developed countries, as shown in the UK, electrolyte derangement is rare, with 1% of admissions having hypernatremia and no reports of hypokalemia or hyponatremia.[28] Awareness of typical signs of hypernatremia, including doughy, velvety skin, dry and beefy red mucous membranes, muscular signs such as twitching and hyper-reflexia and central nervous system symptoms such as lethargy, confusion, irritability, rigidity, generalized convulsions and coma, is of particular importance, although there are no published studies on the reliability of these signs in diagnosing hypernatremia. In most moderate-to-severe cases of diarrhea there is some degree of metabolic acidosis. In malnourished children hypoglycemia may be a serious complication contributing to increased case fatality.[31,32] Persistent diarrhea is a serious complication in young children in developing countries, since it results in severe malnutrition and increased risk of death.[31,33,34] Pathogens such as EPEC, EAggEC, *Shigella*, *Cryptosporidium* and *Giardia* are significantly correlated with persistent infectious diarrhea.[35,36] Some bacterial causes of diarrhea result in other serious long-term sequelae: EHEC (or Shiga-toxin-producing *E. coli*; STEC) infection may be followed by hemolytic uremic syndrome[37] and *C. jejuni* infection by Guillain–Barré syndrome.[38]

Diagnosis

Clinical features

Rapid onset of liquid stools with or without accompanying symptoms or signs such as nausea, vomiting, fever and abdominal pain comprise the clinical picture of acute diarrhea. As mentioned previously, for practical reasons, clinical syndromes of non-inflammatory and inflammatory diarrhea may be distinguished.[1,3,25] Watery diarrhea, sometimes with more prominent vomiting, and no blood or signs of an inflammatory response in the stool (leukocytes or lactoferrin) are features of the first diarrheal syndrome, whereas gross blood (dysentery) and an increased number of stool leukocytes and/or presence of lactoferrin, usually accompanied by fever and prominent, cramping abdominal pain and/or tenesmus, are characteristic of the second syndrome. The presence of gross blood or an inflammatory response in the stool significantly increases the chance for isolation of invasive enteric bacteria.[39–41]

Differential diagnosis

If there are no signs and/or symptoms suggesting an alternative diagnosis (Table 39.2), an episode of acute diarrhea is considered presumably to be infectious. If symptoms and signs persist beyond 10–14 days, the diagnosis should be revised, and a more detailed work-up is indicated focusing on complications and chronic conditions.

Table 39.2 List of conditions that should be considered in the differential diagnosis of acute diarrhea in children

Acute appendicitis
Intussusception
Hypertrophic pyloric stenosis
Malrotation
Hirschsprung's disease (enterocolitis variant)
Ileus
Necrotizing enterocolitis
Inflammatory bowel disease
Food allergy or intolerance
Malaria
Measles (particularly in malnourished children)
Sepsis
Jejunal and ileal diverticula
Diabetic ketoacidosis
Staphylococcal toxic shock syndrome
Celiac disease and other malabsorption syndromes
Irritable bowel syndrome
Pneumonia
Meningitis
Urinary tract infection (pyelonephritis)
Acute otitis media, mastoiditis
Drugs (laxatives, antibiotics, potassium salts, antineoplastic agents)
Congenital adrenal hyperplasia
Münchausen and Münchausen per proxy syndromes
Radiotherapy
Lead intoxication
Mushroom poisoning (*Amanita*)

Estimation of dehydration

Assessment of dehydration is an essential step in evaluation of a child presenting with diarrhea, since the degree of dehydration is the criterion for deciding upon the route of rehydration (oral or intravenous), thus determining also the need for hospital admission. The gold standard is to compare the current body weight of a patient with a recent measurement before the onset of the disease. Dehydration is usually quantified from the percentage of total body weight loss, and categorized as mild (< 5%), moderate (5–10%) or severe (> 10%). Unfortunately, this method is not always possible in practice, especially in infants and young children who grow relatively fast. Therefore, the World Health Organization (WHO) has proposed a set of clinical symptoms and signs, which helps to approximate the degree of dehydration (volume of fluid loss; Table 39.3)[1] and to decide about an appropriate treatment plan (see below). In one prospective cohort study performed in a developing country, prolonged 'skinfold' (skin pinch going back slowly), altered neurological status, sunken eyes and dry oral mucosa were found to correlate best with the percentage of dehydration in infants.[42] A study in American children reported the capillary refill time to be closely correlated with the degree of dehydration,[43] although this was not confirmed subsequently by others.[42,44,45] In another small prospective study performed in hospitalized American children conventional laboratory blood tests were found to be poorly predictive of fluid deficits.[46]

Table 39.3 Assessment for dehydration in a patient with diarrhea (from reference 1)

Degree of dehydration	Condition	Eyes	Tears	Mouth and tongue	Thirst	Skin pinch	Total body weight loss (%)	Estimated fluid deficit (ml/kg)
None or mild	well, alert	normal	present	moist	drinks normally, not thirsty	goes back quickly	<5	<50
Moderate	restless, irritable*	sunken	absent	dry	thirsty, drinks eagerly*	goes back slowly*	5–10	50–100
Severe	lethargic or unconscious; floppy*	very sunken and dry	absent	very dry	drinks poorly or not able to drink*	goes back slowly *	>10	>100

*'Major' signs; to classify a patient into a particular category, at least two signs must be present, including one 'major'

Laboratory testing

Microbiological testing

The majority of episodes of acute infectious diarrhea in children are mild and resolve spontaneously without any specific antimicrobial treatment, hence no in-depth diagnostic testing is usually required for managing an individual case. Antimicrobials are beneficial only in a small, selected proportion of cases (see below), and empirical antibiotic treatment should generally be avoided in acute diarrhea.[3] Routine stool cultures in acute diarrhea have a very low yield (1.5–5.6%) and relatively high cost.[3] On the other hand, organism-specific diagnosis may have great public health importance, allowing for outbreak detection and control, and prevention of spread of infection in the community. Selective testing is therefore recommended, since it improves the yield and cost-effectiveness of stool cultures.[3]

In cases of bloody (dysenteric) or inflammatory (see below) community-acquired or traveler's diarrhea (especially if accompanied by fever) testing for *Salmonella, Shigella, Campylobacter, E. coli* 0157:H7 (and other STEC) and *Clostridium difficile* toxin A and B is recommended, the latter particularly if the diarrhea is severe and the child was treated with antibiotics during the few preceding weeks. History suggesting food-borne disease should also prompt appropriate stool cultures.[3]

In children most cases of nosocomial diarrhea are of viral (mainly rotaviral) or non-bacterial etiology.[47–49] In older children with nosocomial diarrhea, *Clostridium difficile* may be more prevalent than in infants and toddlers.[50] Therefore, older children with nosocomial diarrhea (i.e. with onset after 3 days in hospital), especially when disease is severe, should be tested for *Clostridium difficile* toxins. Routine stool cultures for standard bacterial pathogens are discouraged for episodes occurring after the third day in hospital, since the yield is very low, except for epidemics of bloody diarrhea or suspected food-borne disease.[3,51]

In diarrhea that persists for longer than 10–14 days, especially in an immunocompromised patient, testing for *Giardia, Cryptosporidium, Cyclospora* and *Isospora belli* should be considered.[3] In almost all cases of pediatric diarrheal diseases a single stool test is diagnostic, regardless of the type of pathogen isolated.[3,52]

Fecal screening tests

Initial screening for inflammatory diarrhea may be helpful in identifying patients requiring stool cultures or tests. One systematic review evaluated several methods for the identification of patients with inflammatory bacterial diarrhea: Wright's or methylene blue stain of fresh stool for fecal leukocytes, a test for fecal occult blood, an immunoassay for fecal lactoferrin (a neutrophil marker) and a stain for fecal leukocytes combined with clinical data. It was concluded that fecal lactoferrin appeared to be the most accurate and useful diagnostic test for initial screening for inflammatory diarrhea.[53] Five subsequent studies confirmed the utility of lactoferrin testing to determine patients infected with invasive enteric pathogens.[54–58] Disadvantages of lactoferrin testing include its additional cost and false-positive results in breast-fed infants.[3] Lactoferrin is often negative, despite blood in stool, in STEC infection and *Entamoeba histolytica* colitis.[3]

Electrolyte measurement

Serum electrolyte measurements are generally unnecessary, as most episodes of dehydration caused by diarrhea are isonatremic (see above). The American Academy of Pediatrics recommends that electrolyte levels should be measured in moderately dehydrated children whose histories are inconsistent with straightforward diarrheal episodes and in all severely dehydrated children. Furthermore, electrolytes should be measured in children with features of hypernatremic dehydration that can result from ingestion of hypertonic liquids or the loss of hypotonic fluids in the stool or urine.[27]

Management

The main objectives in the therapeutic approach to a child with acute diarrhea are: to prevent or treat dehydration; to promote weight gain following rehydration; and to reduce the duration of diarrhea and quantity of stool output.

Rehydration

Oral versus intravenous rehydration in mild to moderate dehydration

One systematic review of six randomized controlled trials of unequal methodological quality in 371 children in developed countries with acute gastroenteritis, mostly with mild-to-moderate dehydration, found no significant difference between oral versus intravenous fluids in duration of diarrhea, duration of hospitalization, or weight gain at discharge.[59] Furthermore, patients treated with oral rehydration therapy were not found to be at higher risk of iatrogenic hypernatremia or hyponatremia. Failure of oral treatment defined as the need for intravenous treatment was reported in 3.6% of patients. Similar findings were reported in two additional randomized controlled trials not included in the systematic review.[60,61] In view of the evidence from these clinical trials, oral rehydration therapy is generally recommended to replace fluid and electrolyte losses caused by diarrhea in infants and children with mild-to-moderate dehydration.[1,27,28,62]

Oral versus intravenous rehydration in severe dehydration

One randomized controlled trial in 470 children with severe acute gastroenteritis aged 1–18 months found that oral rehydration compared with intravenous therapy reduced the duration of diarrhea and increased weight gain at discharge, and was associated with fewer adverse effects.[63] Failure of oral treatment occurred in 0.4%. No significant differences in the death rate were found. Although oral rehydration may be used even in severe dehydration, intravenous therapy is generally recommended if the patient is more than 10% dehydrated, as well as in case of shock, failure of oral rehydration therapy, if the patient is unconscious or ileus is present.[27,28,62]

Nasogastric tube versus intravenous fluids

One randomized controlled trial comparing nasogastric and intravenous methods of rehydration in young children with acute dehydration due to vomiting and/or diarrhea found that rehydration through a nasogastric tube was equally efficacious as intravenous rehydration, and was associated with fewer complications and was cost-effective.[64] The nasogastric route of rehydration may be suitable, particularly outside facility-based treatment centers when intravenous fluids are difficult to administer.

Scientific background for using oral rehydration solutions

Oral rehydration therapy, hailed as potentially the most important medical discovery of the 20th century,[65] is the mainstay of treatment of acute diarrhea in patients of all ages provided they are able to drink and that the dehydration is not severe.[1,27,62,66] The effectiveness of oral rehydration solutions depends on co-transport of sodium ions and glucose (or other organic solutes) across the brush-border membranes of enterocytes,[67] which results in passive absorption of water and other electrolytes. It is now well established that this glucose–sodium co-transport system remains largely intact during nearly all kinds of acute infectious gastroenteritis, irrespective of their cause. The integrity of this mechanism during any diarrheal disease makes oral rehydration therapy appropriate for treatment of diarrhea associated with dehydration. Today, a number of different oral rehydration solutions (ORSs) are available. The major differences in these solutions are related to sodium concentration and the source of carbohydrates that affects osmolality (Table 39.4).[68]

Despite the proven efficacy of oral rehydration therapy, it remains underused.[68,69] The main reason for this is that an ORS neither reduces the frequency of bowel movements and fluid loss nor shortens the duration of illness, which decreases its acceptance. Parents, but also health-care professionals, demand safe, effective and inexpensive agents as an additional treatment that will visibly reduce the rate of stool loss and the duration of diarrhea. Such a product could, perhaps, be helpful in efforts to reduce the common practice of treating diarrhea with ineffective antidiarrheal

Table 39.4 Composition of World Health Organization (WHO) and European Society for Paediatric Gastroenterology, Hepatology and Nutrition (ESPGHAN) oral rehydration solutions

	WHO	ESPGHAN
Sodium (mmol/l)	90	60
Potassium (mmol/l)	20	20
Chloride (mmol/l)	80	60
Base (mmol/l)	30 (bicarbonate)	10 (citrate)
Glucose (mmol/l)	111	74–111
Osmolality (mOsm/l)	331	225–260

drugs or unnecessary antibiotics. In the following section we briefly summarize the results of clinical trials of improved oral rehydration solutions.

Reduced-osmolarity oral rehydration solutions

There is a significant body of literature indicating that osmolality is a major factor in determining ORS efficacy.[70] The reduction of the osmolarity of the ORS may be achieved either by reducing the concentration of sodium and glucose or by replacing glucose with a complex carbohydrate.

The optimum sodium concentration of an ideal ORS that would preserve and/or correct the electrolyte balance in a child with acute diarrhea without carrying the risk of inducing hypo- or hypernatremia is controversial. For many years, WHO has recommended the standard formulation of a glucose-based ORS with 90 mmol/l of sodium and 111 mmol/l of glucose and a total osmolarity of 311 mmol/l. This original WHO standard ORS was designed for patients with cholera or cholera-like (toxigenic) diarrhea associated with large stool sodium losses. However, in developed countries, where diarrheal diseases are rarely associated with large stool sodium losses, the use of WHO standard ORS has led to hypernatremia, especially in infants < 3 months of age.[71,72] In these settings, a number of controlled clinical trials have shown the effectiveness of an ORS with a lower sodium concentration, such as 50–60 mmol/l in infants < 3 months and in older children.[73–77] Consequently, based on these studies, the American Academy of Pediatrics (AAP) and the European Society for Paediatric Gastroenterology, Hepatology and Nutrition (ESPGHAN) recommend the use of an ORS with a reduced concentration of sodium for children in developed countries.[27,78]

A recent systematic review of 12 randomized controlled trials has shown that a reduced-osmolarity ORS has beneficial effects over the WHO standard ORS in reducing the needs for unscheduled intravenous infusions, and is associated with smaller stool volume after randomization, and less vomiting. The incidence of hyponatremia was not significantly increased in children receiving a reduced-osmolarity ORS compared with WHO standard ORS. Based on these data, reduced-osmolarity ORS should be the first-line treatment of dehydration in children with non-cholera diarrhea. At present, there are no sufficient data on cholera to change recommendations for this condition.[79]

Cereal-based oral rehydration solutions

Cereal-based ORSs, using various carbohydrate staples such as rice-starch or wheat, are thought to reduce diarrhea by adding more substrate to the gut lumen without increasing osmolality, thus providing additional glucose molecules for glucose-mediated absorption. A meta-analysis of 22 clinical trials of rice-based ORSs compared with the standard ORS found that these solutions appear to be effective in reducing the 24-h stool output in children and adults with cholera, but not in children with non-cholera diarrhea. Contrary to reduced-osmolarity ORS, rice-based ORS did not reduce the need for intravenous infusions.[80]

Maltodextrin-based oral rehydration solutions

Maltodextrins are glucose polymers with low osmotic activity and easy solubility in water without cooking. Several trials have demonstrated that maltodextrin-based ORS formulations (50 g/l) and WHO standard ORS are equally effective in reducing total stool output and duration of diarrhea in children with acute non-cholera gastroenteritis.[81,82] Since maltodextrin-based ORSs are not superior to WHO standard ORS, these are not recommended in the management of acute gastroenteritis.

Amino acid oral rehydration solutions

Another approach to developing an improved ORS formulation was based on adding certain neutral amino acids (glycine, alanine, glutamine) or their dipeptides to WHO standard ORS, as they enhance the absorption of sodium ions and water (independently of other organic solutes). At present, amino acid-containing ORSs are not recommended for either non-cholera or cholera diarrhea, since they are more costly and did not demonstrate clinical advantage over WHO ORS for children with acute non-cholera diarrhea or over rice-based ORS for patients with cholera.[83]

Amylase resistant starch oral rehydration solutions

A novel approach to enhancing the clinical effectiveness of ORSs is the addition of ingredients that utilize the absorptive capacity of the human colon. When undigested carbohydrates, such as an amylase-resistant starch or guar gum, reach the colon they are fermented into short-chain fatty acids, which induce colonic absorption of sodium and water from both the normal and the secreting colon.[84] A small randomized trial in 48 adolescents and adults with watery diarrhea due to *Vibrio cholerae* showed that amylase-resistant starch added to the standard WHO ORS reduced stool output. Furthermore, the mean duration of diarrhea was shorter in the amylase-resistant starch group than in the rice-flour group and the standard WHO ORS group.[85] In a similarly designed trial in 150 children, partially hydrolyzed guar gum added to the standard WHO ORS compared with the control group substantially reduced the duration of diarrhea and modestly reduced stool output in acute non-cholera diarrhea in young children. In contrast, a recent multicenter study by the ESPGHAN in 144 boys with acute non-cholera diarrhea with mild-to-moderate dehydration showed that a mixture of non-digestible carbohydrates (soy polysaccharide 25%, α-cellulose 9%, gum arabic 19%, fructo-oligosaccharides 18.5%, inulin 21.5%, resistant starch 7%) was ineffective as an adjunct to oral rehydration therapy.[86] Further trials are therefore needed.

Other fluids

A recent survey suggested that in some countries fluids other than ORS are used for oral rehydration, including tea, cola drinks, fruit juices or chicken broth.[69] Such beverages contain inappropriate electrolyte (low sodium and potassium) and glucose concentrations, are very often hyperosmotic, and are potentially dangerous as treatments in a dehydrated child. Homemade ORS prepared by parents is also not an optimal treatment, because its preparation may involve significant errors in composition and osmolality.[87,88]

Recommendations on management of dehydration

See Table 39.5 for a summary of practical recommendations for management of dehydration in children with acute diarrhea.

Criteria for hospital admission

No studies were found in which out-patient and in-patient management of children with acute diarrhea was compared. However, in some clinical practice guidelines experts recently reached consensus and specified indications for hospital admission.[1,28,89] Management in the hospital is generally required in: severely dehydrated children; children whose parents are unable to manage oral rehydration at home; patients intolerant of oral rehydration; in case of failure of treatment, e.g. worsening diarrhea and/or progression of dehydration despite oral rehydration therapy; bloody or persistent diarrhea in a severely malnourished child; and other concerns, e.g. diagnosis uncertain, potential for surgery, child at risk, child irritable or drowsy, or child younger than 2 months.

Nutritional management

Early versus late feeding

For many decades it has been an established practice that children with acute diarrhea should be fasted for 24–48 h.[90,91] In various forms, these erroneous practices persist today in many communities.[69] However, several controlled trials have clearly shown the beneficial effect of early feeding in malnourished[92] as well as in adequately nourished children.[93–102] Based on these studies, the ESPGHAN recently recommended, in line with AAP and WHO recommendations, that the optimal management of mild-to-moderately dehydrated children should consist of oral rehydration with an ORS over 3–4 h, and rapid reintroduction of normal feeding thereafter.[1,26,27] Early feeding may decrease the intestinal permeability induced by infection, minimize protein and energy deficits, and thereby maintain growth, reduce functional and morphological hypotrophy associated with bowel rest and maintain disaccharidase activity.[103,104]

Breast feeding

For infants who are breast fed exclusively, continuation of breast feeding at all times results in

Table 39.5 Practical approach to management of a child with acute diarrhea based on published clinical practice guidelines (references 1, 26–28)

Management of dehydration

Estimate severity of dehydration (see Table 39.3).

In mildly to moderately dehydrated children, initial oral rehydration with an oral rehydradtion solution (ORS) given over 3–4 h should be the preferred treatment of fluid and electrolyte losses caused by acute gastroenteritis

In developed countries use of a hypotonic ORS (sodium 60 mmol/l, glucose 74–111 mmol/l), instead of WHO standard ORS, is recommended

Suggested intake of the ORS depends on the degree of dehydration:
- mild dehydration (<5%): 30–50 ml/kg over 3–4 h
- moderate dehydration (5–10%): 50–100 ml/kg over 3–4 h
- severe dehydration (10%): 100–150 ml/kg over 3–4 h)

In severe dehydration, intravenous rehydration might be necessary. Indications for intravenous therapy include:
- >10% dehydration
- signs of shock
- unconsciousness
- presence of ileus
- failure of oral replacement therapy
- inability to tolerate an ORS

Prevention of further dehydration could be accomplished by supplementing maintenance fluids with an ORS for ongoing losses (10 ml/kg per watery stool or approximate volume of vomits)

Nutritional management

Rapid reintroduction of an age-appropriate normal diet (including solids) should take place after successful rehydration for 3–4 h with an ORS is accomplished

Routine use of a special formula is unjustified

Routine use of a diluted formula is unjustified

Continuation of breast feeding at all times is recommended

Pharmacological therapy

Antiemetics and antidiarrheal drugs should not be routinely given to infants and children with acute gastroenteritis

Stool cultures and tests should be performed selectively

Antimicrobial therapy is generally recommended for:
- shigellosis
- suspected cases of cholera
- symptomatic infection with invasive intestinal *Entamoeba histolytica*
- laboratory-proven symptomatic infection with *Giardia intestinalis*
- suspected infection with enteroinvasive bacteria in patients with an increased risk of invasive disease, including infants younger than 6 months and persons with malignant neoplasms, hemoglobinopathies, HIV infection or other immunosuppressive illness or therapy, chronic gastrointestinal tract disease, or severe colitis

decreased stool output, and is generally recommended.[105,106] Importantly, as demonstrated by the results of three randomized controlled trials[107–109] and some observational studies,[110–113] breast feeding protects against diarrhea, thereby this practice in addition may decrease the risk of recurrent diarrheal disease.

Lactose-containing versus reduced lactose or lactose-free feeds

Recurring diarrhea has been attributed to lactose intolerance that can occur for a short period of time after gastroenteritis, because of mucosal damage and temporary lactase deficiency. One systematic review of 13 randomized controlled trials has found that lactose-free feeds versus lactose-containing feeds reduced the duration of diarrhea in children with mild-to-severe dehydration.[114] Subsequent trials found conflicting results. Two found that lactose-free versus lactose-containing feeds significantly reduced the duration of diarrhea,[115,116] and the other two found no significant difference.[117,118] In Europe, where lactose intolerance appears to be uncommon, the ESPGHAN recommends that the normal diet can be resumed without restriction of lactose intake in most cases. However, if diarrhea worsens on the reintroduction of standard milk or formula, stool pH and/or reducing substances should be checked and lactose content reduced only if the stool is acid and contains $>0.5\%$ reducing substances.[26]

Diluted or full-strength milk or formula

There is concern that feeding full-strength formula or animal milk to infants aged less than 6 months with diarrhea may have adverse consequences, although one randomized controlled trial has shown that diluting formula or milk as opposed to using full-strength formula over 48 h did not reduce complications.[119] More recently, one randomized, unblinded, controlled study demonstrated that, in infants aged 3–12 months with acute diarrhea, decreasing the volume of each feed and increasing the frequency of feedings to 12 times per day (while maintaining the same total daily energy intake) speeded recovery, reduced fecal frequency and fecal weight, and increased weight gain during the recovery period.[120]

Recommendations on nutritional management

See Table 37.5 for a summary of practical recommendations on nutritional management of a child with acute diarrhea.

Pharmacological therapy

Rational use of antibacterial drugs

In the vast majority of children, acute infectious diarrhea is self-limited and antibacterial drugs are generally unnecessary, even when a bacterial cause is suspected. WHO recommends routine use of antibacterial agents only for shigellosis, suspected cases of cholera, symptomatic infection with invasive intestinal *Entamoeba histolytica* and laboratory-proven symptomatic infection with *Giardia intestinalis*.[1] Although of unproven benefit, anitmicrobial therapy is generally recommended for suspected infection with enteroinvasive bacteria (e.g. *Salmonella* gastroenteritis) in patients with an increased risk of invasive disease, including infants younger than 6 months of age and persons with malignant neoplasms, hemoglobinopathies, HIV infection or other immunosuppressive illness or therapy, chronic gastrointestinal tract disease, or severe colitis.[121] Furthermore, patients with bloody or inflammatory diarrhea accompanied by high fever, especially when the disease is moderate to severe, may benefit from empirical antibacterial treatment, modified subsequently on the basis of results of stool culture.[3] Antimicrobial treatment should be preceded by appropriate stool cultures or pathogen detection tests. One situation in which empirical antibiotics are commonly recommended without obtaining a fecal specimen is in cases of traveler's diarrhea, in which ETEC or other bacterial pathogens are usually the likely cause. Prompt treatment with trimethoprim–sulfamethoxazole in children or fluorochinolone in adolescents and adults can reduce the duration of illness from 3–5 days to less than 1–2 days.[3] Most of these episodes are self-limiting, and antimicrobial use should always be preceded by careful weighing of the benefits and potential harms of such treatment.[3] Details of treatment of specific infections are summarized in Table 39.6. Because of changing patterns of antimicrobial resistance, recent local patterns are critical in making decisions about antimicrobial therapy.[3] Irrational prescribing of antibiotics may cause more harm than good (for example, it prolongs the excretion of *Salmonella*, leads to the emergence of drug resistance among some bacterial strains, and increases the risk of antibiotic-associated diarrhea and pseudomembranous colitis).[122,123]

Antiemetic drugs

Vomiting is a common symptom in children with gastroenteritis. Metoclopramide, prochlorprezine and promethazine hydrochloride are effective

Table 39.6 Drugs for treatment of enteric pathogens (adapted from reference 3)

Pathogen	Recommended treatment in immunocompetent patients
Shigella species	TMP–SMZ 5 and 25 mg/kg, respectively, twice daily for 3 days (if susceptible) OR fluoroquinolone* for 5 days[185–190] OR nalidixic acid 55 mg/kg per day in four doses for 3 days[191] OR ceftriaxone 100 mg/kg per day in one or two doses[192] OR azithromycin[189]
Non-typhi species of *Salmonella*	not recommended routinely,[122,193,194] but advised if severe infection or in infants <6 months of age and persons with malignant neoplasms, hemoglobinopathies, HIV infection or other immunosuppressive illness or therapy, chronic gastrointestinal tract disease, or severe colitis TMP–SMZ (as above, if susceptible) OR fluoroquinolone* for 5–7 days[25,195,196] OR ceftriaxone 100 mg/kg per day in one or two doses[197]
Campylobacter species	erythromycin† 20–50 mg/kg per day in 2–4 doses for 5–7 days[198,199]
Enterotoxigenic *E. coli*	TMP–SMZ 5 (as above, if susceptible) OR fluoroquinolone* for 3 days[200–202]
Enteropathogenic *E. coli*	as above[203]
Enteroinvasive *E. coli*	as above[204,205]
Enteroaggregative *E. coli*	unknown
Enterohemorrhagic *E. coli* (STEC)	avoid antimotility drugs[206]; role of antibiotics unclear, and administration should be avoided[207–212]
Aeromonas/ Plesiomonas	TMP–SMZ (as above, if susceptible) OR fluoroquinolone*[213–217]
Yersinia species	antibiotics are not usually required;[218–220] deferoxamine therapy should be withheld;[221] for severe infections or associated bacteremia treat using combination therapy with doxycycline, aminoglycoside, TMP–SMZ, or fluoroquinolone*[222]
Vibrio cholerae O1 or O139	single dose doxycycline (>8 years of age) 6 mg/kg OR TMP–SMZ 5 and 25 mg/kg, respectively, twice daily for 3 days; OR single-dose fluoroquinolone*[223–227] OR single-dose azithromycin (20 mg/kg)[228]

Continued

Table 39.6 Continued

Pathogen	Recommended treatment in immunocompetent patients
Toxigenic *Clostridium difficile*	offending antibiotic should be withdrawn if possible[229–231] metronidazole 30 mg/kg per day in four doses for 10 days[232–234]
Giardia	metronidazole 15 mg/kg per day in three doses for 5 days[235–237] OR tinidazole 50 mg/kg single dose (maximum 2 g)[238] OR furazolidone 6 mg/kg per day in four doses for 7–10 days OR paromomycin 25–35 mg/kg per day in three doses for 7 days
Cryptosporidium species	if severe, consider paromomycin 25–35 mg/kg per day in two or four doses for 7 days
Isospora species	TMP-SMZ 5 and 25 mg/kg, respectively, twice daily for 7–10 days
Cyclospora species	TMP-SMZ 5 and 25 mg/kg, respectively, twice daily for 7–10 days[239,240]
Microsporidium species	not determined
Entamoeba histolytica	metronidazole 35–50 mg/kg per day in three doses for 7–10 days plus either diloxanide furoate 20 mg/kg per day in three doses for 10 days OR paromomycin 25–35 mg/kg per day in two or four doses for 7days[241–243]

TMP-SMZ trimethoprim–sulfamethoxazole
*Fluoroquinolones (i.e. ciprofloxacin, ofloxacin, norfloxacin) are not approved for treatment of children in some countries
†Antibiotics are most effective if given early in the course of illness

antiemetics. However, troublesome side-effects, including sedation and extrapyramidal reactions, occur frequently with standard doses.[124–126] Therefore, these drugs should be avoided in young children with vomiting associated with acute diarrhea. Two recent studies have suggested that intravenous or oral ondansetron, a specific serotonin ($5HT_3$) antagonist, decreases vomiting in children with gastroenteritis managed in the emergency room and reduces the need for intravenous fluid administration and hospital admission, and thus may have a valuable role as an antiemetic therapy.[127,128]

Antimotility or antiperistaltic drugs

There is a wide variety of drugs that alter intestinal motility, including loperamide hydrochloride, diphenoxylate with atropine, tincture of opium, camphorated tincture of opium and codeine. These drugs are widely used for the relief of symptoms during diarrheal episodes and are regarded as safe for adults and older children,[129,130] excluding those with bloody diarrhea or documented infection with Shiga toxin-producing *E. coli* (STEC).[3] However, antimotility treatment should not be given for acute diarrhea in infants and young children,[1,27,28] as numerous reports have documented severe and potentially life-threatening adverse effects, including lethargy, ileus, respiratory depression and coma.[131–134]

Adsorbents

In several countries dioctahedral smectite, a natural adsorbent clay capable of adsorbing viruses, bacteria, bacterial toxins and other intestinal irritants, is commonly used for the treatment of acute infectious diarrhea.[69] Three small randomized trials in children[135–137] have suggested that smectite compared with placebo was associated with moderately reduced duration of diarrhea, although there was no significant effect on total stool output. Other adsorbents such as kaolin–pectin, fiber, attapulgite (anhydrous aluminum silicate) and activated charcoal have not been shown to be of value in the treatment of acute diarrhea in children. Adsorbents are not recommended in the routine treatment of acute diarrhea in children.[1,27,28]

Antisecretory drugs

Bismuth subsalicylate, or other bismuth salt preparations, are common constituents of over-the-counter medications for diarrhea. Although the precise mechanism of their action remains unknown, antisecretory and antimicrobial properties have been suggested.[138–140] Three randomized controlled trials that compared bismuth subsalicylate with placebo in infants with acute watery diarrhea found that bismuth subsalicylate modestly reduced the duration and severity of diarrhea.[141–143] In addition to harmless and temporary side-effects (e.g. darkening of the tongue and stool), salicylate toxicity from bismuth subsalicylate use in children has been reported.[144] The routine use of bismuth subsalicylate is not recommended in the management of children with acute diarrhea.[1,27,28]

Racecadotril (acetorphan), is a newer antisecretory drug that exerts its antidiarrheal effects by inhibiting intestinal enkephalinase, thus preventing the breakdown of endogenous opioids (enkephalins) in the gastrointestinal tract, thereby reducing the secretion of water and electrolytes into the gut.[145] In two recent randomized placebo-controlled trials conducted in hospitalized children in developed and developing countries, racecadotril was effective in reducing the volume and frequency of stool output and in reducing the duration of diarrhea (particularly in children with rotavirus or *E. coli* diarrhea).[146,147] Although these data are interesting, the cost-effectiveness as well as safety needs to be defined before this drug is recommended in the routine management of children with acute diarrhea.

Probiotics

Probiotics are living micro-organisms that, upon ingestion in certain numbers, exert health benefits beyond their inherent general nutrition.[148] The most commonly used as probiotics are lactic acid bacteria, such as lactobacilli or bifidobacteria, and the non-pathogenic yeast *Saccharomyces boulardii*. The rationale for the use of probiotics is based on the assumption that they modify the composition of the colonic microflora and act against enteric pathogens. The evidence from two systematic reviews[149,150] and two subsequent randomized controlled trials[151,152] suggest a statistically significant effect and moderate clinical benefit of some probiotic strains in the treatment of acute gastroenteritis, mainly rotaviral, in infants and young children. *Lactobacillus* GG shows the most consistent effect. Other probiotic strains may also be effective, but should be evaluated in randomized controlled trials to prove their clinical utility, since not all products marketed as 'probiotic' are effective.[153] So far, the beneficial effects of probiotics in acute diarrhea in children seem to be: moderate; strain-dependent; dose-dependent (greater for doses $>10^{10}$–10^{11} CFU); significant in watery diarrhea and viral gastroenteritis, but not existing in invasive (inflammatory) bacterial diarrhea; and more evident when treatment with probiotics is initiated early in the course of diarrhea.[154]

Homeopathy

The role of homeopathic remedies in the treatment of acute childhood diarrhea is still controversial. A recent meta-analysis from three randomized controlled clinical trials involving 242 children aged 6 months to 5 years has suggested that some homeopathic treatment decreases the duration of acute diarrhea in children.[155] The exact mechanism by which homeopathic remedies could have exerted their activity is unclear.

Herbal medicine

No systematic review or randomized controlled trial was found on herbal medicine for the treatment of acute diarrhea in children.

Micronutrients (zinc, folic acid)

Zinc deficiency, which is common in young children in the developing world, is associated with impaired water and electrolyte absorption,[156–159] decreased brush-border enzymes,[160–162] and impaired cellular and humoral immunity.[163–166] As intestinal losses of zinc are considerably increased during acute diarrhea,[167,168] a number of trials have evaluated the effect of zinc supplements on diarrheal diseases. The findings suggest that in developing countries zinc supplementation results in clinically important reductions in the duration and severity of acute diarrhea when given as an adjunct to oral rehydration therapy,[169–174] or mixed with an ORS.[175] Further work is needed to clarify whether zinc supplementation would also be of benefit in developed countries in children with diarrhea without pre-existing zinc deficiency.

Previous reports have suggested that there is a therapeutic effect of folic acid in the treatment of acute diarrhea in children.[176] However, a recent well-designed double-blind randomized controlled trial in 106 males aged 6–23 months found no significant effect of folic acid compared with placebo in the treatment of acute watery diarrhea.[177]

Oral immunoglobulins

It has been claimed that oral administration of immunoglobulin-containing preparations of bovine colostrum from immunized cows, egg yolk immunoglobulin from immunized hens or pooled plasma-derived human intravenous immunoglobulins can provide passive immunity.[178] These preparations may inhibit intestinal viral adherence or viral replication and may have a role in the treatment of rotavirus infections. In fact, several randomized controlled trials have confirmed that orally administered immunoglobulins have reduced viral shedding and shortened the duration of rotavirus diarrhea.[179–182] No evidence was found that oral immunotherapy is effective in children with acute diarrhea caused by bacterial pathogens.[183,184] Except for intravenous immunoglobulins given orally in one study,[181] none of the specific preparations mentioned above is available commercially.

Recommendations for drug therapy

See Table 39.5 for a summary of practical recommendations for drug therapy of a child with acute diarrhea.

REFERENCES

1. World Health Organization. *The Treatment of Diarrhea. A Manual for Physicians and Other Senior Health Workers*. WHO/CDR/95.3. Geneva: World Health Organization, 1995.
2. Riedel BD, Ghishan FK. Acute diarrhea. In Walker WA, Durie PR, Hamilton JR, Walker-Smith JA, Watkins JB, eds. *Pediatric Gastrointestinal Disease*, 2nd edn. St. Louis: Mosby Year Book, 1996: 251–262.
3. Guerrant RL, van Gilder T, Steiner TS et al. Practice guidelines for the management of infectious diarrhoea. *Clin Inf Dis* 2001; **32**: 331–350.
4. World Health Organization. *Conquering Suffering, Enriching Humanity*. Report of the Director-General. Geneva: World Health Organization, 1997.
5. Bern C, Glass RI. Impact of diarrhoeal diseases worldwide. In Kapikian AZ, ed. *Viral Infections of the Gastrointestinal Tract*, 2nd edn. New York: Marcel Dekker, 1995.
6. Bern C, Martines J, de Zoysa I, Glass RI. The magnitude of the global problem of diarrhoeal disease: a ten year update. *Bull WHO* 1992; **70**: 705–714.
7. Glass RI, Lew JF, Gangarosa RE et al. Estimates of morbidity and mortality rates for diarrheal diseases in American children. *J Pediatr* 1991; **118**: S27–S33.
8. Kotloff KL, Winickoff JP, Ivanoff B et al. Global burden of *Shigella* infections: implications for vaccine development and implementation of control strategies. *Bull WHO* 1999; **77**: 651–666.
9. World Health Organization. *Fighting Disease, Fostering Development*. Report of the Director-General. Geneva: World Health Organization, 1996.
10. Bresee JS, Glass RI, Ivanoff B et al. Current status and future priorities for rotavirus vaccine development, evaluation and implementation in developing countries. *Vaccine* 1999; **17**: 2207–2222.
11. Glass RI, Bresee JS, Parashar DU et al. First rotavirus vaccine licensed: is there really a need? *Acta Paediatr* 1999; **426** (Suppl): 2–8.
12. Phavichtir N, Catto-Smith AG. Acute gastroenteritis in children. What role for antibacterials? *Pediatr Drugs* 2003; **5**: 279–290.

13. Huilan S, Zhen LG, Matham MM et al. Etiology of acute diarrhoea among children in developing countries: a multicentre study in five countries. *Bull WHO* 1991; **69**: 549–555.
14. Gracey M. Diarrheal disease in perspective. In Gracey M, Walker-Smith JA, eds. *Diarrheal Disease.* Vol 38. Nestle Nutrition Workshop Series Nestec Ltd. and Lippincott-Raven Publishers, Philadelphia, 1991: 1–12.
15. Caeiro JP, Mathewson JJ, Smith MA et al. Etiology of outpatient pediatric nondysenteric diarrhea: a multicenter study in the United States. *Pediatr Infect Dis J* 1999; **18**: 94–97.
16. Caprioli A, Pezzella C, Morelli R et al. Enteropathogens associated with childhood diarrhea in Italy. *Pediatr Infect Dis J* 1996; **15**: 876–883.
17. Abu-Elyazeed R, Wierzba TF, Mourad AS et al. Epidemiology of enterotoxigenic *E. coli* diarrhea in a pediatric cohort in a periurban area of lower Egypt. *J Inf Dis* 1999; **179**: 382–389.
18. Kapikian AZ. Viral gastroenteritis. *JAMA* 1993; **269**: 627–630.
19. Forbes D, Ee L, Camer-Pesci P, Ward PB. Faecal candida and diarrhea. *Arch Dis Child* 2001; **84**: 328–331.
20. Cohen MB. Etiology and mechanisms of acute infectious diarrhea in infants in the United States. *J Pediatr* 1991; **118**: S34–S39.
21. Guandalini S, Pensabene L, Abu Zikri M et al. *Lactobacillus* GG administered in oral rehydration solution to children with acute diarrhea: a multicenter European trial. *J Pediatr Gastroenterol Nutr* 2000; **30**: 54–60.
22. Gastanaduy AS, Begue RE. Acute gastroenteritis. *Clin Pediatr* 1999; **38**: 1–12.
23. Mrukowicz JZ, Krobicka B, Duplaga M et al. Epidemiology and impact of rotavirus diarrhoea in Poland. *Acta Paediatr* 1999; **426** (Suppl): 53–60.
24. Chalmers RM, Salmon RL. Primary care surveillance for acute bloody diarrhea, Wales. *Emerg Infect Dis* 2000; **6**: 412–414.
25. DuPont HL. Guidelines on acute infectious diarrhea in adults. The Practice Parameters Committee of the American College of Gastroenterology. *Am J Gastroenterol* 1997; **92**: 1962–1975.
26. Walker-Smith J, Sandhu B, Isolauri E et al. Recommendation for feeding in childhood gastroenteritis. *J Pediatr Gastroenterol Nutr* 1997; **24**: 619–620.
27. Provisional Committee on Quality Improvement, Subcommittee on Acute Gastroenteritis. Practice Parameter: the management of acute gastroenteritis in young children. *Pediatrics* 1996; **97**: 424–435.
28. Armon K, Stephenson T, MacFaul R et al. An evidence and consensus based guideline for acute diarrhea management. *Arch Dis Child* 2001; **85**: 132–142.
29. Abu-Ekteish F, Zahraa J. Hypernatraemic dehydration and acute gastroenteritis in children. *Ann Trop Paediatr* 2002; **22**: 245–249.
30. Moritz ML, Ayus JC. The changing pattern of hypernatremia in hospitalized children. *Pediatrics* 1999; **104**: 435–439.
31. Uysal G, Sokmen A, Vidinlisan S. Clinical risk factors for fatal diarrhea in hospitalized children. *Indian J Pediatr* 2000; **67**: 329–333.
32. Ahmed T, Ali M, Ullah MM et al. Mortality in severely malnourished children with diarrhoea and use of a standardised management protocol. *Lancet* 1999; **353**: 1919–1922.
33. Victora CG, Huttly SR, Fuchs SC et al. International differences in clinical patterns of diarrhoeal deaths: a comparison of children from Brazil, Senegal, Bangladesh, and India. *J Diarrhoeal Dis Res* 1993; **11**: 25–29.
34. World Health Organization. *Diarrhoeal Disease Control. Persistent Diarrhea in Children.* CCD/DDM/85.1. Geneva: World Health Organization, 1985.
35. Shahid NS, Sack DA, Rahman M et al. Risk factors for persistent diarrhoea. *BMJ* 1988; **297**: 1036–1038.
36. World Health Organization. *Persistent Diarrhea in Children in Developing Countries.* Report of a WHO meeting. WHO/CCD/88.27. Geneva: World Health Organization, 1988.
37. Wong CS, Jelacic S, Habeeb RL et al. The risk of the hemolytic–uremic syndrome after antibiotic treatment of *Escherichia coli* 0157:H7 infections. *N Engl J Med* 2000; **342**: 1930–1936.
38. Nachamkin I, Allos BM, Ho T. *Campylobacter* species and Guillain–Barré syndrome. *Clin Microbiol Rev* 1998 **11**: 555–567.
39. Talan DA, Moran GJ, Newdow M et al. Etiology of bloody diarrhea among patients presenting to US emergency departments: prevalence of *E. coli* 0157:H7 and other enteropathogens. *Clin Inf Dis* 2001; **32**: 573–580.
40. Choi SW, Park CH, Silva TM et al. To culture or not to culture: fecal lactoferrin screening for inflammatory bacterial diarrhea. *J Clin Microbiol* 1996; **34**: 928–932.
41. Huicho L, Campos M, Rivera J et al. Fecal screening tests in the approach to acute infectious diarrhea: a scientific overview. *Pediatr Infect Dis J* 1996; **15**: 486–494.
42. Duggan Ch, Refat M, Hashem M et al. How valid are clinical signs of dehydration in infants? *J Pediatr Gastroenterol Nutr* 1996; **22**: 56–61.
43. Saavedra JM, Harris GD, Li S et al. Capillary refilling (skin turgor) in the assessment of dehydration. *Am J Dis Child* 1991; **145**: 296–298.
44. Schriger DL, Baraff L. Defining normal capillary refill: variation with age, sex, and temperature. *Ann Emerg Med* 1988; **17**: 932–935.
45. Gorelick MH, Shaw KN, Baker MD. Effect of ambient temperature on capillary refill in healthy children. *Pediatrics* 1993; **92**: 699–702.
46. Teach SJ, Yates EW, Feld LG. Laboratory predictors of fluid deficit in acutely dehydrated children. *Clin Pediatr* 1997; **36**: 395–400.
47. Ford-Jones EL, Mindorff CM, Gold R et al. The incidence of viral-associated diarrhea after admission to a pediatric hospital. *Am J Epidemiol* 1990; **131**: 711–718.
48. Szajewska H, Kotowska M, Mrukowicz J et al. *Lactobacillus* GG in prevention of diarrhea in hospitalized children. *J Pediatr* 2001; **138**: 361–365.
49. Mastretta E, Longo P, Laccisaglia A et al. *Lactobacillus* GG and breast feeding in the prevention of rotavirus nosocomial infection. *J Pediatr Gastroenterol Nutr* 2002; **35**: 527–531.
50. Metropol SB, Luberti AA, De Jong AR. Yield from stool testing of pediatric inpatients. *Arch Pediatr Adolesc Med* 1997; **151**: 142–145.
51. Craven D, Brick D, Morrisey A et al. Low yield of bacterial stool culture in children with nosocomial diarrhea. *Pediatr Inf Dis J* 1998; **17**: 1040–1044.
52. Church DL, Cadrain G, Kabani A et al. Practice guidelines for ordering stool cultures in a pediatric population. Alberta Children's Hospital, Calgary, Alberta, Canada. *Am J Clin Pathol* 1995; **103**: 149–153.
53. Huicho L, Campos M, Rivera J et al. Fecal screening tests in the approach to acute infectious diarrhea: a scientific overview. *Pediatr Infect Dis J* 1996; **15**: 486–494.

54. Choi SW, Park CH, Silva TM et al. To culture or not to culture: fecal lactoferrin screening for inflammatory bacterial diarrhea. *J Clin Microbiol* 1996; **34**: 928–932.
55. Huicho L, Garaycochea V, Uchima N et al. Fecal lactoferrin, fecal leukocytes and occult blood in the diagnostic approach to childhood invasive diarrhea. *Pediatr Inf Dis J* 1997; **16**: 644–647.
56. Ruiz-Pelaez JG, Mattar S. Accuracy of fecal lactoferrin and other stool tests for diagnosis of invasive diarrhea at a Colombian pediatric hospital. *Pediatr Inf Dis J* 1999; **18**: 342–346.
57. McIver CJ, Hansman G, White P et al. Diagnosis of enteric pathogens in children with gastroenteritis. *Pathology* 2001; **33**: 353–358.
58. Venkataraman S, Ramakrishna BS, Kang G et al. Faecal lactoferrin as a predictor of positive faecal culture in small Indian children with acute diarrhoea. *Ann Trop Paediatr* 2003; **23**: 9–13.
59. Gavin N, Merrick N, Davidson B. Efficacy of glucose-based oral rehydration therapy. *Pediatrics* 1996; **98**: 45–51.
60. Singh M, Mahmoodi A, Arya LS et al. Controlled trial of oral versus intravenous rehydration in the management of acute gastroenteritis. *Indian J Med Res* 1982; **75**: 691–693.
61. Oritiz A. Rehidratacion oral: experiencia en el manejo de pacientes con gastroenteritis aguda en la sala de emergencia hospital pediatrico. *Bol Asoc Med P R* 1990; **82**: 227–233.
62. Murphy MS. Guidelines for managing acute gastroenteritis based on a systematic review of published research. *Arch Dis Child* 1998; **79**: 279–284.
63. Sharifi J, Ghavami F, Nowrouzi Z et al. Oral versus intravenous rehydration therapy in severe gastroenteritis. *Arch Dis Child* 1985; **60**: 856–860.
64. Nager AL, Wang VJ. Comparison of nasogastric and intravenous methods of rehydration in pediatric patients with acute dehydration. *Pediatrics* 2002; **109**: 566–572.
65. Anonymous. Water with sugar and salt. *Lancet* 1978; **2**: 300–301.
66. Avery ME, Snyder JD. Oral therapy for acute diarrhea. The underused simple solution. *N Engl J Med* 1990; **323**: 891–894.
67. Schultz SA. Sodium coupled solute transport by small intestine: a status report. *Am J Physiol* 1977; **223**: E249–E254.
68. Guarino A, Albano F, Guandalini S, for the ESPGHAN Working Group on Acute Diarrhea. Oral rehydration solution: toward a real solution. *J Pediatr Gastroenterol Nutr* 2001; **33**: S2–S12.
69. Szajewska H, Hoekstra JH, Sandhu B et al. Management of acute gastroenteritis in Europe and the impact of the new recommendations: a multicenter study. *J Pediatr Gastroenterol Nutr* 2000; **30**: 522–527.
70. Thillainayagam AV, Hunt JB, Farthing MJG. Enhancing clinical efficacy of oral rehydration therapy: is low osmolality the key? *Gastroenterology* 1998; **114**: 197–210.
71. Bhargarva SK, Sachder HPS, Das Gupta B et al. Oral rehydration of neonates and young infants with dehydrating diarrhea: comparison of low and standard sodium content in oral rehydration solutions. *J Pediatr Gastroenterol Nutr* 1984; **3**: 500–504.
72. Abdalla S, Helmy N, El Essaily M et al. Oral rehydration for the low birth weight baby with diarrhoea. *Lancet* 1984; **2**: 818–819.
73. Nalin DR, Hanland E, Ramlal A et al. Comparison of low and high sodium and potassium content in oral rehydration solutions. *J Pediatr* 1980; **97**: 848–853.
74. Santosham M, Daum RS, Dillman L et al. Oral rehydration therapy of infantile diarrhoea. A controlled study of well nourished children hospitalized in the United States and Panama. *N Engl J Med* 1982; **306**: 1070–1076.
75. Pizzaro D, Posada G, Villariceucis N et al. Oral rehydration in hypernatremic and hyponatremic diarrheal dehydration. Treatment with oral jejunal electrolyte solution. *Am J Dis Child* 1983; **137**: 730–734.
76. Bhargarva S, Sachder HPS, Das Gupta B et al. Oral therapy of neonates and young infants with dehydrating diarrhea: composition of low and standard sodium in oral rehydration solutions. *J Pediatr Gastroenterol Nutr* 1986; **6**: 416–422.
77. International Study Group on reduced-osmolality ORS solutions. Multicentre evaluation of reduced-osmolarity oral rehydration salts solution. *Lancet* 1995; **345**: 282–285.
78. Booth I, Cunha Ferreira R, Desjeux JF et al. Recommendations for composition of oral rehydration solutions from the children of Europe. Report of an ESPGAN working group. *J Pediatr Gastroenterol Nutr* 1992; **14**: 113–115.
79. Kim Y, Hahn S, Garner P. Reduced osmolarity oral rehydration solution for treating dehydration caused by acute diarrhoea in children (Cochrane Review). *The Cochrane Library*, Issue 2. Oxford: Update Software, 2003.
80. Fontaine O, Gore SM, Pierce NF. Rice-based oral rehydration solution for treating diarrhoea (Cochrane Review). *The Cochrane Library*, Issue 2. Oxford, 2003.
81. Akbar MS, Baker KM, Aziz MA et al. A randomized double-blind clinical trial of a maltodextrin containing oral rehydration solution in acute infantile diarrhoea. *J Diarrhoeal Dis Res* 1991; **9**: 33–37.
82. Santos Ocampo PD, Bravo LC, Rogacion JM et al. A randomized double-blind clinical trial of a maltodextrin containing oral rehydration solution in acute infantile diarrhea. *J Pediatr Gastroenterol Nutr* 1993; **16**: 23–28.
83. Bhan MK, Mahalanabis D, Fontaine O, Pierce NF. Clinical trials of improved oral rehydration salt formulations: a review. *Bull WHO* 1994; **72**: 945–955.
84. Binder HJ, Mehta P. Short-chain fatty acids stimulate active sodium and chloride absorption *in vitro* in the rat distal colon. *Gastroenterology* 1989; **96**: 989–996.
85. Ramakrishna BS, Venkataraman S, Srinivasan P et al. Amylase-resistant starch plus oral rehydration solution for cholera. *N Engl J Med* 2000; **342**: 308–313.
86. Hoekstra JH, Szajewska H, Abu Zikri M et al. Oral rehydration solution with a mixture of non-digestible carbohydrates in the treatment of acute diarrhea. A multicenter randomised placebo controlled study on behalf of the ESPGHAN Working Group on Intestinal Infections. *J Pediatr Gastroenterol Nutr* 2004; in press.
87. Santosham M, Foster S, Garrett S et al. Outpatient use of oral rehydration solutions in an Apache population: effects of instructions on preparation and contamination. *J Pediatr Gastroenterol Nutr* 1984; **3**: 687–691.
88. Snyder JD, Molla M, Cash RA. Home-based therapy for diarrhea. *J Pediatr Gastroenterol Nutr* 1990; **11**: 438–447.
89. Sandhu BK, for the European Society of Paediatric Gastroenterology, Hepatology and Nutrition Working Group on Acute Diarrhoea. Practical guidelines for the management of gastroenteritis in children. *J Pediatr Gastroenterol Nutr* 2001; **33**: S36–S39.
90. Powers GF. A comprehensive plan of treatment for the so-called intestinal intoxication of infants. *J Dis Child* 1926; **32**: 232–257.
91. Goodburn E, Mattosinho S, Mongi P et al. Management of childhood diarrhoea by pharmacists and parents: is Britain lagging behind the Third World? *BMJ* 1991; **302**: 440–443.

92. Brown KH, Gastanaduy AS, Saavedra JM et al. Effect of continued oral feeding on clinical and nutritional outcomes of acute diarrhoea in children. *J Pediatr* 1988; **112**: 191–200.
93. Sandhu B, Isolauri E, Walker-Smith JA et al. Early feeding in childhood gastroenteritis. A multicentre study on behalf of the European Society of Paediatric Gastroenterology and Nutrition Working Group on Acute Diarrhea. *J Pediatr Gastroenterol Nutr* 1997; **24**: 522–527.
94. Vesikari T, Isolauri E. Oral rehydration, rapid feeding and cholestyramine for treatment of acute diarrhoea. *J Pediatr Gastroenterol Nutr* 1986; **4**: 366–374.
95. Isolauri E, Vesikari T, Saha P et al. Milk versus no milk in rapid refeeding after acute gastroenteritis. *J Pediatr Gastroenterol Nutr* 1986; **5**: 254–261.
96. Placzek M, Walker-Smith JA. Comparison of two feeding regimens following acute gastroenteritis in infancy. *J Pediatr Gastroenterol Nutr* 1984; **3**: 245–248.
97. Dugdale A, Lovell S, Gibbs V et al. Refeeding after acute gastroenteritis: a controlled study. *Arch Dis Child* 1982; **57**: 76–79.
98. Rees L, Brook CGD. Gradual reintroduction of full strength milk after acute gastroenteritis in children. *Lancet* 1979; **2**: 770–771.
99. Hoghton MAR, Mittal NK, Mahdi G et al. Continuous modified feeding in acute gastroenteritis. *J Gen Pract* 1996; **46**: 173–175.
100. Dugdale A, Lovell S, Gibbs V et al. Refeeding after acute gastroenteritis: a controlled study. *Arch Dis Child* 1982; **57**: 76–78.
101. Haque KN, Al-Frayh A, El-Rifai R. Is it necessary to regraduate milk after acute gastroenteritis in children? *Trop Geogr Med* 1983; **35**: 369–373.
102. Rajah R, Pettifor JM, Noormohamed M et al. The effect of feeding four different formulae on stool weights in prolonged dehydrating infantile gastroenteritis. *J Pediatr Gastroenterol Nutr* 1988; **7**: 203–207.
103. Isolauri E, Juntunen M, Wiren S et al. Intestinal permeability changes in acute gastroenteritis: effects of clinical factors and nutritional management. *J Pediatr Gastroenterol Nutr* 1989; **8**: 466–473.
104. Levine GM, Deren JJ, Steiger E et al. Role of oral intake in maintenance of gut mass and disaccharide activity. *Gastroenterology* 1974; **67**: 975–982.
105. Brown KH, Lake A. Appropriate use of human and non-human milk for the dietary management of children with diarrhoea. *J Diarrhoeal Dis Res* 1991; **9**: 168–185.
106. Khin MU, Nyunt-Nyunt W, Myokhin AJ et al. Effect of clinical outcome of breast feeding during acute diarrhoea. *BM J* 1985; **290**: 587–589.
107. Morrow AL, Guerrero ML, Shults J et al. Efficacy of home-based peer counselling to promote exclusive breastfeeding: a randomised controlled trial. *Lancet* 1999; **353**: 1226–1231.
108. Kramer MS, Chalmers B, Hodnett ED et al. Promotion of breastfeeding intervention trials (PROBIT): a randomized trial in the Republic of Belarus. *JAMA* 2001; **285**: 413–420.
109. Bhandari N, Bahl R, Mazumdar S et al. Effect of community-based promotion of exclusive breastfeeding on diarrhoeal illness and growth: a cluster randomised controlled trial. *Lancet* 2003; **361**: 1418–1423.
110. Cunningham A, Jelliffe D, Jelliffe E. Breastfeeding and health in the 1980s: a global epidemiologic review. *J Pediatr* 1991; **118**: 659–666.
111. Dewey K, Heinig M, Nommsen-Rivers L. Differences in morbidity between breastfed and formula fed infants. *J Pediatr* 1995; **126**: 696–702.
112. Howie P, Forsyth J, Ogston S et al. Protective effects of breastfeeding against infection. *BMJ* 1990; **300**: 11–16.
113. Oddy WH. Breastfeeding protects against illness and infection in infants and children: a review of the evidence. *Breastfeed Rev* 2001; **9**: 11–18.
114. Brown KH, Peerson JM, Fontaine O. Use of nonhuman milks in the dietary management of young children with acute diarrhea: a meta-analysis of clinical trials. *Pediatrics* 1994; **93**: 17–27.
115. Allen UD, McLeod K, Wang EE. Cow's milk versus soy-based formula in mild and moderate diarrhea: a randomized, controlled trial. *Acta Paediatr* 1994; **83**: 183–187.
116. Fayad IM, Hashem M, Hussein A et al. Comparison of soy-based formulas with lactose and with sucrose in the treatment of acute diarrhea in infants. *Arch Pediatr Adolesc Med* 1999; **153**: 675–680.
117. Clemente YF, Tapia CC, Comino AL et al. Lactose-free formula versus adapted formula in acute infantile diarrhoea. *An Esp Pediatr* 1993; **39**: 309–312.
118. Lozano JM, Cespedes JA. Lactose vs. lactose free regimen in children with acute diarrhoea: a randomized controlled trial, *Arch Latinoam Nutr* 1994; **44**: 6–11.
119. Chew F, Penna FJ, Peret Filho LA et al. Is dilution of cows' milk formula necessary for dietary management of acute diarrhoea in infants aged less than 6 months? *Lancet* 1993; **341**: 194–197.
120. Wan C, Phillips MR, Dibley MJ et al. Randomised trial of different rates of feeding in acute diarrhoea *Arch Dis Child* 1999; **81**: 487–491.
121. American Academy of Pediatrics. *2000 Red Book: Report of the Committee on Infectious Diseases*, 25th edn. Elk Grove Village, IL: American Academy of Pediatrics, 2000.
122. Sirinavin S, Garner P. Antibiotics for treating salmonella gut infections (Cochrane Review). In *The Cochrane Library*, Issue 2. Oxford: Update Software, 2003.
123. Periman P. Antibiotic-associated diarrhea. *N Engl J Med* 2002; **346**: 334–339.
124. DeGrandi T, Simon JE. Promethazine-induced dystonic reaction. *Pediatr Emerg Care* 1987; **3**: 91–92.
125. Bateman DN, Darling WM, Boys R et al. Extrapyramidal reactions to metoclopramide and prochlorperazine. *Q J Med* 1989; **71**: 307–311.
126. Boulloche J, Mallet E, Mouterde O et al. Dystonic reactions with metoclopramide: is there a risk population? *Helv Paediatr Acta* 1987; **42**: 425–432.
127. Reeves JJ, Shannon MW, Fleisher GR. Ondansetron decreases vomiting associated with acute gastroenteritis: a randomized, controlled trial. *Pediatrics* 2002; **109**: e62.
128. Ramsook C, Sahagan-Carreon I, Kozinetz CA et al. A randomized clinical trial comparing oral ondansetron with placebo in children with vomiting from acute gastroenteritis. *Ann Emerg Med* 2002; **39**: 397–403.
129. Manatsathit S, Dupont HL, Farthing M et al. Working Party of the Program Committee of the Bangkok World Congress of Gastroenterology 2002. Guideline for the management of acute diarrhea in adults. *J Gastroenterol Hepatol* 2002; **17** (Suppl): S54–S71.
130. Ericsson CD, Johnson PC. Safety and efficacy of loperamide. *Am J Med* 1990; **88** (Suppl 6A): 10–14.
131. Bhutta TI, Tahir KI. Loperamide poisoning in children. *Lancet* 1990; **335**: 363.
132. Minton NA, Smith PGD. Loperamide toxicity in a child after a single dose. *BMJ* 1987; **294**: 1383.
133. Herranz J, Luzuriaga C, Sarralle R et al. Neurological symptoms precipitated by loperamide. *An Esp Pediatr* 1980; **13**: 1117–1120.

134. Schwartz RH, Rodriquez WJ. Toxic delirium possibly caused by loperamide. *J Pediatr* 1991; **118**: 656–657.
135. Gilbert B, Lienhardt A, Palomera S et al. [A study of the effectiveness of smectite versus placebo or loperamide in acute infantile diarrhea]. *Ann Pediatr* (Paris) 1991; **38**: 633–636.
136. Madkour AA, Madina EMH, El-Azzouni OEZ et al. Smectite in acute diarrhea in children: a double-blind placebo-controlled clinical trial. *J Pediatr Gastroenterol Nutr* 1993; **17**: 176–181.
137. Lachaux A, Danzon A, Collet JP et al. Acute infantile diarrhea. Role of treatment with smectite as complement to rehydration. Randomised double-blind study. *International Rev Pediatr* 1986; **163**: 29–31.
138. Ericsson CD, Tannenbaum C, Charles TT. Antisecretory and antiinflammatory properties of bismuth subsalicylate. *Rev Infect Dis* 1990; **12** (Suppl 1): S16–S20.
139. Ericsson CD, Evans DG, DuPont HL et al. Bismuth subsalicylate inhibits activity of crude toxins of *Escherichia coli* and *Vibrio cholerae*. *J Infect Dis* 1977; **136**: 693–696.
140. Manhart MD. *In vitro* antimicrobial activity of bismuth subsalicylate and other bismuth salts. *Rev Infect Dis* 1990; **12** (Suppl 1): S11–S15.
141. Soriano-Brucher H, Avendano P, O'Ryan M et al. Bismuth subsalicylate in the treatment of acute diarrhea in children: a clinical study. *Pediatrics* 1991; **87**: S18–S27.
142. Figueroa-Quintanilla D, Salazar-Lindo E, Sack RB et al. A controlled trial of bismuth subsalicylate in infants with acute watery diarrheal disease. *N Engl J Med* 1993; **328**: 1653–1658.
143. Chowdhury HR, Yunus M, Zaman K et al. The efficacy of bismuth subsalicylate in the treatment of acute diarrhoea and the prevention of persistent diarrhoea. *Acta Paediatr* 2001; **90**: 605–610.
144. Pickering LK, Feldman S, Ericsson CD et al. Absorption of salicylate and bismuth from a bismuth subsalicylate-containing compound (Pepto-Bismol). *J Pediatr* 1981; **99**: 654–656.
145. Primi MP, Bueno L, Baumer P et al. Racecadotril demonstrates intestinal antisecretory activity *in vivo*. *Aliment Pharmacol Ther* 1999; **13**: 3–7.
146. Salazar-Lindo E, Santisteban-Ponce J, Chea-Woo E et al. Racecadotril in the treatment of acute watery diarrhea in children. *N Engl J Med* 2000; **343**: 463–467.
147. Cézard JP, Duhamel JF, Meyer M et al. Efficacy and tolerability of racecadotril in acute diarrhea in children. *Gastroenterology* 2001; **120**: 799–805.
148. Guarner F, Schaafsma GJ. Probiotics. *Int J Food Microbiol* 1998; **39**: 237–238.
149. Szajewska H, Mrukowicz J. Probiotics in the treatment and prevention of acute infectious diarrhea in infants and children: a systematic review of published randomized, double-blind, placebo controlled trials. *J Pediatr Gastroenterol Nutr* 2001; **33**: S17–S25.
150. Van Niel C, Feudtner C, Garrison MM et al. *Lactobacillus* therapy for acute infectious diarrhea in children: a meta-analysis. *Pediatrics* 2002; **109**: 678–684.
151. Rosenfeldt V, Michaelson KF, Jakobsen M et al. Effect of probiotic *Lactobacillus* strains in young children hospitalized with acute diarrhea. *Pediatr Infect Dis J* 2002; **21**: 411–416.
152. Rosenfeldt V, Michaelson KF, Jakobsen M et al. Effect of probiotic *Lactobacillus* strains on acute diarrhea in a cohort of nonhospitalized children attending day-care centers. *Pediatr Infect Dis J* 2002; **21**: 417–419.
153. Kowalska-Duplaga K, Strus M, Heczko P et al. Lactobif®, a marketed probiotic product containing *Bifidobacterium ruminantium*, was not effective in the treatment of acute rotavirus diarrhea in infants. *J Pediatr Gastroenterol Nutr* 2002; **34**: 4 (ESPGHAN abstr).
154. Szajewska H, Mrukowicz J. Probiotics and acute gastroenteritis in children. Critical review of published evidence. *Ann Nestle* 2003; **61**: 66–78.
155. Jacobs J, Jonas WB, Jimenez-Perez M et al. Homeopathy for childhood diarrhea: combined results and metanalysis from three randomized, controlled clinical trials. *Pediatr Infect Dis J* 2003; **22**: 229–234.
156. Ghisham FK. Transport of electrolytes, water and glucose in zinc deficiency. *J Pediatr Gastroenterol Nutr* 1984; **3**: 608–612.
157. Patrick J, Golden BE, Golden MHN. Leucocyte sodium transport and dietary zinc in protein energy malnutrition. *Am J Clin Nutr* 1980; **33**: 617–620.
158. Patrick J, Michael J, Golden MN et al. Effect of zinc on leukocyte sodium transport *in vivo*. *Clin Sci Mol Med* 1978; **54**: 585–587.
159. Roy SK, Behrens RH, Haider R et al. Impact of zinc supplementation on intestinal permeability in Bangladeshi children with acute diarrhea and persistent diarrhea syndrome. *J Pediatr Gastroenterol Nutr* 1992; **15**: 289–296.
160. Elmes ME, Jones JG. Ultrastructural changes in the small intestines of zinc deficient rats. *J Pathol* 1980; **130**: 37–43.
161. Gebhard RL, Karouani R, Prigge WF et al. Effect of severe zinc deficiency on activity of intestinal disaccharidases and 3-hydroxy-3-methylglutaryl coenzyme A reductase in the rat. *J Nutr* 1983; **113**: 855–859.
162. Jones PE, Peters TJ. Oral zinc supplements and non-responsiveness coeliac syndrome: effect on jejunal morphology, enterocyte production, and brush border disaccharidase activities. *Gut* 1981; **22**: 194–198.
163. Cunningham-Rundles C, Cunningham-Rundles S, Garofalo J. Increased T lymphocyte function and thymopoietin following zinc repletion in man. *Fed Proc* 1979; **38**: 1222.
164. Fenwick PK, Aggett PJ, McDonald D et al. Zinc deficiency and zinc depletion effect on the response of rats to infection with *Trichinella spiralis*. *Am J Clin Nutr* 1996; **52**: 166–172.
165. Schlesinger L, Arevalo M, Arredondo S et al. Effects of a zinc fortified formula on immunocompetence and growth of malnourished infants. *Am J Clin Nutr* 1992; **56**: 491–498.
166. Shankar AH, Prasad AS. Zinc and immune function: the biological basis of altered resistance to infection. *Am J Clin Nutr* 1998; **68**: 447S–463S.
167. Wolman SL, Anderson GH, Marliss EB et al. Zinc in total parenteral nutrition: requirements and metabolic effects. *Gastroenterology* 1979; **76**: 458–467.
168. Castillo-Duran C, Vial P, Uauy R. Trace mineral balance during acute diarrhea in infants. *J Pediatr* 1988; **113**: 452–457.
169. Sachdev HPS, Mittal NK, Mittal SK et al. A controlled trial on utility of oral zinc supplementation in acute dehydrating diarrhea in infants. *J Pediatr Gastroenterol Nutr* 1988; **7**: 877–881.
170. Roy SK, Tomkins AM, Akramuzzaman SM et al. Randomized controlled trial of zinc supplementation in malnourished Bangladeshi children with acute diarrhea. *Arch Dis Child* 1997; **77**: 196–200.
171. Hidayat A, Achadi A, Sunoto, Soedarma SP. The effect of zinc supplementation in children under three years of age with acute diarrhea in Indonesia. *Med J Indonesia* 1998; **7**: 237–241.

172. Faruque ASG, Mahalanabis D, Haque SS et al. Double blind, randomized controlled trial of zinc or vitamin A supplementation in young children with acute diarrhea. *Acta Pediatr* 1999; **88**: 154–160.
173. Sazawal S, Black RE, Bhan MK et al. Zinc supplementation in young children with acute diarrhea in India. *N Engl J Med* 1995; **333**: 839–844.
174. Dutta P, Mitra U, Datta A et al. Impact of zinc supplementation in malnourished children with acute diarrhoea. *J Trop Pediatr* 2000; **46**: 259–263.
175. Bahl R, Bhandari N, Saksena M et al. Efficacy of zinc-fortified oral rehydration solution in 6- to 35-month-old children with acute diarrhea. *J Pediatr* 2002; **141**: 677–682.
176. Haffejee IE. Effect of oral folate on duration of acute infantile diarrhoea. *Lancet* 1988; **2**: 334–335.
177. Ashraf H, Rahman MM, Fuchs GJ et al. Folic acid in the treatment of acute watery diarrhoea in children: a double-blind, randomized, controlled trial. *Acta Paediatr* 1998; **87**: 1113–1115.
178. Bogstedt AK, Johansen K, Hatta H et al. Passive immunity against diarrhoea. *Acta Paediatr* 1996; **85**: 125–128.
179. Sarker SA, Casswall TH, Mahalanabis D et al. Successful treatment of rotavirus diarrhea in children with immunoglobulin from immunized bovine colostrums. *Pediatr Infect Dis J* 1998; **17**: 1149–1154.
180. Mitra AK, Mahalanabis D, Ashraf H et al. Hyperimmune cow colostrum reduces diarrhoea due to rotavirus: a double-blind, controlled clinical trial. *Acta Paediatr* 1995; **84**: 996–1001.
181. Guarino A, Canani RB, Russo S et al. Oral immunoglobulins for treatment of acute rotaviral gastroenteritis. *Pediatrics* 1994; **93**: 12–16.
182. Sarker SA, Casswall TH, Juneja LR et al. Randomized, placebo-controlled, clinical trial of hyperimmunized chicken egg yolk immunoglobulin in children with rotavirus diarrhea. *J Pediatr Gastroenterol Nutr* 2001; **32**: 19–25.
183. Casswall TH, Sarker SA, Faruque SM et al. Treatment of enterotoxigenic and enteropathogenic *Escherichia coli*-induced diarrhoea in children with bovine immunoglobulin milk concentrate from hyperimmunized cows: a double-blind, placebo-controlled, clinical trial. *Scand J Gastroenterol* 2000; **35**: 711–718.
184. Ashraf H, Mahalanabis D, Mitra AK et al. Hyperimmune bovine colostrum in the treatment of shigellosis in children: a double-blind, randomized, controlled trial. *Acta Paediatr* 2001; **90**: 1373–1378.
185. Bennish ML, Salam MA, Haider R et al. Therapy for shigellosis. II. Randomized, double-blind comparison of ciprofloxacin and ampicillin. *J Infect Dis* 1990; **162**: 711–716.
186. Bhattacharya SK, Bhattacharya MK, Dutta P et al. Randomized clinical trial of norfloxacin for shigellosis. *Am J Trop Med Hyg* 1991; **45**: 683–687.
187. Bennish ML, Salam MA, Khan WA et al. Treatment of shigellosis: III. Comparison of one- or two-dose ciprofloxacin with standard 5-day therapy. A randomized, blinded trial. *Ann Intern Med* 1992; **117**: 727–734.
188. Bassily S, Hyams KC, el-Masry NA et al. Short-course norfloxacin and trimethoprim–sulfamethoxazole treatment of shigellosis and salmonellosis in Egypt. *Am J Trop Med Hyg* 1994; **51**: 219–223.
189. Khan WA, Seas C, Dhar U et al. Treatment of shigellosis: V. Comparison of azithromycin and ciprofloxacin. A double-blind, randomized, controlled trial. *Ann Intern Med* 1997; **126**: 697–703.
190. Tauxe RV, Puhr ND, Wells JG et al. Antimicrobial resistance of *Shigella* isolates in the USA: the importance of international travelers. *J Infect Dis* 1990; **162**: 1107–1111.
191. Salam MA, Bennish ML. Antimicrobial therapy for shigellosis. *Rev Infect Dis* 1991; **13** (Suppl): 41.
192. Eidlitz-Marcus T, Cohen YH, Nussinovitch M et al. Comparative efficacy of two- and five-day courses of ceftriaxone for treatment of severe shigellosis in children. *J Pediatr* 1993; **123**: 822–824.
193. Neill MA, Opal SM, Heelan J et al. Failure of ciprofloxacin to eradicate convalescent fecal excretion after acute salmonellosis: experience during an outbreak in health care workers. *Ann Intern Med* 1991; **114**: 195–199.
194. Nelson JD, Kusmiesz H, Jackson LH et al. Treatment of *Salmonella* gastroenteritis with ampicillin, amoxicillin, or placebo. *Pediatrics* 1980; **65**: 1125–1130.
195. Pegues DA, Hohmann EL, Miller SI et al. *Salmonella*, including *S. typhi*. In Blaser MJ, Smith PD, Ravdin JI, Greenberg HB, Guerrant RL, eds. *Infections of the Gastrointestinal Tract*. New York: Raven Press, 1995: 785–809.
196. Mandal BK. Treatment of multiresistant typhoid fever. *Lancet* 1990; **336**: 1383.
197. Soe GB, Oversturf GD. Treatment of typhoid fever and other systemic salmonelloses with cefotaxime, ceftriaxone, cefoperazone and other newer cephalosporins. *Rev Infect Dis* 1987; **9**: 719–736.
198. Mandal BK, Ellis ME, Dunbar EM et al. Double-blind placebo-controlled trial of erythromycin in the treatment of clinical *Campylobacter* infection. *J Antimicrob Chemother* 1984; **13**: 619–623.
199. Salazar-Lindo E, Sack RB, Chea-Woo E et al. Early treatment with erythromycin of *Campylobacter jejuni*-associated dysentery in children. *J Pediatr* 1986; **109**: 355–360.
200. DuPont HL. Treatment of travelers' diarrhea with trimethoprim/sulfamethoxazole and with trimethoprim alone. *N Engl J Med* 1982; **307**: 841–844.
201. Ericsson CD, Johnson PC, DuPont HL et al. Ciprofloxacin or trimethoprim–sulfamethoxazole as initial therapy for travelers' diarrhea. A placebo-controlled, randomized trial. *Ann Intern Med* 1987; **106**: 216–220.
202. Mattila L, Peltola H, Siitonen A et al. Short-term treatment of traveler's diarrhea with norfloxacin: a double-blind, placebo-controlled study during two seasons. *Clin Infect Dis* 1993; **17**: 779–782.
203. Thoren A, Wolde-Mariam T, Stintzing G et al. Antibiotics in the treatment of gastroenteritis caused by enteropathogenic *Escherichia coli*. *J Infect Dis* 1980 **141**: 27–31.
204. Murphy GS, Bodhidatta L, Echeverria P et al. Ciprofloxacin and loperamide in the treatment of bacillary dysentery. *Ann Intern Med* 1993; **118**: 582–586.
205. Prado D, Lopez E, Liu H et al. Ceftibuten and trimethoprim–sulfamethoxazole for treatment of shigella and enteroinvasive *Escherichia coli* disease. *Pediatr Infect Dis J* 1992; **11**: 644–647.
206. Cimolai N, Morrison BJ, Carter JE. Risk factors for the central nervous system manifestations of gastroenteritis-associated hemolytic–uremic syndrome. *Pediatrics* 1992; **90**: 616–621.
207. Pavia AT, Nichols CR, Green DP et al. Hemolytic–uremic syndrome during an outbreak of *Escherichia coli* 0157:H7 infections in institutions for mentally retarded persons: clinical and epidemiologic observations. *J Pediatr* 1990; **116**: 544–551.
208. Cimolai N, Carter JE, Morrison BJ et al. Risk factors for the progression of *Escherichia coli* 0157:H7 enteritis to

hemolytic–uremic syndrome. *J Pediatr* 1990; **116**: 589–592.
209. Ostroff SM, Kobayashi JM, Lewis JH. Infections with *Escherichia coli* 0157:H7 in Washington State: the first year of statewide disease surveillance. *JAMA* 1989; **262**: 355–359.
210. Proulx F, Turgeon JP, Delage G et al. Randomized, controlled trial of antibiotic therapy for *Escherichia coli* O157:H7 enteritis. *J Pediatr* 1992; **121**: 299–303.
211. Carter AO, Borczyk AA, Carlson JA et al. A severe outbreak of *Escherichia coli* O157:H7-associated hemorrhagic colitis in a nursing home. *N Engl J Med* 1987; **317**: 1496–1500.
212. Riley LW, Remis RS, Helgerson SD et al. Hemorrhagic colitis associated with a rare *Escherichia coli* serotype. *N Engl J Med* 1983; **308**: 681–685.
213. Brenden RA, Miller MA, Janda JM. Clinical disease spectrum and pathogenic factors associated with *Plesiomonas shigelloides* infections in humans. *Rev Infect Dis* 1988; **10**: 303–316.
214. Holmberg SD, Farmer JJD. *Aeromonas hydrophila* and *Plesiomonas shigelloides* as causes of intestinal infections. *Rev Infect Dis* 1984; **6**: 633–639.
215. Holmberg SD, Wachsmuth IK, Hickman-Brenner FW et al. Plesiomonas enteric infections in the United States. *Ann Intern Med* 1986; **105**: 690–694.
216. Nathwani D, Laing RB, Harvey G et al. Treatment of symptomatic enteric *Aeromonas hydrophila* infection with ciprofloxacin. *Scand J Infect Dis* 1991; **23**: 653–654.
217. Reinhardt JF, George WL. *Plesiomonas shigelloides*-associated diarrhea. *JAMA* 1985; **253**: 3294–3295.
218. Cover TL, Aber RC. *Yersinia enterocolitica. N Engl J Med* 1989; **321**: 16–24.
219. Ostroff SM, Kapperud G, Lassen J et al. Clinical features of sporadic *Yersinia enterocolitica* infections in Norway. *J Infect Dis* 1992; **166**: 812–817.
220. Pai CH, Gillis F, Tuomanen E et al. Placebo-controlled double-blind evaluation of trimethoprim–sulfamethoxazole treatment of *Yersinia enterocolitica* gastroenteritis. *J Pediatr* 1984; **104**: 308–311.
221. Robins-Browne RM, Prpic JK. Effects of iron and desferrioxamine on infections with *Yersinia enterocolitica*. *Infect Immun* 1985; **47**: 774–779.
222. Scavizzi M. *Yersinia enterocolitica*. In Yu VL, Merlgan TC, Barriere SL, eds. *Antimicrobial Therapy and Vaccines*. Baltiomore: Williams & Wilkins, 1999: 481–488.
223. Alam AN, Alam NH, Ahmed T et al. Randomised double blind trial of single dose doxycycline for treating cholera in adults. *BMJ* 1990; **300**: 1619–1621.
224. Bhattacharya SK, Bhattacharya MK, Dutta P et al. Double-blind, randomized, controlled clinical trials of norfloxacin for cholera. *Antimicrob Agents Chemother* 1990; **34**: 939–940.
225. Gotuzzo E, Seas C, Echevarria J et al. Ciprofloxacin for the treatment of cholera: a randomized, double-blind, controlled clinical trial of a single daily dose in Peruvian adults. *Clin Infect Dis* 1995; **20**: 1485–1490.
226. Khan WA, Begum M, Salam MA et al. Comparative trial of five antimicrobial compounds in the treatment of cholera in adults. *Trans R Soc Trop Med Hyg* 1995; **89**: 1036.
227. Khan WA, Bennish ML, Seas C et al. Randomised controlled comparison of single-dose ciprofloxacin and doxycycline for cholera caused by *Vibrio cholerae* 01 or 0139. *Lancet* 1996; **348**: 296–300.
228. Khan WA, Saha D, Rahman A et al. Comparison of single-dose azithromycin and 12-dose, 3-day erythromycin for childhood cholera: a randomised, double-blind trial. *Lancet* 2002; **360**: 1722–1727.
229. Fekety R. Guidelines for the diagnosis and management of *Clostridium difficile*-associated diarrhea and colitis. American College of Gastroenterology Practice Parameters Committee. *Am J Gastroenterol* 1997; **92**: 739–750.
230. Gerding DN, Johnson S, Peterson LR et al. *Clostridium difficile*-associated diarrhea and colitis. *Infect Control Hosp Epidemiol* 1995; **16**: 459–477.
231. Teasley DG, Olson MM, Gebhard RL et al. Prospective randomised trial of metronidazole versus vancomycin for *Clostridium difficile*-associated diarrhoea and colitis. *Lancet* 1983: 1043–1046.
232. Olson MM, Shanholtzer CJ, Lee JT Jr, Gerding DN. Ten years of prospective *Clostridium difficile*-associated disease surveillance and treatment at the Minneapolis VA Medical Center, 19821991. *Infect Control Hosp Epidemiol* 1994; **15**: 371–381.
233. Teasley DG, Olson MM, Gebhard RL et al. Prospective randomised trial of metronidazole versus vancomycin for *Clostridium difficile*-associated diarrhoea and colitis. *Lancet* 1983; **2**: 1043–1046.
234. Wenisch C, Parschalk B, Hasenhundl M et al. Comparison of vancomycin, teicoplanin, metronidazole, and fusidic acid for the treatment of *Clostridium difficile*-associated diarrhea [published erratum appears in *Clin Infect Dis* 1996; **2**: 423]. *Clin Infect Dis* 1996; **22**: 813–818.
235. Bassily S, Farid Z, Mikhail JW et al. The treatment of *Giardia lamblia* infection with mepacrine, metronidazole and furazolidone. *J Trop Med Hyg* 1970; **73**: 1518.
236. Lerman SJ, Walker RA. Treatment of giardiasis: literature review and recommendations. *Clin Pediatr (Phila)* 1982; **21**: 409–414.
237. Levi GC, de Avila CA, Amato NV. Efficacy of various drugs for treatment of giardiasis. A comparative study. *Am J Trop Med Hyg* 1977; **26**: 564–565.
238. Zaat JOM, Mank ThG, Assendelft WJJ. Drugs for treating giardiasis (Cochrane Review). In *The Cochrane Library*, Issue 2. Oxford: Update Software.
239. Gerding DN, Johnson S, Peterson LR et al. Clostridium difficile associated diarrhea and colitis. *Infect Control Hosp Epidemiol* 1995; **16**: 459–477.
240. Madico G, McDonald J, Gilman RH et al. Epidemiology and treatment of Cyclospora cayetanensis infection in Peruvian children. *Clin Infect Dis* 1997; **24**: 977–981.
241. Rubidge CJ, Scragg JN, Powell SJ. Treatment of children with acute amoebic dysentery. Comparative trial of metronidazole against a combination of dehydroemetine, tetracycline, and diloxanide furoate. *Arch Dis Child* 1970; **45**: 196–197.
242. Scott F, Miller MJ. Trials with metronidazole in amebic dysentery. *JAMA* 1970; **211**: 118–120.
243. Haque R, Huston CD, Hughes M et al. Amebiasis. *N Engl J Med* 2003; **348**: 1565–1573.

40 Approach to the child with acute abdomen

Luigi Dall'Oglio, Paola De Angelis and Giovanni Federici di Abriola

Introduction

'Acute abdomen' is a loose concept, referring to a medical emergency involving signs and symptoms pertaining to the abdomen and whose therapeutic option is usually surgery.

In this chapter we review the clinical signs and symptoms of various gastrointestinal disorders that have an acute onset and can progress dramatically to involve the parietal or visceral peritoneum. Our aim is to help the pediatrician realize when a gastrointestinal condition changes from an indolent to an acute course, and when a surgeon should be consulted. We also describe some simple but important strategies that are helpful in reaching a diagnosis without delay, and in adequately preparing patients for either surgery or for one of the newer effective and less invasive non-surgical treatments.

Symptoms and signs

The symptoms and signs of an acute abdomen vary widely depending on the patient's age and the clinical course of the disease. An early, efficient and accurate diagnosis depends crucially on a meticulous review of the patient's medical history, focusing on the symptoms, their time of onset, and their intensity and character. To avoid a misdiagnosis of other extraintestinal diseases, the history taking must include symptoms apparently unrelated to the digestive tract. For example, a history of excessive thirst, increased urination and lack of appetite preceding the abdominal pain, accompanied by deep sighing and rapid breathing, and severe dehydration, may suggest diabetic ketoacidosis mimicking an acute abdomen.[1]

The most important elements to evaluate in a patient with an acute abdomen are:

(1) Abdominal pain;

(2) The presence and characteristics of vomiting;

(3) The presence and characteristics of fever;

(4) The characteristics of the stools;

(5) The findings from a detailed physical examination.

Abdominal pain

Whereas in older, co-operative children, close observation and a detailed diagnostic work-up of abdominal pain will usually identify various possible causes of an acute abdomen, in infants and newborns, abdominal pain is often a poorly specific symptom. Young infants with functional abdominal colic, at times very painful, need only be kept under clinical observation, whilst those with abdominal pain of organic origin should undergo aggressive diagnostic and therapeutic procedures. In newborns and infants, a true acute abdomen is rare and is generally related to congenital malformation. It should be suspected when the patient presents with abdominal tension, paradoxical diarrhea and vomiting, sometimes accompanied by a surprisingly rapid decline in general condition followed by shock. Circumstances such as these require therapy for shock, along with diagnostic investigations.

In older children, a complete medical history and description of the symptoms can generally be obtained. The suspected diagnosis can then be confirmed with standard clinical examinations and laboratory tests.

The assessment of abdominal pain should include the intensity of pain, the type (continuous or colic) and the site – whether the pain affects a specific site or the entire abdomen, and whether it irradiates to the back, chest, or shoulders. The chronological pattern of the pain, the rapidity of onset and the progression and duration of symptoms can be useful in the diagnosis; pain with sudden and severe onset is generally due to perforation or mesenteric infarction. In gastroenteritis, pain is self-limited; in appendicitis, or in other peritoneal inflammations, pain is progressive. Infants with bowel occlusion typically have evident colicky pain and even more evident postcolic seediness.

As a general rule, visceral pain (noxious stimuli in the intestinal wall) is located in the epigastrium, mid-abdomen and hypogastrium; the pain is generally crampy, burning or gnawing in quality. Parietal pain (noxious stimuli in the parietal peritoneum) is generally more intense and more precisely localized to the site of the lesion, and it is often aggravated by movement or coughing. The onset of pain differs in the various diseases. For example, in patients with perforated ulcers or ruptured abscess, pain has a sudden (instantaneous) onset; in strangulated bowel and intussusception, it has a rapid onset (minutes); and in appendicitis, bowel obstruction, cholecystitis, and Meckel's diverticulitis, it has a gradual onset (a few hours).[2] Close observation, absolutely crucial in infants to gain information on the pain, is also necessary in the older child. A patient lying still in bed, in the fetal position, neither moving nor speaking, with a distressed facial expression, is likely to have peritonitis; conversely, a patient who has short periods free of pain, recognizable by normal appearance and behavior, could have visceral pains due to gastroenteritis or bowel occlusion.[3] Intestinal volvulus generally starts with intense abdominal pain and, after possible vascular torsion, the most important symptom is the worsening of the general condition; vomiting and blood in stools are frequent, without other characteristic clinical indications.

Vomiting

An important symptom in clarifying the severity and type of disease, vomiting is an early sign of peritoneal inflammation or bowel obstruction. Initially, vomit is mixed with food; after minutes or hours, it can become bile-stained, as in intestinal obstruction. Vomiting can be highly dangerous, owing to the risk of aspiration; especially in newborn or in unconscious infants, a nasogastric tube must be inserted for adequate gastric suction.

Fever

An unspecific symptom, fever, when present, can be helpful in suspected peritonitis. As a general rule, a temperature that rises slowly and progressively in parallel with the abdominal signs indicates peritoneal infection. Conversely, a temperature that rises rapidly, despite acute abdominal pain, indicates other, and often self-limited, non-surgical diseases.

Characteristics of the stools

The rule that adults with acute abdomen usually have no passage of stools does not hold true in infants and young children. The important signs to note in infants are: mucousy or bloody diarrhea, and the time elapsing after the last bowel movement and flatus. Bloody diarrhea is a common symptom of bowel occlusion with vascular damage due to strangulation. Diarrhea often accompanies peritoneal inflammation in small children. Older children with pelvic abscess also often have repeated small bowel movements. Complete information about stool habits before the onset of the acute abdominal symptoms is useful. For instance, a history of alternating diarrhea and constipation may be an indication of aganglionosis, while a history of bloody and mucousy stools could raise a suspicion of inflammatory bowel disease (IBD).

Findings from the physical exam of the abdomen

A careful physical examination, looking for the various signs of extra-abdominal systemic disease, is of paramount importance. For example, cutaneous petechiae can raise a suspicion of Henoch–Schönlein purpura and possible bowel involvement with intussusception. The abdomen must be meticulously inspected, looking for distension; visible veins; visible loops of bowel, with or without peristaltic waves; superficial non-abdominal breathing; and flexion of lower limbs over the abdomen. All these signs can be more or less evident, and can differ in intensity, depending on the patient's age, the disease and its severity. The same problems arise during abdominal palpation. In a newborn, insufficient muscular mass and muscle activity makes rigidity from muscular guarding difficult to detect. The only way to obtain information from abdominal palpation in a child is to approach the child carefully, and begin palpation at the least tender site; light finger percussion over an area of tenderness often elicits the same information as deep palpation and is less disturbing to infants and children.[4] Abdominal palpation with the child lying on the side, with one or both legs on the abdomen itself, is a helpful maneuver for obtaining muscular relaxation, thus gaining more information. Percussion can be useful to elicit tympany from intraluminal abdominal gas, as in obstruction, or from extraluminal gas, as in intestinal perforation.

Careful rectal examination yields a great deal of information about anal or rectal malformations, stools, gas, blood, mucus and pelvic tenderness or masses.

Laboratory examination, imaging and other techniques

Laboratory examination

All patients with suspected acute abdomen should have a complete blood count with differential, C-reactive protein (CRP) and urinalysis. Analysis of serum electrolytes, blood urea nitrogen, creatinine and glucose levels is useful in determining fluid and acid–base status, renal function and metabolic status. In newborns and infants the standard laboratory tests sometimes have poor sensitivity and specificity, but they are important for identifying pre-shock signs early, before the clinical status becomes critical.

The patient's clinical history and physical examination may indicate the need for special tests (e.g. liver function tests and amylase in patients with upper abdominal symptoms).

Imaging

Symptoms of acute abdomen generally arise from bowel occlusion or peritoneal inflammation. Plain abdominal X-rays and ultrasonography are the two most common imaging techniques. Plain abdominal X-rays visualize free air, as in perforation, and the possible presence of air–fluid levels, pathognomonic for occlusion. They also provide evidence of various pre-surgical problems, such as pneumatosis in necrotizing enterocolitis, and toxic megacolon which need to be recognized early, in order to avoid delaying surgery.

Plain abdominal series must always be taken in supine, upright and side views; in patients unable to stand in this position, a lateral decubitus film with the left side down (or cross-table lateral) can be useful to identify abnormal gas distribution. A chest X-ray must be obtained to exclude possible respiratory disease; lung-base pneumonia is a well-known cause of acute abdominal symptoms, whereas acute abdominal disease can give rise to chest problems, as it does in pancreatitis or subphrenic abscess. No recently published trials have addressed the diagnostic value of plain series, but in accordance with Glasgow and Mulvihill,[3] 'it is a readily available and inexpensive examination and in most circumstances should be obtained'.

Ultrasound gives rapid, non-invasive, accurate, repeatable and inexpensive information. Unlike plain series, the ultrasound technique needs an experienced examiner who knows precisely which information to seek in the abdomen and how to look for it. Ultrasound allows accurate detection of localized or diffuse liquid and its density; it also defines the morphology of other structures, including the biliary and pancreatic tree. This technique accurately estimates the intestinal wall thickness, and visualizes peristaltic activity. In conjunction with color and pulsed Doppler imaging, ultrasound provides a new tool for diagnosing an acute abdomen, depending on the child's age.[5] It has a well-known role in IBD and in other inflammatory diseases, including intestinal localizations in Henoch–Schönlein purpura. It also visualizes hydrostatic reduction of intussusception with saline enema.[6] The primary imaging procedure[7] in abdominal emergency in childhood is: plain X-ray film of the abdomen followed by ultrasound. The findings from these initial studies dictate the need for further imaging.

The role of computed tomography (CT) and magnetic resonance imaging (MRI) remains less clear. These techniques are expensive and, in uncooperative children, deep sedation is needed to obtain the clear images necessary for a meaningful assessment.

In suspected biliary or pancreatic disease, MRI cholangiography gives full information about morphology[8,9] and, with secretin stimulus, about pancreatic activity.[10] Other invasive diagnostic procedures, including peritoneal lavage or diagnostic laparoscopy, are occasionally useful but are more often used in post-trauma acute abdomen. Digestive endoscopy is generally contraindicated in acute abdomen, although it may have a diagnostic or therapeutic role in special circumstances. These include decompression, reduction and sigmoidopexy of sigmoid volvulus,[11,12] or clip closure of cardia perforation in Mallory–Weiss tears, after dilatations[13,14] or after a lap Nissen procedure.

General considerations about treatment

A good strategy for avoiding misdiagnosis or surgical delay is to contact the surgeon as soon as an acute abdomen develops and maintain full and timely collaboration. While awaiting the surgeon, the pediatrician must complete the diagnostic work-up and start medical treatment. Recent advances in diagnosis and therapy mean that many patients who hitherto would have undergone surgery can now be treated medically. Surgical intervention must be scheduled only after the patient's status has been fully stabilized and only if the non-surgical therapeutic strategy is unsuccessful. In doubtful circumstances, the pediatrician along with the surgeon should observe how the disease evolves clinically, in order to identify the correct timing for diagnostic procedures and to decide between conservative therapeutic options or surgical intervention. Should the diagnosis remain unclear and a life-threatening risk develop, then the surgeon may proceed to an exploratory laparotomy or, as in recent years and in selected cases, laparoscopy.

The management of an acute abdomen also has to be cost-effective. Therefore, surgeons must be involved early in the evaluation phase of patients with an acute abdomen, and follow the patient during the observation period, so that unnecessary laboratory or diagnostic tests can be avoided and the costs reduced.[15,16] The goal in treating an acute abdomen is to reach an early diagnosis and to establish the correct surgical indications and timing to allow effective surgery.

Unfortunately, these goals are not always achieved. Far more often, the clinical presentation and the indications for surgery are unclear. In these cases, the pediatrician must, in strict collaboration with the surgeon, do everything necessary to reach a diagnosis, and at the same time start supportive therapy before the patient's general clinical status takes a downhill course. The following simple but essential procedures can help.

Evaluation of fluid loss

This is obtained by the use of nasogastric suction with a tube of adequate caliber. A simple report on the number of vomits and the presumed amount vomited does not give a precise evaluation of fluid loss. The evaluation requires adequate urine collection and diaper weight for fecal volume.

Placement of an adequate intravenous line

Especially in newborns and infants, a vein catheter must be installed in time to avoid difficult venous puncture under conditions of collapse. In patients whose clinical status is more severe, a central venous catheter can be useful, not only for infusion but also for measuring central venous pressure. This measurement is essential in ensuring a proper fluid intake.

Consideration of pharmacological therapy

Antibiotic therapy is always necessary in patients with clinically evident sepsis and is useful in those with well-diagnosed peritonitis before surgery. In other less clear circumstances, antibiotics might hide the clinical evolution of the disease, thus delaying the definitive diagnosis and proper surgical therapy, and should therefore be avoided.

The usefulness of H_2-antagonists or proton pump inhibitors in the prevention of acute peptic disease is unclear in children and debated in adults. Persistent vomiting attempts can provoke prolapse of the gastric wall through the cardia, thus causing blood in the vomit, despite the absence of a specific gastric disease.[17,18] In patients whose clinical status worsens, 10 mg/kg per day of ranitidine or 1–1.5 mg/kg per day of omeprazole are useful in preventing acute peptic disease.

Specific diseases

Some specific diseases resulting in acute abdomen (such as appendicitis, intussusception, Meckel's diverticulum, Hirschsprung's disease or chronic intestinal pseudo-obstruction) are discussed in detail in their respective chapters. Here we focus only on some conditions that may atypically present the clinical picture of acute abdomen, offering some suggestions pertinent to their diagnosis and treatment.

Foreign body ingestion

Foreign body ingestion is rarely described as a cause of acute abdomen; children can ingest everything and these objects,[19] even button batteries,[20] often pass naturally.

Acute abdomen was described in patients who had ingested bezoars[21,22] especially in mentally retarded children, or in cases where multiple magnets were attracted to each other across the bowel wall, leading to pressure necrosis, perforation, fistula or intestinal obstruction.[23] Ingestion of pins has been described as a cause of gastric perforation.[24]

In our experience of ingested foreign bodies, an acute abdomen occurred twice: duodenal perforation from a hairpin and sigmoid perforation from a fragment of glass from the top of a cola bottle. The first patient, who presented in the pre-endoscopy period, with the foreign bodies embedded in the third duodenal portion, died of pancreatitis and septic complications. In the second case, the foreign bodies passed naturally with a small amount of blood in the stools as a lucky warning sign, in a patient without abdominal pain; radiological evidence of free abdominal gas suggested the surgical direct suture of the 3-cm long sigmoid lesion, with a good outcome. Refer to Chapter 41 for further information.

Inflammatory bowel disease

Acute surgical emergencies in children with IBD need a team approach, involving gastroenterologists and surgeons, avoiding an unnecessary or delayed surgical strategy. If the team chooses the correct time for surgery, acute abdomen from toxic colitis with megacolon, perforation, abdominal abscesses and bowel obstructions can have a good outcome, with morbidity and mortality rates of 15% in childhood.[25] The goal of this team is to make sure that unduly prolonged medical therapy does not result in an emergency operation. Emergency surgery, not being planned in advance, may be performed by a surgical team to which the patient is unknown, and often involves a multistep operation.

Toxic colitis

Toxic colitis is an emergency life-threatening complication of IBD. Crohn's disease was once thought to be secondary only to ulcerative colitis, but we now know that it may cause up to 50% of the cases.[26]

The pathophysiology in Crohn's disease and ulcerative colitis is similar, with transmural vascular congestion, muscular disintegration with consequent colon atony and dilatation, and with very thin, deeply ulcerated walls. Histologically, the inflammation involves all layers of the colon, with myocyte degeneration, necrosis and the formation of granulation tissue, infiltrated by neutrophils, lymphocytes and plasma cells.[27] The etiology seems to be related to colonic muscle paralysis, secondary to the inflammatory infiltrate and destruction of the myenteric plexus. More recent case reports have described toxic megacolon involving nitric oxide, generated by macrophages and smooth muscle cells.[27,28] Once the diagnosis is suspected for worsening general conditions, abdominal distension and tenderness, plain abdominal series may confirm the colonic distension and must be repeated every 12 h in order to provide a close monitoring of its evolution. Medical treatment consists of antibiotics (ciprofloxacin, metronidazole), to avoid bacterial translocation through the bowel wall, high-dose intravenous corticosteroids and cyclosporin or, more recently, tacrolimus. A higher incidence of postoperative complications was described in non-deferrable surgery and high-dose corticosteroid therapy.[25,29,30] If the dilated colon persists, free perforation develops, or the clinical conditions fail to improve within 2 or 3 days, prompt surgery is indicated.[31] Mortality related to perforation may exceed 40%, but if surgery is completed before perforation, the mortality decreases to 2–8%.[27]

Perforation

Perforation occurs in approximately 2% of patients with ulcerative colitis, and is generally associated with toxic colitis and megacolon. In a patient with toxic colitis without megacolon, Crohn's disease must be suspected.[32] The diagnosis may be delayed because high-dose corticosteroids may mask the signs of peritonitis. The transmural damage in Crohn's disease creates an inflammatory adhesion between the affected bowel segments and local structures with consequent sealed perforation.[32] Owing to these adhesions, pneumoperitoneum is present in only 20% of patients with perforated Crohn's disease, and in a smaller percentage of those with ileal perforations.[33,34] The surgical procedure in colon perforation with or without toxic colitis must be limited to total colectomy and terminal ileostomy, avoiding proctectomy because of the risk of blood loss, pelvic sepsis and pelvic nerve damage.[26] This strategy removes the diseased bowel and avoids anastomosis in critically ill patients.[35]

In Crohn's disease, gastroduodenal perforations need debridement and primary repair; jejunal–ileal perforations require resection and primary anastomosis with associated intestinal diversion in unfavorable conditions.[36]

Intra-abdominal abscess

Characteristic of Crohn's disease, intra-abdominal abscess can give rise to an acute abdomen if the abscess ruptures into the peritoneal cavity. Often the abscesses are associated with a fistula, secondary to a distended loop of proximal bowel, to a distal stricture or to transmural ulceration of the diseased bowel. Ultrasound and CT are useful for identifying the type of abscess and its location. Because surgical drainage of an abscess leads to numerous severe complications, it should be avoided. The best options are medical treatment or percutaneous drainage guided by ultrasound or CT. If surgery cannot be deferred, and in patients with intestinal damage, it should aim only at draining the abscess and diverting the fecal stream, avoiding resection or other useless and dangerous maneuvers.[37]

Intestinal obstruction

Intestinal obstruction, generally in the small bowel, is the most common complication requiring surgical correction in Crohn's disease, but is rarely related to acute abdomen; improved medical and nutritional treatment has now reduced the indications for surgical emergencies for bowel obstruction. If acute obstruction cannot be managed otherwise, surgery must be as conservative as possible, avoiding wide resection. In accordance with the conservative strategy for surgery in Crohn's disease, the newer strictureplasty techniques are providing increasingly good results and fewer complications than resective surgery, avoiding the risk of short-bowel syndrome due to repeated resections.[38–42]

Biliary and pancreatic diseases

Biliary diseases

Biliary diseases are uncommon in children and especially rare as a possible cause of acute abdomen. Suppurative cholecystitis or cholangitis, from malformations and cholelithiasis, must be suspected in patients who present with acute abdomen and pain in the right upper quadrant that irradiates to the right shoulder, and laboratory blood findings indicating biliary stasis. Also, jaundice is not an early symptom of biliary and pancreatic disease. Ultrasound, in skilled hands, can be useful in showing common bile duct or gallbladder dilatation with stones or biliary sludge; it will also identify choledochal malformations.

MRI cholangiography gives full information about morphology.[8,9] Endoscopic retrograde cholangiopancreatography (ERCP) can be helpful for morphological evaluation of the biliary and pancreatic ducts and for therapeutic options such as sphincterotomy, stone removal and drainage.[43–45] Percutaneous transhepatic cholangiography, drainage and stenting of the biliary tree is another non-surgical diagnostic and therapeutic option. However, an urgent surgical strategy for biliary drainage must be considered if antibiotic, endoscopic or radiological treatment fails. Depending on the degree of inflammation, surgery generally involves simple biliary drainage through a cholecystotomy. In patients with choledochal malformation, definitive surgery must be postponed until the peritoneal infection has resolved, because of the high risk of complications (including anastomosis leak) in patients with active biliary peritonitis.

Spontaneous perforation of the bile duct

This is a rare pediatric cause of biliary peritonitis[46,47] that has been described in newborns and infants, frequently associated with a choledochal cyst or anomalous pancreaticobiliary union.[48,49] In the absence of a dilated biliary duct, diagnosis is difficult; sometimes, biliary peritonitis is an occasional finding at exploratory laparotomy. The presence of bile-like fluid at abdominal puncture nevertheless suggests this disorder. Patients without malformations or peritonitis should undergo primary repair, with biliary and abdominal drainage. Otherwise, the best choice is simple biliary and abdominal drainage, postponing definitive surgery.

Acute pancreatitis

Acute pancreatitis is a dramatic cause of acute abdomen; it is uncommon in children and, in the past, has been an occasional finding in acute abdomen operated upon for suspected appendicitis.[50] In acute pancreatitis, abdominal pain, referred to the middle or epigastric abdomen, has an acute onset and is deep-seated, requiring adequate analgesic treatment; abdominal parietal tenderness is generally evident. A major decision in the management of severe acute pancreatitis is whether and when surgery is necessary for pancreatic necrosis (see Chapter 21). ERCP, sphincterotomy and drainage can be useful as diagnostic and therapeutic options if hepatic enzyme abnormalities suggest biliary pancreatitis due to stones or sludge.[51,52] Somatostatin and octreotide are widely used but their efficacy is not proven.[53–55] The course of pancreatitis can be assessed by monitoring the patients' general condition, fever, hematological variables (white blood cell (WBC) count, CRP, lactate dehydrogenase, calcium and albumin), and imaging findings (ultrasound, CT).[56] In patients with necrosis and, in particular, septic necrosis, surgical intervention must be considered for drainage of the peripancreatic space.[57]

Infectious and parasitic disease

Typhoid perforation

Typhoid perforation is a well-known surgical complication of *Salmonella typhi* infection,[58–61] whose outcome is related to the number of perforations and to the severity of peritonitis.[58] This last point is obviously related to the timeliness of diagnosis.

Because no specific warning signs are known for identifying a pre-perforation state, the diagnosis rests on close clinical observation. Unspecific laboratory indexes include elevated WBC count and CRP; plain abdominal series will usually identify pneumoperitoneum. Multiple therapeutic protocols and surgical strategies have been proposed, depending on the intensity of peritoneal involvement. Antibiotic therapy consists of aminoxide, metronidazole and the third-generation cephalosporins.[60] In patients without advanced peritonitis, and with a single perforated lesion, excellent results can be achieved by excising the edges followed by direct suture and, in multiple perforations, by segmental resection followed by end-to-end anastomosis. Patients presenting with severe peritonitis must be invariably treated by bowel diversion.[59] The most common postoperative complications are wound infection and enterocutaneous fistula. In a prospective study, the ideal treatment for typhoid enteric perforation was found to be resection anastomosis with copious peritoneal lavage.[62]

Non-typhi *Salmonella*

In this intestinal infection, toxic megacolon can occur. Patients with toxic megacolon have a toxic appearance, diarrhea, high fever (>39°C) and marked colon dilatation with maximal diameter >1.5 times the width of the vertebral body of the first lumbar vertebra (L1-VB). A retrospective analysis identified as the most significant factors associated with intestinal perforation: age >1 year, serum CRP >200 mg/l; colon diameter >2.5 times the width of L1-VB; inadequate early hydration; and delay in inserting a rectal tube.[63]

Entamoeba histolytica

Entamoeba histolytica is another infectious cause of colonic involvement; acute abdomen due to perforation is rarely reported and related to perforated appendicitis. The most frequent manifestations are acute intestinal symptoms and bleeding.[64] In severely ill patients, with acute bleeding and general septic signs, misdiagnosis of fulminant-onset IBD could result in unnecessary colectomy.

Intestinal tuberculosis

This is now widespread and must be suspected in patients who present with perforation or occlusion-like symptoms, as well as in cases of suspected Crohn's disease, given the similarities between these two conditions. Intestinal perforation and fistulae were described in 7% of tuberculosis patients in a large retrospective series.[65] The diagnosis of perforation, due to adhesion between the bowel loops, is not easy. In a retrospective series, most patients presented with non-specific clinical features; pneumoperitoneum on abdominal radiographs was present in only 48.3% of cases.[66] Surgery consists of resection, end-to-end anastomosis and peritoneal drainage.

Intestinal parasites

Intestinal parasites (besides *Entamoeba histolytica*) are rarely a cause of perforation or occlusion. Anisakiasis can be a surprising finding at surgery for bowel obstruction; these parasites can be suspected in children with acute abdomen caused by bowel obstruction, who have eaten raw or undercooked fish. Typical ultrasound findings in patients with suspected anisakiasis are ascites, small-bowel dilatation, focal edema of Kerckring folds,[67] markedly thickened bowel loops associated with luminal narrowing and decreased peristalsis.[68] Cytological examination of a specimen obtained from ascites by abdominal puncture showed a dense infiltration of eosinophils.[68] If the foregoing ultrasound features are found, the diagnosis of intestinal anisakiasis must be considered, because medical treatment has a good outcome and will avoid unnecessary surgery.

Mucormycosis

Mucormycosis is an increasing concern in immunocompromised patients, in whom mortality exceeds 60%. The multiple mycotic localizations (intestinal wall, liver, kidneys, sinuses, lower respiratory tract, or skin) give a dramatic clinical picture with acute abdomen secondary to occlusion and multiple perforations. The last are due to vessel thrombosis.[69,70] The standard treatment is amphotericin B combined with surgical debridement if necessary, depending on occlusion or perforations. In our experience, in one patient with fourth-degree neuroblastoma, after the histological diagnosis of mucormycosis in the gastrointestinal tract (surgical treatment for multiple perforations) and the echographic detection of multiple mycotic localizations in the liver and kidneys, the treatment was high-dose amphotericin B. At the same time, to prevent the growth of hyphae, we avoided the development of anaerobiosis and/or acidosis, as well as hyperglycemia. This therapeutic strategy successfully prevents spreading of the infection and encourages complete healing.[70]

Acute abdomen caused by endoscopic and other diagnostic procedures

Endoscopic procedures, even in skilled hands, can be dangerous and provoke complications sometimes resulting in acute abdomen. Many of these events can be prevented by using strictly pediatric instruments, by suspecting a complication before it becomes irreversible and by instituting specific treatments without delay.

Polypectomy

Simple rules can help in preventing perforation that may become manifest during the procedure or some hours later. Delayed perforation is caused by deep scalding of the intestinal wall due to the use of an inappropriate blend of cutting and hemostatic current and excessively high current intensities.

Incomplete snare closure with its tip hidden by the polyp can perforate the intestinal wall. Sometimes the perforation becomes evident during the procedure because of bleeding and, moreover, because insufflation of air fails to distend the bowel, thus causing abdominal tension with respiratory distress. In cases like this, the complication can be resolved by immediate surgical intervention with direct suture and drainage. Deep scalding can occur during multiple polypectomies or during resection of polyps with a large pedicle, especially those sited in the right colon or jejunum, where the wall is thinner than the gastric or left colon wall. Abdominal pain, fever, leukocytosis and abdominal wall tenderness can be evident even without perforation. In patients with radiological evidence of a large, increasing quantity of free abdominal gas, surgery might be necessary. If surgery is avoided, the lesion may still have a good outcome in 2 or 3 days, after treatment with broad-spectrum antibiotics, metronidazole (22 mg/kg per day) and strict observation with fasting.

Colonoscopy in inflammatory bowel disease

In IBD, an attempted total colonoscopy can be hazardous for the patient, owing to the fragility of the colonic wall. In our experience, in an infant with acute ulcerative colitis careful insufflation into the sigma caused perforation of the transverse colon. In order to prevent peritoneal infection, the patient must undergo emergency surgery to attempt a direct suture of the lesion; if the colon is extensively damaged a fecal diversion (ileostomy) may be required, with or without colectomy.

In colonic strictures from Crohn's disease, surgical resection or stricturoplasty is increasingly avoided in favor of palliative therapy with pneumatic endoscopic dilatations.[71,72] Because of the wall thickness, perforations are rare and the surrounding scar tissue hinders the diffusion of gas and intestinal contents into the peritoneal cavity. Peritoneal involvement is therefore less severe but the diagnosis can be delayed. Helpful ways of preventing further peritoneal complications include diagnostic ultrasound or CT scans, and conservative treatment with antibiotic prophylaxis and strict observation.

Percutaneous endoscopic gastrostomy

To avoid complications related to percutaneous endoscopic gastrostomy (PEG), the operator must be familiar with its contraindications, relative and absolute. The most frequent cause of a PEG-related acute abdomen is air, gastric juice or food in the peritoneal cavity due to incomplete adhesion of the gastric to the abdominal wall.[73–75] During the procedure, especially in infants with bowel distension, inserting the needle can provoke an intestinal perforation that might require surgical intervention.[76] In psychiatric and neurologically impaired children, premature tube removal can provoke peritonitis requiring surgery for peritoneal drainage. In patients without peritonitis, surgical intervention can be avoided by carefully inserting a pigtail wire and replacing the drainage tube, under radiographic control, with a slimmer gastrostomy Foley catheter (Medical Innovation Corporation, Milpitas, CA; Bard Interventional Products, Tewksbury, MA, USA). During substitution of the PEG with a low-profile device, the gastric wall can become detached from the abdominal wall. In our experience, in a patient with cystic fibrosis, this complication developed after a sports injury to the abdomen, which caused dramatic invasion of food into the peritoneum and required open surgery.

In certain clinical settings, such as peritoneal dialysis, this type of complication can be avoided by placing the gastrostomy surgically[77] or by using a special kit (Cliny, Create Medic Co, Ltd, Yokohama, Japan) which, under endoscopic control, allows adhesion between the gastric and abdominal wall. Previous abdominal surgery can expose patients to a high risk of gastrocolic fistula, and surgery is necessary only in cases of dramatic disruption of the gastric or colonic wall, with peritoneal fecal contamination; otherwise antibiotic therapy and gastric drainage resolves the problem within days.

Cardia and esophageal dilatations

Pneumatic or semi-rigid endoscopic dilatations in achalasia, or congenital esophageal strictures, can provoke perforation of the cardia or of the abdominal esophagus and possible acute abdomen. In children with esophageal perforation and mediastinum involvement, current opinion favors the following standard management protocol: nasogastric and pharyngeal suction, wide-spectrum antibiotics, proton pump inhibitors, total parenteral nutrition and daily testing of CRP and WBCs. Endoscopic clip closure of the perforation and transesophageal drainage can be attempted to avoid surgery[13,14] (and D. Fregonese, personal communication). The main indications for surgery are worsening sepsis and insufficient drainage, with diffuse or localized multiple purulent collections. The general rule that purulent infection of the peritoneum contraindicates resections and reanastomosis is even more applicable in these cases. In cardia or abdominal esophageal perforation, an attempt to suture the lesion may require gastrostomy (in order to obtain full gastric drainage), jejunostomy (for early enteral nutrition) and multiple drainage in the subphrenic and posterior mediastinum on both sides of the abdomen. In non-responders, esophagostomy and esophagogastric disconnection can be life-saving maneuvers.

Duodenal hematoma

Symptomatic intramural duodenal hematoma secondary to duodenal biopsies obtained at endoscopy is a rare but sometimes dramatic complication leading to possible perforation, pancreatitis and occlusion-like symptoms.[78,79] The resulting obstruction is self-limited and typically resolves spontaneously within a week. Conversely, perforation and pancreatitis progress to acute abdomen. In a patient with suspected perforation, because the posterior duodenal wall lies in the retroperitoneal cavity, plain abdominal series cannot show free abdominal gas. Nor are abdominal pain and muscular tenderness as obvious as they are in children with gastric or anterior duodenal wall perforation. Ultrasound shows the hematoma and, if present, improvement in pancreatic thickness, and a CT scan allows the diagnosis of perforation to be made. In patients with massive infected necrosis of the pancreatic parenchyma or retroperitoneal infection, surgical drainage is required.

Endoscopic cholangiopancreatography

Complications after ERCP are well known in children as in adults; their incidence, in diagnostic ERCP, is higher in children.[43] The therapeutic options are the same in both age groups.[44] Post-ERCP pancreatitis is also more frequent in children than in adults (8% vs. 3–7%).[45] Its main causes are papillary swelling owing to repeated cannulations; and pancreatic parenchymography due to excessive contrast injection.[80] A transient rise in serum amylase level, unaccompanied by pain or elevated WBC count or CRP level, is not diagnostic of pancreatitis. True pancreatitis with acute abdomen generally responds to conservative management; in our experience we have observed only one case of severe pancreatitis, which was conservatively managed but complicated by a pancreatic pseudocyst.

Biliary tree or duodenal perforation is a rare complication that can be managed conservatively but needs strict clinical surveillance. In a newborn with suspected biliary hypoplasia we observed a post-ERCP duodenal perforation, near the papilla, that responded well to non-surgical therapy.

Rectal suction biopsy

This well-known diagnostic procedure is the reference standard in the diagnosis of Hirschsprung's disease. The diagnostic role of rectal suction biopsy, first described by Noblett,[81] has improved with the availability of acetylcholinesterase staining. Complications of this procedure are bleeding and, especially in newborns, rectal perforation. Rectal perforation was described in 0.2% of 1340 consecutive rectal suction biopsy procedures, including one case of buttock gangrene.[82] In our experience, we have observed one case of bleeding in a patient who received a blood transfusion, and a case of rectal perforation in a patient with acute abdomen and pneumoperitoneum that needed laparotomy, surgical suture and drainage. If a deep suction biopsy specimen has to be taken below the peritoneal reflection, apart from the risk of perirectal septic cellulites, it poses no peritoneal problems.

REFERENCES

1. Valerio D. Acute diabetic abdomen in childhood. *Lancet* 1976; **10**: 66–68.
2. Way LW. Abdominal pain and the acute abdomen. In Sleisenger MH, Fortran JS, eds. *Gastrointestinal Disease*, 2nd edn. Philadelphia: WB Saunders, 1978: 394–410.
3. Glasgow RE, Mulvihill SJ. Abdominal pain, including the acute abdomen. In Feldman M, Scharschmidt BF, Sleisenger MH, eds. *Gastrointestinal Disease*, 6th edn. Philadelphia: WB Saunders, 1998: 80–89.
4. Liebman WM, Thaler MM. Pediatric considerations of abdominal pain and the acute abdomen. In Sleisenger MH, Fortran JS. *Gastrointestinal Disease*, 2nd edn. Philadelphia: WB Saunders, 1978: 411–436.
5. Babcock DS. Sonography of acute abdomen in the pediatric patient. *J Ultrasound Med* 2002; **21**: 887–899.
6. Rohrschneider WK, Troger J. Hydrostatic reduction of intussusception under US guidance. *Pediatr Radiol* 1995; **25**: 530–536.
7. Carty HM. Paediatric emergences: non traumatic abdominal emergences. *Eur Radiol* 2002; **12**: 2835–2848.
8. Shimizu T, Suzuki R, Yamashiro Y et al. Magnetic resonance cholangiopancreatography in assessing the cause of acute pancreatitis in children. *Pancreas* 2001; **22**: 196–199.
9. Hiroashi S, Hiroashi R, Uchida H et al. Pancreatitis: evaluation with MR cholangiopancreatography in children. *Radiology* 1997; **203**: 411–415.
10. Manfredi R, Lucidi V, Gui B et al. Idiopatic chronic pancreatitis in children: MR cholangiopancreatography after secretin administration. *Radiology* 2002; **224**: 675–682.
11. Gonzalez RA, Lopez-Roses L, Lancho SA et al. Strangulated volvulus of the sigmoid colon with inviable mucosal appareance in a non-surgical patient. Endoscopic devolvulation. *Rev Esp Enferm Dig* 2002; **94**: 221–225.
12. Pinedo G, Kirberg A. Percutaneous endoscopic sigmoidopexy in sigmoid volvulus with T-fasteners: report of two cases. *Dis Colon Rectum* 2001; **44**: 1867–1869.
13. Hurlstone DP. Successful endoscopic haemoclipping in Mallory–Weiss syndrome with concurrent closure of esophageal perforation: further prospective evaluation of the technique is required. *Scand J Gastroenterol* 2002; **37**: 866.
14. Cipolletta L, Bianco MA, Rotondano G. Endoscopic clipping of perforation following pneumatic dilatation of esophagojejunal anastomotic strictures. *Endoscopy* 2000; **32**: 720–722.
15. Gill BD, Jenkins JR. Cost-effective evaluation and management of the acute abdomen. *Surg Clin North Am* 1996; **76**: 71–82.
16. Wilkinson AH Jr. Acute abdomen. How to balance costs and quality care. *Semin Pediatr Surg* 1997; **6**: 88–91.
17. Bishop PR, Nowicki MJ, Parker PH Vomiting-induced hematemesis in children: Mallory–Weiss tear or prolapse gastropathy? *J Pediatr Gastroenterol Nutr* 2000; **30**: 436–441.
18. Montes H, Dolfo W, Venezuela M et al. Coexistence of gastric mucosal prolapse and Mallory Weiss tear. *J Gastroenterol Hepatol* 2001; **16**: 1172–1174.
19. Panieri E, Bass DH. The management of ingested foreign bodies in children – a review of 663 cases. *Eur J Emerg Med* 1995; **2**: 83–87.
20. Litovitz T, Schmitz BF. Ingestion of cylindrical and button batteries: an analyisis of 2382 cases. *Pediatrics* 1992; **89**: 747–757.
21. Burstein I, Steinberg R, Zer M. Small bowel obstruction and covered perforation in childhood caused by bizarre bezoars and foreign bodies. *Isr Med Assoc J* 2000; **2**: 129–131.
22. Jiledar, Singh G, Mitra SK. Gastric perforation secondary to recurrent trichobezoar. *Indian J Pediatr* 1996; **63**: 689–691.
23. Cauchi JA, Shawis RN. Multiple magnet ingestion and gastrointestinal morbidity. *Arch Dis Child* 2002; **87**: 539–540.
24. Stricker T, Kellenberger CJ, Neuhaus TJ et al. Ingested pins causing parforation. *Arch Dis Child* 2001; **84**: 165–166.
25. Fonkalsand EW, Loar N. Long term results after colectomy and endorectal pull-through procedure in children. *Ann Surg* 1992; **215**: 57–62.
26. Fazio VW. Toxic megacolon in ulcerative colitis and Crohn's colitis. In Farmer RG, eds. Clinics in gastroenterology. Philadelphia: WB Saunders, 1980: 389–407.
27. Sheth SG, LaMont JT. Toxic megacolon. *Lancet* 1998; **351**: 509–12.
28. Mourelle M, Casellas F, Guarner F et al. Induction of nitric oxide synthase in colonic smooth muscle from patients with toxic megacolon. *Gastroenterology* 1995; **109**: 1497–1502.
29. Ferzoco SJ, Becker JM. Does aggressive medical therapy for acute ulcerative colitis result in a higher incidence of staged colectomy? *Arch Surg* 1994; **129**: 420–423.
30. Furst MB, Stromberg BV, Blatchford GJ et al. Colonic anastomoses: bursting strength after corticosteroid treatment. *Dis Colon Rectum* 1994; **37**: 12–15.
31. Berg DF, Bahadursingh AM, Kaminki DL et al. Acute surgical emergencies in inflammatory bowel disease. *Am J Surg* 2002; **184**: 45–51.
32. Nicholls RJ, Dozois RR. Surgery for ulcerative colitis, Crohn's disease. In Nicholls RJ, Dozois RR, eds. *Surgery*

of the Colon and Rectum. New York: Churchill Livingstone, 1997: 593–644.

33. Nordlinger B, Saint-Mark O. Free perforation. In Michelassi F, Milsom JW. *Operative Strategies in Inflammatory Bowel Disease*. New York: Springer-Verlag, 1999: 369–373.
34. Greenstein AJ, Mann D, Heimann T et al. Spontaneous free perforation and perforated abscess in 30 patients with Crohn's disease. *Ann Surg* 1987; **205**: 72–76.
35. Tjandra JJ. Toxic colitis and perforation. In Michelassi F, Milsom JW, eds. *Operative Strategies in Inflammatory Bowel Disease*. New York: Springer-Verlag, 1999: 234–245.
36. Menguy R. Surgical management of free perforations of the small intestine complicating regional enteritis. *Ann Surg* 1972; **175**: 178–189.
37. Nichols RJ. Intraabdominal mass and/or abscess. In Michelassi F, Milsom JW, eds. *Operative Strategies in Inflammatory Bowel Disease*. New York: Springer-Verlag, 1999: 360–368.
38. Fazio V, Tiandra JJ. Strictureplasy for Crohn's disease with multiple long strictures. *Dis Colon Rectum* 1993; **36**: 71–72.
39. Michelassi F. Side-to side isoperistaltic strictureplasty for multiple Crohn's strictures. *Dis Colon Rectum* 1996; **39**: 345–349.
40. Dietz DW, Fazio VW, Laureti S et al. Strictureplasty in diffuse Crohn's jejunoileitis: safe and durable. *Dis Colon Rectum* 2002; **45**: 764–770.
41. Oliva L, Wyllie R, Alexander F et al. The results of strictureplasty in pediatric patients with multifocal Crohn's disease. *J Pediatr Gastroenterol Nutr* 1994; **18**: 306–310.
42. Federici di Abriola G, De Angelis P, Dall'Oglio L, Di Lorenzo M. Strictureplasty: an alternative approach in long segment bowel stenosis in pediatric Crohn's disease. *J Pediatr Surg* 2003; **38**: 814–818.
43. Prasil P, Laberge JM, Barkun A, Flageole H. Endoscopic retrograde cholangiopancreatography in children: a surgeon's perspective. *J Pediatr Surg* 2001; **36**: 733–735.
44. Freeman ML, Nelson DB, Sherman S et al. Complication of biliary sphincterotomy. *N Engl J Med* 1996; **335**: 909–918.
45. Fox VL, Werlin SL, Heyman MB et al. Endoscopic retrograde cholangiography in children. *J Pediatr Gastroenterol Nutr* 2000; **30**: 335–342.
46. Hasegawa T, Udatsu Y, Kamiyama M et al. Does a pancreatico-biliary maljunction play a role in spontaneous perforation of the bile duct in children? *Pediatr Surg Int* 2002; **18**: 565–566.
47. Kasat LS, Borwankar SS, Jain M, Naregal A. Spontaneous perforation of the extrahepatic bile duct in an infant. *Pediatr Surg Int* 2001; **17**: 463–464.
48. Ando K, Miyano T, Kohno S et al. Spontaneous perforation of choledochal cyst: a study of 13 cases. *Eur J Pediatr Surg* 1998; **8**: 23–25.
49. Shenoy VG, Jawale SA, Oak SN, Kulkarni BK. Anomalous pancreatobiliary union and chronic pancreatitis: rare presentation with biliary peritonitis. *Pediatr Surg Int* 2001; **17**: 549–551.
50. Tam PK, Saing H, Irving IM, Lister J. Acute pancreatitis in children. *J Pediatr Surg* 1985; **20**: 58–60.
51. Yachha SK, Chetri K, Saraswat VA et al. Management of childhood pancreatic disorders: a multidisciplinary approach. *J Pediatr Gastroenterol Nutr* 2003; **36**: 206–212.
52. Zargar SA, Javid G, Khan BA et al. Endoscopic sphincterotomy in the management of bile duct stones in children. *Am J Gastroenterol* 2003; **98**: 586–589.
53. Nikou GC, Arnautis TP, Giamarellos-Bouboulis EJ et al. The significance of the dosage adjustment of octreotide in the treatment of acute pancreatitis of moderate severity. *Hepatogastroenterology* 2001; **48**: 1754–1757.
54. Uhl W, Buchler MW, Malfertheiner P et al. A randomized, double blind, multicentre trial of octreotide in moderate to severe acute pancreatitis. *Gut* 1999; **45**: 97–104.
55. Paran H, Mayo A, Paran D et al. Octeotride treatment in patients with severe acute pancreatitis. *Dig Dis Sci* 2000; **45**: 2247–2251.
56. DeBanto JR, Goday PS, Pedroso MR et al. Acute pancreatitis in children. *Am J Gastroenterol* 2002; **97**: 1726–1731.
57. Jackson WD. Pancreatitis: etiology, diagnosis and management. *Curr Opin Pediatr* 2001; **13**: 447–451.
58. Onen A, Dokucu AI, Cigdem MK et al. Factors affecting morbidity in typhoid intestinal perforation in children. *Pediatr Surg Int* 2002; **18**: 696–700.
59. Mallick S, Klein JF. Management of typhoid perforation of the small bowel: a case series in Western French Guiana. *Med Trop* 2001; **61**: 491–494.
60. Kouame BD, Ouattara O, Dick RK et al. Diagnostic, therapeutic and prognostic aspects of intestinal typhoid perforations in children of Abidjan, Cote d'Ivoire. *Bull Soc Pathol Exot* 2001; **94**: 379–382.
61. Rahman GA, Abubakar AM, Johnson AW, Adeniran JO. Typhoid ileal perforation in Nigerian children: an analysis of 106 operative cases. *Pediatr Surg Int* 2001; **17**: 628–630.
62. Shah AA, Wani KA, Wazir BS. The ideal treatment of the typhoid enteric perforation – resection anastomosis. *Int Surg* 1999; **84**: 35–38.
63. Chao HC, Chiu CH, Kong MS et al. Factors associated with intestinal perforation in children's non-typhi *Salmonella* toxic megacolon. *Pediatr Infect Dis J* 2000; **19**: 1158–1162.
64. Ciftci AO, Karnak I, Senocak ME et al. Spectrum of complicated intestinal amebiasis through resected specimens: incidence and outcome. *J Pediatr Surg* 1999; **34**: 1369–1373.
65. Nagi B, Lal A, Kochhar R et al. Perforations and fistulae in gastrointestinal tuberculosis. *Acta Radiol* 2002; **43**: 501–506.
66. Talwar S, Talwar R, Prasad P. Tuberculous perforations of the small intestine. *Int J Clin Pract* 1999; **53**: 514–518.
67. Ido K, Yuasa H, Ide M et al. Sonographic diagnosis of small intestinal anisakiasis. *J Clin Ultrasound* 1998; **26**: 125–130.
68. Shirahama M, Konga T, Ishibashi H et al. Intestinal anisakiasis: US in diagnosis. *Radiology* 1992; **185**: 789–793.
69. Herbrecht R, Letscher-Bru V, Bowden RA et al. Treatment of 21 cases of invasive mucormycosis with amphotericin B colloidal dispersion. *Eur J Clin Microbiol Infect Dis* 2001; **20**: 460–466.
70. Villani A, Vacca P, Onofri A, Cori M. Disseminated mucormycosis. A rare case in pediatric intensive care. *Minerva Anesthesiol* 1997; **63**: 249–252.
71. Legnani PE, Kornbluth A. Therapeutic options in the management of strictures in Crohn's disease. *Gastrointest Endosc Clin North Am* 2002; **12**: 589–603.
72. Thomas-Gibson S, Brooker JC, Hayward CM, Shah SG. Colonoscopic balloon dilatation of Crohn's strictures: a review of long-term outcomes. *Eur J Gastroenterol Hepatol* 2003; **15**: 485–488.
73. Segal D, Michaud L, Guimber D et al. Late-onset complications of percutaneous endoscopic gastrostomy

in children. *J Pediatr Gastroenterol Nutr* 2001; **33**: 495–500.

74. Fox VL, Abel SD, Malas S et al. Complications following percutaneous endoscopic gastrostomy and subsequent catheter replacement in children and young adults. *Gastrointest Endosc* 1997; **45**: 64–71.
75. Pofahl WE, Ringold F. Management of early dislodgment of percutaneous endoscopic gastrostomy tubes. *Surg Laparosc Endosc Percutan Tech* 1999; **9**: 253–256.
76. Meng Boey CC, Goh KL, Sithasanan N, Goh DW. Jejunal perforation complicating PEG insertion in a child. *Gastrointest Endosc* 2002; **55**: 607–608.
77. Ledermann SE, Spitz L, Moloney J et al. Gastrostomy feeding in infants and children on peritoneal dialysis. *Pediatr Nefrol* 2002; **17**: 246–250.
78. Warngard O, Stenhammar L, Ascher H et al. Small bowel biopsy in Swedish paediatric clinics. *Acta Paediatr* 1996; **85**: 240–241.
79. Guzman C, Bousvaros A, Buonuomo C, Nurko S. Intraduodenal hematoma complicating intestinal biopsy: case reports and review of the literature. *Am J Gastroenterol* 1998; **93**: 2547–2550.
80. Dall'Oglio L, De Angelis P, Federici di Abriola G et al. La colangiopancreatografia retrograda per via endoscopica in età pediatrica. In De Angelis GL, ed. *L'endoscopia digestiva in età pediatrica e giovanile*, 1st edn. Rome: Edizioni Medico Scientifiche Internazionali, 2002: 95–109.
81. Noblett HR. A rectal suction biopsy tube for use in the diagnosis of Hirschsprung's disease. *J Pediatr Surg* 1969; **4**: 406–409.
82. Teitelbaum DH, Coran AG, Weitzman JJ et al. Hirschsprung's disease and related neuromuscular disorders of the intestine. In O'Neill JA, Rowe MI, Grosfeld JL et al. eds. *Pediatric Surgery*, 5th edn. St. Louis: Mosby-Year Book, 1998: 1381–1424.

41 Management of ingested foreign bodies

Yvan Vandenplas, Said Hachimi-Idrissi and Bruno Hauser

Introduction

The first report of a foreign body in a child dates from 1692 when Frederick the Great who, at the age of 4 swallowed a shoe buckle that passed without incident.[1] Accidental ingestion of a foreign body occurs frequently in children, and accounts for a significant number of emergency room visits. In general, accidental ingestion causes little or no morbidity.[2–4] In the majority of cases that come to medical attention, the ingestion was witnessed or is strongly suspected by the child's caretaker. A significant number of accidental ingestions are likely to remain asymptomatic, since most objects pass without any incident. Sometimes the foreign object is discovered by accident in the stools[5].

Epidemiology

Ingestion of foreign bodies is mainly a pediatric problem, since about 80% of cases occur in children between the ages of 6 and 36 months.[6–9] In our series of 325 children, the median age of the children was 2.8 years (Table 41.1).[6] According to reported series, the median age is less than 5 years. In adults, ingestion of foreign bodies may be intentional, as can be the case in adolescents. Intentional ingestion occurs most frequently in psychiatrically impaired individuals and prisoners.[10] The largest series ingested by one individual was reported by Chalk and Foucour in 1928 and was an assortment of 2533 pins, needles and bobbins.[11] We had an adolescent girl who was a pencil-swallowing recidivist (unpublished). Amongst the miscellaneous foreign bodies observed in our series, one developmentally retarded child managed to ingest a large plastic bag (the type used in supermarkets); the plastic bag caused decreased food intake as single symptom.[6]

During recent years, a number of large pediatric series have been reported in the literature. The series of Weissberg included 70 patients (children and adults),[12] Kim et al reported 104 Korean pediatric cases,[13] and Olives report a series of 395 children.[8] Athanassiadi et al reported a series of 400 cases,[14] and Lam and et al reported as many as 5240 ingested foreign bodies.[15] In the USA, about 200 000 accidental ingestions occur yearly in children and adolescents.[16] In 1997, there were more than 21 000 emergency room visits by children in the USA for coin ingestions alone.[17] The incidence

Table 41.1 Age distribution of 325 children with foreign body ingestion

Age (years)	No. of patients	%
0–1	36	11
1–2	64	20
2–3	78	24
3–4	55	17
4–5	27	8
5–6	29	9
6–7	12	4
7–8	10	3
8–10	6	2
10–18	8	2
Total	**325**	**100**

Mean age 2.8 years (range 5 months to 18 years)
Boys/girls, 58/42%

Table 41.2 Nature and number of foreign bodies ingested

	n	%
Coins	89	27
Sharp objects (needles, pins, etc.)	51	16
Batteries	43	13
Toy parts	38	12
Bones (fish, chicken)	38	12
Large food bags	37	12
Jewellery	19	6
Miscellaneous	10	3
Total	**325**	**100**

Table 41.3 Comparison between our data and the study reported by Olives[8]

	Present study	Olives[8]
Number of patients	325	395
Age distribution	5 months to 18 years	2 months to 18 years
Boy/girl ratio (%)	58/42	60/40
Radio-opaque foreign body (%)	60	64
Asymptomatic (%)	46	20
Dysphagia, restrosternal pain (%)	24	59
Coins	most frequent (27%)	most frequent (40%)
Endoscopic removal (%)	25	85
Success rate (%)	99	64
Perforation (*n*)	0	0

and type of foreign body ingested depends on the geographic region (and reports depending on the specialty of the author). In our department, during a period of 15 years, 325 pediatric cases were seen because of ingestion of a foreign body or symptoms of acute esophageal obstruction. In general, coins are the most common foreign bodies ingested, and account for 27–70% of all cases[6,10,18-21] (Tables 41.2 and 41.3, and Figure 41.1). History in determining coin denomination is unreliable.[22] In seaside regions, fish bones tend to be the most important.[23] The incidence of accidental ingestion of fish bones in China seems very high, with an incidence reaching 84%.[24] In the children of this series, fish bones accounted for 43% and coins for 39%.[24] Other frequently ingested objects are sharp objects such as needles and pins, batteries, toy parts, chicken or fish bones. Each accounts for 5–30%, depending on the series.[6,10,23] In adults, unintentional ingestions most frequently involve meat or fish bones. Gastric (tricho-) bezoars can be considered as a special group of foreign bodies, most of the time needing surgical removal.[25] In young infants, lactobezoars can cause gastric outlet obstruction.[26] Some candies contain a gel that may become compact in the intestinal lumen and cause obstruction.[27]

In our series of 325 children, 12 children had ingested more than one foreign body. Ten children were 'recidivists', and were seen twice because of ingestion of a foreign body.[6] Overall, natural elimination occurred in 46% of the patients.[6]

Clinical signs and symptoms

Location of the object

Most swallowed foreign bodies do not come to medical attention as they do not cause symptoms. Sometimes foreign bodies are discovered by coincidence, on a standard X-ray that was performed for other indications.[6] The majority of coin ingestions are asymptomatic.[6,23] The symptoms of obstruction caused by a foreign body depend on patient age, object size and its location. Symptoms in young children are non-specific and can include choking, drooling and poor feeding. There may be

History of radio-opaque foreign body (FB)

Fluoroscopy or X-ray neck, chest, stomach (abdomen)

Symptomatic

endoscopy and

- FB trapped in esophagus: push into stomach
- attempt at removal

(fasting if symptoms allow waiting time)

Asymptomatic

FB In pharynx, esophagus: removal/push into stomach

FB in stomach: removal if sharp, battery, large (>3–4 cm in length)

(magnet probe vs. endoscopy)

FB beyond stomach: wait and see if after 1–2 weeks, FB not observed in stools: control X-ray

History of radiolucent swallowed foreign body

Symptomatic

endoscopy and

- FB trapped in esophagus: push into stomach and in pharynx, esophagus: removal/push into stomach
- attempt at removal

(fasting if symptoms allow waiting time)

Asymptomatic

X-ray with contrast (visualizes FB if trapped in esophagus, diagnostic possibly therapeutic)

if FB remains in esophagus: endoscopy when fasting

if FB not in esophagus: wait and see (observe stools) if after 1–2 weeks, FB not observed in stools: control X-ray

History of choking spell (acute onset of severe onset cough, difficulty breathing, anxiety)

Physical examination

Normal

X-ray neck, chest (anterior–posterior, lateral) normal: wait and see

FB: removal

Abnormal

X-ray neck, chest (anterior–posterior, lateral)

FB: removal

Figure 41.1 Proposed recomendations for a child who has possibly swallowed a foreign body or presents the symptoms suggesting esophageal obstruction.

a time interval between ingestion and development of (respiratory) symptoms in infants.[10] Children may alter their diet to consume liquids or a soft diet. Older children and teenagers with a foreign body in the esophagus typically complain of dysphagia, odynophagia and chest pain.

Depending on the organization of medical care, approximately 5–10% of patients will have the foreign body located in the oropharynx, 20% in the esophagus, 60% in the stomach and 10% distal to the stomach.[28] Where fish bone ingestion is common, a higher percentage of patients will have the foreign body located in the oropharynx. In general, foreign bodies in the oropharynx are symptomatic and cause dysphagia.[6–10] In our series, 22 of the 28 (79%) foreign bodies in the oropharynx were bones from fish or poultry. The rest were glass and there was one metal object.[6] These foreign bodies were visible on physical examination of the oropharynx.[6] Additionally, it should be mentioned that there were 17 children who became symptomatic during the eating of fish or poultry, but with a negative inspection and no visualization of a bone on X-ray. Because symptoms persisted in these children, endoscopy was performed and a (small) laceration of the pharyngeal or esophageal mucosa could be observed in eight of them.[6]

In our experience, 54% of the children had transient symptoms immediately after the ingestion.[6] In the patients in whom the ingestion was not witnessed (32 out of 176; 18%), the sudden onset of symptoms (such as acute and severe coughing, pain, etc.) and the circumstances of this sudden onset made the diagnosis of accidental ingestion suspected. Symptoms were in almost all cases pain or discomfort at the pharyngeal or retrosternal region, excessive saliva production, nausea and vomiting, acute coughing and difficulties in breathing. In 28 out of 325 patients (9%), the event was accompanied by more severe manifestations such as cyanosis or severe dysphagia.[6]

Approximately 60–70% of foreign bodies that become stuck in the esophagus are located in the proximal esophagus at the level of the upper esophageal sphincter.[10,28] Twenty per cent of the obstructions occur at the lower esophageal sphincter; the rest occur in the mid-esophagus at the level of the aortic notch. Patients with underlying esophageal disease are at greater risk for the foreign body being entrapped in the esophagus. Especially children with congenital esophageal atresia, tracheoesophageal fistula or fundoplication are at risk. Coins are relatively frequently trapped in the esophagus, although the reported incidence varies from 5 to 60%, mostly at the level of the upper or lower esophageal sphincter.[29,30] The history of the child does not help to understand the pathophysiological reason of this trapping. Manometric measurements of the sphincters have not been performed in these patients.

Respiratory symptoms such as wheezing, stridor and speech impairment may be the only symptoms of a foreign body in the esophagus. Respiratory symptoms can be the consequence of paraesophageal soft tissue swelling[10]. Isolated respiratory symptoms are more frequent in infants and toddlers.

In our published series, the vast majority of the foreign bodies (196; 60%) were located in the stomach at the time of presentation.[6] Thirty-six (11%) foreign bodies were already located in the small intestine at first presentation.[6] All these, except three, were eliminated spontaneously. Three foreign bodies were very long sharp metal objects (screws of >5 cm) located in the duodenum at presentation. In order to avoid complications, they were endoscopically removed under anesthesia. Gastric and intestinal foreign bodies may cause obstruction and perforation.

Complications

Yearly, approximately 1500 deaths occur in the USA secondary to foreign body ingestion[31]. Foreign bodies impacted in the oropharynx are usually sharp and cause symptoms, and may cause life-threatening complications such as retropharyngeal abscess and perforation.[23,32–35]

Perforation is one of the most dangerous complications, but occurs in less than 1% of cases. Sharp objects are associated with a much higher perforation rate than dull objects.[36] Pins can cause gastric perforation and migrate into the thorax.[36] The notion that 'advancing points perforate and trailing points do not' dates back to 1937, based on the evidence provided by analysis of 3266 accidental ingestions and inhalations.[37] A foreign body entrapped in the esophagus may initially be asymptomatic, but cause ulceration of the esophageal mucosa due to pressure necrosis in case of a dull object. Sharp objects may perforate, and cause aortic–esophageal fistula, mediastinitis, tracheo-esophageal fistula and broncho-esophageal fistula.[23] Esophageal diverticula or pseudodiverticula may develop secondary to pressure by a dull object.

Death because of multiple perforations occurred within 2 months in an individual who had swallowed over 500 pins.[38] No child in our series or in Olives' series presented with perforation.[6,8] In the series reported by Weissberg, 15 perforations occurred in 70 patients.[12] Differences and similarities between the reported series are likely to be related to the selection of the patients.[39] Perforation can result in extraluminal migration of the foreign body. Perforations occur most frequently in the region of the ileocecal valve. Congenital malformations such as Meckel's diverticulum or prior intestinal surgery are sites of increased risk for foreign body entrapment and perforation.[28]

Foreign bodies only rarely cause jejunal, ileal or colic obstruction, although it has been reported to occur.[40] Obstruction of the appendix with a foreign body is extremely rare.[41]

Metallic foreign bodies such as coins that remain for several weeks in the stomach could cause toxicity, especially with zinc-predominant coins.[17]

Diagnosis and differential diagnosis

Rapid diagnosis and treatment of foreign bodies trapped in the gastrointestinal tract will decrease morbidity and length of hospital stay.[42] A foreign body not discovered in all patients with symptoms suggests the presence of an object in the oropharynx. In the series of Olives, 11% of the swallowed foreign bodies were not found in the gastrointestinal tract.[8]

Oral fluids make coins move easily into the stomach.[30] Therefore, a 5-day observation at home is advised.[30] Whether X-ray is recommended in every child who is suspected of having swallowed a foreign body has been a topic of controversy for many years.[43] Between 60 and 90% of ingested foreign bodies are radio-opaque.[6,10,18] Although most foreign body ingestions remain asymptomatic, when ingestion is witnessed it is recommended to perform a roentgenogram because the object may be lodged in the esophagus and pose a risk to the patient even if asymptomatic.[28] An anterior–posterior X-ray demonstrates the location of a coin. A lateral radiograph may be helpful in case of ingestion of a sharp object such as a needle or a pin to exclude asymptomatic location in the airways. Since esophageal trapping of a foreign body may remain asymptomatic, and since chronic impaction may cause ulceration and necrosis of the mucosa, fluoroscopy or X-ray is advised. Unnecessary exposure to radiation is less harmful than the consequence of chronic impaction. A simple X-ray or fluoroscopy (smaller irradiation than X-ray) is much easier than the use of metal detectors.[44,45]

In 6% of our patients, the foreign body was radiolucent, with five cases with a fish or chicken bone that penetrated the esophageal mucosa and 16 cases of impaction of a food bolus[6]. Three of these children were psychomotor retarded, and the other children had been operated upon previously because of an esophageal atresia and were known to have a residual esophageal stenosis.[6] Non-radio-opaque foreign bodies represent a much more difficult diagnostic challenge than radio-opaque bodies. A negative radiographic analysis does not rule out the presence of a foreign body in the gastrointestinal tract.[42] Indeed, non-radio-opaque foreign bodies such as plastic bag clips seem to be relatively frequently swallowed, and may cause obstruction and perforation.[46] If a non-radio-opaque foreign body is not observed in the stools after a period of 2 weeks, control investigations should be performed. We perform contrast X-ray to detect a gastric foreign body, because we consider this less invasive than endoscopy.

Chronic unexplained respiratory disease necessitates the exclusion of a foreign body in the gastrointestinal tract or airways. This object can be radiolucent and therefore difficult to diagnose. In such a case, the majority of centers recommend diagnostic and immediate therapeutic bronchoscopy.[47]

Treatment options

Over 80% of foreign body ingestions that come to medical attention are naturally eliminated spontaneously. Ten to twenty per cent require endoscopic removal, and less than 1% require surgery.[6]

Foreign bodies located in the oropharynx may be visible on physical examination, and if this is the case, the foreign body can be removed with the help of a Magill's forceps or similar equipment.[48] In our experience, the foreign body was impacted in 28 (9%) of the patients in the oropharynx on presentation, and could be extracted with a Magill forceps.[6]

Symptomatic patients who are unable to swallow their secretions and those with respiratory symptoms should undergo emergency endoscopy.[49] The first endoscopic extraction dates from 1972.[50] Different forceps and baskets used for removal are shown in Figure 41.2. Sharp objects and batteries should be removed whenever possible.[21] Straight pins are the exception to the perforation risk, because the blunt-ended head passes first through the gastrointestinal tract. (However, sharp metal objects can also be removed safely with a magnet.)

The incidence of endoscopic removal is as low as 25% in our series, but is 77% and 85% in other series,[8,23] and with a success rate of 99% in our experience and that of Kim et al,[6,13] whereas Olives reported a failure rate of 36%.[8] The timing of the extraction of the body from the esophagus depends on the severity of the symptoms and the fasting state of the patient.[6] Sedation and anesthesia, or esophageal introduction of the endoscope or magnet probe, in half of our patients caused relaxation of the sphincter, resulting in a spontaneous passage of the foreign body into the stomach. If the patient was under anesthesia, the foreign body was removed. If the patient was only sedated, endoscopy was stopped and the management for gastric foreign bodies was applied (Figure 41.3).[6] Intravenous administration of glucagons dilates the esophagus and has been successfully used in adults, but has not been effective in children.[51]

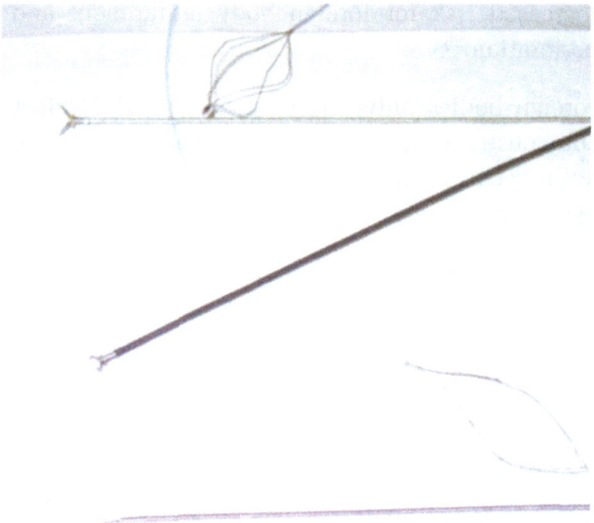

Figure 41.2 Alligator jaw forceps, tripod or pentapod forceps and baskets used for endoscopic removal.

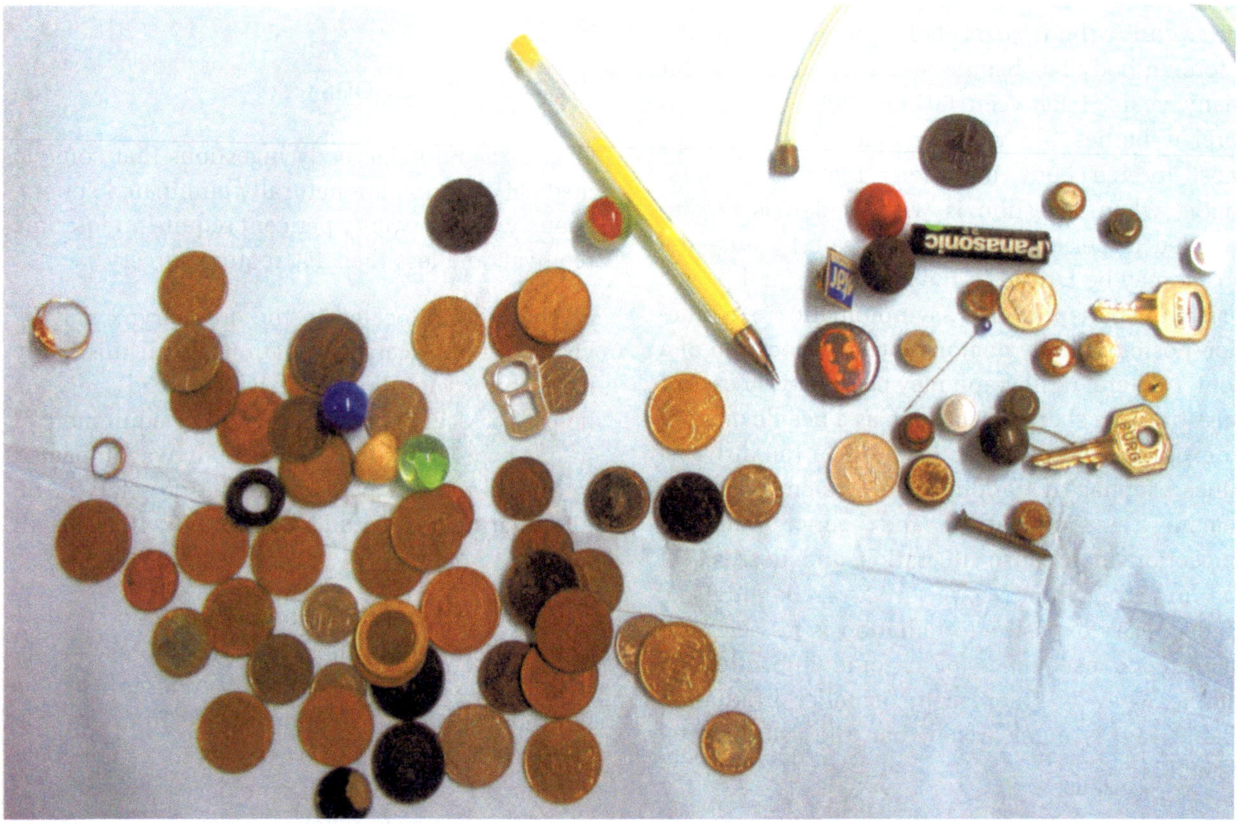

Figure 41.3 Foreign bodies that have been extracted from the gastrointestinal tract in our unit.

Esophageal extraction with a Foley catheter was already reported in 1966 by Bigler.[52] Smooth foreign bodies can be removed from the esophagus with a Foley catheter.[10] This technique has been reported to be 95% successful.[53] Fluoroscopically guided Foley catheter extraction of retained coins in pediatric patients who lack evidence of significant esophageal edema causing tracheal compromise is a safe and efficacious technique.[54] However, the procedure has also been said to be potentially dangerous, because a foreign body can flip out with catheter removal, and cause immediate respiratory complications.[55]

If the foreign body is in the stomach at the moment of presentation, the recommended attitude is to 'wait and observe', except for long sharp objects such as needles and pins (>3 to 4 cm).[6] Gastric coins do not have to be extracted, since the majority of them will be eliminated spontaneously.[30] However, extraction is recommended if, after several weeks, the object is still in the stomach.[6] Also, administration of prokinetics has been reported in this indication,[7] although this is not recommended. Objects greater than 10 cm in length in the stomach of an adult-size patient cannot pass the duodenum.[49] An ovoid object greater than 5 cm in length or with a thickness greater than 2 cm is unlikely to pass the pylorus.[56] Objects of the size of toothbrushes[1] or pencils (own experience) should be removed from the stomach. Anecdotally, in one of our cases, when a child had swallowed a ring worth over $2000 in a jeweler's shop, the ring was removed immediately.

In our department, magnetic foreign bodies are removed with a magnet probe.[6] In the series we reported, extraction of batteries was attempted with a magnet probe, but failed in four cases out of 36.[6] The largest series of battery ingestions reported was from a national survey registry reporting 2382 ingestions in 2320 patients.[57] Button batteries from hearing aids are frequently ingested. Children imitate body piercing by using small powerful magnets across parts of their body including nose, ears, penis and tongue.[58] Some swallowed the magnets while attempting to use them, resulting in at least one near fatal complication.[58] There have been 25 reported cases of batteries dislodged in the esophagus, causing development of fistula, strictures and even death.[57] Batteries impacted in the esophagus should be immediately removed.[49,59] Severe complications have occurred even with small batteries, and esophageal perforation was reported within 6 h after ingestion. The caustic material in the battery, and perhaps discharge of current, may be responsible for the rapid development of severe complications.[60] Batteries contain corrosive substances and may cause necrosis of the mucosa in case of leakage.[4,21,61] Ingestion of 12 small magnets caused perforation; the magnets were attracted to each other and caused pressure necrosis.[62] As a consequence, according to some authors, batteries cause a dilemma between a 'wait-and-see' attitude and an urgent laparoscopy.[59,63] Therefore, the development of a magnet probe is a useful tool, since it enables easy extraction in safe conditions.[9,61,64,65] In our series, all gastric needles and pins could be removed with the magnet probe, except for two patients who had swallowed open safety pins. In these cases, endoscopic extraction under anesthesia was performed.[6]

Prevention is preferable to treatment. Modification of toy manufacturing practices and labeling standards may decrease the relative incidence of toy part ingestion. The US Consumer Product Safety Commission considers the toys within eggs to violate the small parts regulation of this Commission with respect to children under 3, and therefore these chocolate eggs are not allowed to be marketed in the USA, although no injuries involving these toys have been reported to date.[66]

Appropriate equipment and personnel for emergency resuscitation should be present when removing a foreign body without general anesthesia and intubation.[6]

Food impaction

Impaction of food, usually meat, is the most common obstruction in adolescents and in toddlers after esophageal repair for congenital atresia.[67,68] Contrast radiography is not indicated because of the risk of aspiration.[49] If the symptoms are not too serious, tenderizers can be help.[67] Cola drinks in small amounts can also help in digesting impacted food (own experience).

Cocaine ingestion

This phenomenon occurs primarily in adolescents and young adults who act as a 'mule' and ingest cocaine-filled condoms as a method of smuggling.[49] Absorption of 1–3 g of cocaine following condom rupture is fatal, but one condom contains 3–5 g.

Follow-up

A telephone survey 2 weeks after ingestion of the foreign body did not reveal any unexpected complication.[6] In our experience, with a gastric foreign body that was not extracted, we advise the parents to observe the stools for 2 weeks.[6] If the foreign body was not observed in the stools, which was the case in as much as 62% of our patients, a control X-ray was performed.[6] In our series, in about two-thirds of the cases, the foreign body appeared to be eliminated spontaneously, despite being undetected by the parents.[6] This finding is in accordance with those of Macgregor and Ferguson stating that almost 50% of the foreign bodies were not recovered in the stools.[7] In about one-third, the foreign body was still present in the stomach. In that case, the foreign body was actively removed.[6] Kim et al[13] reported a spontaneous elimination of the foreign body in only 22% of cases, whereas we observed this phenomenon in almost half of our patients (46%). Amin et al reported a gastric passage of only 19% of ingested coins.[22] The transit time is variable and unpredictable; the mean transit time in the series of children who presented at our emergency department was 3.8 days.[6,7,39]

Because gastric foreign bodies are frequently eliminated naturally, esophageal bougienage pushing a foreign body from the esophagus into the stomach has been recommended.[69] Whether esophageal extraction or passage into the stomach should be attempted depends largely on the local possibilities and on the condition of the patient, fasting or not. If, after a 'reasonable long period' such as 4–6 weeks, the foreign body is still present in the stomach, endoscopic removal is proposed.[6]

Conclusions

Only a minority of the accidental foreign body ingestions in children are witnessed by a bystander, and as a consequence it can be hypothesized that the majority of accidental ingestions remain asymptomatic. However, experience shows that esophageal trapping may be asymptomatic and that a foreign body can remain in the stomach for several weeks. Severe complications such as obstruction or perforation have been reported. Therefore, management should be balanced, not neglecting the small risk for severe morbidity but also avoiding over-investigation. In Figure 41.1, a practical attitude is proposed. These recommendations are limited to swallowed foreign bodies, and do not discuss foreign bodies in the respiratory tract.

REFERENCES

1. Kirk AD, Bowers BA, Moylan JA, Meyers WC. Toothbrush swallowing. *Arch Surg* 1988; **123**: 382–384.
2. Harris LS, Baker SP, Smith GA. Childhood asphyxiation by food: a national analysis and overview. *J Am Med Assoc* 1984; **251**: 2231–2235.
3. Litovitz T, Schmitz BF. Ingestion of cylindral and button batteries: an analysis of 2382 cases. *Pediatrics* 1992; **89**: 747–757.
4. Vandenplas Y, de Pont S. Foreign bodies in the upper gastrointestinal tract. *Acta Endosc* 1994; **24**: 363–370.
5. Bendig DW, Mackie GG. Management of smooth–blunt gastric foreign bodies in asymptomatic patients. *Clin Pediatr* 1990; **29**: 642–645.
6. Arana A, Hauser B, Hachimi-Idrissi S, Vandenplas Y. Management of ingested foreign bodies in childhood and review of the literature. *Eur J Pediatr* 2001; **160**: 458–472.
7. Macgregor D, Ferguson J. Foreign body ingestion in children: an audit of transit time. *J Accid Emerg Med* 1998; **15**: 371–373.

8. Olives JP. Ingested foreign bodies. *J Pediatr Gastroenterol Nutr* 2000; **31** (Suppl 2): S188.
9. Webb WA. Management of foreign bodies of the upper gastrointestinal tract. *Gastroenterology* 1988; **94**: 204–216.
10. Macpherson RI, Hill JG, Othersen HB. Esophageal foreign bodies in children: diagnosis, treatment and complications. *Am J Roentgenol* 1996; **166**: 919–924.
11. Chalk SG, Foucour HO. Foreign bodies in the stomach: report of a case in which more than 2,500 foreign bodies were found. *Arch Surg* 1928; **16**: 494–500.
12. Weissberg D. Foreign bodies in the gastro-intestinal tract. *S Afr J Surg* 1991; **29**: 150–153.
13. Kim JK, Kim SS, Kil JI et al. Management of foreign bodies in the gastrointestinal tract: an analysis of 104 cases in children. *Endoscopy* 1999; **31**: 302–304.
14. Athanassiadi K, Gerazounis M, Metaxas E, Kalantzi N. Management of esophageal foreign bodies: a retrospective review of 400 cases. *Eur J Cardio-Thorac Surg* 2002; **21**: 653–656.
15. Lam HC, Woo JK, van Hasslet CA. Management of ingested foreign bodies: a retrospective review of 5240 patients. *J Laryngol Otol* 2001; **115**: 954–7.
16. Litovitz TL, Keliin-Schwartz W, White S. 1999 Annual report of the American Association of Poison Control Centers Toxic Exposure Surveillance System. *Am J Emerg Med* 2000; **18**: 517–574.
17. Jefferson T. A thought for your pennies. *J Am Med Assoc* 1999; **281**: 122.
18. Darrow DH, Holinger LD, Lemberg PS. Aerodigestive tract foreign bodies in the older child and adolescent. *Ann Otol Rhinol Laryngol* 1996; **105**: 267–271.
19. Campbell JB, Quattromani FL, Foley LC. Foley catheter removal of blunt esophageal foreign bodies. Experience with 100 consecutive children. *Pediatr Radiol* 1983; **13**: 116–118.
20. Paul RI, Christoffel KK, Binns HJ, Jaffe DM. Foreign body ingestions in children: risk for complication varies with site on initial health care contact. Pediatric Practice Research Group. *Pediatrics* 1993; **91**: 121–127.
21. Webb WA. Management of foreign bodies of the upper gastrointestinal tract: update. *Gastrointest Endosc* 1995; **41**: 39–51.
22. Amin MR, Buchinsky FJ, Gaughan JP, Szeremeta W. Predicting outcome in pediatric coin ingestion. *Int J Pediatr Otorhinolaryngol* 2001; **59**: 201–206.
23. Cheng W, Tam PK. Foreign body ingestion in children: experience with 1,265 cases. *J Pediatr Surg* 1999; **34**: 1472–1476.
24. Nandi P, Ong GB. Foreign body in the oesophagus: review of 2,394 cases. *Br J Surg* 1978; **65**: 5–9.
25. De Backer A, van Nooten V, Vandenplas Y. Huge gastric trichobezoar in a 10-year old girl: case report with emphasis on endoscopy in diagnosis and therapy. *J Pediatr Gastroenterol Nutr* 1999; **28**: 513–515.
26. DuBose T, Southgate WM, Hill JG. Lactobezoars: a patient series and literature review. *Clin Pediatr* 2001; **40**: 603–606.
27. Seidel JS, Gausche-Hill M. Lychee-flavored gel candies: a potentially lethal snack for infants and children. *Arch Pediatr Adolesc Med* 2002; **156**: 1120–1122.
28. Panieri E, Bass DH. The management of ingested foreign bodies in children – a review of 663 cases. *Eur J Emerg Med* 1995; **2**: 83–87.
29. Binder L, Anderson WA. Pediatric gastro-intestinal foreign body ingestions. *Ann Emerg Med* 1984; **13**: 112–117.
30. Caravati EM, Bennett DL, McElwee NE. Pediatric coin ingestion. A prospective study on the utility of routine roentgenograms. *Am J Dis Child* 1989; **143**: 549–551.
31. Schwartz GF, Polsky HS. Ingested foreign bodies of the gastrointestinal tract. *Am Surg* 1976; **42**: 236–238.
32. Bizakis JG, Segas J, Haralambas S. Retropharyngeal abscess associated with a swallowed bone. *Am J Otolaryngol* 1993; **14**: 354–357.
33. Gostout C, Bowyer B, Alhquist D. Mucosal malformation of the gastrointesinal tract. Clinical observations and results of the endoscopic neodymium-YAG laser therapy. *Mayo Clin Proc* 1988; **63**: 894–899.
34. Knight LC, Lesser TH. Fish bones in the throat. *Arch Emerg Med* 1989; **6**: 13–16.
35. Simic MA, Budakov BM. Fatal upper esophageal hemorrhage caused by a previously ingested chicken bone: case report. *Am J Forensic Med Pathol* 1998; **19**: 166–168.
36. Stricker T, Kellenberger CJ, Neuhaus TJ et al . Ingested pins causing perforation. *Arch Dis Child* 2001; **84**: 165–166.
37. Jackson C, Jackson CL. *Disease of the Air and Food Passages of Foreign Body Origin*. Philadelphia: WB Saunders, 1937.
38. Henderson CT, Engel J, Schlesinger P. Foreign body ingestion: review and suggested guidelines for management. *Endoscopy* 1987; **19**: 68–71.
39. Hachimi-Idrissi S, Corne L, Vandenplas Y. Management of ingested foreign bodies in childhood: our experience and review of the literature. *Eur J Emerg Med* 1998; **5**: 461–463.
40. Da Silva EJ, Golakai VK. Foreign body causing chronic subacute small bowel obstruction: an unusual case from Harare hospital. *Centr Afr J Med* 1998; **44**: 16–18.
41. Klinger PJ, Seeling MH, de Vault KR et al. Ingested foreign bodies within the appendix: a 100 year review of the literature. *Dig Dis* 1998; **16**: 308–314.
42. Messner AH. Pitfalls in the diagnosis of aerodigestive tract foreign bodies. *Clin Pediatr* 1998; **37**: 359–365.
43. Hodge D, Tecklenburg F, Fleisher G. Coin ingestion: does every child need a radiograph? *Ann Emerg Med* 1985; **4**: 443–446.
44. Bassett KE, Schunk JE, Logan L. Localizing ingested coins with a metal detector. *Am J Emerg Med* 1999; **17**: 38–41.
45. Seikel K, Primm PA, Elizondo BJ, Remley KL. Handheld metal detector localization of ingested metallic foreign bodies: accurate in any hands? *Arch Pediatr Adolesc Med* 1999; **153**: 853–857.
46. Newell KJ, Taylor B, Walton JC, Tweedie EJ. Plastic bread-bag clips in the gastrointestinal tract: report of 5 cases and review of the literature. *CMAJ* 2000; **162**: 527–529.
47. Dunn GR, Wardrop P, Lo S, Cowan DL. Management of suspected foreign body aspiration in children. *Clin Otolaryngol* 2002; **27**: 384–387.
48. Mahafza TM. Extracting coins from the upper end of the esophagus using a Magill forceps technique. *Intern J Pediatr Otorhinolaryngol* 2002; **62**: 37–39.
49. Wahbeh G, Wyllie R, Lay M. Foreign body ingestion in infants and children: location, location, location. *Clin Pediatr* 2002; **41**: 633–640.
50. Morrissey JF. Gastrointestinal endoscopy. *Gastroenterology* 1972; **62**: 1241–1268.
51. Mehta D, Attia M, Quintana E, Cronan K. Glucagon use for esophageal coin dislodgment in children: a prospective, double-blind, placebo-controlled trial. *Acad Emerg Med* 2001; **8**: 200–203.
52. Bigler FC. The use of a Foley catheter for removal of blunt foreign bodies from the esophagus. *J Thorac Cardiovasc Surg* 1966; **51**: 759–760.

53. Campbell JB, Condon VR. Catheter removal of blunt esophageal foreign bodies in children. Survey of the Society for Pediatric Radiology. *Pediatr Radiol* 1989; **19**: 361–365.
54. Harned RK 2nd, Strain JD, Hay TC, Douglas MR. Esophageal foreign bodies: safety and efficacy of Foley catheter extraction of coins. *Am J Roentgenol* 1997; **169**: 443–446.
55. Myer CM III. Potential hazards of esophageal foreign body extraction. *Pediatr Radiol* 1991; **21**: 97–98.
56. Koch H. Operative endoscopy. *Gastrointest Endosc* 1977; **24**: 65–68.
57. Litovitz T, Schimitz BF. Ingestion of cylindrical and button batteries: an analysis of 2,382 cases. *Pediatrics* 1992; **89**: 747–757.
58. McCormick S, Brennan P, Yassa J, Shawis R. Children and mini-magnets: an almost fatal attraction. *Emerg Med J* 2002; **19**: 71–73.
59. Chan YL, Chang SS, Kao KL et al. Button battery ingestion: an analysis of 25 cases. *Chang Gung Med J* 2002; **25**: 169–174.
60. McDermott VG, Taylor T, Wyatt JP. Orogastric magnet removal of ingested disc batteries. *J Pediatr Surg* 1995; **30**: 29–32.
61. Volle E, Beyer P, Kaufmann HJ. Therapeutic approach to ingested button-type batteries. Magnetic removal of ingested button-type batteries. *Pediatr Radiol* 1989; **19**: 114–118.
62. Cauchi JA, Shawis RN. Multiple magnet ingestion and gastrointestinal morbidity. *Arch Dis Child* 2002; **87**: 539–540.
63. Namasivayam S. Button battery ingestion: a solution to management dilemma. *Pediat Surg Int* 1999; **15**: 383–384.
64. Kuhns DW, Dire DJ. Button battery ingestion. *Am Emerg Med* 1989; **18**: 293–300.
65. McDermott VG, Taylor T, Wyatt JP. Oro-gastric magnet removal of ingested disc batteries. *J Pediatr Surg* 1995; **30**: 29–32.
66. Kehrt R, Niggeman B, Klaue S, Wahn U. Small toys contained in chocolate eggs – good or bad surprise? *Resp Med* 2002; **96**: 955–956.
67. Ginsburg GG. Management of ingested foreign objects and food bolus impactions. *Gastrointest Endosc* 1995; **41**: 33–38.
68. Mamel JJ, Weiss D, Pouagare M, Nord HJ. Endoscopic suction removal of food boluses from the upper gastrointestinal tract using Stiegmann–Goff friction-fit adaptor: an improved method for removal of food impactions. *Gastrointest Endosc* 1995; **41**: 593–597.
69. Calkins CM, Christianes KK, Sell LL. Cost analysis in the management of esophageal coins: endoscopy versus bougienage. *J Pediatr Surg* 1999; **34**: 412–414.

42 Medical aspects of intestinal transplantation

Olivier Goulet

Introduction

Intestinal transplantation was first demonstrated to be technically feasible in humans in the early 1960s.[1] The initial excitement, however, rapidly decreased when post-transplant rejection and severe sepsis resulted in high morbidity and mortality rates.[1] After extensive experimental reports, and despite very encouraging clinical results for heart and liver transplantation, the use of cyclosporin A did not enable, except in one child,[2] long-term survival after isolated small-bowel transplantation for short-bowel syndrome.[3] In the early 1990s, two advances made intestinal transplantation a promising option for the treatment of end-stage intestinal failure: the combination with liver transplantation[4] and the development of FK506 (tacrolimus).[5] Recent advances in immunosuppressive treatment and the better monitoring and control of acute rejection have brought intestinal transplantation into the realm of standard treatment for intestinal failure. The results from the Intestinal Transplant Registry (www.intestinaltransplant.org) indicate that intestinal transplantation is currently an acceptable clinical modality for selected patients with irreversible intestinal failure.[6,7]

Irreversible intestinal failure

Intestinal failure is a condition in which gastrointestinal function is insufficient to satisfy body nutrient and fluid requirements. Parenteral nutrition (PN) and home PN remain the mainstay of therapy for intestinal failure, whether it is partial or total, provisional or permanent. Since its introduction, PN has improved greatly, especially with the development of home PN.[8–12] Data from the European Registry indicate that the long-term survival of non-malignant patients on home PN is currently higher than the 1–3-year survival after isolated intestinal transplantation.[9] The North American Home Parenteral and Enteral Nutrition Registry reported 1- and 4-year survival rates of all children receiving PN at home as a result of short-bowel syndrome of 94 and 80%, respectively.[12] The survival rates of patients with chronic intestinal pseudo-obstruction are inferior, being 87 and 70%, respectively. Although long-term PN is associated with complications such as liver impairment, bone disease, vascular thrombosis and sepsis, innovative therapeutic modalities are required. Indeed, some patients develop complications while receiving standard therapy for intestinal failure and are considered for intestinal transplantation. Indications for intestinal transplantation involve mostly pediatric patients and may be divided into three main group: short-bowel syndrome, intestinal motility disorders and congenital diseases of the epithelial mucosa.

Short-bowel syndrome

Short-bowel syndrome (see also Chapter 29) caused by extensive resection of the small bowel has logically been the first indication for intestinal transplantation. After extensive resection of the small bowel, most neonates now survive and acquire gastrointestinal autonomy after a period depending on the extent and site of resection, the preservation of the ileocecal valve and the quality of the remaining gut.[13,14] Two groups are potential candidates for intestinal transplantation. Infants left with only a duodenum or at most 10 cm of jejunum and no ileocecal valve will remain permanently dependent on PN. A small number of infants, approximately 10–15% in our experience, who have undergone massive intestinal resection in the neonatal period are at high risk of permanent intestinal failure when a stereotypical combination of features are present: small-bowel length of less than 30–40 cm, absence of ileocecal valve, resection of some colon, minimal tolerance of enteral feeding within the first months after intestinal resection, dilated intestinal loop and bacterial overgrowth, and multiple surgical procedures.[15] Older children or adolescents have a lesser degree of growth potential of the bowel compared with neonates who have extensive intestinal resection. Intestinal adaptation and intestinal absorption sufficient to meet growth requirements can only be obtained if the length of remaining small bowel is more than 50–60 cm beyond the angle of Treitz. Some children do not become autonomous even after more than 10 years of home-based PN, and are thus candidates for intestinal transplantation.[16]

In patients with short-bowel syndrome on long-term PN, intestinal transplantation can only be envisaged once it has been formally shown that the remnant bowel cannot adapt. Surgical approaches such as lengthening of the small bowel, loop interposition or assembly of a 'reverse' intestinal loop should be attempted.[17–21]

Trophic factors such as recombinant human growth hormone (rhGH) might be helpful in some patients and might contribute to decreasing the need for intestinal transplantation in the near future. Studies have indicated that pituitary hormones modulate small-bowel growth in animals.[22–24] Clinical studies have provided controversial results.[25–30] Recent data in adults as well as in pediatric patients demonstrated that rhGH treatment sometimes allows improvement in intestinal function.[27–30] Glucagon-like peptide-2 (GLP2) might, in the near future, be very helpful in enhancing gut mucosa trophicity and in reducing delay for achieving intestinal autonomy.[31]

Therefore, only a small number of patients with short-bowel syndrome are candidates for intestinal transplantation in the absence of life-threatening complications, especially progressive liver disease which raises another problem. The prevalence of complicated home PN-related liver disease increases with a longer duration of PN. This condition is one of the main causes of death in patients with permanent non-malignant intestinal failure.[32]

Some pediatric patients were reported to have received an isolated liver transplantation for end-stage liver disease complicating short-bowel syndrome.[33–35] Some of them became intestinally autonomous after liver transplantation. However, it is important to stress that to be obliged to transplant the liver to achieve intestinal autonomy is clearly not the most logical or the easiest procedure. Thus, the primary aim must remain to prevent end-stage liver disease in short-bowel patients by using appropriate and long-term PN especially in the patients at high risk of liver disease.

Intestinal motility disorders

Motility disorders in childhood include total aganglionosis (extensive Hirschsprung's disease) and chronic intestinal pseudo-obstruction syndrome. The first causes the same problems as short-bowel syndrome, with two main differences. The non-functioning colon is excluded and the ganglionic small bowel has motility disorders. Therefore, when normally innervated small bowel is shorter than 60 cm the probability of long-term PN dependency is high. Logically, this situation requires a combined colon transplantation.[36,37] Chronic intestinal pseudo-obstruction syndrome (see Chapter 18) is a very heterogeneous condition with regard to clinical presentation, histopathological features, severity of motility disorders and outcome.[38–40] In our experience, 20–25% of patients will become dependent on long-term PN.[38] Recent data reported that intestinal transplantation or multivisceral transplantation have been performed in these patients, including some with associated urinary tract involvement.[41,42] Munchäusen syndrome by proxy causing intestinal pseudo-obstruction must be recognized, even if difficult, and never justifies intestinal transplantation, as previously reported.[43]

Congenital enteropathies

Two congenital intractable epithelial mucosal diseases are responsible for permanent intestinal failure and are currently recognized as requiring intestinal transplantation: microvillus inclusion disease and epithelial dysplasia (see Chapter 1). Both are autosomal recessive inherited disorders with neonatal onset of severe watery diarrhea and total malabsorption. Microvillus inclusion disease involves the intracellular pathway of brush-border development,[44] whereas epithelial dysplasia is associated with abnormal enterocytes and basement membrane.[45] The primary inherited defect is not currently known for either of these diseases. Some children with one of these two mucosal diseases have undergone successful small-bowel transplantation in isolation or in combination with the liver.[46–52]

Clinical results after intestinal transplantation

Immunosuppressive treatment

The current immunosuppression we use is based on tacrolimus (Prograf®), steroids and monoclonal antibodies directed against interleukin-2 (IL-2) receptors (anti R-IL2 mAb). Tacrolimus is started intraoperatively to maintain whole blood levels using microparticle enzyme immunoassay technology, around 15–20 ng/ml during the first month, 10–15 ng/ml during the following month and 5–10 ng/ml thereafter. Methylprednisolone is given as an initial bolus (20–25 mg/kg over 6 hours), then 2 mg/kg per day during the first month and then progressively tapered to 0.5 mg/kg every other day.

Rapamycin (sirolimus) is now used in children, but follow-up is too short, even if encouraging results have been reported.[53] However, no randomized trial using this drug for intestinal transplant recipients is yet available. Azathioprine (Imuran®) is now rarely used and has mainly been replaced in some programs by mycophenolate mofetil. Caution is recommended with the use of mycophenolate mofetil because it has been shown to induce diarrhea.[54] A new monoclonal antibody Campath® was recently reported to improve survival after intestinal transplantation.[55]

Other procedures have been proposed for decreasing immunogenicity of the graft such as irradiation or for enhancing the natural microchimerism by infusing recipients with donor bone marrow during the perioperative period.[56] Combined bone marrow augmentation did not significantly improve graft survival[57] and was reported to favor the occurrence of graft-versus-host disease (GVHD) in animals.[58]

Survival after intestinal transplantation

Current clinical results come from the data collected through the International Intestinal Transplant Registry (www.intestinaltransplant.org). To date, approximately 1000 intestinal transplantations have been performed throughout the world, mostly in the USA, Canada, France and the UK. The current available data from the registry include 989 transplantations in 923 patients from 61 intestinal transplantation programs. Among recipients, 61% were children or adolescents. The transplants involved the isolated small-bowel transplantation with or without the colon (37%), the liver + small-bowel transplantation (50%) and multivisceral grafts (13%), including the stomach, pancreas, liver and small-bowel.

The main indications in 563 children were short-bowel syndrome (63%), chronic intestinal pseudo-obstruction syndrome (10%), severe intractable diarrhea (10%), total aganglionosis/Hirschsprung's disease (7%), and in 360 adults: ischemia (23%), Crohn's disease (14%), trauma (16%), desmoid tumor (9%) or tumors (8%). The main immunosuppression included tacrolimus (97%) and steroids in association with a variety of immunosuppressive agents including mycophenolate mofetil, rapamycin, azathioprine and IL-2 blockers.

Overall 3-year patient survival is around 50–60% depending on several factors related to the type of transplanted organ (e.g. isolated intestine or combined with liver), the experience of the center, the immunosuppressive regimen including rapamycin or not, and the period from 1991 to now (Figure 42.1). Post-transplant death was due mainly to infections (46%), multiorgan failure (2.5%) or lymphoma (10%). Full nutritional autonomy with complete discontinuation of PN has been achieved in 81% of survivors and partial recovery was documented in another 10% giving a total rehabilitation rate of 85% in survivors, 8% of the intestinal grafts being removed.

It is clear from the intestinal transplantation registry and from individual programs that prognosis has improved during the past 10 years. Surgical procedures are well described and adapted to each organ combination.[59] Patient survival is associated with the type of organ transplanted, with better survival after small-bowel

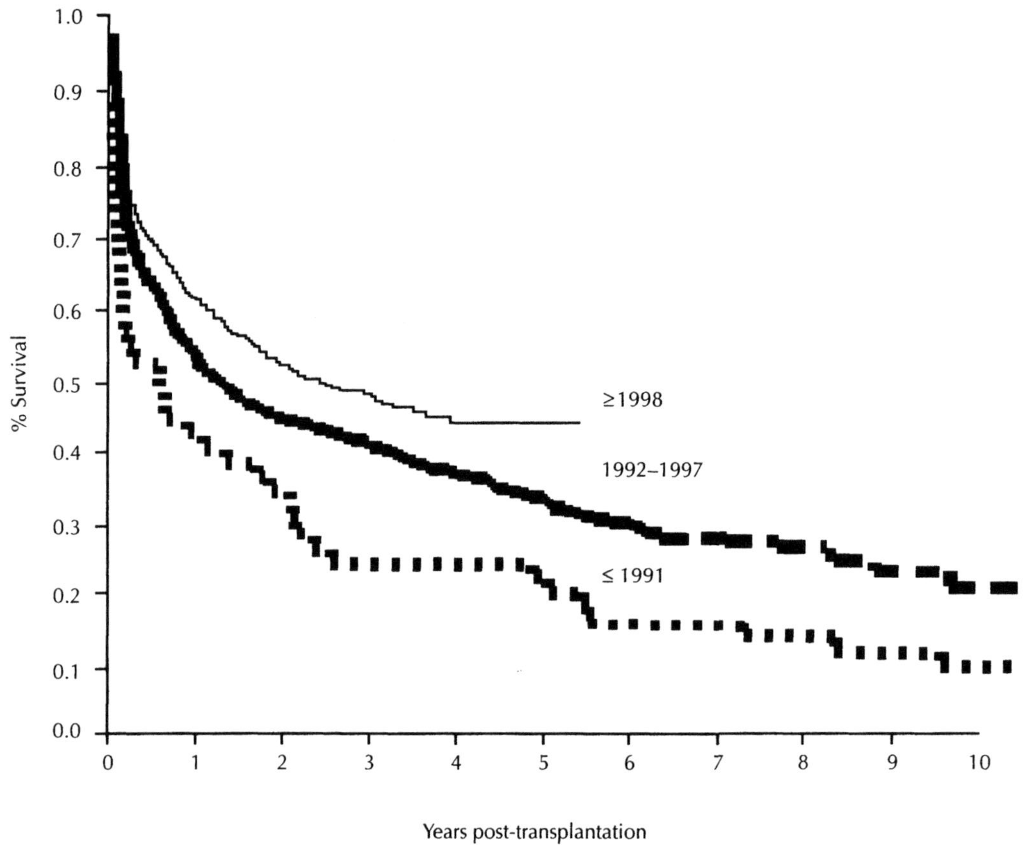

Figure 42.1 Actuarial graft survival according to the era of intestinal transplantation (data available from the International Intestinal Transplantation Registry, www.intestinaltransplant.org).

transplantation. Nevertheless, these results must be interpreted with care because they represent the first 12 years' experience of a large number of programs in children and adults, using different immunosuppressive regimens. The results from the largest of these centers reflect the current situation more closely.[60–65] In addition, programs that have performed at least ten transplants have better graft and patient survival rates compared with those that have performed less than ten.[7]

At the University Hospital Necker in Paris, 25 isolated intestinal transplantations and 30 combined intestine–liver transplantations were performed from November 1994 in 51 children (17 girls) ranging in age between 2.5 and 15 years (median 5 years). Associated right colon transplantation was performed 37 times (21 intestine–liver transplants). All patients were on long-term PN for a median duration of 4.5 years (range 18 months–13 years) for congenital enteropathy ($n = 18$), short-bowel syndrome ($n = 14$), extensive Hirschsprung's disease ($n = 13$) and intestinal pseudo-obstruction ($n = 6$). Immunosuppression included tacrolimus, methylprednisolone, azathioprine and IL-2 blockers. With a follow-up ranging between 6 months and 8.5 years, 36 patients are alive (patient survival 70.5%; graft survival 65%). The following factors are significantly related to poor outcome (death or graft loss) age >7 years ($p < 0.01$), pretransplant multiple surgery ($p < 0.01$), intestinal failure-related complications ($p < 0.01$), intestinal pseudo-obstruction ($p < 0.01$), steroid-resistant intestinal rejection ($p < 0.01$) and fungal sepsis ($p < 0.01$). Right colon grafting did not affect patient or graft survival whatever the type of transplantation. Feeding was introduced at a median of 9 days post-transplant (range 6–62 days). All the children have been weaned from PN 3 weeks to 4 years after transplantation, and they continue to gain weight and most have recovered normal growth velocity.

Liver-induced immune tolerance

It is currently difficult to analyze the difference in intestinal graft survival rates between isolated and combined liver–intestine transplant. In general, the clinical status of liver–small bowel recipients is poor at the time of transplantation and contributes to the high post-transplant rate of morbidity and mortality. This is suggested by the 1- and 2-year survival of patients, who have not undergone transplantation, being 30 and 22%, respectively, and the number of deaths on the waiting list.[66] On the other hand, the isolated small-bowel graft not only has the highest incidence of rejection, but also requires more intense immunosuppression to control it. It appears from our experience that the most encouraging results have been with combined small bowel–liver transplantation. Intestinal graft rejection was less frequent and less severe in small bowel–liver transplant recipients. Simultaneous liver grafting might reduce the risk of intestinal rejection as supported by experimental data[67,68] and clinical results.[60,69]

The mechanism by which the liver induces tolerance is still under debate. The deletion of donor alloreactive T cells was initially suggested but remains controversial.[70] Other mechanisms such as anergy or the generation of regulatory cells might contribute to liver-induced tolerance, as suggested by the decreased expression of CD25 or CD8 T cells infiltrating tolerated intestinal graft and the reversal of tolerance by IL-2.[71] Currently, the role of liver-derived dendritic cells in inducing tolerance is stressed.[72] A better insight into the mechanisms involved in liver-induced tolerance is important in the design of immunosuppressive regimens for small bowel–liver transplant recipients, because there is experimental evidence that immunosuppressive drugs may inhibit the tolerogenic effect of the liver.[73,74]

Complications after intestinal transplantation

The singularities of the gut may impede intestinal transplantation for several reasons:

(1) The gut-associated lymphoid tissue can induce GVHD and may enhance allograft rejection and the subsequent risk of Gram-negative sepsis;
(2) The secretion of lymphokines or the production of cytotoxic T cells in response to intraluminal pathogens may impede the induction of tolerance and thereby favor allograft rejection;
(3) The need for heavy immunosuppressive treatment increases the risk of developing opportunistic infection and post-transplant lymphoproliferative disorders (PTLD).

Graft-versus-host-disease

GVHD has been extensively studied in animal models of intestinal transplantation.[1] In humans, despite the presence of circulating donor-derived lymphocytes during the first few weeks after transplantation, clinical signs of GVHD have rarely been reported.[75] GVHD is not therefore a major complication after intestinal transplantation, unlike graft rejection.

Intestinal rejection

Intestinal allograft rejection remains the major complication after intestinal transplantation. As a result of increased immunosuppressive treatment, graft rejection may further precipitate opportunistic infections that become additive factors in patient and graft losses. As rejection can occur rapidly and can be life-threatening, close monitoring is required. This has led to the development of numerous diagnostic methods, which have not been validated in human intestinal transplantation or have limited value.[76–78] Therefore, regular biopsies of the proximal and distal ends of the graft for histological or immunohistochemical analysis are required[79–83] (Figure 42.2). Clinical signs of rejection occur later than histological and immunohistochemical signs and correspond to a relatively advanced rejection process with marked histological lesions. Rejection and sepsis can be intimately related after small-bowel transplantation when rejection compromises normal intestinal barrier mechanisms and bacterial translocation results with consequent multiorgan failure. Graft rejection may be reversed by using methylprednisolone pulses. Severe exfoliative rejection leaves the intestine totally denuded of its mucosa and does not respond to methylprednisolone or to anti-

(a)

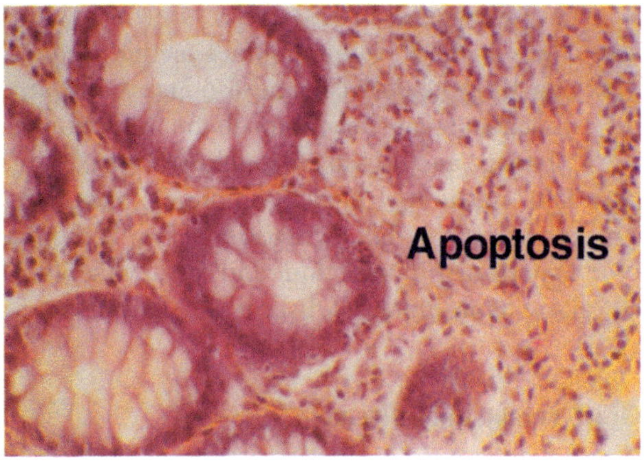

(b)

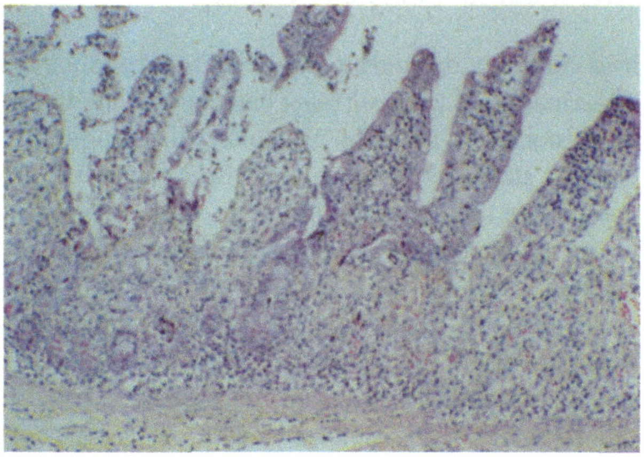

(c)

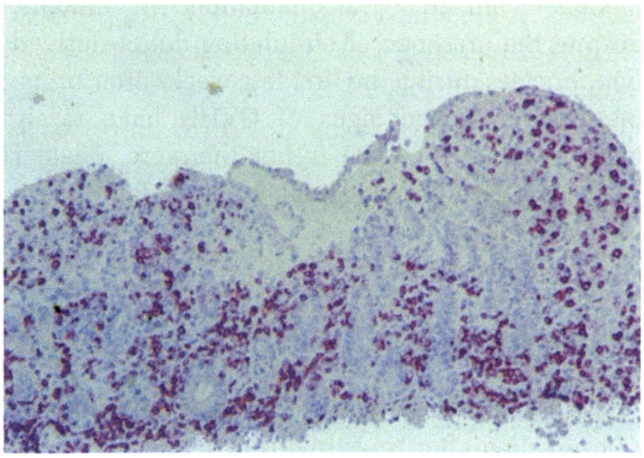

Figure 42.2 (a) Mild intestinal graft rejection showing only pictures of apoptosis in the gland (HES x1200); (b) severe intestinal graft rejection showing epithelial blunting and disappearance of glands (HES x200); (c) severe 'exfoliative' intestinal graft rejection with total villous atrophy, epithelium disappearance, absence of glands and T-cell infiltration (HES x800).

lymphoglobulins or anti-CD3 mAb. Recovery may sometimes occur after exfoliative rejection but with a very high cost related to severe protracted protein-losing enteropathy during which albumin and hemoglobin replacement is needed and malnutrition may occur. In case of unresponsive exfoliative graft rejection, subepithelial fibrosis may appear, leading to severe hypomotility and subsequent intraluminal bacterial overgrowth.[81–83] In our experience, we do consider that a rejection unresponsive to methylprednisolone pulses is a matter of discussing intestinal graft removal instead of dramatic increase of immunosuppression with the risk of infection and PTLD. This decision is difficult and is based on the specific experience of each program with the mandatory input of the pathologist.

Infectious complications

Clinical manifestations of allograft rejection are non-specific. It is obviously very important to differentiate other sources of potential intestinal allograft disease that may clinically mimic rejection, such as cytomegalovirus (CMV), adenovirus, Epstein–Barr virus (EBV) or other bacterial/viral enteritis. Viral infections are frequent, such as CMV primo-infection or reactivation, which is not always prevented by the use of pre-emptive treatment (ganciclovir). The diagnosis of CMV infection improved with the use of the polymerase chain reaction (PCR), which has been shown to be a sensitive method for the early detection of CMV infection in solid-organ and intestinal graft recipients.[84] The incidence of CMV infection has been reported to be as high as 29% in pediatric recipients of intestinal grafts.[84] It is recommended to avoid using a seropositive graft in a seronegative recipient. Nevertheless, patients who are awaiting composite grafts are frequently too sick to await a CMV-seronegative donor. CMV prophylaxis is now well established with the wide use of ganciclovir.[85]

EBV infection in association with immunosuppressive drugs used for solid-organ transplantation can produce a spectrum of illnesses. Donor selection and the prevention of EBV infection remain unsolved problems. Indeed, a high incidence of EBV-induced PTLD has been reported.[86] The incidence increases with the degree of immunosuppression. Because of the high rates of morbidity and mortality associated with EBV disease, a pre-emptive therapy based on serial monitoring of the EBV viral load is required. Quantitative EBV–PCR in the peripheral blood has recently enabled early diagnosis as well as the follow-up of patients with EBV infection.[87] This may allow the diagnosis of EBV infection before the development of PTLD. In the case of established EBV-related PTLD, therapeutic changes based on quantitative PCR are helpful in preventing the end phases of this disease.[84] In addition, in the case of documented PTLD, the use of anti-CD20 monoclonal antibodies has proved to be efficient in reversing the disease.[88]

Other severe life-threatening complications have been reported, such as diffuse adenovirus enterocolitis or hemophagocytosis.[89–91] The early identification of viral infections, based on the repeated use of appropriate methods, may help in avoiding the misdiagnosis of rejection leading to an unnecessary increase of immunosuppressive treatment with consequent exacerbation of the underlying infectious condition.

Intestinal graft function

Provided that the small intestine survives ischemia and reperfusion injury, long-term graft function is dependent on the effects of denervation, lymphatic disruption, immunosuppressive treatment, rejection and infection. These factors may explain impaired function of the intestinal graft and a delay in achieving intestinal autonomy.

Intestinal motor function after intestinal transplantation

The experimental study of small-bowel allografts provides a unique opportunity to develop insights into the impact of manipulation, preservation, ischemia/reperfusion injury, extrinsic denervation and immunological injury on intestinal function. However, very few data exist on these injuries to transplanted human small intestine. Ischemia-reperfusion injury or intestinal manipulation evokes an inflammatory response within the intestinal muscularis that is associated with intestinal dysmotility. It was shown from human intestinal graft specimens obtained during transplantion that manipulation during organ harvesting initiates a functionally relevant molecular and cellular inflammatory response within the graft muscularis that is potentiated during the reperfusion period.[92]

The loss of extrinsic innervation of the small bowel severely impairs intestinal motor function. It has been shown in animal models that extrinsic denervation with maintenance of intestinal continuity only alters the regularity of the interdigestive myoelectric complex.[93] However, autotransplantation causes complete disruption of the orderly, sequential migration of the interdigestive myoelectric complex from the innervated to the denervated intestine, and food intake no longer inhibits the myoelectric complex.[94] Studies have observed the changes of the transplanted intestine itself in order to evaluate the effects of intestinal transplantation on the intrinsic nervous system. Taguchi et al found that the contractile properties of small-bowel smooth muscle and its sensitivity to drugs were unaltered by transplantation.[95] Although the excitatory response was comparable with that of normal intestine, the inhibitory response was modified by the loss of the extrinsic adrenergic inhibitory innervation. They also studied the temporary additional loss of intrinsic inhibition caused by prolonged graft storage, which recovers within 7–8 days after transplantation.[96] An increase was also shown of the intestinal contractile motility after intestinal transplantation, associated with a marked increase of non-adrenergic, non-cholinergic (NANC) neural components, with the dominant intrinsic neural component changing from cholinergic to NANC over 4 weeks.[97] Autotransplantation as well as isotransplantation in dogs or rats has allowed the study of the reinnervation process after small-bowel transplantation.[98,99] Reinnervation of the graft intestinal wall does occur but requires a prolonged period. The major route of reinnervation is along the arterial axis of the intestinal graft, not beyond the enteric anastomosis.[100] On the other hand, Taguchi et al studied immunohistochemically the distribution of neurons in a syngeneic model of transplantation in Lewis rats. Both the nitric oxide (NO) and peptidergic neurons markedly decreased just after transplantation, and the NO neurons recovered faster than peptidergic neurons suggesting an important role in the adaptation process in the early period after transplantation.[101] After transplantation of the entire jejuno-ileum, isotransplanted rat intestine has qualitatively normal myoelectrical activity but decreased absorptive capacity.[102–104] If rejection is controlled and ischemic time is kept to a minimum, allografts of small intestine will exhibit a normal propagated motor myoelectric complex. In humans, the intrinsic motor activity of the small intestine is preserved for the most part, although there is some discoordination between proximal and distal elements in the fed state.[105,106]

Acute allograft rejection provokes intestinal paralysis before mucosal destruction is established.[107] In animals, chronic rejection causes thickening of muscularis propria by both hyperplasia and hypertrophy accompanied by inflammatory cell infiltrate.[108] Chronic allograft rejection severely impairs the enteric nerve with subsequent alteration of myoelectrical activity.[108–110] Functional impairment partially regresses after FK506 rescue.[109] In clinical practice, chronic rejection is very rare but its expression is dominated by severe intestinal obstruction.

Very few data regarding intestinal motility are available in humans.[106] Most knowledge comes from the observations of recovery of intestinal transit and contrast examination of the transplanted intestine.[111]

Absorptive function after intestinal transplantation

Studies performed in animals have shown that intestinal tranates, lipids, glutamine, water and electrolytes, but there is no evidence in humans.[112–120] Feeding must resume as early as possible after transplantation because this ensures optimal mucosasplantation disturbs the absorption of carbohydrl trophicity and reduces gastrointestinal stasis, which causes intraluminal bacterial overgrowth. Clinical experience has demonstrated that because of water–electrolyte malabsorption, abnormal motility and impaired lymphatic drainage it may take several weeks to achieve normal intestinal transit and reduced stool volume. If the recipient has no colon, associated colon transplantation has physiological advantages in terms of water and electrolyte re-absorption, slowing intestinal transit and trophic factors, through colonic synthesis of short-chain fatty acids. Finally, it is currently considered that intestinal transplantation restores an enteral axis capable of ensuring digestion and absorption. Intestinal function sufficient to withdraw PN completely may be achieved with adequate nutritional management. In our experience, colon grafting does not impede survival after intestinal transplantation and improves the patient's condition with early PN weaning. The colon water–electrolyte absorption capacity reduces the need for compensation by the parenteral route.

Post-transplant practice and procedures

Initial post-transplant period

Total PN is administered continuously, with modifications made to the electrolyte and macronutrient content of the solution based upon serum and urine laboratory parameters. Hyperglycemia may result from initial high steroid doses and steroid recycles during early rejection episodes and/or from tacrolimus. Post-transplant pancreatitis may also affect glucose metabolism. Thus, insulin may be required in patients with severe hyperglycemia to maintain adequate caloric balance. Impaired renal function may require the limitation of nitrogen intake required for post-transplant wound healing and fluid restrictions may prohibit the ability to provide enough total PN volume to supply adequate calories. Use of intravenous lipid emulsion whenever possible according to metabolic tolerance and infectious state is recommended to achieve adequate calorie intake and essential fatty acid provision. The type of emulsion has never been evaluated in such situations and might be controversial. In our practice, we preferentially use medium-chain/long-chain triglyceride (MCT/LCT) emulsion without overpassing 1.5 g/kg per day.

Initiation of enteral and oral feeding

Continuous enteral feeding through a gastrostomy or, for others, from proximal jejunostomy is started once intestinal motility occurs, generally within 1 week. Enteral feeding is initiated and advanced slowly unless contraindicated, as in the presence of severe diarrhea or vomiting and, of course, in the presence of an acute graft rejection. In our experience and elsewhere, the patients initially receive a low-antigenic and low-fat formula and are subsequently transferred over a period of weeks and months to a more complex product with intact macronutrients. The use of an amino acid- versus a peptide-based enteral product remains a controversial issue in the non-transplant critically ill patient with impaired gastrointestinal function.[121] However, in the presence of carbohydrate and fat, nitrogen absorption has been reported to be greater with a 100% elemental free amino acid-protein source.[122] Moreover, the presence of free glutamine in powdered amino acid-based formulas has been shown to be beneficial in protecting gastrointestinal mucosa and reducing bacterial translocation.[123] Conversely, peptide-based elemental formulas are generally lower in osmolality which may make them more suitable for use in the presence of increased stool output. Finally, it is impossible to identify significant differences in outcome as measured by the length of time until the patient is completely weaned from total PN, length of hospital stay, ileostomy output or time until transition to oral intake alone, by the type of enteral formula used, peptide or hydrolyzed casein-based enteral formula versus an amino acid preparation. Post-transplant-impaired lymphatic drainage with either chylous ascites or intestinal lymphangiectasia, limits lipid intake. Low-fat formulas and MCT-rich formulas are recommended at initiation of enteral feeding. In our experience, children with inferior vena cava thrombosis are at high risk of chylous ascites and must be fed very slowly with MCT-rich formulas. More complex products with intact macronutrients are progressively introduced according to graft status, digestive tolerance and capacity of eating.

Parenteral nutrition weaning

PN weaning is a crucial objective, allowing the intestinal transplantation to be considered successful. Full nutritional autonomy with complete discontinuation of PN has been achieved in 81% of cases and partial recovery was documented in another 11%, for a total rehabilitation rate of 92% in survivors. In the absence of major complications, recipients of an isolated intestinal allograft are weaned from PN relatively quickly, the median time ranging between 4 and 6 weeks[60,65] Patients are weaned from PN as enteral feeding is progressively increased according to the tolerance of the child. It can take several weeks or months depending on the pre-transplant nutritional status, post-transplant complication rate, and intestinal graft recovery and function. In our experience, among 31 survivors after isolated ($n = 11$) or combined intestine–liver transplantation ($n = 20$), all patients were weaned from PN after a delay ranging from 4 weeks to 3 years. In the absence of major complications, recipients of an isolated intestinal allograft can be weaned from PN relatively quickly within 4–6 weeks. The longer time to achieve full enteral nutrition after small bowel–liver transplantation reflects a more prolonged recovery from the surgical procedure compared with isolated small-bowel transplantation.

Eating disorders

Chronically ill infants and children are at risk for oral aversion caused by the loss of the sucking or swallowing reflex in those maintained on total PN or tube feeding for an extended period of time without oral intake. Further oral-associated problems, including delayed speech and language development, may also result from this aversion. Pre-transplant management of eating disorders and early and adequate post-transplant stimulation of oral feeding can reduce food aversion. It is essential to insert a digestive access (gastrostomy or proximal jejunostomy) at the time of transplant surgery, especially in patients felt to have eating disorders. Full enteral feeding can be progressively achieved by using a polymeric diet. Psychological evaluation and assistance are of course required in each case. In our experience, all patients achieved oral feeding, sometimes up to 2 years after transplantation.

Monitoring of intestinal function

The D-xylose absorption test provides basic information regarding mucosal integrity, but is influenced by a number of factors, such as impaired gastric emptying or accelerated intestinal transit. This test is never used in our clinical practice.

Mucosal enzyme activities, especially disaccharidase activity, can be assayed from a biopsy specimen obtained from endoscopy. Enzyme levels correlate with mucosal injury due to allograft rejection or viral infection.[124] Thus, the relevance of this assessment for monitoring of intestinal function in a stable patient is a matter of debate.

Recipients with an ileostomy, during the 2–3 months following transplant procedure, or continent older patients, can benefit from stool analysis. We used to perform a stool balance as measured by a comparison of 72-h fecal output with oral or enteral intake. Since multiple variables may affect fat absorption, including intestinal transit, lymphatic integrity, exocrine pancreas function and mucosal injury, assessment of fat balance is very relevant. However, as most patients receive a mixture of LCTs and MCTs, the measurement of fat excretion by using the Van de Kamer assay is not relevant. It is thus preferable to use the Jeejeebhoy method that extracts and detects both LCTs and MCTs.[125] In our practice we also used to measure energy balance by performing bomb calorimetry analysis. Stool balance analysis in 20 PN-weaned transplanted children, showed that lipid absorption rate was decreased, ranging between 70 and 88%.

Nutritional outcome after intestinal transplantation

Besides the enteral or oral feeding approach, nutritional evaluation following intestinal transplantation is mandatory. However, few nutritional data are available in children after intestinal transplantation.[126–128] We studied 20 children (8.8 ± 3.5 years) with at least 12 months follow-up (median 27 months).[128] PN was stopped 110 ± 84 days after grafting. They were on unrestricted oral feeding, with enteral supplementation in six patients with varying degrees of eating disorders. At 12 months post-transplant, body weight-for-age and height-for-age were decreased, being 89 ± 13% and 93 ± 5%, respectively. Body weight-for-height was increased (105 ± 9%) with a fat body mass (FBM) of 20.1 ± 4.3% of body weight. Growth velocity was decreased 6 months before and after grafting by 67 ± 38% and 57 ± 46% of the normal for age, respectively, but was increased by 142 ± 64% of the normal for age during the last 6 months of follow-up. Bone mineral density (BMD), measured by using dual X-ray absorptiometry (DEXA), was decreased in all children according to age. Nutritional parameters showed normal albumin and pre-albumin plasma levels as well as plasma tocopherol. Conversely, both vitamin A and RBP plasma levels were decreased, as well as serum iron and ferritine.

Weight gain with excessive FBM and catch-up growth is observed after intestinal transplantation in most cases, in our experience. However, in some cases, there is evidence of severe inhibition of linear growth at the time of transplantation with no evidence of catch-up after transplantation.[127,128] Growth velocity is severely altered both before and just after transplantation due to liver disease and high-dose steroid thereafter. Thus catch-up growth is delayed. A follow-up period of 6 months is too short to observe positive trends in height/length. Despite normal growth, BMD is low and some nutritional biological parameters are altered, such as vitamin A plasma levels. Monitoring should not be restricted to growth parameters but include body composition and biological parameters recording nutritional supplementation if required. Post-intestinal transplantation nutritional management should include BMD assessment on a longitudinal basis. Insufficient BMD may be due to previous long-term PN worsened with high-dose steroids.

Potential candidates for intestinal transplantation

In order to improve the risk–benefit ratio and cost-effectiveness of intestinal transplantation it is mandatory to select appropriate candidates and to decide the adequate time for performing the procedure. The number of potential candidates for intestinal transplantation is very difficult to establish according to the heterogeneity of patients included in home-PN programs, and in general, to the mostly well-tolerated long-term PN.[8–12] The number of patients will never be as high as the number of kidney or liver transplant recipients.

However, intestinal transplantation is theoretically indicated for all patients permanently dependent on PN. Functional grafts lead to gastrointestinal autonomy (weaning off PN) while maintaining satisfactory nutritional status and normal growth in children. However, as PN is generally well tolerated, even for long periods, each indication for transplantation must be carefully weighed in terms of survival rate, morbidity and quality of life.[129–133] By excluding malignant disease and immune deficiency, survival rates of patients with chronic intestinal failure on long-term home PN remain higher than after intestinal transplantation, even with the most optimistic interpretation of available data.[8–12] Intestinal transplantation is often accompanied by numerous life-threatening complications such as those briefly reviewed above, leading to recurrent or long-term hospitalization and sometimes a poor outcome. An evaluation of the quality-of-life after intestinal transplantation among home PN was recently performed in adult patients using a quality-of-life instrument in the form of a self-administered questionnaire.[131] Intestinal transplant recipients with functioning grafts reported a significant improvement in the quality of their life and function. This information is encouraging and should be used towards future advancement in intestinal transplantation.

Thus, when long-term PN is effective and well tolerated, it can thus be used pending further progress in intestinal transplantation. In contrast, when PN has reached its limits, especially in those cases associated with extensive thrombosis, recurrent sepsis, severe metabolic disorders or advanced liver disease, intestinal transplantation must be undertaken.

Intestinal transplantation: isolated or combined with liver

Patients with irreversible intestinal failure and end-stage liver disease (liver cirrhosis and complicated portal hypertension) are certainly candidates for a life-saving procedure such as combined small bowel–liver transplantation. Patients with severe hepatic fibrosis are more difficult to manage. Repeated liver biopsies within 6–12 months and careful assessment for portal hypertension are mandatory. It is difficult to predict the liver damage related to the persistent need for PN or to rejection or infection during the first weeks or months after transplantation. In addition, it is difficult to assess the amount of functioning liver necessary to withstand the insult of portal diversion during the transplantation procedure. Those patients with severe hepatic fibrosis or cirrhosis are thus usually listed for small bowel–liver transplantation.

Patients with irreversible intestinal failure and PN dependency without consistent liver disease must satisfy rigorous criteria to be considered as candidates for isolated small-bowel transplantation. They must fulfill at least one of the following criteria: extensive thrombosis impeding the ability to administer PN, recurrent life-threatening sepsis, severe metabolic disorders preventing nutritional requirements from being met, with consequent failure to thrive in children, underlying disease with high water–electrolyte losses with the risk of life-threatening dehydration in the case of PN disruption. Some patients with severe chronic intestinal pseudo-obstruction may be disabled because of chronic, massive gastrointestinal dilation refractory to stomal decompression or partial enterectomy. They might be considered for intestinal transplantation, although the usual indications, including progressive liver disease, the threatened loss of vascular access and recurring life-threatening sepsis, have not developed.

Contraindications to intestinal transplantation

Contraindications to intestinal transplantation do not differ from those pertaining to other solid organs.[134] According to the high morbidity and mortality rates after intestinal transplantation and the donor pool size, the concept that the patient must have the potential to derive an obvious benefit from the procedure must remain paramount. Other contraindications include congenital or acquired neurological disabilities, life-threatening extradigestive illnesses, congenital or acquired immune disorders, non-resectable malignancy, and insufficient vascular patency to guarantee easy central venous access for up to 6 months after intestinal transplantation.

Timing for referral and prevention of liver disease

Intestinal failure management

Unfortunately, few centers manage all the stages of intestinal failure from onset to intestinal transplantation, including the home-PN program. Beath et al[135] reported a marked discrepancy in clinical status between children referred for intestinal transplantation from centers with and without nutritional care teams. It was shown that the mortality rate, death within 6 months of evaluation for transplantation, was 90% in children with short guts, 50% in those with mucosal disease and 40% in those with chronic intestinal pseudo-obstruction syndrome.[136] Factors impacting the survival of children with intestinal failure referred for intestinal transplantation have been studied in a series of 257 patients (mean age 3.4 ± 0.26 years) evaluated for intestinal transplantation.[66] Only 82 (32%) underwent intestinal transplantation (68 small bowel–liver transplantation) with a mean waiting time of 10.1 ± 1.3 months. Of the 175 patients who were not transplanted, 120 died. The main factors associated with poor prognosis were: age below 1 year, surgical disease, bridging fibrosis or cirrhosis, bilirubin levels of over 3 mg/dl and thrombocytopenia.

Combined small bowel–liver transplantation

It is sometimes difficult to decide on liver transplantation. Indeed, some PN-dependent patients with advanced liver dysfunction in the setting of short-bowel syndrome may experience functional and biochemical liver recovery which appears to parallel autologous gut salvage.[137] On the other hand, we reported consecutive cases of severe cholestasis that totally resumed after discontinuation of intravenous lipid administration.[138] Histology is not always predictive of functional liver recovery. However, in our experience, in the absence of biological change and PN administration, the time taken to go from portal fibrosis to cirrhosis is approximately 12 months, similar to the waiting time.[139] Once cirrhosis has been established, survival at 1 year is only 30%.[66,135]

It is well established that patients referred for small bowel–liver transplantation are more debilitated, have multiple complications, and have prolonged stays in the intensive care unit.[140] It may explain the lower patient and graft survival rate compared with isolated small-bowel transplantation reported from several programs.[60–62,64,65] It was suggested that early isolated small-bowel transplantation with such a short period of postoperative hospitalization could well prove to be cost-effective compared with the intensive use of resources that characterizes the short-bowel patient with liver failure.[141]

Financial considerations

Financial issues are now considered in managing intestinal failure patients. Provision of basic home PN is associated with charges. Actual costs for total PN, including the pharmacist's time for compounding, are different according to home-PN programs and countries. The costs for transplant evaluation, the transplant and postoperative care, and post-transplant follow-up are not currently available for comparison.[142,143]

Short-bowel syndrome

Patients with short-bowel syndrome can lead a productive, lengthy, happy and useful life if educated and managed appropriately. It is possible to reduce or even eliminate PN requirements over time in many of these patients using the evidence-based techniques of dietary and PN management (see Chapter 29). Hormonal therapy may eventually be available to augment the intestinal adaptation process as this becomes better understood. For patients with irreversible intestinal failure who do require total PN, it is essential that the therapy be prescribed appropriately. PN is associated with several potentially serious complications, many of which can be prevented when both the patient and the caring professional have the appropriate expertise.

Early referral for irreversible intestinal failure

As pediatric patients represent almost two-thirds of the indications for small-bowel tranplantation, appropriate therapeutic strategies should be developed for all phases of intestinal failure. It is first necessary to recognize, as early as possible, the patient with irreversible intestinal failure, such as extreme short-bowel syndrome or congenital disease of the intestinal mucosa. These patients should be referred at an early stage to multidisciplinary teams involved in small-bowel transplantation in optimal nutritional status. For other patients, attempts at achieving intestinal autonomy (PN weaning) require appropriate management as previously emphasized. Intestinal transplantation thus requires a strategy based on a long-term multidisciplinary approach, aimed at demonstrating the irreversibility of intestinal failure, to avoid the complications of long-term PN and to refer early selected patients requiring this procedure.[141–145]

Particular procedures

Because of the reduced size of the donor pool, strategies have been developed to enhance it and to perform transplantation without delay to avoid death on the waiting list, if the patient is in need of a combined liver–intestine transplantation.

Living related donors

Intestinal grafts are usually obtained from size-matched brain-dead adults or children. The ABO identity is necessary to avoid hemolysis related to circulating antibodies. It is difficult to obtain HLA compatibility, mainly for logistical reasons (the graft poorly tolerates ischemia). However, the longest survival time before the advent of cyclosporin A was observed after intrafamilial transplantation. Long-term survival has since been obtained in intrafamilial transplantation with cyclosporin A or FK506 immunosuppression.[146–149] A unique case of a successful isolated intestinal transplantation without immunosuppressive treatment between identical twins was recently reported.[149] However, living-related intestinal transplantation should remain very limited.

Reduced-size composite liver–intestinal allograft

Strict donor selection to prevent factors that may adversely affect the intestinal graft and size-matching have limited donor availability.[66] These factors contribute to the long waiting time for pediatric patients. Reduced-sized orthotopic composite liver–intestinal allografts are technically feasible and may increase the donor pool.[150,151]

Multivisceral transplantation

Multivisceral or 'cluster' transplantation of organs from the celiac region (liver, stomach, duodenum–pancreas and small bowel) was reported for the first time in 1989. From the Registry, it represents 13% in children and 24% in adults of all intestinal grafts. This procedure raises specific technical problems, but immunosuppressive treatment is no different. The Miami group performed multivisceral transplantation in very small children as an alternative to *en bloc* liver–intestine transplantation due to its advantage in creating more room in the abdominal space.[152] They reported improved survival rates with an excellent functional outcome of the stomach and the pancreas.

Conclusion

During the past decade, intestinal transplantation has gone from being an experimental procedure to one that is being increasingly accepted and performed. Further improvements depend on several factors, including the early and adapted management of patients with intestinal failure, refractory or likely to become refractory, by trained medico-surgical teams, improvements of immunosuppression by using new-generation drugs or monoclonal antibodies targeting receptors involved in T-cell activation, and the better prevention of post-transplant infectious complications by using appropriate antiviral therapy.[153–156] Constant progress in immunosuppression provides the hope of continuing to improve outcome after intestinal transplantation in selected patients. Indeed, when successful, intestinal transplantation allows patients surviving with their graft a recovery of intestinal function sufficient to discontinue a mostly long-term dependency on parenteral nutrition.

REFERENCES

1. Schraut W. Current status of small bowel transplantation. *Gastroenterology* 1988; **94**: 525–535.
2. Goulet O, Révillon Y, Brousse N et al. Successful small bowel transplantation in an infant. *Transplantation* 1992; **53**: 940–943.
3. Schroeder P, Goulet O, Lear P. Small bowel transplantation: European experience. *Lancet* 1990; **336**: 110–111.
4. Grant D, Wall W, Mimerault R. Successful small bowel–liver transplantation. *Lancet* 1990; **335**: 181–184.
5. Todo S, Tsakis A, Abu-Elmagd K et al. Cadaveric small bowel and small bowel–liver transplantation in humans. *Transplantation* 1992; **53**: 369–376.
6. Grant D. Intestinal Transplantation Registry on behalf of the current results of intestinal transplantation. *Lancet* 1996; **347**: 1801–1803.
7. Grant D. Intestinal transplantation: 1997 Report of the International Registry. *Transplantation* 1999; **15**: 1061–1064.
8. Colomb V, Goulet O, Ricour C. Home enteral and parenteral nutrition. *Baillière's Clin Gastroenterol* 1998; **122**: 877–894.
9. Messing B, Lemann M, Landais P et al. Prognosis of patients with chronic intestinal failure receiving long-term home parenteral nutrition in France and Belgium. *Gastroenterology* 1995; **108**: 1005–1010.
10. Howard L, Ament M, Fleming R et al. Current use and clinical outcome of home parenteral and enteral nutrition therapies in the United States. *Gastroenterology* 1995; **109**: 355–365.
11. Howard L, Hassan N. Home parenteral nutrition: 25 years later. *Clin Nutr* 1998; **27**: 418–512.
12. Howard L, Malone M. Current status of home parenteral nutrition in the United States. *Transplant Proc* 1996; **28**: 2691–2695.
13. Goulet O, Baglin-Gobet S, Jais JP et al. Outcome and long-term growth after extensive small bowel resection in the neonatal period: a survey of 87 children. *Eur J Pediatr Surg* 2004; in press.
14. Sondheimer JM, Cadnapaphornchai M, Sontag M, Zerbe GO. Predicting the duration of dependence on parenteral nutrition after neonatal intestinal resection. *J Pediatr* 1998; **132**: 80–84.
15. Goulet O, Révillon Y, Jan D et al. Which patients need small bowel transplantation for neonatal short bowel syndrome. *Transplant Proc* 1992; **24**: 1058–1059.
16. Goulet O, Ricour C. The short bowel syndrome. In Buts JP, Sokal EM, eds. Elsevier Science Publishers BV, 1993: 307–318.
17. Bianchi A. Longitudinal intestinal lengthening and tailoring: results in 20 children. *J R Soc Med* 1997; **90**: 429–432.
18. Thompson JS, Langnas AN, Pinch LW et al. Surgical approach to short-bowel syndrome. Experience in a population of 160 patients. *Ann Surg* 1995; **222**: 600–605.
19. Berger DL, Malt RA. Management of the short gut syndrome. *Adv Surg* 1996; **29**: 43–57.
20. Vanderhoof JA. Short bowel syndrome in children and small intestinal transplantation. *Pediatr Clin North Am* 1996; **43**: 533–546.
21. Panis Y, Messing B, Rivet P et al. Segmental reversal of the small bowel as an alternative to intestinal transplantation in patients with short bowel syndrome. *Ann Surg* 1997; **225**: 401–407.
22. Shulman DI, Shih Hu C, Duckett G, Lavallee-Grey M. Effects of short-term growth hormone therapy in rats undergoing 75% small intestinal resection. *J Pediatr Gastroenterol Nutr* 1992; **14**: 3–11.
23. Ulshen MA, Dowling RH, Fuller CR et al. Enhanced growth of small bowel in transgenic mice overexpressing bovine growth hormone. *Gastroenterology* 1993; **104**: 973–980.
24. Benhamou PH, Canarelli JP, Leroy C et al. Stimulation by recombinant human growth hormone of growth and development of remaining bowel after subtotal ileojejunectomy in rat. *J Pediatr Gastroenterol Nutr* 1994; **18**: 446–452.
25. Byrne TA, Persinger RL, Young LS et al. A new treatment for patients with short-bowel syndrome: growth hormone, glutamine and a modified diet. *Ann Surg* 1995; **22**: 243–255.
26. Scolapio JS, Camilleri M, Fleming CR et al. Effect of growth hormone, glutamine, and diet on adaptation in short-bowel syndrome: a randomized, controlled study. *Gastroenterology* 1997; **113**: 1074–1081.
27. Seguy D, Vahedi K, Kapel N et al. Low-dose growth hormone in adult home PN-dependent short bowel patients: a positive study. *Gastroenterology* 2003; **124**: 293–302.
28. Dabbas-Tyan M, Colomb V, Rosilio M et al. Evaluation of the effect of recombinant human growth hormone (rhGH) treatment of children with short bowel syndrome. *J Pediatr Gastroenterol Nutr* 2000; **31**: 5165–5166.
29. Ellegard L, Bosaeus I, Nordgren S, Bengtsson BA. Low-dose recombinant human growth hormone increases body weight and lean body mass in patients with short bowel syndrome. *Ann Surg* 1997; **225**: 88–96.
30. Szkudlarek J, Jeppesen P-B, Mortensen P-B. Effect of high dose growth hormone with glutamine and no change in diet on intestinal absorption in short bowel patients: a randomised, double blind, crossover, placebo controlled study. *Gut* 2000; **47**: 199–205.
31. Jeppesen PB, Mortensen AP. Enhancing bowel adaptation in short bowel syndrome. *Curr Gastroenterol Rep* 2002; **4**: 338–347.
32. Beath SV, Davies P, Papadopoulou A et al. Parenteral nutrition-related cholestasis in postsurgical neonates: multivariate analysis of risk factors. *J Pediatr Surg* 1996; **31**: 604–606.
33. Lawrence J P, Dun SP, Billmire DF et al. Isolated liver transplantation for liver failure in patients with short bowel syndrome. *J Pediatr Surg* 1994; **29**: 751–753.
34. Horslen SP, Sudan DL, Iyer KR et al. Isolated liver transplantation in infants with end-stage liver disease associated with short bowel syndrome. *Ann Surg* 2002; **235**: 435–439.
35. Hassan OK, Beath SV, McKlerman PJ et al. Difficult management choices for infants with short bowel syndrome and liver failure. *J Pediatr Gastroenterol Nutr* 2002; **35**: 216–219.
36. Sharif K, Beath SV, Kelly DA et al. New perspective for the management of near-total or total intestinal aganglionosis in infants. *J Pediatr Surg* 2003; **38**: 25–28.
37. Révillon Y, Aigrain Y, Jan D et al. Improved quality of life by combined transplantation in Hirschsprung's disease with a very long aganglionic segment. *J Pediatr Surg* 2003; **38**: 422–424.
38. Goulet O, Jobert-Giraud A, Michel JL et al. Chronic intestinal pseudoobstruction syndrome in pediatric patients. *Eur J Pediatr Surg* 1999; **9**: 83–90.

39. Rudolph CD, Hyman PE, Altschuler SM et al. Diagnosis and treatment of chronic intestinal pseudoobstruction in children: report of consensus workshop. *J Pediatr Gastroenterol Nutr* 1997; **24**: 102–112.
40. Faure C, Goulet O, Ategbo S et al. Chronic intestinal pseudoobstruction syndrome: clinical analysis, outcome and prognosis in 105 children. *Dig Dis Sci* 1999; **44**: 953–959.
41. Sigurdsson L, Reyes J, Kocoshis SA et al. Intestinal transplantation in children with chronic intestinal pseudo-obstruction. *Gut* 1999; **45**: 570–574.
42. Masetti M, Rodriguez MM, Thompson JF et al. Multivisceral transplantation for megacystis microcolon intestinal hypoperistalsis syndrome. *Transplantation* 1999; **68**: 228–232.
43. Kosmach B, Tarbell S, Reyes J, Todos S. 'Munchausen by proxy' in a small bowel transplant recipient. *Transplant Proc* 1996; **28**: 2790–2791.
44. Phillips A, Schmitz J. Congenital microvillus atrophy: a clinico-pathological survey of 23 cases. *J Pediatr Gastroenterol Nutr* 1992; **14**: 380–396.
45. Goulet O, Kedinger M, Brousse N et al. Intractable diarrhea of infancy with epithelial and basement membrane abnormalities. *J Pediatr* 1995; **127**: 212–219.
46. Oliva MM, Perman JA, Saavedra JM et al. Successful intestinal transplantation for microvillous inclusion disease. *Gastroenterology* 1994; **106**: 771–774.
47. Lacaille F, Cuenod B, Colomb V et al. Combined liver and small bowel transplantation in a child with epithelial dysplasia. *J Pediatr Gastroenterol Nutr* 1998; **27**: 230–233.
48. Sudan DL, Kaufman SS Shaw BW Jr et al. Isolated intestinal transplantation for intestinal failure. *Am J Gastroenterol* 2000; **95**: 1506–1515
49. Herzog D, Atkinson P, Grant D et al. Combined bowel-liver transplantation in an infant with microvillus inclusion disease. *J Pediatr Gastroenterol Nutr* 1996; **22**: 405–408.
50. Randak C, Langnas AN, Kaufman SS et al. Pretransplant management and small bowel-liver transplantation in an infant with microvillus inclusion disease. *J Pediatr Gastroenterol Nutr* 1998; **27**: 333–337.
51. Ruemmele F, Révillon Y, Jan D et al. New perspectives for children with microvillous inclusion disease: early small bowel transplantation. *Transplantation* 2004; **77**: 1024–1028.
52. Paramesh AS, Fishbein T, Tschernia A et al. Isolated small bowel transplantation for tufting enteropathy. *J Pediatr Gastroenterol Nutr* 2003; **36**: 138–140.
53. Fishbein TM, Florman S, Gondolesi G et al. Intestinal transplantation before and after the introduction of sirolimus. *Transplantation* 2002; **73**: 1538–1542.
54. Berribi C, Loirat C, Jacqz-Aigrain E. Mycophenolate mofetil may induce apoptosis in duodenal villi. *Pediatr Nephrol* 2000; **14**: 177–178.
55. Tzakis AG, Kato T, Nishida S et al. Preliminary experience with campath 1H (C1H) in intestinal and liver transplantation. *Transplantation* 2003; **75**: 1227–1231.
56. Reyes J, Mazariegos GV, Bond GM et al. Pediatric intestinal transplantation: historical notes, principles and controversies. *Pediatr Transplant* 2002; **6**: 193–207.
57. Wekerle T, Kurtz J, Sykes. Mixed hematopoietic chimerism and transplantation tolerance: insights from experimental models. *Curr Opin Organ Transplant* 1999; **4**: 44–49
58. Pirenne J, Gruessner AC, Beneditti E. Donor-specific unmodified bone marrow transfusion does not facilitate intestinal engraftment after bowel transplantation in a porcine model. *Surgery* 1997; **121**: 79–88.
59. De Roover A, Langnas AN. Surgical methods of small bowel transplantation. *Curr Opin Organ Transplant* 1999; **4**: 335–342.
60. Reyes J, Bueno J, Kocoshis S et al. Current status of intestinal transplantation in children. *J Pediatr Surg* 1998; **33**: 243–254.
61. Farmer DG, McDiarmid SV, Smith C et al. Experience with combined liver–small intestine transplantation at the University of California, Los Angeles. *Transplant Proc* 1998; **30**: 2533–2534.
62. Atkison P, Williams S, Wall S, Grant D. Results of pediatric small bowel transplantation in Canada. *Transplant Proc* 1998; **30**: 2521–2522.
63. Nishida S, Levi D, Kato T et al. Ninety-five cases of intestinal transplantation at the University of Miami. *J Gastrointest Surg* 2002; **6**: 233–239.
64. Goulet O, Lacaille F, Colomb V et al. Intestinal transplantation in children: Paris experience. *Transplant Proc* 2002; **34**: 1887–1888.
65. Iyer KR, Srinath C, Horslen S et al. Late graft loss and long-term outcome after isolated intestinal transplantation in children. *J Pediatr Surg* 2002; **37**: 151–154.
66. Bueno J, Ohwada S, Kocoshis S et al. Factors impacting the survival of children with intestinal failure referred for intestinal transplantation. *J Pediatr Surg* 1999; **34**: 27–33.
67. Sarnacki S, Révillon Y, Cerf-Bensussan N et al. Long term small bowel graft survival induced by spontaneously tolerated liver allograft in inbred rat strains. *Transplantation* 1992; **54**: 383–385.
68. Zhong R, He G, Sakai Y et al. Combined small bowel and liver transplantation in the rat: possible role of the liver in preventing intestinal allograft rejection. *Transplantation* 1991; **52**: 550–552.
69. Goulet O, Jan D, Lacaille F et al. Intestinal transplantation in children: preliminary experience in Paris. *J Parenter Enter Nutr* 1999; **23**: S121–S125.
70. Kamada N, Shinomiya T. Clonal deletion as the mechanism of abrogation of immunological memory following liver grafting in rats. *Immunology* 1985; **55**: 85–90.
71. Tu Y, Arima T, Flye MW. Rejection of spontaneously accepted rat liver allografts with recipient interleukin 2 treatment or donor irradiation. *Transplantation* 1997; **63**: 177–181.
72. Thomson AW. Are dendritic cells the key to liver transplant tolerance. *Immunol Today* 1999; **20**: 27–32.
73. Sarnacki S, Nakai H, Calise D et al. Decreased expression of CD25 on CD8+ recipient T cells in intestinal grafts tolerated after liver transplantation in rats. *Gut* 1998; **43**: 849–855.
74. Bishop GA, Sharland AF, McCaughan GW. High-dose/activation associated tolerance model for allografts: lesson from spontaneous tolerance of transplanted livers. *Curr Opin Organ Transplant* 1999; **4**: 58–64.
75. Iwaki Y, Starzl TE, Yagihasni A et al. Replacement of donor lymphoid tissue in small bowel transplantation. *Lancet* 1991; **337**: 818–819.
76. Goulet O. Recent studies on small intestinal transplantation. *Gastroenterology* 1997; **13**: 500–509.
77. Kaufman SS, Wisecarver JL, Ruby EI et al. Correlation of mucosal disaccharidase activities with histology in evaluation of rejection following intestinal transplantation. *Pediatr Transpl* 1998; **2**: 134–138.
78. Goulet O, Brousse N, Révillon Y, Ricour C. Pathology of human intestinal transplantation. In Grant D, Wood RFM, eds. *Small Bowel Transplantation*. London: Edward Arnold, 1993: 112–120.
79. Lee RG, Nakamura K, Tsamandas AC et al. Pathology of human intestinal transplantation. *Gastroenterology* 1996; **110**: 1820–1834.

80. Sigurdsson L, Reyes J, Todo S et al. Anatomic variability of rejection in intestinal allografts after pediatric intestinal transplantation. *J Pediatr Gastroenterol Nutr* 1998; **27**: 403–406.
81. Nogushi Si S, Reyes J, Maeariegos GV, Parizhskaya M, Jaffe R. Pediatric intestinal transplantation: the resected allograft. *Pediatr Dev Pathol* 2002; **5**: 3–21.
82. Parizhskaya M, Redondo C, Demetris A et al. Chronic rejection of small bowel grafts: pediatric and adult study of risk factors and morphologic progression. *Pediatr Dev Pathol* 2003; **6**: 240–250
83. Wu T, Abu-Elmagd K, Nalesnik MA et al. A schema for histologic grading of small intestine allograft acute rejection. *Transplantation* 2003; **75**: 1241–1248.
84. Green M, Bueno J, Sigurdsson L et al. Unique aspects of the infectious complications of intestinal transplantation. *Curr Opin Organ Transplant* 1999; **4**: 361–367.
85. Patel R, Snydman DR, Rubin RH et al. Cytomegalovirus prophylaxis in solid organ transplant recipients. *Transplantation* 1996; **61**: 1279–1289.
86. Finn L, Reyes J, Bueno J, Yunis E. Epstein-Barr virus infection in children after transplantation of the small intestine. *Am J Surg Pathol* 1998; **22**: 299–309.
87. Green M, Reyes J, Jabbour N et al. Use of quantitative PCR to predict onset of Epstein–Barr viral infection and post-transplant lymphoproliferative disease after intestinal transplantation in children. *Transplant Proc* 1996; **28**: 2759–2760.
88. Berney T, Delis S, Kato T et al. Successful treatment of posttransplant lymphoproliferative disease with prolonged rituximab treatment in intestinal transplant recipients. *Transplantation* 2002; **74**: 1000–1006.
89. Furukawa H, Kusne S, Sutton DA et al. Acute invasive sinusitis due to trichoderma longibrachiatum in a liver and small bowel transplant recipient. *Clin Infect Dis* 1998; **26**: 487–489.
90. Muiesan P, Dhawan A, Wendon J et al. Hemophagocytosis: a potential complication in small bowel transplantation. *Transplantation* 1998; **66**: 794–796.
91. Berho M, Torroella M, Viciana A et al. Adenovirus enterocolitis in human small bowel transplants. *Pediatr Transplant* 1998; **2**: 277–282.
92. Turler A, Kalff JC, Heeckt P et al. Molecular and functional observations on the donor intestinal muscularis during human small bowel transplantation. *Gastroenterology* 2002; **122**: 1886–1897.
93. Sarr MG, Kelly KA. Myoelectric activity of the autotransplantation canine jejuno-ileum. *Gastroenterology* 1981; **81**: 303–310.
94. Sugitani A, Bauer AJ, Reynolds JC et al. The effects of small bowel transplantation on the morphology and physiology of intestinal muscle – a comparison of autografts versus allografts in dogs. *Transplantation* 1997; **63**: 186–194.
95. Taguchi T, Zorychta E, Sonnino RE, Guttman FM. Small intestinal transplantation in the rat: effect on physiological properties of smooth muscle and nerves. *J Pediatr Surg* 1989; **24**: 1258–1263.
96. Taguchi T, Zorychta E, Sonnino RE, Guttman FM. Function of smooth muscle and nerve after small intestine transplantation in the rat: effect of storing donor bowel in Eurocollins. *J Pediatr Surg* 1989; **24**: 634–638.
97. Ishii H, Kusunoki M, Fujita S et al. Changes of intestinal motility after small bowel transplantation in the rat. *Transplantation* 1994; **57**: 1149–1152.
98. Kusunoki M, Ishii H, Nakao K et al. Long-term effects of small bowel transplantation on intestinal motility. *Transplantation* 1995; **60**: 897–899.
99. Lu G, Sarr MG, Szurszewski JH. Effect of extrinsic denervation in a canine model of jejunoileal autotransplantation on mechanical and electrical activity of jejunal circular smooth muscle. *Dig Dis Sci* 1997; **42**: 40–46.
100. Suginati A, Reynolds JC, Tsuboi M, Todo S. Extrinsic intestinal reinnervation after canine small bowel autotransplantation. *Surgery* 1998; **123**: 25–35.
101. Taguchi T, Guo R, Masumoto K et al. Chronological change of distribution in nitric oxide and peptidergic neurons after rat small intestinal transplantation. *J Pediatr Surg* 1999; **34**: 341–345.
102. Murr MM, Miller VM, Sarr MG. Contractile properties of enteric smooth muscle after small bowel transplantation in rats. *Am J Surg* 1996; **171**: 212–217.
103. Hamada N, Hutson WR, Nakada K et al. Intestinal neuromuscular function after preservation and transplantation. *J Surg Res* 1996; **63**: 460–466.
104. Lu G, Sarr MG, Szurszewski JH. Effect of intrinsic denervation in a canine model of jejunoileal autotransplantation on mechanical and electrical activity of jejunal circular smooth muscle. *Dig Dis Sci* 1997; **42**: 40–46.
105. Johnson CP, Sarna SK, Zhu YR et al. Effects of intestinal transplantation on postprandial motility and regulation of intestinal transit. *Surgery* 2001; **129**: 6–14.
106. Mousa H, Bueno J, Griffiths J et al. Intestinal motility after small bowel transplantation. *Transplant Proc* 1998; **30**: 2535–2536.
107. Pernthaler H, Kreczy A, Plattner R et al. Myoelectric activity during small bowel allograft rejection. *Dig Dis Sci* 1994; **39**: 1216–1221.
108. Klaus A, Klima G, Margreiter R, Pernthaler H. Myoelectric activity during chronic small bowel allograft rejection in rats. *Dig Dis Sci* 2002; **47**: 2506–2511.
109. Kenneth KWL, Heeckt PF, Halfter WM et al. Functional impairment of enteric smooth muscle and nerves caused by chronic intestinal allograft rejection regresses after FK506 rescue. *Transplantation* 1995; **59**: 159–164.
110. Telford GL, Nemeth MA, Sarna SK et al. Myoelectric activity and absorptive capacity of rat small intestinal isografts. *Dig Dis Sci* 1996; **41**: 1082–1087.
111. Campbell WL, Abu-Elmagd K, Federle MP et al. Contrast examination of the small bowel in patients with small-bowel transplants: findings in 16 patients. *Am J Roentgenol* 1993; **161**: 969–974.
112. Yanchar NL, Riegel TM, Martin G et al. Tacrolimus [FK 506] – its effects on intestinal glucose transport. *Transplantation* 1996; **61**: 630–634.
113. Oishi AJ, Inoue Y, Souba WW, Sarr MG. Alterations in carrier-mediated glutamine transport after a model of canine jejunal autotransplantation. *Dig Dis Sci* 1996; **41**: 1915–1924.
114. Sun SC, Katz SM, Schechner RS et al. Effect of tacrolimus on hemodynamics and absorption of experimental small intestinal transplants. *Transplantation* 1996; **61**: 1447–1450.
115. Sigalet DL, Kneteman NN, Fedorak RN et al. Small intestinal function following syngeneic transplantation in the rat. *J Surg Res* 1996; **61**: 379–384.
116. Kato Y, Hamada Y, Ito S et al. Epidermal growth factor stimulates the recovery of glucose absorption after small bowel transplantation. *J Surg Res* 1998; **80**: 315–319.
117. Kim J, Fryer J, Craig RM. Absorptive function following small intestinal transplantation. *Dig Dis Sci* 1998; **43**: 1925–1930.
118. Kellersman R, Zhong R, Kiyochi H et al. Reconstruction of the intestinal lymphatic drainage after small bowel transplantation. *Transplantation* 2000; **69**: 10–16.

119. Sigalet DL, Williams DC, Garola R et al. Impact of FK506 and steroids on adaptation after intestinal resection or segmental transplantation. *Pediatr Transplant* 2000; **4**: 12–20.
120. Libsch KD, Zyromski NJ, Tanaka T et al. Role of extrinsic innervation in jejunal absorptive adaptation to subtotal small bowel resection: a model of segmental small bowel transplantation. *J Gastrointest Surg* 2002; **6**: 240–247.
121. Tsiotos GG, Kendrick ML, Libsch K et al. Ileal absorptive adaptation to jejunal resection and extrinsic denervation: implications for living-related small bowel transplantation. *J Gastrointest Surg* 2001; **5**: 217–224.
122. Raimundo AH, Grimble GK, Rees RG et al. The effect of carbohydrate and fat on the absorption of amino acids and peptides in the normal human small intestine [abstract]. *J Parenter Enteral Nutr* 1989; **13** (Suppl): 9S.
123. Van Der Hulst RRJ, Van Kreel BK, Von Meyenfeldt MF et al. Glutamine and the preservation of gut integrity. *Lancet* 1993; **341**: 1363–1365.
124. Kaufman SS, Lyden ER, Brown CR et al. Disaccharidase activities and fat assimilation in pediatric patients after intestinal transplantation. *Transplantation* 2000; **15**: 362–365.
125. Caliari S, Vantini I, Sembenini C et al. Fecal fat measurement in the presence of long- and medium-chain triglycerides and fatty acids. *Scand J Gastroenterol* 1996; **31**: 863–867.
126. Iyer K, Horslen S, Iverson A et al. Nutritional outcome and growth of children after intestinal transplantation. *J Pediatr Surg* 2002; **37**: 464–466.
127. Nucci AM, Barksdale EM Jr, Beserock N et al. Long-term nutritional outcome after pediatric intestinal transplantation. *J Pediatr Surg* 2002; **37**: 460–463.
128. Goulet O, Allegri A, Colomb V et al. Growth and nutritional status after intestinal transplantation in children. *J Pediatr Gastroenterol Nutr* 2000; **31** (Suppl 2): S165 [A]
129. Brook G. Quality of life issues: parenteral nutrition to small bowel transplantation – a review. *Nutrition* 1998; **14**: 813–816.
130. Rovera GM, Di Martini A, Schoen RE et al. Quality of life of patients after intestinal transplantation. *Transplantation* 1998; **66**: 1141–1145.
131. Tarbell SE, Kosmach B. Parenteral psychosocial outcomes in pediatric liver and/or intestinal transplantation: pretransplantation and the early postoperative period. *Liver Transpl Surg* 1998; **4**: 378–387.
132. Iyer K, Kaufman S, Sudan D et al. Long-term results of intestinal transplantation for pseudo-obstruction in children. *J Pediatr Surg* 2001; **36**: 174–177.
133. Sudan D, Iyer K, Horslen S et al. Assessment of quality of life after pediatric intestinal transplantation by parents and pediatric recipients using the child health questionnaire. *Transplant Proc* 2002; **34**: 963–964.
134. Kaufman S, Atkinson JB, Bianchi A et al. Indications for pediatric intestinal transplantation: a position paper of the American society of transplantation. *Pediatr Transplant* 2001; **5**: 80–87.
135. Beath SV, Booth IW, Murphy MS et al. Nutritional care and candidates for small bowel transplantation. *Arch Dis Child* 1995; **73**: 348–350.
136. Beath SV, Brook GA, Kelly DA et al. Demand for pediatric small bowel transplantation in the United Kingdom. *Transplant Proc* 1998; **30**: 2531–2532.
137. Iyer K, Horslen S, Torres C et al. Histology is not predictive of functional liver recovery in parenteral-nutrition associated liver dysfunction. *Pediatr Transplant* 2003; **7**: 69(A).
138. Colomb V, Jobert-Giraud A, Lacaille F et al. Role of lipid emulsions in cholestasis associated with long-term parenteral nutrition in children. *J Parenter Enteral Nutr* 2000; **24**: 345–350.
139. Colomb V, Jobert A, Lacaille F et al. Parenteral nutrition-associated liver disease in children : natural history and prognosis. *Clin Nutr* 1999; **18 (Suppl 1)**: 36.
140. Filston HC, Colombani PM. Preliminary experience with intestinal transplantation in infants and children. *Pediatrics* 1996; **97**: 583–584.
141. Goulet O, Ruemmele F, Lacaille F, Colomb V. Irreversible intestinal failure. *J Pediatr Gastroenterol Nutr* 2004; **38**: 250–269.
142. Buchman AL, Scolapio J, Fryer J. AGA technical review on short bowel syndrome and intestinal transplantation. *Gastroenterology* 2003; **124**: 1111–1134.
143. Kaufman SS. Small bowel transplantation: selection criteria, operative techniques, advances in specific immunosuppression, prognosis. *Curr Opin Pediatr* 2001; **13**: 425–428.
144. Fishbein TM, Shciano T, LeLeiko N et al. An integrated approach to intestinal failure. Results of a new program with total parenteral nutrition, bowel rehabilitation, and transplantation. *J Gastrointest Surg* 2002; **6**: 554–562.
145. Martin D, Ezzelarab M, Bond G et al. Patient profile and candidacy for intestinal transplantation at the University of Pittsburgh. *Transplant Proc* 2002; **34**: 1897–1898.
146. Jaffe BM, Beck R, Flint L et al. Living-related small bowel transplantation in adults – a report of two patients. *Transplant Proc* 1997; **29**: 1851–1852.
147. Fujimoto Y, Uemoto S, Inomata Y et al. Living-related small bowel transplant: management of rejection and infection. *Transplant Proc* 1998; **30**: 1149.
148. Ding J, Guo CC, Li CN et al. Postoperative endoscopic surveillance of human living-donor small bowel transplantations. *World J Gastroenterol* 2003; **9**: 595–598.
149. Genton L, Raguso CA, Berney T et al. Four year nutritional follow up after living related small bowel transplantation between monozygotic twins. *Gut* 2003; **52**: 659–662.
150. Reyes J, Fishbein T, Bueno J et al. Reduced-size orthotopic composite liver-intestinal allograft. *Transplantation* 1998; **66**: 489–492.
151. Bueno J, Abu-Elmagd K, Mazariegos G et al. Composite liver–small bowel allografts with preservation donor duodenum and hepatic biliary system in children. *J Pediatr Surg* 2000; **35**: 291–295; discussion 295–296.
152. Mittal N, Kato T, Miller B et al. Multivisceral transplantation in children – functional outcomes of the transplanted pancreas and stomach in en-bloc graft. *Pediatr Transplant* 2003; **7**: 51(A).
153. Abu-Elmagd K, Bond G. The current status and future outlook of intestinal transplantation. *Minerva Chir* 2002; **57**: 543–560.
154. Sigalet DL, Thorne PC, Martin GR et al. Combined immunosuppression with cyclosporine, rapamycin, and mycophenolate mofetil controls rejection with minimal nutritional impact in experimental small intestinal transplantation. *Transplant Proc* 2002; **34**: 1121–1123.
155. Pirenne J, Koshiba T, Geboes K et al. Complete freedom from rejection after intestinal transplantation using a new tolerogenic protocol combined with low immunosuppression. *Transplantation* 2002; **73**: 966–968.
156. Starzl TE, Murase N, Abu-Elmagd K et al. Tolerogenic immunosuppression for organ transplantation. *Lancet* 2003; **361**: 1502–1510.

43 Intussusception

Adolfo Bautista Casasnovas

Introduction

Intussusception is a form of intestinal obstruction, due to the telescoping or prolapse of one section of the intestine (the intussusceptum) into an adjacent section (the intussuscipiens). In most cases, the terminal ileum telescopes into the colon. Intussusception occurs most frequently before the age of 2 years; the incidence is highest in the first year, during which it is the most frequent cause of intestinal obstruction.

This disorder has been known since the time of Aristotle, but the first detailed description was that of Paul Barbette, who in 1676 proposed surgical treatment.[1] Until the mid-19th century, however, intussusception remained almost invariably fatal. The first successful surgical treatment (of a 2-year-old boy) was reported in 1873 by Jonathan Hutchinson.[2] In 1876, Hirschsprung described the treatment of a series of patients with hydrostatic enema, marking the start of a period of progress in treatment.[3] In 1905 Hirschsprung published a new series of 107 cases, with 35% mortality in patients treated by enema and 80% mortality in patients treated surgically.

In 1948 Ravitch and McClure published their experience with barium contrast radiography, and established indications and contraindications for hydrostatic reduction.[4] Subsequent publications helped generalize the use of hydrostatic reduction, typically with high success rates (94%) and low mortality (0.02%).[5–7] In the 1980s, ultrasonography was introduced as an innocuous and reliable method for diagnosis.

Current standard treatment practice is based on careful early diagnosis, generally by contrast radiography and/or ultrasonography. Treatment usually involves hydrostatic or pneumatic reduction, with surgery reserved for a specific small subset of cases. When this approach is followed, morbidity is less than 1% and mortality close to zero.

Epidemiology

Intussusception is the predominant cause of intestinal obstruction between 5 months and 5 years of age, with incidence differing between countries and races. In the UK and USA, for example, reported mean incidences range from 1.5–4.3 per 1000 liveborn children,[8–10] versus 2.7–6.1 per 1000 in Spain.[11,12]

Prevalence is typically about three times higher in boys than in girls, and indeed about eight times higher in boys from age 4 years onwards.

It can present at any age, but as already noted it is most common in the first 2 years of life, with incidence peaking between 3 and 12 months (mean 7–8 months). Two-thirds of cases present in the first year of life.

Some studies have reported different patterns of seasonal variation in incidence, but large-sample and long-series studies suggest that there is no consistent seasonal pattern. Certainly, however, the incidence clearly increases during epidemics of gastroenteritis, respiratory infection and adenovirus infection, and during periods of vaccination against rotavirus.[13–16]

Etiopathology

Primary idiopathic intussusception

Despite numerous publications, the etiology of intussusception remains poorly understood. In 90% of cases there is no detectable organic lesion acting as the lead point.[17] The high incidence during the first year of life appears to be related to the abundant lymphoid tissue of the terminal ileum at this age, with lymphoid tissue hypertrophy being detected in most surgical interventions, and often apparent on ultrasonography. However, some authors have suggested that these adenopathies are a consequence, not a cause, of the intussusception.[18]

As noted, the most commonly intussuscepted section is the terminal ileum, telescoped into the colon (i.e. ileocolic intussusception). The intussusception extends a variable distance along the colon, and may even reach the rectum, where it can be detected by rectal palpation. Occasionally, ileoileal intussusceptions are observed, extending to the ileocecal valve.

In ileocolic intussusception, the intussusceptum is a section of the proximal part of the ileum, which telescopes into the adjacent distal colon, causing compression of the mesentery and strangulation of mesenteric blood vessels, with rapid edema of the intestinal wall, leading to impairment of venous return, edema of surrounding tissues, hemorrhage, blood infiltration and intestinal obstruction. The venous engorgement and ischemia lead to mucus secretion and bleeding, resulting in the classic 'currant jelly' stool. If the venous obstruction and ischemia continue, the patient will develop gangrene, intestinal perforation due to necrosis of the intussusceptum and peritonitis.

Secondary/organic intussusception

With increasing age of the patient, it is increasingly likely that the intussusception will have an organic origin. About 5–10% of intussusceptions are caused by an organic lesion. Above the age of 4 years, this percentage increases to 50%.

The most frequent organic cause is Meckel's diverticulum, followed by enteric duplications, intestinal polyps (whether isolated or forming part of Peutz–Jeghers syndrome), hemangiomas, traumatic hematomas and, less frequently, Henoch–Schönlein purpura, foreign bodies and trichobezoars, Crohn's disease, cystic fibrosis, leukemias, lymphomas, and intestinal lymphosarcomas.[11,12,19]

Postoperative intussusception may appear after any type of surgery (thoracic, abdominal, otorhinolaryngological, etc.), although it is most frequent after surgery to the digestive tract. Such intussusceptions make up about 1% of the total, and are related to postoperative motility alterations and paralytic ileus, or anesthetic medication. They typically present in the first 15–20 days after surgery and are often difficult to diagnose, since they are generally ileoileal or jejunoileal, and not revealed by contrast enema. They are rarely diagnosed in the immediate postoperative period, during which the signs and symptoms of intussusception are typically masked by postoperative pain and other consequences of the surgery. Treatment is surgical: usually surgical reduction is sufficient, without any need for intestinal resection.[20,21]

Clinical manifestations

Intussusception typically presents in thriving and otherwise healthy nursing infants, and starts with a sudden crisis of crying and screaming, with knees drawn up to the abdomen. After a few minutes these responses generally subside, and the child appears normal, but the crises then recur at regular intervals of 10–20 min, and may often be dramatic in that the child cannot be calmed. Sometimes the child has suffered a similar crisis during the preceding days or months. Vomiting of undigested food typically occurs a short time after onset of the pain crises; bilious vomiting generally occurs only if the disorder is left untreated for a long period. Stools of normal appearance may be passed (i.e. feces already present distal to the intussusception), but at later stages (generally not before 8–12 h after onset of the pain crises) the patient will discharge the characteristic blood-and-mucus clots known as 'currant jelly' stools.

It should be stressed that the 'typical' symptom triad of abdominal pain, vomiting and blood in stools is rarely seen early. In other words, Ombredanne's criterion (i.e. intussusception=ileal signs+blood in stools), which was widely used in the past, is in fact valid only for the late course. Occasionally, other symptoms (such as fever, diarrhea and prostration) may appear. Diarrhea may suggest gastroenteritis and delay diagnosis, as may constipation, which occurs in up to 20% of cases.[22]

Repeated occurrence of the typical crises over a period of days or weeks may indicate chronic intussusception with spontaneous reduction, presenting at intervals as acute crises.

Patients may show lethargy (i.e. apathy, sleepiness, prostration) during the early stages. Lethargy most commonly occurs between the pain crises, but in some cases may be the first symptom noted, before the pain crises, possibly suggesting encephalitis. Indeed, intussusception initially presenting as lethargy alone is typically problematic for diagnosis, since lethargy is normally associated with structural, toxic or metabolic disorders of the central nervous system; in such cases, central nervous system-related diagnostic procedures are typically applied before it becomes clear that the problem is in fact intussusception, with consequent diagnostic delay.[23,24] In this connection, it has been suggested that intussusception be included in mnemotechnics for diagnosis of patients with coma, with the letter 'i' being used to indicate 'insulin' and 'intussusception'.[25] Various hypotheses have been put forward to explain the lethargy arising in association with intussusception, including secretion of endogenous opioids and cytokines during the pain crises, absorption of toxins into the bloodstream and association with rapid dehydration and shock. In almost all cases in which lethargy is observed, some other symptoms are present, such as vomiting, abdominal distension, or irritability. It may also appear in association with other neurological symptoms such as convulsions, coma, pinpoint pupils, opisthotonos and hypotonia.

Occasionally, intussusception is not diagnosed until rectal bleeding occurs. This occurs most commonly in patients aged more than 1 year.

If untreated, the patient's condition is likely to worsen rapidly, with dehydration and possible shock. Early diagnosis is thus essential.

Some years ago we reviewed the symptoms observed in cases of intussusception treated at our hospital over the period 1969–84.[11] The most common symptoms were cramping abdominal pain (87% of patients), rectal bleeding (82%) and vomiting (78%) (Table 43.1).

Physical examination

In the early stages physical examination is in most cases normal, with the infant typically appearing well-fed and healthy. During pain crises, and if the crying permits, hyperperistaltic noise may be heard, with the abdomen tense and painful to palpation. Between the crises the right lower quadrant may appear strangely empty if the intussusception is ileocecal, with a mass palpable in practically any part of the abdomen; this mass is typically sausage-shaped and curved, owing to the traction exerted by the mesentery on the intestine.

In rectal examination, the examining finger may appear covered with bloody mucus or blood, but direct contact between the examining finger and the intussuscepted mass is rare. Rectal hemorrhage, together with fever and tachycardia, become increasingly likely over time. In the past, when intussusceptions were typically diagnosed late, the intussusceptum was often detectable on rectal examination, and indeed there are

Table 43.1 Signs and symptoms observed in intussusception patients seen at the Santiago de Compostela Clinical Hospital over the period 1969–84

Signs and symptoms	Patients	
	n	%
Cramping abdominal pain	61	87
Rectal bleeding	58	82.8
Vomiting	55	78.5
Abdominal distension	30	42.8
Abdominal mass	27	35.8
Respiratory illness	16	22.8
Lethargy	12	17
Gastroenteritis	10	14.3
Previous intussusception	2	3

descriptions of prolapse through the anus, with consequent ischemic damage (an extremely severe sign, generally associated with severe illness). If the intussusception has remained untreated for a long period, the patient may present with symptoms of hypovolemic shock.

Diagnosis

All pediatricians are well aware that persistent crying and abdominal pain in a nursing infant, particularly if associated with vomiting, needs to be carefully evaluated to confirm or rule out intussusception. Cramping pain with vomiting is sufficient grounds for continuous monitoring.

Complementary examinations should follow a systematic order. Initially, simple abdominal radiography and ultrasonography should be performed, which together will reveal intussusception and possible repercussions for intestinal transit. In the absence of contraindications, hydrostatic enema or pneumoenema should then be performed, to confirm the diagnosis and, when appropriate, to achieve reduction.

Simple abdominal radiography

This will reveal about 50% of intussusceptions, allowing evaluation of the degree of intestinal obstruction and exclusion of perforation due to pneumoperitoneum. The radiographic signs are not in themselves fully diagnostic, and a normal radiograph does not allow intussusception to be ruled out; nevertheless, in my opinion it should be performed routinely.

The most characteristic radiographic findings in ileocolic intussusception (Figure 43.1) are as follows:

(1) Reduced or absent intestinal gas in the right quadrant;

(2) Air–fluid levels;

(3) Diffuse radiolucent image, generally located in the right hypochondrium;

(4) Circle sign: two concentric circles and fat density, superimposed over the kidney to the right of the vertebral column;

(5) Convex mass effect with interruption of air at the level of the transverse colon;

(6) Obstruction of the small intestine.[26–28]

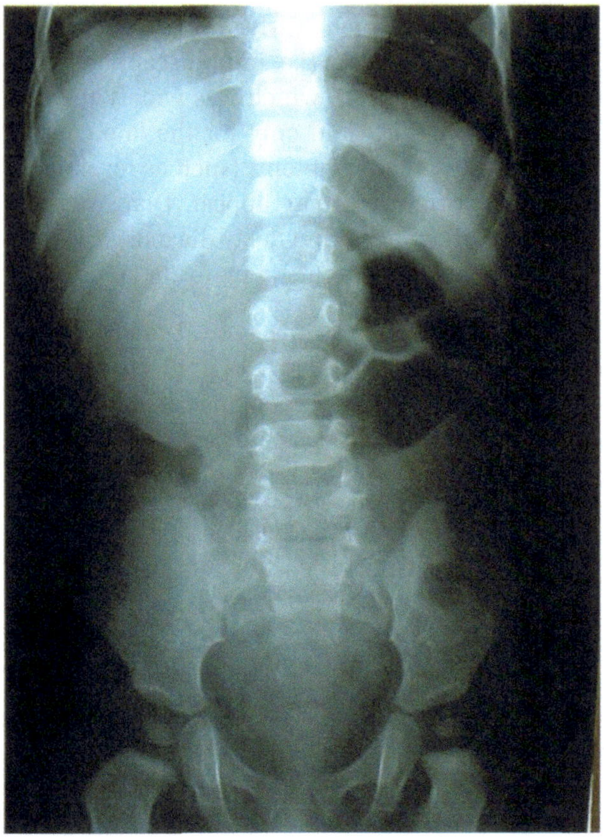

Figure 43.1 Simple abdominal radiograph showing abnormal distribution of intestinal gas, with subhepatic mass.

Ultrasonography

Since the first report of the diagnosis of intussusception in adult patients by ultrasonography in 1977, this technique has become the imaging method of choice, and nowadays emergency ultrasonography will detect most cases of intussusception, particularly if the abdomen is not greatly distended by gas.[29]

There have been numerous descriptions of the ultrasonographic signs of intussusception, which habitually show a donut or 'target' image, with a hypoechoic peripheral ring representing the edematous walls of the intussusceptum, and a hyperechoic central zone made up of areas of compressed mucus. In longitudinal section the hypoechoic walls on both sides of the hyperechoic center show a tubular 'pseudokidney' or 'sandwich' appearance[30] (Figure 43.2).

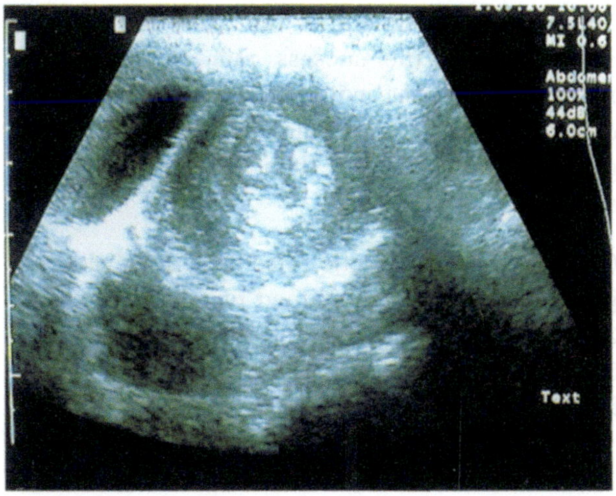

Figure 43.2 Ultrasonogram showing typical 'pseudokidney' image in subhepatic location, indicative of intussusception.

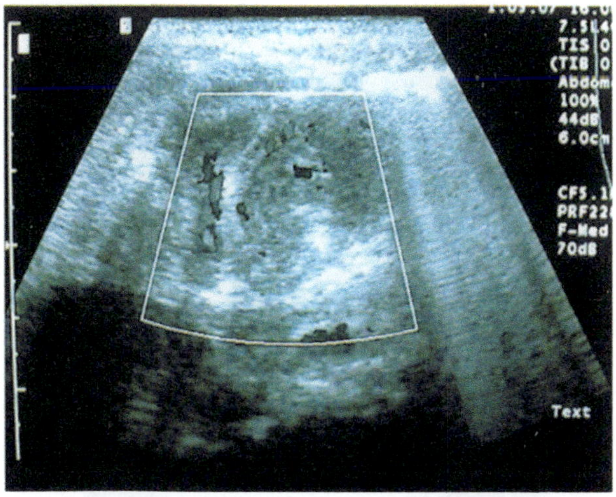

Figure 43.3 Doppler sonogram showing good vascularization of the intussusceptum, so that enema reduction is not contraindicated.

Ultrasonograms are not entirely pathognomonic for intussusception, but most published series indicate sensitivity and negative predictive value of close to 100%.[31,32]

Ultrasonography also offers a number of other important advantages: it is fast, cheap, non-invasive, innocuous (no ionizing radiation) and capable of detecting intussusceptions that are difficult to detect by conventional clinical examination and radiography, notably ileoileal and post-surgical intussusceptions. Ultrasonography facilitates assessment of reducibility and of the feasibility of non-surgical reduction, in view of the existing amount of intraperitoneal liquid, the thickness of the intestinal wall and the degree of distension and peristalsis of the intussusceptum. Doppler sonography (Figure 43.3) facilitates assessment of the degree of vascularization or ischemia of the intussusceptum, which is important for treatment selection.[33,34]

Ultrasonography may also detect pathological lead points such as Meckel's diverticulum, lymphomas of the small intestine, or cysts.[35] In addition, it allows the examiner to rule out other causes of abdominal pain, such as appendicitis, ovarian pathology or anomalies of the urinary tract.

Since the introduction and widespread use of hydrostatic reduction under ultrasonographic guidance, reduction success rates of up to 95.5% have been reported,[36] with reduction confirmed by disappearance of the characteristic image, saline and air reflux through the ileocecal valve and distension of the ileum by the saline. The principal advantages are lack of exposure to ionizing radiation and absence of significant complications. Indeed, the only complication reported to date is perforation, easily recognized during reduction, and with fewer associated risks than escape of barium into the abdominal cavity. In short, hydrostatic reduction under ultrasound guidance is as effective as, or more effective than other reduction techniques, and has the obvious advantage of avoiding radiation exposure.[37]

Barium enema

As a purely diagnostic method, barium enema is nowadays of little value. It may be useful for confirming the diagnosis in doubtful cases, showing a concave image at the head of the barium column corresponding to the apex of the intussusceptum; the image may be delimited by barium between the intussusceptum and the intussuscipiens, and is clearer when some of the barium is evacuated from the colon distal to the intussusception (Figure 40.4). However, possible organic causes of intussusception are rarely detected by this method.

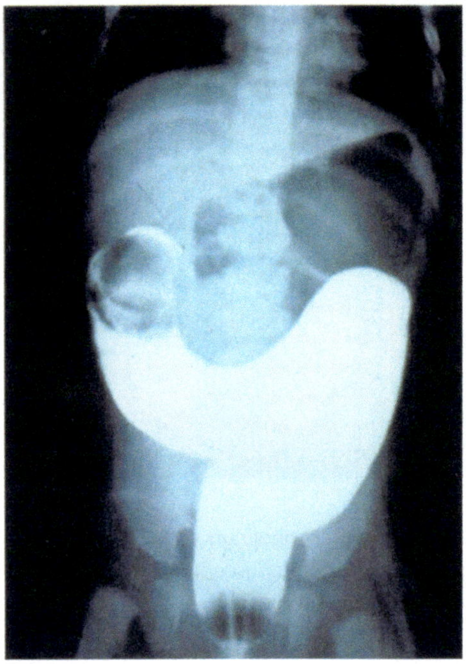

Figure 43.4 Diagnostic barium contrast enema: radiograph showing non-passage of barium beyond the level of the hepatic angle, and with barium extending between intussusceptum and intussuscipiens.

Treatment

Medical treatment

Once intussusception has been diagnosed, a nasogastric tube should be inserted, and peripheral endovenous fluid therapy should be started. Blood tests, including coagulation and electrolytes, should be done. Routine antibiotic treatment is not recommended, and should be reserved for complicated cases. Sedation and analgesia are recommended (with drugs including diazepam, midazolam, meperidine, thiopental sodium, ketamine, phenobarbital sodium and atropine) to avoid pain, reduce spasm, shorten the time required for reduction, and increase the likelihood of success. Glucagon is not currently used, in view of its doubtful efficacy.[38,39]

We consider non-surgical reduction to be contraindicated if the patient shows poor general status, with signs of shock, dehydration or peritoneal irritation, or clinical, radiographic or ultrasonographic signs of perforation or advanced intestinal obstruction, or when the patient is attended a long time after the onset of intussusception, since the success rate of hydrostatic reduction declines with increasing time since onset. In such cases, the aim should be to recover good general status and then perform emergency surgery.

Once successful reduction has been achieved, the patient should be maintained on observation for 24h with nothing *per os*, and discharged after re-introduction and confirmed tolerance of oral feeding.

Hydrostatic reduction

The publication of Ravitch's series in 1948 led to the widespread adoption of hydrostatic barium enema as a standard treatment method.[4] As noted, hydrostatic reduction under ultrasonographic guidance offers high diagnostic sensitivity together with high treatment success rates.

Various contrast materials are available, the most widely used being barium sulfate, dissolved in physiological saline to avoid water intoxication and hyponatremia, or alternatively non-barium hydrosoluble contrasts (which have fewer negative effects) (Figures 43.5 and 43.6).

It is important to note that the column height of the enema should be between 1 and 1.2 m never exceeding 1.5 m. The anus should not be fully occluded, permitting reflux of contrast medium if excessive pressure develops. The abdomen should not be manipulated during reduction. Each reduction attempt should not exceed 10 min, and if no progress is made the attempt should be abandoned. If progress is detected, further attempts may be made, at intervals of 5–15 min.

Pneumatic reduction

Intussusception reduction using pressurized air under radiographic guidance was described by Fiorito and Recalde Cuesta,[5] although apparently techniques of this type were traditionally used in China.[40]

Within the colon, pressurized air 'pushes' the intussusceptum, and at the same time enters into

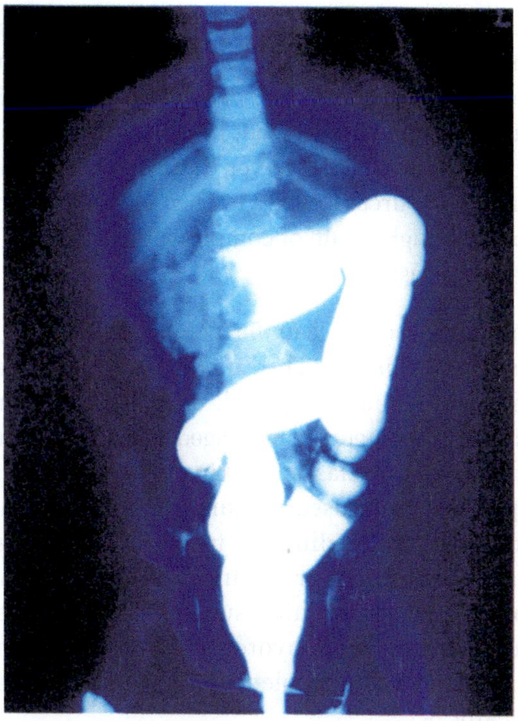

Figure 43.5 Barium contrast radiograph showing an ileocecal intussusception in the transverse colon.

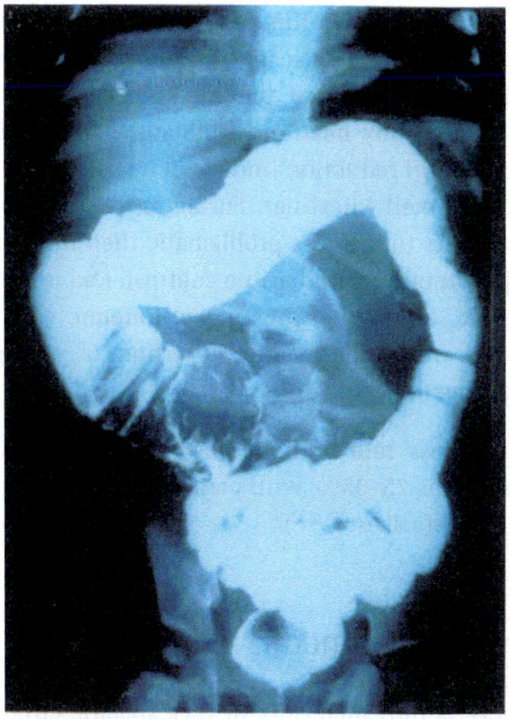

Figure 43.6 Barium contrast radiograph showing an ileocecal intussusception in the ileocecal valve.

the space between the intussusceptum and the intussuscipiens, facilitating reduction (Figure 43.7). The reduction can be guided either by contrast radiography or by ultrasonography.[7,41]

Various devices for the introduction of air have been described, all including some sort of pump, a manometer and an intracolic pressure regulator. Pressure can be controlled with a sphygmomanometer to control pressure, and any sort of expulsion pump can be used (Richardson's bulb, syringe pump, etc.). It has been shown that CO_2 is more readily absorbed than air in the intestinal lumen, but reduction efficacy does not seem to be any higher.[42]

With the child in the prone position, an 18–20 Fr Foley catheter is inserted into the rectum, with an initial pressure of 60 mmHg, gradually increased to no more than 80–100 mmHg in infants and 120 mmHg in older children. Intestinal perforation is thought not to be a result of excessive pneumatic pressure, but of inappropriate application of this technique in cases in which the intestine is ischemic or necrotic.

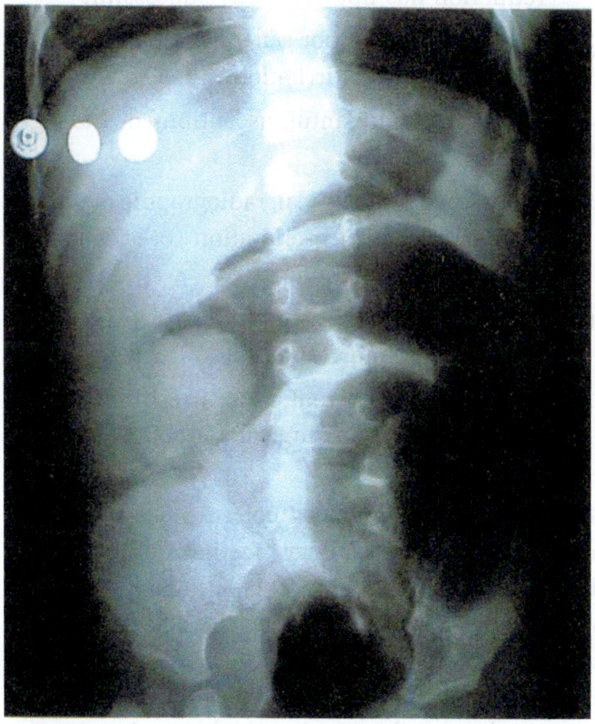

Figure 43.7 Air contrast radiography of an ileocecal intussusception extending as far as the hepatic angle. The intussusception is visible as a radiopaque mass that prevents the passage of air.

We currently prefer this technique to hydrostatic reduction, since it is easier to perform, and permits ready visualization of the intussusceptum, does not absorb body heat and facilitates confirmation of successful reduction (indicated by passage of air into the small intestine). Furthermore, if perforation occurs this is less problematic than in hydrostatic reduction with barium contrast, and is easier to treat, since the pneumoperitoneum can be drained immediately after insertion of a large-gauge needle.[41,43,44]

The success rate with hydrostatic or pneumatic reduction is 75–95%, with perforation occurring in 0.11–2% of cases.[6,7,38,39]

Surgical treatment

Surgery is indicated only in very specific circumstances:

(1) Whenever there are signs of shock or peritonitis;

(2) In patients in whom hydrostatic or pneumatic reduction has not been fully successful;

(3) In patients with poor general status, dehydration or peritoneal irritation;

(4) In patients with intussusceptions of the sigmoid or rectum;

(5) When there are clinical, radiographic or sonographic signs of perforation or advanced intestinal obstruction;

(6) When the intussusception is not diagnosed until a long time after onset;

(7) In cases of recurrent intussusception, with two or three non-surgical reductions previously per-formed.

Successful reduction does not rule out the existence of organic pathology, so that any residual defect is an indication for laparotomy. Patients older than 2–3 years have been the object of some controversy, since the possibility that a lead point exists is much higher; in our series, 50% of children aged more than 2 years had organic causes, and some surgeons argue that in these patients exploratory laparotomy should be performed, even after successful non-surgical reduction.

Surgery has certain advantages: any organic pathology will invariably be detected, the intussusception reduction will be complete and the recurrence rate is somewhat lower than with non-surgical reduction. However, it also has a higher financial/resources cost, longer hospitalization time and a higher rate of complications (up to 17% in some series).[45]

Comfortable access can be achieved by a right transverse incision. The affected intestine can generally be readily exposed, enabling the intussusceptum to be gently massaged out of the intussuscipiens, using classic 'milking' movements, and not pulling the intussusceptum. Reduction in fact often tends to be difficult in surgically treated cases, and resections are required rather often; this probably reflects the high success rates obtained with pneumatic and hydrostatic reduction, and the fact that only problematic cases are treated surgically.

Once complete reduction has been achieved, the viability of the intestine should be assessed, to identify possible regions of necrosis or doubtful viability, and to detect possible organic causes. After reduction, the cecal region and terminal ileum show a highly characteristic appearance, with thickening of the intestinal walls, and in some cases presence of a hard edematous plaque at the level of the terminal ileum; this should not be confused with an organic cause and does not require any sort of surgical response, which indeed would only cause complications. When intestinal resection is necessary, this should be as conservative as possible, aiming to maintain the ileocecal valve. Appendectomy should be performed routinely if the edema of the ileocecal region permits, although some authors have questioned its utility. Surgical treatment does not exclude the possibility of recurrence, which in one study was reported in 3.2% of cases.[46]

Intestinal fixation techniques (e.g. fixation of the cecum, suture of the terminal ileum to the ascending colon, Noble's plication) were in the past widely used to prevent recurrence, but are now generally regarded as being ineffective and unnecessary.

Recurrent intussusception requires a personalized treatment program: characteristically, surgery is not required in patients aged less than 2 years, when they show a second or third crisis over a short period of time. In older patients, radiographic and sonographic findings should be assessed, since the higher frequency of organic causes at these ages obliges us to consider the need for exploratory laparotomy, which of course will not always detect any organic lesion.

REFERENCES

1. Barbette P. *Oeuvres chirugiques at anatomiques*. Geneva: Francois Miege, 1674: 522.
2. Hutchinson J. A successful case of abdominal section for intussusception. *Proc R Med Chir Soc* 1873; **7**: 195–198.
3. Hirschsprung H. Et Tilfaetde af suakut Tarminvagination. *Hospitals-Tidende* 1876; **3**: 321–327.
4. Ravitch MM, McClure RM. Reduction of intussusception by barium enema: a clinical and experimental study. *Ann Surg* 1948; **728**: 904.
5. Fiorito ES, Recalde Cuesta LA. Diagnosis and treatment of acute intestinal intussusception with controlled insufflation of air. *Pediatrics* 1959; **24**: 241–244.
6. YaXiong She. Traitement de l'invagination intestinale avec regard spécial sur la reduction par insufflation du clan. Expérience de 5110 cases. *Chir Pédiatr* 1982; **23**: 373–378.
7. Guo J, Ma X, Zhou Q. Results of air pressure enema reduction of intussusception: 6396 cases in 13 years. *J Pediatr Surg* 1986; **21**: 1201–1203.
8. Stringer MD, Pablot SM, Brereton RJ. Paediatric intussusception. *Br J Surg* 1992; **79**: 867–876.
9. Smith IM. Incidence of intussusception and congenital hypertrophic pyloric stenosis in Edinburgh children. *BMJ* 1960; **1**: 551–552.
10. Shah BR, Laude TA. Intussusception. In Shah BR, Laude TA, eds. *Atlas of Pediatric Clinical Diagnosis*. Philadelphia: W.B. Saunders, 2000: 338–341.
11. Bautista Casasnovas A, Varela Cives R, Nieto Vázquez B et al. Evaluación del tratamiento medico y quirúrgico de la invaginación intestinal en el niño. *An Esp Pediatr* 1988; **29**: 279–283.
12. Eizaguirre I, Morras I, Jimenez J, Tovar J. Invaginación intestinal. Revisión de 110 casos. *Rev Esp Pediatr* 1985; **41**: 339–344.
13. Bruce J, Huh YS, Cooney DR et al. Intussusception: evolution of current management. *J Pediatr Gastroenterol Nutr* 1987; **6**: 663–674.
14. Simonsen L, Morens D, Elixhauser A et al. Effect of rotavirus vaccination programme on trends in admission of infants to hospital for intussusception. *Lancet* 2001; **358**: 1224–1229.
15. DiFiore JW. Intussusception. *Semin Pediatr Surg* 1999; **84**: 214–220.
16. Meier DE, Coln CE, Rescorla FJ et al. Intussusception in children: international perspective. *World J Surg* 1996; **20**: 1035–1040.
17. Ong NT, Beasley SW. The leadpoint in intussusception. *J Pediatr Surg* 1990; **25**: 640–643.
18. Luks FI, Yazbeck S, Brandt ML, Desjardins JG. Fievre transitoire associée a la réduction de l'invagination intestinale. *Chir Pédiatr* 1990; **37**: 157–159.
19. Ducharme JC, Perreault G, Cyr R, Medoux L. L' invagination intestinale, 188 malades traites au course d' une periode de 22 ans. *Chir Pediatr* 1982; **23**: 23–27.
20. de Vries S, Sleeboom C, Aronson DC. Postoperative intussusception in children. *Br J Surg* 1999; **86**: 81–83.
21. Linke F, Eble F, Berger S. Postoperative intussusception in childhood. *Pediatr Surg Int* 1998; **14**: 175–177.
22. Yazbeck S. Intestinal obstruction in infancy and childhood. In Roy CC, Silverman MA, Alagille D, eds. *Pediatric Clinical Gastroenterology*, 4th edn. Boston: Mosby, 1993: 106–110.
23. Singer J. Altered consciousness as an early manifestation of intussusception. *Pediatrics* 1979; **64**: 93–95.
24. Villanueva Jeremias A, Bautista Casasnovas A. Niño de 11 meses con letargia. *Casos Clínicos Pediatría* 2002; **1**: 10–15.
25. McCabe JB, Singer JL, Love T, Roth R. A supplement to the mnemonic for coma. *Pediatr Emerg Care* 1987; **3**: 118–119.
26. Ratcliffe JF, Fong S, Cheong I, O'Conell PO. The plain abdominal film in intussusception: the accuracy and incidence of radiographic signs. *Pediatr Radiol* 1992; **22**: 110–111.
27. Bisset GS, Kirks DR. Intussusception in infants and children: diagnosis and treatment. *Radiology* 1998; **168**: 141–145.
28. Daneman A, Alton DJ. Intussusception. Issues and controversies related to diagnosis and reduction. *Radiol Clin North Am* 1996; **34**: 743–756.
29. Weissberg DL, Scheible W, Leopold GR. Ultrasonographic appearance of adult intussusception. *Radiology* 1977; **124**: 791–792.
30. Bhisitkul DM, Listernick R, Shikolnik A et al. Clinical application of ultrasonography in the diagnosis of intussusception. *J Pediatr* 1992; **727**: 182–186.
31. Woo SK, Kim JS, Suh SI et al. Childhood intussusception: US-guided hydrostatic reduction. *Radiology* 1992; **782**: 77–80.
32. Yoon CH, Kim HJ, Goo HW. Intussusception in children: US-guided pneumatic reduction initial experience. *Radiology* 2001; **218**: 85–88.
33. Mirilas P, Koumanidou C, Vakaki M et al. Sonographic features indicative of hydrostatic reducibility of intestinal intussusception in infancy and early childhood. *Eur Radiol* 2001; **11**: 2576–2580.
34. Britton I, Wilkinson AG. Ultrasound features of intussusception predicting outcome of air enema. *Pediatr Radiol* 1999; **29**: 705–710.
35. Navarro O, Dugougeat F, Kornecki A et al. The impact of imaging in the management of intussusception owing to pathologic lead points in children. A review of 43 cases. *Pediatr Radiol* 2000; **30**: 594–603.

36. Wang GD, Liu SI. Enema reduction of intussusception by hydrostatic pressure under ultrasound guidance: a report of 377 cases. *J Pediatr Surg* 1988; **23**: 814–818.
37. Shehata S, El Kholi N, Sultan A, El Sahwi E. Hydrostatic reduction of intussusception: barium, air, or saline? *Pediatr Surg Int* 2000; **16**: 380–382.
38. Katz ME, Kolm P. Intussusception reduction 1991: an international survey of pediatric radiologists. *Pediatr Radiol* 1992; **22**: 318–322.
39. Meyer IS. The current radiologic management of intussusception: a survey and review. *Pediatr Radiol* 1992; **22**: 323–325.
40. Jinzhe Z, Yenxia W, Linchi W. Rectal inflation reduction of intussusception in infants. *J Pediatr Surg* 1986; **21**: 30–32.
41. Gu L, Zhu H, Wang S et al. Sonographic guidance of air enema for intussusception reduction in children. *Pediatr Radiol* 2000; **30**: 339–342.
42. Palder SB, Ein SH, Stringer DA, Alton D. Intussusception: barium or air? *J Pediatr Surg* 1991; **26**: 271–275.
43. Heenan SD, Kyriou J, Fitzgerald M, Adam EJ. Effective dose at pneumatic reduction of paediatric intussusception. *Clin Radiol* 2000; **55**: 811–816.
44. Stringer DA, Ein SH. Pneumatic reduction: advantages, risks and indications. *Pediatr Radiol* 1990; **20**: 475–477.
45. Leonidas JC. Treatment of intussusception with small bowel obstruction: application of decision analysis. *Am J Reotgenol* 1985; **145**: 665–669.
46. Aubrespy P, Derlon S, Alessandrini P et al. Invagination intestinale aigue du neurrison et de l' enfant. Analyse de 125 observations traitées chirurgicalement. *Chir Pédiatr* 1983; **24**: 392–395.

44 Meckel's diverticulum

Richard G Azizkhan

Introduction

Meckel's diverticulum is the most common congenital anomaly of the gastrointestinal tract and the most common cause of serious gastrointestinal bleeding in children. Anatomically, it is an outpouching on the antimesenteric border of the small bowel (Figure 44.1). Although first reported by Fabricus Hildanus in 1598, this abnormality derives its name from Johann Friedrich Meckel, who in 1809 detailed its embryological origin and identified it as a potential cause of disease.[1,2] Reports estimate that Meckel's diverticulum affects 2% of the general population. However, it is usually clinically silent, identified only as an incidental finding during laparotomy, laparoscopy, or at autopsy. Estimates of the lifetime risk of complications occurring range from 4 to 6%.[3–5] These complications are usually due to ectopic tissue within the diverticulum or to omphalomesenteric or mesodiverticular bands. The clinical presentation of Meckel's diverticulum is diverse. Symptoms often mimic those associated with other more common abdominal disorders, making preoperative diagnosis quite difficult. This chapter focuses on the major complications of this anomaly, describing its pathogenesis, diagnosis and management. Relevant embryology, histology and epidemiology will set the stage for this discussion.

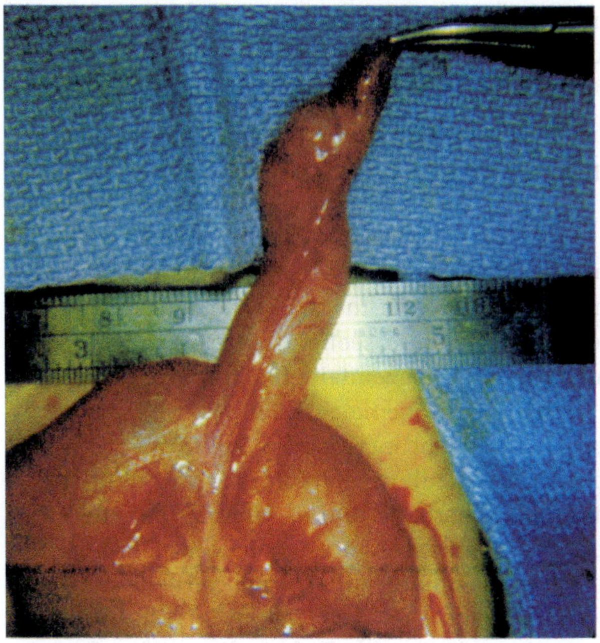

Figure 44.1 Operative view of a Meckel's diverticulum. The distal tip had heterotopic gastric mucosa.

Pathoembryology

Meckel's diverticulum is one of a spectrum of congenital anomalies of the midgut that are embryological remnants of the vitelline (omphalomesenteric) duct. During week 3 of gestation, the yolk sac communicates with the gut through this duct. Between weeks 5–9 of gestation, the duct is normally obliterated, as the functioning placenta replaces the yolk sac as the source of fetal nourishment. Failure of this normal obliteration process can result in a number of developmental anomalies, of which Meckel's diverticulum is the most common. The diverticulum may remain completely attached to the abdominal wall at the umbilicus, may remain attached as a fibrous cord as the distal portion of the vitelline duct involutes, or may remain unattached and free within the peritoneal cavity. The last presentation is the most common, occurring in 74% of cases.[6] Other anomalies related to the disturbance of vitelline duct involution include persistence of a patent omphalomesenteric duct (Figure 44.2) or the development of an omphalomesenteric sinus or cyst. Such a cyst may form when both proximal

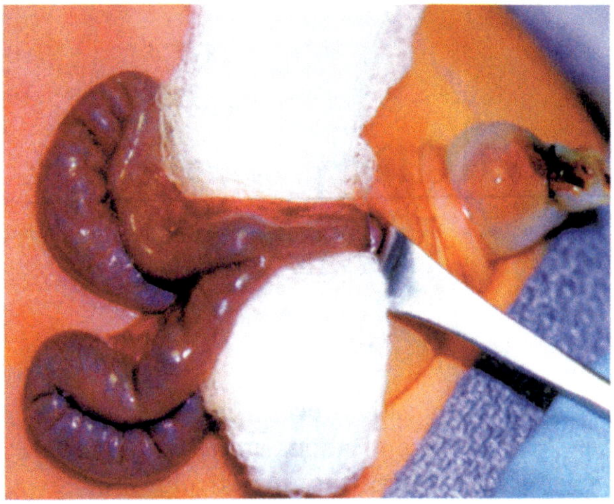

Figure 44.2 Patent omphalomesenteric duct in a neonate. The mucosa can be visualized in the transected umbilical cord. The omphalomesenteric duct communicates from the distal ileum to the umbilicus.

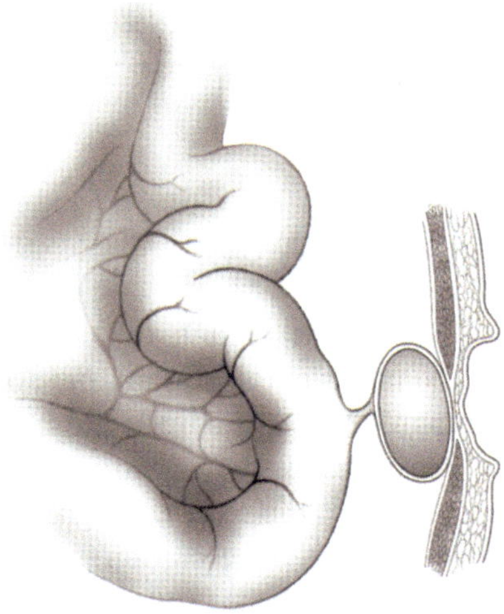

Figure 44.3 Drawing depicting an omphalomesenteric cyst attached to the umbilical region as well as to a fibrous band to the terminal ileum.

and distal obliteration occurs while the central portion of the duct remains patent (Figure 44.3).

The blood supply to Meckel's diverticulum is derived from the paired vitelline arteries. The left vitelline artery involutes, whereas the right persists as the superior mesenteric artery. A remnant of the primitive right vitelline artery arises directly from the mesentery to supply the diverticulum. The blood supply is anatomically unique in that the vessels to the diverticulum pass over the serosa of the ileum, terminating on the antimesenteric rather than the mesenteric side of the bowel. Although these vessels usually terminate at the tip of the diverticulum, they may continue on to the abdominal wall. They may also persist as a fibrous cord connecting the ileum to the umbilicus after obliteration of the diverticulum. The tip of the diverticulum may remain attached to the base of the mesentery by a fibrous remnant of the vitelline vessels, creating a mesodiverticular band through which loops of small bowel may pass and become incarcerated.

Histology

Meckel's diverticulum is usually located within 100cm (3 feet) of the ileocecal junction on the antimesenteric border of the ileum. It is a true diverticulum, containing all layers of the intestinal wall. Heterotopic mucosa is found in up to 55–60% of Meckel's diverticula[7–9] and is found predominantly in symptomatic patients.[5,10–12] Gastric and pancreatic tissue predominate, with corresponding incidences of 60–90% and 5–16%[5,10–13] (Figure 44.4); both ectopic tissue types may be found together within the diverticulum. Although colonic, duodenal, jejunal, hepatic and endometrial ectopic tissues have been found,[11,14–17] these are rare and are not generally associated with complications.

Epidemiology

Of symptomatic Meckel's diverticula, 50–60% occur in children younger than 2 years of age. A significant increase in the 1–2% incidence in the general population is seen in association with a number of other congenital anomalies. In a series of nearly 6000 pediatric autopsies, authors reported significant increases in the incidence of Meckel's diverticulum in children born with a cleft palate, bicornuate uterus, annular pancreas, esophageal or anorectal atresia, or gross malformation of the central nervous or cardiovascular systems.[18] Meckel's diverticulum is also more common in patients with Crohn's disease[19] and in patients with omphalocele, approximately 25% of whom exhibit some form of omphalomesenteric

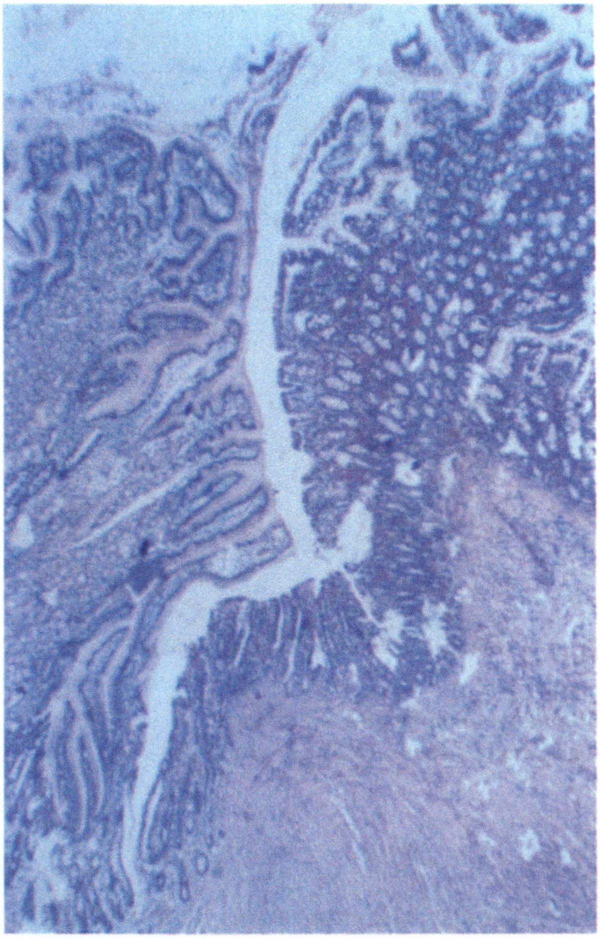

Figure 44.4 Histology of a Meckel's diverticulum demonstrating gastric and ileal mucosa. The deep cleft is an ulcer separating the two types of mucosa.

remnant.[20] Although rare, carcinoid tumors have been found to arise from the diverticulum.[21–23] Other tumors have also been reported, but these have occurred primarily in adult patients.[7]

Clinical presentations

Predisposing factors

While heterotopic tissue within the diverticula is the most significant predisposing factor to complications, several other factors also appear to be associated with an increased likelihood of complications. The reported predominance of symptomatic Meckel's diverticulum in males (ratios ranging from 2 : 1 to 5 : 1) indicates that gender may play a role.[11,13] Studies have also shown that diverticular length[11] and base diameter[24] are predisposing factors. Long, narrow-based diverticula are thought to be more prone to obstruction or inflammation, whereas short, large-based diverticula are subject to foreign body entrapment. Whether or not age can be correlated with the incidence of complications is currently controversial. Although the risk of complications has historically been thought to decline with age,[3,11,24] two relatively recent studies have demonstrated an even age distribution in patients with complications.[13,26]

Complications

The most common complications are gastrointestinal bleeding, intestinal obstruction and inflammation. Clinical presentation is generally associated with the presence of ectopic gastric mucosa within the diverticulum or fixation of omphalomesenteric duct remnants to the abdominal wall. The ectopic mucosa may cause ulceration, which can result in inflammation, bleeding, or perforation. Fixation of omphalomesenteric duct remnants to the abdominal wall may result in intestinal obstruction from torsion of small-bowel loops around the point of fixation (Figure 44.5). The Meckel's diverticulum may be recognized on preoperative studies or at operation, or it may be found unexpectedly in a resected specimen. The likelihood of the presence of heterotopic mucosa in surgically resected Meckel's diverticula depends on the clinical presentation. It is found in approximately 50% of all symptomatic patients who have gastrointestinal bleeding, obstruction or inflammation (diverticulitis).

Gastrointestinal bleeding

Gastrointestinal bleeding occurs in 22% of all children with Meckel's diverticula and 40–60% of symptomatic children.[12,26] It is the most common presenting symptom in children younger than age 4, and the mean age of presentation is 2.8 years.[12] Painless rectal bleeding is the usual manifestation. Although the bleeding may be significant, it is often episodic. The color of blood may vary from bright red to dark red or maroon to black and tarry, and may even appear as the 'currant jelly stool' typically associated with intussusception.[26] Bleeding is sometimes massive, transfusions are often required and life-threatening hemorrhage

(a)

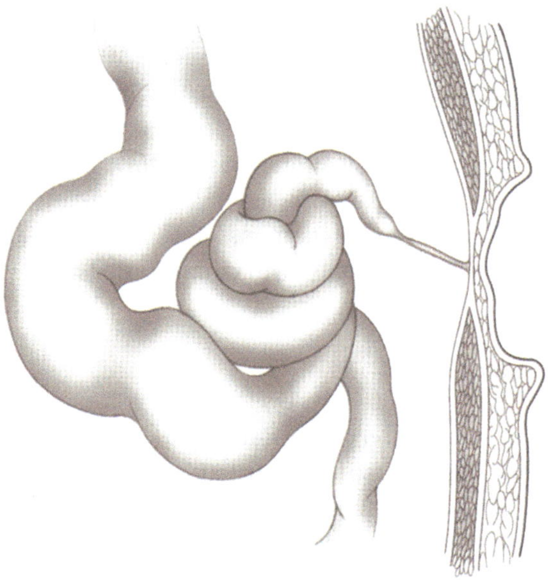

(b)

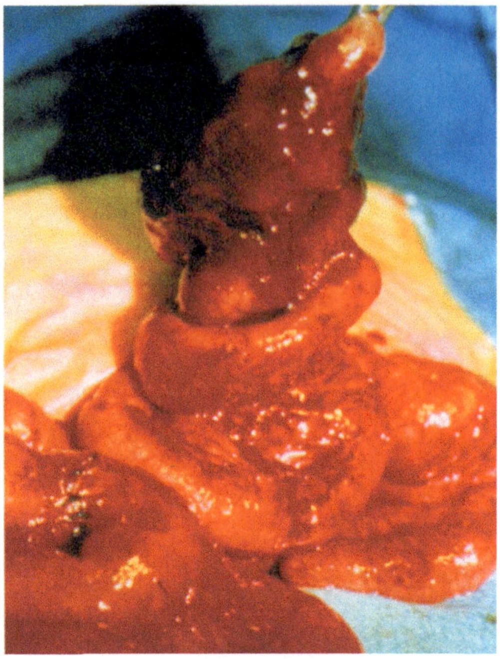

Figure 44.5 (a) Drawing depicting a segmental ileal volvulus around an omphalomesenteric band. (b) Intraoperative photograph showing a segmental ileal volvulus around a Meckel's diverticulum and omphalomesenteric band.

occasionally occurs. This requires rapid resuscitation and stabilization and early diagnosis and treatment.

Bleeding is thought to occur as a result of peptic ulceration caused by secretion of hydrochloric acid from parietal cells within the ectopic gastric mucosa located in the diverticulum. In patients who show bleeding only, the prevalence of heterotopic gastric mucosa approaches 100%.[7] Unlike the stomach, the ileum cannot buffer the resulting low pH and is thus more prone to ulceration. The ulceration may be small, visible only to the pathologist. It is generally located at the base of the diverticulum, at the junction of ectopic gastric mucosa and normal ileal mucosa. It may, however, also be found within the ectopic gastric mucosa itself or on the mesenteric side of the ileum, opposite the diverticulum (Figure 44.6). Ectopic gastric mucosa and ulceration are identified in about 95% and 98%, respectively, in specimens resected for bleeding.[5]

Although *Helicobacter pylori* plays a major role in ulcerogenesis elsewhere, it does not appear to be a significant factor in the pathogenesis of bleeding and inflammatory complications from the ectopic gastric mucosa in Meckel's diverticula, and has only rarely been isolated from specimens.[27–29]

Differential diagnosis includes inflammatory bowel disease, intestinal polyps, duplications and arteriovenous malformations. Peptic ulcer disease and variceal bleeding may also present in a similar fashion, but can be distinguished through bloody nasogastric aspirates or with upper endoscopy. Occult bleeding with anemia is an infrequent presentation of Meckel's diverticulum.

Intestinal obstruction

Bowel obstruction in any previously healthy child merits a high index of suspicion for Meckel's diverticulum. When this anomaly is present, the obstruction is usually due to intussusception (46%) or volvulus (24%).[7] In children with intussusception, Meckel's diverticulum often serves as the lead point of the intussusception (Figure 44.7). The clinical presentation of intussusception includes vomiting, intermittent abdominal pain, bloody stools, a palpable lower abdominal mass and eventual progression to dehydration and

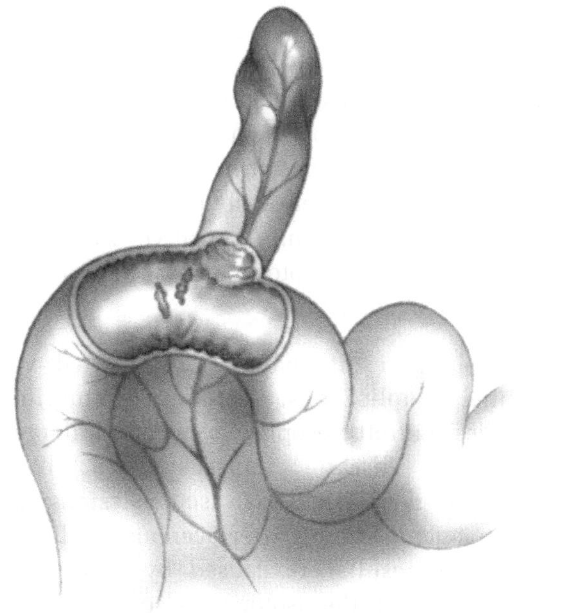

Figure 44.6 Drawing demonstrating two ileal ulcers on the mesenteric side of the ileum which may be seen in patients with bleeding related to heterotopic gastric mucosa in the Meckel's diverticulum.

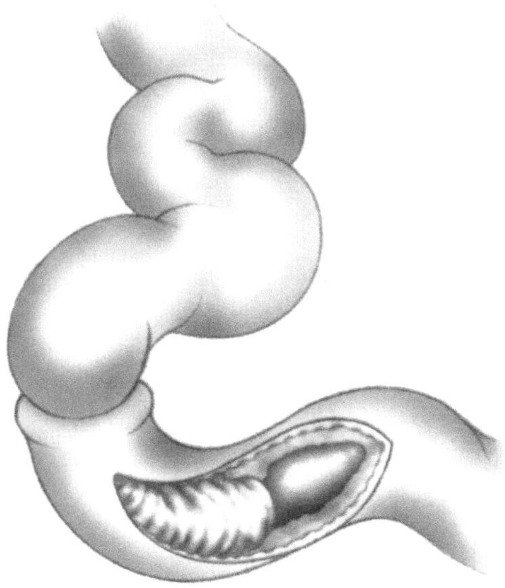

Figure 44.7 Drawing demonstrating an ileo-ileal intussusception caused by a Meckel's diverticulum.

lethargy.[7] Ultrasonography, as well as pneumatic or barium enema are useful in establishing the diagnosis of intussusception. Rarely, complete reduction is obtained with enema and if Meckel's diverticulum is visualized by imaging, an elective diverticulectomy can be performed. Most patients, however, have incomplete reduction of their ileoileal/ileocolonic intussusception, and require surgery to reduce the intussusception and resect the Meckel's diverticulum.

Volvulus can occur through several mechanisms. It is usually an acute event, and if allowed to progress, may result in strangulation of the involved bowel. Vitelline remnants or the omphalomesenteric duct may attach to the abdominal wall and form an anchor around which the bowel twists. The intestine may herniate under mesodiverticular bands, kinking or obstructing (Figure 44.8). Rarely, a long diverticulum twists on itself (axial torsion), causing obstruction. Also rare, intestinal obstruction may result from incarceration of a Meckel's diverticulum within a hernia sac (Littre's hernia). In neonates, an inverted Meckel's diverticulum has been associated with intestinal obstruction and microcolon.[30]

Resuscitation for bowel obstruction consists of intravenous hydration, correction of electrolytic abnormalities, administration of broad-spectrum antibiotics, intestinal decompression and definitive operation.

Inflammation

In contrast to bleeding and intestinal obstruction, diverticulitis occurs more commonly in adolescents and adults. It is generally indistinguishable from appendicitis and, as with appendicitis, failure to diagnose the diverticulitis promptly may lead to perforation, peritonitis and death. The role of the ectopic mucosa in this process is suggested by its high incidence in resected inflamed mucosa. Thus, when appendicitis is suspected but not found at operation, it is critical to inspect the distal ileum for a symptomatic Meckel's diverticulum.

Other clinical presentations

Inflammation and perforation of a Meckel's diverticulum by a foreign body in the gastrointestinal tract has been reported.[12,16] Although rarely seen

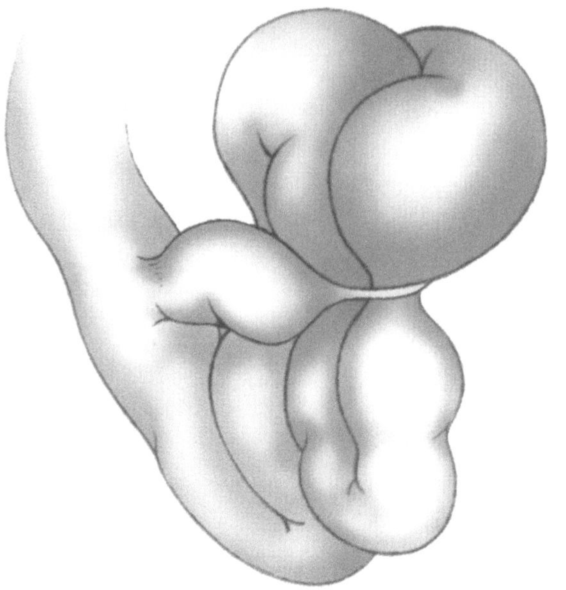

Figure 44.8 Herniation and obstruction of small intestine through a Meckel's band adhering to the base of the ileal mesentery.

in pediatric patients, malignancies,[9] stone formation within the diverticulum, and even parasitic infections have also been documented.[31,32] Additionally, a recent report described the atypical presentation of recurrent urinary tract infections caused by an infected Meckel's diverticulum that displaced the urinary bladder.[33]

Diagnostic evaluation

Abdominal scintigraphy (Meckel's scan) using Tc-99m pertechnetate is a well-established diagnostic technique to evaluate children with lower gastrointestinal bleeding and is considered the diagnostic procedure of choice when there is a suspicion of Meckel's diverticulum (Figure 44.9). Reported results of a 10-year pediatric review of this type of scan revealed a sensitivity for detection of Meckel's diverticulum of 85%, a specificity of 95% and accuracy of 90%. False-negative results occurred in 1.7% of cases, and false-positive results in only 0.05% of cases.[34]

The high affinity of Tc-99m pertechnetate for gastric mucosa is what makes this radiopharmaceutical such a valuable tool. Tc-99m pertechnetate is taken up and secreted by the tubular glands of the gastric mucosa. The remainder of the isotope is concentrated within the urinary bladder. Sequential 1-min anterior abdominal images are obtained for 30–60 min. A positive scan shows abnormal uptake of isotope outside the stomach and urinary bladder.[35]

False-positive results have been reported with intestinal duplications, certain genitourinary anomalies, Barrett's esophagus, ulcers, inflammatory bowel disease, intussusception, bowel obstruction, neoplasms and vascular lesions such as hemangiomas and arteriovenous malformations; these results are caused by non-specific accumulation of the isotope. False-negative Tc-99m pertechnetate scintigraphy may result from a small diverticulum or hemorrhage washing out the isotope. Also, residual contrast in the bowel from previous barium studies may hinder its detection, or tracer in the urinary bladder may obscure visualization of heterotopic gastric mucosa if it is located near the bladder.[35] Several pharmacological agents, including pentagastrin, histamine-2 blockers (e.g. cimetidine), and glucagon have been used to enhance the diagnostic accuracy of the scan. Pentagastrin stimulates gastric mucosal uptake, histamine-2 blockers inhibit excretion of the isotope once it is taken up and glucagon inhibits peristalsis, thereby increasing retention of the isotope in the diverticulum. While some authors maintain that pharmacological enhancement is necessary only when results of a non-pharmacologically enhanced study are inconclusive,[35] I feel that enhancement reduces the need for repeated radionuclide studies and therefore use it routinely. Fasting, nasogastric suctioning, and bladder catheterization may also increase the diagnostic yield of the scan.

Although Tc-99m pertechnetate scintigraphy is the diagnostic procedure of choice, there are limitations to its use in clinical decision-making. According to a recent study,[36] in patients with gastrointestinal bleeding and a serum hemoglobin level of less than 11 g/dl, the Meckel's scan has a relatively low negative predictive value (0.74). Authors suggest that replacing the scan with early operative evaluation may be cost-effective,

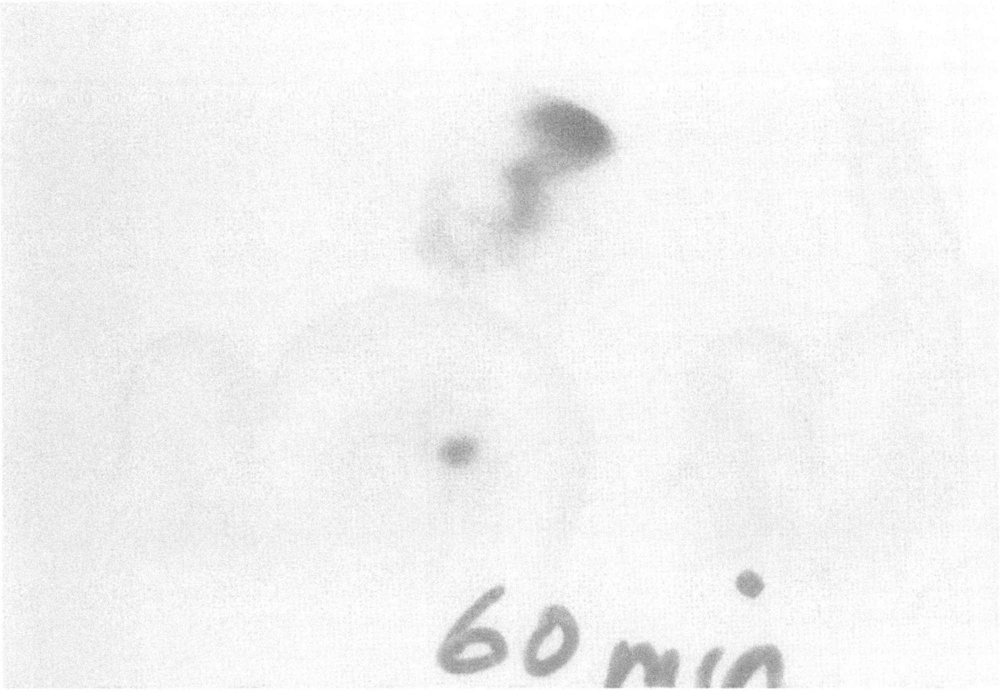

Figure 44.9 Positive Tc-99m pertechnetate radionuclide scan at 60 min demonstrating abnormal uptake of the radionuclide in the lower abdomen in a child with a Meckel's diverticulum. Note the normal gastric uptake in the upper abdomen.

especially in patients in whom there is a high index of suspicion for a bleeding Meckel's diverticulum. The known advantages of minimally invasive laparoscopy have led others to advocate this operative approach as a means of identifying the presence of a bleeding Meckel's diverticulum. They have suggested that it may replace the Meckel's scan in the diagnostic evaluation of pediatric patients with clinically significant gastrointestinal bleeding and high suspicion for this disease process.[37,38]

Visceral angiography is rarely needed, but is occasionally useful as a diagnostic tool in the actively bleeding patient (more than 0.5–1 ml/min) when the Meckel's radionuclide scan is negative. In this instance, the angiogram may show extravasation of contrast from the ileocolic branch of the superior mesenteric artery. A superselective superior mesenteric artery angiogram may show a non-branching, elongated artery originating from the ileal artery and a group of dilated tortuous vessels at the distal portion of this artery in patients with Meckel's diverticulum.[39] This technique allows visualization of Meckel's diverticulum, even in the absence of bleeding.

Management

Management of the asymptomatic patient with an incidentally discovered Meckel's diverticulum has long been controversial. The debate focuses on the probability of the diverticulum becoming symptomatic in the future as opposed to the likelihood of complications associated with resection. To date, there are no definitive intraoperative anatomic or biological features that enable the surgeon to predict the probability of future complications. While predisposing factors for symptomatic Meckel's diverticula have been identified, these factors are only of limited value to the surgeon in deciding whether or not to resect an asymptomatic diverticulum.

In some clinical situations, there is a degree of consensus that helps in making an intraoperative judgment. Resection is clearly indicated in patients with a long, narrow-based Meckel's diverticulum or in those in whom the diverticulum is palpably thickened at its terminal portion; in patients who have vitellointestinal remnants or abdominal wall attachments; and in patients with a history of unexplained abdominal pain. These

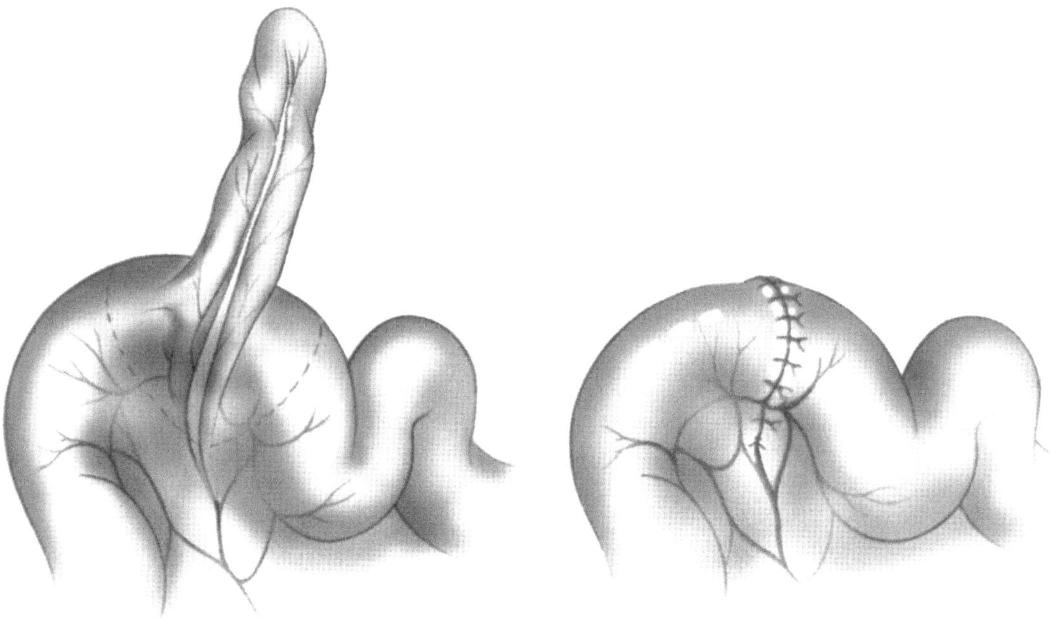

Figure 44.10 Drawing demonstrating the concept of segmental ileal resection and anastomosis.

factors all increase the likelihood of bleeding, obstruction, or diverticulitis. Because Meckel's diverticulum can become symptomatic at any age, the age of the patient is not the primary factor in the decision to resect the asymptomatic diverticulum. In general, this decision must be made after careful consideration of the risks and benefits for each patient. Owing to the risk of suture line disruption, an elective diverticulectomy is contraindicated if a Meckel's diverticulum is identified during repair of gastroschisis.[7]

Symptomatic Meckel's diverticulum must be resected, and resection should be preceded by prompt and aggressive fluid resuscitation and blood transfusion when necessary. In patients with intestinal obstruction and possible intestinal ischemia, the patient's physiology should be stabilized to the degree possible prior to operation. When a laparotomy is performed, the diverticulum is generally approached through a transverse right lower quadrant incision. Visual inspection and palpation to identify the location of ectopic gastric mucosa and ulceration is critical. If one is confident that the ulceration is confined to the diverticulum, simple diverticulectomy may be performed with either sutures or a stapling device. To prevent luminal narrowing, especially with broader-based diverticula, the defect may be closed transversely in a Heineke–Mikulicz fashion. If the base of the diverticulum is too broad, or if ulceration is identified on the mesenteric side of the ileum opposite the diverticulum, segmental resection of the ileum containing the diverticulum with an end-to-end anastomosis is preferred (Figure 44.10). Care must be taken to separately ligate the blood supply to the Meckel's diverticulum. When a right lower quadrant incision is used, an appendectomy should be concomitantly performed to prevent future diagnostic dilemmas.

Laparoscopic resection performed either intracorporeally or extracorporeally has increasingly been reported.[40–42] With intracorporeal resection, the diverticulum is identified and grasped, and a diverticulectomy is performed using a stapling device if the diverticulum is deemed anatomically suitable for such an approach (Figure 44.11). The disadvantage of this technique with a bleeding Meckel's diverticulum is the inability to exclude ulceration on the mesenteric side of the ileum opposite the diverticulum, which could result in continued bleeding after resection. Also, it is technically more difficult to perform a segmental small-bowel resection if indicated. With extracorporeal resection, the

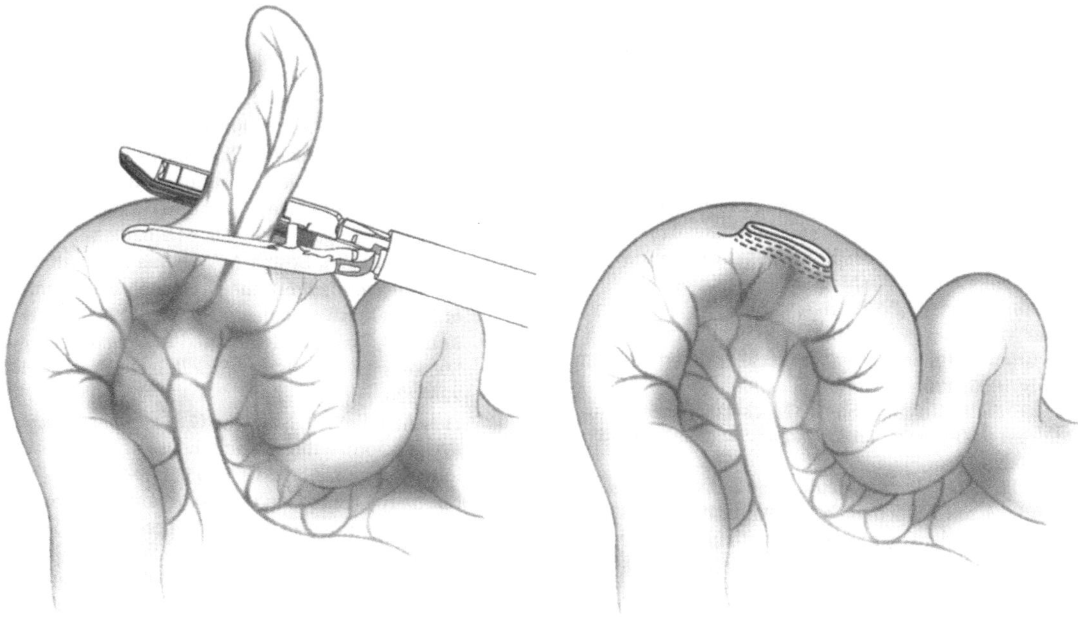

Figure 44.11 Laparoscopic stapling and removal of a Meckel's diverticulum.

diverticulum is identified, grasped and brought out through the umbilical or other trocar site. Once the diverticulectomy or segmental small bowl resection is performed, the bowel is returned to the peritoneal cavity. The advantage of this technique is that it allows the surgeon to inspect and palpate the bowel, and to perform an intestinal anastomosis, easily.

One limitation of laparoscopic resection is that it does not allow for the management of a giant Meckel's diverticulum, which may be difficult to resect through small laparoscopic incisions. Although theoretical advantages of a laparoscopic approach include improved cosmesis and less post-operative pain, prospective studies that demonstrate these advantages are warranted.

Outcomes

Since the 1980s, incidental diverticulectomy for patients with asymptomatic Meckel's diverticulum has been associated with morbidity and mortality rates ranging from 0–9% to 0–1%, respectively.[13,24,26,43] In a comprehensive Mayo Clinic study including both children and adults, the overall rate of morbidity of incidental removal of Meckel's diverticulum was 2%, while the postoperative mortality rate was 1%. The risk of developing long-term complications by 20 years after an incidental diverticulectomy was only 2%. In view of the 4–6% lifetime risk of complications[3–5] from a Meckel's diverticulum, these combined findings suggest that incidental Meckel's diverticulectomy is justified in select cases in which the anatomical features of the diverticulum put patients at higher risk for future complications.

Reported morbidity and mortality rates for diverticulectomy in symptomatic patients vary widely, ranging between 0–18% and 0–9%, respectively.[11,13,24,26,43] The Mayo Clinic study[13] reported a 12% incidence of early postoperative complications; these were mainly wound infection (3%), prolonged ileus (3%) and anastomotic leak (2%). The mortality rate was 1.5%. The incidence of late postoperative complications during a 20-year follow-up was 7%. In our own institution, operation in symptomatic pediatric patients has yielded excellent long-term outcomes. The perioperative complication rate has been less than 6%, with the most common complications being wound infection and prolonged ileus. We have had no reported deaths in over a decade.

REFERENCES

1. Meckel JF. Uber die divertikel am daemkanal. *Archiv Physiol* 1809; **9**: 421–453.
2. Meckel JF. *Handbuch der Pathologischen Anatomie.* vol 1. Leipzig, Germany: Reclam, 1812
3. Soltero JM. Bill AH. The natural history of Meckel's diverticulum and its relation to incidental removal. A study of 202 cases of diseased Meckel's diverticulum found in King County, Washington, over a fifteen year period. *Am J Surg* 1976; **132**: 168–173.
4. Matsagas MI, Fatouros M, Koulouras B et al. Incidence, complication and management of Meckel's diverticulum, *Arch Surg* 1995; **130**: 143–146.
5. St-Vil D, Brandt ML, Panic S et al. Meckel's diverticulum in children: a 20-year review. *J Pediatr Surg* 1991; **26**: 1289–1292.
6. Soderlund S. Meckel's diverticulum: a clinical and histologic study. *Acta Chir Scand Suppl* 1959; **248**: 213–233.
7. Amoury RA, Snyder CL. Meckel's diverticulum. In O'Neill JA, Rowe MI, Grosfeld JL et al. eds. *Pediatric Surgery*, 5th edn. St Louis, MO: Mosby; 1998: 1173–1184.
8. Haubrich WS, Schaffner F, Berk JE, Bockus HL. *Gastroenterology*, 5th edn, vol 2. Philadelphia: WB Saunders, 1995: 912–914.
9. Yachouchy EK, Marano AF, Etienne JCF et al. Meckel's diverticulum. *J Am Coll Surg* 2001; **192**: 658–662.
10. DeBartolo HM Jr, van Heerden JA. Meckel's diverticulum. *Ann Surg* 1976: **183**: 30–33.
11. Mackay WC, Dineen PA. Fifty-year experience with Meckel's diverticulum. *Surg Gynecol Obstet* 1983; **156**: 56–64.
12. Vane DW, West KW, Grosfeld JL. Vitelline duct anomalies. Experience with 217 childhood cases. *Arch Surg* 1987; **122**: 542–547.
13. Cullen JJ, Kelly KA, Moir CR et al. Surgical management of Meckel's diverticulum. An epidemiologic, population-based study. *Ann Surg* 1994; **220**: 564–569.
14. Yamaguchi M, Takeuchi S, Awazu S. Meckel's diverticulum investigation of 600 patients in the Japanese literature. *Am J Surg* 1978; **136**: 247–249.
15. Weinstein EC, Cain JC, ReMine WH. Meckel's diverticulum: 55 years of clinical and surgical experience. *JAMA* 1962; **182**: 131–133.
16. Moses WR. Meckel's diverticulum. Report of two unusual cases. *N Engl J Med* 1947; **237**: 118–122.
17. Baker AL, Marshall SF. Meckel's diverticulum: a report on ninety three cases. *Am Surg* 1955; **21**: 1173–1181.
18. Simms M, Corkery J. Meckel's diverticulum: its association with congenital malformation and the significance of atypical morphology. *Br J Surg* 1980; **67**: 216–219.
19. Andreyev HJN, Owen RA, Thompson I et al. Association between Meckel's diverticulum and Crohn's disease: a retrospective review. *Gut* 1994; **35**: 788–790.
20. Nicol JW, MacKinlay GA. Meckel's diverticulum in exomphalos minor. *J R Coll Surg Edinb* 1994; **39**: 6–7.
21. Moyana TN. Carcinoid tumors arising from Meckel's diverticulum: a clinical, morphologic, and immunohistochemical study. *Am J Clin Pathol* 1989; **91**: 52–56.
22. Nies C, Zielke A, Hasse C et al. Carcinoid tumors of Meckel's diverticula. Report of two cases and review of the literature. *Dis Colon Rectum* 1992; **35**: 589–596.
23. Silk YN, Douglass HO Jr, Penetrante R. Carcinoid tumor in Meckel's diverticulum. *Am Surg* 1988; **54**: 664–667.
24. Leijonmarck CE, Bonman-Sandelin K, Frisell J et al. Meckel's diverticulum in the adult. *Br J Surg* 1986; **73**: 146-149.
25. Arnold JF, Pellicane JV. Meckel's diverticulum: a ten-year experience. *Am Surg* 1997; **63**: 354–355.
26. Rutherford RB, Akers DR. Meckel's diverticulum: a review of 148 pediatric patients, with special reference to the pattern of bleeding and to mesodiverticular vascular bands. *Surgery* 1966; **59**: 618–626.
27. Bemelman WA, Bosma A, Wiersma PH et al. Role of *Helicobacter pylori* in the pathogenesis of complications of Meckel's diverticula. *Eur J Surg* 1993; **159**: 171–175.
28. Kumar S, Small P, Mohammed R. *Helicobacter pylori* and Meckel's diverticulum. *J R Coll Surg Edinb* 1991; **36**: 225–226.
29. Fich A, Talley NJ, Shorter RG et al. Does *Helicobacter pylori* colonize the gastric mucosa of Meckel's diverticulum? *Mayo Clin Proc* 1990; **65**: 187–191.
30. Donnelly LF, Johnson JF. Case report: inverted Meckel's diverticulum with associated microcolon. *Clin Radiol* 1988; **53**: 226–227.
31. Pujari BD, Deodhare SG. Ascarideal penetration of Meckel's diverticulum. *Int Surg* 1978; **63**: 113–114.
32. Hangloo VK, Koul I, Safaya R et al. Primary ascaridial perforations of small intestine and Meckel's diverticulum. *Indian J Gastroenterol* 1990; **9**: 287–288.
33. Oğuzkurt P, Arda S, Kayaselcuk F et al. Cystic Meckel's diverticulum: a rare cause of cystic pelvic mass presenting with urinary symptoms. *J Pediatr Surg* 2001; **36**: 1855–1858.
34. Sfakianakis GN, Conway JJ. Detection of ectopic gastric mucosa in Meckel's diverticulum and in other aberrations by scintigraphy: II. Indications and methods – a 10-year experience. *J Nucl Med* 1981; **22**: 732–738.
35. Emamian SA, Shalaby-Rana E, Majd M. The spectrum of heterotopic gastric mucosa in children detected by Tc-99m pertechnetate scintigraphy. *Clin Nucl Med* 2001; **26**: 529–535.
36. Swaniker F, Soldes O, Hirschl RB. The utility of technetium 99m pertechnetate scintigraphy in the evaluation of patients with Meckel's diverticulum. *J Pediatr Surg* 1999; **34**: 760–765.
37. Stylianos S, Stein J, Flanigan LM et al. Laparoscopy for diagnosis and treatment of recurrent abdominal pain in children. *J Ped Surg* 1996; **31**: 1158–1160.
38. Teitelbaum DH, Polley TZ Jr, Obeid F. Laparoscopic diagnosis and excision of Meckel's diverticulum. *J Pediatr Surg* 1994; **29**: 495–497.
39. Okazaki M, Higashihara H, Saida Y et al. Angiographic findings of Meckel's diverticulum: the characteristic appearance of the vitelline artery. *Abdom Imaging* 1993; **18**: 15–19.
40. Echenique M, Dominguez A, Echenique I et al. Laparoscopic diagnosis and treatment of Meckel's diverticulum complicated by gastrointestinal bleeding. *J Laparoendosc Surg* 1993; **3**: 145–148.
41. Sanders LE. Laparoscopic treatment of Meckel's diverticulum. Obstruction and bleeding managed with minimal morbidity. *Surg Endosc* 1995; **9**: 724–727.
42. Huang CS, Lin LH. Laparoscopic Meckel's diverticulectomy in infants: report of three cases. *J Pediatr Surg* 1993; **281**: 1486–1489.
43. Ludtke FE, Mende V, Kohler H et al. Incidence and frequency of complications and management of Meckel's diverticulum. *Surg Gynecol Obstet* 1989; **169**: 537–542.

45 Acute appendicitis

Adolfo Bautista Casasnovas

Introduction

Acute appendicitis is a common pediatric surgical disease requiring urgent attention. In many cases it shows characteristic clinical manifestations, but in others it may simulate several other syndromes, leading to delays in diagnosis and thus increased morbidity and mortality. It is the most frequent cause of emergency surgery in infancy, and one of the most frequent causes of abdominal pain.

In 1731, Aymand reported in *Philosophical Transactions of the Royal Society* the first successful appendectomy, performed in a child with a very large inguinoscrotal hernia, the sac of which contained an appendix perforated by a needle and giving rise to a stercoral fistula. The intervention lasted 30 min, and the patient survived.

The term 'appendicitis' was coined in 1886 by the American pathological anatomist Reginald Fitz, who stressed the need for early diagnosis and surgery in cases of acute inflammation of the appendix.[1] In 1889, McBurney declared that 'In every case the seat of greatest pain, determined by the pressure of one finger, has been very exactly between an inch and a half and two inches from the anterior spinous process of the ilium on a straight line drawn from that process to the umbilicus'.[2] Since that time this manifestation has been known as the McBurney sign, marking the start of a period of greater scientific rigor in the diagnosis and treatment of acute appendicitis, with early diagnosis and treatment being recognized as essential.

Epidemiology

The incidence of acute appendicitis in the USA has been estimated at about 11 cases per 10 000 people per year, rising to 23 per 10 000 per year in the 10–19-year-old age group, with slightly higher incidence among boys. Incidence among preschool children is lower, but in this age group delayed diagnosis and complications are more frequent.[3,4] About a quarter of operated acute appendicitis cases are found to be perforated at surgery.

In fact, only about 0.5–2% of cases of acute appendicitis appear in children aged less than 2 years. Heredity seems to be important: children who have appendicitis are twice as likely to have a positive family history as children who present lower abdominal quadrant pain not due to appendicitis, and almost three times as likely to have a positive family history as surgical controls without abdominal pain.[5]

In recent decades, as a consequence of the development of new and more effective antibiotics, and of advances in postoperative treatment, a marked reduction in morbidity and mortality has been achieved, but early diagnosis continues to be the most important factor for a good prognosis.[6] To reduce the incidence of complications and perforated appendicitis, practitioners should err on the side of caution: it is considered acceptable for up to 10% of laparotomies for suspected acute appendicitis to prove unnecessary (i.e. normal appendix).

Anatomy

The development of the cecum and appendix commences in the cecal diverticulum on the antimesenteric side of the caudal end of the medial intestine, around the 5th week of gestation. During its descent, the cecoappendiceal complex may locate in a retrocecal or retrocolonic position (about 75% of cases) or inferomedial to the cecum (about 20% of cases). The infant cecum is located in the right iliac fossa in about 55% of individuals.[7] In newborn children it is funnel-shaped with the 'base' oriented upwards and the vertex continuous with the appendix. The proximal end of the appendix is narrower, and its muscle layers thicker, which explains why perforations occur most frequently at the tip. Both cecum and appendix are irrigated by the ileocecal trunk, the ileocolic artery. The arterial supply is terminal, so that thrombosis leads to rapid necrosis. The veins drain to the superior mesenteric vein, which is a common route for propagation of infections from the appendix to the liver.

The lymphatics of the cecum and appendix drain into a group of five or six lymph nodes located in the area of the terminal ileum, so that infections of the appendix may reach the peritoneum or even the thorax.[8]

The cecum and appendix are innervated by the solar plexus via the superior mesenteric plexus, from thoracic sympathetic nerves IX–XI. The autonomic innervation is provided by a small number of ganglion cells irregularly distributed in the submucosa and muscular layers, without forming a plexus.[9]

Pathophysiology

The function of the appendix is unknown: it possibly plays some immunological role in the identification of foreign proteins and bacteria, and in the manufacture of IgA. It has been demonstrated experimentally that mucus secretion (1–2 ml/day) when drainage is blocked increases intraluminal pressure with consequent vascular compromise. The appendix shows independent irregular peristaltic activity, detectable on radiography.[9]

Obstruction is a fundamental factor in the development of acute appendicitis. The position of the blind sac of the appendix favors obstruction of the lumen (by foreign bodies, fecaliths, doubling of the lumen upon itself, lymphoid hyperplasia, infection or tumor), which increases intraluminal pressure leading to ischemia, bacterial invasion, necrosis and perforation.[10] In the early phases, activation of receptors in the intestinal wall leads to perception of pain in the periumbilical region; in later phases, pain is perceived in the right iliac fossa, as a result of irritation due to purulent secretion or contact between the appendix and the parietal peritoneum.

The bacteriological causes of appendiceal infection/inflammation are highly varied. For some authors, infection almost always occurs via the blood,[11] while others consider that intraluminal bacteria are generally responsible.[12–14] The characteristic bacteria are those present in the human colon, predominantly anaerobic, including *Escherichia coli*, *Enterococcus*, *Bacterioides fragilis*, *Pseudomonas*, *Klebsiella* and *Clostridium*.

The higher incidence of acute appendicitis at certain times of the year suggests that respiratory and/or digestive infections showing similar seasonal trends may predispose to lymphoid hyperplasia and resulting narrowing of the appendiceal lumen.

The apparent etiological relationship with certain infections (whether exanthematous or not) probably reflects lymphoid hyperplasia and resulting inflammation and obstruction, as observed in measles, infectious mononucleosis and infections with HIV, adenovirus or coxsackievirus B. The incidence of acute appendicitis is abnormally high in patients with such infections, and with a higher incidence of perforation because of the difficulty of early diagnosis.[15,16]

Likewise, it has been suggested that intestinal parasites may contribute to appendicitis, although a study in the USA found that parasites were present in less than 10% of 100 extirpated appendices.[17]

Carcinoid tumors may cause acute appendicitis in children, especially when close to the tip; in such cases simple appendectomy is generally sufficient treatment.[18]

Clinicopathological course

The course of appendicitis – from the normal state to gangrene – follows a series of clinicopathological states, classifiable as follows:

Simple appendicitis

The first clinical manifestation is congestion of the subserous blood vessels and inflammatory exudate, together with loss of the characteristic shininess of the serous layer. Parietal thickening and luminal obstruction are typically manifested by swelling of the appendix and particularly its tip, with appearance of fibrin. Microscopy reveals small intraluminal groupings of pyocytes, scaling plaques in the mucosa, cryptic abscesses and scarce polymorphonuclear lymphocytes in the lamina propria. At this stage the patient typically begins to feel periumbilical pain, which gradually shifts towards the right iliac fossa.

Phlegmonous appendicitis

Suppurative areas are seen on the wall of the appendix, and venous thromboses in the meso-appendix. Microperforations are observed, generally in large numbers. The appendix is typically covered with omentum. Microscopy reveals an inflammatory infiltrate, together with evident signs of thrombosis and necrosis.

Ulceronecrotic appendicitis

The appendix has become a soft, friable, purplish red structure, with very evident signs of necrosis, including in some cases macroscopic perforation and purulent exudate.[19]

Fibrin increases the adherence of the appendix to neighboring structures, above all in older children. Initially, the peritoneal cavity is seen to contain a clear sterile liquid, due to increased pressure within the lumen. Later, the cavity is invaded by fibrin, leukocytes and pathogens, forming an exudate which, when invaded by bacteria (from the intestine, or due to perforation of the appendix) leads to abdominal abscess formation, generally in the right iliac fossa, close to the cecum and usually foul-smelling; this typically occurs in the phlegmonous or necrotic stages of acute appendicitis.

Diagnosis

The incidence of acute appendicitis gradually increases from age 1 year onwards, peaking at around age 12 years, when the number of lymphatic follicles in the appendix is maximal, favoring its obstruction.[7] Appendicitis is rare during the first year of life, although an association has been reported between Hirschsprung's disease and appendiceal perforation.[20]

Diagnosis of acute appendicitis may be easy or difficult, depending on the patient. All clinicians are familiar with the classic course of acute appendicitis, but early diagnosis is necessary to minimize complications and ensure successful treatment. Diagnosis can almost always be achieved on the basis of a brief history and physical exploration of the abdomen. Difficulties of diagnosis may arise with obese patients (particularly pre-adolescent girls), and with girls younger than 2 years. Except in these two patient categories, analytical and imaging studies are not usually necessary, since they provide relatively little additional information.

Clinical manifestations

The classic sequence (fever, persistent abdominal pain and localized pain on palpation at McBurney's point) starts with periumbilical pain, preceded by appetite loss in about 50–60% of children. Over a varying period of time, this pain gradually shifts to the right iliac fossa, with a corresponding increase in pain on palpation. The pain may be constant, colic or stabbing, or a dull ache. Characteristically the pain is implacable and is exacerbated by movements and pressure, making deambulation painful and difficult.[21]

The change in location of pain is an important diagnostic sign, related to parietal peritoneal irritation, which as it intensifies leads to disappearance of the periumbilical pain.

Nausea and vomiting are also important for diagnosis. They appear after the onset of pain. Indeed, if vomiting appears *before* the onset of pain, other diagnoses (notably enteritis) should be considered.

During the early stages of appendicitis, diarrhea simulating that occurring in the early stages of gastroenteritis is not infrequent; furthermore, in very advanced stages, diarrhea is characteristic. Urological symptoms (dysuria, urine retention) may be similarly misleading, even when urine analysis reveals high white blood cell (WBC) counts, given the proximity of the appendix to the bladder and the ureter. In other words, the clinician should not allow diarrhea or urological symptoms to distract from the possibility of acute appendicitis.

A child with acute appendicitis typically walks bent over and slowly, taking care not to make brusque movements. Often, he or she finds it difficult or impossible to get up onto the examination table.

Fever, which appears after pain and vomiting, is generally not very high; indeed, patients typically have low-grade fever. In many cases there is a marked difference (up to about 1°C) between axillary and rectal temperature. Early-onset high fever argues against acute appendicitis, but late-onset high fever with generalized abdominal pain suggests peritonitis, which is also accompanied by general malaise.

Children with appendicitis are typically anorexic. When a child with abdominal pain shows strong appetite, appendicitis can generally be ruled out, although there are exceptions. Symptoms may be influenced by the anatomic location of the appendix. For example, a retrocecal appendix may cause flank pain or back pain. If the inflamed tip contacts the ureter, pain may be experienced in the inguinal region or testes, and may cause urinary symptoms. Pelvic appendicitis with the inflamed tip contacting the bladder may cause pollakiuria and/or dysuria, or ureteral compression with hydronephrosis (Figure 45.1).

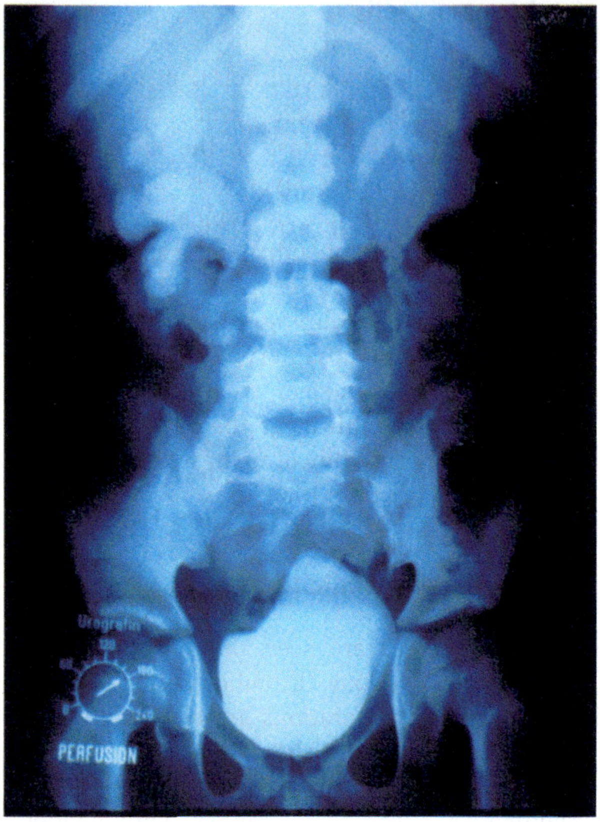

Figure 45.1 Urography showing a mass in the right iliac fossa compressing the bladder and obstructing the ureter, giving rise to hydronephrosis, with an abscess secondary to undiagnosed acute appendicitis.

Approximately two-thirds of appendices are retrocecal or retrocolic. In some cases the appendix may cross the abdomen, with the tip extending into the other quadrant. In cases of incomplete rotation of the intestine, the appendix may be found in the right upper quadrant of the abdomen, or less frequently on the left side.[22]

In pre-weaning and young weaned infants, the diagnosis of acute appendicitis is more difficult, and from 24h after onset the risk of perforation increases considerably.[23] This is particularly problematic, given the still immature immunity of young infants. The omentum is also not fully developed, so that the effects of the appendicitis (e.g. fluid release into the peritoneal cavity) are typically less localized. Early diagnosis is thus imperative, and is complicated by the difficulty of clinical examination. Infants with acute appendicitis typically show vomiting and irritability, and draw up their legs to reduce pain. Other common manifestations include abdominal distension, diarrhea, lethargy and anorexia, together with fever. In 50% of cases an abdominal mass is detectable on palpation.[24]

In conclusion, all patients with abdominal pain, vomiting and moderate fever should be considered as suffering acute appendicitis until otherwise demonstrated.

Physical examination

Physical examination performed with empathy, patience and experience is more valuable than a well-equipped laboratory.[25] A good start for the physical examination is to take the patient's pulse, for at least 30 s; indeed, the pulse rate may be a more useful diagnostic clue than temperature. Observations of features such as general condition, mucocutaneous wetness or dryness, posture, and frequency and type of respiration (in small children with diaphragmatic respiration, immobility of the diaphragm due to peritoneal irritation may lead to respiratory compromise) may all be useful for achieving the diagnosis. Excessively hasty and brusque examinations may of course lead to incorrect diagnosis. Inspection of the throat and rectal examination are uncomfortable for the patient, and should be left for last. A distended bladder is painful and may lead to false diagnosis; the child should therefore urinate before the examination.

Abdominal auscultation should be performed routinely, and should precede palpation. The examiner should take advantage of the stethoscope to auscultate suspected areas. A silent abdomen suggests inflammatory pathology, while hyperperistaltism is more indicative of gastroenteritis or intestinal obstruction.

If the patient is asleep, an initial abdominal palpation should be performed above the clothing, since a sleeping patient is easier to examine. Some maneuvers, such as slight bending of the hips, improve relaxation. In some patients, abdominal palpation may be so difficult that it necessitates sedation to suppress voluntary contractions.[17]

Palpation should always be first superficial and then deep. Involuntary reflex contractions and guarding are very important. To locate pain in response to deep palpation, the palpation should start in an area without pain, and the patient's face should be watched for signs of discomfort.

In addition to McBurney's point, other palpation points have been described (Morris's, Gray's, Loeper's, Lanz's, Kelly's, etc.), together with maneuvers aimed at localization of pain (psoas maneuver, obturator test, etc.).[10–13,17] In fact, the important thing to look for during examination is *any* localized area of abdominal pain.

Rebound tenderness or Blumberg's sign (i.e. pain felt on sudden release of steady pressure in the right iliac fossa region) simply reflects irritation of the parietal peritoneum of the inflamed appendix, and associated fluid secretion.

Rectal examination invariably causes discomfort to children, but is necessary for detection of possible pelvic abscess, right-sided pain, or pain on movement of the bladder.

Laboratory tests

WBC counts are of limited diagnostic value. It is increasingly clear that diagnosis of acute appendicitis is basically clinical. However, a WBC count may be useful to confirm the diagnosis. Acute appendicitis leads to an increased WBC count (generally between 10000 and 20000 per mm^3), with increased polymorphonuclear leukocytes, neutrophils and immature neutrophils. The WBC count will generally be higher in cases of peritonitis or perforation.

Some patients with acute appendicitis may, however, show a normal or low WBC count. This may reflect retrocecal or occult appendicitis. In such cases toxic granulations should be looked for. Determination of C-reactive protein level helps improve diagnostic certainty, but only when pain has been present for over 12–14 h.[26,27]

Experience indicates that neutrophilia is more decisive for diagnosis than leukocytosis. In doubtful cases it is useful to monitor WBCs, as long as the patient is not receiving antibiotics.[28,29]

Urine sediment analyses are useful for detecting diseases of the urinary tract, ranging from infection to lithiasis; such analyses can be considered more important than WBC counts. However, it should be borne in mind that irritation of the ureter or the bladder by a retrocecal or pelvic appendix may lead to the appearance of leukocytes or blood in the urine, confusing the diagnosis.[30,31]

Diagnostic imaging

It is currently accepted that simple radiography is both inadequately sensitive and inadequately specific for diagnosis of acute appendicitis; in addition, the cost–benefit relationship is poor. It thus seems probably that we will see a decline in the use of simple radiography as a primary diagnostic approach in patients with acute pain in the right iliac fossa; however, it will probably remain useful for detecting secondary problems associated with inflammation. The signs most frequently encountered are a dilated cecum with air–fluid level, antalgic scoliosis of the right concavity, obscuration of the right psoas muscle, free peritoneal fluid, minimal pneumoperitoneum and appendiceal fecalith.[30] The presence of a fecalith is highly suggestive of acute appendicitis if clinical characteristics are observed; however, an appendicolith (Figure 45.2) is observed in only 10% of cases.

Ultrasonography has constituted a significant advance in the diagnosis of acute appendicitis, in view of its rapidity, innocuity, sensitivity of 85–90% and specificity of 92–96%. It is of particular value in adolescent and prepubertal girls, since it helps to identify other possible causes of abdominal pain. It should be the first approach in doubtful cases. It is worth mentioning that the examiner must be an expert in pediatric ultrasound. The normal appendix is not usually visualized on ultrasonography. The most characteristic signs are the presence of free liquid and a distended non-compressible tubular structure corresponding to the inflamed appendix, with a size greater than 6 mm. Other useful signs are pericecal inflammatory changes and an appendix located in the retrocecal position or in front of the psoas (Figure 45.3).[32–34]

In recent years, abdominal computed tomography (CT) has become the most informative imaging technique in the study of patients with atypical manifestations, with sensitivity and specificity of 98% according to Rao et al.[35] In the future, it seems likely that continued development of helical CT

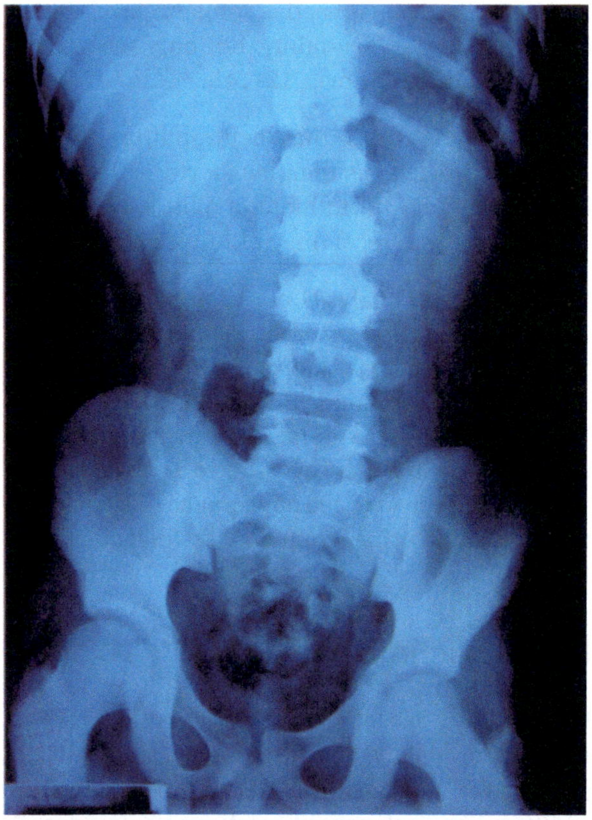

Figure 45.2 Simple radiography of the abdomen in a patient with acute appendicitis, showing anomalous distribution of gas with scoliosis of the right concavity and an appendicolith in the right iliac fossa.

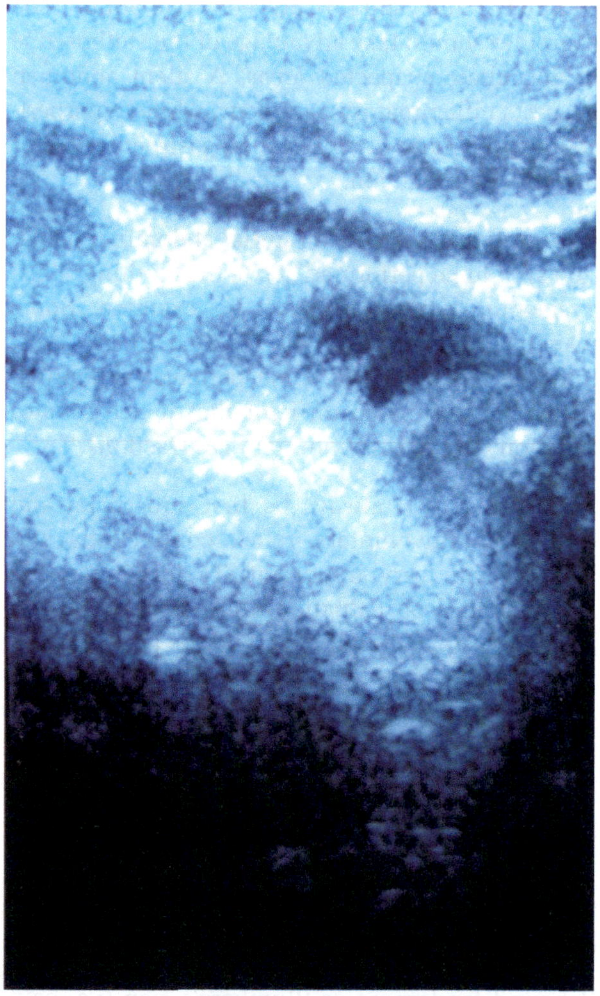

Figure 45.3 Ultrasonography of a patient with acute appendicitis, showing a distended non-compressible tubular structure, with size greater than 6 mm, an appendicolith and surrounded by free fluid.

technology will make this the diagnostic method of choice.[35] It is accepted that the sensitivity and specificity of diagnosis by CT is greater than that of ultrasound, with the following criteria: fluid-filled tubular structure measuring >6 mm in maximum diameter, fat stranding, abscess or phlegmon in adjacent tissue, appendicolith and focal cecal apical thickening.[32,36,37]

Recent studies suggest that imaging should be performed even in cases where the diagnosis of acute appendicitis is clinically likely, as the procedure would enable the detection of a high percentage of normal appendices and the detection of other diagnoses.[38,39]

Differential diagnosis

The disorders most frequently confused with acute appendicitis are urinary diseases (infections, hydronephrosis, lithiasis), basal pneumonias, constipation and gastroenteritis.[17,22,30,40] It should here be stressed that repeated examination is of key importance for differential diagnosis, with careful monitoring of the patient during the first few hours of abdominal symptoms.

Pollakiuria with dysuria and an increased pyocyte count in the urine suggests a urinary tract infection, but these signs may also be observed in pelvic appendicitis, or in appendicitis with the appendix close to the ureter or bladder. It may be helpful to note that flank pain is more commonly associated with renal infection, in which fever and leukocytosis may be observed despite minimal abdominal symptoms. Other urological pathologies to be borne in mind are obstructive disorders such as pyeloureteral or ureterovesical stenosis, as well as vesicoureteral reflux, all of which may cause acute abdominal pain.[41]

Infectious pathologies of the lower lobe of the right lung may cause abdominal pain and generalized abdominal muscular spasm, but such cases do not show localized hypersensitivity in the right iliac fossa; in addition, these children are typically drowsy and sleep a great deal, with high fever and sometimes cough. In rarer cases, the pneumonia is secondary to appendicitis. This occurs when the inflamed appendix is in the retrocecal or subhepatic location, and develops an abscess that invades the subphrenic area with pleural effusion and radiological images suggestive of pulmonary pathology.

Constipation is common in older children, and may involve crises with abdominal pain, fever, vomiting and leukocytosis. There are not always clear antecedents of constipation. In these cases there is no migration of pain from the epigastric region to McBurney's point, and in addition there are no signs of peritoneal irritation. Hard packed feces may be palpated through the abdominal wall.

Gastroenteritis is probably the most common cause of acute abdominal pain, and is frequently confused with appendicitis. Early-onset vomiting accompanied by abdominal pain is the most reliable feature of gastroenteritis, while in appendicitis vomiting appears late after the onset of abdominal pain. Abundant foul-smelling diarrhea is likewise indicative of gastroenteritis, by contrast with the scant mucosal secretions appearing in pelvic appendicitis. Nevertheless, it should be stressed that frequent bowel movements do not rule out appendicitis.[42]

In pubertal girls, premenstrual syndrome and dysmenorrhea are common causes of unnecessary surgery, and their differential diagnosis is not always easy. Ovarian cysts can be diagnosed by rectal examination or ultrasonography; they cause acute pain when ruptured or torsioned, and the patient typically shows vomiting. In doubtful cases, laparoscopy is of key value.

In primary peritonitis due to pneumococcus or streptococcus, the severe effects on general well-being call for emergency surgery; in any case, acute appendicitis and peritonitis are often not distinguishable without surgery.

Differential diagnosis with respect to mesenteric lymphadenitis may be very difficult, because of the close clinical similarities with acute appendicitis. Criteria indicative of adenitis include initial high fever, severe spasmodic abdominal pain, absence of anorexia and, in some cases, a history of respiratory infection. As noted in the classic texts, careful monitoring of the patient is extremely important.[12]

Inflammatory bowel diseases, notably Crohn's disease, may sometimes be first detected during acute appendicitis, but generally the patient will present with a prolonged history of abdominal pain, diarrhea attacks and growth restriction, in some cases with a positive family history.

Patients with severe leukopenia due to cancer or chemotherapy may show invasive infection of the entire wall of the cecal region (i.e. typhlitis), with pain and guarding of the right iliac fossa. If there is no improvement on antibiotic treatment, or if symptoms are suggestive of irritation or perforation of the bowel, surgery should be performed.

Other differential diagnoses to be taken into account are viral hepatitis (especially in the preicteric phase), as a result of lymphoid–appediceal involvement by viral infections (hepatitis B, Herpes, coxsackievirus, adenovirus); intussusception; viral exanthematous diseases; sickle cell anemia; cholecystitis; pancreatitis; omentum infarction; and duodenal ulcer (Table 45.1).

Table 45.1 Main differential diagnosis of acute appendicitis

Urological pathology
Urinary tract infections
Pneumonia
Constipation
Gastroenteritis
Premenstrual syndrome
Ovarian pathology
Primary peritonitis
Mesenteric adenitis
Meckel's diverticulitis
Henoch–Schönlein purpura
Viral hepatitis
Inflammatory bowel disease
Intussusception
Typhlitis
Viral exanthematous diseases
Sickle cell anemia
Cholecystisis
Pancreatitis
Omentum infarction
Duodenal ulcer
Abdominal migraine
Acute porphyria
Familial Mediterranean fever
Hemolytic uremic syndrome

Treatment

The treatment of choice for acute appendicitis is of course early appendectomy. Rapid administration of intravenous fluid and electrolytes (to restore acid–base balance) is fundamental for a good course. Depending on the clinical characteristics (degree of dehydration, fasting status, presence of vomiting), the rehydration fluid may be physiological saline with glucose, or lactate Ringer's solution, in either case with supplementary potassium if necessary. In cases of peritonitis, losses to the third space should be taken into account, since this will increase the rehydration requirement.

Once surgical intervention has been decided upon, intravenous antibiotic treatment should be started.[43]

In cases of intestinal obstruction or distension, the insertion of a nasogastric tube facilitates decompression of the abdomen and minimizes the risk of aspiration during anesthesia induction.

If the appendix is gangrenous with peritonitis and the patient is seriously ill, intensive reanimation will be required before appendectomy, with immediate intravenous administration of antibiotics together with rehydration. In some cases, a vesical drainage will be necessary as well as nasogastric drainage, but generally the patient can undergo surgery within 6–8 h of the start of reanimation.

The type of antibiotic therapy used varies among different centers. Some authors have recommended prophylactic administration of one dose of cefotoxin before surgery and three doses after surgery.[44] However, cefotoxin may be less effective than a combination of aminoglycosides, synthetic penicillin and metronidazole in the treatment of a perforated appendix. Other authors have suggested the use of piperacillin and tazobactam.[30] Presurgery treatment with ampicillin, gentamycin and clindamycin has been successfully used in some countries since the 1970s.[45] In the Pediatric Surgery Service of our hospital (the Santiago de Compostela University Hospital in northwest

Spain), we currently use treatment with tobramycin plus metronidazole, with a low incidence (<4%) of postoperative infections and abscesses. It is certainly clear that presurgery antibiotic treatment reduces the incidence of complications.[46] In children with peritonitis, the administration of antibiotics should be continued for at least 5–8 days after surgery.[21]

The surgical approach of choice in children is the Rockey–Davis approach, for esthetic reasons, although the McBurney approach is still widely used. Both approaches allow the peritoneum to be reached with minimal contamination, a better exposure in the event of unexpected findings, the possibility of lateral extension, a low incidence of eventrations and satisfactory scar esthetics[47] (Figure 45.4).

Once the peritoneum has been reached, a sample of peritoneal fluid should be obtained for anaerobic and aerobic culture, necessary for effective choice of antibiotics.

Laparoscopic appendectomy is an alternative to conventional open appendectomy, but its advantages are still widely debated. Some randomized studies have found that laparoscopic appendectomy is at least as effective as conventional appendectomy, with the advantage that the initial laparoscopy reduces the risk of incorrect diagnosis.[48,49] Other apparent advantages are reduction of postoperative pain, faster recovery and discharge

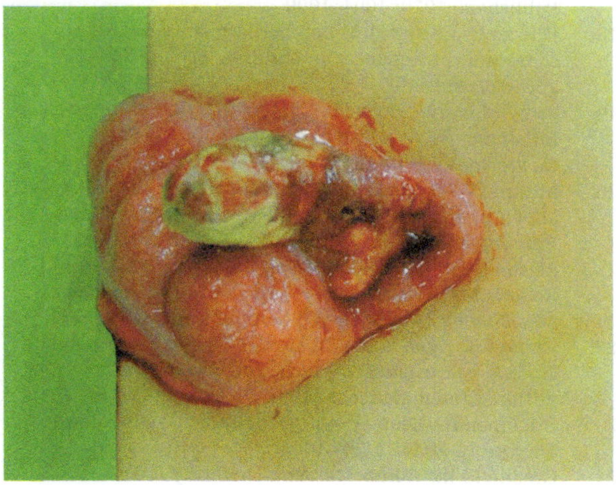

Figure 45.4 Typical appearance of acute appendicitis during surgery.

from hospital, and lower surgical wound infection rates. However, the operation takes longer, has a higher cost and requires pediatric surgeons with experience in this technique.[50–52]

The course after surgery depends on whether there is bacterial contamination, abscess formation, and recovery of intestinal mobility. In cases of peritonitis, antibiotic treatment should be maintained for at least 5 days post-surgery; if the patient has a normal temperature and tolerates food, he or she can be discharged on day 6. In cases of simple appendicitis, antibiotic treatment need be maintained for only 24–72 h, and discharge can be sooner.

Complications

Without doubt the most frequent complication of acute appendicitis is infection, and the risk of infection is increased when the appendix is perforated. The most frequent site of infection is the operative wound. Wound infection typically presents in the first week post-surgery as localized pain, reddening, hypersensitivity and tumefaction; spontaneous suppuration may also occur, accompanied by fluctuating fever and leukocytosis.[30]

When the patient's condition does not improve despite surgery, with persistence of pain and ileus, together with fever and leukocytosis, we should suspect an intra-abdominal abscess (most frequently located in the pelvis, sometimes in the subphrenic space or medial zone of the abdomen). When located in Douglas' pouch, a painful fluctuant mass can be palpated on rectal examination. Sometimes infectious complications arise weeks after the patient's apparent complete recovery (and thus discharge). In the past decade, antibiotic therapies and percutaneous drainage guided by ultrasonography or CT have made surgery rarely necessary for drainage of these abscesses.

Prolonged intestinal paralysis (ileus) is directly related to peritoneal infection; the more severe the peritonitis, the longer the period required for recovery of normal intestinal transit. Prolonged ileus should make us suspect an intra-abdominal abscess; however, an abscess may also present as intestinal obstruction. More rarely, intestinal obstruction may be secondary to adherences.

After surgery of any type, late adherences may be observed, but a large proportion of adherence-related obstructions are secondary to surgery for acute appendicitis, even though they first present months or even years later. Adherences and infections of this type have also been implicated in the sterility observed in some girls after surgery for acute appendicitis;[53] however, other studies have not been able to detect any raised incidence of sterility in patients of this type.[54]

Summary

The large series to date have suggested that mortality in acute appendicitis is about 1%, and rather higher in children aged less than 2 years.[55,56] The incidence of postoperative complications has previously been reported to be about 5–10%. Over the past 25 years in our hospital, the incidence of complications has been about 0.5%. This low incidence is perhaps attributable to the use of efficient broad-spectrum antibiotics, to progress in pre- and postoperative care, and to improved anesthesia techniques.

Efforts to reduce morbidity and mortality further in acute appendicitis will require improved early diagnosis on the basis of anamnesis and physical examination, improved preoperative care and well-trained surgeons.

REFERENCES

1. Fitz RH. Perforating inflammation of the vermiform appendix with special reference to its early diagnosis and treatment. *Am J Med Sci* 1886; **7**: 321–346.
2. McBurney C. Experience with early operative interference in cases of diseases of the vermiform appendix. *NY State J Med* 1889; **50**: 676–684.
3. Harmatz P. Acute apendicitis. In Finberg L, Kleinman RE, 2nd edn. *Saunder Manual of Pediatric Practice*. New York: WB Saunders, 2002: 590–592.
4. Bratton SL, Haberrrkern CM, Waldhausen JH. Acute appendictis risks of complications: age and medicaid insurance. *Pediatrics* 2000; **106**: 75-78
5. Gauderer MW, Crane MM, Green JA et al. Acute appendictis in children: the importance of family history. *J Pediatr Surg* 2001; **36**: 1214–1217.
6. Helmer KS, Robinson EK, Lally KP et al. Standardized patient care guidelines reduce infectious morbidity in appendectomy patients. *Am J Surg* 2002; **183**: 608–613.
7. Testut L, Latarjet A. *Tratado de anatomía humana*, vol IV, 4th ed. Barcelona: Salvat, 1964: 396–432.
8. Skandalakis JE, Gray SW. *Embryology for Surgeons*, 2nd edn. Baltimore: Williams and Wilkins, 1994: 224–245.
9. Morson BC, Dawson IMP. The normal appendix. In Morson BC, Dawson IMP, eds. *Gastrointestinal Pathology*. Oxford: Blackwell Scientific Publications, 1972: 391–407.
10. Drachter R, Gossmann JR. *Chirurgie des Kindesalter*, 3rd edn. Leipzig: Van FCW Vagel, 1930: 231–257.
11. Ombredanne L. *Precis clinique et opératoire de chirurgie infantile*, 12th edn. Paris: Masson, 1925: 532–561.
12. Gross RE. Appendicitis. In Gross RE, ed. *The Surgery of Infancy and Childhood*. Philadelphia: WB Saunders, 1953: 253–280.
13. Ein SH. Appendicitis. In Ashcraft KW, Murphy JP, Sharp RJ, Sigalet DL, Snyder CL, Eds. *Pediatric Surgery*, 3rd edn. Philadelphia: WB Saunders Company, 2000: 571–579.
14. Rautio M, Saxen H, Siitonen A et al. Bacteriology of histopathologically defined appendicitis in children. *Pediatr Infect Dis J* 2000; **19**: 1078–1083
15. Lawrence KB, Waring GW. Acute appendicitis complicating the acute infectious diseases of childhood. *N Engl J Med* 1949; **247**: 1–6.
16. Pancharoen C, Ruttanamongkol P, Suwangool P et al. Measles-associated appendicitis: two case reports and literature review. *Scand J Infect Dis* 2001; **33**: 632–633.
17. Folkman J. Appendicitis. In Ravitch MM, Welch KJ, Benson CD, Aberdeen E, Randolph JG, eds. *Pediatric Surgery*, 3rd edn. Chicago: Year Book Medical Publishers, 1979: 1004–1009.
18. Pelizzo G, La Riccia A, Bouvier R et al. Carcinoid tumors of the appendix in children. *Pediatr Surg Int* 2001; **17**: 399–402.
19. Tsujy M, Puri P, Reen DJ. Characterization of the local inflammatory response in appendicitis. *J Pediatr Gastroenterol Nutr* 1993; **76**: 43–48.
20. Martin LW, Perring EW. Neonatal perforation of the appendix in association with Hirschsprung's disease. *Ann Surg* 1967; **766**: 799–802.
21. Mason Cobb L, Lelli JL. Appendicitis. In Reisdorff EJ, Roberts MR, Wiegenstein JG, eds. *Pediatric Emergency Medicine* Philadelphia: WB Saunders, 1993: 314–321.
22. Cloud DT. Apendicitis. In Holder TM, Ashcraft KW, eds. *Tratado de Cirugía Pediátrica*, 2nd edn. Madrid: Editorial Interamericana–McGraw Hill, 1995: 484–491.
23. Brickman ID, Leon W. Acute appendicitis in childhood. *Surgery* 1960; **60**: 1083–1089.
24. Grosfffeld JL, Weinberger M, Clatworthy HW. Acute appendicitis in the first two years of life. *J Pediatr Surg* 1973; **8**: 285–293.

25. Raffensperger JC. *El abdomen agudo en lactantes y niños*, 2nd edn. Buenos Aires: Bernardes Ediciones, 1969: 121–141.
26. Wetzman M. Diagnostic utility of white blood cell and differential counts. *Am J Dis Child* 1973; **129**: 1183–1189.
27. Gronroos JM, Gronoos P. Leucocyte count and C-reactive protein in the diagnosis of acute appendicitis. *Br J Surg* 1999; **86**: 501–504.
28. Andersson RE, Hugander A, Ravn H. Repeated clinical and laboratory examinations in patients with an equivocal diagnosis of appendicitis. *World J Surg* 2000; **24**: 479–485.
29. Schwartz MZ, Bulas D. Acute abdomen. Laboratory evaluation and imaging. *Semin Pediatr Surg* 1997; **6**: 65–73.
30. Lund DP, Folkman J. Appendicitis. In Walker WA, Durie PR, Hamilton JR, Walker-Smith JA, Watkins JB, eds. *Pediatric Gastrointestinal Disease: Pathophysiology, Diagnosis and Management*, 3rd edn. Hamilton, Ontario: BC Decker, 2000: 821–829.
31. Rothrock SG, Pagane J. Acute appendicitis in children: emergency department diagnosis and management. *Ann Emerg Med* 2000; **36**: 39–51.
32. Garcia Pena BM, Mandl KD, Kraus SJ. Ultrasonography and limited computed tomography in the diagnosis and management of appendicitis in children. *JAMA* 1999; **282**: 1041–1046.
33. Crady SK, Jones JS, Wyn T, Luttenton CR. Clinical validity of ultrasound in children with suspected appendicitis. *Ann Emerg Med* 1993; **22**: 1125–1129.
34. Sivit JS, Applegate KE, Stallion A et al. Imaging evaluation of suspected appendicitis in a pediatric population: effectiveness of sonography versus CT. *Am J Roentgenol* 2000; **175**: 977–980.
35. Rao PM, Rhea JT, Novelline RA et al. Helical CT combined with contrast material administered only through the colon for imaging of suspected appendicitis. *Am J Roentgenol* 1997; **169**: 1275–1280.
36. Kaiser S, Frenckner B, Jorulf HK. Suspected appendicitis in children: US and CT – a prospective randomized study. *Radiology* 2002; **223**: 633–638.
37. Lowe LH, Perez R Jr, Scheker LE et al. Appendicitis and alternate diagnoses in children: findings on unenhanced limited helical CT. *Pediatr Radiol* 2001; **31**: 569–577.
38. Rettenbacher T, Hollerweger A, Gritzmann N et al. Appendicitis: should diagnostic imaging be performed if the clinical presentation is highly suggestive of the disease? *Gastroenterology* 2002; **123**: 992–998.
39. Pena BM, Taylor GA, Fishman SJ, Mandl KD. Costs and effectiveness of ultrasonography and limited computed tomography for diagnosing appendicitis in children. *Pediatrics* 2000; **106**: 672–676.
40. Hecker WCH. Zur Einweisung Diagnose Appendicitis in Kindesalter. *Arztl Wschr* 1954; **9**: 1149–1153.
41. Bertin P, Tovar JA, Pellerin D. L'appendicitis avant trois ans. A propos de 77 observations en 12 ans. *Rev Pediatr* 1973; **9**: 121–128.
42. Ferre M. *Chirurgie infantile de urgencie*, 2nd edn. Paris: Masson, 1958: 146–159.
43. Neilson IR, Laberge JM, Nguyen LT et al. Appendicitis in children: current therapeutic recomendations. *J Pediatr Surg* 1990; **25**: 1113–1116.
44. Kaiser AB. Antimicrobial prophylaxis in surgery. *N Engl J Med* 1986; **315**: 1129.
45. Gilbert SR, Emmens RW, Putnam TC. Appendicitis in children. *Surg Gynecol Obstet* 1985; **161**: 261.
46. Andersen BR, Kallehave FL, Andersen HK. Antibiotics versus placebo for prevention of postoperative infection after appendectomy. *Cochrane Database Syst Rev* 2001: **3**: CD001439.
47. Shackelford RT. Surgery of the Alimentary Tract. Philadelphia: WB Saunders, 1955: 2562–2567.
48. Reiertsen O, Larsen S, Trondsen E et al. Randomized controlled trial with sequential design of laparoscopic versus conventional appendicectomy. *Br J Surg* 1997; **84**: 842–847.
49. Chung RS, Rowland DY, Li P, Diaz J. A meta-analysis of randomized controlled trials of laparoscopic versus conventional appendectomy. *Am J Surg* 1999; **177**: 250–256.
50. Moir CR. Appendectomy: open and laparoscopic approaches. In Spitz L, Coran AC, eds. *Pediatric Surgery*. London: Chapman, 1995: 408–410.
51. Meguerditchian AN, Prasil P, Cloutier R et al. Laparoscopic appendectomy in children: a favorable alternative in simple and complicated appendicitis. *J Pediatr Surg* 2002; **37**: 695–698.
52. Little DC, Custer MD, May BH et al. Laparoscopic appendectomy: an unnecessary and expensive procedure in children? *J Pediatr Surg* 2002; **37**: 310–317.
53. Puri P, McGuinness EP, Guiney EJ. Fertility following perforated appendicitis in girls. *J Pediatr Surg* 1989; **24**: 547–549.
54. Andersson R, Lambe M, Bergstrom R. Fertility patterns after appendicectomy: historical cohort study. *Br Med J* 1999; **318**: 963–967.
55. Flum DR, Koepsell T. The clinical and economic correlates of misdiagnosed appendicitis: nationwide analysis. *Arch Surg* 2002; **137**: 799–804.
56. Blomqvist PG, Andersson RE, Granath F et al. Mortality after appendectomy in Sweden, 1987–1996. *Ann Surg* 2001; **233**: 455–460.

46 Vascular lesions of the gastrointestinal tract in childhood

Steven R Allen and Richard G Azizkhan

Introduction

Over the years, various histopathological systems combined with descriptive vernacular have been used to describe vascular lesions. Changes in nomenclature and inconsistencies in terminology have led to confusion and misunderstanding among medical specialists, making it difficult to compare published literature describing pathology, treatment and outcomes. A comprehensive biological classification system proposed in 1982 correlated endothelial and mast cell kinetics of vascular lesions with their clinical characteristics and natural history.[1] With minor modifications, this classification system is now universally accepted by those at the forefront of this specialized field and is used to classify all vascular lesions in infancy and childhood.

According to the current system, there are two main types of vascular lesion: tumors and malformations. Within the category of vascular tumors, hemangiomas are by far the most common. Lesions in the two classifications differ in their clinical, radiological, histopathological and hemodynamic presentations.[2,3] However, both types of lesion can permeate any organ system. Although they generally present cutaneously, they can also develop in multiple anatomic sites, and often involve the extremities, thoracoabdominal walls and cavities, solid organs, hollow viscera and brain.[4] Clinical symptoms are diverse, ranging from minor cervicofacial manifestations to serious and potentially life-threatening symptoms that may be difficult to identify (e.g. pain, bleeding, mass effect and congestive heart failure). Because management approaches and prognostic assessment for various lesions are different, accurate, precise and consistent terminology is essential.

To clarify long-held misconceptions and to ensure that readers share common terminology and a common knowledge base, we will first describe the key clinical and biological features that distinguish hemangiomas from vascular malformations. Our discussion will then focus on the clinical presentation, diagnosis and management of vascular lesions of the gastrointestinal tract. We will briefly describe similar cutaneous vascular lesions. Since they are often associated with gastrointestinal manifestations, familiarity with them provides a useful framework for establishing a correct diagnosis.

Clinical differences between vascular tumors and malformations

Hemangiomas are benign tumors. They are characterized by endothelial hyperplasia with multilamination of the basement membrane and increased numbers of mast cells. After a period of rapid postnatal proliferation beginning shortly after birth, hemangiomas typically undergo slow, spontaneous involution. As involution is completed, mast cells fall to normal levels. Involution occurs in 50% of lesions by the age of 5 and in 70% by the age of 7. Other lesions continue to regress until the ages of 10–12. Because of this clinical course, most hemangiomas do not require treatment.

In contrast to hemangiomas, vascular malformations are not neoplastic lesions. Rather, they result from errors of vascular morphogenesis, and usually exhibit normal endothelial turnover and normal numbers of mast cells. Typical microscopic findings show progressive ectasia of structurally abnormal blood vessels. The blood-filled channels are lined by a thin, flat endothelium, overlying a thin basal lamina. Additionally, there is a paucity or absence of smooth muscle within the vessel walls of vascular malformations. Although present at birth, these lesions may not manifest until childhood, adolescence, or even adulthood. Unlike hemangiomas, malformations generally grow commensurately with the child. They encompass a wide spectrum of anomalies, appearing with unique presentation and varying pathophysiology. Malformations are subcategorized by their predominant channel type as capillary, venous, arterial, lymphatic, or some combination of these. Lesions that have an arterial component are termed 'fast-flow' malformations, while capillary, venous and lymphatic lesions are slow-flow malformations. Fast-flow malformations are associated with high-output cardiac states, cardiac failure and disproportionate growth of involved organs and extremities.

Whereas proliferating hemangiomas rarely cause bone distortion or hypertrophy, slow-flow malformations are frequently associated with diffuse bone hypertrophy, distortion, or elongation. Fast-flow malformations can cause destructive interosseous changes.

Vascular malformations also show hematological dissimilarities with vascular tumors. Hemangioendothelioma and tufted angioma, both of which are rare types of vascular tumors, can cause platelet trapping, shortened platelet half-life and profound thrombocytopenia. Vascular malformations, particularly the venous type, induce a true intravascular coagulation defect with only mild thrombocytopenia and slightly decreased platelet survival (Table 46.1).

In most cases, the type of vascular anomaly can be correctly diagnosed by correlating physical

Table 46.1 Clinical differences between vascular tumors and malformations (modified from reference 5)

Vascular tumors	Vascular malformations
Neoplasm	Congenital abnormality
Generally apparent during first few weeks of life	May not become apparent until months or even years after birth
Female/male ratio of 3:1	No gender predilection
Rapid postnatal growth followed by slow involution	Slow steady growth; sepsis, trauma, or hormonal change may cause rapid expansion; no involution
Endothelial cell hyperplasia	Normal endothelial cell turnover
Increased mast cells	Normal mast cell count
Multilaminated basement membrane	Normal basement membrane
Infrequent mass effect on adjacent bone; hypertrophy rare	Slow-flow: frequent bone hypertrophy, distortion, or elongations Fast-flow: destructive interosseous changes
Hemangioendothelioma and tufted angioma associated with platelet trapping and thrombocytopenia	Mild thrombocytopenia and only slightly decreased platelet survival
Angiographic findings: well circumscribed, intense lobular–parenchymal staining with equatorial vessels	Angiographic findings: diffuse, no parenchyma Low-flow: phleboliths, ectatic channels High-flow: enlarged, tortuous arteries with arteriovenous shunting
Response to corticosteroids and antiangiogenic agents	No response to corticosteroids or antiangiogenic agents

findings and case history. Nevertheless, deep cutaneous and visceral lesions can be difficult to identify without radiological evaluation. Also, overlapping of clinical characteristics of the two classifications does occur, and because distinctive histopathological features of hemangiomas diminish during their evolution from the proliferative to the involutive phase, their differentiation from vascular malformations becomes increasingly difficult.[5] Doppler ultrasonography is often used to distinguish between these two types of lesion and to detect arterial flow. Depending on clinical circumstances, computerized tomography, magnetic resonance imaging, blood cell scintigraphy and angiography may also be required to determine the type, location and extent of lesions.

Common errors in nomenclature

Fishman and Fox[6] describe several important errors and inconsistencies in nomenclature that are readily apparent in the literature and are important for clinicians to be aware of. The term 'hemangioma' is ubiquitously misused to label a wide spectrum of vascular lesions with different etiologies and natural histories. Moreover, some authors add misleading and incorrect descriptors such as 'capillary' or 'cavernous'. Lesions with large blood-filled spaces, often referred to as 'cavernous hemangiomas' are generally not hemangiomas, but are rather venous malformations. Also important to note, the suffix 'oma' in modern medical parlance implies a neoplastic process with rapid cellular turnover. Since vascular malformations are non-neoplastic lesions with quiescent endothelium, terms that are often seen in the literature such as 'lymphangioma', 'cystic hygroma', and 'angioma' are misnomers that should be avoided. Lesions that are commonly referred to as 'lymphangiomas', should be classified as lymphatic malformations. Cystic hygromas are more accurately classified as cystic lymphatic malformations, usually of the head and neck.

Hemangiomas

Hemangiomas are the most common tumor in infancy and are more common in girls than in boys, with a ratio of 3:1. They range in appearance from small, hardly noticeable birthmarks to large grotesque tumors that can destroy tissue, obstruct the airway, or impair vision. Cutaneous hemangiomas generally become apparent early in the neonatal period, beginning as a faint discoloration. During proliferation, they typically turn bright red or crimson, and may ulcerate and/or bleed. After spontaneous regression, the lesion may become unnoticeable or may leave a fibrofatty residuum without much color.[6] A hemangioma that has ulcerated during proliferation can, however, leave wrinkling, telangiectasia, a yellowish inelastic patch, or a scar.[5]

Gastrointestinal hemangiomas can occur anywhere in the gastrointestinal tract. Although the liver is the most common visceral site, specific and adequate discussion of hepatic lesions is beyond the scope of the present chapter. Unlike cutaneous hemangiomas, gastrointestinal hemangiomas are rarely seen. They become evident only when lesions are symptomatic, and are often associated with multifocal cutaneous lesions (Figure 46.1). Mild to life-threatening gastrointestinal bleeding may occur, the later requiring repeated blood transfusions. Since an intestinal hemangioma rarely

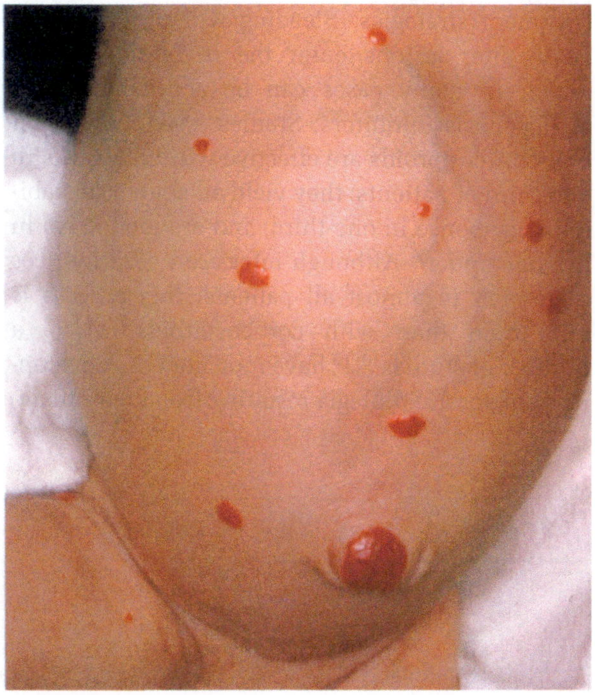

Figure 46.1 A 2-month old infant with multiple cutaneous hemangiomas.

bleeds after the proliferative phase has ended, such a lesion would not, however, be a likely cause of bleeding beyond the first year or two of age. Another possible presenting symptom, though even less commonly seen, is intestinal obstruction.

Treatment for hemangiomas is based on the degree and severity of symptoms. A small isolated hemangioma of the stomach or colon can be banded endoscopically, although not without risk of perforation or increased hemorrhage.[7] Occasionally, a focal lesion may be amenable to treatment with other endoscopic techniques such as multipolar thermocoagulation or argon plasma coagulation. For lesions visible by endoscopy, intralesional injection with corticosteroid may also be considered.[6] Indications for excision include complications such as intussusception or obstruction, uncontrollable ulceration with hemorrhage or perforation, or infection (Figure 46.2). A surgical approach is not indicated when there is diffuse multifocal involvement of the gastrointestinal tract. Such lesions are more appropriately treated with corticosteroids, interferon α-2a, or other antiangiogenic agents (Table 46.2).

In summary, if symptoms can be managed with persistent and aggressive blood replacement and pharmacotherapy, these are often the most prudent treatment strategies. Bleeding will diminish and cease after lesions enter the involution phase, which in many cases can be accelerated with angiogenesis inhibitors. Studies have shown that oral corticosteroids are effective within 2 weeks in one-third of patients; they yield an equivocal stabilizing response in one-third; and are ineffective in the remainder.[8] Although interferon α-2a induces regression in almost all patients, this process is less rapid than with corticosteroids.[9] Also, a number of studies[10–12] have indicated the development of spastic diplegia resulting from neurotoxicity during the course of interferon therapy; this is more commonly seen in infants younger than 1 year of age. Although the condition generally reverses with the termination of therapy, careful monitoring of neurodevelopmental status is required. In light of the potential side-effects, interferon therapy is used only when hemangiomas are unresponsive to steroids or are life threatening.

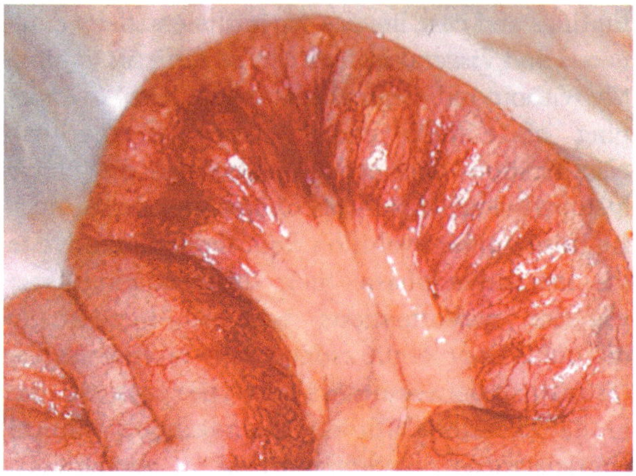

Figure 46.2 Jejunoileal hemangioma associated with significant gastrointestinal hemorrhage in a 5-month-old infant.

Vascular malformations

Gastrointestinal vascular malformations parallel the four main malformation groups described earlier: capillary, venous, lymphatic and arteriovenous (and complex combined lesions). Severity varies greatly both among malformations within each clinical group and among the four general group classifications.

Table 46.2 Pharmacotherapy options for problematic hemangiomas

	Dosage	Duration
Oral prednisone	3-4 mg/kg per day (initial dosage)	gradual tapering over several months
Interferon α-2a	1–3 million units/m^2 per day	12–18 months
Vincristine	0.05 mg/kg weekly	4–12 weeks

Capillary malformations

Capillary malformations of the skin include port wine stain (also known as nevus flammeus) and congenital telangiectasias. These are present at birth and remain throughout life. With aging, the surface of the red vascular stain becomes raised and studded with nodular lesions. Lesions can be localized or can occur extensively on the face, trunk or limbs, and can be isolated or associated with other congenital malformations or vascular anomalies. Sturge–Weber syndrome consists of facial capillary malformation in association with ipsilateral leptomeningeal and ocular anomalies. Malformations on the trunk or extremities may coexist with venous and lymphatic abnormalities (Klippel–Trénaunay syndrome) (Figure 46.3). They may also overlie a deep arteriovenous malformation anywhere in the body. A facial lesion may indicate a unilateral arteriovenous malformation of the retina and intracranial optic pathway (Wyburn–Mason's syndrome).

Symptomatic capillary malformations of the gastrointestinal tract are extremely rare in childhood. Patients with hereditary hemorrhagic telangiectasia (Osler–Weber–Rendu syndrome) may experience gastrointestinal bleeding, but this rarely occurs before adulthood[13] and is generally preceded by pulmonary manifestations, which include arteriovenous malformations and cerebrovascular lesions. Diagnosis is usually established by endoscopic evaluation. Treatment for identified bleeding sites can readily be accomplished by endoscopic laser photocoagulation.

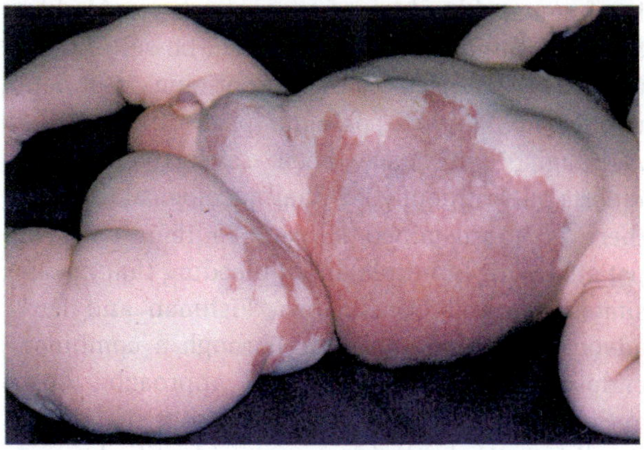

Figure 46.3 Complex combined capillary venous and lymphatic malformation involving the left lower extremity and trunk of an infant with Klippel–Trénaunay syndrome.

Two published case reports[14,15] describe an association between hereditary hemorrhagic telangiectasia and juvenile polyposis. These reports are, however, inconclusive as to the actual cause of bleeding, since colonic polyps themselves are highly vascular and thus a common source of bleeding in childhood.

Venous malformations

These slow-flow lesions appear as a faint blue patch or a soft blue mass. Because of their coloration and soft, spongy consistency, they are frequently mislabeled as 'cavernous hemangiomas'. Venous malformations are not tumors, do not regress spontaneously and do not respond to antiangiogenesis inhibitors. Lesions can be localized or extensive, and can range from miniscule to massive and disfiguring. Phleboliths are pathognomonic and, if present, can easily distinguish a venous malformation from a hemangioma. While cutaneous and soft tissue lesions are often asymptomatic, they may cause pain; this is probably due to congestion and/or low-grade thrombosis.

Venous malformations are the most commonly symptomatic vascular anomalies of the gastrointestinal tract in childhood.[7] They generally present with either chronic or acute upper or lower gastrointestinal bleeding, which is often not identified until the patient is found to be severely anemic. Less commonly, malformations of the gut may cause pain or obstruction.

Gastrointestinal lesions appear in the varying patterns described below.[5] Diagnostic and management approaches are best tailored according to these patterns.

Focal venous malformations

Focal venous malformations can occur anywhere in the gastrointestinal tract. These lesions may vary in size and may be mucosal, mural, or transmural. Endoscopic ultrasound may be helpful in making this determination. A small focal lesion that is clearly not transmural may be treated nonoperatively. Such a lesion can be managed with endoscopic sclerotherapy using sclerosing agents such as absolute ethanol or 1% sodium tetradecyl sulfate, which are generally effective in obliterating abnormal venous channels. Because of the danger of systemic intravascular migration of the sclerosing agent, clinicians should consider performing pretreatment angiography or a direct intralesional contrast study to identify any anomalous or large vessels communicating with the lesion. Another treatment option for small mucosal venous lesions is endoscopic banding.[7] However, since perforations can occur after endoscopic treatment of small, unsuspected transmural lesions, it is best to provide for surgical back-up should complications arise.[5] Surgical excision is required for large or transmural gastrointestinal venous malformations.

Multifocal venous malformations (blue rubber bleb nevus syndrome)

Blue rubber bleb nevus syndrome is a rare multifocal syndrome of cutaneous and gastrointestinal venous malformations. Cutaneous lesions can be found over the entire body surface and usually become apparent by 2 years of age. They typically vary in size from 1–2 mm to 2 cm, and range in number from a single lesion to several hundred lesions that grow in proportion to the growth of the child. Skin lesions are most commonly flat or minimally raised and are deep blue or purple. They are often most dense on the plantar aspect of the feet.[5] Lesions may be tender to palpation and may become spontaneously painful. They may be partially emptied of blood if firm pressure is applied.[16]

Gastrointestinal manifestations can occur anywhere from the mouth to the rectum and may become symptomatic years after the appearance of cutaneous lesions. The number of intestinal lesions in a patient generally tends to parallel the number of cutaneous lesions, varying from a few to several hundred. Large gastrointestinal lesions may cause intussusception, resulting in the onset of acute abdominal pain and vomiting. Oral and esophageal lesions may compress the airway. Blood loss tends to be most prominent from small bowel lesions. Almost all patients have multiple lesions in the liver, but lesions can be present in the subcutaneous tissues, muscles, or almost any organ. A total body survey can be obtained using Tc-99m-labeled red blood cell scintigraphy.[5] Characteristically, there is pooling of the Tc-99m red blood cells within the lesions. Lesions have a pathognomonic endoscopic appearance, presenting as discrete purple, berry-like protuberances from several millimeters to several centimeters in size. Most lesions are sessile. A broad rim of normal mucosa is often at the base of the lesion and encircles its reddish blue apex.[5]

Patients inevitably develop chronic gastrointestinal bleeding and anemia, beginning early in infancy or in young adulthood. They eventually require ongoing transfusions and iron replacement supplemented with the administration of erythropoietin. Melena is common. Some patients also experience intermittent bouts of severe abdominal cramping secondary to recurrent small-bowel intussusceptions.[5,16]

Treatment varies depending on the degree of gastrointestinal tract involvement and the severity of symptoms. Patients with mild or moderate anemia usually do not require transfusions or surgical intervention. Acid reduction therapy with proton pump inhibitors is used to reduce bleeding from gastric lesions. Patients are advised to eat a diet rich in iron and to take iron supplements as well as multivitamins. Also, to reduce the chance of trauma and bleeding from lesions in the left colon, stool softeners are sometimes advised. While patients with moderate anemia require occasional blood transfusions, they are treated similarly. Additionally, endoscopic ablation may be used to treat problematic gastric or colonic lesions. Patients with persistent or severe anemia require multiple interventions over time, including frequent blood transfusions, endoscopic ablation and surgical excision of small-bowel lesions. Octreotide is used as a temporizing treatment method to stabilize patients prior to surgery.[16] Although there have been several published reports of treatment with pharmacological therapy, there is no sustained efficacy in their use. For patients with life-threatening bleeding that necessitates repeated transfusions, Fishman and Fox[6] advocate surgical excision. Through a combined endoscopic and open surgical approach, these authors inspect the entire gastrointestinal tract. Small-intestinal lesions are identified and resected. If superficial, lesions of the esophagus, stomach, duodenum, colon and rectum are eradicated by endoscopic band ligation. If not amenable to this approach, such lesions are surgically excised. The authors have reported that, with up to a 7-year follow-up, none of the nine patients who had undergone surgery developed anemia or required a transfusion after hospital discharge.[6]

Diffuse venous malformations

Diffuse venous malformations involve large adjacent segments of bowel and extraintestinal structures, including mesentery, retroperitoneum, pelvic space, muscles, subcutaneous tissue and skin. Diffuse upper visceral malformations may warrant treatment only if there is symptomatic portal hypertension. Selective portosystemic shunts may be beneficial in that they reduce portal–venous pressure in the malformation. Malformations of the lower gastrointestinal tract typically extend from the anorectum proximally, involving the left colon or the entire colon. Most of these lesions are transmural and may extend into the pelvic structures. Imaging studies often reveal thickening of the colonic and rectal wall. Colonoscopic examination reveals engorged purple mucosa with varix-like projections. These lesions often cause chronic hemorrhage that requires transfusions throughout life. Endoscopic therapy is often futile and may exacerbate hemorrhage and cause perforation. Depending on the extent of involvement, a variety of surgical options are used. These include partial or subtotal colectomy with end ileostomy or colostomy, or colectomy with anorectal mucosectomy and endorectal pull-through.[17] In most cases, full-thickness resection of the rectum should be avoided because of the risk of uncontrollable hemorrhage from the extrarectal pelvic venous malformation.

Lymphatic malformations

Lymphatic malformations (often incorrectly referred to as 'lymphangiomas') include a wide spectrum of anomalies that can vary from simple cutaneous lymphatic lesions to severe lymphatic malformations that involve different organs and anatomic regions. These malformations can be seen in any anatomic region but are more commonly seen in rich lymphatic areas, such as the neck, axilla, mediastinum, groin and retroperitoneum. They present in many forms, from tiny cutaneous or mucosal blebs to large channel or multilocular lesions. There are two morphological types of lymphatic malformation: microcystic and macrocystic. The former present as clear, tiny cutaneous vesicles that permeate the skin and muscles; these vesicles are often firm and may give the impression of a brawny edema. Macrocystic lesions are large, soft, smooth, translucent masses under normal or bluish skin. Capillary or venous malformations are frequently seen in association with lymphatic malformations.

Mesenteric cysts

Mesenteric cysts are rare macrocystic lesions that are thought to be lymphatic malformations (Figure 46.4). They may be malformations of the lacteals and major mesenteric lymphatic vessels, including the cisterna chyli, or may be more diffuse, involving retroperitoneum and mesentery. Lesions are occasionally associated with chylous ascites and protein-losing enteropathy. Although they can be found anywhere from the duodenum to the rectum, they most commonly occur in the mesentery of the small bowel; the retroperitoneum is the second most frequent site.[18] Children tend to present acutely, requiring urgent admission and surgical intervention. Complaint at presentation is commonly abdominal pain due to hemorrhage or obstruction. Intestinal obstruction may occur from volvulus or acute enlargement from hemorrhage into the cyst, or from compression of the adjacent bowel. Diagnosis is primarily made with ultrasonography, often followed by a computed tomography scan to confirm the cystic nature of the lesions (Figure 46.5). Ultrasonography also

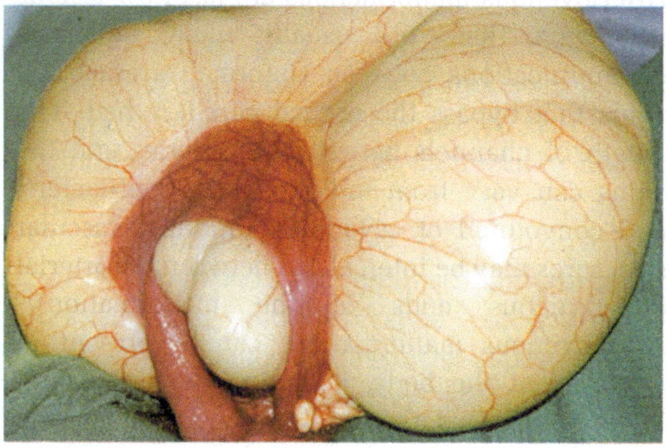

Figure 46.4 A mesenteric cyst seen at laparotomy in a 4-year-old with partial intestinal obstruction.

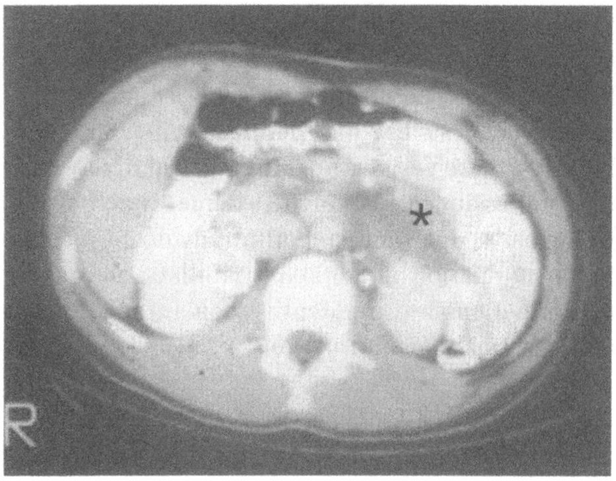

Figure 46.5 Computed tomography scan demonstrating a mesenteric cyst (asterisk).

provides preoperative measurements and is valuable for postoperative monitoring. When lesions are localized, small portions of the intestine can be resected with a good prognosis. In children in whom there is a diffuse process involving most of the intestinal mesentery, unroofing of major cysts to allow drainage of lymphatic fluid into the abdomen provides long-term relief of symptoms. In some patients with unremitting chylous ascites, oversewing of leaking retroperitoneal lymphatics is reportedly effective.[19] When there is respiratory compromise from massive chylous ascites or when other efforts are unsuccessful, peritoneovenous shunting is useful, although it carries significant risks.[20]

Arteriovenous malformations

Arteriovenous malformations are fast-flow lesions in which there are usually many abnormal communications between abnormal arteries and veins that bypass the normal capillary bed. The length of channels between the arteries and the veins can vary from millimeters to centimeters, and convoluted or cavernous abnormal vascular structures may be intercalated between the arterial and venous ends of the malformations.[6] Arteriovenous malformations can be present in any part of the body, including the upper and lower extremities, the head and neck, the gut, the liver, the lungs and the central nervous system. Cutaneous lesions become evident in infancy or childhood and are often initially mistaken for hemangioma or port wine stain. Puberty, pregnancy and trauma tend to trigger expansion, causing lesions to exhibit the cutaneous signs of its fast-flow nature. The skin becomes red or purplish, a mass appears beneath the vascular stain and there is local warmth, thrill and bruit.[4] This inevitably results in ischemic skin changes, ulceration, intractable pain and intermittent bleeding. In severe cases, lesions can result in high-output cardiac failure.

Symptomatic arteriovenous malformations of the gastrointestinal tract are extremely rare in childhood. Typically, patients develop massive hematochezia or chronic melena with iron deficiency anemia. A case of intestinal perforation secondary to an arteriovenous malformation has also been reported.[21] As with cutaneous arteriovenous malformations, some patients present with pain and, in severe cases, with high-output cardiac failure. Endoscopic examination of the bowel may reveal a pulsatile vascular lesion. Endoscopic ultrasonography demonstrates high flow through the lesion.

Traditional angiography or magnetic resonance imaging help in localizing the arteriovenous malformation and are essential for diagnosis and treatment planning. Angiography frequently shows characteristic enlargement and an increased number of arteries; on the venous phase, there is early venous return and venous dilatation in the region of the malformation.

Embolization alone may lead to intestinal necrosis and perforation. Embolization combined with surgical excision is, however, the treatment of choice. Amenability of lesions to complete excision depends upon their extent and location. Specific localization in the gastrointestinal tract before resection can be enhanced by tattooing during selective angiography.[22] When resection is possible, it is curative. Proximal vessel ligation alone or embolization combined with incomplete surgical resection may result in the re-establishment of additional feeding vessels, and lead to re-expansion of the arteriovenous malformation.[5]

Complex combined vascular malformations

While various combinations of anomalous vessel channel types can occur, the most common gross vascular abnormalities to affect the gastrointestinal tract are evidenced in Klippel–Trénaunay syndrome. This condition results from a combination of capillary, lymphatic and venous malformations and is characterized by purple capillary stains, limb hypertrophy, congenitally abnormal veins and lymphatic vesicles that often protrude through the skin. It is not uncommon for lesions to extend into the pelvis, involving both the bowel and the bladder. As with lower visceral diffuse venous malformations, these lesions typically extend from the anus proximally to involve part of or the entire colon (Figure 46.6).[5] Colonoscopic appearances differ, showing varying degrees of mural thickening and vascular discoloration. Patients with severe chronic anemia due to hemorrhage or with recurrent cellulitis of the buttock or thigh require therapeutic intervention. Such infections are sometimes attributed to the translocation of enteric organisms from the feces through the abnormal mucosal barrier into the malformation. These symptoms may be minimized or eliminated by partial colectomy with a diverting colostomy, or by colectomy with anorectal mucosectomy and a coloanal pull-through procedure.[23] Extensive perineal malformations may preclude performing the pull-through procedure.[5]

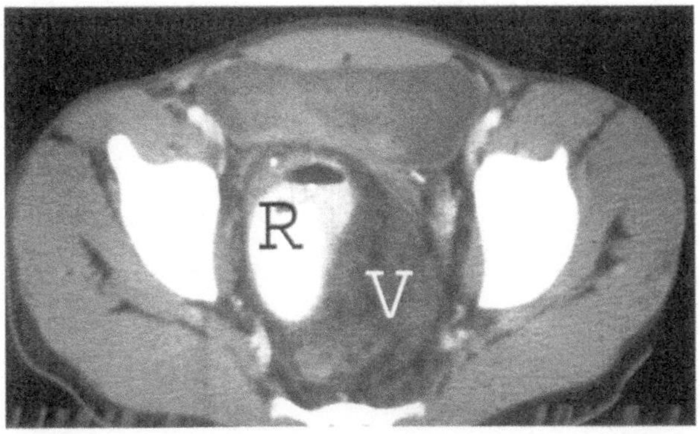

Figure 46.6 Computed tomography scan in a patient with Klippel–Trénaunay syndrome and profuse rectal bleeding demonstrating a complex venous malformation (V) adjacent to the rectum (R).

Summary

Although bleeding is the most common symptom of both vascular tumors and vascular malformations, diagnostic and treatment approaches are entirely different. Understanding the biological classifications and natural history of these lesions is thus essential. In light of the varied etiologies and complexity of vascular lesions, particularly those with visceral components, an individualized and interdisciplinary approach is frequently required. The importance of using current nomenclature to ensure optimal communication and understanding cannot be overemphasized.

REFERENCES

1. Mulliken JB, Glowacki J. Hemangiomas and vascular malformations in infants and children: a classification based on endothelial characteristics. *Plast Reconstr Surg* 1982; **69**: 412–422.
2. Martinez-Perez D, Fein NA, Boon LM et al. Not all hemangiomas look like strawberries: uncommon presentations of the most common tumor of infancy. *Pediatr Dermatol* 1995; **12**: 1–6.
3. Meyer JS, Hoffer FA, Barnes PD. Biological classification of soft-tissue vascular anomalies: MR correlation. *Am J Roentgenol* 1991; **157**: 559–564.
4. Mulliken JB, Fishman SJ. Vascular anomalies: hemangiomas and malformations. In O'Neill JA, Rowe MI, Grosfeld JL et al., eds. *Pediatric Surgery*, 5th edn. St Louis, MO: Mosby, 1998: 1939–1951.
5. Azizkhan RG. Vascular lesions in childhood. In Fischer JE, Baker RJ, eds. *Mastery of Surgery*, 4th edn. Philadelphia, PA: Lippincott, Williams & Wilkins, 2001: 389–403.
6. Fishman SJ, Fox VL. Visceral vascular anomalies. *Gastrointest Endosc Clin North Am* 2001; **11**: 813–834.
7. Fishman SJ, Burrows PE, Leichtner AM et al. Gastrointestinal manifestations of vascular anomalies in childhood: varied etiologies require multiple therapeutic modalities. *J Pediatr Surg* 1998; **33**: 1163–1167.
8. Enjolras O, Riche MC, Merland JJ et al. Management of alarming hemangiomas in infancy: a review of 25 cases. *Pediatrics* 1990; **85**: 491–498.
9. Ezekowitz RA, Mulliken JB, Folkman J. Interferon alfa-2a therapy for life-threatening hemangiomas of infancy. *N Engl J Med* 1992; **326**: 1456–1463.
10. Vesikari T, Nuutila A, Cantell K. Neurologic sequelae following interferon therapy of juvenile laryngeal papilloma. *Acta Paediatr Scand* 1988; **77**: 619–622.
11. Worle H, Maass E, Kohler B et al. Interferon alpha-2a therapy in haemangiomas of infancy: spastic diplegia as a severe complication. *Eur J Pediatr* 1999; **158**: 344.

12. Barlow CF, Priebe CJ, Mulliken JB et al. Spastic diplegia as a complication of interferon Alfa-2a treatment of hemangiomas of infancy. *J Pediatr* 1998; **132**: 527–530.
13. Guttmacher AE, Marchuk DA, White RI Jr. Hereditary hemorrhagic telangiectasia. *N Engl J Med* 1995; **333**: 918–924.
14. Ballauff A, Koletzko S. Hereditary hemorrhagic telangiectasia with juvenile polyposis – coincidence or linked autosomal dominant inheritance? *Z Gastroenterol* 1999; **37**: 385–388.
15. Inoue S, Matsumoto T, Iida M et al. Juvenile polyposis occurring in hereditary hemorrhagic telangiectasia. *Am J Med Sci* 1999; **317**: 59–62.
16. Andersen JM. Blue rubber bleb nevus syndrome. *Curr Treat Options Gastroenterol* 2001; **4**: 433–440.
17. Fishman SJ, Shamberger RC, Fox VL et al. Endorectal pull-through abates gastrointestinal hemorrhage from colorectal venous malformations. *J Pediatr Surg* 2000; **35**: 982–984.
18. Kurtz RJ, Heimann TM, Holt J et al. Mesenteric and retroperitoneal cysts. *Ann Surg* 1986; **203**: 109–111.
19. Unger SW, Chandler JG. Chylous ascites in infants and children. *Surgery* 1983; **93**: 455–461.
20. Chang JHT, Newkirk J, Carlton G et al. Generalized lymphangiomatosis with chylous ascites – Treatment by peritoneo-venous shunting. *J Pediatr Surg* 1980; **15**: 748–750.
21. Munn J, Hussain AN, Castelli MJ et al. Ileal perforation due to arteriovenous malformation in a premature infant. *J Pediatr Surg* 1990; **25**: 701–703.
22. Frémond B, Yazbeck S, Dubois J et al. Intestinal vascular anomalies in children. *J Pediatr Surg* 1997; **32**: 873–877.
23. Telander RL, Ahlquist D, Blaufuss MC. Rectal mucosectomy: a definitive approach to extensive hemangiomas of the rectum. *J Pediatr Surg* 1993; **22**: 379–381.

47 The role of minimally invasive surgery in pediatric gastrointestinal disease

Stig Somme and Donald C Liu

Introduction

Traditionally, large incisions have been considered necessary for adequate surgical exposure. However, these wounds frequently result in significant perioperative stress and postoperative pain and morbidity, not to mention poor cosmesis. The concept of avoiding large incisions to perform invasive surgery forms the basis for the revolution of minimally invasive surgery. In this chapter, we focus on and describe minimally invasive procedures that are performed in infants and children with gastrointestinal disease.

Background

With advances in microchip technology and micro-instrumentation, as well as the development of sophisticated video equipment with supreme optics, the stage was set for the rapid development of minimally invasive surgery in the form of intracavitary endoscopic surgery, better known as laparoscopy in adults. The first significant minimally invasive surgery performed in adults was the laparoscopic cholecystectomy.[1] This sentinel event in general surgery, however, had little initial impact on the practice of pediatric surgery in children with gastrointestinal disease.

Several factors are thought to be responsible for the slow development of the practice of minimally invasive surgery in children. Unfortunately, physicians, particularly surgeons, typically have underappreciated postoperative pain and surgical stress in young children, who essentially are unable adequately to verbalize their discomfort. Furthermore, the advantages of smaller incisions were underestimated by pediatric surgeons, because they already use 'small incisions' in their patients. However, in reality, when incision length is compared with body size, pediatric incisions for open procedures are proportional to adult incisions for comparable procedures.

The need to develop endoscopic techniques further deters their use in children. Minimally invasive surgery demands that the surgeon acquire not only an entirely new set of surgical skills, but often requires an entirely different way of thinking about common pediatric surgical problems. The lack of depth perception and tactile sensation required during endoscopic procedures necessitate major changes in operative technique. The operative choreography for minimally invasive surgery often deviates from the routine fixated in the mind of the pediatric surgeon from years of traditional training. Increasingly, however, reports and the literature are documenting the safety, efficacy and cost-effectiveness of minimally invasive surgery in children and are showing a rapid evolution in instrumentation and the performance of such procedures.[2,3]

Minimally invasive surgery in children has become a highlight and focus of many general pediatric surgery practices across the world. At the present time, the number of minimally invasive procedures being performed for pediatric gastrointestinal diseases is growing rapidly. Current practice techniques for various pediatric gastrointestinal diseases are listed in Table 47.1 and are categorized under laparoscopy.

Technical considerations

The key concepts behind laparoscopic surgery are to obtain safe access to the abdominal cavity and create an 'operating dome' through establishment of pneumoperitoneum. Small trocars ranging from 2 to 12 mm in size are subsequently placed

Table 47.1 Pediatric gastrointestinal diseases treatable via minimally invasive surgery

Disease	Laparoscopy
Achalasia	Heller myotomy
Appendicitis	appendectomy
Chronic abdominal pain	diagnostic laparoscopy
Constipation	appendicostomy (ACE procedure)
Crohn's disease	enterectomy
Gallstone disease	cholecystectomy
Gastroesophageal reflux disease	fundoplication
Hirschsprung's disease	endorectal pull-through
Imperforate anus	anal reconstruction
Pyloric stenosis	pyloromyotomy
Ulcerative colitis	colectomy, ileoanal reconstruction

strategically to facilitate placement of miniaturized endoscopic instruments to perform surgery. Initial access to the peritoneum via the umbilicus is generally obtained by two different methods: direct puncture via the Veress needle or direct vision through the Hasson technique.[4] The skin is bluntly grasped, a small incision through the dermis made and the spring-loaded Veress needle advanced into the abdominal cavity. Gas insufflation is started using low gas flow and pneumoperitneum achieved. The Hasson technique mandates direct vision of the fascia and peritoneum before a blunt trocar is passed into the abdominal cavity, and is the technique preferred for patients with a history of previous abdominal surgery. Some surgeons advocate the use of the Hasson technique on a routine basis because of some support in the literature for a lowered risk of major complications compared with the Veress needle technique.[5]

The intra-abdominal pressure is adjusted according to the size of the patient with intra-abdominal pressures ranging from 5 to 15 mmHg.[6] For example, in infants of < 2 kg, an intra-abdominal pressure of 5 mmHg would suffice, compared to 15 mmHg in an adult-sized adolescent.

Gastroesophageal reflux disease

Pathological gastroesophageal reflux in infants and children is occurring in almost epidemic proportions.[7] The use of laparoscopic techniques to treat severe gastroesophageal reflux disease (GERD) in children has gained much popularity among pediatric surgeons, with successful surgical outcome described in several large series.[8,9] In cases of severe GERD that are refractory to medical therapy, almost all pediatric surgeons perform fundoplication as the surgical treatment of choice.[10] In most series, laparoscopic Nissen fundoplication was the most commonly performed procedure, although there have been various modifications, including the Rossetti modification, where the short gastric vessels are not routinely divided, and partial fundoplication techniques theoretically minimize the risk of intra- and postoperative difficulties.[8–10] In any event, the operation traditionally performed has been completed via laparotomy through a long midline or subcostal incision. With minimally invasive surgery, fundoplication is performed laparoscopically via five small (2–5 mm) puncture sites and typically is completed in less than 1 h (Figure 47.1). The child is often discharged by postoperative day 1 or 2, with minimal morbidity. Compared with the open procedure (laparotomy), perioperative morbidity consisting of incisional pain and related complications such as atelectasis or pneumonia appears to decrease. The incidence of known complications of fundoplication including postoperative dysphagia and/or gas bloat syndrome appears to be similar if not less in minimally invasive surgery series presented thus far compared to historical results of open

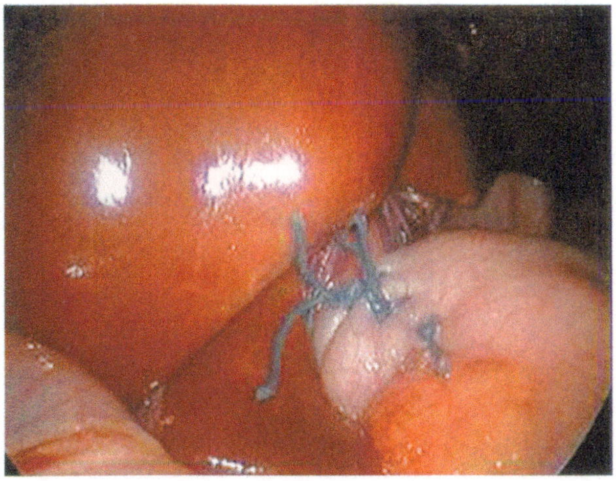

Figure 47.1 Laparoscopic Nissen fundoplication: 360° fundic wrap.

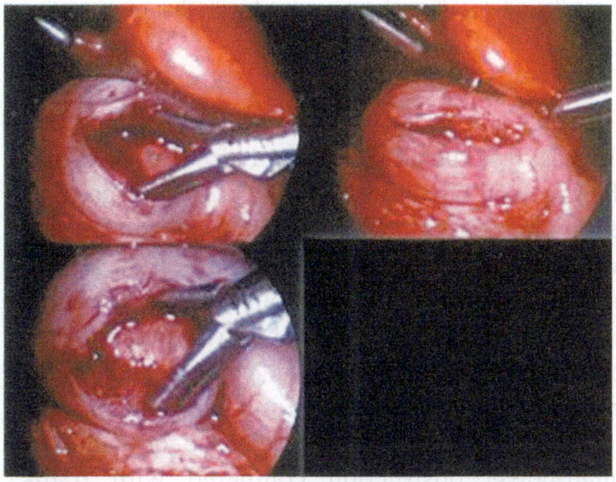

Figure 47.2 Laparoscopic pyloromyotomy. The pylorus is incised sharply with a sheathed blade and the pyloric muscle is then carefully split and spread along the hypertrophic pylorus.

fundoplication.[8,9] Importantly, strict postoperative dietary regimen enforcement and manipulation appears to contribute significantly to the avoidance of the necessity of esophageal dilatation in a population expected to have varying degrees of dysphagia secondary to the nature of the operation. Results in preventing GERD thus far have been excellent with recurrence rate less than 10% at 5 years, similar to if not in some cases lower than historical controls obtained from the 'open' operation.[8–10] Longer follow-up, however, would be needed to establish the rate of recurrence in children undergoing laparoscopic fundoplication for GERD.

It is likely that new treatment modalities, that are even less invasive, will be used to a larger extent in the treatment of GERD. One such techniquo that has recently been introduced is Stretta.[11] This utilizes an endoscopic device with several perpendicular probes that are launched by the operator under videoscopic guidance. The probes are advanced into the mucosa of the lower esophageal sphincter and an electrical current is applied through the probes. This creates fibrosis in the area that, in cases of mild-to-moderate GERD, is enough to obviate gastroesophageal reflux. Data from the adult patient population indicates that Stretta is safe and that it relieves the symptoms of GERD.[12,13] No published follow-up data exists for pediatric patients.

Pyloric stenosis

In infants with pyloric stenosis, laparoscopic pyloromyotomy is performed through three puncture wounds (approximately 2 mm in length each) in the upper abdomen. The pylorus is incised sharply with a sheath blade, and the pyloric muscle is then carefully split and spread along the length of the hypertropic pylorus (Figure 47.2). Children typically are discharged the following day with complete resolution of symptoms. Several studies have demonstrated the safety and efficacy of this procedure, although improvements in relevant surgical outcome parameters such as operating time and length of hospital stay have not been demonstrated when compared to the open procedure.[14,15] However, cosmesis is excellent and can be compared with that of an open pyloromyotomy (Figure 47.3).

Inflammatory bowel disease

Several series reporting the results of laparoscopic procedures for the treatment of inflammatory bowel disease have clearly demonstrated the feasibility of minimally invasive surgery in the pediatric population. Laparoscopic colectomy was first described in 1991 and, since then, laparoscopic colorectal procedures in adults ranging from simple ileocolic resection for Crohn's disease to complex total colectomy with ileal/anal reconstruction for ulcerative colitis have been well

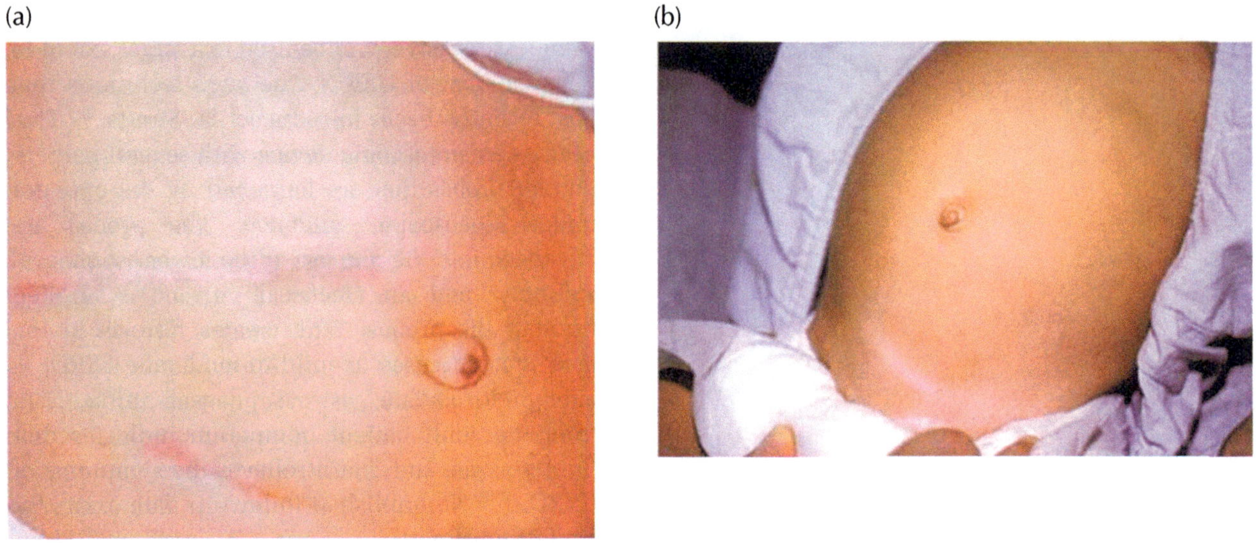

Figure 47.3 Children who have undergone laparoscopic pyloromyotomy (a) and (b) typically are discharged the following day with complete resolution of symptoms. Cosmesis is excellent (b) and can be compared with that of an open pyloromyotomy (a).

described.[16–18] However, acceptance of minimally invasive surgery as a standard surgical technique for Crohn's disease remains controversial. Theoretically, the gross inflammation and phlegmon characteristic of Crohn's disease can simulate landmines to the inexperienced laparoscopic surgeon. Nevertheless, these complications, plus their severe sequelae, can be effectively addressed by the careful, experienced laparoscopic surgeon. This, and the fact that Crohn's disease affects a predominately younger group of patients who are likely to require re-resection, lends support to the application of minimally invasive surgery in Crohn's disease. The pan-enteric and recurrent nature of Crohn's disease renders a surgical cure impossible and results in re-operation in 70–90% of all patients and multiple procedures in more than 30%.[19] Ileocolic disease comprises the majority of surgical morbidity and predicts a high probability for surgical intervention. Furthermore, patients with ileocolic disease have the highest risk of recurrence, contributing to >40% probability for re-operation at 15 years. Laparoscopic ileocecectomy, the most common minimally invasive surgery procedure in children with Crohn's disease, can be performed without complications and with excellent cosmesis (Figures 47.4 and 47.5).[16] Furthermore, in children with intra-abdominal abscesses, minimally invasive surgery techniques can be used successfully to drain the abscess, lyse the adhesions and also ascertain that the involved bowel was healthy enough according to the surgeon's judgement to warrant or not warrant resection, keeping in mind that bowel preservation is the hallmark of surgery for Crohn's disease.[20] Thus, minimally invasive surgery with its advantages of decreased postoperative pain from small wound sites, low incidence of hernias, better cosmesis and decreased rate of adhesive small-bowel obstruction compared with traditional laparotomy seem ideal in this patient population, who more often than not will require re-operation in the future. Laparoscopy reduces the need for surgical procedures not related to disease in this population and preserves the abdominal wall should stomas be needed in the future. Also, tiny, nearly invisible, strategically placed scars improve the perception of cosmesis in this younger population with already significant body image issues.

Children with acute ulcerative colitis are generally referred for surgery on an emergency basis after failing to respond to aggressive medical therapy, including high-dose steroids and other immunosuppressants.[17] In these often acutely ill children, we favor a staged surgical approach highlighted by initial subtotal colectomy and ileostomy followed by completion proctectomy and ileoanal pouch reconstruction several months later. From a

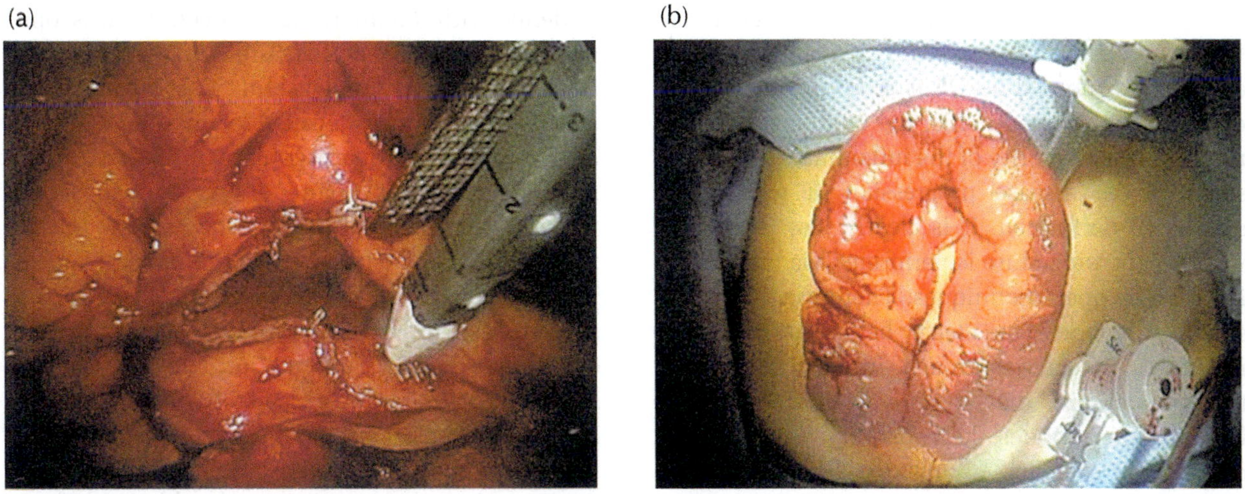

Figure 47.4 (a) Laparoscopically dissected diseased terminal ileum of Crohn's disease; (b) exteriorized diseased bowel segment after laparoscopic dissection.

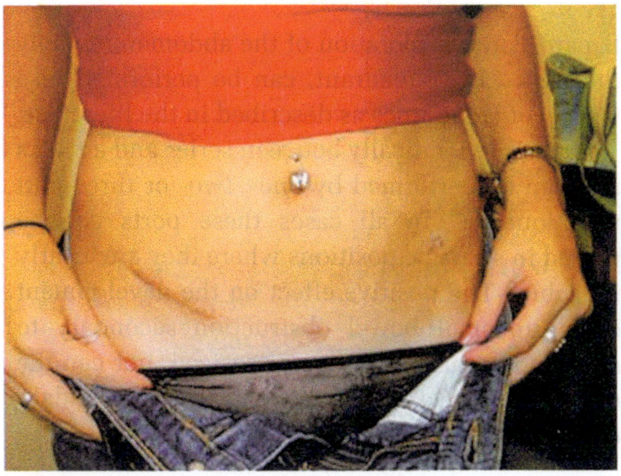

Figure 47.5 Excellent cosmesis following laparascopic colectomy for Crohn's disease.

technical standpoint, a mini-Pfannenstiel incision of 2–3 cm is a critical addition to our procedure because it facilitates safer dissection and subsequent transection at the rectosigmoid junction and, in addition, facilitates removal of the entire specimen. Laparoscopic subtotal colectomy in several series has been shown to be a safe procedure with acceptable blood loss.[17,21–27] Subsequent proctectomy and ileoanal reconstruction can be successfully completed with excellent results.

The most common criticism of laparoscopic intestinal surgery in patients with inflammatory bowel disease has been increased operative time with resultant increased morbidity due to length of surgery. With increasing operative experience, it is fair to assume that operating times will decrease as surgeons gain experience and will be comparable to traditional open surgery.

Although larger numbers of patients, longer-term follow-up, and a prospective, randomized, controlled study are necessary to determine the advantages of minimally invasive surgery in children with inflammatory bowel disease, preliminary results from several studies have demonstrated at the very least that minimally invasive surgery is a safe and viable surgical option. We are of the opinion that, with improving technology, increased surgeon expertise and better selection of patient populations, minimally invasive surgery may well become the standard approach when surgery for inflammatory bowel disease becomes necessary.

Appendicitis

Appendicitis is the most common diagnosis in children that requires emergency surgical intervention. Several randomized studies have compared open versus laparoscopic appendectomy and the results show a slight, but significant, reduction in postoperative wound infections.[28,29] However, all other parameters compared, including length of stay, need for re-exploration, cost and pain showed no significant difference between the two groups. Some studies have even indicated that the laparoscopic/minimally invasive surgery operation takes more time.[2,30] It is apparent that, in children with appendicitis, the outcome depends mainly on the severity of the inflammation and the stage of the disease progression at which the surgery is performed. It is clearly less important whether the procedure is performed via minimally invasive or open techniques. There are, however, some patients who are clearly better served with a minimally invasive approach, in particular when the preoperative diagnosis is in question. The laparoscope provides the capability of looking at other organ systems, e.g. ovaries, Fallopian tubes and even the gallbladder, to investigate various pathologies. Patients who often fall into this category are adolescent females or obese patients.

In cases where the appendix has perforated, as documented via radiological studies, a decision can be made regarding the practice of 'interval' appendectomy.[29] In these cases intravenous antibiotics or a combination of intravenous and oral antibiotics are initiated in the patient and carried out for 4–6 weeks, at which time the appendix is subsequently removed ('interval appendectomy') on an out-patient basis via minimally invasive surgery.

In summary, laparoscopic appendectomy is a good, albeit sometimes unnecessary, option in uncomplicated appendicitis. In the cases that are difficult to diagnose, and where exposure would be difficult, minimally invasive surgery is the technique of choice, resulting in better cosmesis.

Chronic abdominal pain of unknown origin

In children with complaints of non-specific abdominal pain and where an extensive work-up including abdominal ultrasonography, computerized tomography, upper gastrointestinal series and/or upper and lower endoscopy cannot identify any pathology, laparoscopic exploration of the abdomen has been shown to be useful.[31] The laparoscope provides an optimal tool for visualizing the entire abdominal cavity. Particularly in females, the adnexa and uterus can be inspected and manipulated atraumatically. The bowel can be inspected in its entire intraperitoneal length. In patients with Mediterranean fever, laparoscopic evaluation of the abdomen and elective appendectomy have been found useful, to rule out perforated appendicitis as a cause for peritonitis. Some surgeons believe laparoscopic exploration for ill-defined abdominal pain or abdominal sepsis provides the ability to identify the problem and in most cases also the possibility of immediate repair. Importantly, unusual causes of abdominal pain such as Meckel's diverticulum and related pathology (diverticulitis), obstruction, intussusception secondary to various lead points including Meckel's, perforated duodenal ulcer, or inflammatory bowel disease, notably Crohn's disease, can be discovered at laparoscopy and addressed from both a diagnostic and therapeutic perspective. Furthermore, unnecessary large disfiguring incisions can be avoided with the same postoperative result.

Laparoscopic exploration of the abdomen, notably the right lower quadrant, can be performed in a variety of techniques as described in the literature. These vary specifically between series and authors and can be performed by one-, two- or three-port technique.[28,29] In all cases these ports can be placed in strategic positions where they are 'nearly invisible'. The positive effect on the development of future small-bowel obstruction secondary to adhesions cannot be overemphasized, nor can the theoretical affect of preserving fertility secondary to minimizing adhesions in a female child.

Cholecystectomy

Etiologies for gallbladder disease in children are many and have been extensively reviewed elsewhere in this text. When cholecystectomy becomes necessary, laparoscopic cholecystectomy can be performed safely and effectively with excellent cosmetic results. Laparoscopic cholecystectomy has for more than a decade been considered a standard of care for removal of the gallbladder in uncomplicated cases.[1] Important adjuncts to biliary track surgery including performance of intraoperative cholangiogram and common bile duct exploration for choledocholithiasis can also be performed via minimally invasive techniques. Laparoscopic cholecystectomy is generally performed through four ports (2–5 mm) and the gallbladder is removed through the umbilicus. Both automatic and single reloadable stapling devices are used to ligate the cystic duct and artery. Important considerations in laparoscopic cholecystectomy include consideration of potential aberrant anatomy of the hepatic arteries specifically the right hepatic artery coming off the superior mesenteric artery (10% of occasions). Sometimes, the superior mesenteric artery can be mistaken for the cystic artery, especially in a small child. The greatest complication that can occur in laparoscopic cholecystectomy is injury to the common bile duct, which can be devastating, notably in a small child where biliary reconstruction can be prohibitive.[1] Thus, it is important to identify clearly the common bile duct, cystic duct and cystic artery prior to ligation and division of any of these structures. If there is any doubt as to the anatomy of the biliary tract, an intraoperative cholangiogram should be performed and conversion to laparotomy considered to prevent a devastating common bile duct injury.

Constipation

Constipation in children is 90% from functional causes versus 10% from mechanical causes. Hirschsprung's disease is the most common surgical cause of constipation in children. Endorectal pull-through for Hirschsprung's disease was first described by Soave in 1963.[32] In this technique, a ganglionic segment of colon is pulled down to the muscular cuff in the rectal canal after transabdominal mucosectomy of the distal sigmoid colon. The technique was modified by Boley, who performed a coloanal anastomosis to complete the operation.[33] Common to these techniques is the fact that the rectal mucosectomy was performed via laparotomy. Today, advancements in minimally invasive techniques and instrumentation permit surgeons to mobilize the colon and perform a pull-through operation by minimally invasive techniques. Furthermore, rectal mucosectomy, aganglionic colectomy and normal ganglionic pull-through are performed by some surgeons entirely through the anus without the aid of laparotomy or laparoscopy, a truly minimally invasive approach.[32,33]

A critical step in any minimally invasive surgery technique for Hirschsprung's disease is transanal mucosectomy.[34] Transanal mucosectomy provides several advantages, as follows. In open cases, it allows for shorter operating times, because a mucosectomy can be performed simultaneously and even completed during laparotomy. Transanal mucosectomy in conjunction with laparoscopic techniques theoretically confers all the advantages of laparoscopy versus laparotomy, including reduced hospital stay, less postoperative ileus and better cosmesis. Favorable postoperative outcomes with an acceptable rate of constipation, strictures, no reported incontinence of stools and an acceptable incidence of enterocolitis, the most significant complication of Hirschsprung's disease, have been reported by several authors.

In cases were children have been deemed to have functional constipation and where no surgical causes can be found, few surgical options exist. One option, however, that has been shown to be effective is the appendicostomy enema or so-called ACE procedure.[35] In this technique, the appendix is used as a conduit for daily enemas to relieve symptoms of constipation. This procedure can be performed laparoscopically; the appendix is mobilized and brought out to the skin and used effectively as the entry site for enemas. The minimally invasive techniques used to complete the ACE procedure allow for easier postoperative recovery, less postoperative ileus and, importantly, better cosmesis, especially in children who already have self-image issues, such as children with spinal dysraphism syndromes.

Ladd's procedure

As part of the work-up for recurrent emesis in children, an upper gastrointestinal series is performed generally to assess for gastroesophageal reflux disease. Occasionally during these studies, however, malrotation is found to be present and thought to be the etiology. In order to address emesis surgically in cases of malrotation, and importantly lower the future incidence of midgut volvulus, an elective Ladd's procedure is performed. Surgeons today have described performing this procedure through minimally invasive techniques where division of Ladd's bands, appendectomy and placement of the cecum in the left side of the abdomen can be performed laparoscopically.[36] Clearly, the advantages of performing this procedure via minimally invasive techniques are less postoperative pain, shorter time until recovery from the postoperative ileus and a much improved cosmetic result. A longer follow-up period will be necessary to compare the incidence of midgut volvulus in the two groups receiving the open versus minimally invasive procedure.

Complications

In addition to the complications that are specific for each procedure, there are complications uniquely associated with laparoscopic procedures in general.[5] The most feared complications are the major vascular injuries. These injuries are not common, with an incidence of 0.05% in the adult literature, but have a high mortality when they occur, ranging from 8 to 17%. The most common major complication is perforation of hollow-organ viscera during insertion of the Veress needle or trocar, the most commonly injured being the small bowel. Dissection-related hollow- or solid-organ injuries may also occur, though with lower frequency. Most safety studies have clearly demonstrated a higher incidence of complications early in the learning curve of the surgeon, with significant decrease coinciding with increasing experience. Most complications do not result in conversion to laparotomy (< 30%).[5] Importantly, keeping in mind that patient safety is foremost, the surgeon should not hesitate to convert to traditional laparotomy at a moment's notice.

Conclusion

As more pediatric surgeons become involved in performing minimally invasive surgery in children with pediatric gastroenterological diseases, the application of these techniques will expand. It is beyond the scope of this chapter to describe several other successful applications, such as minimally invasive surgery for achalasia or anorectal malformations such as imperforate anus. However, it is clear that minimally invasive surgery can be performed safely in children with gastrointestinal disease and can be of significant benefit. The reduction in pain, wound complications and length of stay combined with improved cosmesis fuels the drive of surgeons today to expand the application of minimally invasive surgery to children with gastrointestinal diseases.

REFERENCES

1. Miller TA. Laparoscopic cholecystectomy; passing fantasy or legitimate treatment option? *Gastroenterology* 1990; **5**: 1527–1529.
2. Ure BM, Bax NM, van der Zee DC. Laparoscopy in infants and children: a prospective study on feasibility and the impact on routine surgery. *J Pediatr Surg* 2000; **35**: 1170–1173.
3. Reissman P, Durst AL, Rivkind A et al. Elective laparoscopic appendectomy in patients with familial Mediterranean fever. *World J Surg* 1994; **18**: 139–141.
4. Champault G, Cazacu F, Taffinder N. Serious trocar accidents in laparoscopic surgery: a French survey of 103,852 operations. *Surg Laparosc Endosc* 1996; **6**: 367–370.
5. Esposito C, Mattioli G, Monguzzi GL et al. Complications and conversions of pediatric videosurgery: the Italian multicentric experience on 1689 procedures. *Surg Endosc* 2002; **16**: 795–798.
6. Bax NM, van der Zee. DC. Trocar fixation during endoscopic surgery in infants and children. *Surg Endosc* 1998; **12**: 181–182.
7. Blewett CJ, Hollenbeak CS, Cilley RE, Dillon PW. Economic implications of current surgical management of gastroesophageal reflux disease. *J Pediatr Surg* 2002; **37**: 427–430.
8. Collins JB, Georgeson KE, Vicente Y et al. Comparison of open and laparoscopic gastrostomy and fundoplication in 120 patients. *J Pediatr Surg* 1995; **30**: 1065–1071.
9. Liu DC, Flattman GJ, Karam MT et al. Laparoscopic fundoplication in children with previous abdominal surgery. *J Pediatr Surg* 2000; **35**: 334–337.
10. Watson DI, Pike GK, Baigrie, RL et al. Prospective double-blind randomized trial of laparoscopic Nissen fundoplication with division and without division of short gastric vessels. *Ann Surg* 1997; **226**: 642–652.
11. Triadafilopoulous G. Stretta. An effective minimally-invasive treatment for gastroesophageal reflux disease. *Am J Med* 2003; **115** (Suppl 3A).
12. Triadafilopoulous G. Clinical experience with the Stretta procedure. *Gastrointest Endosc Clin North Am* 2003; **13**: 145–155.

13. Richards WO, Houston HL, Torquati A et al. Paradigm shift in the management of gastroesophageal reflux disease. *Ann Surg* 2003; **37**: 638–649.
14. Caceres M, Liu D. Laparoscopic pyloromyotomy: redefining the advantages of a novel technique. *JSLS* 2003; **7**: 123–127.
15. Campbell BT, McLean K, Barnhart DC et al. A comparison of laparoscopic and open pyloromyotomy at a teaching hospital. *J Pediatr Surg* 2002; **37**: 1068–1071.
16. Falk PM, Beart RW Jr, Wexner SD et al. Laparoscopic colectomy: a critical appraisal. *Dis Colon Rectum* 1993; **36**: 28–34.
17. Jacobs M, Verdeja JC, Goldstein HS. Minimally invasive colon resection (laparoscopic colectomy). *Surg Laparosc Endosc* 1991; **1**: 144–150.
18. Hunter JG. The case for fellowships in gastrointestinal and laparoendoscopic surgery. *Surgery* 2002; **132**: 523–525.
19. Lock MR, Farmer RG, Fazio VW et al. Recurrence and reoperation for Crohn's disease. A role of disease location in prognosis. *N Engl J Med* 1981; **304**: 1586–1588.
20. Geis WP, Kim HC. Use of laparoscopy in the diagnosis and treatment of patients with surgical abdominal sepsis. *Surg Endosc* 1995; **9**: 178–182.
21. Gurland BH, Wexner SD. Laparoscopic surgery for inflammatory bowel disease: results of the past decade. *Inflamm Bowel Dis* 2002; **8**: 46–54.
22. Chen HH, Wexner SD, Iroatulam AJN et al. Laparoscopic colectomy compares favorably with colectomy by laparotomy for reduction of postoperative ileus. *Dis Colon Rectum*, 2000; **43**: 61–65.
23. Duepree HJ, Senagore AJ, Delaney CP et al. Advantages of laparoscopic resection for ileocecal Crohn's disease. *Dis Colon Rectum* 2002; **45**: 605–610.
24. Milsom JW, Bohm B, Hammerhofer KA et al. A prospective, randomized trial comparing laparoscopic versus conventional techniques in colorectal cancer surgery: a preliminary report. *J Am Coll Surg* 1998; **187**: 46–57.
25. Paik PS, Beart RW Jr. Laparoscopic colectomy. *Surg Clin North Am* 1997; **77**: 1–3.
26. Proctor ML, Langer JC, Gerstle JT et al. Is laparoscopic subtotal coloctomy better than open subtotal colectomy in children? *J Ped Surg* 2002; **37**: 706–708.
27. Ramos JM, Beart RW Jr, Goes R et al. Role of laparoscopy in colorectal surgery: a prospective evaluation of 200 cases. *Dis Colon Rectum* 1995; **38**: 494–501.
28. Morfesis FA, Ahmad F. Use of laparoscopy in the treatment of acute and chronic right lower quadrant pain. *J Ky Med Assoc* 1996; **94**: 16–21.
29. Nowzaradan Y, Barnes JP Jr, Westmoreland J, Hojabri M. Laparoscopic appendectomy: treatment of choice for suspected appendicitis. *Surg Laparosc Endosc* 1993; **3**: 411–416.
30. Lujan Mompean JA, Robles Campos R, Parrilla Paricio P et al. Laparoscopic versus open appendicectomy: a prospective assessment. *Br J Surg* 1994; **81**: 133–135.
31. Schier F, Waldschmidt J. Laparoscopy in children with ill-defined abdominal pain. *Surg Endosc* 1994; **8**: 97–99.
32. Georgeson KE, Inge TH, Albanese CT. Laparoscopically assisted anorectal pull-through for high imperforate anus – a new technique. *J Pediatr Surg* 2000; **35**: 930–931.
33. Georgeson KE, Fuenfer MM, Hardin WD. Primary laparoscopic pull-through for Hirschsprung's disease in infants and children. *J Pediatr Surg* 1995; **30**: 1017–1021.
34. Liu DC, Rodriguez J, Hill CB, Loe WA Jr. Transanal mucosectomy in the treatment of Hirschsprung's disease. *J Pediatric Surg* 2000; **35**: 235–238.
35. Lynch AC, Beasley SW, Robertson RW, Morreau PN. Comparison of results of laparoscopic and open antegrade continence enema procedure. *Pediatr Surg Int* 1999; **15**; 343–346.
36. Bass KD, Rothenberg SS, Chang JH Laparoscopic Ladd's procedure in infants with malrotation. *J Pediatr Surg* 1998; **33**: 279–281.

48 Polyps and other tumors of the gastrointestinal tract

Warren Hyer and John Fell

Introduction

Gastrointestinal polyps in children most commonly present with rectal bleeding and may have potential for malignant change if part of a polyposis syndrome. This chapter reviews the polyposis syndromes, the genetics of these conditions, their malignant potential and their management algorithms. Other tumors of the gastrointestinal tract are discussed.

Gastrointestinal polyps

Histopathological classification

Gastrointestinal polyps in children fall into two major categories: hamartomas and adenomas (Table 48.1). Solitary polyps in children are most commonly hamartomas, predominantly of the juvenile type. Of the familial syndromes, familial adenomatous polyposis is more common than juvenile polyposis or Peutz–Jeghers polyposis. Table 48.2 outlines the different histological features.

Table 48.1 Polyps and polyposis syndromes seen in childhood

Adenomatous polyposis syndromes
familial adenomatous polyposis
Turcot's syndrome
Hamartomatous polyps
solitary juvenile polyp
juvenile polyposis syndrome
Peutz–Jeghers syndrome
Bannayan–Riley–Ruvalcaba syndrome
Gorlins's syndrome
Cowden's syndrome
Lymphoid nodular hyperplasia
Inflammatory polyps
Mixed polyposis syndrome

Clinical management

The most common manifestation of a large-bowel polyp is painless rectal bleeding. Other symptoms attributed to polyps include abdominal pain, altered bowel habit, or prolapse of the polyp or rectum. Some children are completely asymptomatic – their polyps may be found as part of a screening program for a familial polyposis syndrome.

Diagnosis is made at full colonoscopy and polypectomy. Apart from biopsying for histology, polypectomy serves to remove the symptomatic polyp, e.g. source of bleeding or intussusception (Table 48.3).

In order to plan management appropriately, the pediatrician treating a child with a gastrointestinal polyp must know the histopathological type, the number and site of polyps, and whether or not there is a family history of polyps or colorectal cancer. The clinician should direct his history and examination towards complications related to polyposis syndromes (Table 48.4).

Juvenile polyp (solitary at diagnosis)

Clinical presentation and diagnosis

Children with a solitary juvenile polyp present at a mean age of 4 years with painless rectal bleeding or peranal polyp protrusion. Up to 40% of children

Table 48.2 Pathological features of polyps seen in children

Polyp type	Macroscopic appearance	Microscopic appearance	Dysplasia
Juvenile	pedunculated 1–3 cm in size, rarely larger with smooth red surface, 'Swiss cheese' cut surface	dilated cysts filled with mucin, abundant lamina propria with prominent inflammatory infiltrate; ulcerated surface with underlying granulation tissue, glands branched, haphazardly arranged	rare, approximately <5%
Peutz–Jeghers	sessile or pedunculated with lobulated surface 0.5–3 cm in size, pink or tan cut surface with or without ulceration	elongated branching glands lined by epithelium native to polyp location; arborizing strands of smooth muscle; less stroma and cysts than juvenile polyps	rare, <5%
Tubular adenoma	pedunculated smooth, red lobulated surface 0.5–5 cm in size	glands and tubules with or without inflammatory infiltrate	always present; graded mild, moderate or severe
Villous adenoma	sessile, broad-based papillary surface 1–5 cm in size	villous structures with or without inflammatory infiltrate	always present; graded mild, moderate or severe

Table 48.3 Endoscopic polypectomy in children

Only skilled endoscopists should be performing colonoscopic polypectomy in children – if experienced, the risk of perforation and significant bleeding should be <1%.

Modern video endoscopes provide unrivalled views of the colonic mucosa and most polyps of >1mm are readily visible.

Tiny adenomas, <1 mm in size, confirm the diagnosis of familial adenomatous polyposis, and can be seen more easily by spraying 0.2% indigo carmine dye onto the colonic surface either via specially designed spray-catheters or directly down the biopsy channel.

Position change and endoscopic rotation are important to place the polyp in the convenient 5 o'clock position prior to attempting polypectomy.

Small polyps <5 mm can be removed using the hot biopsy forceps. This technique is relatively easy and almost always ensures adequate histology. Great care must be taken to minimize heat damage to the bowel wall, and the procedure is probably best avoided in the thin-walled right colon.

Polyps of >5 mm should be removed by snare polypectomy.

Pedunculated polyps, in which larger vessels may be present within the stalk are best removed using coagulating diathermy (15 W) in preference to pulsed cutting therapy.

Newer non-contact techniques such as argon plasma coagulation offer safe and rapid destruction of multiple polyps, but do not provide histology.

The risk of removing larger (>1 cm) sessile polyps is considerable, particularly in the right colon, and requires more advanced polypectomy techniques such as submucosal injection of 1 : 10000 adrenaline (epinephrine) or hypertonic saline to lift the mucosa away from the underlying muscle layer.

Table 48.4 History and examination in a child with possible gastrointestinal (GI) polyps

History
Nature of bleeding and frequency
Painful or painless rectal bleeding
History of GI obstructive symptoms
Detailed family history, exploring early deaths or diagnosis of GI cancer
Weight loss, anorexia (tumor)
Learning difficulties (JPS)
Examination
Mucosal pigmentation (PJS)
Dysmorphic features (JPS)
Edema (hypoalbuminemia in infantile JPS)
Extraintestinal manifestations of FAP – see Table 45.6 – e.g. subcutaneous cysts, exostosis, congenital hypertrophy of the retinal pigmented epithelium
Hepatic mass (FAP)
Thyroid mass (FAP or Cowden's syndrome)

JPS, juvenile polyposis syndrome; PJS, Peutz–Jeghers syndrome; FAP, familial adenomatous polyposis

with a juvenile polyp have multiple polyps; 60% are proximal to the rectosigmoid, confirming the need for full colonoscopy even if a polyp is found in the rectum.[1] Although the risk of developing malignancy in a solitary juvenile polyp is very small, such polyps should be removed even when discovered incidentally by endoscopic polypectomy. If a polyp is found to be solitary after full colonoscopy, and there is no relevant family history, endoscopic polypectomy is sufficient treatment.

Complications and follow-up

The risk of malignant change for a solitary juvenile polyp is almost negligible, although neoplastic change has been documented.[2] In patients with a solitary juvenile polyp, there appears to be no increased risk of colorectal cancer or of dying as a result of the polyp.[3]

If the polyp was solitary and the patient is discharged, parents must be aware that juvenile polyps may be the first feature of juvenile polyposis. If fresh symptoms arise, the child should be reinvestigated. When, however, there is a positive family history, or when multiple juvenile polyps are found, the possibility of juvenile polyposis syndrome (JPS) is raised and a different management strategy should be employed.

Juvenile polyposis syndrome

Clinical signs and diagnosis

JPS is a rare autosomal dominant condition characterized by the occurrence of multiple juvenile polyps in the gastrointestinal tract. In children, the most common presentation is at a mean age of 9 years with rectal bleeding, anemia or prolapse of either the polyp or the rectum. A significant proportion of patients with juvenile polyposis have been reported to have other morphological abnormalities, including digital clubbing, macrocephaly, alopecia, cleft lip or palate, congenital heart disease, genitourinary abnormalities or mental retardation.[4]

Compared to patients with solitary juvenile polyps, patients with JPS have more polyps, and are more likely to have right-sided polyps (hence the need for full colonoscopy), polyps with adenomatous change and anemia.[5] As the condition progresses, the number of polyps rises to 50–200. Polyps are found primarily in the colon, but also in the stomach and small intestine.[6] The number of polyps needed to make the diagnosis remains controversial (between three and five).[2,7]

Less commonly, the condition presents in infancy with anemia and hemorrhage, diarrhea, protein-losing enteropathy and rectal bleeding.[8] In this scenario the entire gastrointestinal tract is usually affected and there may be mild dysmorphic features (e.g. macrocephaly, clubbing, nail dystrophy); the prognosis appears to be related to the severity and extent of gastrointestinal involvement. The course in such infants is fulminant and death frequently occurs before the age of 2 years in severe cases despite colectomy.[9]

Genetics of juvenile polyposis

A family history is found in 20–50% of patients, the inheritance apparently being autosomal dominant. There is evidence for genetic heterogeneity in JPS. Subsets of families have mutations in the tumor-suppressor gene *PTEN* located at 10q23.3, but these patients may have features suggestive of other polyposis syndromes, e.g. Cowden's syndrome.[10,11] A proportion of JPS patients (especially those without stigmata of other polyposis syndromes) do not have germline mutations in *PTEN* – instead they have mutations in *SMAD4/DPC4* located at 18q21.[12] It would appear that germline *SMAD4* mutations predispose to hamartomas and cancer through disruption of the transforming growth factor (TGF)-β signaling pathway. Multiple genetic alterations (including *APC* mutations and *K-ras* mutations) appear to play a role in the neoplastic transformation of juvenile polyps of JPS patients.

Complications

There is little doubt that juvenile polyposis is a premalignant condition. There is a 15% incidence of colorectal carcinoma occurring in patients under the age of 35 years, leading to a cumulative risk of colorectal cancer of 68% by the age of 60 years.[7] Neoplastic changes have been documented both in the polyps and in flat apparently normal colonic mucosa. Malignancies in the stomach, duodenum and pancreas have been described in adults.

Treatment and follow-up

Patients with features suggestive of JPS should have surveillance colonoscopy with random biopsies of polyps and flat mucosa every 2 years (see Management algorithm, Figure 48.1). When the number of polyps is small, endoscopic polypectomy and follow-up may suffice, but it is not clear whether endoscopic surveillance is adequate to prevent malignancy. When there are numerous polyps, or symptoms such as bleeding and diarrhea persist, prophylactic colectomy should be considered after adolescence. As yet, there are insufficient data to justify prophylactic colectomy solely for the risk of colorectal carcinoma.

With a risk of polyps in close relatives, first-degree relatives of patients with JPS should be screened by colonoscopy starting at age 12 years, even when the subject is asymptomatic.[13]

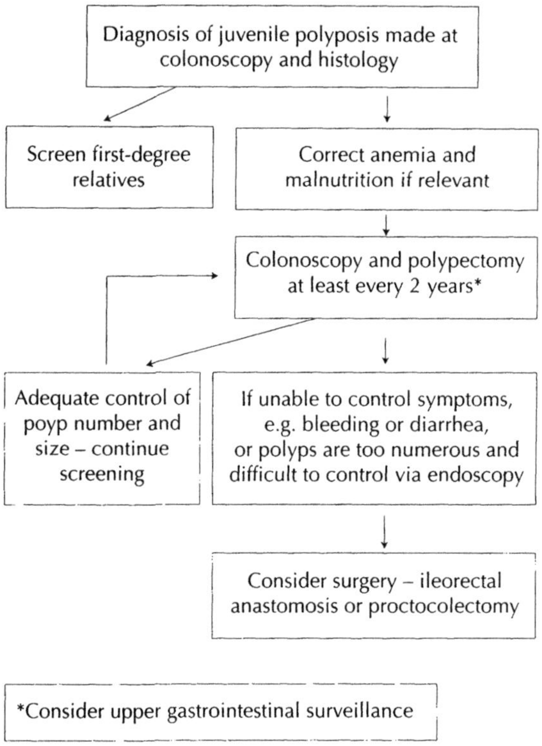

Figure 48.1 Management of juvenile polyposis in childhood.

Peutz–Jeghers syndrome

Clinical features and diagnosis

Peutz–Jeghers syndrome (PJS) is a rare autosomal dominant condition in which gastrointestinal polyps occur in association with macular melanin pigmentation. A definitive diagnosis of PJS can be made if a person fulfills one of the following criteria:

(1) Two or more PJS polyps in the gastrointestinal tract;
(2) One PJS polyp in the gastrointestinal tract, together with either the classical PJS pigmentation, or a family history of PJS.

Presumptive diagnosis can be made in those with a positive family history and typical PJS freckling.[14]

Polyps arise primarily in the small bowel, and to a lesser extent in the stomach and colon. Pigmentation occurs in most, although not all,

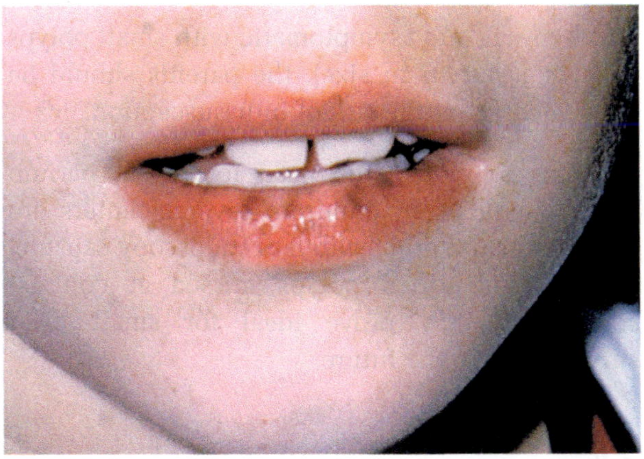

Figure 48.2 Macular pigmentation of the lips in a child with Peutz–Jeghers syndrome.

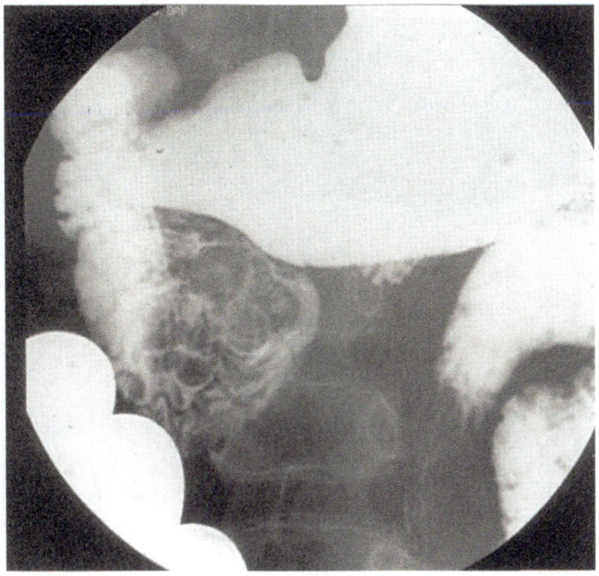

Figure 48.3 Small-bowel barium study showing a massive Peutz–Jeghers syndrome polyp in the second part of the duodenum.

patients and is seen most frequently on the lips and buccal mucosa (Figure 48.2) and occasionally on the hands, feet and eyelids. Clinicians should be aware that buccal mucosa pigmentation can occur in the normal population. The primary concern to the pediatrician is the risk of small-bowel intussusception causing intestinal obstruction (Figure 48.3), vomiting and pain. In addition, intestinal bleeding leading to anemia can occur.

Genetics of Peutz–Jeghers syndrome

The gene for this condition has recently been identified. The mutated gene *LBK1/STK11* located on chromosome 19p13.3 is associated with PJS and encodes a serine/threonine kinase.[15,16] It appears that *STK11* is a tumor-suppressor gene that might act as a gatekeeper regulating the development of hamartomas and adenocarcinomas in PJS.[17,18] Allelic imbalance (allele loss and loss of heterozygosity) has previously been reported in a number of PJS cases, suggesting the existence of a hamartoma–carcinoma sequence in tumorigenesis.[19]

There is marked inter- and intra-family phenotypic variability in PJS. Therefore, the availability of predictive genetic testing may have some value, but cannot determine the likely severity of phenotype.[20] In addition, not all PJS patients have the demonstrated *LKB1/STK11* gene,[21] there remain potential loci for alternative mutated genes predisposing to PJS. If the gene mutation is known for previous affected cases in the family, it might have a role in presymptomatic testing in those patients with no pigmentation (or even potential prenatal diagnosis).

Management and complications

Controversy exists over the management of the young child with mid-gut polyps. There is a high re-operation rate after initial laparotomy for small-bowel obstruction; this rate might be reduced in skilled hands by intraoperative enteroscopy (possibly through a surgical enterotomy) to remove other polyps. Intraoperative small-bowel endoscopy picked up 38% more polyps at laparotomy (17 additional polyps) compared with external palpation and small-bowel transillumination[22] (Figure 48.4). Surgery for small-bowel complications in children with PJS is common (65% of patients <18 years) and the majority of these laparotomies were performed as an emergency procedure.[23]

At present it is not possible to be prescriptive about management of polyps of different sizes. The advantages and disadvantages of prophylactic polypectomy for asymptomatic patients should be discussed with the family. Management is influenced by the size of the polyps and their location (Figure 48.5). This protocol is adapted from adult practice, and therefore the size of polyps requiring resection may be smaller in young children. Symptomatic children with sizable mid-gut polyps (larger than 1.5 cm in size) should be referred for laparotomy and intraoperative enteroscopy. For

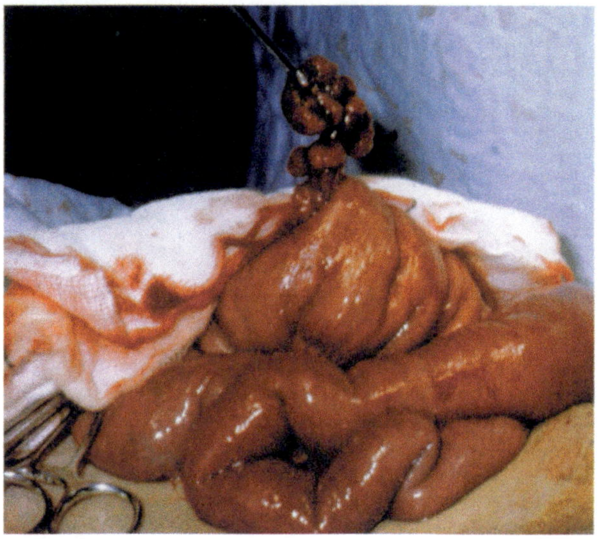

Figure 48.4 A 2-cm pedunculated polyp in Peutz–Jeghers syndrome at resection after intraoperative endoscopic surveillance.

children who are asymptomatic with small polyps (less than 1.0 cm in size), the parents should be counseled about the risk of intussusception.[24,25]

In order to reduce the need for repeat barium contrast studies in children, several centers are piloting the use of the wireless endoscopy capsule. This has identified polyps missed at contrast study, and may prove ideal for small-bowel surveillance in the future.

Follow-up

The risk of neoplasia is well documented in young adults and includes development of unusual tumors such as Sertoli cell tumor of the ovary and testicular tumors in prepubescent boys.[26] A meta-analysis of the existing literature to assess the risk of cancer in PJS identified a relative risk for all cancers in PJS patients (aged 15–64) of 15.2 compared to the normal population, with tumors reported throughout the gastrointestinal tract, and extraintestinal tumors of the lung, testis, breast, uterus, ovary and cervix.[27] Clinicians caring for

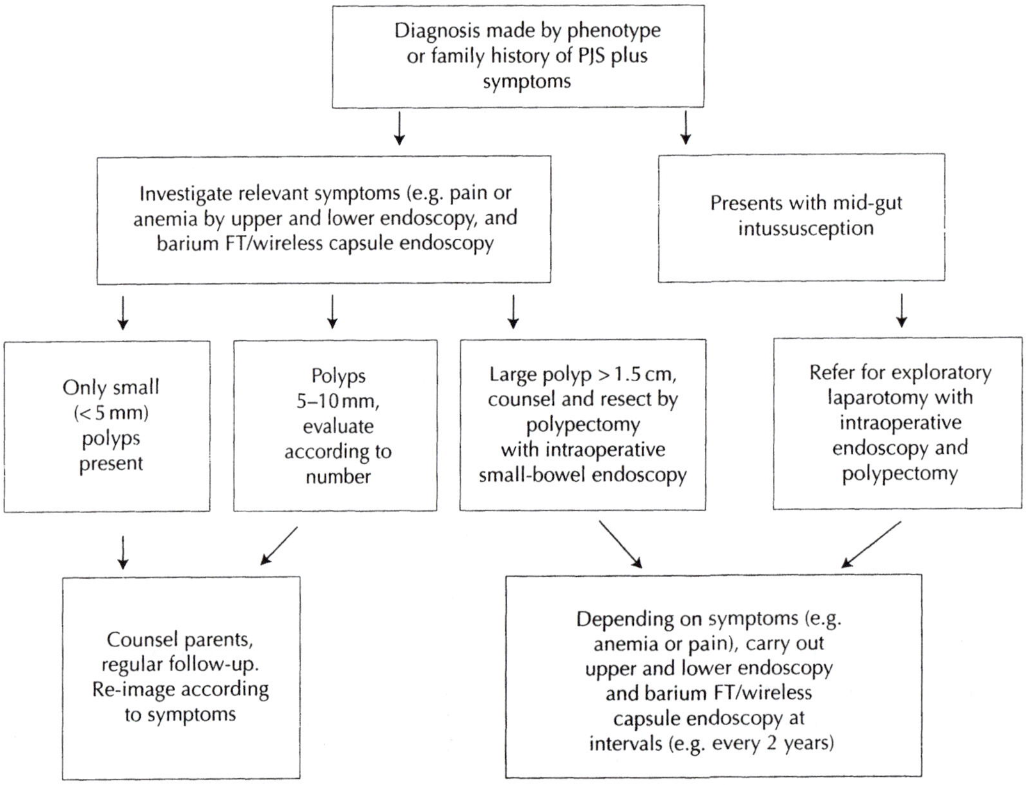

Figure 48.5 Management of Peutz–Jeghers syndrome (PJS) in childhood. Barium FT, barium follow-through.

adolescents with PJS should be aware of unusual symptoms, e.g. those due to a feminizing testicular tumor, and have a low threshold for investigating potential malignancies. A recommended screening program for PJS patients after adolescence is shown in Table 48.5, but it is not clear that such a program will reduce morbidity or mortality.

Familial adenomatous polyposis

In children, gastrointestinal adenomas are almost always associated with hereditary adenomatous polyposis syndromes. Therefore, whenever a colorectal adenoma is found in a child, total colonoscopy with dye spray is mandatory. Familial adenomatous polyposis (FAP) is the most common of the adenomatous polyposis syndromes.

Clinical features

Patients with FAP typically develop multiple adenomas throughout the large bowel, usually more than 100 and sometimes more than 1000 (Figure 48.6). Polyps begin to appear in childhood or adolescence and increase in number with age. By the fifth decade colorectal cancer is almost inevitable if colectomy is not performed. Adult patients with FAP are also at increased risk of malignancies of the duodenum, ampulla of Vater, thyroid and pancreas. Papillary carcinoma of the thyroid has been reported in adolescence.[28] Children under 5 years of age may develop hepatoblastoma.[29] It may be advisable to measure serum α-fetoprotein levels and/or carry out abdominal ultrasound examination in children at risk.

There are three ways in which a patient with FAP may present to the pediatrician.

(1) Most will be called for screening because of a positive family history.

(2) Some will present with colorectal symptoms such as bleeding or diarrhea.

(3) A minority present with extracolonic manifestations (Table 48.6). General pediatricians treating a child with an unusual lesion such as maxillary osteoma or a rare tumor such as hepatoblastoma should consider the possibility of FAP, particularly if there are multiple tumors or another sibling is affected.[30]

Genetics of familial adenomatous polyposis

The prevalence of FAP is estimated at 1:10000. It is inherited as an autosomal dominant trait with high penetrance but with a variable age of onset. The rate of spontaneous mutations is relatively high – reported as 10–30%.[31]

Table 48.5 Program for screening for malignancies in Peutz–Jeghers syndrome after adolescence

Annual investigations
Hemoglobin
Pelvic ultrasound, gynecological and breast examinations (in females)
Testicular ultrasound examinations (in males)

Two-yearly investigations
Upper and lower endoscopy
Small bowel contrast X-ray

Other investigations
Cervical smear 3-yearly
Breast mammography 5-yearly from age 25 years

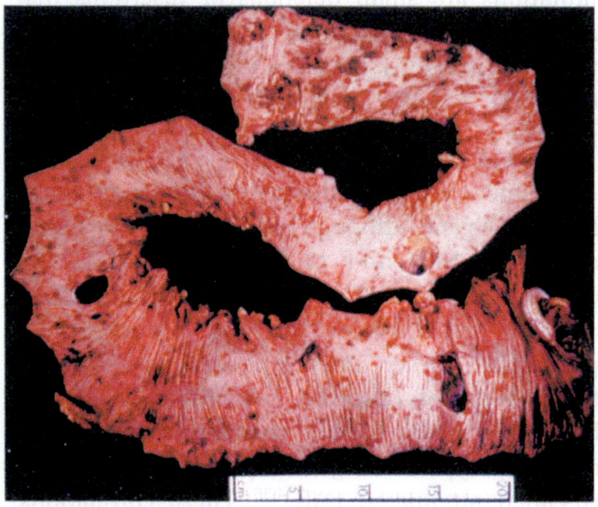

Figure 48.6 Colectomy specimen demonstrating carpeting with dense polyposis in an adolescent with familial adenomatous polyposis.

Table 48.6 Extracolonic manifestations of familial adenomatous polyposis in children and young adults

Site	Examples
Bone	osteomas, mandibular and maxillary exostosis sclerosis
Dental abnormalities	impacted or supernumerary teeth unerupted teeth
Connective tissue	desmoid tumors excessive intra-abdominal adhesions fibroma subcutaneous cysts
Eyes	congenital hypertrophy of the retinal pigmented epithelium
Central nervous system	glioblastomas, e.g. Turcot's syndrome
Adenomas	stomach duodenum small intestine adrenal cortex thyroid gland
Carcinomas	thyroid gland adrenal gland
Liver	hepatoblastoma

The gene responsible for FAP, *APC* (adenomatous polyposis coli), is located on chromosome 5q21 and appears to be a tumor-suppressor gene.[32] Most mutations are small deletions or insertions that result in the production of a truncated APC protein. In FAP a germline mutation inactivates one of the two *APC* alleles that underlie the predisposition to adenoma formation.

Mutations are widely distributed throughout the 5′ half of the gene, although two 'hot spots' are found at codons 1061 and 1309 (Figure 48.7). These account for around one-third of all mutations detected and are associated with a more severe phenotype. Other phenotype–genotype correlations have been observed.[33] A variant of FAP has been described which is characterized by fewer colonic polyps and a generally milder phenotype, so-called attenuated FAP.[34,35] These correlations are not absolute and there may be considerable intrafamilial variation suggesting that there are other factors involved in the pathogenesis of the disease. Some of the phenotypic variability seen in patients cannot be explained by the location of their *APC* mutation. Environmental factors and other genes – often termed modifier genes – may have critical effects on *APC* function and disease expression.[36]

More than 300 different germline mutations have been described; finding the mutation may be a formidable task. Families need to be aware that the mutation may be detected in only 60–80% of cases. It is only in these cases that a predictive test can be offered to individuals at risk.

Diagnosis – interpretation of the genetic test and clinical screening in familial adenomatous polyposis

In order to define which screening protocol is appropriate for a given family, the first step is to determine, where possible, which mutation is present in the FAP-affected index case. At this stage, if a mutation cannot be found, the genetic

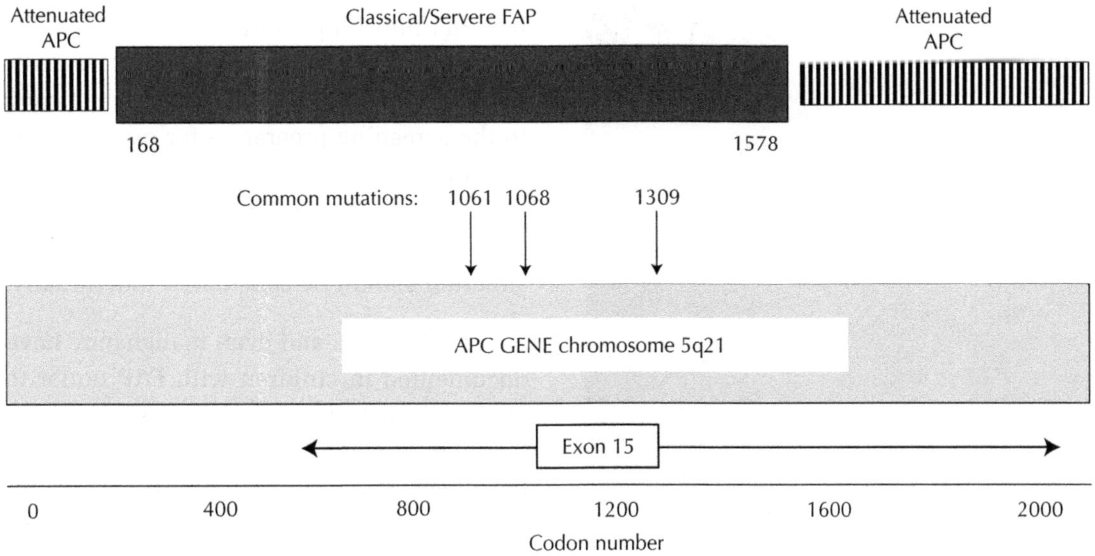

Figure 48.7 Structure of the *APC* gene. FAP, familial adenomatous polyposis.

testing is non-informative and it will not be possible to offer predictive testing to asymptomatic at-risk relatives (Figure 48.8).

For the 60–80% in whom a mutation is detected, at-risk relatives can be tested. A negative test is considered accurate in excluding FAP and the subject should be considered to hold an average population risk for the subsequent development of adenomas and cancer. Such genotype-negative individuals can be discharged from follow-up. Those patients where the deletion has not been sequenced, but has been excluded by linkage analysis with intragenic markers alone (a less reliable method for determining the risk of carrying the *APC* gene mutation) should not be discharged and they should undergo endoscopic surveillance.

A positive test confirms the diagnosis of FAP and patients should undergo endoscopic assessment. The diagnosis is confirmed by finding polyps at flexible sigmoidoscopy, histologically confirmed as adenomas (Figure 48.9). Affected individuals undergo annual flexible sigmoidoscopy from the age of 10–14 years until adenomas are found.[37–39] Most gene-positive children will have had a full colonoscopy by the age of 16 years to determine polyp density and location, and degree of dysplasia.

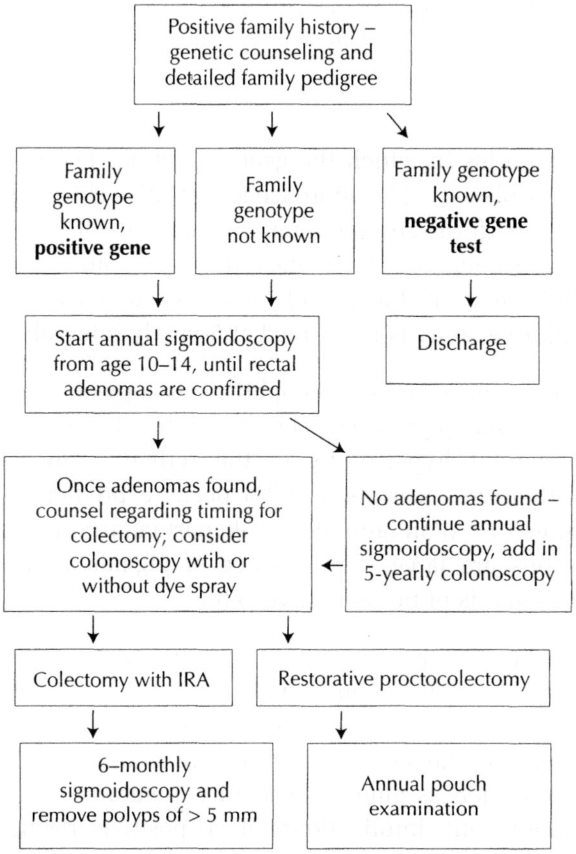

Figure 48.8 Management protocol for screening children and adolescents at risk of familial adenomatous polyposis. IRA, ileorectal anastomosis.

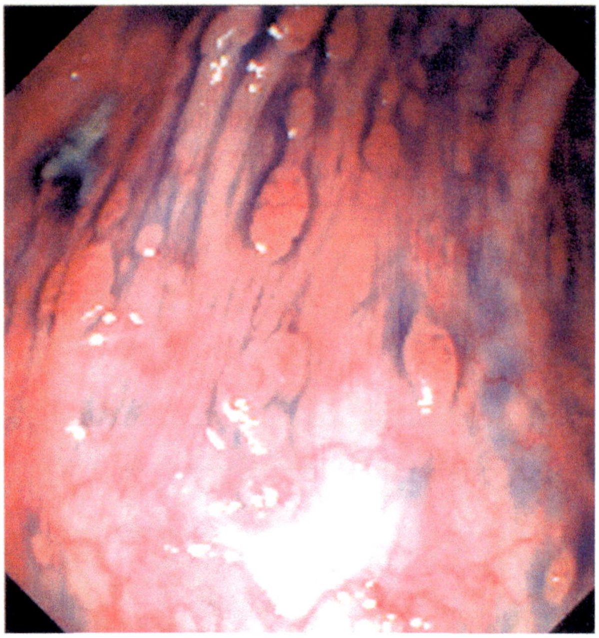

Figure 48.9 Endoscopic appearance of colon showing occasional adenomas in a 10-year-old with familial adenomatous polyposis. Dye spray emphasizes small polyps down to < 0.5 mm.

In families in which the genotype is not known, protocols vary. The approach at St Mark's Hospital is to perform annual sigmoidoscopy in all first-degree relatives until adenomas are found. In addition, from the age of 20 years, colonoscopy with dye spray is performed at 5-yearly intervals.

The presence on indirect ophthalmoscopy of more than four pigmented ocular fundus lesions – congenital hypertrophy of the retinal pigment epithelium – carries a 100% positive predictive value for FAP in families at risk, particularly if the lesions are large. The absence of pigmentation, however, is of no predictive value.

No patient should undergo screening for FAP without detailed counseling. It is essential that the individual being screened understand the nature of the test and its possible outcomes.[40] Issues such as emotional, family, insurance and employment implications of a positive result should be discussed prior to testing and there should be a clear protocol for post-test management.[41]

Controversy surrounds the issue of screening in childhood for a condition that will cause few problems before adolescence.[42] Many authorities feel that the child should be involved in the decision-making process, and the diagnosis be delayed until the child is old enough to contribute to the screening program – for example, from the age of 11 years onwards.[43,44] Some children understand the genetic screening and its consequences at a younger age, e.g. 8 years; each family situation should be considered individually.

Severe dysplasia and even malignancy have been documented in children with FAP under the age of 12 years. Consequently, those children from families in which severe dysplasia or carcinomas have been found at a young age should undergo screening at an earlier age.[45] This is particularly so if the family has one of the mutations associated with a severe phenotype, e.g. 1309 in exon 15. Those children with symptoms such as diarrhea or rectal bleeding/anaemia should be investigated early, as this may signify severe colonic disease.[38]

Duodenal and ampullary cancers are currently the most common cause of cancer deaths in adults who have had a colectomy for FAP. Upper endoscopic surveillance of the stomach, duodenum and periampullary region with a side-viewing endoscope is recommended after the age 20 years, unless the patient has symptoms such as upper abdominal pain, which warrant earlier investigation.[46]

Management of familial adenomatous polyposis

Colectomy is the only effective therapy that eliminates the inevitable risk of colorectal cancer. In the absence of severe dysplasia, colectomy is usually performed in the mid- to late teens or early twenties to accommodate work and school schedules. Some clinicians advocate colectomy before puberty so that the patient can adapt to life without a colon before adolescence – each case should be considered on its own merits. Almost all FAP screen-detected adolescents are asymptomatic and may not contemplate interruptions in their schooling or effects on relationships. The surgical option, therefore, must not only be carefully timed but also have low morbidity and an excellent functional result.

The timing of primary preventative surgery may be influenced by knowledge of the mutation site and the likely severity of the polyposis. For example, patients with a deletion at exon 15 at codon 1309 may be offered earlier surgery since this phenotype is characterized by a large number of polyps and a higher risk of cancer.[47] Even though a low polyp density suggests a lower risk of developing malignancy,[48] it is unsafe to delay surgery on the grounds of polyp density alone.[49]

Surgical options include subtotal colectomy with ileorectal anastomosis, or restorative proctocolectomy with ileo-anal anastomosis (pouch procedure). The ileorectal anastomosis is a low-risk operation with good functional results, but the rectum remains at risk of cancer. Six-monthly surveillance of the rectum is needed postoperatively; despite this, inexperience can result in early cancers being missed.[50] A pouch procedure removes the colorectal cancer risk almost completely, but is more complicated than an ileorectal anastomosis, carrying a higher morbidity and often requiring a temporary ileostomy. The pouch procedure may carry a higher risk of complications, reoperations, longer hospital stays, night evacuation and influence on later sexual function.[51,52] Other authors have differing experience and claim acceptable morbidity following pouch construction for FAP[53,54] or total colectomy with rectal mucosectomy and straight endorectal pull-through.[55] Pouch creation is associated with an as yet unknown risk of pouch neoplasia; the pouch should be examined regularly.[56]

The advantages of a pouch with a lower risk of cancer must be compared against the higher operative morbidity; the patients and parents must be carefully counseled. Conversion to an ileoanal pouch can be carried out when the patient is much older.[57] Patients with a large number of rectal polyps, or those with high-risk genotypes, may be better with a pouch procedure in the first instance, owing to the greater risk of malignancy.[58–60]

Desmoid disease

Desmoids are locally aggressive but non-metastasizing myofibroblastic lesions which occur with disproportionate high frequency in patients with FAP. Associated etiological factors include germline mutation, estrogens and surgical trauma.[61] Desmoids occur most commonly in the peritoneal cavity (Figure 48.10), and may infiltrate locally leading to small-bowel, ureteric or vascular obstruction. These lesions may progress rapidly or may resolve spontaneously, their unpredictable nature making them difficult to treat.[62] Attempted surgical resection carries a high morbidity and mortality (10–60%) and usually stimulates further growth.[63] Medical treatments including non-steroidal anti-inflammatory drugs (NSAIDs) and antiestrogens have limited success. Cytotoxic chemotherapy is used as a last resort. Pediatricians treating children with extraintestinal desmoid tumors should consider the possibility of FAP in the family.

Other polyposis syndromes

Infrequently, juvenile polyposis may occur as part of the Bannayan–Riley–Ruvalcaba syndrome. This is characterized by macrocephaly, intestinal juvenile polyposis, pigmentation of the genitalia, psychomotor delay in childhood and occasionally lipid storage myopathy.[64] Cowden's disease is the

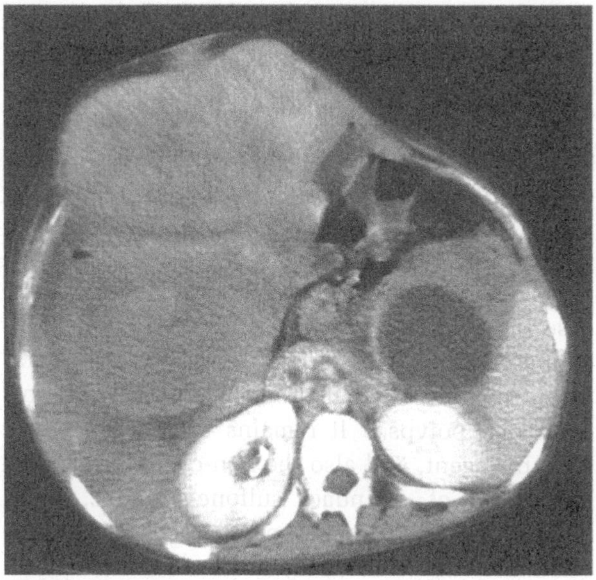

Figure 48.10 Abdominal computed tomography scan showing a massive intra-abdominal desmoid tumor in a 14-year-old with familial adenomatous polyposis.

association of multiple hamartomas of the stomach, small intestine or colon with macrocephaly, fibrocystic disease and cancer of the breast and thyroid. Germline mutations in the tumor-suppressor gene *PTEN* have been found in Cowden's and Bannayan–Riley–Ruvalcaba pedigrees.[65] Gorlin's syndrome is an autosomal dominant condition comprising upper gastrointestinal hamartomas and pink or brown macules in exposed areas such as the face and hands. In addition, patients may have frontal and parietal bossing, hypertelorism and variable skeletal abnormalities and intracranial calcification and are at risk of medulloblastoma.

Turcot's syndrome is characterized by concurrence of a primary brain tumor and multiple colorectal adenomas. Patients with a polyposis syndrome and neurological symptoms should undergo thorough neurological examination and investigation for possible brain tumor. The management of the colonic polyps in Turcot's syndrome is the same as for FAP.

In the vast majority of patients with polyposis, a clear-cut diagnosis can be made, e.g. FAP or PJS. However, there are some rare cases where distinctions cannot be made on histology – the mixed polyposis syndromes.[66]

Future chemoprevention

Studies have suggested that NSAIDs may be protective against colon cancer. NSAIDs inhibit prostaglandin synthesis via their effects on cyclooxygenase (COX). Several trials have shown regression of adenomas using the NSAID sulindac,[67,68] but widespread use of sulindac has been limited by concerns regarding gastrointestinal side-effects with prolonged administration and case reports of rectal cancer despite treatment.[69] Clinical trials using selective COX-2 inhibitors have reported a reduction in the number of colorectal polyps.[70] It remains to be seen what role this agent, and also the non-cyclo-oxygenase metabolite of sulindac, sulfone-sulindac, may have in the future management of colorectal and duodenal adenomas. They may have a role prior to surgery in young patients, but sulindac administered before polyps developed in genotype-positive adolescents did not prevent the development of adenomas.[71] Primary chemoprevention with an NSAID may not prevent polyp formation.

Intestinal neoplasia

In pediatric practice, colonic carcinoma and lymphoma are very rare, yet an awareness of these conditions is still important since a delay in diagnosis adversely affects outcome.

Carcinoma of the colon

Colorectal cancer is a major cause of morbidity and mortality in adult practice but its incidence in younger individuals is very low, with fewer than 200 pediatric cases reported in the literature by 1994.[72] Compared to adults, where sporadic cases of cancer predominate, in children there is an over-representation of cases with pre-existing polyposis or colitis (10%).[73]

Pathogenesis

Colorectal carcinoma is believed to result from several sequential genetic mutations known as the adenoma–carcinoma sequence. Although the pattern of mutation is not consistent in all colorectal cancers, it is proposed that progress to malignant transformation occurs following the accumulation of a combination of four or five defects including mutational activation of oncogenes and inactivation of tumor-suppressor genes.[74,75]

Pathology

The pathology of colonic carcinoma in children when compared to adult cases is characterized by more right-sided disease, with 50% located in the cecum to transverse colon.[76] Colorectal cancers grow locally, eventually penetrating the bowel wall. They can spread to regional lymphatics and subsequently to distant lymph nodes, and also to the liver, lungs and vertebrae. Cases are staged according to the degree of local spread and the presence or absence of transmural penetration, the degree of lymph node involvement and presence of distant metastases. In a review of younger patients with colonic cancer, 82% of these cases had either distant metastases, lymph node involvement, or transmural penetrating disease, significantly higher than in adult patients.[77,78]

The usual histological appearance of colorectal cancers in adults is of a moderate to well differentiated adenocarcinoma. In children the proportion of tumors with mucinous (30%) and signet-ring (10%) histological appearances, associated with a poorer prognosis, is greater, and together with the tendency towards a more advanced stage at presentation may account for the poorer outcome of the disease in children.

Clinical presentation

Abdominal pain is the main presenting symptom, occurring in over 90% of cases, although other symptoms – weight loss, vomiting, rectal bleeding and altered bowel habit – may also be present. The clinical presentation is influenced by the site of the lesion, with constipation, obstruction and bleeding more common with left-sided disease, whereas right-sided disease may not present with obstruction, for example, until the lesion is larger, and a mass is palpable.

Diagnosis is by colonoscopy in most cases, although the lesion can also be identified by other imaging modalities such as ultrasound or magnetic resonance imaging. Although serological markers such as carcinoembryonic antigen (CEA) are available, their role in establishing this rare diagnosis in children has not been fully evaluated.[79]

Treatment and outcome

Surgery is the main treatment for colonic carcinoma, with complete resection of the primary lesion and draining lymphatics being the primary objective. Complete resection is often not possible in children, owing to the advanced stage at presentation. Chemotherapy for metastatic disease has in general been disappointing, and the role of radiotherapy or combination therapies awaits further study in the pediatric age group.

The prognosis for children with colon cancer is poor, with 5-year survival rates of 10–20% reported.[80] These poor results are due to a combination of unfavorable histology and delayed presentation.

Lymphoma

Compared to adults, in younger patients there is a significant difference in the preponderance of the various histological types of lymphoma and also in the frequency of disease at different intestinal sites.

Epidemiology and classification

In the developed world, lymphoma accounts for 10% of all cancers in children under 15 years of age.[81] In central Africa there is a very high incidence of Burkitt's lymphoma (small non-cleaved B-cell lymphoma), accounting for up to 50% of all childhood cancers, whilst in North Africa and the Middle East there is a high rate of immunoproliferative small intestinal disease (IPSID).

Etiology

Non-Hodgkin's lymphoma is associated in some cases with immunodeficiency syndromes, both inherited (e.g. ataxic-telangiectasia) and acquired (e.g. HIV infection), and also with immune suppressive therapy (e.g. after organ transplantation). An infectious agent (Epstein–Barr virus) may play a role in disease pathogenesis in some cases. This appears particularly to be the case for endemic Burkitt's lymphoma, although the geographical association with malaria infection implies that co-infection may be important in promoting B-cell activation as part of the process leading to malignant change. Other conditions that give rise to chronic mucosal inflammation have also been linked to lymphoma. T-cell non-Hodgkin's lymphoma is associated with celiac disease, whilst both lymphoma and adenocarcinoma are associated with both Crohn's disease, where the lesion is typically in the small bowel, and ulcerative colitis.[82,83]

Pathology

Intra-abdominal non-Hodgkin's lymphoma in children typically is of an undifferentiated histological type – only around 50% have a primary intestinal origin[84] – most common intestinal primary sites are the distal ileum, cecum and appendix. Bone-marrow involvement occurs in up to 40% of undifferentiated lymphoma, whilst central nervous system involvement is uncommon. In endemic Burkitt's lymphoma 60% have abdominal disease, 60% have characteristic involvement of the mandible.[84]

Clinical presentation

Disease may present with non-specific symptoms such as abdominal distension, nausea, vomiting, altered bowel habit and abdominal pain. Disease primarily in the intestinal tract, typically localized to the distal ileum and cecum in children, may present with a mass, an ileo-cecal intussusception, obstructive symptoms or bleeding.

The diagnosis of non-Hodgkin's lymphoma depends on histological examination with immunophenotyping and cytogenetics. Staging of disease with chest and abdominal imaging, lumbar puncture and bone-marrow examination are also required, and may allow treatment to start if there is a delay in undertaking a laparotomy.

Treatment and outcome

Surgical resection of local disease is indicated where it is possible, although such fully resectable disease accounts for only 60–75% of cases.[84] The high mortality associated with intestinal perforation in more advanced disease has led to debate as to the role of partial resection as opposed to simple biopsy to establish histological type. Subsequent chemotherapy is required in all cases. For more localized disease the overall outcome is relatively good. In the 30% of childhood non-Hodgkin's lymphoma cases with localized disease, cure rates as high as 95% have been reported following surgical resection and combination chemotherapy.[84]

REFERENCES

1. Mestre JR. The changing pattern of juvenile polyps. *Am J Gastroenterol* 1986; **81**: 312–314.
2. Giardiello FM, Hamilton SR, Kern SE et al. Colorectal neoplasia in juvenile polyposis or juvenile polyps. *Arch Dis Child* 1991; **66**: 971–975.
3. Nugent KO, Talbot IC, Hodgson SV et al. Solitary juvenile polyps: not a marker for subsequent malignancy. *Gastroenterology* 1993; **105**: 698–700.
4. Desai DC, Murday V, Phillips RKS. A survey of phenotypic features in juvenile polyposis. *J Med Genet* 1998; **35**: 476–481.
5. Hoffenberg EJ, Sauaia A, Malttzman T et al. Symptomatic colonic polyps in childhood: not so benign. *J Pediatr Gastroenteral Nutr* 1999; **28**: 175–181.
6. Desai DC, Neale KF, Talbot IC et al. Juvenile polyposis. *Br J Surg* 1995; **82**: 14–17.
7. Jass JR, Williams CB, Bussey HJR et al. Juvenile polyposis – a precancerous condition. *Histopathology* 1988; **13**: 619–630.
8. Sachatello CR, Hahn IS, Carrington CB. Juvenile gastrointestinal polyposis in a female infant: a report of a case and review of the literature of a recently recognised syndrome. *Surgery* 1974; **75**: 107–114.
9. Scharf GM, Becker JHR, Laage NJ. Juvenile gastrointestinal polyposis or the infantile Cronkhite–Canada syndrome. *J Pediatr Surg* 1986; **21**: 953–954.
10. Lynch ED, Ostermeyer EA, Lee MK et al. Inherited mutations in PTEN that are associated with breast cancer, cowden disease, and juvenile polyposis. *Am J Hum Genet* 1997; **61**: 1254–1260.
11. Woodford-Richens K, Bevan S, Churchman M et al. Analysis of genetic and phenotypic heterogeneity in juvenile polyposis. *Gut* 2000; **46**: 656–660.
12. Howe JR, Roth S, Ringold JC et al. Mutations in the *SMAD4/DPC4* gene in juvenile polyposis. *Science* 1998; **280**: 1086–1088.
13. Stemper TJ, Kent TH, Summers RW. Juvenile polyposis and gastrointestinal carcinoma. A study of a kindred. *Ann Intern Med* 1975; **83**: 639–646.
14. Tomlinson IPM, Houlston RS. Peutz Jeghers syndrome. *J Med Genet* 1997; **34**: 1007–1011.
15. Hemminki A, Markie D, Tomlinson I et al. A serine/threonine kinase gene defective in Peutz–Jeghers syndrome. *Nature* 1998; **391**: 184–187.
16. Jenne DE, Reimann H, Nezu J et al. Peutz–Jeghers syndrome is caused by mutations in a novel serine threonine kinase. *Nature Genetics* 1998; **18**: 38–43.
17. Entius MM, Keller JJ, Westerman AM et al. Molecular genetic alterations in hamartomatous polyps and carcinomas of the patients with Peutz Jeghers syndrome. *J Clin Pathol* 2001; **54**: 126–131.
18. Gruber SB, Entius MM, Petersen GM et al. Pathogenesis of adenocarcinoma in Peutz–Jeghers syndrome. *Cancer Res* 1998; **58**: 5267–5270.
19. Wang ZJ, Ellis I, Zauber P et al. Allelic imbalance at the LKB1 (STK11) locus in tumours from patients with Peutz–Jeghers' syndrome provides evidence for a hamartoma-(adenoma)-carcinoma sequence. *J Pathol* 1999; **188**: 9–13.

20. McGarrity TJ, Kulin HE, Zaino RJ. Peutz–Jeghers syndrome. *Am J Gastroenterol* 2000; **95**: 598–604.
21. Olschwang S, Markie D, Seal S et al. Peutz–Jeghers disease: most, but not all, families are compatible with linkage to 19p13.3. *J Med Genet* 1998; **35**: 42–44.
22. Spigelman AD, Thomson JPS, Phillips RKS. Towards reducing the relaparotomy rate in Peutz Jeghers syndrome: the role of a peroperative small bowel endoscopy. *Br J Surg* 1990; **77**: 301–302.
23. Hyer W, Fell JM, Philp C, Phillips RK. Peutz–Jeghers syndrome – a case for luminal surveillance in childhood. *J Pediatr Gastroenteral Nutr* 2002; **34**: P452.
24. Pennazio M, Rossini FP. Small bowel polyps in Peutz–Jeghers syndrome: management by combined push enteroscopy and intra operative enteroscopy. *Gastrointest Endosc* 2000; **51**: 304–308.
25. Edwards DP, Stafforton R, Phillips RKS et al. The long term results of polyp clearance in Peutz Jeghers syndrome by intra operative endoscopy. Abstract of the *Third Joint Meeting, Leeds Castle Polyposis Group.* Venice, Italy, 26–28 April 2001.
26. Young RH, Welch WR, Dickerson GR, Scully RE. Ovarian sex cord tumour with annular tubules: review of 74 cases including 27 with Peutz–Jeghers syndrome and four with adenoma malignum of the cervix. *Cancer* 1982; **50**: 1384–1402.
27. Giardiello FM, Brensinger JD, Tersmette AC et al. Very high risk of cancer in familial Peutz Jeghers Syndrome. *Gastroenterology* 2000; **119**: 1447–1453.
28. Bulow C, Bulow S. Is screening for thyroid carcinoma indicated in familial adenomatous polyposis? The Leeds Castle Polyposis Group. *Int J Colorectal Dis* 1997; **12**: 240–242.
29. Bala S, Wunsch PH, Ballhausen WG. Childhood hepatocellular adenoma in familial adenomatous polyposis: mutations in adenomatous polyposis coli gene and p53. *Gastroenterology* 1997; **112**: 919–922.
30. Clark SK, Pack K, Pritchard J et al. FAP presenting with childhood desmoid tumours. *Lancet* 1997; **349**: 471.
31. Rustin RB, Jagelman DG, McGannon E et al. Spontaneous mutation in familial adenomatous polyposis. *Dis Colon Rectum* 1990; **33**: 52–55.
32. Kinzler KW, Nilbert MC, Su LK et al. Identification of FAP locus genes from chromosome 5q21. *Science* 1991; **253**: 661–665.
33. Nugent KP, Phillips RK, Hodgson SV et al. Phenotypic expression in familial adenomatous polyposis: partial prediction by mutation analysis. *Gut* 1994; **35**: 1622–1623.
34. Brensinger JD, Laken SJ, Luce MC et al. Variable phenotype of familial adenomatous polyposis in pedigrees with 3' mutation in the APC gene. *Gut* 1998; **43**: 548–552.
35. Lynch HT, Smyrk T, McGinn T et al. Attenuated familial adenomatous polyposis (AFAP). A phenotypically and genotypically distinctive variant of FAP. *Cancer* 1995; **76**: 2427–2433.
36. Houlston R, Crabtree M, Phillips R et al. Explaining differences in the severity of familial adenomatous polyposis and the search for modifier genes. *Gut* 2001; **48**: 1–5.
37. Vasen HF. When should endoscopic screening in familial adenomatous polyposis be started? *Gastroenterology* 2000; **118**: 808–809.
38. Church JM, McGannon, Burke C et al. Teenagers with familial adenomatous polyposis. *Dis Colon Rectum* 2002; **45**: 887–889.
39. Church J, Burke C, McGannon E. Predicting polyposis severity by proctoscopy. *Dis Colon Rectum* 2001; **44**: 1249–1254.
40. Giardiello F. Genetic testing in hereditary colorectal cancer. *JAMA* 1997; **278**: 1278–1281.
41. Giardiello FM, Brensinger JD, Petersen GM et al. The use and interpretation of commercial APC gene testing for familial adenomatous polyposis. *N Engl J Med* 1997; **336**: 823–827.
42. Harper P, Clarke A. Should we test children for 'adult' genetic diseases? *Lancet* 1990; **335**: 1205–1206.
43. Kodish ED. Testing children for cancer genes: the rule of the earliest onset. *J Pediatr* 1999; **135**: 390–395.
44. Hyer W, Fell J. Screening for familial adenomatous polyposis. *Arch Dis Child* 2001; **84**: 377–380.
45. Eccles DM, Lunt PW, Wallis Y et al. An unusually severe phenotype for FAP. *Arch Dis Child* 1997; **77**: 431–435.
46. Working Group on Endoscopic and Diagnostic Techniques. *World Congress of Paediatric Gastroenterology, Hepatology and Nutrition*, 2000: 205–218.
47. Caspari R, Friedl W, Mandl M et al. FAP: mutation at codon 1309 and early onset of colon cancer. *Lancet* 1994; **343**: 629–632.
48. Debinski HS, Love S, Spigelman AD et al. Colorectal polyp counts and cancer risk in FAP. *Gastroenterology* 1996; **110**: 1028–1030.
49. Mills SJ, Chapman PD, Burn J, Gunn A. Endoscopic screening and surgery for familial adenomatous polyposis: dangerous delays. *Br J Surg* 1997; **84**: 74–77.
50. Vasen HF, Van Duijvendijk P, Buskens E et al. Decision analysis in the surgical treatment of patients with familial adenomatous polyposis: a Dutch–Scandinavian collaborative study including 659 patients. *Gut* 2001; **49**: 231–235.
51. Madden MV, Neale KF, Nicholls RJ et al. Comparison of morbidity and function after colectomy and ileo rectal anastomosis or restorative proctocolectomy for FAP. *Br J Surg* 1991: **78**; 789–792.
52. Bjork J, Akerbrabt H, Iselius L et al. Outcome of primary and secondary pouch–anal anastomosis and ileorectal anastomosis in patients with familial adenomatous polyposis. *Dis Colon Rectum* 2001; **44**: 984–992.
53. Parc YR, Moslein G, Dozois RR. Familial adenomatous polyposis: results after ileal pouch–anal anastomosis in teenagers. *Dis Colon Rectum* 2000; **43**: 893–902.
54. Soravio C, Klein L, Berk T et al. Comparison of ileal pouch–anal anstomosis and ileorectal anastomosis in patients with familial adenomatous polyposis. *Dis Colon Rectum* 1999; **42**: 1028–1034.
55. Shilyansky J, Lelli JL, Drongowski R, Coran A. Efficacy of the straight endorectal pull-through in the management of familial adenomatous polyposis – a 16 year experience. *J Pediatr Surg* 1997; **32**: 1139–1143.
56. Wu J, McGannon BSW, Church JM. Incidence of neoplastic polyps in the ileal pouch of patients with familial adenomatous polyposis after restorative proctocolectomy. *Dis Colon Rectum* 1998; **41**: 552–557.
57. Soravia C, O'Connor BI, Berk T et al. Functional outcome of conversion of ileorectal anastomosis to ileal pouch–anal anastomosis in patients with familial adenomatous polyposis and ulcerative colitis. *Dis Colon Rectum* 1999; **42**: 903–907.
58. Cetta F, Gori M, Baldi C et al. APC genotype, polyp number, and surgical options in familial adenomatous polyposis. *Ann Surg* 1999; **229**: 445–446.

59. Vasen HF, van der Luijt RB, Slors JF et al. Molecular genetic tests as a guide to surgical management of FAP. *Lancet* 1996; **348**: 433–435.
60. Wu JS, McGannon PP, Church JM. APC genotype, polyp number, and surgical options in familial adenomatous polyposis. *Ann Surg* 1988; **227**: 57–62.
61. Farmer KCR, Hawley PR, Phillips RKS. Desmoid disease. In Phillips RKS, Spigelman AD, Thomson JPS, eds. *FAP and other Polyposis Syndromes*. London: Edward Arnold, 1994: 128–142.
62. Clark SK, Smith TG, Katz DE et al. Identification and progression of desmoid precursor lesion in patients with FAP. *Br J Surg* 1998; **85**: 970–973.
63. Clark SK, Phillips RK. Desmoids in FAP. *Br J Surg* 1996; **83**: 1494–1504.
64. Gorlin RJ, Cohen MM Jr, Condon LM, Burke BA. Bannyan–Riley–Rulcaba syndrome. *Am J Med Genet* 1992; **44**: 307–314.
65. Liaw D, Marsh D, Li J et al. Germline mutations of the PTEN gene in Cowden disease, an inherited breast and thyroid cancer syndrome. *Nature Genet* 1997; **16**: 64–67.
66. Whitelaw SC, Murday VA, Tomlinson IPM. Clinical and molecular features of the hereditary mixed polyposis syndrome. *Gastroenterology* 1997; **112**: 327–324.
67. Giardiello FM, Hamilton SR, Krush AJ, et al. Treatment of colonic and rectal adenomas with sulindac in familial adenomatous polyposis. *N Engl J Med* 1993; **328**: 1313–1316.
68. Hawk E, Lubet R, Limberg P. Chemoprevention in hereditary colorectal cancer syndromes. *Cancer* 1999; **86** (Suppl): 2551–2563.
69. Niv Y, Fraser GM. Adenocarcinoma in the rectal segment in familial polyposis coli is not prevented by sulindac therapy. *Gastroenterology* 1994; **107**: 854–857.
70. Steinbach G, Lynch PM, Phillips RKS et al. The effect of celecoxib, a cyclooxygenase-2 inhibitor, in familial adenomatous polyposis. *N Engl J Med* 2000; **342**: 1946–1952.
71. Giardiello FM, Yang VW, Hylind LM et al. Primary chemoprevention of familial adenomatous polyposis with sulindac. *N Engl J Med* 2002; **346**: 1054–1058.
72. Steele GD. The national cancer data base report on colorectal cancer. *Cancer* 1994; **74**: 1979–1989.
73. Chabalko JJ, Fraumeni JF. Colorectal cancer in children: epidemiologic aspects. *Dis Colon Rectum* 1975; **18**: 1–3.
74. Midgley R, Kerr D. Colorectal cancer. *Lancet* 1999; **353**: 391–399.
75. Ho JW, Yuen ST, Chung LP et al. Distinct clinical features associated with microsatellite instability in colorectal cancers of young patients. *Int J Cancer* 2000; **89**: 356–360.
76. Griffin PM, Liff JM, Greenberg RS, Clark WS. Adenocarcinomas of the colon and rectum in persons under 40 years of age: a population-based study. *Gastroenterology* 1991; **100**: 1033–1040.
77. Enker WE, Palovan E, Kirsner JB. Carcinoma of the colon in adolescents: a report of survival and an analysis of the literature. *Am J Surg* 1977; **133**: 737–741.
78. LaQuaglia MP, Heller G, Filippa DA et al. Prognostic factors and outcome in patients 21 years and under with colorectal carcinoma. *J Pediatr Surg* 1992; **27**: 1085–1090.
79. Angel CA, Pratt CB, Rao BN et al. Carcinoembryonic antigen and carbohydrate 19-9 antigen as markers for colorectal carcinoma in children and adolescents. *Cancer* 1992; **69**: 1487–1491.
80. Rao BN, Prall CB, Fleming ID et al. Carcinoma in children and adolescents. *Cancer* 1985; **55**: 1322–1326.
81. Shad A, Magrath I. Malignant non-Hodgkin's lymphomas in children. In Pizzo PA, Poplack DG, eds. *Principles and Practice of Pediatric Oncology*, 3rd edn. Philidelphia: Lippincott-Raven, 1997: 545–587.
82. Shepherd NA, Hall PA, Williams GT et al. Primary malignant lymphoma of the large intestine complicating chronic inflammatory bowel disease. *Histopathology* 1989; **15**: 325–337.
83. Greenstein AJ, Mullin GE, Strauchen JA et al. Lymphoma in inflammatory bowel disease. *Cancer* 1992; **69**: 1119–1123.
84. LaQuaglia MP, Stolar CJ, Krailo M et al. The role of surgery in abdominal non-Hodgkin's lymphoma: experience from the children's cancer study group. *J Pediatr Surg* 1992; **27**: 230–235.
85. Goldsby RE, Carroll WL. The molecular biology of pediatric lymphomas. *J Pediatr Hematol Oncol* 1998; **20**: 282–296.

Index

9781841843155